The Surgical Review

AN INTEGRATED BASIC AND CLINICAL SCIENCE STUDY GUIDE

SECOND EDITION

Compliments of

GLAXOSMITHKLINE
Oncology & *Acute Care*

The Surgical Review

AN INTEGRATED BASIC AND CLINICAL SCIENCE STUDY GUIDE

SECOND EDITION

EDITED BY

▬ PAVAN ATLURI, MD

Resident in Surgery
Department of Surgery
University of Pennsylvania
Philadelphia, Pennsylvania

▬ GIORGOS C. KARAKOUSIS, MD

Resident in Surgery
Department of Surgery
University of Pennsylvania
Philadelphia, Pennsylvania

▬ PAIGE M. PORRETT, MD

Resident in Surgery
Department of Surgery
University of Pennsylvania
Philadelphia, Pennsylvania

▬ LARRY R. KAISER, MD

John Rhea Barton Professor and Chairman
Department of Surgery
University of Pennsylvania
Philadelphia, Pennsylvania

LIPPINCOTT WILLIAMS & WILKINS
A **Wolters Kluwer** Company

Philadelphia • Baltimore • New York • London
Buenos Aires • Hong Kong • Sydney • Tokyo

Acquisitions Editor: Brian Brown
Managing Editor: Michelle LaPlante
Project Manager: Nicole Walz
Senior Manufacturing Manager: Ben Rivera
Senior Marketing Manager: Adam Glazer
Design Coordinator: Holly Reid McLaughlin
Cover Designer: Karen Quigley
Production Services: Laser Words Pvt. Limited
Printer: Edwards Brothers

2nd Edition
© 2006 by Lippincott Williams & Wilkins
© 2001 by Lippincott Williams & Wilkins
530 Walnut Street
Philadelphia, PA 19106

The surgical review : an integrated basic and clinical science study guide/edited by Pavan Atluri ... [et al.]. — 2nd ed.
   p. ; cm.
Includes bibliographical references and index.
ISBN 0-7817-5641-3 (alk. paper)
1. Surgery—Examinations, questions, etc. I. Atluri, Pavan.
[DNLM: 1. Surgery. 2. Surgical Procedures, Operative—methods.
WO 100 S9628 2005]
RD37.2.S9749 2005
617'.0076—dc22

2005016028

Care has been taken to confirm the accuracy of the information presented and to describe generally accepted practices. However, the authors, editors, and publisher are not responsible for errors or omissions or for any consequences from application of the information in this book and make no warranty, expressed or implied, with respect to the currency, completeness, or accuracy of the contents of the publication. Application of this information in a particular situation remains the professional responsibility of the practitioner.

The authors, editors, and publisher have exerted every effort to ensure that drug selection and dosage set forth in this text are in accordance with current recommendations and practice at the time of publication. However, in view of ongoing research, changes in government regulations, and the constant flow of information relating to drug therapy and drug reactions, the reader is urged to check the package insert for each drug for any change in indications and dosage and for added warnings and precautions. This is particularly important when the recommended agent is a new or infrequently employed drug.

Some drugs and medical devices presented in this publication have Food and Drug Administration (FDA) clearance for limited use in restricted research settings. It is the responsibility of health care providers to ascertain the FDA status of each drug or device planned for use in their clinical practice.

The publishers have made every effort to trace copyright holders for borrowed material. If they have inadvertently overlooked any, they will be pleased to make the necessary arrangements at the first opportunity.

To purchase additional copies of this book, call our customer service department at (800) 638-3030 or fax orders to (301) 824-7390. Lippincott Williams & Wilkins customer service representatives are available from 8:30 am to 6:30 pm, EST, Monday through Friday, for telephone access. Visit Lippincott Williams & Wilkins on the Internet: http://www.lww.com.

10 9 8 7 6 5 4 3 2 1

Contents

Contributing Authors

IBRAHIM ABDULLAH, MD Resident in Surgery, Department of Surgery, University of Pennsylvania School of Medicine, Philadelphia, Pennsylvania

MICHAEL A. ACKER, MD Professor of Surgery, Chief, Cardiothoracic Surgery, Department of Surgery, University of Pennsylvania School of Medicine, Philadelphia, Pennsylvania

PAVAN ATLURI, MD Resident in Surgery, Department of Surgery, University of Pennsylvania School of Medicine, Philadelphia, Pennsylvania

THOMAS J. BADER, MD Assistant Professor of Obstetrics and Gynecology, Department of Obstetrics and Gynecology, University of Pennsylvania School of Medicine, Philadelphia, Pennsylvania

STEPHEN M. BAUER, MD Resident in Surgery, Department of Surgery, University of Pennsylvania School of Medicine, Philadelphia, Pennsylvania

MARK F. BERRY, MD Resident in Surgery, Department of Surgery, University of Pennsylvania School of Medicine, Philadelphia, Pennsylvania

ROBERT J. CANTER, MD Chief Resident in Surgery, Department of Surgery, University of Pennsylvania School of Medicine, Philadelphia, Pennsylvania

JEFFREY P. CARPENTER, MD Professor of Surgery, Director, Vascular Laboratory , Division of Vascular Surgery, Department of Surgery, University of Pennsylvania School of Medicine, Philadelphia, Pennsylvania

ARA A. CHALIAN, MD Associate Professor, Director of Facial Plastic/Reconstructive Surgery, Department of Otolaryngology-Head/Neck Surgery, University of Pennsylvania School of Medicine , Philadelphia, Pennsylvania

RAFFI ARA CHALIAN, MD Resident in Obstetrics and Gynecology, Department of Obstetrics and Gynecology, University of Pennsylvania School of Medicine, Philadelphia, Pennsylvania

JEFFREY A. DREBIN, MD, PHD Professor of Surgery, Vice Chairman for Research, Chief, Division of Gastrointestinal Surgery, Department of Surgery, University of Pennsylvania School of Medicine, Philadelphia, Pennsylvania

KRISTOFFEL DUMON, MD Resident in Surgery, Department of Surgery, University of Pennsylvania School of Medicine, Philadelphia, Pennsylvania

JOHN L. ESTERHAI, JR, MD Professor of Orthopaedic Surgery, Department of Orthopaedic Surgery, University of Pennsylvania School of Medicine, Philadelphia, Pennsylvania

RONALD M. FAIRMAN, MD Associate Professor of Surgery and Radiology, Chief, Division of Vascular Surgery, Department of Surgery, University of Pennsylvania School of Medicine, Philadelphia, Pennsylvania

MARK B. FARIES, MD Director, Translational Tumor Immunology, John Wayne Cancer Institute, Santa Monica, California

DOUGLAS L. FRAKER, MD Jonathan E. Rhoads Associate Professor of Surgical Science, Vice Chairman of Clinical Affairs, Chief, Division of Endocrine and Oncologic Surgery, Department of Surgery, University of Pennsylvania School of Medicine, Philadelphia, Pennsylvania

ROBERT FRY, MD Emilie & Roland deHellebranth Professor of Surgery, Chief, Division of Colon and Rectal Surgery, Department of Surgery, University of Pennsylvania School of Medicine, Philadelphia, Pennsylvania

STEPHEN C. GALE, MD Fellow in Trauma Surgery, Division of Trauma and Surgical Critical Care, Department of Surgery, University of Pennsylvania School of Medicine, Philadelphia, Pennsylvania

THOMAS G. GLEASON, MD Assistant Professor of Surgery, Division of Cardiothoracic Surgery, Department of Surgery, Northwestern University Feinberg School of Medicine; Director, Thoracic Aortic Surgery Program, Bluhm Cardiovascular Institute, Chicago, Illinois

LEE J. GOLDSTEIN, MD Resident in Surgery, Department of Surgery, University of Pennsylvania School of Medicine, Philadelphia, Pennsylvania

VICENTE H. GRACIAS, MD Assistant Professor of Surgery, Co-Medical Director, Surgical Critical Care, Division of Trauma and Surgical Critical Care, Department of Surgery, University of Pennsylvania School of Medicine, Philadelphia, Pennsylvania

C. WILLIAM HANSON III, MD Professor of Anesthesia, Surgery and Internal Medicine, Departments of Anesthesia, Surgery, and Medicine, Section Chief, Critical Care, Department of Anesthesia, University of Pennsylvania School of Medicine, Philadelphia, Pennsylvania

GREGORY G. HEUER, MD, PHD Resident in Neurosurgery, Department of Neurosurgery, University of Pennsylvania School of Medicine, Philadelphia, Pennsylvania

JAMES H. HOLMES, IV, MD Fellow in Trauma Surgery, Division of Trauma and Surgical Critical Care, Department of Surgery, University of Pennsylvania School of Medicine, Philadelphia, Pennsylvania

BENJAMIN M. JACKSON, MD   Resident in Surgery, Department of Surgery, University of Pennsylvania School of Medicine, Philadelphia, Pennsylvania

VASANT JAYASANKAR, MD   Chief Resident in Surgery, Department of Surgery, University of Pennsylvania School of Medicine, Philadelphia, Pennsylvania

KEVIN D. JUDY, MD   Associate Professor of Neurosurgery, Department of Neurosurgery, University of Pennsylvania School of Medicine, Philadelphia, Pennsylvania

LARRY R. KAISER, MD   The John Rhea Barton Professor and Chairman, Chief, Department of Surgery, Department of Surgery, University of Pennsylvania School of Medicine, Philadelphia, Pennsylvania

GIORGOS C. KARAKOUSIS, MD   Resident in Surgery, Department of Surgery, University of Pennsylvania School of Medicine, Philadelphia, Pennsylvania

JAGAJAN KARMACHARYA, MD, FRCS   Chief Resident in Surgery, Department of Surgery, University of Pennsylvania School of Medicine, Philadelphia, Pennsylvania

RACHEL RAPAPORT KELZ, MD, MSCE   Assistant Professor of Clinical Surgery, Division of Endocrine and Oncologic Surgery, Department of Surgery, University of Pennsylvania School of Medicine, Philadelphia, Pennsylvania

SUSAN B. KESMODEL, MD   Chief Resident in Surgery, Department of Surgery, University of Pennsylvania School of Medicine, Philadelphia, Pennsylvania

PATRICK K. KIM, MD   Assistant Professor of Surgery, Division of Trauma and Surgical Critical Care, Department of Surgery, University of Pennsylvania School of Medicine, Philadelphia, Pennsylvania

LISA D. KHOURY, MD   Resident in Orthopaedic Surgery, Department of Orthopaedic Surgery, University of Pennsylvania School of Medicine, Philadelphia, Pennsylvania

LAURA KRUPER, MD, MSCE   Resident in Surgery, Department of Surgery, University of Pennsylvania School of Medicine, Philadelphia, Pennsylvania

JOHN C. KUCHARCZUK, MD   Assistant Professor of Surgery, Division of Thoracic Surgery, Department of Surgery, University of Pennsylvania School of Medicine, Philadelphia, Pennsylvania

BRADLEY G. LESHNOWER, MD   Resident in Surgery, Department of Surgery, University of Pennsylvania School of Medicine, Philadelphia, Pennsylvania

JAMES F. MARKMANN, MD, PHD   Associate Professor of Surgery, Director of Pancreas Transplantation, Division of Transplant Surgery, Department of Surgery, University of Pennsylvania School of Medicine, Philadelphia, Pennsylvania

MIREILLE ASTRID MOISE, MD   Resident in Surgery, Department of Surgery, University of Pennsylvania School of Medicine, Philadelphia, Pennsylvania

MICHAEL J. MOROWITZ, MD   Chief Resident in Surgery, Department of Surgery, University of Pennsylvania School of Medicine, Philadelphia, Pennsylvania

JON B. MORRIS, MD   Professor of Surgery, Division of Gastrointestinal Surgery, Department of Surgery, University of Pennsylvania School of Medicine, Philadelphia, Pennsylvania

RICHARD J. MYUNG, MD   Resident in Surgery, Department of Surgery, University of Pennsylvania School of Medicine, Philadelphia, Pennsylvania

MICHAEL L. NANCE, MD   Associate Professor of Surgery, Department of Surgery, University of Pennsylvania School of Medicine; Director, Pediatric Trauma Program, Department of Surgery, Children's Hospital of Philadelphia, Philadelphia, Pennsylvania

APRIL ESTELLE NEDEAU, MD   Resident in Surgery, Department of Surgery, University of Pennsylvania School of Medicine, Philadelphia, Pennsylvania

KIM M. OLTHOFF, MD   Associate Professor of Surgery, Director, Liver Transplantation, Division of Transplant Surgery, Department of Surgery, University of Pennsylvania School of Medicine, Philadelphia, Pennsylvania

PAIGE M. PORRETT, MD   Resident in Surgery, Department of Surgery, University of Pennsylvania School of Medicine, Philadelphia, Pennsylvania

JIN HEE RA, MD   Resident in Surgery, Department of Surgery, University of Pennsylvania School of Medicine, Philadelphia, Pennsylvania

STEVEN E. RAPER, MD   Associate Professor of Surgery, Division of Gastrointestinal Surgery, Department of Surgery, University of Pennsylvania School of Medicine, Philadelphia, Pennsylvania

G. TIMOTHY REITER, MD   Assistant Professor of Neurosurgery, Department of Neurosurgery, Penn State College of Medicine, Hershey, Pennsylvania

JOHN L. ROMBEAU, MD   Professor of Surgery, Division of Colon and Rectal Surgery, Department of Surgery, University of Pennsylvania School of Medicine, Philadelphia, Pennsylvania

ERNEST F. ROSATO, MD   Professor of Surgery, Division of Gastrointestinal Surgery, Department of Surgery, University of Pennsylvania School of Medicine, Philadelphia, Pennsylvania

C. WILLIAM SCHWAB, MD   Professor of Surgery, Chief, Division of Trauma and Surgical Critical Care, Department of Surgery, University of Pennsylvania School of Medicine, Philadelphia, Pennsylvania

C. WILLIAM SCHWAB, II, MD   Resident in Urology, Department of Urology, University of Pennsylvania School of Medicine, Philadelphia, Pennsylvania

JEFFREY M. SHAARI, MD   Resident in Otorhinolaryngology, Department of Otorhinolaryngology—Head and Neck Surgery, University of Pennsylvania School of Medicine, Philadelphia, Pennsylvania

JOSEPH B. SHRAGER, MD   Associate Professor of Surgery, Chief, General Thoracic Surgery, Department of Surgery, University of Pennsylvania School of Medicine, Philadelphia, Pennsylvania

SEEMA S. SONNAD, PHD Associate Professor of Surgery, Director of Outcomes Research, Department of Surgery, University of Pennsylvania School of Medicine, Philadelphia, Pennsylvania

FRANCIS R. SPITZ, MD Assistant Professor of Surgery, Division of Endocrine and Oncologic Surgery, Department of Surgery, University of Pennsylvania School of Medicine, Philadelphia, Pennsylvania

MICHAEL F. STIEFEL, MD, PHD Resident in Neurosurgery, Department of Neurosurgery, University of Pennsylvania School of Medicine, Philadelphia, Pennsylvania

LEONARD T. SU, MD Chief Resident in Surgery, Department of Surgery, University of Pennsylvania School of Medicine, Philadelphia, Pennsylvania

JULIA C. TCHOU, MD, PHD Assistant Professor of Surgery, Division of Endocrine and Oncologic Surgery, Department of Surgery, University of Pennsylvania School of Medicine, Philadelphia, Pennsylvania

LISA D. UNGER, MD Assistant Professor of Clinical Surgery, Attending Physician, Clinical Nutrition Support Service, Department of Surgery, University of Pennsylvania School of Medicine, Philadelphia, Pennsylvania

KEITH N. VAN ARSDALEN, MD Professor of Urology and Radiology, Departments of Urology and Radiology, University of Pennsylvania School of Medicine, Philadelphia, Pennsylvania

OMAIDA C. VELAZQUEZ, MD Assistant Professor of Surgery, Division of Vascular Surgery, Department of Surgery, University of Pennsylvania, Philadelphia, Pennsylvania

WILLIAM J. VERNICK, MD Assistant Professor of Anesthesia, Department of Anesthesia, University of Pennsylvania School of Medicine, Philadelphia, Pennsylvania

MICHAEL J. WILDERMAN, MD Resident in Surgery, Department of Surgery, University of Pennsylvania School of Medicine, Philadelphia, Pennsylvania

Y. JOSEPH WOO, MD Assistant Professor of Surgery, Director, Minimally Invasive and Robotic Cardiac Surgery Program, Division of Cardiothoracic Surgery, Department of Surgery, University of Pennsylvania School of Medicine, Philadelphia, Pennsylvania

HEIDI YEH, MD Fellow in Transplant Surgery, Division of Transplant Surgery, Department of Surgery, University of Pennsylvania School of Medicine, Philadelphia, Pennsylvania

Preface

This edition of *The Surgical Review* has been rewritten in its entirety to provide the most up-to-date knowledge on which surgical practice is based. Each chapter was written following an extensive review of the current literature in order to integrate the changes occurring in the rapidly evolving field of surgery. Each chapter is co-authored by a senior surgical resident and an attending surgeon expert with the intent to provide a comprehensive and readable source of knowledge for those at all levels of surgical training. There have been many significant changes incorporated into this edition including a focused section on resuscitation and management of the traumatically injured patient, an extensive chapter on pediatric surgery, numerous updated and focused illustrations, and a summary of key points at the end of each chapter for rapid review of high-yield facts.

When we began this project, we set out to achieve several goals based on our own experience as medical students and surgical residents. This concise text of surgical practice provides a solid foundation of both basic and clinical surgical knowledge that should be useful for medical students and residents alike. Furthermore, for those who have completed their surgical training, this book can serve as a review for the American Board of Surgery Qualifying Examination, as well as for those completing the cognitive examination portion of the Maintenance of Certification process.

The authors have worked earnestly to create a first rate product. We strongly believe that we have met these objectives and hope that you share our enthusiasm for this book.

Pavan Atluri, MD
Giorgos C. Karakousis, MD
Paige M. Porrett, MD
Larry R. Kaiser, MD

Neurosurgery

Gregory Heuer   *G. Timothy Reiter*
Michael F. Stiefel   *Kevin D. Judy*

In the beginning of the 20th century, most neurosurgical procedures were still performed by general surgeons. Harvey Cushing first recognized the need for surgeons dedicated solely to this field and defined neurosurgery as a distinct subspecialty. Although the broad knowledge base of neuroanatomy, neurophysiology, and neuropathophysiology necessary for a complete understanding of this field is constantly evolving, familiarity with these concepts is a must for all physicians.

MICROSCOPIC ANATOMY

The central nervous system (CNS) is composed of neurons and supporting neuroglial cells. The neuron is the functional unit of the CNS. It has a cell body, axon, and multiple dendrites. The axon carries impulses away from the cell body. A bundle of axons is a nerve fiber. Dendrites are neuronal cell processes that carry impulses to the cell body.

Neuroglial cells, such as astrocytes, oligodendrocytes, ependymocytes, and microglia, surround and support the neurons. Astrocytes contain rigid gliofilaments that provide physical support to the CNS. Astrocytes have foot processes that surround capillaries and contribute to the blood–brain barrier (BBB). Gliosis is the overgrowth of the cytoplasmic processes of astrocytes in an injured area of the CNS, similar to a scar. Oligodendrocytes produce and maintain myelin in the CNS, whereas in the peripheral nervous system (PNS), Schwann cells produce and maintain myelin. Each oligodendrocyte can myelinate many axons in the CNS; however, each Schwann cell can myelinate only one axon in the PNS. Ependymocytes form the simple cuboidal epithelial lining of the ventricular system. Resting microglial cells are present within the gray and white matter of the CNS and are analogous to the resident macrophages found in other tissues of the body. A mass of neuronal cell bodies and supporting glial cells is referred to as gray matter. A group of many axons traveling together with their supporting glial cells is called *white matter*.

The BBB is formed primarily at the level of the capillaries. It consists of three layers: the vascular endothelium with tight junctions between cells, a basal lamina, and the perivascular foot processes of astrocytes that encircle the capillaries. The functional component of the BBB is the tight junctions between the endothelial cells, which impede many substances from moving into the CNS from the bloodstream. Substances can cross the BBB by diffusion, by carrier-mediated transport, or by energy-requiring active transport. With disease and after injury, the BBB can break down, thereby making it more permeable. The neurohypophysis (posterior pituitary), median eminence, pineal gland, organum vasculosum of the lamina terminalis, subfornical organ, subcommissural organ, and area postrema all lack a BBB and are called the *circumventricular organs*.

Action potentials (APs) are signals that are transmitted along axons. In the resting state, the inside of the neuron has a net negative charge, whereas the extracellular fluid has a net positive charge. This charge differential creates an electrical gradient across the cell membrane, which normally equals -70 mV and is called the *resting membrane potential*. This gradient is produced by the sodium pump by active transport of potassium into the cell and sodium out of the cell using one molecule of adenosine triphosphate (ATP) for every three sodium ions exchanged. This scenario produces a high intracellular concentration of potassium compared to the extracellular fluid concentration and a high extracellular concentration of sodium compared to the intracellular fluid concentration. Excitation of the neuron, owing to chemical or mechanical stimuli, results in the opening of voltage-gated sodium channels, and an AP is initiated by the large influx of sodium down its gradient into the cell. This process is termed *depolarization*. The AP is transmitted down the axon by sequential depolarization. Myelin encircles some of the axons and acts like an insulator around an electric wire. The voltage-gated sodium channels are located only at intermittent gaps in the myelin sheath called *nodes of Ranvier*. This configuration allows the AP to propagate much faster down the axon via a process referred to as a saltatory conduction. A myelinated axon can conduct an AP at a rate of up to 120 m per second, whereas an unmyelinated axon can conduct an AP at a rate of up to only 2 m per second.

Neurons communicate with one another through synapses, which are the gaps between the end of the axon of one neuron and the cell body of another neuron. Most synapses in humans are chemical synapses. Chemical synapses have neurotransmitters stored in synaptic vesicles located at the end bulbs of axons. Neurotransmitters are released from the presynaptic membrane and travel across the gap to the postsynaptic membrane where they bind to receptors. If an excitatory neurotransmitter binds to a receptor on the postsynaptic membrane, the membrane potential becomes less negative. If enough excitatory neurotransmitters bind, a threshold is reached and the cell is depolarized, thereby producing an AP. If an inhibitory neurotransmitter is released and binds to a receptor on the postsynaptic membrane, the membrane potential becomes more negative, termed *hyperpolarization,* making an AP more difficult to generate.

ANATOMY

The scalp consists of five layers. The most superficial layer is the skin, with a thin layer of underlying connective tissue. Underneath the connective tissue is the galea aponeurotica (galea). The large blood vessels of the scalp are located in the connective tissue layer just overlying the galea. The galea retracts when lacerated, which decreases the bleeding. A deep layer of sutures is needed during surgical repair of the scalp to approximate the galea. Beneath the galea is a layer of loose connective tissue and deep to that layer is the periosteum of the skull. A subgaleal hematoma forms from bleeding into the loose connective tissue layer underlying the galea and most commonly occurs in children after traumatic injuries.

The skull is a protective bony case for the brain, which is composed of multiple bones including the frontal, nasal, lacrimal, parietal, sphenoid, temporal, ethmoid, and occipital. The junction between the frontal and parietal bones is the coronal suture, the junction between the two parietal bones is the sagittal suture, and the junction between the parietal and occipital bones is the lambdoid suture. The pterion is the area where the frontal, parietal, temporal, and sphenoid bones come together on the side of the skull forming an *H.*

The spinal cord is surrounded by the bony vertebral column. There are seven cervical vertebrae, 12 thoracic vertebrae, five lumbar vertebrae, five fused sacral vertebrae, and four fused coccygeal vertebrae, totaling 33 vertebrae (Fig. 1-1). Each vertebra, except C1, has a body, paired pedicles, paired transverse processes, paired laminae, and a spinous process. C1 through C6 have bilateral transverse foramina through which the vertebral arteries pass. C1 is called the *atlas* and C2 is called the *axis.* The odontoid process, also called the *dens,* is a superiorly projecting process that comes off the body of the axis. The odontoid process articulates with the atlas and allows for rotation of the head. Between the vertebral bodies are intervertebral disks. They consist of a fibrous outer ring, called the *annulus fibrosis,* and an inner elastic portion, called the *nucleus pulposus.* The disk has a limited blood supply, often making it a nidus for infection.

The meninges form a cover over the brain and spinal cord and consist of three layers: the dura mater, the arachnoid membrane, and the pia mater. The dura mater is the outermost layer and is composed of two layers around the brain, but only one layer around the spinal cord. Surrounding the brain, there is an outer periosteal layer and an inner

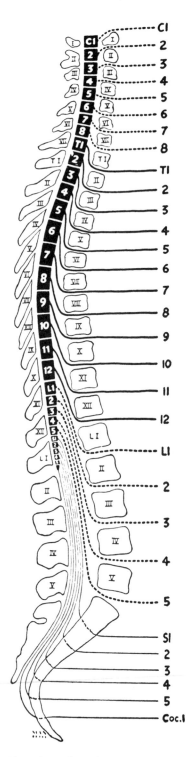

Figure 1-1   The relationship of the spinal cord segments to the vertebrae and spinal roots to the intervertebral foramina. (From Carpenter MB, Sutin J. *Human neuroanatomy.* Baltimore: Williams & Wilkins, 1983, with permission.)

meningeal layer of dura. These layers lie mostly adjacent to each other but separate at certain locations to form the venous dural sinuses. The meningeal layer of the dura has several reflections. These include the falx cerebri, which separates the cerebral hemispheres; the tentorium cerebelli (tentorium), which separates the occipital and temporal lobes from the cerebellum and brainstem; the diaphragma sellae through which the pituitary stalk passes; and the falx cerebelli, which separates the cerebellar hemispheres.

Beneath the dura is the thin, delicate arachnoid membrane. Between the dura mater and arachnoid membrane is the subdural space. Underlying the arachnoid membrane is the pia mater, which lies on the surface of the brain and spinal cord. Between the arachnoid membrane and the pia mater is the subarachnoid space. At the base of the brain, these spaces are substantial and are filled with cerebrospinal fluid (CSF). These fluid-filled structures are called the *basal cisterns* and are seen surrounding the brainstem on computerized tomography. Major arteries are located in the subarachnoid space. The arachnoid membrane and pia mater collectively are called the *leptomeninges*.

The right and left cerebral hemispheres consist of gray matter on the surface of the gyri, white matter deep to the gyri, and deep central neuronal masses called the *basal ganglia*. On the cerebral surface are multiple gyri and sulci. Each hemisphere is divided into frontal, parietal, temporal, and occipital lobes. The central sulcus (of Rolando) separates the frontal lobe from the parietal lobe. The lateral fissure (of Sylvius) separates the temporal lobe from the frontal and parietal lobes (Fig. 1-2). The parietooccipital sulcus, seen on the medial surface of the hemisphere, separates the parietal lobe from the occipital lobe. The lobes of the brain are located in different fossae. The anterior cranial fossa contains the frontal lobes, the middle cranial fossa contains the temporal lobes, and the posterior cranial fossa contains the cerebellum and the brainstem. Specific functions can be assigned to the different lobes of the brain. The frontal lobes are involved in personality, emotion, and movement. The parietal lobes process sensory information, and the occipital lobes are concerned with vision. The dominant temporal lobe (usually the left side) contains the language areas of the brain. The basal ganglia comprises the caudate nucleus, the putamen, the globus pallidus, and the amygdaloid nuclear complex. The caudate, putamen, and globus pallidus are called the *corpus striatum* and play an important role in the motor system. The putamen and globus pallidus together are called the lentiform nuclei.

Blood to the brain is supplied by the paired internal carotid arteries and by the paired vertebral arteries. The vertebral arteries come together to form the basilar artery, which lies on the anterior surface of the brainstem. The internal carotid arteries and the basilar artery form an anastomotic loop called the *circle of Willis*, which is located at the base of the brain just anterior to the brainstem. Each internal carotid artery bifurcates into an anterior cerebral artery and a middle cerebral artery. The basilar artery bifurcates into the paired posterior cerebral arteries. Communicating arteries join the carotid and basilar arteries to form the circle of Willis. The anterior communicating artery connects the left and right anterior cerebral arteries. The paired posterior communicating arteries join the internal carotid artery to the posterior cerebral artery on the same side (Fig. 1-3). The internal carotid arteries and their branches supply the frontal and parietal lobes and most of the temporal lobes. The basilar artery and its branches supply the brainstem, the cerebellum, the occipital lobes, and the inferior temporal lobes. Eighty percent of the blood flow to the brain is supplied by the internal carotid arteries.

The venous anatomy of the brain consists of a deep and a superficial system of drainage. The superficial system is composed of superficial veins on the convexity of the cortex, which drain into the superior sagittal sinus. The deep system drains into the internal cerebral veins, which join to form the great cerebral vein (of Galen). The great cerebral vein becomes the straight (rectus) sinus, which runs along the midline of the tentorium. The systems meet at the confluens sinuum (torcular herophili), where the superior sagittal sinus joins the rectus sinus. The paired

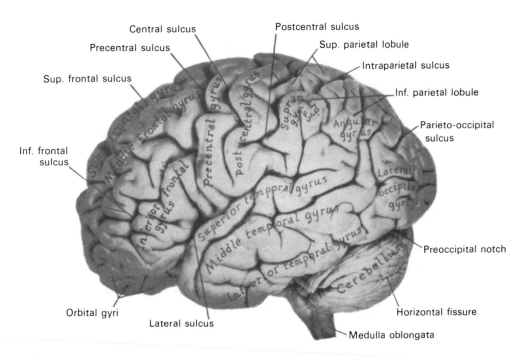

Figure 1-2 The lateral surface of the brain. (From Carpenter MB, Sutin J. *Human neuroanatomy.* Baltimore: Williams & Wilkins, 1983, with permission.)

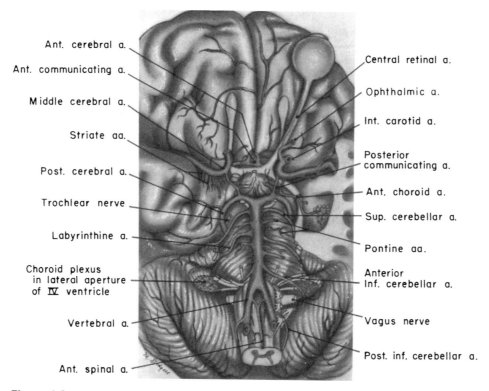

Figure 1-3   The ventral surface of the brain illustrating the arterial anatomy. (From Carpenter MB. *Core text of neuroanatomy.* Baltimore: Williams & Wilkins, 1991, with permission.)

transverse sinuses carry blood from the confluens sinuum to the sigmoid sinuses, which become the internal jugular veins (Fig. 1-4).

Within the brain are CSF-filled spaces called *ventricles*. There are a pair of lateral ventricles, and there is a midline third ventricle and a midline fourth ventricle. Each lateral ventricle connects to the third ventricle through the interventricular foramen (Monro foramen). The third ventricle connects to the fourth ventricle through the cerebral (sylvian) aqueduct. The fourth ventricle connects

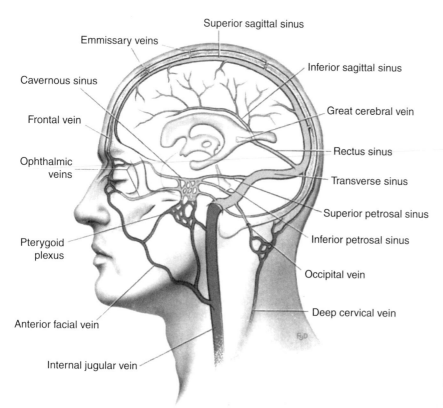

Figure 1-4   The venous drainage of the brain. (From Carpenter MB. *Core text of neuroanatomy.* Baltimore: Williams & Wilkins, 1991, with permission.)

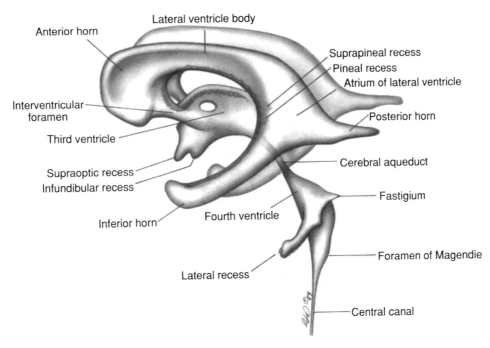

Anterior horn

Lateral ventricle body

Suprapineal recess

Pineal recess

Atrium of lateral ventricle

Interventricular foramen

Third ventricle

Posterior horn

Supraoptic recess

Infundibular recess

Cerebral aqueduct

Fastigium

Inferior horn

Fourth ventricle

Foramen of Magendie

Lateral recess

Central canal

Figure 1-5   The ventricular system of the brain. Cerebrospinal fluid flow is from lateral to third to fourth ventricle. (From Carpenter MB. *Core text of neuroanatomy*. Baltimore: Williams & Wilkins, 1991, with permission.)

to the subarachnoid space around the brainstem by the midline foramen of Magendie and the paired lateral foramina of Luschka. CSF is produced by the choroid plexus, which is found in all of the ventricles. In general, the flow of CSF goes from the lateral ventricles to the third ventricle and then to the fourth ventricle. From the fourth ventricle, CSF enters the subarachnoid space surrounding the brain and the spinal cord (Fig. 1-5). CSF passes from the subarachnoid space to the venous system through the arachnoid villi (granulations), which are located in the walls of the dural sinuses. This is a dynamic system in that the choroid plexus produces approximately 500 mL of CSF per day, but only about 150 mL of CSF is present within the CNS at one time.

The cerebellum is located dorsal to the brainstem and inferior to the tentorium in the posterior fossa. The structure is divided into a midline portion called the *vermis* and two lateral hemispheres. The cerebellum has three paired connections to the brainstem: the superior cerebellar peduncles connect to the midbrain, the middle cerebellar peduncles connect to the pons, and the inferior cerebellar peduncles connect to the medulla. The paired deep cerebellar nuclei lie within the cerebellar white matter. From medial to lateral, they are the fastigial, globose, emboliform, and dentate nuclei.

The brainstem is divided into four parts (Fig. 1-6). From rostral to caudal, these are the diencephalon, the midbrain (mesencephalon), the pons (metencephalon), and the medulla oblongata (myelencephalon). The largest subdivision of the diencephalon is the thalamus. Both sensory input to the cerebrum and motor output from the cerebrum pass through the thalamus. The midbrain is the smallest division of the brainstem. It is divided into the tectum, the tegmentum, and the crura cerebri. The substantia nigra lies between the crura cerebri and the tegmentum and has efferent and afferent connections to the basal ganglia. Loss of dopaminergic neurons in the substantia nigra is seen in Parkinson disease. The pons consists of a large ventral part containing descending motor fibers and the pontine nuclei that project to the cerebellum via the middle cerebellar peduncle, and a smaller dorsal portion in which the pontine reticular formation and various cranial nerve nuclei are located. Anteriorly, the basilar artery runs along the surface of the pons in the basilar sulcus. The medulla is the most caudal portion of the brainstem, which inferiorly becomes the spinal cord. It can be divided into the dorsal medullary reticular formation, which is associated with arousal and wakefulness, and the ventral medullary pyramids, which contain the motor output from the cerebrum. Dorsal to the medulla and the pons lies the fourth ventricle.

At the base of the brain, anterior to the brainstem and just posterior to the optic chiasm, is the hypophysis (pituitary gland). The infundibulum (stalk of the hypophysis) descends from the inferior surface of the hypothalamus, passes through the diaphragma sellae (a dural reflection with a central hole), and enters the sella turcica, where it becomes the hypophysis. The hypophysis is divided into an anterior and a posterior lobe. The hypothalamus communicates with the adenohypophysis (anterior lobe) by a portal system of blood vessels. Adrenocorticotropic hormone (ACTH), thyrotropin, prolactin, growth hormone, follicle-stimulating hormone, and luteinizing hormone are produced in the adenohypophysis and released into the bloodstream under the control of releasing hormones from the hypothalamus. The hypothalamus also contains neurons that project axons to the neurohypophysis (posterior hypophysis). These axons transport hormones, such as antidiuretic hormone (vasopressin) and oxytocin—which are made in the hypothalamus—to the posterior hypophysis where they are released into the bloodstream (Fig. 1-7).

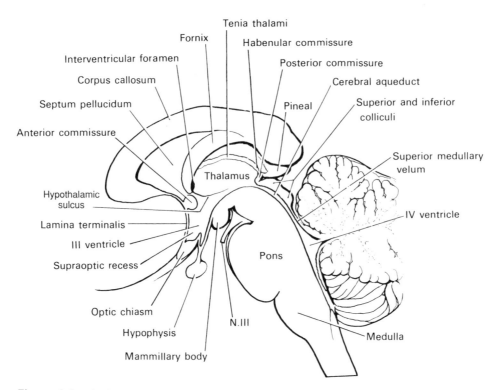

Figure 1-6 The brainstem in a midsagittal section. (From Carpenter MB, Sutin J. *Human neuroanatomy.* Baltimore: Williams & Wilkins, 1983, with permission.)

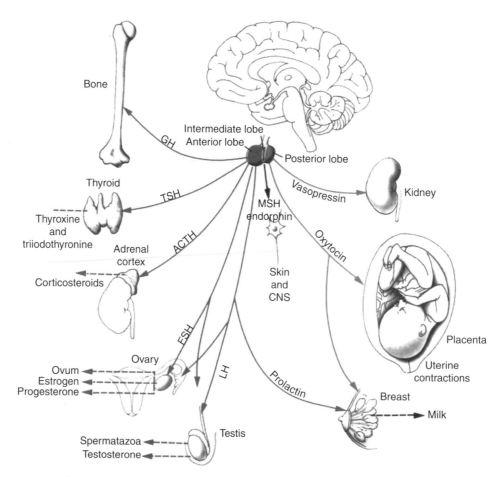

Figure 1-7 The actions of the pituitary hormones on their target organs. (From Carpenter MB, Sutin J. *Human neuroanatomy.* Baltimore: Williams & Wilkins, 1983, with permission.)

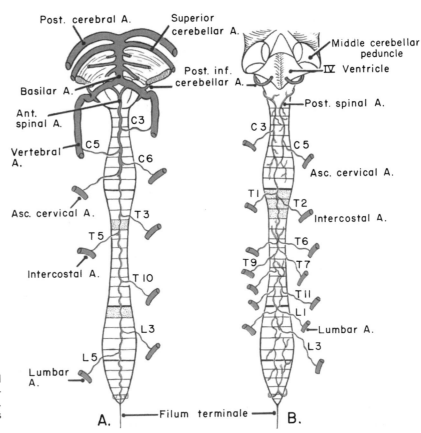

Figure 1-8 The arterial supply to the spinal cord. The watershed zones are stippled. **A:** anterior view; **B:** posterior view. (From Carpenter MB. *Core text of neuroanatomy.* Baltimore: Williams & Wilkins, 1991, with permission.)

The spinal cord is the continuation of the brainstem as it passes through the foramen magnum. The cord ends as the conus medullaris near the L1 vertebral body. The lumbar and sacral nerve roots travel caudally in the spinal canal as the cauda equina before they reach their respective vertebral body and exit to the periphery. The filum terminale is a condensation of pia mater that extends from the conus medullaris and becomes the coccygeal ligament, which attaches to the coccyx. The thecal sac refers to the dural tube within the spinal canal. The denticulate ligaments arise laterally from the pia mater between the ventral and dorsal spinal roots and attach to the adjacent dura mater to stabilize the cord.

The spinal cord has eight pairs of cervical roots, 12 pairs of thoracic roots, five pairs of lumbar roots, five pairs of sacral roots, and one pair of coccygeal roots. The cervical roots exit over the pedicle of the same-numbered vertebra, with the eighth cervical root exiting over the first thoracic pedicle. The thoracic and lumbar roots exit below the pedicle of the same-numbered vertebral body (Fig. 1-1). The spinal roots leave the cord as an anterolateral ventral root (motor) and a posterolateral dorsal root (sensory). These unite in the intervertebral (neural) foramina to form the spinal nerve, which is composed of afferent sensory fibers and efferent motor fibers. Sensory fibers from the periphery enter the spinal nerve, travel to the dorsal root ganglion located in the intervertebral foramen, become the dorsal root, and enter the spinal cord. The white matter of the cord, composed mostly of axons, is located on the periphery. Tracts within the cord include the lateral corticospinal tract, the lateral spinothalamic tract, and the posterior columns. The centrally located anterior and posterior horns of the spinal cord contain gray matter, the location of neuronal cell bodies.

The arterial blood supply of the spinal cord comes from the anterior and posterior spinal arteries, which are branches of the vertebral arteries. As spinal arteries descend along the spinal cord, they receive additional feeding branches from multiple radicular arteries. In the neck, the radicular arteries are branches of the vertebral arteries and the thyrocervical trunks. In the thorax, the radicular arteries branch from the intercostal arteries. In the low back, the radicular arteries are branches of lumbar arteries. An important radicular artery, the artery of Adamkiewicz, usually arises on the left side between T10 and L2 and supplies the lower thoracic spinal cord and the conus medullaris (Fig. 1-8). Damage to the arterial system of the spinal cord leads to ischemia and stroke, which may result in paralysis, sensory loss, or loss of bowel and bladder function. A spinal cord stroke may occur during the repair of a thoracic or abdominal aortic aneurysm if a radicular artery (which feeds the spinal cord) is compromised. A strategy to avoid spinal cord ischemia includes the preoperative placement of a lumbar drain to decrease the intraspinal pressure and, therefore, increase intraspinal blood flow during the procedure.

FUNCTIONAL ORGANIZATION

The motor system is located anteriorly or ventrally in most parts of the CNS. The upper motor neuron (UMN) is a pyramidal neuron with its cell body in the precentral gyrus of the frontal lobe. The motor homunculus is a representation of the body in the primary motor area located in the

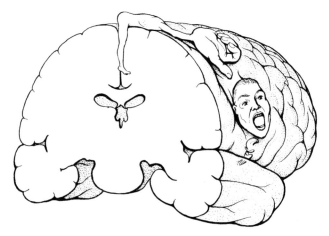

Figure 1-9 The sensory or motor homunculus. The representation of the body in the precentral (motor) or postcentral (sensory) gyri. (From Carpenter MB. *Core text of neuroanatomy.* Baltimore: Williams & Wilkins, 1991, with permission.)

precentral gyrus (Fig. 1-9). The axon of the UMN travels through the genu (muscles of the face) or posterior limb (muscles of the body) of the internal capsule, down the crura cerebri, through the medullary pyramids where the axon crosses over to the contralateral side (decussation of the pyramids), and finally down the lateral corticospinal tract in the spinal cord. The UMN axon synapses on the lower motor neuron (LMN) cell body (anterior horn cell) in the spinal cord. The LMN sends its axon ipsilaterally to the muscle it innervates. The ventral roots of the spinal cord are composed of LMN axons. If a UMN is damaged, its inhibitory effect on the LMN is lost and the LMN becomes hyperactive, resulting in a spastic paralysis. When an LMN is damaged, the muscle loses its innervation, resulting in a flaccid paralysis.

The sensory system is located, for the most part, in the posterior or dorsal portion of the CNS. The postcentral gyrus in the parietal lobe contains the primary somesthetic areas. The secondary somesthetic areas lie adjacent to the primary areas. The sensory homunculus is a representation of the body in the somatosensory cortex (Fig. 1-9). The cortical sensory areas receive input from the ventral posterior nuclei of the thalamus, which relays impulses from the posterior columns, spinothalamic tract (body), and trigeminothalamic tract (face). The paired posterior columns contain afferent fibers that transmit information regarding kinesthetic sense (position and movement) and tactile sense (touch and pressure). In the spinal cord the posterior columns are divided into the fasciculus gracilis, which contains afferent fibers from the leg, and the fasciculus cuneatus, which contains afferent fibers from the arm. The fibers of the posterior columns enter the spinal cord and ascend, without crossing the midline, to the nucleus cuneatus and nucleus gracilis, both of which are located in the medulla. Fibers from the nucleus cuneatus and nucleus gracilis cross the midline in the medulla and ascend in the contralateral medial lemniscus to the thalamus. The paired lateral spinothalamic tracts are formed by afferent pain and temperature fibers from peripheral receptors. These fibers synapse in the dorsal root ganglia and then enter the spinal cord as the dorsal roots. The lateral spinothalamic tract crosses in the anterior white commissure of the spinal

cord within two to three levels after entering the cord and ascends in the contralateral half of the spinal cord. The trigeminothalamic tract carries pain and temperature fibers from receptors in the face.

The input to the visual system is light entering the eye. The image of an object is represented on the retina upside down and backward. Therefore, the superior temporal (lateral) visual field of one eye is represented on the inferior nasal (medial) portion of the retina of the same eye. The retinal fibers travel in the optic nerves (cranial nerve II) to the optic chiasm. Here, the fibers from temporal halves of visual fields (the nasal halves of the retinas) cross, but the fibers from the nasal halves of the visual fields (temporal halves of the retinas) do not cross. The fibers then leave the chiasm and form the optic tracts. The temporal half of the visual field of one eye and the nasal half of the visual field of the other eye travel together in one optic tract. In other words, the left half of the visual field of both eyes is in the right optic tract and the right half of the visual field of both eyes is in the left optic tract. The optic tracts travel to the lateral geniculate bodies of the thalamus. The optic radiations leave the thalamus and travel to the occipital lobes. The primary visual area is in the calcarine sulcus of the occipital lobe. Stereoscopic vision first occurs in the occipital cortex. In general, only lesions between the retina and the chiasm can produce a unilateral visual loss. Lesions between the chiasm and the occipital lobes produce ipsilateral visual-field deficits in both eyes, called a *homonymous hemianopsia.* The closer the lesion is to the occipital lobe, the more congruent are the field cuts of the homonymous hemianopsia (Fig. 1-10).

Other brainstem structures concerned with vision include the superior colliculus and the Edinger-Westphal nucleus. The superior colliculus receives visual input from the retina and sends impulses indirectly to the motor neurons of the upper spinal cord (tectospinal tract) involved in reflex head and neck movements initiated by visual stimuli. The Edinger-Westphal nucleus supplies the parasympathetic fibers to the constrictor muscle fibers in the iris. The sympathetic fibers to the dilator muscle fibers in the iris come from the superior cervical ganglion. The movement of the eyes are controlled by the extraocular muscles. The oculomotor nerve (cranial nerve III) innervates the superior rectus, the medial rectus, the inferior rectus, the inferior oblique, and the levator palpebrae muscles. This nerve carries parasympathetic fibers to the ciliary muscle and the sphincter muscle of the pupil. The trochlear nerve (cranial nerve IV) supplies the superior oblique muscle. The abducens nerve (cranial nerve VI) supplies the lateral rectus muscle.

The input to the auditory system is sound that travels as a wave to the ear. The sound wave causes movement of the tympanic membrane, which transmits the impulse to the bones in the middle ear (malleus, incus, and stapes). The impulse is converted to a fluid wave in the perilymph of the cochlea. Hair cells in the cochlea transform the fluid wave into an electrical impulse that travels down the cochlear nerve (a division of cranial nerve VIII, vestibulocochlear nerve). In the brainstem, the cochlear nerve fibers synapse in the inferior colliculus. From here, projections go to the medial geniculate body of the thalamus and then to the transverse gyrus of Heschl located in the temporal lobe. Each temporal lobe receives input from both ears.

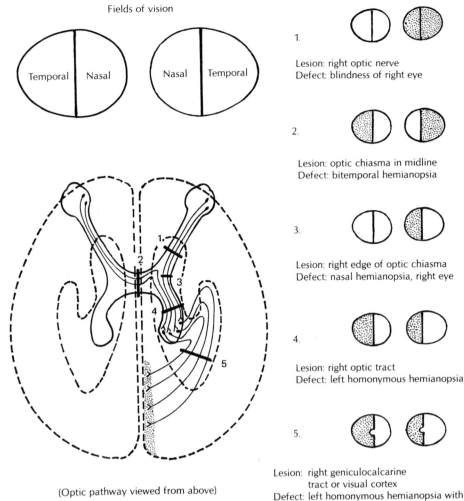

Fields of vision

1.

Lesion: right optic nerve
Defect: blindness of right eye

2.

Lesion: optic chiasma in midline
Defect: bitemporal hemianopsia

3.

Lesion: right edge of optic chiasma
Defect: nasal hemianopsia, right eye

4.

Lesion: right optic tract
Defect: left homonymous hemianopsia

5.

Lesion: right geniculocalcarine
tract or visual cortex
Defect: left homonymous hemianopsia with
sparing of macular vision

Figure 1-10 Visual deficits caused by lesions at different points along the visual pathway. (From Barr ML, Kiernan JA. *The human nervous system.* Philadelphia: JB Lippincott Co, 1993, with permission.)

(Optic pathway viewed from above)

Several areas of the brain are involved with language. The area involved in speech comprehension is the Wernicke area, located in the temporal lobe of the dominant hemisphere. The area involved in speech production is the Broca area, located in the frontal lobe of the dominant hemisphere. Patterns of aphasia include Wernicke aphasia, Broca aphasia, global aphasia, and conduction aphasia. Wernicke aphasia is a problem with the comprehension of speech. The patient can speak fluently, but the sentences produced have no meaning and do not make sense. Broca aphasia is a motor aphasia in which the patient can comprehend speech but cannot produce speech and is not fluent. The speech muscles are not paralyzed, but they cannot be coordinated to produce meaningful speech (apraxia). A global aphasia is caused by a lesion that destroys almost all of the language areas, leaving patients unable to speak, comprehend, read, write, or repeat what is said to them. A conduction aphasia occurs when the connection between Broca and Wernicke areas is disrupted. The most striking feature of a conduction aphasia is the difficulty patients have repeating what is said to them.

The autonomic nervous system (ANS) is divided into the sympathetic nervous system and the parasympathetic nervous system. The fibers of the autonomic nervous system run in the lateral portions of the spinal cord. The sympathetic nervous system is a global activating system concerned with fight or flight reactions, and the parasympathetic nervous system is a more precise regulator of bodily functions and homeostasis. The ANS is not under voluntary control and its input is not required for the viscera to function. Both systems are able to change the activity of the viscera and carry sensory information from the viscera to the CNS.

NEURORADIOLOGY

Plain x-rays, computerized tomographic (CT), and magnetic resonance imaging (MRI) are diagnostic studies that are used frequently in neurosurgery. Anteroposterior, lateral, and oblique plain films show bony detail of the skull and spinal column and can demonstrate traumatic and degenerative disease. Computerized tomography is more sensitive than plain films for visualizing fractures.

A CT scan displays a true image of CNS structures. The various tissues of the body attenuate radiation differently, owing to different tissue densities, and are assigned different values of Hounsfield units (HU). Tissue attenuation spans are between +1,000 HU, signifying total attenuation, and −1,000 HU, signifying no attenuation. Water is assigned the value of 0 HU and air is assigned the value of −1,000 HU. Fat has a value between −40 and −100 HU. White and gray matter have similar densities, with values between 30 and 50 HU. Calcified structures (bone) have values of approximately 150 HU.

A gray scale is used to view the images with endpoints chosen anywhere between +1,000 and −1,000 HU. The width of the window is the difference between these endpoints. The smaller the window, the greater the difference in shades of gray between two similar HU values. The drawback of a small window is that more tissue lies outside the chosen window. Differently windowed images are sensitive to particular processes. Common window algorithms include brain windows, subdural windows, and bone windows. A brain window is a narrow window that allows differentiation of white and gray matter. Unfortunately, bony detail is lost because it usually lies outside of this window. To see bony detail, a wider window (bone window) is used. A subdural window is an intermediate window between brain and bone windows that helps differentiate acute blood from bone (Fig. 1-11).

When tissue attenuates very little radiation (low HU value), it is referred to as *hypodense* and appears dark gray to black on a CT image. Tissue and fluid with high water content will be hypodense in relation to normal brain tissue

on CT. Examples are areas of brain edema and the ventricular system, which is filled with CSF. Other hypodense substances are air and fat. When a tissue attenuates a significant amount of radiation (high HU value), it is referred to as *hyperdense* and appears bright or white on the CT image. Hyperdense substances include bone, acute blood, and iodinated contrast. Very dense tissue, such as a highly cellular tumor, may also appear hyperdense relative to normal brain tissue; however, it will not appear as hyperdense as bone.

When intravenous (i.v.) contrast is given, an area where the BBB has broken down will appear white, referred to as an *area of enhancement*. Some enhancing chronic processes include tumors, infections, and abscesses. In addition, contrast will opacify the lumina of vessels. With correct timing, the large cerebral vessels can be imaged while contrast is passing through them and three-dimensional (3D) reconstructions can be created, a technique called *CT angiography*.

Computed tomography is effective for imaging acute processes that necessitate an emergent neuroradiologic evaluation such as a hemorrhage from a trauma, a brain tumor, a stroke, or an aneurysm. Furthermore, computerized tomography is useful for detecting pathologic conditions in bone, such as vertebral fractures. Acute hemorrhage is hyperdense to normal brain tissue on computerized tomography when viewed using brain windows. In an emergent situation, contrast is not given because acute hemorrhage can be confused with an area of enhancement. One acute process not well imaged by computerized tomography is an ischemic stroke. An infarcted area of the brain will become hypodense on computerized tomography after 6 to 12 hours. However, computerized tomography is still useful for ruling out hemorrhage. When a stroke becomes hypodense on CT, it involves both the gray matter on the surface of the brain and the underlying white matter. This is because of cytotoxic edema, which results in increased intracellular water and cell death. An abscess or metastatic tumor usually appears on computerized tomography as a sharply demarcated ring-enhancing mass surrounded by white matter edema. A primary brain tumor typically has less distinct margins and irregular enhancement compared to an abscess or metastatic tumor.

MRI is another CNS imaging modality. Tissues are described as having different intensities (CT, density; MRI, intensity). A tissue is described as *hypointense* (darker), *isointense* (the same), or *hyperintense* (brighter) to a reference tissue. Different sequences are used to evaluate different tissues and processes. A T1-weighted sequence is used to demonstrate anatomic detail. With this sequence, tissue and fluid with a high water content (edema and CSF) are hypointense, whereas fat is hyperintense. T1-weighted scans are obtained with and without gadolinium (an i.v. contrast agent), to look for areas where the BBB has broken down. These areas will appear hyperintense and are referred to as *areas of enhancement*. A T2-weighted sequence is sensitive to focal changes in tissue-water content, which is of value in differentiating normal brain tissue from abnormal tissue. In this sequence, tissue and fluid with a high water content are hyperintense. Magnetic resonance angiography (MRA) can be used to evaluate the blood flow in the extracranial carotid arteries and in the arteries of the circle of Willis. Magnetic resonance venography (MRV) is used to evaluate the blood flow in the cerebral venous sinuses.

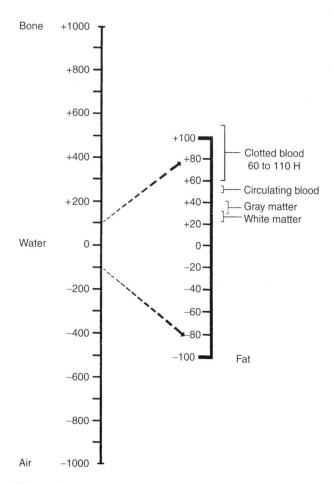

Figure 1-11 Hounsfield number scale with values of certain body tissues. This determines the appearance of the tissue on computerized tomographic (CT) scan. (From Taveras JM. *Neuroradiology*. Baltimore: Williams & Wilkins, 1996, with permission.)

Chronic processes not needing an emergent neuroradiologic evaluation are better evaluated by using MRI. These processes include tumors of the brain and spinal cord, congenital abnormalities, vascular malformations, degenerative disk disease of the spine, and inflammatory processes of the CNS such as multiple sclerosis. MRI is also superior as a technique for imaging soft tissue at the base of skull, which includes the sellar (pituitary) region and the posterior fossa. The enhancement patterns on MRI are similar to what is seen on CT.

Currently, angiography and myelography are rarely performed in the initial diagnostic work-up of a neurosurgical patient. Instead, these techniques are used to gain additional information once a diagnosis is made. Angiography is used in the head, neck, and spine. It is an invasive procedure, and cerebral angiography carries a risk of stroke from 0.5% to 3%. Most commonly, cerebral angiography is used to evaluate a patient with a nontraumatic subarachnoid hemorrhage (SAH) or a patient suspected of having a carotid stenosis, carotid dissection, traumatic arterial injury, arteriovenous malformation (AVM), or vasculitis. Therapeutic procedures can be performed during angiography including coiling of an aneurysm, embolization of a vessel that is bleeding or part of a pathologic process, thrombolysis of an acute ischemic stroke, and stenting of stenotic vessels.

Myelography is an invasive procedure that has been largely replaced by MRI as the primary mode of imaging the spinal cord. Computed tomography has enhanced the utility of myelography by adding axial images. There are still occasions when a myelogram can add important information by showing excellent detail of spinal column anatomy in relation to the outline of the spinal cord and roots within the thecal sac. Two clinical situations when myelography is useful include diffuse disease of the subarachnoid space, such as tumor seeding and arachnoiditis, and a complex spinal case in which the patient has had previous surgery or has had a nondiagnostic CT scan and MRI.

BASIC PROCEDURES

Basic intracranial procedures include burr holes, intracranial pressure (ICP) monitoring, ventriculostomy, stereotactic biopsy, craniectomy, craniotomy, and insertion of a ventriculoperitoneal shunt. Burr holes are drilled in the skull to gain access to the epidural and subdural spaces and are used as starting points for a craniectomy or craniotomy. They are also used to drain chronic subdural hematomas (SDHs). An ICP monitor (bolt) is passed through a hole in the skull to measure the ICP but it cannot be used to drain CSF. A ventriculostomy is a catheter placed through a hole in the skull and into the ventricular system. It can be used to measure the ICP and therapeutically drain CSF to lower the pressure. A stereotactic biopsy can be done under computed tomographic or MRI guidance. It can be used to obtain tissue for diagnosis in a patient with an unresectable intracranial mass or masses, or for drainage of a brain abscess. A craniectomy is performed by removing a portion of bone to gain intracranial access and not replacing that piece of bone at the end of the operation. A craniectomy may be performed to relieve elevated intracranial pressure in a case of traumatic head

injury with severe brain swelling. Leaving the resected bone off gives the brain room to expand. A craniotomy is performed by removing a portion of the skull to gain intracranial access and replacing that portion of bone at the end of the operation. A ventriculoperitoneal shunt is a catheter that connects the ventricular system to the peritoneal cavity. The flow of CSF in the shunt is regulated by a pressure-responsive one-way valve. CSF is allowed to flow only from the ventricle to the peritoneum. A shunt is used to treat hydrocephalus.

Basic spinal procedures include posterior and anterior approaches. The posterior approaches provide access to the dorsal and lateral aspects of the thecal sac and include laminectomy and microdiskectomy. A laminectomy is performed through a midline incision in the back, parallel to the spinal axis. The lamina are exposed and then removed to expose the posterior aspect of the thecal sac. A microdiskectomy is done for a ruptured lumbar disk. The ruptured disk is approached from a small midline incision in the back. A portion of the lamina on the side of the ruptured disk usually needs to be removed to gain access to the space around the thecal sac where the fragment of disk is located. An anterior approach to the spine provides exposure of the vertebral bodies, intervertebral disks, and anterior aspect of the thecal sac. Removal of the entire vertebral body, called a *corpectomy*, can be done from an anterior approach in the cervical, thoracic, and lumbar spine. An anterior cervical diskectomy is the removal of an intervertebral disk in the cervical spine. Discectomies in the thoracic and lumbar spine can also be accomplished with an anterior approach. After removal of a vertebral body and disk, a piece of bone, usually fibula or iliac crest, is placed in the defect, and this procedure is referred to as a *fusion*.

ABNORMALITIES OF THE CEREBROSPINAL FLUID SPACES

Hydrocephalus is an increase in the total amount of CSF in the ventricular system, resulting either from the restriction of the bulk flow of CSF or from the overproduction of CSF. As a result, the ventricular system dilates and the ICP increases. When the bulk flow of CSF is disturbed, either noncommunicating or communicating hydrocephalus results. Noncommunicating hydrocephalus, also called *internal* or *obstructive*, results from an obstruction within one of the ventricles, the foramen, or the aqueduct. The ventricular system proximal to the obstruction becomes dilated. Most frequently, the obstruction occurs where the ventricular system is narrow, such as in the aqueduct of Sylvius, the foramen of Monro, or the outlets of the fourth ventricle (the foramina of Luschka and Magendie). Obstructions are created by tumors, intraventricular clots, parasites, and various other mass lesions. Communicating hydrocephalus, also referred to as *external hydrocephalus*, results when there is an impediment to CSF flow in the subarachnoid space, a failure of adequate resorption of CSF, or the overproduction of CSF. Dilation of the entire ventricular system occurs. Communicating hydrocephalus may occur after meningitis, and it is caused by the blockage of CSF flow within the basal cisterns, part of the subarachnoid space. After an SAH, communicating hydrocephalus is caused by inadequate resorption of CSF at the arachnoid villi. Communicating hydrocephalus can also occur after trauma, encephalitis, and intraventricular hemorrhage. Hydrocephalus, caused by the overproduction of CSF, may occur with a choroid plexus papilloma or carcinoma.

Hydrocephalus may be present at birth—present in three to four newborns per 1,000 live births—or may develop after a child is born. Infants between birth and 2 years of age frequently develop hydrocephalus secondary to a congenital lesion. Two congenital malformations associated with hydrocephalus are Chiari II and Dandy-Walker malformations. The Chiari II malformation is described further in the "Congenital Malformations" section of this chapter. The Dandy-Walker syndrome is noncommunicating hydrocephalus, a posterior fossa cyst, and cerebellar dysgenesis. The posterior fossa cyst is in communication with the fourth ventricle, but the normal outflow of the fourth ventricle, the foramina of Magendie and Luschka, is atretic. Other lesions that cause noncommunicating hydrocephalus in infants include aqueductal atresia or stenosis, developmental cysts, encephaloceles, neoplasms, arachnoid cysts, and vascular abnormalities such as a vein of Galen aneurysm. In a hydrocephalic infant with open cranial sutures, the skull expands along with the ventricles and the infant develops a large head (macrocrania) and widened cranial sutures. Without dysgenesis of the brain, there are no early neurologic symptoms. As the ventricles expand and the ICP increases, the superficial scalp veins become prominent and the anterior fontanelle bulges. Neurologic signs of increased ICP include papilledema and bilateral abducens palsies, which result in a loss of lateral gaze. With long-standing elevated ICP, optic atrophy occurs, resulting in visual deterioration and the development of spastic paralysis of the lower extremities secondary to motor fibers being stretched over the enlarged lateral ventricles. The infant may develop Parinaud syndrome, which is paralysis of upward gaze (setting sun sign), paralysis of accommodation, and the failure of the pupils to react to light.

In children older than 2 years, frequent causes of hydrocephalus include brain tumors, meningitis, intracerebral hemorrhage, and aqueductal stenosis. In this age-group, the presentation is often acute because the cranial sutures are closed. Symptoms include headache, vomiting, and lethargy. With acute hydrocephalus, progression to unresponsiveness and even death may be rapid. With chronic hydrocephalus, a slow progressive onset of symptoms from the elevated ICP occurs and symptoms include slowed cognitive function, behavior changes, or deteriorating school performance. In addition, the child may have endocrine or hypothalamic disorders. In adults, hydrocephalus generally has an insidious onset. Common causes include infectious meningitis, ventriculitis, late-onset aqueductal stenosis, intraventricular hemorrhage, SAH, and neoplasm. The elderly can develop normal-pressure hydrocephalus in which the patient has large ventricles, but the ICP is not elevated. Normal-pressure hydrocephalus is characterized by a triad of symptoms: ataxia, urinary incontinence, and progressive cognitive decline (dementia). Clinical improvement after a high volume lumbar puncture can be diagnostic of normal-pressure hydrocephalus.

When imaging hydrocephalic patients with MRI or CT, enlarged ventricles are seen. The tissue surrounding the frontal horns of the lateral ventricles may be hypodense, a process called *transependymal flow* of CSF. In these areas,

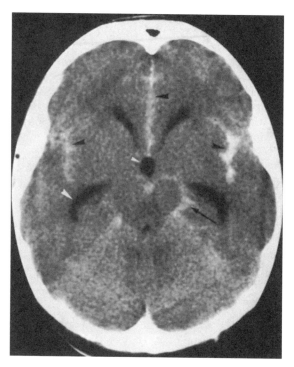

Figure 1-12 A noncontrast computerized tomographic (CT) scan of the brain. Early hydrocephalus is demonstrated by the prominence of the temporal horns of the lateral ventricles and a rounded third ventricle. Subarachnoid hemorrhage is present in both sylvian (lateral) fissures and the interhemispheric fissure. (From Greenfield LJ. *Surgery: scientific principles and practice.* Philadelphia: JB Lippincott Co, 1993, with permission.)

CSF is being forced through the ventricular walls by the increased intraventricular pressure. The temporal horns of the lateral ventricles are prominent and the third ventricle is more rounded than usual (Fig. 1-12).

Acute hydrocephalus is an emergency and is treated with a ventriculostomy or ventriculoperitoneal shunt. Chronic hydrocephalus is treated with a shunt. The ventricular portion can be inserted through either a frontal or a parietal burr hole. The distal end of a shunt can be placed in the peritoneum (ventriculoperitoneal shunt), the pleura (ventriculopleural), or the right atrium of the heart (ventriculoatrial). Most shunts are inserted on the right side of the head to avoid the dominant hemisphere. After the insertion of a shunt, children must be followed closely for motor development, intellectual function, and ventricular size. Complications of shunt placement include infections, malfunctions of the hardware, and perforation of abdominal viscera. An alternative way to treat communicating hydrocephalus is insertion of a lumboperitoneal shunt. The catheter is inserted into the thecal sac of the lumbar spine, and CSF is drained into the peritoneal cavity. Whenever possible, the underlying cause of the hydrocephalus should be treated.

An arachnoid cyst is a CSF-filled cavity that is not in continuity with the ventricular system. These cysts are congenital lesions commonly found in the temporal fossa and are frequently asymptomatic. When they do present with accompanying neurologic symptoms, it usually occurs in childhood. These cysts can act as mass lesions causing signs of increased ICP (headache, vomiting, and lethargy) or focal signs (hemiparesis and aphasia).

In the spinal cord, a cystic dilation within the parenchyma of the cord filled with CSF is called a syrinx. Syringomyelia is a syrinx lined by glial tissue within the substance of the spinal cord. Hydromyelia is a dilation of the central canal of the spinal cord that is lined by ependymal tissue, like the ventricular system. Hydromyelia is commonly seen with Chiari malformations. Both syringomyelia and hydromyelia may be asymptomatic or they may cause weakness, sensory loss, or myelopathy.

CONGENITAL MALFORMATIONS

Two percent of infants are born with a congenital abnormality, and 60% of these abnormalities involve the CNS. Most of the CNS defects occur during the closure of the dorsal midline structures. Normally the neural groove closes in the midline to form the neural tube. At each end of the newly formed neural tube are openings called the *anterior* and *posterior neuropores*. The anterior neuropore typically closes before closing of the posterior neuropore. The neural tube becomes encircled in bone and is covered by skin. Defects occurring at the posterior end of the neural tube cause spinal dysraphism, and defects occurring at the anterior end of the neural tube cause cranial dysraphism. Spinal dysraphism is the failure of ectodermal and mesodermal midline structures to fuse. Abnormal closure of the neural groove, failure of bony fusion, and maldevelopment of the ectoderm are all possible. Spina bifida is the failure of the bony structures to fuse in the midline. When the spinal cord is not affected, this condition is usually not symptomatic and is found incidentally. Spinal dysraphism can be divided into occult spinal dysraphism and open spinal dysraphism.

Open spinal dysraphism (spina bifida aperta or spina bifida cystica) occurs when the bone and overlying skin fail to fuse in the midline, thereby allowing meninges and sometimes neural tissue to herniate through the defect. Two forms of open spinal dysraphism are meningocele and myelomeningocele. When the neural tissue is not involved and only CSF-filled meninges (dura) herniate through the defect in the bone and skin, it is called a *meningocele*. Even though the spinal cord is not involved, one third of affected neonates still have a neurologic deficit. Surgical treatment involves excision of the meningocele, closure of the dura in a watertight manner over the posterior defect, and closure of the skin defect.

When bone, dura, and neural tissue all fail to fuse, the malformation is called a *myelomeningocele*, which is the most common CNS birth defect. There is incomplete closure of the posterior neuropore, causing a mass of unfused neural tissue to protrude from the back of the neonate. Unfortunately, there is complete motor, sensory, and autonomic failure below the lesion, which includes the loss of bowel and bladder function. Families who have had a child with a myelomeningocele or who have a close relative who has had a child with a myelomeningocele, particularly if it is a maternal relative, are at a greater risk of having a child with a myelomeningocele. A mother who is deficient in folic acid is also at a greater risk of having an affected child. Because the neural tube closes at 3 to 4 weeks of gestation, frequently before a pregnancy is confirmed, women planning to become pregnant should take a dietary supplement with folic acid. A myelomeningocele is fixed as soon as possible after birth (usually within 36 hours) to prevent infection (meningitis). In utero repair is currently being investigated. The operative goals are to preserve as much neural tissue as possible, to release the tethering of the spinal cord by the surrounding soft tissue, and to achieve a watertight dural closure.

Almost all neonates with a myelomeningocele have a Chiari II (Arnold-Chiari) malformation and hydrocephalus. The Chiari II malformation is manifested by the caudal displacement of cerebellar vermis, fourth ventricle, and medulla through the plane of the foramen magnum. It is also associated with supratentorial abnormalities, such as hydrocephalus and microgyria, and myelodysplasia (developmental abnormalities of the spinal cord). The Chiari I malformation has less brain herniation than the Chiari II malformation. Only the cerebellar tonsils are displaced caudally through the plane of the foramen magnum.

Myeloschisis is similar to a myelomeningocele, but the exposed neural tissue is uncovered by meninges (dura). It is a more severe, but less common, defect than a myelomeningocele. The unfused spinal cord lies on the surface of the back uncovered by meninges or skin. Most commonly, this occurs in the thoracolumbar region, resulting in paraplegia and absence of bladder function. It is also associated with a Chiari II malformation and hydrocephalus. Treatment is similar to that for myelomeningocele.

When a spinal dysraphic condition is covered by skin, making it not obvious on gross inspection of the back, the condition is usually discovered later in life and is referred to as *occult spinal dysraphism* (spina bifida occulta). Lipomyelomeningocele, split cord malformation, and neurenteric cysts are all forms of occult spinal dysraphism. Lipomyelomeningocele is a subcutaneous lipoma that extends through a defect in the dura and blends with the substance of the spinal cord or attaches to the conus medullaris. A split cord malformation is the presence of two hemicords in one or two dural sacs, separated by a septum within the spinal canal. Neurenteric cysts are rests of endodermal tissue in the CNS. Affected infants commonly present with midline cutaneous stigma or a malformation of the foot or leg. The midline cutaneous stigmata may be a tuft of hair, a capillary hemangioma, a subcutaneous mass, a rudimentary appendage, or an atretic meningocele, which is a small discolored area of thinned skin. A midline tuft of hair on the back over the thoracolumbar region is almost always associated with some form of spina bifida occulta. Older children and adults more commonly present with pain, progressive neurologic dysfunction, or scoliosis. Neurologic deficits include bladder dysfunction and weakness of the lower extremities. Diagnosis is determined by MRI. Treatment includes early surgery before the progression of any neurologic deficits.

A congenital dermal sinus is a dysraphic condition that begins as an opening in the skin and continues as an epithelial-lined tract that can end outside the dura or extend through it. The sinuses can be found anywhere along the neural axis but are most commonly found in the lumbosacral region. A dermal sinus can be associated with recurrent bouts of meningitis, a meningitis from an unusual organism, or a meningitis from a mixture of organisms. An opening in the skin over the coccyx, in the intergluteal cleft, is not a congenital dermal sinus. Instead, it is a coccygeal pit, which is benign and requires no further workup.

Tethering of the spinal cord is associated with spinal dysraphism. A tethered cord is attached tightly to a surrounding nonneural structure, causing the spinal cord to be abnormally stretched as the child grows, which may result in a neurologic deficit. A tethered cord needs to be released at the same time the spinal dysraphic state is repaired.

Cranial dysraphism results from the failure of the anterior end of the neural tube to close properly, which occurs much less commonly than spinal dysraphism. Anencephaly is the failure of the anterior neuropore to close and is not compatible with life. An encephalocele is a midline skull defect with a cystic protrusion of the meninges and brain, which is usually covered by skin and frequently associated with hydrocephalus.

TRAUMA

The pathophysiology of head injury is divided into a primary and secondary phase. The primary injury occurs at the time of the traumatic event, consists of the irreversible damage sustained by neurons and axons in the brain, and cannot be changed by subsequent treatment. Following the primary injury, a secondary injury to the brain may occur. Therapeutic intervention is targeted at preventing or minimizing secondary injury to the brain. Mechanisms of secondary injury include metabolic abnormalities, hypoxia, and hypovolemia. These can be caused by hypoventilation, blood loss, hypotension, and endocrine disturbances. Ischemia can lead to cell death, thereby causing cytotoxic edema and an increase in ICP. The goal of treatment is to prevent secondary injury by supporting blood pressure and controlling ICP.

The evaluation of a traumatically injured patient, whether there is a suspected head or spinal cord injury (SCI), proceeds with a rapid clinical assessment, starting with the airway, breathing, and circulation (ABCs) of Advanced Trauma Life Support (ATLS). After the patient is stabilized, efficient neurologic history taking and examination are undertaken, including the determination of the Glasgow coma scale (GCS) (Table 1-1). Prehospital personnel should be asked whether a patient had any loss of consciousness. The examination should include the evaluation of the size and function of the pupils, noting whether the patient is awake or can be aroused easily; whether the patient follows commands; whether the patient is confused; and whether the patient has any pain in the head, neck, or back. All four extremities should be evaluated for motor function and sensation. If the patient is unresponsive or does not follow commands, movement of the extremities can be produced by painful central stimuli (e.g., sternal rub). Any eye opening or verbal response produced by a painful stimulus applied to an unresponsive patient should be noted. Initial radiologic evaluation consists of a lateral cervical spine film and a head CT scan.

Head injury can be stratified by severity into mild, moderate, and severe. A mild head injury (GCS 13 to 15) usually does not result in any significant primary brain injury. There may be a transient loss of consciousness, commonly referred to as a *concussion*. Other common symptoms of mild head injury are headache, nausea, lethargy, and, at

TABLE 1-1
THE GLASGOW COMA SCALE

Parameter	Response	Score
Eye opening	Spontaneous	4
	To voice	3
	To pain	2
	None	1
Motor response	Follows commands	6
	Localizes to pain	5
	Withdraws from pain	4
	Flexor posturing to pain	3
	Extensor posturing to pain	2
	None	1
Verbal response	Oriented	5
	Confused	4
	Inappropriate words	3
	Incomprehensible sounds	2
	None	1
	Total	15

times, restlessness. Management includes a CT scan of the head, which is positive for a hemorrhage less than 10% of the time, and x-rays of the cervical spine because neck injuries are commonly associated with head injuries. The patient may be admitted to the hospital for observation and frequent neurologic examinations. A patient with a moderate head injury (GCS 9 to 12) usually presents as lethargic and possibly combative. The initial evaluation includes a lateral cervical spine film and a CT scan of the head. The patient is admitted to the hospital for observation and frequent neurologic monitoring. Approximately 10% of moderately head-injured patients will have a discrete lesion on CT. A patient with a severe head injury presents with a GCS of 8 or less. Such a patient is not awake and needs to be intubated for protection of the airway. If possible, a neurologic examination should be performed before the patient is sedated and paralyzed for intubation. A lateral cervical spine film and a CT scan of the head should be part of the initial evaluation. Up to 40% of those with a severe head injury have a large epidural, subdural, or intraparenchymal hematoma (IPH) on CT and need an emergent craniotomy to evacuate the clot and stop the bleeding.

A traumatic head injury may result in a scalp laceration, skull fracture, epidural hematoma (EDH), SDH, or IPH. A *scalp laceration* may hemorrhage profusely. As long as there is not an adjacent skull fracture, the initial management includes holding pressure on the edges of the laceration to decrease the bleeding. As soon as possible, the wound should be débrided and irrigated. Scalp lacerations through the galea should be closed in two layers. First, the galea needs to be approximated, and then the overlying skin is approximated.

Skull fractures can be classified into different types. A skull fracture with overlying skin intact is a closed fracture. If the skin is disrupted, it is an open (compound) fracture and the patient is at risk for a CNS infection. If a fracture extends into a sinus or a mastoid air cell, it is considered open. A linear fracture has a single fracture line. A stellate fracture has several fracture lines radiating from a central point. If there is fragmentation of the bone, it is a comminuted fracture. A diastatic fracture, which is more common in young children, extends into and causes separation of a suture. If the outer table of at least one edge of a fracture fragment lies below the normal anatomic level of the inner table of the adjacent skull, it is a depressed skull fracture.

The treatment of skull fractures depends on the type of fracture, the location of the fracture, and the presence of any associated pathology. Most closed skull fractures that are not depressed require no specific treatment. If the fracture line crosses a vascular channel, for example, the middle meningeal artery in the temporal bone or the sagittal sinus at the vertex of the skull, it can be associated with an EDH or an SDH. Large hematomas need to be removed surgically. Open fractures are treated in the operating room with débridement, irrigation, and closure of the galea and skin. A dural laceration may be seen with a comminuted skull fracture and needs to be repaired. A depressed skull fracture requires surgery to elevate the fragments if it is causing a neurologic deficit, is an open fracture, is associated with a CSF leak, or is depressed a distance greater than the thickness of the skull (generally 8 to 10 mm). However, a depressed skull fracture over a dural sinus may be dangerous to elevate, and these indications do not apply.

Basilar skull fractures have distinct clinical presentations, they can cause cranial nerve palsies, and they commonly have associated CSF leaks. Fractures in the floor of the anterior cranial fossa frequently produce raccoon eyes (periorbital ecchymosis). Battle sign (ecchymosis behind the ear) is associated with a fracture in the petrous portion of the temporal bone, which forms the floor of the middle cranial fossa. A facial nerve palsy can occur with a fracture

of the temporal bone. Facial weakness may begin immediately if the nerve has been lacerated by the fracture or may be delayed if the facial nerve has only been contused. A contused nerve will progressively swell and become compressed within its bony canal. If a basilar skull fracture extends into a paranasal sinus or mastoid air cell, a traumatic CSF leak is possible. Fluid may drain from the nose (CSF rhinorrhea) or the ear (CSF otorrhea), or it may drain down the back of the throat. Antibiotics are not routinely given by neurosurgeons for traumatic CSF leaks because they usually seal spontaneously in 7 to 10 days and infectious complications are uncommon. Traumatic CSF leaks are treated initially with elevation of the head—to decrease the ICP—and observation. If the leak fails to stop after 7 to 10 days, a lumbar drain may be placed or a surgical repair can be undertaken.

An EDH arises between the inner table of the skull and the dura. It does not cross suture lines, because the dura is attached tightly to the inner surface of the skull at the suture lines and, therefore, has a characteristic convex shape. An EDH is a high-pressure bleed from a lacerated epidural artery. The most common source is a lacerated middle meningeal artery or one of its branches, which results in a temporal EDH. Less commonly, an EDH can also occur after a tear in the wall of a venous sinus secondary to a depressed skull fracture. The classic, but uncommon, scenario of a patient with an EDH involves a victim with an initial brief loss of consciousness immediately after an accident, followed by a lucid interval and then a progressive decrease in the level of consciousness. More commonly, patients have only a progressive decrease in their level of consciousness. Focal signs, such as a hemiparesis, are often associated with this injury (Fig. 1-13).

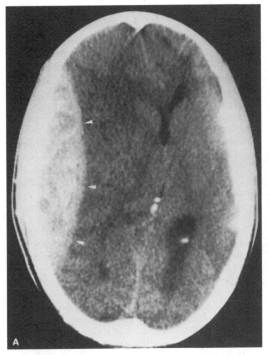
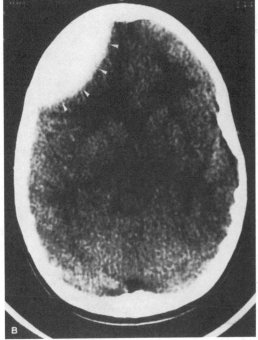

Figure 1-13   Two noncontrast computerized tomographic (CT) scans of the brain. **A:** A large epidural hematoma with marked midline shift. **B:** A smaller epidural hematoma. Note the lenticular shape of both. (From Greenfield LJ. *Surgery: scientific principles and practice.* Philadelphia: JB Lippincott Co, 1993, with permission.)

An SDH arises between the dura mater and the arachnoid membrane. It is caused by the laceration of a subdural bridging vein that runs from the cortex to the dura, which results in a low-pressure venous hemorrhage. An SDH is crescent-shaped over the surface of the cerebral hemisphere and is bounded by the falx cerebri and tentorium (dural reflections). An SDH may also be caused by a tear in the subdural wall of a venous sinus or the extension of an IPH into the subdural space. SDHs are often subdivided according to their duration into acute, subacute, and chronic. An acute SDH is found at the time of injury. Treatment for small asymptomatic acute SDH is observation, frequent neurologic examinations, and a follow-up CT scan of the brain to ensure that the hemorrhage is not enlarging. Treatment for a large, symptomatic, acute SDH entails an emergent craniotomy to evacuate the clot and stop the bleeding. An acute SDH is often associated with a severe head injury, and even after the evacuation of the hematoma a patient may have a residual neurologic deficit resulting from the widespread neuronal injury (Fig. 1-14). A subacute SDH occurs after a minor blow to the head. The symptoms begin a few days to weeks after the injury and include headache, progressive lethargy, hemiparesis, or double vision (cranial nerve VI nerve palsy). Treatment entails drainage of the subacute SDH by burr holes if it is liquid or a craniotomy if it is an organized clot. Postoperative patients usually recover well. A chronic SDH also occurs after a minor blow to the head. Often, the patient does not remember the injury. A chronic SDH is believed to start as a small SDH, which slowly becomes encased in fibrous membrane. It then liquefies and gradually enlarges. Headache, lethargy, and focal neurologic deficits can occur

with increasing size of the SDH. Papilledema, from increased ICP, may be seen on ophthalmologic examination. Chronic SDHs are commonly seen in infants and the elderly. A subdural hygroma presents as a chronic SDH but occurs secondary to a tear in arachnoid membrane. This defect allows CSF to flow into the subdural space from the subarachnoid space. Burr holes can be used to drain the hygroma fluid from the subdural space.

Other forms of traumatic intracranial hemorrhage include an IPH and a traumatic SAH. An IPH results from tearing of intraparenchymal capillaries. It is associated with a cerebral contusion and subarachnoid hemorrhage. A traumatic SAH occurs when a vessel in the subarachnoid space is damaged and bleeds. Trauma is the most common cause of all SAHs (the most common cause of a nontraumatic SAH is rupture of a cerebral aneurysm).

Diffuse axonal injury (DAI) is commonly seen with severe blunt head trauma. In DAI, many axons within the brain are injured as a result of shearing forces. DAI is best diagnosed using MRI, which shows multiple hemorrhages in deep white matter structures such as the corpus callosum and hemorrhages within the brainstem.

In 1995, the Brain Trauma Foundation published the *Guidelines for the Management of Severe Head Injury*, which outlines how to manage a patient with a GCS between 3 and 8. This is an evidence-based approach to head injury management, with each recommendation assigned a degree of certainty. The three degrees of certainty are standards, guidelines, and options, which reflect a high, moderate, and unclear degree of clinical certainty of the management principle. The following is a summary of these guidelines.

The guidelines make recommendations about blood pressure and oxygenation goals during the initial resuscitation of a patient with a head injury. There is no standard of treatment because of insufficient data, but there is a guideline that recommends maintaining a systolic blood pressure of greater than 90 mm Hg and an arterial partial pressure of oxygen (PaO_2) of greater than 60 mm Hg. The option presented is to keep the mean arterial pressure (MAP) greater than 90 mm Hg so that the cerebral perfusion pressure (CPP) is maintained at greater than 70 mm Hg. The CPP is calculated by subtracting the ICP from the MAP, or mathematically, $CPP = MAP - ICP$ and $MAP = (2DBP+SPB)/3$, where *DBP* is the diastolic blood pressure and *SBP* is the systolic blood pressure.

The best method for ICP monitoring, the indications for ICP monitoring, when to treat elevated ICP, and when to treat a low CPP are all addressed. The best way to monitor ICP is with a ventricular catheter, when possible, because it is the most accurate method and can be used to lower ICP by draining CSF. There is no standard for when to monitor ICP, but there are guidelines. Any patient with a GCS of 3 to 8 after cardiopulmonary resuscitation and an abnormal CT scan of the head showing a contusion, hematoma, edema, or swelling of the brain should be monitored. In a patient with a GCS of 3 to 8 and a normal CT of the head, monitoring is indicated if the patient is older than 40 years, is decerebrate or has decorticate posturing, or has a systolic blood pressure less than 90 mm Hg. The treatment of elevated ICP is also not governed by a standard, but a guideline of treating ICP of greater than 20 to 25 mm Hg is recommended. The options of corroborating the ICP treatment threshold with the clinical examination and CPP

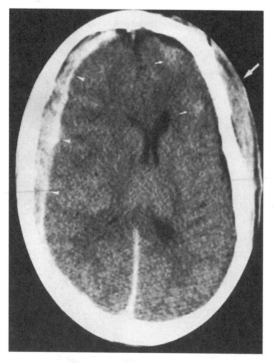

Figure 1-14 A noncontrast computerized tomographic (CT) scan of the brain. An acute subdural hematoma with marked midline shift. Note the crescent shape. The large white area depicts the point of impact. (From Greenfield LJ. *Surgery: scientific principles and practice.* Philadelphia: JB Lippincott Co, 1993, with permission.)

measurement and maintaining the CPP at or greater than 70 mm Hg are presented.

The topic of hyperventilation in the head-injured patient is governed by recommendations of what not to do. The standard of treatment is that a severely head-injured patient should not be hyperventilated below a arterial partial pressure of carbon dioxide ($PaCO_2$) of 25 mm Hg for a prolonged period. The recommended treatment guideline is that a severely head-injured patient should not be hyperventilated to lower than a $PaCO_2$ of 35 mm Hg for the first 24 hours after the injury. Two options are as follows: brief periods of hyperventilation can be used with acute neurologic deterioration, or hyperventilation therapy may be instituted with jugular venous oxygen saturation and cerebral blood flow monitoring.

The use of mannitol and high-dose barbiturate therapy in the severely head-injured patient is addressed. There are not sufficient data to outline standards for the use of either of these agents. The guideline concerning the use of mannitol states that it is an effective means of lowering elevated ICP in a severely head-injured patient at a dose between 0.25 and 1 g per kilogram of body weight. Mannitol is probably most effective if given in intermittent boluses rather than as an i.v. drip. The options for mannitol use are as follows: It can be used emergently before ICP monitoring is instituted if there are signs of transtentorial herniation not secondary to systemic pathology and if hypovolemia is avoided. In a patient at risk for renal failure, the serum osmolality should be kept below 320 mOsmol and the patient being treated with mannitol needs to have a Foley catheter. The guideline set forth for the use of high-dose barbiturate therapy (pentobarbital coma) states that the agent can be used in a severely head-injured patient with elevated ICP that is refractory to other methods of management, but the patient should be hemodynamically stable and capable of making a meaningful recovery.

The standard concerning antiseizure drugs after severe head injury is that their prophylactic use does not prevent late posttraumatic seizures. There is not a guideline for antiseizure drugs, but the option of using them to prevent early posttraumatic seizures is given. When phenytoin is given prophylactically, it should be given for 7 days after the injury and then discontinued unless the patient develops a seizure disorder. Glucocorticoid therapy after severe head injury is not recommended.

Finally, a critical pathway for treatment of the severely head-injured patient is outlined. The expert opinions of the committee members who wrote the *Guidelines for the Management of Severe Head Injury* are used to formulate this pathway. Early management interventions to minimize ICP include elevating the head of the patient, repositioning the neck into a neutral position to improve the venous drainage from the brain, treating hyperthermia aggressively, beginning prophylactic treatment against seizures, sedating the patient with or without pharmacologic paralysis, avoiding hypoxia, and resuscitating the volume status of the patient. If the patient has ICP elevations after the institution of these therapies and has a ventriculostomy, intermittent drainage of CSF should be used to lower the ICP. If this is not effective or if the patient does not have a ventriculostomy, mannitol should be used. The patient can also be ventilated to keep the $PaCO_2$ at or greater than 35 mm Hg. If mannitol is being used, the serum osmolality should be

maintained below 320 mOsmol. If all of these treatments are unsuccessful, further hyperventilation directed by jugular venous saturation measurements or cerebral blood flow monitoring should be considered. If ineffective, second-tier therapy, such as high-dose barbiturate therapy should be considered. It must be remembered that an acute elevation in ICP could also be caused by a newly developed hemorrhage. Therefore, a low threshold for repeat of the CT scan of the head should be maintained.

The outcome after head injury depends on several factors. The potential for recovery is inversely proportional to age and proportional to the GCS score on admission. Other determinants of poor outcome include elevated ICP that is refractory to surgical and medical management, abnormal brainstem reflexes on initial examination, preexisting illnesses, penetrating trauma (especially gunshot wounds), intracranial hemorrhage, SDH, delay in treatment, multiple system trauma, and systemic insults (including acidosis, hypoxia, and hypotension). Patients with both an SDH and an IPH have a very poor prognosis.

There are several mechanisms of supratentorial brain herniation that can occur with elevated ICP. One important mechanism is transtentorial (central) herniation, which presents with the classic triad of lethargy that progresses to unresponsiveness (coma), a fixed and dilated ipsilateral pupil, and a contralateral hemiplegia. With increased ICP, Cushing triad is seen, which consists of hypertension, bradycardia, and respiratory irregularity. If treated unsuccessfully, transtentorial herniation results in death. Another form of brain herniation is uncal herniation, which is similar to transtentorial herniation but a decrease in consciousness occurs late and decorticate posturing rarely occurs. Subfalcine herniation is the forced displacement of a cingulate gyrus under the falx and to the contralateral side. Infratentorial herniation of the cerebellum can involve the upward movement of the cerebellum into the supratentorial compartment or the downward herniation of the cerebellar tonsils.

Patients with loss of brain function are declared brain-dead. They must meet strict criteria on physical examination and diagnostic testing. During testing for brain death, a patient must have an adequate blood pressure, an adequate body temperature, and cannot be pharmacologically impaired. A brain-death examination includes a neurologic test of the brainstem reflexes, an apnea test, and a confirmatory study showing no blood flow to the brain (cerebral angiography or cerebral radionuclide angiogram).

Finally, it is important to remember that intracranial hemorrhage can be the cause, not the result, of a traumatic injury. For example, a patient may sustain an intracranial bleed from an aneurysm or an AVM and then fall or be involved in an automobile accident. In these situations, the location of hemorrhage may provide clues to the etiology.

All trauma patients are initially assumed to have an unstable spinal column and are treated with spinal precautions by placement on a backboard in a rigid cervical collar. On initial clinical assessment, any tenderness of the neck or back is noted. On neurologic examination, sensation and voluntary motor strength in all extremities is evaluated, along with perianal sensation and voluntary contraction of the external anal sphincter. X-rays of the cervical spine are obtained, which include a lateral view showing the skull base to the top of the T1 vertebral body, an anteroposterior view, and an odontoid view. Additional radiographs of the thoracic and lumbar spine can be obtained to view areas that are tender, have palpable deformities, or are involved in penetrating trauma. Thoracic and lumbar spine films are also obtained if the patient has a neurologic deficit. An area of the spine suspicious for a fracture can be further evaluated with a CT scan including reconstructed sagittal and coronal images. An acute disk rupture or an epidural hematoma can also be seen on CT. The x-ray and CT findings need to be correlated with those of the neurologic examination. In a patient with an SCI, a discrepancy between the radiologic level and the neurologic level needs to be further evaluated in an emergent manner. An MRI can evaluate the spinal cord and look for compressive lesions away from the site of bony injury, which may require emergent surgery if associated with progressive neurologic deficits. In a patient without any neurologic deficits or bony fractures, ligamentous injury must be ruled out as this could make the cervical spine unstable. Lateral flexion and extension cervical spine x-rays in the awake, nonimpaired patient show instability if there is movement between the vertebral bodies. Flexion-extension films should not be done if palpation or movement of the neck is painful. In this case, the patient should be kept in a hard cervical collar until the resolution of his or her neck pain, at which time flexion-extension x-rays should be performed. Neck pain may cause neck muscle spasms, which could mask instability.

Neck fractures can be divided into upper (C1-2) and subaxial (C3-7) cervical spine fractures. Injuries of the upper cervical spine include atlantooccipital dislocations, Jefferson fractures, hangman's fractures, and odontoid fractures. Atlantooccipital dislocation occurs when the ligaments that hold the skull to the spinal column are disrupted. Often, this is a fatal cervical spine injury because of a respiratory arrest. A Jefferson fracture consists of bilateral fractures through the arches of C1, which usually result from axial compression. This fracture usually causes instability of the patient's cervical spine, but the patient commonly does not have any neurologic deficits. It is treated with immobilization of the neck. A hangman's fracture consists of bilateral fractures through the pars interarticularis of C2. The pars interarticularis is the junction of the pedicle and lamina in the ring of C2. Classically, with hangings associated with capital punishment, it is caused by hyperextension and distraction of the neck (therefore, during a hanging, the noose needs to be anterior to the neck to cause this fracture), but it is more commonly caused by hyperextension and axial loading of the neck as a result of a motor vehicle accident. Often, there is anterior subluxation (traumatic spondylolisthesis) of C2 on C3. The patient's cervical spine with an isolated hangman's fracture is usually stable and neurologic deficits are infrequent. Hangman's fractures are also treated with immobilization of the neck. The most common fracture of C2 is an odontoid fracture (dens). Odontoid fractures are classified into three types. A type I fracture is through the odontoid process and it does not involve the junction of the odontoid process with the body of C2. This is a rare fracture that is usually unstable and may need surgical treatment. A type II fracture is through the base of the odontoid process at its junction with the body of C2. This is the most common odontoid fracture and usually causes instability of the patient's cervical spine.

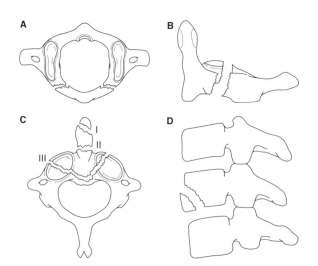

Figure 1-15 Cervical spine fractures. **A:** A Jefferson fracture. Superior view of the atlas (C1). **B:** A hangman's fracture. Lateral view of the axis (C2). **C:** The three types of odontoid fractures—I, II, III. Superior view of the axis (C2). **D:** A teardrop fracture. Lateral view of the lower cervical spine.

Most type II fractures in adults can be treated with halo immobilization, but in certain instances surgical fusion is needed. A type III fracture extends through the odontoid process into the body of C2 (Fig. 1-15). The cervical spine of the patient is usually stable and the patient is treated by immobilization of the neck.

Subaxial cervical spine injuries include subluxations, locked facets, teardrop fractures, and clay shoveler's fractures. Subluxation of one vertebral body on another is caused by a flexion injury to the cervical spine. A horizontal subluxation of greater than 3.5 mm or angular subluxation of greater than 11 degrees on a lateral cervical spine film indicates ligamentous instability. Locked facets can be either unilateral or bilateral. Both are a severe form of subluxation and are caused by flexion injuries. The initial treatment of locked facets is to emergently put the patient in traction (Gardner-Wells tongs) to reduce the dislocation and realign the spinal column. Usually, 10 lb of traction for each cervical level higher than that of the dislocation is the maximum amount of weight applied. Frequent neurologic examinations need to be performed during the application of traction, and the procedure should be aborted with any neurologic deterioration. In addition, frequent x-rays to evaluate the degree of reduction and alignment of the spinal column should be obtained and reviewed. When traction is unsuccessful or there is neurologic deterioration, surgical reduction is indicated. A teardrop fracture results from hyperflexion of the neck and is named because of its appearance on x-ray. A lateral cervical spine film will show a small bone chip anterior and inferior to the fractured vertebral body. This vertebral body is usually wedged anteriorly and a fragment of it is displaced posteriorly into the spinal canal (Fig. 1-15). A teardrop fracture makes the patient's cervical spine unstable and the patient is frequently quadriplegic. Surgical stabilization of the cervical spine is needed.

Fractures at the thoracolumbar junction are seen with traumatic injuries, and when these occur the possibility of spinal instability needs to be addressed. A three-column model has been proposed by Denis, which divides the structural components of the thoracolumbar spinal column into anterior, middle, and posterior columns. The anterior column consists of the anterior longitudinal ligament and the anterior two thirds of the vertebral body. The middle column consists of the posterior one third of the vertebral body and the posterior longitudinal ligament. The posterior column contains the posterior elements, the facet joints, and the associated ligaments (Fig. 1-16). When two or more of these columns are injured, the spine is considered unstable. Instability alone is not an indication for surgery. Most thoracolumbar fractures without neurologic deficits can be treated with bed rest, and, if unstable, can be immobilized in a clamshell orthosis.

The timing of surgery with spinal fractures remains a controversial topic. Some general guidelines of when early surgery is appropriate for traumatic injuries of the cervical, thoracic, and lumbar spine include progressive neurologic deterioration; severe compression of the spinal cord seen on MRI or CT scan and consistent neurologic deficits; an open wound that requires débridement; and the need for early mobilization and rehabilitation. The goals of surgical intervention are to decompress the neural structures, correct the alignment of the bony elements, and stabilize the spinal column.

SCI can be associated with a fracture of the vertebral column, a herniation of an intervertebral disk, a ligamentous injury of the spine, or a penetrating traumatic injury. Head injury is commonly associated with SCI. Lesions at C3 or higher are associated with respiratory failure. Patients with lesions between C4 and C6 have borderline respiratory function and commonly have insufficient tidal volumes. If the level of injury is higher than T5, the patient can go into neurogenic shock. The output of the sympathetic nervous system to the body is cut off, which leads to the loss of vascular tone and hypotension. Because the parasympathetic output is now unopposed, the patient becomes bradycardiac. Other common systemic problems associated with SCI include an ileus of the gastrointestinal tract and bladder distention, which can cause compression of the pelvic veins and impede the venous return to the heart. With a complete SCI, a patient will acutely go into spinal shock, which is characterized by a flaccid paralysis and loss of spinal reflexes below the level of the lesion. Spinal shock occurs because of the loss of supraspinal excitatory input

to the injured portion of the cord and lasts on average from 3 to 4 weeks. After this period the patient gradually gets increased muscle tone with hyperactive reflexes.

SCI can be divided into complete and incomplete injuries. In a complete injury there is a total loss of motor, sensory, and autonomic function below the level of the injury. This includes the loss of motor and sensory function in the lowest sacral segment (S4-5), which consists of perianal sensation and voluntary external anal sphincter contraction. An incomplete injury has sparing of some sensory or motor function below the level of injury, which needs to include sparing of sensory function in the lowest sacral segment (perianal sensation). Incomplete SCIs have a better prognosis for neurologic recovery than complete SCIs do.

Several classic patterns of incomplete SCI are described. The Brown–Sequard syndrome occurs with an anatomic or functional hemisection of the spinal cord. Clinically, the patient has an ipsilateral motor paralysis, ipsilateral loss of light touch, ipsilateral loss of position sense, and contralateral loss of pain and temperature sensation. A patient with central cord syndrome has a more profound weakness of the upper extremities than the lower extremities, particularly affecting fine finger movements in the hand. Both the motor (corticospinal) and the pain and temperature (spinothalamic) tracts are affected. Frequently, this syndrome is seen after an elderly individual with a narrow spinal canal from cervical spondylosis sustains a face-first fall, causing the neck to hyperextend. It is also seen in people with congenitally narrow cervical spinal canals. The anterior spinal artery syndrome is caused by the occlusion of the anterior spinal artery, resulting in an infarction of the anterior and lateral funiculi of the spinal cord. Clinically, it presents with a bilateral motor paralysis, from infarction of the corticospinal tracts, and a bilateral loss of pain and temperature sensation, from infarction of the spinothalamic tracts, below the level of the injury. The dorsal columns, which carry position sense and light touch, are not affected. An acute disk rupture may cause anterior spinal artery syndrome by directly compressing the anterior spinal artery.

A patient with a traumatic SCI is given high-dose corticosteroids, which have been shown to improve neurologic recovery after a blunt injury to the spinal cord. The dosing regime is an initial i.v. bolus of methylprednisolone at 30 mg per kg over 15 minutes followed by a 45-minute pause. Then a continuous i.v. infusion of 5.4 mg/kg/min is given for 24 or 48 hours. If steroids are administered within 3 hours of the injury, they should be given for a total of 24 hours. If steroids are initiated between 3 and 8 hours after the injury, then a total of 48 hours should be given. If begun more than 8 hours after the injury, steroids have not been proven beneficial. In addition, high-dose steroids have not been shown to improve neurologic outcome after an injury to the cauda equina or after a penetrating injury to the spinal cord. Proposed beneficial mechanisms of high-dose steroids include the inhibition of lipid peroxidation and the augmentation of blood flow to the injured portion of the spinal cord.

In the United States, child abuse is the most frequent cause of severe head injuries in infants younger than 1 year of age. Either a blow to the infant's head, even with a soft object, or shaking the infant can have catastrophic results.

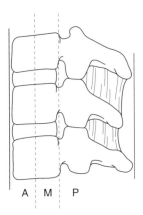

Figure 1-16 The three-column model of the thoracolumbar spine. Lateral view. A, anterior column; M, middle column; P, posterior column.

In toddlers, a significant proportion of hospitalizations for traumatic injuries are the result of abuse. Any suspected case of child abuse needs to be reported immediately to a child abuse investigation team. When the child is medically stable a skeletal survey can be done to look for long bone or rib fractures at different stages of healing. This may indicate previous abusive episodes.

PERIPHERAL NERVE INJURY

Both Seddon and Sunderland have established classification schemes for peripheral nerve injury. Seddon stratified injuries into three tiers: neurapraxia, axonotmesis, and neurotmesis. Neurapraxia is the transient loss of function secondary to local conduction block, usually after a mild traction or compression injury. The motor fibers are affected more often than the sensory fibers, and the autonomic fibers are usually spared. The neurologic deficit is frequently incomplete and there is little, if any, muscle atrophy. If demyelination of large fibers occurs, the recovery time may be prolonged. Surgery is not indicated. Recovery can occur within hours but most commonly occurs within 6 to 8 weeks. Anatomic continuity and electrical conductivity are preserved.

In axonotmesis, the axon and its myelin sheath are disrupted; this is usually caused by a stretch injury or a prolonged compressive injury. The connective tissue stroma is preserved and the portion of the axon distal to the injury undergoes wallerian degeneration. The result is complete motor, sensory, and autonomic paralysis, along with progressive muscle atrophy. Surgery is not indicated because a path for distal nerve regeneration is still present within the intact connective tissue stroma. The nerve regrows at an average rate of approximately 1 mm per day or 1 inch per month. Recovery is usually good and innervation occurs from proximal to distal.

Neurotmesis is the complete disruption of all components of a nerve, making spontaneous recovery impossible. The axons, myelin sheaths, and connective tissue stroma are all disrupted, and the portion of the axons that is distal to the injury undergoes wallerian degeneration. Neurotmesis can result from transection of a nerve or a severe crush, traction, or ischemic injury that causes massive internal disruption of a nerve, even though it may still be in continuity. Complete muscle, sensory, and autonomic paralysis result and are accompanied by progressive muscle atrophy. If untreated, scar tissue blocks the nerve from regenerating and may cause a painful neuroma, which is a mass of misdirected axons. Even with surgery, recovery is usually incomplete.

The Sunderland classification has five degrees of injury. First-degree injury is a reversible local conduction block, similar to neurapraxia. Second-degree injury is a disruption of the axon and myelin sheath only, equivalent to axonotmesis. Third-degree injury is the disruption of the axons, myelin sheaths, and endoneurium, but the fascicular pattern of the nerve is preserved; if it is a mild injury, it is similar to axonotmesis, and if it is a severe injury, it is similar to neurotmesis. In fourth-degree injuries, the fascicular pattern of the nerve is disrupted, but the epineurium is still intact. Fifth-degree injury is the transection of the nerve. Both fourth-degree and fifth-degree injuries are equivalent to neurotmesis.

Part of the clinical examination in a patient with a peripheral nerve injury is eliciting a Tinel sign, which is useful for following regrowth of nerves. By lightly tapping over a regenerating nerve, the patient will experience tingling paresthesia in the cutaneous distribution of the regenerating nerve. The point at which this is first elicited is the most distal point of small fiber regeneration. This point will move distally along the extremity as the nerve regenerates. Helpful clinical tests in the evaluation of a peripheral nerve injury include plain films and electromyography (EMG). When a peripheral nerve injury is diagnosed, plain films to rule out a foreign body or fracture should be obtained. EMG evaluates the electrical activity in muscles. Immediately after a normal muscle is denervated, electromyographic results will be normal. A few weeks after the injury, changes consistent with denervation, such as fibrillation potentials and the absence of voluntary APs, will be seen on EMG. Early reinnervation changes include a decrease in the amount of fibrillation potentials and nascent polyphasic potentials. However, electromyographic reinnervation changes do not guarantee recovery.

Treatment of peripheral nerve injuries depends on the continuity of the nerve and the type of wound. A nerve in continuity that has lost function distal to an injury should initially be observed for spontaneous recovery. If its time for recovery is longer than expected, an external neurolysis may be indicated, to free the nerve from surrounding scar tissue. If there is no evidence of recovery after several weeks, the injured portion of the nerve can be excised and the cut ends repaired with an end-to-end anastomosis, with or without a graft. If the injured nerve is not in continuity, the type of wound needs to be considered. If the nerve was sharply cut and the wound is relatively clean, the nerve can be immediately repaired with an end-to-end anastomosis. If the wound is dirty or there is extensive tissue damage, a secondary repair a few weeks after injury is indicated. A surgically repaired nerve should not be under any tension. To keep tension at a minimum after the operation, the joints of the extremity can be flexed, the nerve can be freed from local attachments, and a nerve graft may be used. A nerve graft is simply a conduit for distal regeneration of a nerve when a gap in the nerve needs to be bridged. Commonly, the sural nerve is used as a graft. Poor prognostic factors in a peripheral nerve injury include an associated bony fracture, older age, proximal nerve injury, extensive neural tissue loss, and associated soft tissue injury. A worse prognosis is also seen with injuries to nerves that have mixed sensory and motor function and in injured extremities with severe muscle denervation. If a nerve graft is used, the additional suture line worsens the prognosis.

Injury to a peripheral nerve can also be secondary to chronic compression. The most frequent example in the upper extremity is carpal tunnel syndrome, which is median nerve entrapment within the carpal tunnel of the wrist. Other structures that pass through the carpal tunnel include the tendons of the flexor digitorum profundus and superficialis muscles. The patient with carpal tunnel syndrome complains of paresthesia and loss of sensation in the radial half of the palm, the thumb, the index finger, the middle finger, and the radial half of the ring finger. In more severe cases, weakness of the first and second lumbrical, opponens pollicis, abductor pollicis brevis, and flexor pollicis brevis muscles may occur. Surgical treatment consists of dividing the transverse carpal ligament to relieve the compression. A tardy ulnar palsy is the compression of the ulnar nerve at the elbow.

Causalgia is a rare syndrome of burning pain, autonomic dysfunction, and trophic changes in an extremity after a major peripheral nerve injury. Symptoms begin in the distribution of the affected nerve and progress to involve the entire limb. The syndrome begins as a swollen limb with erythema that is very sensitive to tactile stimulation and may exhibit hyperhidrosis. The extremity later becomes pale, cool, and atrophic. Reflex sympathetic dystrophy is similar to causalgia but does not involve a major peripheral nerve injury. In both of these, the affected limb is not used, owing to the constant burning pain that may intensify with touch or movement of the limb. The limb eventually becomes useless. The joint creases disappear, the skin becomes smooth, and the bones become osteopenic. Treatments include a sympathectomy or a transcutaneous peripheral nerve stimulator.

VASCULAR DISORDERS

An intracranial hemorrhage is a common reason for a neurosurgical consultation and can be the result of SAH, intraventricular hemorrhage, IPH, SDH, EPH, or a combination of these. Nontraumatic lesions that cause intracranial bleeding are cerebral aneurysms, AVMs, hypertensive arteriopathy, and amyloid angiopathy. The patient with an intracranial hemorrhage may present with various symptoms and signs including headache, lethargy, photophobia, stiff neck, or a focal neurologic deficit such as a hemiparesis or cranial nerve palsy. When a nontraumatic intracranial hemorrhage is suspected, an emergent CT scan of the head should be obtained. The etiology of the hemorrhage can often be postulated on the basis of its location.

Cerebral aneurysms (Berry aneurysms) are the most common cause of nontraumatic SAH, accounting for 75% to 80% of these hemorrhages. Cerebral aneurysms usually occur at a point where an artery is branching from a parent artery close to the circle of Willis and develop where the vessel wall is abnormal as a result of a congenital defect or a degenerative change, producing a thin-walled outpouching. The aneurysm is named for the origin of the branching vessel. The wall of an aneurysm lacks an internal elastic lamina and muscularis layer. Only the intimal layer and adventitia of the artery form the dome of the aneurysm. Eighty-five percent of cerebral aneurysms occur in the anterior (carotid) circulation, with the most common locations at the origin of the anterior communicating artery, the origin of the posterior communicating artery, and the bifurcation of the middle cerebral artery. Other locations for anterior circulation aneurysms include the carotid bifurcation and the origin of the anterior choroidal artery. Locations of posterior circulation aneurysms include the basilar artery bifurcation, the origin of the posterior inferior cerebellar artery, and the vertebrobasilar junction.

An unruptured cerebral aneurysm is usually discovered incidentally on CT scan, MRI, or angiography obtained for an unrelated reason, or may present with symptoms of local mass effect. A symptomatic unruptured posterior communicating artery aneurysm may compress the oculomotor nerve and cause an ipsilateral third nerve palsy.

Giant cerebral aneurysms, those larger than 2.5 cm, can present as intracerebral mass lesions.

Cerebral aneurysms most commonly present after they rupture and produce an SAH. The peak ages for rupture of a cerebral aneurysm are between 55 and 60 years, but these aneurysms may occur in younger adults. Clinically, a patient complains of the sudden onset of an explosive headache, which is described as the worst headache of his or her life. With the onset of the headache, there is a change in the level of consciousness, owing to transient elevation of the ICP, which may be limited to transient confusion or could result in prolonged unresponsiveness (coma). Nausea and vomiting, seizures, and focal deficits may accompany the sudden headache. Blood in the subarachnoid space causes a sterile meningitis, resulting in a stiff neck, photophobia, and a low-grade fever. The headache lasts for days, until the subarachnoid blood is cleared. The hemorrhage may occur during sleep or physical stress. It may be the cause of a fall or motor vehicle accident; therefore, an SAH in a distribution similar to an aneurysmal bleed in a trauma patient warrants further workup. Recognizing the signs and symptoms of an aneurysmal SAH is important because approximately one third of patients have a sentinel bleed, a small warning bleed, days to weeks before a large SAH. If recognized early, a catastrophic hemorrhage can be prevented. Unfortunately, a sentinel bleed is not always recognized. Approximately 10% of patients die before reaching the hospital.

A patient with an SAH from an aneurysm is graded based on the most recent clinical examination using the Hunt-Hess grading scale. Grade 0 corresponds to a patient with an unruptured aneurysm. Grades 1 to 5 describe patients with ruptured cerebral aneurysms. Grade 1 is assigned to a patient with a mild headache and mild nuchal rigidity. Grade 2 corresponds to a patient with a moderate-to-severe headache and nuchal rigidity. These patients may also have a cranial nerve palsy. Grade 3 is a lethargic or confused patient who may have mild focal neurologic deficit. Grade 4 patients are unresponsive (comatose) and may have a moderate-to-severe hemiparesis. Grade 5 corresponds to an unresponsive patient with decerebrate posturing.

The initial diagnostic study for a patient with a suspected SAH is a CT scan of the head. Subarachnoid blood may be seen in the sylvian fissures, the basal cisterns, or the interhemispheric fissure (Fig. 1-12). An intracerebral hematoma or an SDH may also occur with ruptured aneurysm when the powerful jet of blood dissects into the parenchyma of the brain or the subdural space. If there is a high clinical suspicion for an SAH, but the CT scan does not reveal subarachnoid blood and does not demonstrate a mass intracranial lesion, a lumbar puncture is indicated. If the CSF is xanthochromatic or if it is bloody and does not clear as it is drained into successive collection tubes, the patient has sustained an SAH. When an SAH has occurred, four-vessel (bilateral carotid and bilateral vertebral arteries) cerebral arteriography is performed to identify a cerebral aneurysm. Seventy-five to eighty percent of patients with nontraumatic SAH will be found to have a ruptured aneurysm. Approximately 20% of these patients will have multiple cerebral aneurysms. Much less commonly, a patient will have an AVM associated with an aneurysm. In approximately 15% of patients with a nontraumatic SAH, no cause will be found.

The goals of treatment are to prevent rebleeding, which is the greatest cause of morbidity and mortality in the first few days after an aneurysmal rupture, and to minimize the risk of vasospasm. All patients with a ruptured cerebral aneurysm are admitted to the intensive care unit (ICU). Measures to prevent rebleeding include strict bed rest with head elevation, systolic blood pressure controlled (usually lower than 150 mm Hg), and minimal stimulation. Frequent neurologic examinations are performed by the nursing staff. Medications administered to the patient may include an anticonvulsant (phenytoin) and a calcium channel blocker (nimodipine), which has been shown to reduce the incidence of poor outcome that is the result of cerebral vasospasm. Corticosteroids may be given in the perioperative period.

Further treatment depends on the Hunt-Hess grade of the patient. To prevent rebleeding in grade 1, 2, and 3 patients, early surgery is performed to place a clip across the neck of the aneurysm and exclude it from the cerebral circulation. Surgical clipping of the aneurysm is done within 72 hours of the bleed to avoid the high-risk period for vasospasm. If a patient has gone into vasospasm, the brain does not tolerate surgery well. Grade 4 and 5 patients may have hydrocephalus secondary to the SAH, and treating this with an emergent ventriculostomy may allow the patient to awaken, improve his or her Hunt-Hess grade, and undergo surgery. Grade 4 and 5 patients who do not improve are medically managed. In a Hunt-Hess grade 4 or 5 patient or a patient with a preexisting medical condition, which makes surgery riskier, a ruptured aneurysm can be thrombosed by the endovascular placement of coiled wires into its dome. A microcatheter is passed from the femoral artery into the aneurysm and detachable coils are placed within the aneurysm. The coils promote clots to form within the aneurysm, thereby isolating it from the circulation.

During postbleed days 3 and 14, vasospasm is the major cause of morbidity and mortality. Vasospasm is an idiopathic narrowing of the intracranial vessels, commonly occurring after aneurysmal SAH and lasting 3 to 4 weeks. Vasospasm is observed in more than 50% of arteriograms from patients with aneurysmal SAH, but only about 30% of patients have symptomatic vasospasm. Decreased blood flow in the narrowed vessels causes focal ischemia of the brain and focal neurologic deficits, such as aphasia and hemiparesis. Treatment (triple-H therapy) is aimed at increasing the cerebral blood flow by increasing the systemic blood volume (hypervolemia), increasing the systemic blood pressure (hypertension), and decreasing the rheology of the blood (hemodilution). The goal hematocrit to optimize the rheologic properties of blood and not sacrifice the oxygen-carrying capacity is 30%. If medical management fails, vessels in spasm can be treated with endovascular techniques, such as the direct intraarterial injection of papaverine and arterial balloon dilatation. Unsuccessfully treated symptomatic vasospasm leads to ischemic stroke and even death.

Other types of aneurysms that affect the cerebral circulation are mycotic, traumatic, and fusiform atherosclerotic aneurysms. Aneurysms secondary to infection or trauma are usually located more distally on the cerebral vasculature. Mycotic aneurysms are caused by bacterial or fungal infections and may result as a complication of infectious endocarditis when an infectious embolus enters the cerebral circulation. The embolus travels predominantly into a distal branch of the middle cerebral artery because it receives the greatest percentage of blood flow to the brain of all cerebral arteries. Local infectious and inflammatory processes lead to the development of the aneurysm. Traumatic aneurysms occur at distal locations in the cerebral vasculature, usually near a fixed structure such as the falx cerebri. A traumatic pericallosal artery aneurysm is thought to result from the relatively mobile pericallosal artery being torn by the immobile falx. Fusiform atherosclerotic aneurysms occur in the proximal internal carotid artery and in the vertebrobasilar complex. They are difficult lesions to treat, because they are a dilation of the entire circumference of the vessel wall. An extracranial to intracranial arterial bypass procedure (EC–IC bypass) may be valuable in treating these lesions when symptomatic. Several variations of this operation are performed, including connecting the superficial temporal artery to the middle cerebral artery or using a vein graft to connect the extracranial internal carotid or vertebral artery to an intracranial artery such as the middle cerebral artery.

An extradural ophthalmic artery aneurysm may form if the ophthalmic artery branches off the internal carotid artery within the cavernous sinus before it enters the dura. If this aneurysm ruptures, it hemorrhages into the cavernous sinus, which results in a carotid-cavernous fistula (CC fistula). This is a direct arterial-to-venous shunt. A CC fistula may also occur with a traumatic injury of the intracavernous carotid artery. If a CC fistula has a high flow or is causing visual deterioration, it is treated by endovascular balloon occlusion.

An *AVM* is a congenital abnormality consisting of a collection of abnormal blood vessels. By definition, there is a direct arterial-to-venous connection without intervening capillaries. As a result there is decreased resistance to blood flow compared to normal brain. An AVM frequently presents in the third or fourth decade of life as either a ruptured or unruptured lesion. Common symptoms of an unruptured AVM include headaches, seizures, or progressive neurologic deficits, which may be secondary to ischemia from the AVM shunting blood from the adjacent normal cortex because of its lower resistance to blood flow than normal brain (steal syndrome). Focal deficits may also occur from the mass effect of the AVM on the surrounding brain. An unruptured AVM is believed to have a risk of hemorrhage of about 1% per year. A patient with a ruptured AVM may present with a headache, loss of consciousness, seizure, or focal neurologic deficit. On CT scan of the head, a ruptured AVM commonly produces an intracerebral hematoma within the parenchyma of the brain. Less frequently, intraventricular hemorrhage or SAH may occur. The hematoma is most commonly located within a cerebral hemisphere.

The goal of acute treatment is to help the patient survive the initial hemorrhage. Large life-threatening hematomas causing unresponsiveness (coma) and impending herniation need to be evacuated emergently. Awake and responsive patients can be observed in the ICU because a previously ruptured AVM has a hemorrhage rate of approximately 5% per year, with no substantial increase in this rate during the period immediately following a bleed. After the patient recovers from the hemorrhage, cerebral angiogram and MRI of the head are used to define the anatomy of the AVM. Angiographic features of an AVM include a nidus of abnormal vessels and early draining veins. A cerebral aneurysm on a feeding artery is observed in 10% of AVMs. Abnormal flow voids are seen on MRI. Successful surgical resection of an AVM depends on its location, size, and complexity. Endovascular embolization of the feeding arteries is frequently performed preoperatively. Rarely, embolization may totally obliterate the AVM. Stereotactic radiosurgery is frequently used for smaller AVMs (less than 3 cm), particularly when they are deep within the brain. It takes 6 months to 2 years for the AVM to be obliterated after radiosurgery, and unfortunately the risk of rebleeding is not decreased during this time.

According to National Stroke Association statistics, a stroke occurs in the United States every minute. This year, stroke will afflict more than 750,000 Americans. Approximately 150,000 will die; many will be left permanently disabled or neurologically impaired. Alarmingly, stroke is the third leading cause of death in the United States, and it is the number one cause of adult disability. Strokes may have either an ischemic or hemorrhagic etiology. Hemorrhagic stroke may be further classified as a hypertensive hemorrhage or the result of amyloid angiopathy. Hypertensive hemorrhages occur in patients with a long-standing history of hypertension, and the presenting signs and symptoms varying according to the location of the hemorrhage. Commonly, hemorrhage occurs in the putamen or external capsule when there is rupture of a deep perforating artery that has undergone chronic degenerative hypertensive-related changes. Other common hemorrhagic sites include the thalamus, cerebellum, and brainstem. Less frequently a lobar hemorrhage in the cerebral cortex may be associated with hypertension. A patient who has bled into the putamen, external capsule, or thalamus presents with a progressive focal neurologic deficit and progressive lethargy. A headache may or may not be associated. On examination, the patient may have one or more of the following symptoms and signs: a contralateral hemiparesis, a contralateral hemisensory loss, or a contralateral hemianopsia. A hemorrhage in this location is usually caused by the rupture of a lenticulostriate or thalamoperforating artery. A patient who sustains a cerebellar hypertensive hemorrhage complains of the sudden onset of a headache, nausea and vomiting, and dizziness. Ataxia may be found on examination. The hematoma may compress the brainstem directly, resulting in the loss of upward gaze and progressive lethargy until the patient is unresponsive. A hypertensive hemorrhage in the pons results from the rupture of a pontine artery, a branch of the basilar artery. Unfortunately, the patient usually presents as unresponsive and quadriparetic with pinpoint pupils; these hemorrhages are almost always fatal.

A hypertensive hemorrhage is diagnosed with use of an emergent noncontrast CT scan of the head according to the location of the hematoma. Intraventricular hemorrhage may accompany the intraparenchymal clot and both may cause hydrocephalus. Coagulation studies including a platelet count, prothrombin time, and partial prothrombin time should be ordered emergently and these parameters should be corrected if abnormal. For supratentorial hematomas, surgical evacuation is reserved for large, life-threatening clots that have not resulted in a neurologically devastated patient. For cerebellar hematomas, immediate treatment is required, which includes an emergent suboccipital craniectomy and

evacuation of the hematoma. Surgery is not needed to stop the hemorrhage or prevent further hemorrhages. Once the patient has bled, blood pressure control is important to prevent another hemorrhage. There is a good prognosis if the patient survives the bleed and is not neurologically devastated. The hematoma frequently dissects along axonal planes and causes minimal tissue destruction. Some of the initial neurologic deficits may be secondary to edema and to direct compression of surrounding cortex by the hematoma. These deficits will improve as the hematoma resolves. The best treatment for a hypertensive hemorrhage is to prevent it from occurring by controlling chronic hypertension.

Another vascular disorder of the brain is ischemic cerebrovascular disease. Ischemic strokes occur most commonly in the distribution of the carotid arteries because they are responsible for nearly 80% of the brain's blood supply. Ischemic events can be classified according to their duration into transient ischemic attacks, reversible ischemic neurologic deficits, and completed strokes. A transient ischemic attack (TIA) usually lasts less than 30 minutes but by definition can last for up to 24 hours with complete neurologic recovery. A TIA of the retina is called *amaurosis fugax*, which is described by patients as a shade being pulled down or up across one eye causing the transient loss of vision. A TIA of the brain may cause a transient hemiparesis, hemisensory deficit, or aphasia. A reversible ischemic neurologic deficit (RIND) lasts 24 hours to 3 days with full recovery of neurologic function. A completed stroke occurs when a neurologic deficit associated with brain ischemia lasts longer than 3 days.

A stroke can be caused by the formation of a thrombus in a large cerebral artery or the passage of an embolus into a cerebral arteriole. When an occlusive or nonocclusive thrombus forms in a large artery, the blood flow to a portion of the brain may be completely impaired or decreased below a critical threshold, with resulting ischemia. Most commonly this is caused by thrombus superimposed on a vessel lumen narrowed by atherosclerosis. The region of the brain supplied by the occluded artery depends entirely on collateral flow from other cerebral vessels. If there is adequate collateral blood supply to the region in jeopardy, no ischemia results. If not, this region becomes ischemic and a neurologic deficit may occur. A frequent extracranial site of atherosclerotic disease is the carotid bifurcation and origin of the internal carotid artery. Intracranial atherosclerosis commonly occurs in the carotid siphon, in the distal internal carotid artery, and in the proximal middle cerebral artery. Complete cutoff of the blood supply to an area of the brain results from the embolic occlusion of a cerebral arteriole. An embolus may originate from an atherosclerotic ulceration at the carotid bifurcation, a mural thrombus in the heart, or a valvular lesion in the heart. Heart-derived emboli are associated with atrial fibrillation and myocardial infarctions. Emboli most frequently pass into the middle cerebral arteries. Clinically, the patient presents with a focal, sometimes progressive, neurologic deficit and may be lethargic.

Clinical studies clearly show that the best long-term treatment of stroke is its prevention. Risk factors need to be identified and treated or modified. Risk factors for ischemic stroke include hypertension, diabetes, hypercholesterolemia, obesity, smoking, as well as a family history of stroke. Medical treatment of ischemic cerebrovascular disease includes antiplatelet therapy and anticoagulation. Surgical treatment may complement medical therapy and consists of carotid endarterectomy for common carotid and proximal internal carotid artery atherosclerotic disease. Multiple randomized trials have shown a benefit in recently symptomatic patients with a significant carotid stenosis contralateral to their symptoms, as long as the patient has not had a recent major stroke and does not have any comorbid medical conditions that would greatly increase the risk of surgery. In asymptomatic patients, several randomized studies have also shown a benefit for carotid artery endarterectomy. When selecting a patient for surgery, it is important to rule out, with cerebral angiography or MRA, more distal stenotic lesions in the internal carotid artery, which may be the cause of the ischemic symptoms.

Carotid endarterectomy can be performed using local anesthesia to allow for frequent neurologic examinations, or general anesthesia, utilizing electroencephalogram (EEG) monitoring. If the neurologic examination of the patient or the EEG changes while the carotid artery is clamped, a temporary shunt from the common carotid artery to the internal carotid artery is needed during the surgery. The shunt is a plastic tube that the surgeon is able to work around to remove the plaque. When releasing the arteries, the clamp on the common carotid artery is released first, then the external carotid is opened prior to the internal carotid so any emboli dislodged by the restoration of blood flow will enter the external circulation. An acceptable mortality rate for carotid artery endarterectomy is 1%, with an acceptable morbidity rate between 1% and 5%.

When the internal carotid artery stenosis is higher up in the neck, it is inaccessible to an endarterectomy procedure. With this and other surgically inaccessible ischemic cerebrovascular disease, a microvascular bypass from the external carotid artery to the internal carotid artery (EC–IC bypass) may be helpful.

The spinal cord is affected by the same vascular disorders that affect the brain; however, they occur much less commonly.

TUMORS

Brain tumors account for approximately 10% of all neoplasms and can be either primary CNS tumors or metastases. Primary tumors arise from the various cells in the cerebral cortex, the coverings of the brain, as well as from the pituitary gland. Metastatic tumors can spread by local extension or through the blood, lymph, or CSF. The location of brain tumors varies with age. In adults, approximately 70% of brain tumors are supratentorial (located superior to the tentorium cerebelli). The most common brain tumor in adults is a metastatic lesion. In children, about 70% of brain tumors are infratentorial (in the posterior fossa) and account for 15% to 20% of all childhood tumors. In fact, brain tumors are the second most common childhood cancer overall (leukemia is the most common) and the most common solid tumor of childhood.

Patients with brain tumors may present with signs and symptoms of increased ICP, a focal deficit, or a seizure. The increased ICP is a result of the tumor adding tissue mass within the skull. The modified Monro-Kellie hypothesis states that the skull is a nonexpansile structure that can hold only a finite volume of blood, brain, CSF, and any abnormal components (tumor, hematoma, etc.). If the amount of one of these increase, the amount of a different one must decrease. Therefore, elevated ICP results when mechanisms that compensate for the additional volume from the tumor are overwhelmed. Adding to the increased ICP may be associated edema, hydrocephalus, or tumor hemorrhage. Symptoms of increased ICP include chronic headaches, which are worse upon awakening in the morning and with dependent head positions. Headaches are typically exacerbated during straining, that is, nausea or vomiting. Elevated ICP is also associated with slowed cognitive function and will lead to progressive lethargy and eventually unresponsiveness. The signs of increased ICP include papilledema and a unilateral or bilateral abducens (cranial nerve IV) palsy. Because of its long intracranial course, the abducens nerve can be compressed by the elevated ICP and this is referred to as a *false localizing sign.* Patients with brain tumors also present with neurologic deficits. With supratentorial tumors, deficits include monoparesis, hemiparesis, hemisensory deficit, visual deficit, aphasia, and cranial nerve palsies. With infratentorial tumors, neurologic deficits include ataxia, nystagmus, and cranial nerve palsies.

A patient with a supratentorial brain tumor may present with a seizure, either partial or generalized. A partial seizure may be a simple partial seizure with focal motor or sensory symptoms but no loss of consciousness, a complex partial seizure with some alteration of consciousness and an associated automatism, or a partial seizure with secondary generalization, which is a seizure that begins focally and progresses to involve the entire body, including a loss of consciousness. A generalized seizure starts on both sides of the body simultaneously and consciousness is lost at the onset. A brain tumor should be suspected in any patient older than 20 years who has his or her first idiopathic seizure.

Patients with suspected intracranial masses are best evaluated with a CT scan or MRI of the head. With an acute presentation—for example, a new onset seizure, progressive neurological deficit, or lethargy—an unenhanced CT scan is indicated because it is a quick method for identifying large lesions with mass effect or acute hemorrhage that may be life threatening. If the patient is awake and there is no sense of urgency, an MRI with and without contrast should be obtained because it is a more sensitive imaging modality for the soft tissues of the CNS.

Primary brain tumors can be divided into tumors that are derived from elements that are normally present in the CNS and tumors derived from embryonic remnants. The tumors that arise from cells normally found in the CNS can be further divided into tumors that arise from neural tube derivatives (astrocytomas, glioblastomas, oligodendrogliomas, ependymomas, and choroid plexus papillomas), tumors that arise from neurons (medulloblastomas and gangliomas), tumors that arise from neural crest derivatives (meningiomas and acoustic neuromas-vestibular schwannoma), and tumors that arise from other cells present in the CNS (primary CNS lymphoma, hemangioblastomas, glomus jugulare tumors, and pituitary adenomas). Tumors that are derived from embryonic remnants include craniopharyngiomas, germinomas, teratomas, epidermoids, and dermoids.

Glioma is a general term for any tumor arising from a stromal cell of the CNS, which is a derivative of the neural tube. A glioma frequently has indistinct borders and infiltrates the surrounding brain by spreading along white matter tracts. However, a glioma will rarely metastasize outside of the CNS but may spread to other areas within the CNS through the CSF. Over time, a glioma may transform from a "relatively" benign tumor into a malignant tumor. Types of gliomas include low-grade astrocytomas, anaplastic astrocytomas, glioblastomas, oligodendrogliomas, ependymomas, and choroid plexus papillomas.

Low-grade astrocytomas tend to grow slowly and cause mild symptoms for several years before they are diagnosed; they occur most commonly in individuals between the ages of 30 and 50 years. On MRI or CT scan, a low-intensity or low-density supratentorial mass is identified that may or may not enhance following contrast administration. Histologic sections show brain parenchyma with greater cellularity than normal, with infiltration of the surrounding normal brain. Treatment consists of surgical resection and, for more aggressive tumors, postoperative external beam radiation therapy. The 5-year survival rate has been reported to be up to 50%. Low-grade astrocytomas commonly transform into high-grade anaplastic astrocytomas and glioblastomas.

Anaplastic astrocytomas (AAs) are high-grade lesions that are more cellular and have a more rapid growth rate than low-grade astrocytomas. They commonly present in 45 to 65 year olds. On MRI or CT scan, a hypointense or hypodense mass is seen, which usually enhances. Pathologic section shows increased cellularity and infiltration of the surrounding brain. The cells have more malignant characteristics than do cells of low-grade astrocytomas including nuclear pleomorphism, bizarre-looking nuclei, and mitoses. Treatment is surgical resection and postoperative external beam radiation. If the lesion is not amenable to resection, a stereotactic biopsy can be performed to obtain tissue for a pathologic diagnosis. The average survival is about 2 years.

The most malignant glioma is the glioblastoma multiforme (GBM; glioblastomas), which is also a form of astrocytoma. GBM is the most common primary intracranial tumor. The peak age of occurrence is between 50 and 70 years. The diagnosis is based on the histologic characteristics of the tumor, which include nuclear pleomorphism, mitoses, necrosis, pseudopalisading of cells around the necrotic areas, and neovascularization with endothelial cell proliferation. GBM is often associated with tumor hemorrhage. Treatment is surgical resection or a stereotactic biopsy for diagnosis, followed by external beam radiation and chemotherapy. Average survival is less than 1 year. A subset of GBMs or AAs are called *butterfly gliomas* because they invade the corpus callosum and involve both cerebral hemispheres. These tumors are unresectable and have a poor prognosis.

A benign subset of astrocytomas are the pilocytic astrocytomas, which occur mainly in children and adolescents. Pilocytic astrocytomas commonly occur in the cerebellum. Cerebellar pilocytic astrocytomas have a favorable prognosis, with a 10-year survival rate of 80%; moreover, a complete resection is considered a cure. Pilocytic astrocytomas may also occur around the third ventricle and in the brainstem. Unfortunately, tumors in these locations are difficult

to resect completely without devastating neurologic consequences and are therefore difficult to cure. A much lower 5-year survival rate of 15% to 30% is associated with these tumors. Pilocytic astrocytomas may originate in the optic nerve and are termed *optic nerve gliomas.* A complete resection is possible with unilateral optic nerve involvement, and may be curative. Unfortunately, optic nerve gliomas may invade the optic chiasm or hypothalamus, making total resection impossible.

Oligodendrogliomas are derived from the cells that produce and maintain myelin in the CNS (oligodendrocytes). They occur less frequently than astrocytomas, making up about 5% of gliomas. Oligodendrogliomas are slow-growing neoplasms that usually present with seizures. Most commonly they occur in 40 to 50 year olds and are rare in children. On MRI or CT scan, they are almost always supratentorial, usually located in the frontal lobe, commonly have areas of calcification, and usually enhance with the administration of i.v. contrast. Microscopically, they usually appear benign with cells that resemble "fried eggs," but anaplastic features are possible. In up to one third of cases, neoplastic oligodendrocytes are mixed with neoplastic astrocytes or ependymal cells, called a *mixed glioma.* Treatment consists of surgical resection. With an incomplete resection or for a tumor with malignant histology, postoperative external beam radiation is added. The 5-year survival rate for oligodendrogliomas (not including mixed gliomas) is 50% to 80%, with a 20-year survival rate of approximately 6%.

Ependymocytes, line the ventricular system and are the cell of origin of ependymomas, which comprise approximately 5% of gliomas. The peak incidence occurs in childhood when two thirds of ependymomas are located in the posterior fossa, usually growing in the floor of the fourth ventricle. When they occur in adults, these tumors are usually supratentorial and about one half are intraventricular. They may cause hydrocephalus from obstruction to the flow of CSF, and may metastasize through the CSF. On MRI or CT scan, they appear as enhancing well-circumscribed masses. Treatment consists of surgical resection; however, they frequently recur and are associated with a 5-year survival rate of about 50%.

Choroid plexus papillomas are tumors that arise from the cells that produce CSF. They occur within the ventricular system and are benign. Hydrocephalus is classically considered to be secondary to the overproduction of CSF. Choroid plexus carcinoma refers to the rare malignant variant. In children, choroid plexus papillomas are located frequently in the left lateral ventricle, and, in adults, they often occur in the fourth ventricle. This is opposite of the usual supratentorial brain tumor location in adults and infratentorial location in children. Treatment consists of surgical resection.

Medulloblastomas, also referred to as *primitive neural ectoderm tumors* (PNETs), originate from primitive bipotential cells of the cerebellum. About two thirds of PNETs occur in children and adolescents, and they are rare in people older than 40 years. In addition, 20% of childhood brain tumors are PNETs. Commonly, medulloblastomas present with signs of increased ICP and signs of cerebellar dysfunction, which include ataxia and nystagmus. Primitive neural ectoderm tumors are usually located in the vermis of the cerebellum, which forms the roof of the fourth ventricle (as opposed to ependymomas, which are located in the floor of the fourth ventricle). In patients older than 15 years, they may occur in the cerebellar hemispheres. These tumors are very cellular, malignant lesions that can metastasize through the CSF, but they rarely metastasize outside of the CNS. Once a tumor has been identified by radiologic imaging before surgical manipulation of the tumor, the CSF should be assessed for malignant cells. With gross total resection and craniospinal radiation therapy, the 5-year survival rate is nearly 75%. Chemotherapy may also be used, particularly with recurrent tumors and in young children not amenable to radiation. If gross total resection is not possible, the 5-year survival rate is much lower.

Meningiomas account for nearly 17% of intracranial tumors. They are benign extraaxial primary CNS tumors that arise from cells of the arachnoid granulations located within the meninges. Women are affected more frequently than men and progesterone receptors and estrogen receptors have been isolated on meningioma cells. Meningiomas are most commonly diagnosed in patients between the ages of 30 and 60 years. Common locations for meningiomas are the convexity of the cerebral hemisphere (parasagittal), the floor of the anterior cranial fossa (olfactory groove), the sphenoid wing, the clivus, the falx cerebri, the posterior fossa, the tuberculum sellae, and the middle cranial fossa. Usually, these tumors indent the brain but do not invade it; however, they may invade the adjacent bone. On MRI or CT scan, they enhance brightly with i.v. contrast administration and may have a dural tail, which is the enhancing portion of thickened dura adjacent to the tumor. Treatment involves surgical resection of the tumor and the involved dura. Meningiomas have a good long-term prognosis and a low recurrence rate. Rarely, a meningioma will be classified as atypical or malignant; these tumors recur more frequently and have a worse prognosis.

Acoustic neuromas are tumors composed of Schwann cells, most often arising from the vestibular portion of the eighth cranial nerve (more properly called *acoustic schwannomas*). Adult women are most frequently affected. Acoustic neuromas commonly present with hearing loss or cerebellar dysfunction. Facial numbness, from compression of the facial nerve as it exits the brainstem, and obstructive hydrocephalus from brainstem compression may also occur. Acoustic neuromas are benign lesions, which may be cured with complete resection. The surgery is technically challenging because of the neural structures adjacent to the tumor in the cerebellopontine angle, which include the brainstem and the facial nerve (cranial nerve VII). The preservation of hearing and facial nerve function is related directly to the size of the tumor. Neurofibromatosis type II is associated with bilateral acoustic neuromas. Schwannomas may also grow on other sensory cranial nerves, including the trigeminal nerve.

Primary CNS lymphomas are increasing in incidence. Frequently, they are related to immunosuppression associated with organ transplantation and acquired immunodeficiency syndrome (AIDS). They may have single or, in about one fourth of cases, multiple foci. Most commonly they are of B-cell origin and are radiosensitive. Treatment includes stereotactic biopsy for diagnosis, and radiation and steroids.

Hemangioblastomas are benign tumors that arise from vascular cells. They are uncommon, making up 1% of intracranial tumors. In adults, they are the most common primary intraaxial tumor within the posterior fossa and present in the fourth decade of life. Hemangioblastomas are usually located in the cerebellum and present with cerebellar dysfunction and hydrocephalus. Less commonly, they are located in the brainstem, spinal cord, or cerebral hemisphere. On MRI or CT scan, they may appear as a large cyst with a brightly enhancing mural nodule, or, less frequently, they may be solid tumors that enhance brightly. Polycythemi, is often present from a hematopoietic factor released from the tumor. Complete surgical resection is curative for an isolated lesion with about an 80% survival rate at 10 years. The combination of CNS hemangioblastomas, retinal angiomatosis, renal and pancreatic cysts, and renal cell carcinoma is *von Hippel–Lindau disease,* which is localized to a mutation on the short arm of chromosome 3 and has an autosomal dominant inheritance pattern.

Pituitary adenomas are benign tumors that arise from the anterior lobe of the pituitary gland (hypophysis). They present most commonly in patients between the ages of 20 and 40 years. They can be divided into microadenomas (which are less than 1 cm in diameter) and macroadenomas (measuring greater than 1 cm in diameter). Microadenomas are discovered because of symptoms related directly to overproduction by the tumor of one or more pituitary hormones. Common presentations include amenorrhea and galactorrhea secondary to the overproduction of prolactin by a prolactinoma. Patients may also present with acromegaly from excess growth hormone and Cushing disease from the overproduction of adrenocorticotropic hormone (ACTH). Macroadenomas do not produce active pituitary hormones. Instead, they become symptomatic by compressing surrounding structures or causing visual loss, hypopituitarism, or hyperprolactinemia. In addition to causing headaches, macroadenomas cause bitemporal hemianopsia, which is the typical visual-field deficit associated with the tumor. This results from the compression of the medial portions of both optic nerves anterior to the optic chiasm. Hyperprolactinemia is caused by the compression of the pituitary stalk by the tumor, which blocks dopamine (released from the hypothalamus) from traveling through the stalk to the posterior lobe of the pituitary gland, where it normally inhibits the production of prolactin. Most microadenomas and masses located in the sella are treated surgically via a transsphenoidal approach through the nose and sphenoid sinus. Prolactinomas are treated medically with dopamine agonists, such as bromocriptine. For large macroadenomas with significant suprasellar extension, resection of the tumor can also be accomplished through a craniotomy. Overall, the prognosis is good.

Metastatic brain tumors are the most common brain tumor in adults. They arise from a lung tumor 35% of the time, breast tumor 20%, malignant melanoma 10%, kidney tumor 10%, and gastrointestinal tumor 5% of the time. Testicular cancer may also metastasize to the brain. Metastatic brain tumors most commonly affect older adults. Signs and symptoms of lesions in the cerebral hemispheres include headache, a change in mental status, seizures, and neurologic deficits. Cerebellar lesions may cause ataxia, nystagmus, and vomiting. On CT scan or MRI, metastatic lesions are located at the junction between the gray and white matter, and extensive vasogenic edema is seen in the white matter surrounding the tumor. Treatment includes corticosteroids, which effectively decrease the amount of vasogenic edema and have been shown to prolong survival. Surgical treatment includes either a biopsy for diagnosis in a patient with multiple lesions or a craniotomy for resection of a single lesion in a patient with an expected survival of at least 4 months. In carefully selected patients, multiple metastatic lesions may be surgically resected. Whole brain radiation therapy is used postoperatively and in nonsurgical patients who are expected to survive at least a couple months. A single session of focused radiation, known as *stereotactc radiosurgery,* is now being used for multiple small metastatic lesions. The prognosis depends on the type of primary tumor, with median survival in the 1- to 2-year range. Metastatic lesions also occur within the dura, skull, and posterior pituitary gland.

Meningeal carcinomatosis is the metastatic spread of a systemic cancer to the leptomeninges. This most commonly occurs with childhood leukemia, adult lymphoma, breast cancer, lung cancer, and melanoma. Presenting signs may include a cranial nerve palsy, radiculopathy, obstructive hydrocephalus, and meningeal signs (headache, stiff neck, and photophobia). If there is no mass lesion on CT scan of the head, a lumbar puncture can be performed, which may show an increased opening pressure, elevated protein, and decreased glucose. The CSF should be sent for cytology to look for metastatic cells. MRI reveals diffuse enhancement of the involved subarachnoid spaces. Treatment includes radiation therapy and intrathecal chemotherapy administered via a ventricular catheter or by lumbar puncture. The prognosis is usually poor.

INFECTION

Infections in the CNS can be bacterial, viral, fungal, or parasitic. Bacterial infections can be subgaleal, osseous, epidural, subdural, leptomeningeal, intraventricular, or intraparenchymal. A subgaleal abscess is located between the galea and pericranium and is usually a complication of a traumatic or surgical wound. The skin overlying a subgaleal abscess is tender, warm, and swollen. Treatment consists of surgical drainage and antibiotics. Osteomyelitis is an infection of the bone. When the skull is infected, it is usually the result of the direct spread of an adjacent tissue infection such as a paranasal sinus infection, a subgaleal abscess, a penetrating wound infection, or a postoperative wound infection. Rarely, osteomyelitis of the skull is the result of hematogenous spread. Treatment includes systemic antibiotics, removal of the infected bone, debridement of the surrounding soft tissue, and assessing and treating the underlying cause of the infection. Osteomyelitis also occurs in the spine, where it is usually the result of the hematogenous spread of bacteria. The infection can spread into the epidural space and create a spinal epidural abscess. An epidural abscess is more common in the spine than in the head. A patient will usually present febrile with spine tenderness localized over the infected area of the spine. Clinical evaluation should include blood cultures and an MRI of the spine. Epidural abscesses are treated with i.v. antibiotics and, if the patient has a neurologic deficit, emergent surgical drainage of the abscess and decompression of the spinal cord. A subdural empyema (subdural abscess)

occurs around the brain. It is a purulent infection of the subdural space, which is widespread over the surface of the cerebral hemisphere. The source of a subdural empyema can be from an infection within the CNS, such as a meningitis, or from the spread of an infection from outside of the CNS. An outside source penetrates the CNS via extension through the dura. Sites of origin commonly include sinusitis, an infected traumatic or surgical wound, or a transcranial emissary vein thrombosis. Contrast-enhanced CT scan or MRI reveals an enhancing subdural. Treatment includes emergent surgical drainage and evacuation of the subdural empyema. A subdural empyema is associated with a significant mortality rate.

Meningitis is inflammation of the leptomeninges. Bacterial meningitis is an infection of the leptomeninges. Patients may present with fever, lethargy, headache, nausea and vomiting, nuchal rigidity, seizures, and cranial nerve palsies. A patient suspected of having bacterial meningitis should first undergo a CT scan of the head to rule out a mass lesion. If a CT scan is negative, lumbar puncture can be performed and CSF sent for gram staining, culture, glucose level, protein level, and white blood cell count. CSF results consistent with bacterial meningitis include a low glucose level (less than two thirds of the serum glucose level), a high protein level, and the presence of white blood cells with a predominance of polymorphonuclear lymphocytes (PMLs). In addition, blood should be submitted for cultures, which may yield the causative organism. The treatment of bacterial meningitis is systemic i.v. antibiotics; if a source of the meningitis is found such as a postoperative or traumatic CSF leak, treatment of the underlying cause should be attempted. The initiation of antibiotics should not be delayed until the completion of the CT scan of the head, the lumbar puncture, and blood cultures in a sick patient because untreated cases are almost always fatal. Complications of bacterial meningitis include communicating hydrocephalus, subdural empyema, and cerebritis leading to cerebral abscess formation.

Cerebritis is a focal cerebral inflammation, which immediately precedes the development of an abscess. A cerebral abscess may arise from the direct spread of bacteria from an adjacent non-CNS infection or from the hematogenous spread of bacteria. The direct extension of an infection from the skull can occur with mastoiditis, which leads to a temporal or cerebellar abscess, or frontal sinusitis, which leads to a frontal abscess. Inoculation of bacteria through the meninges via an open skull fracture, gunshot wound, or surgical wound can also occur. Abscesses caused by direct extension are usually solitary. Abscesses caused by the hematogenous spread of bacteria occur with pneumonia, bacterial endocarditis, or diverticulitis. Cerebral abscesses are more common in patients with a right-to-left shunt, such as a cardiac septal defect or a pulmonary AVM, owing to paradoxical emboli. Emboli usually lodge in a branch of the middle cerebral artery, because this vessel receives the largest proportion of cerebral blood flow. When cerebral abscesses are from the hematogenous spread of bacteria, they frequently are multiple. Patients without preceding meningitis may not have systemic signs of infection. Focal signs, such as a hemiparesis or a focal seizure, can occur as the abscess grows and compresses the surrounding brain. Symptoms and signs of increased ICP, such as headache and decreased mental status, occur as the abscess enlarges and the surrounding brain becomes edematous. On CT scan or MRI, a thin-rimmed ring-enhancing lesion is seen. Treatment consists of obtaining blood cultures, administering i.v. antibiotics, and surgically draining the abscess. Corticosteroids may be given to treat the associated brain edema and an anticonvulsant may be used for seizure prophylaxis. Cerebral abscesses are more common in immunocompromised patients.

Viral infections include meningitis and encephalitis. A viral encephalitis may present like a brain tumor or mass lesion. Herpes simplex encephalitis frequently presents as a temporal lobe mass causing aphasia, upper-extremity weakness, seizure, or a combination of these. It may also present with generalized symptoms from increased ICP. MRI or CT scan frequently show a hemorrhagic, necrotic, and sometimes cystic temporal lobe mass. Treatment includes a stereotactic biopsy to obtain a diagnosis or a craniotomy for biopsy and debulking of the mass.

Fungal infections are usually caused by opportunistic organisms in immunocompromised patients. Commonly they are associated with a pulmonary fungal infection. A meningitis or an abscess is possible, and complications include hydrocephalus.

Parasitic infections are uncommon in the United States. Cysticercosis is an infection caused by the pork tapeworm, *Taenia solium*, which can spread through the bloodstream to the meninges, the brain parenchyma, or the ventricular system. A patient may present with seizure, focal deficit, or signs of increased ICP secondary to obstructive hydrocephalus. Cysticercosis also infects the spine and can be located in the intramedullary region (causing a transverse myelitis), or extramedullary (causing a compressive myelopathy). *Echinococcosis*, also called *hydatidosis*, is an infection by *Echinococcus granulosus*, the dog tapeworm, which spreads through the bloodstream to the white matter. These cysts are associated with little if any inflammation. It is possible for a cyst to act like a mass lesion and cause a neurologic deficit. When this occurs, the cyst can be surgically excised.

DEGENERATIVE DISEASES OF THE SPINE

Degenerative changes affect both the cervical and lumbar spine. In the cervical spine, a disk or a fragment of a disk, degenerative changes in the ligaments, or bony growth called *osteophytes* can cause neurologic symptoms. A cervical vertebral disk can herniate along the midline and compress the spinal cord or can herniate to one side of the spinal canal and compress a spinal nerve root. In the cervical spine, the nerve root that is compressed is the one exiting at the level of the disk herniation. For example, a C6-7 disk compresses the C7 root. A C7-T1 disk compresses the C8 root. When a free fragment of disk is extruded into the canal or foramen, it is called a *soft disk* or a *herniation of nucleus pulposus*, which most commonly occurs in the lower cervical spine at C6-7 or C5-6, where most neck flexion and extension occurs. The usual history given by a patient with a herniated cervical disk is that the symptoms began with no history of trauma when he or she awoke in the morning. Patients with herniated cervical disks complain of neck pain, which is exacerbated by movement, particularly extension of

the neck and lateral flexion of the neck toward the side of the herniated disk. Radicular symptoms and signs from a compressed nerve root include pain and hypoesthesia within the dermatome of that root (Fig. 1-17), weakness in the muscles innervated by the nerve root, and loss of a deep tendon reflex mediated by the nerve root. The pain experienced by the patient may be worsened by straining and coughing and improved with bed rest. With severe acute spinal cord compression, quadriparesis and bowel or bladder dysfunction occurs. On examination, the patient will have decreased range of motion of the neck, particularly in extension. MRI is the most effective technique to look for free fragments of disk and cord abnormalities.

Any combination of the following pathologic processes can cause stenosis of the cervical spinal canal (cervical stenosis) or stenosis of the intervertebral foramen: one or more osteophytes (hard disks) located at the posterior edge of the vertebral bodies, hypertrophy or calcification of the posterior longitudinal ligament, hypertrophy of the ligamentum flavum, one or more medial disk bulges, hypertrophy of the dura, hypertrophy of the lamina of the vertebrae, and a congenitally narrow spinal canal. Osteophytes are formed at the superior and inferior end-plates of the vertebral bodies. When cervical stenosis is caused by a long-standing degenerative process, it is called *cervical spondylosis.* The result is narrowing of the bony spinal canal causing chronic compression of the spinal cord, which results in myelopathic symptoms and narrowing of the intervertebral foramen, thereby causing chronic compression of exiting nerve roots and resultant radicular symptoms. Myelopathy is characterized by UMN dysfunction, which includes spasticity, hyperactive deep tendon reflexes, and the presence of a Babinski sign. A patient with spastic legs has difficulty ambulating and may experience frequent falls. Bowel and bladder dysfunction, sexual dysfunction, and decreased sensation may also occur. Radicular symptoms include LMN dysfunction, resulting in weakness of muscles innervated by the compressed root and hypoactive deep tendon reflexes of the same muscles. Radicular symptoms also include sensory loss in the dermatome innervated by the compressed root. Nerve root compression can be worsened by osteoarthritis of zygapophyseal (facet) joints and joints of Luschka, which causes additional narrowing of the intervertebral foramina. On lateral cervical spine films, there is a loss of the normal cervical lordosis and straightening or even kyphosis of the cervical vertebral column, and there are narrowed disk spaces, osteophytes, and narrowing of the anteroposterior diameter of the spinal canal. MRI is the best study to evaluate the spinal cord pathology, including the severity and location of the spinal cord compression and the presence of any signal change in the cord. Computed tomography is the best study for evaluation of the bony pathology.

The management is similar for acute disk rupture and chronic cervical stenosis. If the patient presents with only radicular pain and sensory symptoms, without motor, bowel, or bladder dysfunction, conservative management is initiated, that is, bed rest, pain medication, antiinflammatory medication, application of local heat, muscle relaxants, intermittent immobilization of the neck in a soft or hard collar (for comfort only, not for stability), and physical therapy. If the patient fails an adequate trial of conservative management, surgery is considered. If the patient has motor

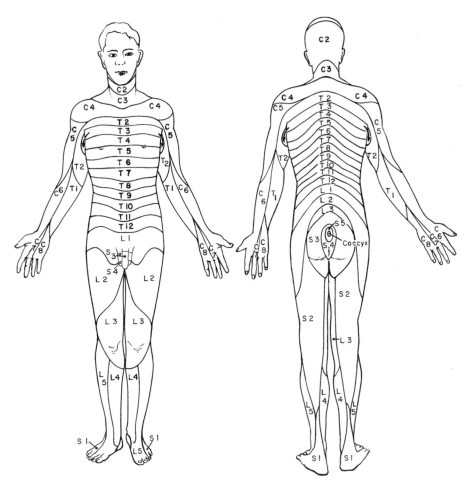

Figure 1-17 Dermatomes. The sensory innervation of the spinal roots. (From Barr ML, Kiernan JA. *The human nervous system.* JB Lippincott Co, 1993, with permission.)

weakness, bowel or bladder dysfunction, or myelopathic symptoms, surgery is necessary. An anterior approach via an anterior cervical diskectomy, or a posterior approach, such as a laminectomy, is performed depending on the location of the pathologic lesion.

Disk pathology occurs much less frequently in the thoracic spine because there is less movement in this portion of the spine. The thoracic bony spinal canal is narrow, leaving little extra space around the spinal cord. Therefore, neurologic deficits are common when a thoracic disk herniates into the spinal canal. Symptoms and signs include pain, sensory changes, and leg weakness. Thoracic disk herniations are seen in trauma and as chronic degenerative lesions usually occurring below T8.

Disk herniations commonly occur in the lumbosacral spine. Herniated disks are pieces of the nucleus pulposus that are extruded into the spinal canal through a defect in the annulus fibrosis. If the disk fragment protrudes partially through the annulus, it will create a bulge in the annulus. If the disk fragment is extruded through the annulus, a free fragment within the spinal canal results. Because the spinal cord usually ends at the L1 vertebral body and most lumbar disk herniations occur at L5-S1 or L4-5, patients will present with radicular symptoms. The compressed nerve root is the one exiting below the disk space with the herniation; for example, L4-5 disk herniation will compress the L5 root. With an L5-S1 disk herniation, the S1 root is compressed. Less commonly, a far lateral herniation of a lumbar disk can

compress the nerve root exiting in the intervertebral foramen of the same level; for example, a far lateral L4-5 disk will compress the L4 nerve root. Most lumbar disk herniations occur at L5-S1 or L4-5 because this is where most of the flexion and extension of the low back occurs. The patient may give a history of hearing or feeling a "pop" in the low back during exertion, after which the radicular symptoms began, or more commonly, the patient may give a history of slowly progressive symptoms. The radicular pain caused by a herniated lumber disk is increased with bending, sitting, standing, lifting, coughing, straining, or extension of the spine. Symptoms are relieved with bed rest, particularly if the patient lies on his or her side with his hips and knees flexed. Sciatica is pain radiating down the posterior or lateral leg to the ankle or foot in the distribution of the sciatic nerve and commonly occurs on the same side of the herniated disk. Signs on examination include sensory loss in the dermatome (Fig. 1-17), weakness in muscles innervated by the compressed nerve root, low back tenderness, paravertebral muscle spasm, and loss of deep tendon reflexes effected by the compressed root. The straight-leg raise test is performed by having the patient lie flat on his or her back as the examiner slowly raises the fully extended legs of the patient one at a time. A positive result is when radicular symptoms are reproduced in the symptomatic leg. Back pain does not constitute a positive finding. Herniated lumbar disks are best imaged by MRI, which shows the fragment or disk bulge and the compressed nerve root. Treatment for a herniated lumbar disk can be conservative if the patient has only pain and sensory symptoms. Medical management includes strict bed rest, pain medications, local application of heat, anti-inflammatory medications, and skeletal muscle relaxants. Physical therapy can be added later for low back strengthening. Surgery, usually a microdiskectomy, is indicated if a patient has weakness, progressive worsening of the neurologic exam, or chronic disabling pain. A herniated disk can recur after medical or surgical treatment.

Lumbar spinal stenosis—narrowing of the lumbar spinal canal, which compresses the cauda equina—is caused by one or more of the following: a congenitally narrow lumbar spinal canal, facet hypertrophy, hypertrophy of the ligamentum flavum, bulging of intervertebral disks, and spondylolisthesis. Spondylolisthesis is the anterior subluxation of a vertebral body on the vertebral body below it, most commonly L5 on S1. In addition to the canal being narrowed, the intervertebral foramina are narrowed, thereby compressing the exiting nerve roots. Patients with lumbar spinal stenosis present with chronic radicular symptoms in the lower extremities. Neurogenic claudication (NC) occurs with lumbar spinal stenosis and can be differentiated from vascular claudication (VC) by history and physical examination. Both occur with walking, but a patient with VC can walk a predictable distance before he or she must stop because of pain, whereas a patient with NC can walk variable distances before the onset of symptoms. The pain with NC is within one or several dermatomes, and the pain with VC is in a stocking distribution. The stenosis of the lumbar spinal canal is worsened by upright postures needed for standing and walking because the lumbar spine is extended. Flexing the lumbar spine relieves the pain, which is accomplished by bending at the waist or sitting. Therefore, the NC patient must sit to get relief after walking, as opposed to a patient with VC who needs only to rest by standing still. In addition, relief with resting usually comes sooner to the patient with VC. On examination, decreased sensation in one or both legs is common, limitation of back movement (particularly forward flexion) is seen, and motor weakness and loss of deep tendon reflexes can occur. Signs of vascular insufficiency on examination, such as absent peripheral pulses and foot pallor with elevation, should not be present in a patient with NC. Plain x-rays may show spondylolisthesis, narrowing of the anteroposterior diameter of the canal, and disk space narrowing. Flexion and extension x-rays may be helpful. MRI is the best study to visualize the cauda equina and the exiting nerve roots, computed tomography is best for evaluating the bony pathology, and a myelogram with a postmyelogram CT scan is helpful with complex cases. Medical treatment is indicated for a patient with lumbar stenosis without weakness. Surgery is indicated if a patient has weakness, progressive worsening of examination results, or chronic disabling pain.

The cauda equina syndrome is caused by a large compressive lesion usually located at L4-5. The signs and symptoms include bowel and bladder dysfunction, saddle anesthesia, motor weakness in multiple nerve root distributions, low back pain, sciatica, absence of both ankle reflexes, and sexual dysfunction. However, all of these symptoms and signs do not need to be present. Saddle anesthesia is numbness of the buttocks, the perineal region, and the posterior superior thighs. Sciatica, when present, may be bilateral. Emergent surgical decompression is needed.

KEY POINTS

▲ Head injury can be stratified by severity into mild [Glasgow coma scale (GCS) 13 to 15], moderate (GCS 9 to 12), and severe (GCS less than 9). Therapeutic interventions are targeted at preventing or minimizing secondary injury to the brain. Mechanisms of secondary injury include metabolic abnormalities, hypoxia, intracranial hypertension, and hypovolemia. The initial evaluation includes a lateral cervical spine film and a CT scan of the head. Computed tomography is used to image acute processes that necessitate an emergent neuroradiologic evaluation. Acute hemorrhage is hyperdense to normal brain.

▲ Acute traumatic injury can result in an epidural hematoma (EDH), subdural hematoma (SDH), intraparenchymal hematoma (IPH), subarachnoid hemorrhage (SAH), cerebral contusion, or diffuse axonal injury (DAI). An EDH arises between the inner table of the skull and the dura from a high-pressure bleed that is caused by a lacerated epidural artery or a tear in the wall of a venous sinus, secondary to a depressed skull fracture. Treatment involves craniotomy, hematoma evacuation, and repair of the lacerated vessel. Epidural hematomas are often not associated with a significant underlying brain injury. An SDH arises between the dura mater and the arachnoid membrane and is caused by the laceration of a subdural bridging, a tear in the subdural wall of a venous sinus, or the extension of an IPH into the subdural space. Treatment for a symptomatic acute SDH entails an emergent craniotomy to evacuate the clot and stop the bleeding. An acute SDH is often associated with a severe head injury.

▲ Spinal cord injury (SCI) can be divided into complete and incomplete injuries. In a complete injury there is a total loss of motor, sensory, and autonomic function below the level of the injury, whereas in an incomplete injury there is sparing of some sensory or motor function below the level of injury. Incomplete SCIs have a better prognosis for neurologic recovery than complete SCIs. After a blunt traumatic SCI, administration of high-dose corticosteroids has been shown to facilitate neurologic recovery. Classic patterns of incomplete SCI include Brown–Sequard syndrome after anatomic or functional hemisection of the spinal cord, central cord syndrome after a hyperextension injury in a patient with cervical spondylosis, and anterior spinal artery syndrome after infarction of the anterior and lateral funiculi of the spinal cord.

▲ Brain tumors can be either primary CNS tumors or metastases. Primary brain tumors include gliomas, oligodendrogliomas, ependymomas, choroid plexus papillomas, medulloblastomas, gangliomas, meningiomas, acoustic neuromas-vestibular schwannoma, primary CNS lymphoma, hemangioblastomas, glomus jugulare tumors, pituitary adenomas, craniopharyngiomas, germinomas, teratomas, epidermoids, and dermoids. Metastatic brain tumors are the most common brain tumors in adults. They commonly arise from lung, breast, malignant melanoma, kidney, and the gastrointestinal tract. Signs and symptoms of lesions include headache or other signs of increased intracranial pressure (ICP), change in mental status, seizures, and neurologic deficits.

SUGGESTED READINGS

American Association of Neurological Surgeons. *Guidelines for the management of severe head injury.* New York: Brain Trauma Foundation, 1995.

Barr ML, Kiernan JA. *The human nervous system, an anatomical viewpoint.* Philadelphia: JB Lippincott Co, 1993.

Bracken MB, Shepard MJ, Collins WF, et al. A randomized controlled trial of methylprednisolone or naloxone in the treatment of acute spinal cord injury. *N Engl J Med* 1990;322:1405–1411.

Bracken MB, Shepard MJ, Holford TR, et al. Administration of methylprednisolone for 24 or 48 hours in the treatment of acute spinal cord injury. *JAMA* 1997;227:1597–1604.

Kaye A. *Essential neurosurgery.* Edinburgh: Churchill Livingstone, 1991.

Immunology and Transplantation

Heidi Yeh   James F. Markmann

INTRODUCTION

The immune system starts with the skin and mucosal surfaces, which form a barrier between the internal environment of the organism and the outside world. Once pathogens have entered the body, the immune system functions to identify, isolate, and eliminate them. Generally, these pathogens are microorganisms such as bacteria, viruses, and fungi, but parasites are also included. In the case of malignancy, mutated "self" cells would also qualify for eradication.

The immune system is divided broadly into two branches: the innate immune system and the adaptive immune system (Table 2-1). *Innate immunity* is phylogenetically older and utilizes components that are present from the time of birth and that are available to attack and sequester pathogens immediately. These components are activated by surface molecules conserved across entire classes of pathogens and are therefore nonspecific. Depending on one's point of view, innate immunity could be said to have no memory or to have "innate" memory that does not require previous exposure to the pathogen. Not unexpectedly, pathogens have developed ways of evading the innate immune system; it is thought that the adaptive immune system evolved as a counter-response, and this idea is supported by the fact that the adaptive immune system uses the effector components of the innate immune system. The *adaptive immune system* revolves around clonal selection of effector cells that are also present from birth, but are neither activated nor circulating in sufficient numbers to mount an effective response. At the first exposure

to an antigen, there is an induction period—the delay resulting from the time required for activation and amplification. Once primed, the response is much faster on subsequent challenges; hence the term, "immunologic memory." This paradigm represents a compromise between the amount of energy and cell mass required to mount an adequate immune response and the vast number of antigens that the immune system must be prepared to recognize specifically. Because clinical transplantation is largely driven by our understanding of adaptive immunity, this chapter mainly concerns the basic concepts of the adaptive immune response.

MAJOR HISTOCOMPATIBILITY COMPLEX

The major histocompatibility complex (MHC) is the crux of the adaptive immune system's ability to identify different antigens; it serves as the scaffold on which all peptides are presented. Peptides sit in a special groove of the MHC molecule; effector cells recognize the three-dimensional structure formed by the MHC molecule and the peptide together as a unit (Fig. 2-1A). Stable binding of a peptide to the MHC molecule does not require contact at every single amino acid, so each MHC molecule can bind many different peptides that are similar at only a few residues. Because different MHC molecules differ in their ability to bind peptide and activate effector cells, the repertoire of MHC determines the effectiveness of antigen presentation and the subsequent immune response. Variation in binding capacity leads to the phenomenon of certain populations being more "susceptible" to particular infections than others. For example, in an area of chronic measles infections, individuals who express MHC molecules that are efficient at presenting measles peptides survive to pass on the genes for those MHC alleles. Eventually, the percentage of the population expressing these alleles is much higher than would be expected by chance and random mutation. In a measles-naïve area, MHC alleles have been selected for their ability to present some other unrelated peptides, and only a small number of individuals will be able to mount an effective response to the measles virus.

TABLE 2-1

ADAPTIVE VERSUS INATE IMMUNITY

	Inducible	Immediate Response	Antigen Specific
Adaptive immunity	Yes	No	Yes
Innate immunity	No	Yes	No

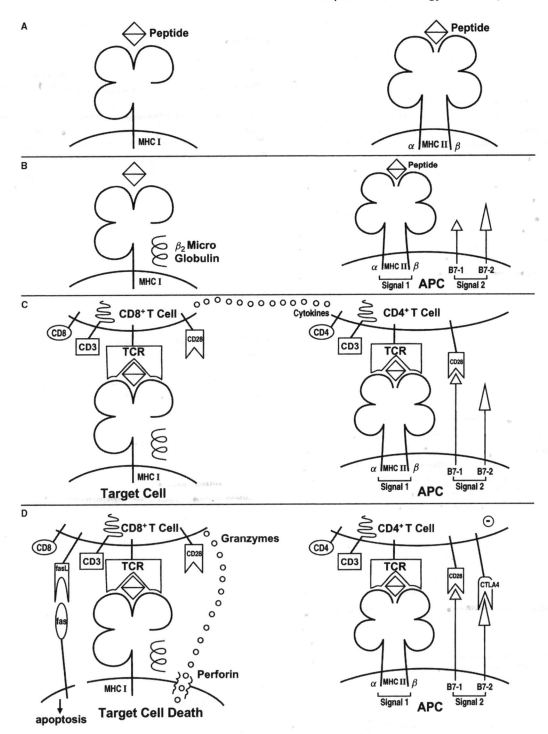

Figure 2-1 Major histocompatibility complex (MHC) and T-cell receptor (TCR) structure. **A:** The peptide binding groove is made of the α chain of the MHC I molecule and the α and β chains of the MHC II molecule. **B:** β_2-Microglobulin stabilizes MHC I. Antigen-presenting cells express MHC II and costimulatory molecules. **C:** The TCR recognizes a complex comprising MHC + peptide. CD4 cells elaborate cytokines, which provide "help" to CD8 T cells. **D:** CD8$^+$ cytotoxic T lymphocytes secrete granzymes that lead to the destruction of the target cell. CTLA-4 transmits an inhibitory signal to T cells.

Therefore, on initial exposure, the virus takes a much more virulent course through the population. Human MHC, known as *human leukocyte antigen* (HLA), has more than 70 alleles at some loci, making the HLA genes the most polymorphic of human genes. Teleologically, this diversity in peptide receptor–presenting molecules may serve to ensure that at least some individuals of a species will respond successfully to a given pathogen.

The human MHC (HLA) region is located on the short arm of chromosome 6 and also encodes a number of other proteins that are not directly related to the immune system. Because the proximity of the different genes results in a low recombination frequency, HLAs are usually inherited *en bloc* from each parent, and the set of closely linked genes is referred to as a haplotype. A child is therefore always 1-haplotype identical with each biologic parent. Siblings have a 50% chance of sharing one haplotype with each other, a 25% chance of being HLA identical (sharing both haplotypes), and a 25% chance of sharing neither haplotype.

There are three classes of MHC. *MHC class I* is expressed on all nucleated cells and is generally loaded with intracellular peptides, either self or viral proteins. *Natural killer (NK) cells*, part of the innate immune system, are inhibited by MHC class I. Malignant transformation results in down-regulation of MHC class I, and this makes cancer cells targets for destruction by NK cells. In humans, there are three Class I loci, HLA-A, -B, and -C, which are expressed codominantly and for which individuals are usually heterozygous. Therefore, every cell could express six different class I molecules. The polymorphic α chain of class I molecules, also known as the heavy chain, is a 45-kDa, transmembrane protein. It is noncovalently bound to β_2-microglobulin, also known as the light chain, a 12-kDa soluble protein that is actually encoded by a gene on chromosome 15. β_2-Microglobulin binds to and stabilizes the extracellular domain of the α chain (Fig. 2-1B).

MHC class II is expressed constitutively on thymic epithelium and antigen-presenting cells (APCs), predominantly dendritic cells, macrophages, and B lymphocytes. MHC class II molecules are generally loaded with proteins, which are phagocytosed or otherwise internalized from the surrounding tissues and body fluids. In humans, there are also three class II loci, HLA-DP, -DQ, and -DR, which are expressed codominantly. MHC class II comprises an α and a β chain, both polymorphic and both spanning the cell membrane, which together form a peptide binding groove (Fig. 2-1A). The DR locus encodes an extra β chain, and α and β chains from different loci can cross-combine (transcomplementation).

The MHC class III region encodes a number of molecules including heat shock proteins, complement, and cytokines, which are involved in the inflammatory response but do not participate directly in antigen presentation and are not polymorphic. Conversely, there are a number of genes that are not involved in immunity or inflammation but that are polymorphic. These general-function, or housekeeping, proteins are encoded throughout the genome and are termed minor histocompatibility antigens; they are equivalent to exogenous foreign peptides in terms of their ability to stimulate an immune response.

ANTIGEN-PRESENTING CELLS

APCs—dendritic cells, macrophages, and B lymphocytes—are defined by their ability to trap and present antigen (signal 1) and to deliver a costimulatory signal (signal 2) to T cells (Fig. 2-1B). Dendritic cells residing in tissues express both class I and class II MHC and are highly effective at ingesting antigen. In response to inflammation, they travel to the lymph nodes, where they lose their phagocytic ability but upregulate expression of adhesion molecules and the

costimulatory molecules B7-1 and B7-2 (CD80 and CD86). B cells take up specific antigens using surface-bound immunoglobulin as a receptor. They express class II MHC constitutively on their surface but display costimulatory molecules only if induced by inflammation. Macrophages take up antigen efficiently through phagocytosis, but expression of both class II MHC and costimulatory molecule depend on inflammatory signals. The separation of antigen presentation and costimulatory molecule expression helps to prevent the activation of T cells in the absence of a pathogenic infection and, in fact, such signals may render T cells anergic, or unable to respond. In addition to the delivery of the additional signals through accessory molecules, APCs secrete cytokines, which influence the response of T lymphocytes.

T CELLS

The antigen (peptide/MHC) recognition molecule on T cells is the T-cell receptor (TCR). TCR diversity is generated by somatic cell gene rearrangement after T-cell progenitors leave the bone marrow to mature in the thymus. The TCR gene is arranged in cassette fashion; variable (V), diversity (D), and joining (J) regions all exist as multiple variable segments in the germline. During maturation, each T cell randomly rearranges its TCR gene to remove all but one segment each of the V, D, and J regions so that each T cell has a slightly different TCR (Fig. 2-2). The TCR is formed by two transmembrane chains, α and β, each of which is encoded in the germline by a large number of V, D, and J segments.

The thymus arises embryologically from the third pharyngeal pouch and the third branchial cleft, and it is fully developed before birth but begins to involute at puberty. *Positive selection* is triggered by epithelial cells in the thymic cortex and involves expansion of T cells expressing TCR that weakly recognize self-peptides bound to self-MHC. Those T cells that do not presumably are not MHC-restricted and undergo programmed cell death, or apoptosis, accounting for about 95% of thymocyte death. *Negative selection* is triggered by bone marrow–derived dendritic cells in the thymic medulla and results in deletion of T cells that have high affinity for self-peptides bound to self-MHC. This is the primary step at which self-reactive T cells are removed from the pool. Mature T lymphocytes that are exported to the periphery express TCRs on their cell surface, which can potentially recognize foreign peptide in the context of self-MHC, but do not recognize MHC loaded with self-peptides.

All T lymphocytes express CD3[1], an accessory molecule stably associated with the TCR on the cell surface (Fig. 2-1C). CD3 is necessary for the cell-surface expression of TCR and, by virtue of its extensive cytoplasmic region, is also responsible for signal transduction to intracellular proteins

---

[1]*CD* stands for clusters of differentiation. In the early days of immunology, cell surface molecules were identified, not by amino acid or DNA sequencing, but by the group of antibodies they would bind. Each molecule was then given the number of the corresponding antibody group. Hence, CD3 was a means of identifying the cell surface molecule on T cells that contained epitopes for antibody group 3.

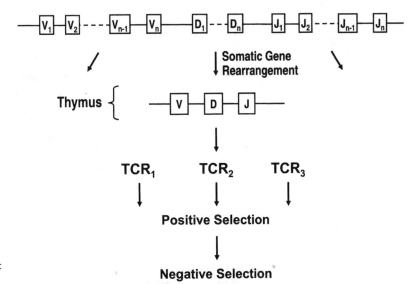

Figure 2-2 Somatic cell gene rearrangement results in T-cell receptor (TCR) diversity.

following binding of the TCR to MHC-peptide. In fact, T cells can be activated nonspecifically through CD3 without binding the TCR at all. CD28, the receptor for the costimulatory molecules B7-1 and B7-2 (CD80 and CD86) is also expressed on all T cells. Engagement of the TCR without a costimulatory signal results in anergy, or inactivation, of T cells. Once activated, T cells upregulate CTLA-4, which also binds CD80 and CD86. However, CTLA-4 ligation results in an inhibitory signal and limits T-cell amplification and activation as a form of negative feedback (Fig. 2-1D).

In addition, T cells express either CD4 or CD8 co-receptor molecules, which bind to the constant regions of MHC class II or class I, respectively (Fig. 2-1C). These interactions stabilize the TCR–MHC complex, but also identify T-cell subsets with different functions. In general, CD4$^+$ T cells synthesize soluble growth factors, or cytokines that support the proliferation of T cells and B cells, and are therefore termed *helper T cells*. CD8$^+$ T cells are also known as *cytotoxic T lymphocytes* (CTLs) and recognize target cells by their class I MHC–peptide complex. They kill target cells by one of two methods: (i) releasing digestive enzymes (granzymes) directly into target cells via transmembrane pores generated by perforin polymers and

(ii) inducing apoptosis by binding Fas receptors on target cells with Fas ligand expressed on the CTL cell surface (Fig. 2-1D). Because CD8$^+$ T-cell effector function is largely cell-contact dependent, T cells are said to mediate the *cellular immune response*.

B CELLS

In contrast to the T-cell-mediated cellular immune response, the *humoral immune response* is mediated by antibody-producing B lymphocytes. *Antibodies* are made up of four protein chains, two heavy chains and two light chains, which are linked by interchain disulfide bonds and have constant regions at their carboxy terminals and variable regions at their amino terminals (Fig. 2-3). The variable amino terminal (F_{ab}) binds antigens and is generated by somatic cell gene rearrangement of V and J regions similar to the TCR. The constant region (F_c) binds complement and Fc receptors on macrophages and NK cells and distinguishes the different classes, or *isotypes*, of antibody: immunoglobulin (Ig)M, IgA, IgE, IgG, and IgD (Table 2-2). Immunoglobulin M is the first class produced during an immune response and is expressed on the B-cell surface

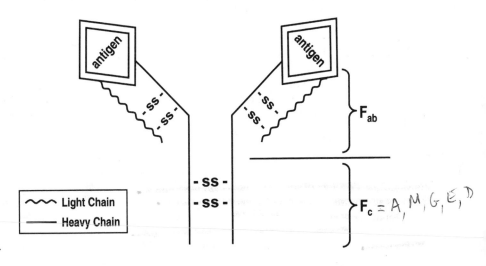

Figure 2-3 Antibody structure.

TABLE 2-2

MAJOR DIFFERENCES IN IMMUNOGLOBULIN ABILITIES ACCORDING TO IMMUNOGLOBULIN CLASS

	IgA	IgD	IgE	IgG	IgM
Cross placenta	−	−	−	+	−
Cross mucosal barriers	+	−	−	−	−
Complement activation	−	−	−	+	+
Binding to mast cells and basophils	−	−	+	−	−
Binding to macrophages	−	−	−	+	−

even before activation. Once B cells bind foreign antigen through their surface receptor, they proliferate and differentiate into antibody-secreting plasma cells or into memory B cells. This process requires help from CD4$^+$ T cells, in the form of cytokines such as interleukin (IL)-4, IL-5, and IL-6, and CD40-CD40 ligand engagement, which is important for the isotype switching from IgM to IgG, IgA, or IgE. IgA is produced at mucosal surfaces and is found in the secretions of the airway and gastrointestinal tract; IgE binds mast cells and basophils, resulting in histamine and serotonin release and the clinical allergic response. Both IgG and IgM can activate complement, but only IgG can cross the placenta and bind macrophages.

The *complement system* is part of the innate immune system and can be activated by infectious microorganisms in the blood, by endotoxin, or by the unnatural surfaces present in extracorporeal perfusion circuits. The complement cascade can also be activated when antibodies of the IgG or IgM isotype specifically bind to foreign antigen. C1q, one of the complement proteins, then binds to the Fc domain of the bound antibody and initiates the complement cascade resulting in formation of C3 convertase and assembly of the membrane-attack complex C5b-C9. This complex actually creates transmembrane channels and disrupts membrane integrity. In addition, binding of antibodies to foreign antigen can lead to opsonization and clearance of the antigen–antibody complex by phagocytes. Antibody-dependent cell-mediated cytotoxicity (ADCC) is effected by NK cells and macrophages and starts with binding of Fc receptors on antibodies bound to target cells.

CYTOKINES

Cytokines are soluble factors that are secreted by lymphocytes, dendritic cells, endothelial cells, macrophages, and other cells of the immune system. They have a short half-life and interact with high-affinity cytokine-specific receptors on target cells in a paracrine fashion. Specific cytokines can have multiple effects, and there is considerable redundancy among the function of different cytokines. Interleukin 1 (IL-1) is produced by macrophages and stimulates proliferation of activated B and T lymphocytes. It is also responsible for the *fever response* mediated by the hypothalamus. Tumor necrosis factor (TNF)-α is produced by monocytes and is thought to play a major role in the

systemic inflammatory response syndrome (SIRS). Another cytokine, IL-2, is critical for expansion of T lymphocytes following their initial activation, and IL-2 receptors are not expressed on resting T lymphocytes. Inhibition of IL-2 production by calcineurin inhibitor drugs (cyclosporine or tacrolimus) is the basis for clinical immunosuppression. Produced by T cells and macrophages, IL-6 is the primary signal for induction of hepatic acute phase proteins and promotes liver regeneration following injury.

REJECTION

After transplantation, the recipient's APCs can present graft allopeptide in a self-MHC-restricted fashion. This is referred to as *indirect presentation* and results in a response of a magnitude similar to that resulting from any other typical foreign antigen. However, the vigor of the immune response to an allograft probably results from another route of antigen presentation, known as *direct presentation*, in which donor APCs expressing donor MHC can migrate from the graft into the recipient's lymphoid organs and directly activate recipient T lymphocytes. These allorestricted T lymphocytes, which recognize the foreign donor MHC complex, greatly outnumber (up to 10% of total T cells) the number of graft-specific self-restricted T lymphocytes (on the order of .01%). This phenomenon is probably responsible for *acute rejection*, the most frequent form of rejection seen clinically. It generally occurs within a few weeks of transplantation, but it can occur episodically at any time during the transplantation course. Its frequency may wane with time, as donor-derived APCs are eliminated and replaced by those from the host. CD8$^+$ CTLs recognize donor MHC class I antigen and kill the cells of the transplant organ. The elaboration of cytokines by CD4$^+$ T helper cells promotes the nonspecific activation of macrophages, neutrophils, mast cells, and NK cells, which also contribute to graft damage. In cases of severe rejection, IgG antibodies may also be involved.

Although there has been substantial progress in the prevention and treatment of acute allograft rejection, *chronic rejection* remains the major cause of late graft failure. Likely examples of chronic rejection include obliterative bronchiolitis, cardiac allograft vasculopathy, and glomerulosclerosis. The liver is generally less susceptible to chronic rejection, although "ductopenic" chronic rejection is well described. Chronic rejection is typically seen months to years after transplantation. Both humoral and cell-mediated immunity have been suggested to participate in producing the damage leading to chronic graft rejection. In addition to histoincompatibility, nonimmune mechanisms such as ischemia–reperfusion injury, infections, and donor-recipient–size mismatching are also thought to contribute to late graft failure.

Hyperacute rejection occurs within minutes of graft revascularization and is the result of preformed antibodies directed against donor antigens. Presensitization can occur following blood transfusions, pregnancy, or previous transplantation. Complement activation injures the graft's endothelium, thereby leading to deposition of fibrin and platelets, vasoconstriction, neutrophil adhesion, and, finally, hemorrhagic necrosis of the graft. Hyperacute rejection can be largely avoided by screening of recipients for antibodies in two ways. Recipient serum can be tested against a panel of cells representing common HLA antigens for reactivity, giving a percentage positive *panel reactive antibody* (PRA). More specifically, the recipient's serum can be tested against donor lymphocytes in a process known as *prospective cross-matching*. A positive crossmatch, that is, the recipient's serum contains antibodies that bind donor lymphocytes, is considered incompatible. Prospective crossmatches are done routinely only for kidney and pancreas transplants, as they are most susceptible to hyperacute rejection and most tolerant of the extra ischemia time resulting from performing the crossmatch. An exceptional circumstance where a crossmatch for a kidney transplant is not required is when the kidney is transplanted together with a liver from the same donor. The liver is known to be relatively resistant to humoral injury; therefore, when the liver alone is transplanted, a prospective crossmatch is not required, even for highly sensitized patients. This is presumably because of the ability of the liver to adsorb donor-specific antibodies from the recipient circulation without sustaining any damage. This process is so efficient that by the time the kidney (from the same donor) is transplanted and perfused, there is no longer sufficient circulating antibody to trigger hyperacute rejection of the kidney. A prospective crossmatch is routine for cardiac transplants in which the recipient in known to have a high PRA.

IMMUNOSUPPRESSION

Steroids

Corticosteroids intervene at many points in the immune system. They inhibit deoxyribonucleic acid (DNA) and ribonucleic acid (RNA) production, and after forming complexes with intracellular receptors, they impair transcription of cytokines such as IL-1, IL-2, IL-6, interferon (IFN)-γ, and (TNF)-α. In addition, they act in an antiinflammatory fashion by inhibiting margination of lymphocytes, decreasing chemotaxis, and impairing function of macrophages and granulocytes. Long-term administration of corticosteroids is associated with multiple side effects including hypertension, hyperlipidemia, hyperglycemia, cataract formation, osteoporosis, psychosis, pancreatitis, gastrointestinal bleeding, ulceration and perforation, poor wound healing, and growth retardation.

Calcineurin Inhibitors

Calcineurin is a Ca$^+$-dependent serine-threonine phosphatase that dephosphorylates a number of DNA transcription factors, including nuclear factor of activated T cells (NFAT). Following dephosphorylation, NFAT localizes to the nucleus and binds to the promoter region of the IL-2 gene, resulting in upregulation of IL-2 expression. Neoral/Sandimmune (cyclosporine), a cyclic peptide drug derived from a fungus, binds to cyclophilin-A, a peptidyl-prolyl isomerase that normally facilitates cellular protein folding. The complex of cyclosporine and cyclophilin, however, binds and inhibits the phosphatase activity of calcineurin, resulting in the failure of IL-2 production (Fig. 2-4). One of the notable complications of cyclosporine use is *nephrotoxicity*, resulting from a combination of vasoconstriction and interstitial nephritis. Other side effects include gingival hyperplasia, hypertension, and hyperkalemia. Cyclosporine is metabolized by the cytochrome P-450 system in the liver, and its dosing must be adjusted when given with other drugs that either compete for the P-450 system or upregulate its activity.

FK506/Prograf (tacrolimus) was first isolated from *streptomyces* and binds to a cellular protein named FK506 binding protein (FKBP). The complex of FK506 and FKBP inhibits calcineurin activity, ultimately inhibiting IL-2 expression, much as cyclosporine does (Fig. 2-4). FK506 also inhibits production of IL-3, IL-4, (IFN)-γ, and expression of the IL-2 receptor. Like cyclosporine, FK506 can cause significant nephrotoxicity, hypertension, and hyperkalemia at high serum levels. Other electrolyte abnormalities include hypomagnesemia. FK506-induced central

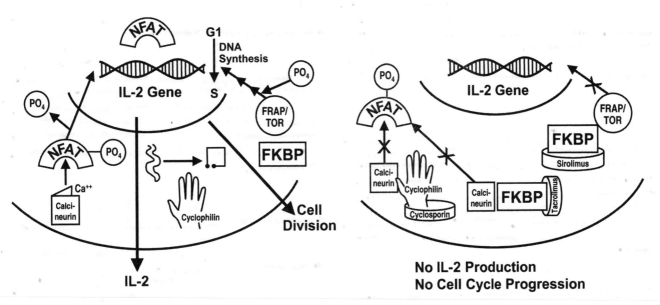

Figure 2-4 Calcineurin inhibitor and rapamycin pathway.

nervous system (CNS) toxicity can manifest as headaches, tremors, mental status changes, or even seizures. Another serious side effect of FK506 is diabetes, which seems to be related to inhibition of insulin gene transcription as well as some degree of beta cell toxicity rather than to insulin resistance, although preexisting insulin resistance obviously increases the patient's risk for requiring insulin. FK506-associated diabetes is sometimes reversible after withdrawal of the drug.

Cell Cycle Inhibitors

Sirolimus (rapamycin/Rapamune) also binds to FKBP but does not exert its immunosuppressive activity via the calcineurin pathway (Fig. 2-4). Rather, the complex of sirolimus and FKBP binds to and inhibits a kinase named FRAP (FKBP-rapamycin/sirolimus-associated protein), which is variably known as "target of Rapamune" (TOR). Kinase activity of FRAP/TOR is required to activate cyclin-dependent kinases necessary for T cells to progress from the G1 to the S phase during the proliferative response to IL-2 and IL-6. Sirolimus is associated with much less nephrotoxicity but does cause hyperlipidemia, hypertension, pneumonitis, acne, and rashes.

Antimetabolites

Mycophenolate mofetil (MMF/Cellcept/myfortec) is a prodrug that is hydrolyzed to mycophenolic acid (MPA), the active form of the drug. MPA inhibits the activity of inosine monophosphate dehydrogenase (IMPDH), an enzyme in the *de novo* guanine synthesis pathway. B and T cells are dependent on *de novo* guanine synthesis for proliferation because they lack the salvage pathway upon which other rapidly dividing cells frequently depend. As a result, MPA inhibits leukocyte proliferation, without the skin, hair, and gastrointestinal side effects that other antimetabolites cause. In addition, MPA blocks glycosylation of adhesion molecules, thereby inhibiting leukocyte recruitment and adhesion to endothelial cells. Although MMF causes no renal toxicity, it does cause bone marrow suppression and gastrointestinal symptoms such as nausea, diarrhea, and vague abdominal pain, and its use is contraindicated in pregnancy. MMF has reduced absorption with magnesium and aluminum hydroxide.

Once the first-line antimetabolite, *azathioprine* (Imuran) is now used only for patients who are intolerant of MMF. It contains an imidazole linked to 6-mercaptopurine, which is converted to its active form, 6-thioguanine, in the liver, by hypoxanthine-guanine phosphoribosyltransferase (HGPRT). The substituted purine resembles a real purine sufficiently to get incorporated into DNA, but not enough to allow for DNA replication and RNA transcription. Its preferential uptake into B and T lymphocytes, hence its selective inhibition of DNA and RNA synthesis in leukocytes, is not well understood. Adverse effects include increased risk of malignancy, hepatitis, myelosuppression (especially leukopenia), cholestasis, alopecia, and pancreatitis. The dose of azathioprine must be decreased if given with allopurinol, because allopurinol inhibits one of the enzymes that degrades azathioprine to its inactive metabolite. Azathioprine, too, is contraindicated in pregnancy. It should not be used with angiotensin-converting enzyme (ACE) inhibitors, as the combination can result in severe anemia and pancytopenia.

Methotrexate is rarely used except for occasional use in pediatric heart transplant recipients. Methotrexate inhibits DNA and RNA synthesis by blocking folic acid metabolism. It also inhibits chemotaxis of macrophages. Adverse effects include myelosuppression, gastrointestinal toxicity, hepatic dysfunction, nephrotoxicity, and dermatitis.

Anti-T-Cell Antibodies

Polyclonal and monoclonal antibodies directed toward cell-surface proteins on T lymphocytes are used as part of immunosuppressive induction therapies or for the treatment of steroid-resistant acute rejection. Rabbit antithymocyte immunoglobulin (Thymoglobulin) is a polyclonal preparation purified from the serum of rabbits that have been repeatedly inoculated with human thymocytes. ATGAM is similar to Thymoglobulin, except that it is isolated from horses. Once T cells are bound by antibody, they are depleted from the circulation through opsonization and complement-assisted, antibody-dependent cell-mediated cytotoxicity. Damaged T cells are cleared by the lymphoreticular system. OKT-3 (muromonab-CD3) is a monoclonal murine IgG2a antibody against the TCR-CD3 complex. Administration of OKT-3 results first in transient activation of T cells and a massive release of cytokines. This is called the "cytokine release syndrome" and is characterized by severe flu-like symptoms (fevers, chills, dyspnea, and bronchospasm), flash pulmonary edema, and CNS complications. Antibody-bound T cells are then removed from the circulation by opsonization in the liver and spleen and cytolysis via ADCC. Although T cells will reappear, they are CD3-negative as a result of receptor downregulation and are not able to be activated.

Anti-IL-2 Receptor Antibodies

Basiliximab (Simulect) is a chimeric murine/human IgG1 produced by a genetically engineered mouse myeloma cell line. It expresses plasmids encoding the human heavy and light chain constant regions fused to the mouse heavy and light chain variable regions that encode an antibody that binds to the IL-2 receptor α chain. Also known as CD25, this component of the high affinity IL-2 receptor is expressed preferentially on activated T lymphocytes. Simulect binds but does not activate the IL-2 receptor and functions as a competitive inhibitor for endogenous IL-2. *Daclizumab* (Zenapax) is another construct that has been humanized to a different degree and has a murine variable region that binds to a different epitope of the IL-2 high affinity receptor. Both are used primarily as induction agents for renal transplantation.

Anti-B Cell Antibodies

Rituximab is another human/murine chimeric antibody with the human IgG1 Fc regions fused to the murine variable light and heavy chain regions that recognize CD20, a surface marker found on B cells. Through binding of complement to the Fc portion, rituximab eliminates B cells via complement and ADCC. Frequently used to treat non-Hodgkin B cell lymphoma, rituximab has recently entered the transplant arena mainly for treatment of steroid-resistant antibody-mediated rejection or rejection with evidence of vasculitis, especially those cases with peritubular C4d-positive immunohistochemical staining as a marker for humoral rejection. The agent is also used to treat post-transplantation lymphoproliferative disorder (PTLD) (see subsequent text). As with other antibody treatments, production of anti-rituximab antibodies (which has been documented in lymphoma patients) results in poor efficacy, since the agent is cleared from circulation before it can bind CD20 and activate complement. In addition, plasma cells do not express high levels of CD20 and are therefore not good targets.

Inhibitors of Lymphocyte Trafficking

FTY720 is a small semisynthetic molecule based on myricin, an immunosuppressive compound isolated from the culture broth of the Chinese herb, *Isaria sinclairii*. Following phosphorylation by sphingosine kinase, FTY720 monophosphate (FTY720-P) becomes a high affinity agonist for the G-protein-coupled sphingosine-1-phosphate (S1P) receptor. Activation of the S1P receptor promotes chemotaxis of naïve T cells to the lymph nodes in a chemokine-dependent manner. Unlike the endogenous ligand, FTY720-P causes S1P receptor internalization. Because lymphocytes require the S1P receptor to escape the lymph node, lymphocytes exposed to FTY720-P become trapped in the lymph nodes and Peyer patches and are no longer available in the circulation or to migrate to the allograft. In animals, FTY720 does not appear to have an effect on the development of antibody or CTL in response to viral challenges, and it does not inhibit cytokine production or development of antigen specific $CD4^+$ cells in response to ovalbumin. FTY720 also seems to have no effect on the circulation of memory cells, since they rely on different homing receptors that are not part of the S1P receptor pathway. In addition, S1P receptors are implicated in the stabilization of capillaries, promoting cell–cell contact and adherens junction assembly between endothelial cells, thereby enhancing endothelial barrier function. As such, FTY720 may also limit ischemia-reperfusion injury. The major side effect of FTY720 is transient bradycardia during the first 24 hours of dosing. This effect may be due to cross-talk between the G proteins coupled to the S1P receptor and those coupled to the muscarinic receptor. S1P receptors are highly expressed on cardiac tissue; fortunately, S1P receptors on heart cells are rapidly desensitized to FTY720, and the bradycardic effect usually passes after the first dose. Studies are now underway to evaluate the safety and efficacy of FTY720.

ORGAN DONORS

The majority of transplanted organs are procured from brain-dead patients. Brain death is determined by two in-hospital examinations, performed 12 hours apart by a neurologist or neurosurgeon, confirming loss of cerebral function (no response to painful stimuli and no movement except for spinal reflexes) and loss of brainstem function (fixed pupils; absence of corneal, oculovestibular, oculocephalic, and gag reflexes; and no respiratory effort

after 3 minutes at a $PaCO_2$ of greater than or equal to 60 mm Hg). Declaration of brain death may be made 6 hours sooner with a nuclear medicine brain scan documenting lack of cerebral blood flow. Because of the potential for conflict of interest, the surgical transplantation team is never involved with the care of the donor or in the determination of brain death.

Patients occasionally have irreversible neurologic injury but do not fulfill the criteria for true brain death. If families decide to withdraw life support, these donors can be used after cessation of circulatory and respiratory function. These donors have a prolonged phase of hypotension followed by cardiac arrest before organ recovery can begin. Historically, only kidneys have been used from non-heart-beating donors, but livers and occasionally other organs (pancreas and heart) are now being used in select cases.

The two main exclusion criteria for cadaveric donors are malignancy and infection. The overall rate of transmission of cancer from a donor to recipient is about 50% and that for melanoma approaches 80%. The organ being transplanted need not be one that is typically a site of metastasis for the primary in order for tumor transmission to occur. Infection with human immunodeficiency virus (HIV) infection excludes patients as donors. Hepatitis virus, cytomegalovirus (CMV), and syphilis serologies are checked, but positive serologies do not preclude organ donation; organs from donors with positive hepatitis serologies are generally allocated only to recipients who are also positive for hepatitis B or C or both. Furthermore, CMV infection and syphilis can be treated, should they occur in the recipient. A history of tuberculosis, active hepatitis B [HBsAg$^+$ (hepatitis virus surface antigen positive)], active herpes simplex virus (HSV) encephalitis, and seropositivity for human T lymphotropic virus (HTLV)-1 or HTLV-2 are also considered exclusion criteria.

BRAIN DEATH PHYSIOLOGY

During the onset of and after brain death, many physiologic aberrations occur, manifesting mainly as hypotension and coagulopathy. As brainstem ischemia progresses, a flood of endogenous catecholamines is released in an attempt to maintain cerebral circulation. Although the blood pressure is high, the resultant vasoconstriction actually impairs circulation to the abdominal organs. Increased left-sided heart pressures can result in pulmonary edema or even alveolar hemorrhage. With the onset of brain death, neurogenic vasodilation and hypotension ensue, further compromising end-organ perfusion. Cardiac function is additionally depressed by low thyroid hormone and cortisol levels in brain death and hypothermia, owing to loss of temperature-regulating centers in the hypothalamus. The development of diabetes insipidus secondary to lack of vasopressin leads to inappropriate water diuresis, which can result in hypernatremia and hypovolemia, further compounding hypotension. Hypovolemia frequently preexists in these patients who may have experienced traumatic hemorrhage or undergone therapeutic dehydration for the control of cerebral edema. Exogenous supplementation of vasoconstrictors, vasopressin, thyroid hormone, and methylprednisolone is frequently used to maintain hemodynamic stability in brain-dead donors. Coagulopathy occurs as a result of the release of large amounts of tissue thromboplastin and plasminogen from ischemic and necrotic brain tissue. Hypothermia also contributes to coagulopathy.

DONOR OPERATION

The abdomen and thorax are entered through a midline incision, extending from the suprasternal notch to the pubis. A sternotomy is performed and the pericardium opened. The chest and abdomen are explored to rule out neoplasia or infection, and the organs are visually inspected for quality. In the thorax, the superior vena cava and aorta are dissected out to allow occlusion of the inflow and outflow tracts. In the abdomen, a right medial visceral rotation is performed, exposing the aorta, inferior vena cava (IVC), and inferior mesenteric vein (IMV). The left triangular ligament of the liver and the gastrohepatic ligament are divided and the supraceliac aorta is prepared for cross-clamping. Heparin is given systemically. Cannulas are placed in the distal abdominal aorta, IMV, and the ascending aorta. The heart is cooled with a potassium-rich cardioplegia solution through the ascending aortic cannula, and cold preservative solution is infused through the distal aortic and IMV cannulas. Ice is packed around the abdominal organs and blood is vented through the IVC into the chest.

Blanching of the heart occurs within a few seconds and the heart is removed first. After inflation of the lungs, the endotracheal tube is removed, and the trachea is stapled in preparation for removal of the lungs. The liver is removed with a diaphragmatic patch around the suprahepatic IVC, and the infrahepatic IVC is divided just above the renal veins. The gastroduodenal artery is divided, the portal vein is divided near the junction of the superior mesenteric vein (SMV) and splenic veins, and the common bile duct is divided near the duodenum. The hepatic artery is traced back to the origin of the celiac axis, where it is removed with a segment of aorta. The pancreas is removed with the duodenum and a short segment of proximal jejunum, the spleen, and a Carrel patch around the superior mesenteric artery. The intestines can be kept in continuity with the liver if they are being used in a composite liver–intestine graft. The ureters are divided at the pelvic brim with their surrounding periureteral tissue. The kidneys can then be removed *en bloc* with the aorta and the IVC kept in continuity or separated. The iliac arteries and veins are taken in the event vascular reconstruction of either the pancreatic or liver vessels is required for successful implantation.

ORGAN PRESERVATION

In order to slow metabolic activity, hypothermia is induced by flushing the organs with 4° C preservation solution and storing the organs on ice. Nevertheless, metabolism continues, and the build-up of lactate, free fatty acids, and nucleotide breakdown products is accompanied by the depletion of glycogen, glutathione, and other reducing agents, making the organ sensitive to reperfusion injury. Cell swelling and loss of intracellular potassium occurs as

TABLE 2-3

PRESERVATION SOLUTIONS

Solution	Component	Concentration
EuroCollins solution (pH 7.4)	KH_2PO_4	15 mmol/L
	K_2HPO_4	42 mmol/L
	KCl	15 mmol/L
	$NaHCO_3$	10 mmol/L
	Glucose	195 mmol/L
UW solution	Lactobionic acid	100 mmol/L
	KOH	20 ml (5M)
(pH 7.4, Na 25, K 100, mOsm 300)	NaOH	5 ml (5M)
	Adenosine	5 mmol/L
	Allopurinol	3 mmol/L
	KH_2PO_4	25 mmol/L
	$MgSO_4$	5 mmol/L
	Glutathione	3 mmol/L
	Raffinose	30 mmol/L
	Hydroxyethyl starch	5 g%
	Insulin	40 U/L
	Dexamethasone	9 mg/L
	Bactrim	2 ml/L

the membrane ion pumps slow down. Loss of membrane gradients releases calcium into the cytosol, thereby activating phospholipases and proteases that degrade proteins and membrane components. University of Wisconsin preservation fluid (UW solution), currently the most commonly used preservation solution, is formulated to counteract these effects (Table 2-3). The cationic composition (high K^+, low Na^+) resembles the intracellular composition to minimize diffusion down electrochemical gradients. Lactobionate is impermeable and acts as an osmotic agent to suppress hypothermia-induced cell swelling. It also chelates calcium, thereby suppressing the activity of calcium-dependent enzymes such as phospholipases and proteases that would otherwise autodigest the cell. By chelating iron, lactobionate may help suppress oxidative damage during reperfusion. Phosphate buffers are included to counteract the accumulated acids, and together with adenosine and dextrose, represent an effort to provide an energy source for the cells.

Each organ can tolerate a different duration of cold ischemia (Table 2-4). Kidneys can be placed on a pump and perfused by machine. Although machine perfusion

TABLE 2-4

COLD STORAGE TIME (HOURS) FOR SOLID ORGANS

Organ	Maximum Ischemic Time	Clinical Practice
Kidney	72	24–30
Kidney on pump	120–168	30
Liver	48	12–20
Pancreas	72	10–20
Heart	4	4
Lung	4	4

leads to a less than 10% delayed graft function (DGF) of kidneys and simple cold storage results in up to 35%, there is no evidence that the savings in temporary dialysis costs would cover the cost of machine perfusion and so the latter is not used routinely.

POSTTRANSPLANTATION COMPLICATIONS

Infections

As a consequence of their dependency on pharmacologic immunosuppression, transplant recipients are at increased risk for the development of a multitude of infections. The potential development of any particular infection is influenced by the time-interval posttransplantation. During the first month following transplantation, patients are at increased risk for bacterial infections in the wound, urinary tract, and lung. Perioperative antibiotics help limit the incidence of wound infection, and every effort should be made to remove Foley catheters as soon as possible. Low grade fevers and elevated white blood cell counts, even in the absence of symptoms, deserve a full culture workup. In the subsequent first 6 months following transplantation, patients are at increased risk of opportunistic infections and viral infections such as those caused by *Pneumocystis carinii*, *Candida* species, and CMV. Infections caused by CMV in immunocompetent individuals frequently pass unnoticed or cause mild flu-like symptoms, but in immunosuppressed individuals, CMV can plague a myriad of organ systems and present as esophagitis, gastrointestinal bleeding and ulceration, colitis, hepatitis, leukopenia, pneumonia, renal insufficiency, and CNS changes, including coma. Patients are frequently placed on Bactrim, nystatin, and acyclovir or ganciclovir as prophylaxis against these infections during the early months following transplantation. Bactrim also helps to prevent urinary tract infections.

Malignancy

The increased risk of neoplasia in transplantation patients has been attributed to suppression of immunologic surveillance mechanisms that would normally destroy malignant cells that express mutant proteins (especially in cancers that are associated with viral pathogenesis) and to the direct carcinogenic effect of immunosuppressive agents. The risk of developing malignancy in transplantation patients is several times greater when compared to healthy age-matched populations. Most common among transplantation patients are cervical cancer [associated with various subtypes human papilloma virus (HPV) infection], carcinoma of the vulva and perineum (HSV), squamous cell carcinomas of the skin and lip (HPV), Kaposi sarcoma [Epstein-Barr virus (EBV)], and lymphomas (HTLV-1), rather than the lung and colon cancers that are most prevalent in the general population. Renal cancers, hepatobiliary carcinomas, and various sarcomas are also more prevalent among transplantation patients.

Most commonly, PTLD represents a spectrum of EBV-related proliferation ranging from polyclonal B-cell hyperplasia to monoclonal B-cell lymphomas. All levels of clonality and histology can be found at different sites in the same patient. The incidence of PTLD—1% to 2% in renal transplants, 2% to 5% in liver and heart, 10% in heart-lung recipients—is related to the intensity of immunosuppression associated with each organ rather than the organ itself. Antilymphocyte antibody therapy in particular is associated with increased risk for development of PTLD. Although the epithelial cells of the upper respiratory tract are the initial site of EBV infection, B lymphocytes become secondarily infected as they travel through the lymphoid tissues of the oropharynx. Proteins expressed from the viral genome inactivate cellular transcription inhibitors that normally promote terminal differentiation and apoptosis and prevent proliferation. Nuclear factor kappa B (NFκB activity is upregulated, leading to the production of inflammatory cytokines, further promoting uncontrolled proliferation. Activation of recombination activation genes (RAGs) promotes chromosomal rearrangements leading to chromosomal instability, increasing the likelihood of malignant transformation. More than 90% of adults in the general population are seropositive for EBV and harbor latently infected B lymphocytes.

As observed with CMV infection, PTLD can present in a variety of manners: as unexplained fevers without other symptoms; as a mononucleosis-like syndrome or hepatitis; as bleeding mesenteric masses or intestinal obstruction; or with CNS symptoms such as seizures, altered mental status, or focal neurologic dysfunction as a consequence of neurologic tumor burden. The absence of adenopathy on radiologic imaging does not rule out PTLD, as the disease can be entirely extranodal. The highest risk for PTLD is during the first year after transplantation and in children. The diagnosis is made by tissue biopsy.

The mainstay of treatment for PTLD is to decrease the level of immunosuppression. Up to 86% of patients have regression of PTLD with reduction of immunosuppression alone, but this is not effective if PTLD has progressed to a true monoclonal B-cell lymphoma. Acyclovir, ganciclovir, and foscarnet have also been used as prophylaxis or in early PTLD, but reports of their success are anecdotal; tumor cells are latently infected and do not express thymidine kinase, so there is no reason to expect PTLD to respond to antiviral agents. Traditional CHOP chemotherapy (cyclophosphamide, doxorubicin, vincristine, prednisolone), similar to that used in the treatment of non-Hodgkin lymphoma, has been used to treat PTLD, and there have been promising results with the anti-B-cell monoclonal antibody rituximab. Occasionally patients will undergo surgical reduction or radiation for debulking of massive local disease.

Posttransplantation T-cell lymphomas are usually related to HTLV-1, not EBV, and tend to develop much later (more than 5 years after transplantation).

RENAL TRANSPLANTATION

Renal transplantation is preferable to long-term dialysis, despite the attendant immunosuppression, because it offers recipients more independence, improves their quality of life, is associated with better survival rates, and transplantation care costs half as much as dialysis. The majority of kidney transplants are performed in patients with insulin-dependent diabetes mellitus, glomerulonephritis, and hypertensive nephrosclerosis. Other causes of renal failure leading to transplantation include polycystic kidney disease, systemic lupus erythematosus, Alport disease, IgA nephropathy, obstructive nephropathy, recurrent pyelonephritis, nephrosclerosis, and interstitial nephritis. A recently growing indication for renal transplantation is chronic calcineurin inhibitor–induced nephrotoxicity following transplantation of other organs. Recent data suggest that end-stage renal disease (ESRD) accumulates in nonrenal transplant patients at a rate of 1% to 1.5% per year, and the development of ESRD is associated with increased mortality. During evaluation of the potential kidney transplant recipient, screening for occult infections at hemodialysis and peritoneal dialysis sites should complement the usual investigation for underlying malignancy or infectious processes that may complicate transplantation. Furthermore, particular care should be taken to evaluate the severity of vascular disease in the coronary, cerebral, and peripheral vessels, given the frequent association of systemic vasculopathy with many of the disease processes that contribute to the development of ESRD.

Although the usual exclusion criteria for active infection and malignancy also apply to cadaveric kidney donors, "expanded criteria donors" who are older than 65 years of age or for whom there is a history of hypertension or diabetes may be utilized under certain circumstances. These donors routinely undergo renal biopsy to look for evidence of histologic damage to the glomeruli, even if their serum markers of kidney function are acceptable. Living donors are generally 18 to 55 years of age and have no other medical problems. The presence of two normal kidneys is confirmed by measuring serum chemistries and creatinine clearance, performing a urinalysis, and by imaging the kidney parenchyma, collecting systems, and vasculature, usually by a combined magnetic resonance imaging/magnetic resonance angiography (MRI/MRA) or computed tomographic (CT) angiography.

Transplantation outcomes with kidneys from living donors are better than those from cadaveric donors. This is because of several factors including the fact that living-donor kidneys are in better condition, the time of transplantation may be optimized for the recipient, and the recipient and donor may be better matched for HLA haplotype. Furthermore, living-donor kidneys are less likely to have delayed graft function or acute tubular necrosis because cold ischemia time is kept to a minimum. In addition, cadaveric kidneys may have sustained multiple physiologic insults while still in the donor because of the previously mentioned derangements that occur during brain death. In terms of timing of transplantation for the recipient, waiting times for a cadaveric kidney depend on blood type and average 3 to 5 years after listing (for which a glomerular filtration rate (GFR) of less than 20 mL per min is required). It has been shown that a longer waiting period translates into an increased risk of death, even after transplantation. It is often possible to avoid dialysis altogether, only with a living-donor transplant. Although patients are fully evaluated and medically optimized for surgery at the time of evaluation, it is difficult to maintain this status during the long waiting period. Finally, the potential for improved HLA matching contributes to a longer half-life for living-donor kidneys, although totally mismatched living-donor grafts still fare better than cadaveric grafts.

The open *living donor nephrectomy* is performed through an oblique flank incision. In living donors, a longer renal vein and easier access to the renal artery make the left kidney the graft of choice. Exceptions to this strategy are donors who have multiple left renal arteries as demonstrated by preoperative imaging. Gonadal and adrenal veins are ligated if necessary. The ureter is divided first, in proximity to the bladder, and the distal stump is ligated. The renal artery is divided as close as possible to its origin from the aorta and then the renal vein is divided near its junction with the vena cava. Blood is flushed from the kidney by instilling cold heparinized preservative solution into the artery, and the kidney is immersed in icy slush during the interval before transplantation. Living-donor nephrectomies are also performed laparoscopically, with or without hand assistance. Although operating room costs are greater for laparoscopic donor nephrectomies, this higher cost is compensated for by quicker return to work and to activities of daily living, shorter hospital stays, and improved quality of life.

The kidney recipient operation is performed through an extraperitoneal approach via an oblique incision in the left or right lower quadrant (Fig. 2-5). The lymphatics overlying the iliac vessels should be ligated to avoid lymphocele formation posttransplantation. Most commonly, the donor renal artery is anastomosed end-to-side to the external iliac artery. The renal vein is anastomosed end-to-side to the external iliac vein. The donor ureter is usually attached to the recipient bladder (ureteroneocystostomy), but urinary tract continuity can also be established by anastomosing recipient ureter to donor renal pelvis (ureteropyelostomy) if there are problems with either the donor's ureter or the recipient's bladder. Before unclamping the vessels, most surgeons administer mannitol and furosemide to promote diuresis.

Acute tubular necrosis (ATN), or *delayed graft function* (DGF), occurs in up to 30% of cadaveric transplants. This is usually caused by the ischemic insult and resulting reperfusion injury and occurs much more rarely in living-donor transplants. This condition is generally self-limiting, but it is important to distinguish it from other causes of low urine output such as rejection or technical complications that require intervention. A radioisotope renal perfusion scan demonstrating adequate blood flow, no ureteral obstruction, and delayed cortical transit time is reassuring with regard to technical complications. However, if serial scans show worsening of function or fail to show improvement, biopsy should be performed to exclude rejection. *Vascular thrombosis*, usually presenting with sudden anuria, can be the result of hypercoagulability, diseased or dissected arteries, or kinking, and requires emergent reexploration to salvage the graft. *Occlusion of the transplant renal vein* can usually be treated by anticoagulation but may occasionally require operative thrombectomy. *Urine leaks* can present as fluid collections or persistently elevated creatinine owing to reabsorption of urine. These can develop secondary to ischemia of the distal ureter and can usually be treated with stenting and percutaneous drainage. Mild ischemia can lead to late strictures in the ureter and may require surgical reconstruction if dilatation and stenting fail. *Renal transplant artery stenosis* (RTAS) usually occurs between 3 months and 2 years after transplantation. This condition presents

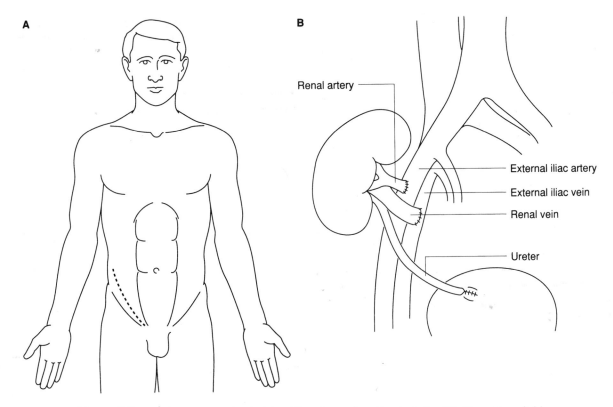

Figure 2-5 Renal transplantation incision **(A)** and completed implantation **(B)**. (From Greenfield LJ. *Surgery: scientific principles and practice*, 1st ed. Philadelphia: JB Lippincott, 1993:517, with permission.)

with hypertension and decreased renal function and can be caused by either technical or immunologic factors. Percutaneous transluminal angioplasty is usually successful in treating RTAS.

A relatively rare complication of renal transplantation is *tertiary hyperparathyroidism*. Chronic renal failure is associated with low vitamin D activity, calcium wasting, and phosphorous retention. Low levels of serum calcium and elevated levels of serum phosphorus lead to increased activity in the parathyroid gland, or secondary hyperparathyroidism. Tertiary hyperparathyroidism occurs when parathyroid hyperfunction continues after renal transplantation and is associated not with hypocalcemia, but with hypercalcemia. Clinical manifestations include bone pain, renal calculi, abdominal pain, pancreatitis, gastrointestinal tract ulcers, and mental status changes. The treatment for tertiary hyperparathyroidism is subtotal parathyroidectomy or total parathyroidectomy and autotransplantation of small portions of one parathyroid gland into the patient's forearm.

Rejection of the graft remains the most frequent cause of early graft failure. Hyperacute rejection is rare because of prospective crossmatching, but if it occurs it becomes evident shortly after revascularization. Alloreactive antibodies fix and activate complement, making the endothelium prothrombotic. Deposition of fibrin thrombi and platelet aggregates cause rapid compromise of perfusion, bluish discoloration of the graft, and cessation of graft function. This devastating complication necessitates removal of the graft. *Acute cellular rejection* is the most common form of

rejection and typically occurs within 3 months of transplantation. Patients may present with fever, graft tenderness, malaise, oliguria, or elevation in serum creatinine level. A renal biopsy, usually obtained percutaneously, is the gold standard for diagnoses of acute graft rejection. If acute rejection is diagnosed, prompt treatment with intravenous high-dose steroids or antilymphocyte preparations is initiated. *Chronic rejection* causes a gradual decline of renal function over years and is an important contributor to late graft loss. Clinical signs include proteinuria and microscopic hematuria, which are usually accompanied by a progressive rise in serum creatinine. The diagnosis of chronic rejection is made by renal biopsy, which shows thickening of the glomerular basement membranes, interstitial fibrosis, and proliferation of arterial smooth muscle cells. There is no current treatment for chronic rejection except the discontinuation of nephrotoxic medications, including converting patients from immunosuppressants such as cyclosporine and tacrolimus to less nephrotoxic agents such as sirolimus.

One-year graft survival for HLA-identical living-related kidney transplants exceeds 95%, 5-year graft survival is 90%, and 10-year graft survival is 65%. One-year graft survival of 1-haplotype matched living-related kidneys is greater than 90%. For cadaveric renal transplants, 1-year graft survival rates are approximately 88% and 5-year graft survival is approximately 66%. Among cadaveric renal grafts, six antigen-matched grafts have a superior 1-year (93%) and 5-year (77%) graft survival; these data provided the impetus for national sharing of such organs.

LIVER TRANSPLANTATION

Indications for liver transplantation include decompensated cirrhosis or intractable portal hypertension resulting from a variety of diseases: fulminant liver failure, genetic defects resulting in failure to produce an essential liver protein, a select population of nonresectable tumors isolated to the liver, and recurrent cholangitis not amenable to conventional surgical treatment. Causes of cirrhosis and portal hypertension include alcoholic liver disease, chronic hepatitis B or C, Wilson Disease, hemochromatosis, rare forms of α_1-antitrypsin deficiency and amyloidosis, Budd-Chiari syndrome, nonalcoholic steatotic hepatitis, congenital hepatic fibrosis, primary sclerosing cholangitis, and primary biliary cirrhosis. Fulminant liver failure can be caused by viral hepatitis (Hep A > Hep B > Hep C), autoimmune hepatitis, drug toxicity (especially acetaminophen), or ingestion of Amanita mushrooms. Liver transplantation for acute liver failure is associated with a higher acute mortality than that for chronic liver disease, although the long-term survival may be superior. Hepatocellular carcinoma (HCC) can be unresectable for anatomic reasons, but, more frequently, resection cannot be undertaken because of insufficient hepatic reserve in a patient with underlying chronic liver disease (i.e., cirrhosis). Patients with early HCC (stages I and II) presenting as a single lesion less than 5 cm in diameter or less than or equal to three lesions, each less than 3 cm in diameter; no macrovascular invasion, and no extrahepatic spread may benefit from liver transplantation and experience long-term survival on par with other indications for transplantation. The treatment of HCC by either transplantation or resection is discussed further in Chapter 15, "The Hepatobiliary System."

Allocation of organs for chronic liver failure is based on the model for end-stage liver disease (MELD), which stratifies patients according to risk of mortality within 3 months. A MELD score is assigned on the basis of a patient's international normalized ratio (INR), and total bilirubin and creatinine levels (Table 2-5). In pediatric patients, the pediatric model for end-stage liver disease (PELD) includes albumin rather than creatinine level, and points are given for children younger than age 1 year and children with growth retardation. "Exception" points are also awarded for nonresectable HCC, recurrent cholangitis, or inborn errors of metabolism. Status 1 designation pertains only to patients with fulminant hepatic failure and to those with primary graft nonfunction or early hepatic artery thrombosis following transplantation. Although donor–recipient pairs are

---

TABLE 2-5

MELD AND PELD CALCULATIONS

MELD = $9.57 \times \log e$ (creatinine) + $3.78 \times \log e \times$ (bilirubin) + $11.2 \times \log e$ (INR) + 6.43

PELD = $4.8 \times \log e$ (bilirubin) + $18.57 \times \log e$ (INR) − 6.87 $\times \log e$ (albumin) + 4.36 (if patients <1 year of age) + 6.67 (if patient has height or weight ≤2 standard deviations below average for age).

Calculated score is rounded to the nearest whole number.

INR, international normalized ratio.

---

usually chosen with ABO blood group compatibility in mind, HLA matching and prospective cross-matching are not performed, as discussed previously.

Uncontrolled infection or cardiovascular instability is the most frequent cause for failure to qualify for liver transplant. Hepatorenal and hepatopulmonary syndrome are not contraindications to liver transplantation, although evaluation by a nephrologist or pulmonologist may determine that the patient's renal or lung dysfunction will not reverse with liver replacement and that the patient therefore needs simultaneous kidney or lung transplantation. Evidence of severe brain edema in fulminant hepatic failure suggests irreversible brain damage and is considered a contraindication to transplantation.

The shortage of donor organs, particularly for pediatric patients, has led to the development of alternatives to the standard orthotopic liver transplantation procedure. The combination of the liver's regenerative capacity and its internal architecture, which provides vascular pedicles that supply hepatic segments individually, makes partial liver transplantation possible. Therefore, two recipients can benefit from one donor and the reduced-size livers can fit into the abdominal cavity of a child.

Another approach to increase the donor pool is *living-related liver transplantation*. Potential advantages of living-related liver transplantation are similar to those of living-related renal transplantation: shortened waiting times, shorter cold ischemic times, improved histocompatibility, and use of an organ from a physiologically normal donor. Because a graft-to-body weight ratio of greater than 1% is generally required for adequate synthetic function, right lobe grafts are usually used for adult recipients, whereas a left lateral segment may be sufficient for pediatric recipients. Of note, the left lobe of a right lobe donor reaches 90% of starting volume by 2 to 4 weeks, whereas the transplanted right lobe has reached standard liver volume by the end of 1 month. Living-donor lobectomies and segmentectomies differ from those done for cancer, in that parenchymal dissection must be completed before interrupting any blood flow in order to limit warm ischemia time. Criteria for living donors of liver transplants are even stricter than those for kidney donation owing to the increased complexity and potential morbidity associated with the procedure. Candidates are healthy, nonobese adults between the ages of 21 and 50 years who have normal serum markers of liver function and a normal liver biopsy results. They must not have a history of hepatotoxic behavior (such as alcoholism).

The *liver transplant recipient operation* (Fig. 2-6) is performed through a bilateral subcostal incision with a midline extension. Bleeding may occur because of portal hypertension and coagulopathy, and this is limited by using electrocautery for the majority of the dissection and by using the argon beam coagulator as needed. The right and left branches of the hepatic artery, the common bile duct (CBD), and the cystic duct are divided at the hilum and trimmed back during implantation. Clamps are placed on the portal vein and suprahepatic vena cava/hepatic veins, and veno-venous bypass may be used to improve blood return and limit mesenteric venous congestion during the anhepatic phase of the procedure, depending on surgeon preference. The suprahepatic IVC anastomosis can be done end-to-end followed by an end-to-end anastomosis at the

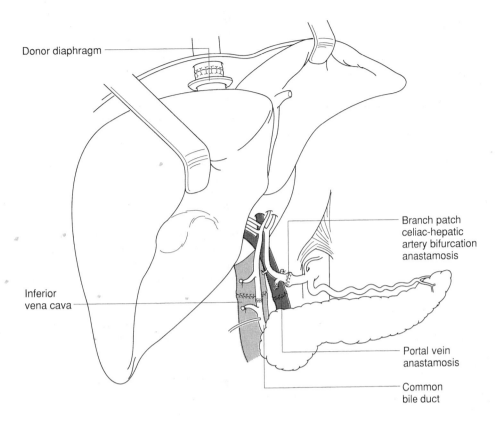

Figure 2-6 Completed liver transplantation. (From Greenfield LJ. *Surgery: scientific principles and practice*, 1st ed. Philadelphia: JB Lippincott, 1993:534, with permission.)

infrahepatic IVC. Alternatively, the recipient hepatectomy can be performed leaving the IVC in place, and an end-to-side anastomosis done to the combined orifices of the recipient's hepatic veins ("piggy-backing") followed by ligation of the donor infrahepatic IVC. The preservative fluid is flushed form the liver by infusing lactated Ringer solution through the portal vein. The portal vein is anastomosed end-to-end, and then the liver is reperfused. Hypotension, cardiac dysrhythmias, and, occasionally, cardiac arrest may occur because of the bolus of cold, hyperkalemic, and acidotic blood-solution mixture traveling from the donor liver to the heart. The arterial anastomosis is usually done with a *Carrel patch* of the aorta around the celiac trunk of the donor to a branch-patch of the recipient hepatic artery. Biliary reconstruction can be performed as an end-to-end anastomosis of donor and recipient CBD or as a Roux-en-Y choledochojejunostomy between donor common bile duct and a defunctionalized limb of recipient jejunum.

Technical complications include intraabdominal bleeding, hepatic artery thrombosis, and biliary leak. Although *postoperative bleeding* is occasionally a result of surgical bleeding from a large varix or one of the vascular anastomoses, it is more common that no site of bleeding is found upon reexploration of the patient. Postoperative coagulopathy and thrombocytopenia result in diffuse oozing from the extensive dissection planes; the intraabdominal clot and blood then promotes fibrinolysis, causing persistent oozing even if the INR and platelet count are corrected. Patients with persistent blood transfusion requirement require re-operation for evacuation of hematoma to interrupt the fibrinolytic cycle, even if there is no source of

surgical bleeding to repair. *Hepatic artery thrombosis* is a particular problem in pediatric patients because of the diminutive size of the vessels involved, but it may occur occasionally in adults as well. Because the vascular supply of the bile duct, particularly the donor CBD, arises from the hepatic artery, these patients may present with a biliary leak or even necrosis and complete dehiscence of the common bile duct accompanied by deteriorating liver function. This complication requires retransplantation. *Biliary leaks* that are the result of overzealous skeletonization of the donor duct or technical errors in the placement of stitches sometimes respond to conservative management if the leaks are adequately drained. Signs of peritonitis, infection, worsening bile leak, and rising serum bilirubin require surgical revision. These patients are at increased risk of developing late strictures because of scar tissue around the duct.

Graft failure from nontechnical causes include primary nonfunction, delayed nonfunction, and early rejection. *Primary nonfunction* occurs in 2% to 5% of liver transplantations and has been attributed to ischemia/re-perfusion injury, steatosis, poor nutritional status of the donor, and an undefined humoral immune response. Clinically, the patient develops a picture of fulminant hepatic failure upon leaving the operating room. Retransplantation is generally required within a few days. If retransplantation can be accomplished within the first week, the results are equivalent to that of a primary transplantation. *Delayed nonfunction* presents after several days of improving graft function, frequently following some minor physiologic insult such as a subclinical infection or relative hypotension from hypovolemia. It is characterized by progressive hyperbilirubinemia and failure to completely correct coagulopathy. It is thought to be caused by a marginal graft that functions well in a stable host, but does not have enough reserve during the early recovery period to withstand any stress. These patients also require retransplantation.

In addition to the infections common to all patients who undergo transplantation, clinicians should understand the infections unique to the liver transplantation population. *Posttransplant cholangitis*, which can present as rising bilirubin and alkaline phosphatase levels with or without fevers and frequently without right upper quadrant (RUQ) pain, can occur even in the absence of biliary obstruction. *Late hepatic artery thrombosis* can present with areas of necrosis in the liver that become superinfected and can present with fever resulting from liver abscesses.

Hepatic allograft rejection remains a major cause of morbidity after liver transplantation. Hyperacute rejection occurs very rarely in hepatic transplantation. Acute rejection occurs most commonly during the first 7 days to 6 months after transplantation. Fever, graft tenderness, leukocytosis, and elevations in serum bilirubin and hepatic enzymes suggest acute rejection, but the gold standard for diagnosing acute hepatic rejection is a liver biopsy. These specimens can be obtained percutaneously, or through the internal jugular vein in patients with ascites or coagulopathy who may be at increased risk for complications following percutaneous transabdominal biopsy. Histologic findings of acute rejection include periportal inflammatory infiltrates, destructive cholangitis or endotheliitis, and minor inflammatory changes in hepatic lobules. Acute rejection is treated with steroids or antilymphocyte therapy with OKT3. *Chronic rejection* has also been referred to as ductopenic rejection or the "vanishing bile duct syndrome." Patients usually experience an asymptomatic rise in alkaline phosphatase and γ-glutamyl transpeptidase and eventually develop jaundice and pruritus. Severe cases of chronic rejection need to be treated with retransplantation.

The current 1-year survival rate after liver transplantation is greater than 85% at most institutions; 10-year survival is 61%. Survival rates are dependent on the indication for the procedure; the best results are obtained in patients who undergo hepatic transplantation for cholestatic liver disease, and the worst results are reported for patients who have hepatitis B, hepatitis C, and advanced malignancy. These patients often experience recurrence of disease and are often not considered candidates for retransplantation. Outcomes are also worse in patients who are older or who have had multiorgan system failure (especially ventilator and dialysis dependence) prior to transplantation.

WHOLE PANCREAS TRANSPLANTATION

For patients with insulin-dependent diabetes, the concept of achieving normoglycemia and avoidance of microvascular complications without the use of insulin seems attractive; however, the risk of the procedure and subsequent immunosuppression are often significant and no conclusive evidence exists to indicate that the procedure is lifesaving. As a result, pancreas transplantation is usually limited to patients with diabetic nephropathy who require immunosuppression to maintain a kidney transplant or to those with labile diabetes

with repeated episodes of life-threatening hypoglycemia, for whom endogenous glucose control could be lifesaving.

Contraindications to pancreas donation include a history of type I or type II diabetes mellitus, history of pancreatic trauma, history of prior pancreatic surgery, and pancreatitis, severe atherosclerosis, and intraabdominal contamination. Although segmental pancreas grafts are being performed, most centers transplant whole pancreaticoduodenal grafts.

The pancreas graft is transplanted ectopically to the iliac fossa with the arterial blood supply coming from the recipient iliac artery (Fig. 2-7). Venous drainage is established by anastomosing the donor portal vein to the recipient iliac vein (systemic drainage) or to the superior mesenteric vein (portal drainage). Exocrine drainage is generally managed through enteric or bladder drainage via the duodenal segment. Advantages of bladder drainage include the ability to diagnose rejection by urinary amylase levels, cystoscopic access for transduodenal needle biopsies, lower rates of infection, and relative technical ease. The main disadvantages are hematuria and cystitis/urethritis secondary to biochemical irritation from the pancreatic exocrine drainage, as well as metabolic acidosis resulting from loss of bicarbonate in the urine.

Glucose levels are followed closely postoperatively, and patients are maintained initially on insulin infusions to keep serum glucose levels lower than 200 mg per dL, if the graft does not produce sufficient insulin initially. Particular attention needs to be paid to fluid balance as well as bicarbonate and electrolyte losses in the initial postoperative period. Serum amylase and lipase are frequently elevated initially as a result of ischemia-reperfusion pancreatitis but should rapidly decrease.

One-year patient survival exceeds 90%, and 1-year pancreas graft survival, as defined by complete insulin

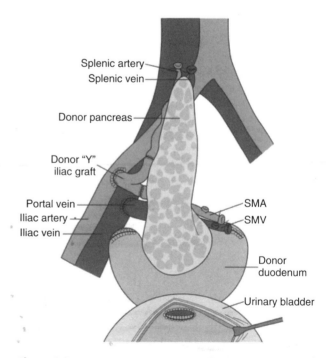

Figure 2-7 Bladder drainage of pancreas via duodenal segment SMA, superior mesenteric artery; SMV, superior mesenteric vein. (From Miller TA. *Modern surgical care*, 2nd ed. St Louis: Quality Medical Publishers, 1998:144, with permission.)

independence, is greater than 70%. One-year pancreas survival for simultaneous pancreas–kidney transplants is higher, at 80% to 83%. Despite the relatively good outcomes associated with pancreas transplantation, clinical vigilance must be maintained to detect and treat potential posttransplantation complications. Because *rejection* is the major etiology for graft loss, early diagnosis and treatment is critical to the outcome of pancreas transplantation. Rejection of the exocrine gland precedes rejection of the endocrine pancreas. Therefore, hyperglycemia indicates advanced rejection and potentially irreversible damage to the graft. Pancreatic graft rejection can be suggested by changes in exocrine and endocrine parameters in the serum (and urine for the bladder-drained pancreas) and is sometimes treated empirically with antilymphocyte antibody therapy if there is high clinical suspicion. In the combined kidney-pancreas recipient, the status of both grafts may be conveniently ascertained by evaluation of the kidney graft alone via serum creatinine level or renal biopsy. Another cause of graft failure is *donor splenic vein thrombosis* progressing into the SMV/portal confluence, preventing venous outflow from the graft. This type of failure, too, can present with pain and elevated serum amylase, lipase, and glucose levels and is best diagnosed by using magnetic resonance venography (MRV). Anticoagulation is sometimes sufficient for nonocclusive thrombi, but percutaneous or surgical thrombectomy is sometimes required.

PANCREATIC ISLET TRANSPLANTATION

Pancreatic islet transplantation is an attractive option for restoring glycemic control as it does not involve major surgery with complex vascular reconstruction and permits a lesser degree of immunosuppression than does whole-organ transplantation. It is currently available as an experimental procedure. In islet transplantation, the pancreas is procured with the same techniques used to procure a pancreas for whole-organ transplantation. The pancreatic duct is then cannulated, and collagenase is infused to digest the stromal tissue so that the exocrine and endocrine components are released. Islets are then separated from exocrine and ductal tissue by density-gradient centrifugation. Typically, patients require two separate infusions of islets from two pancreata to gain insulin independence.

Islets are infused into the liver, either under direct view through a mesenteric vessel via mini laparotomy or percutaneously into the portal vein. In general, steroid-free immunosuppressive protocols are being used to minimize beta-cell toxicity. Complications include bleeding from percutaneous puncture of the liver and partial thrombosis of the portal vein. Some centers report a 1-year graft survival as high as 80%, equivalent to whole-organ results.

SMALL BOWEL TRANSPLANTATION

Candidates for small bowel transplantation are most commonly patients who have short gut syndrome and are dependent on total parenteral nutrition (TPN). Short-gut syndrome can be the result of massive surgical resection secondary to conditions such as embolic or thrombotic events, inflammatory bowel disease, necrotizing enterocolitis,

malrotation, trauma, and certain neoplasms. Rarely, irreversible intestinal failure can be the result of impairments of motility or absorptive capacities. Small bowel transplantation is usually recommended when patients experience loss of access sites for TPN or experience complications of TPN, such as irreversible cholestatic liver failure. In the latter case, a combined small bowel–liver transplant would be performed. There is convincing experimental evidence that liver grafts can act in an immunologically protective fashion and reduce rejection episodes of concomitantly transplanted organs.

Because enterocytes express high levels of class II MHC on their surfaces, small bowel transplants are particularly immunogenic. In addition, small bowel transplant recipients have a propensity to develop graft-versus-host disease (GVHD) owing to the large amount of lymphatic tissue in the gut. The donor and recipient must be ABO blood group compatible and are usually matched for CMV status. Because of the large amount of lymphatic tissue in the small bowel, the graft is considered to harbor a large viral load, and CMV enteritis, in particular, following transplantation is refractory to treatment with antivirals. The abdominal cavity of most recipients is small for total body size because the recipients most often have no intestines, so it is actually preferable for the donor to be slightly smaller than the recipient. Some centers also administer OKT-3 to donors in order to decrease the number of donor lymphocytes transferred with the small bowel. There is no evidence, however, that this is effective in decreasing GVHD.

For isolated small bowel transplants, the entire small bowel and the right colon are removed with vascular pedicles including the superior mesenteric artery (SMA) and origin of the portal vein (PV). The donor SMA can be anastomosed directly to the recipient's SMA or an aortic segment of the donor containing the SMA can be connected to the recipient's infrarenal aorta. The venous drainage via the donor's superior mesenteric vein (SMV) can be performed into the PV or systemically. Portal drainage may be the more physiologic option with first-pass of hepatatrophic substances through the liver. In combined small bowel–liver grafts, the donor PV is anastomosed to the recipient's PV so that the entire gastrointestinal tract drains into the transplanted liver. A donor aortic conduit containing both the celiac artery and the SMA is anastomosed to the recipient's infrarenal aorta. Suprahepatic, infrahepatic, and caval, as well as biliary anastomoses in this procedure are analogous to those employed in liver transplantation. Although the proximal portion of the intestinal graft is anastomosed to the recipient's small bowel, a stoma is created distally to allow access to the graft for mucosal biopsies in the postoperative period (Fig. 2-8).

Acute rejection occurs most often during the first year following transplantation. Fever, increase in stomal output, and gastrointestinal symptoms mandate multiple endoscopic biopsies of the small bowel to rule out rejection. In early rejection, the small bowel mucosa may appear normal, and visual inspection is not sufficient. An unusual infectious complication in small bowel transplants is bacterial translocation associated with rejection. Such episodes are actually controlled by increasing immunosuppression in conjunction with administering broad spectrum antibiotics. The disruption of lymphatic

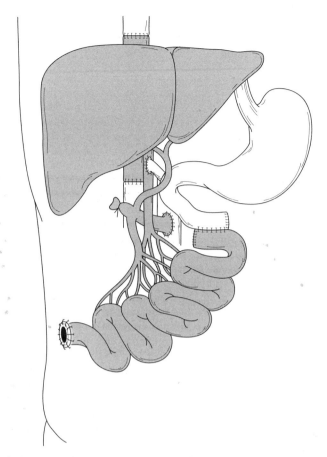

Figure 2-8   Combined small bowel–liver transplant. (From Asfar S, Zhong R, Grant D. *Surgical Clinics of North America.* October 1994. *Horizons in Organ Transplantation.* Philadelphia: WB Saunders, 1203, with permission.)

drainage during the procurement and re-implantation of the small bowel leads to poor absorption of lipids, and small bowel transplant recipients require dietary supplementation with medium chain triglycerides, which are absorbed directly into the portal circulation. Intestinal graft survival is approximately 72% at 1 year, 48% at 3 years, and 41% and 5 years. Patient survival is only marginally better: 75% at 1 year, 55% at 3 years, and 48% at 5 years. Some centers are attempting segmental living-related small bowel transplantation in adults, but the numbers are too small to evaluate whether their outcomes are significantly different.

HEART TRANSPLANTATION

Cardiac transplantation is performed for end-stage heart disease that is refractory to medical management and not amenable to other surgical interventions associated with a life expectancy of less than 1 year without transplantation. One-year survival rates are greater than 80% and 5-year survival rates are much greater than 70%. Improvements in medical management, revascularization techniques, and mechanical ventricular assist devices have decreased the rate of death of patients while on the waiting list. The most common etiologies of heart failure are idiopathic dilated cardiomyopathy and ischemic heart disease. More

unusual etiologies include ventricular dysfunction secondary to valvular or congenital disease, malignant ventricular dysrhythmia, or cardiac allograft vasculopathy. Congenital heart disease is the primary indication for heart transplantation in children. Contraindications to cardiac transplantation include cancer, recent pulmonary embolus, active infection, and fixed pulmonary resistance greater than 6 Wood units that does not respond to vasodilators.

Donors and recipients must be ABO and size (within 20% total body weight) compatible. HLA matching is done only if recipients have a high PRA; sensitization in this population can occur because many have had blood transfusions associated with previous cardiac surgery, including previous transplantation. Contraindications to heart donation include infection, extracranial malignancy, ventricular dysrhythmias (which may occur primarily as a result of the physiologic changes of brain death), and death from carbon monoxide poisoning with a blood carboxyhemoglobin level greater than 20%. Donor management frequently requires a Swan–Ganz catheter to guide hemodynamic monitoring, and donors older than 40 to 45 years of age may get a cardiac catheterization to exclude coronary atherosclerosis. An echocardiogram must show normal anatomy, valvular, and ventricular function.

Most hearts are transplanted orthotopically. The biatrial technique involves four anastomoses: the left and right atrial, the pulmonary artery, and the aorta (Fig. 2-9). The bicaval heart transplantation begins with complete excision of the recipient heart, except for a cuff of left atrial tissue around the ostia of the paired pulmonary veins and small cavoatrial cuffs, and therefore requires

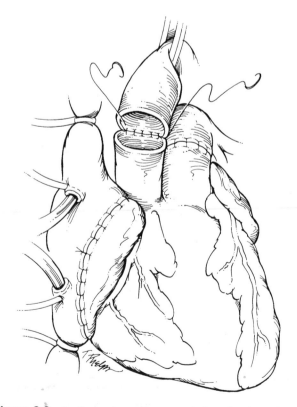

Figure 2-9   Aortic anastomosis at completion of orthotopic cardiac transplantation. (From Kaiser LR, Kron IL, Spray TL. *Mastery of cardiothoracic surgery,* 1st ed. Philadelphia: Lippincott William & Wilkins, 1998:506, with permission.)

five anastomoses. Total orthotopic implantation utilizes pulmonary venous cuffs, necessitating six anastomoses. Proponents of the latter two methods argue that they are associated with improved atrial function, a reduction of atrial dysrhythmias, and improved tricuspid and mitral valve function. However, most surgeons feel that these advantages are marginal and are outweighed by the longer ischemic times and higher risk for anastomotic complications.

Right ventricular dysfunction occurs commonly in the early posttransplantation period, usually as a result of ischemic injury and elevated pulmonary vascular resistance. Inotropic support and pulmonary vasodilators are frequently required during the first 2 to 3 days postoperatively. Loss of vagal innervation to the transplanted heart results in a resting heart rate of about 100 beats per minute and unresponsiveness to digoxin and atropine. Early postoperative bradydysrhythmias are usually the result of donor sinoatrial and atrioventricular dysfunction caused by surgical trauma, ischemic injury, and long bypass time. Most of these bradydysrhythmias respond well to pharmacologic agents such as isoproterenol or to temporary epicardial pacing and resolve spontaneously. Occasionally, permanent pacemakers are required.

Acute rejection is common during the first few months after transplantation, but accounts for less than 10% of early deaths after cardiac transplantation. The most frequent symptom of rejection is fatigue and one of the early signs of rejection is tachydysrhythmia. Endomyocardial biopsy is the gold standard for diagnosing acute rejection, and surveillance biopsies are frequently done during the first year after transplantation. Acute allograft rejection usually responds to steroids. Cytolytic agents are reserved for episodes of severe rejection associated with hemodynamic compromise or episodes resistant to steroids. The major cause of morbidity and mortality after the first year following transplantation is cardiac allograft vasculopathy (CAV). This pathologic process diffusely narrows the epicardial coronary arteries, intramyocardial arterioles, and venous structures. Because reinnervation is incomplete, most cardiac transplantation patients do not experience chest pain, so transplanted cardiac ischemia presents not as angina, but as heart failure or sudden death. Either coronary angiography or intravascular coronary ultrasonography is necessary to diagnose cardiac allograft vasculopathy. Acute rejection ischemia-reperfusion injury, drug toxicity, hyperlipidemia, and hypertension may contribute to the development of CAV. The only definitive treatment for CAV is retransplantation. Infections are responsible for 10% of early deaths and 30% of late deaths. Heart transplant recipients are particularly susceptible to infections with the herpesviruses, namely CMV, EBV, varicella-zoster virus, and HSV types 1, 2, and 6.

LUNG TRANSPLANTATION

Chronic obstructive pulmonary disease (including α_1-antitrypsin deficiency) accounts for 45% of lung transplantations. Other causes of end-stage lung disease treated with transplantation include cystic fibrosis, idiopathic pulmonary fibrosis, primary pulmonary hypertension, Eisenmenger syndrome, sarcoidosis, drug and radiation-induced pulmonary fibrosis, histiocytosis X, bronchiolitis

obliterans–organizing pneumonia, asbestosis, desquamative interstitial pneumonitis, lymphangioleiomyomatosis, eosinophilic granuloma, and collagen-vascular disorders. Septic diseases such as cystic fibrosis and bronchiectasis are treated with double-lung replacement in order to remove septic foci and avoid contamination of the donor allograft by the native lung. Lung and combined heart–lung transplants are performed for end-stage pulmonary parenchymal and vascular disorders. Each disease process has specific guidelines [e.g., values for forced expiratory volume in 1 second (FEV_1), vital capacity, or pulmonary artery pressure] for the timing of referral for transplantation, but the general criteria are failure of other therapies, high risk of death within 2 years, and functional disability without loss of the ability to ambulate. Active cigarette smokers are not considered candidates for lung transplantation. High-dose steroid therapy and ventilator dependence are relative contraindications to transplantation. One-year survival after lung transplantation is 80%, 2-year survival is 70%, and 5-year survival is 50%, the lowest of all solid-organ transplants.

Donor and recipient must be ABO and size compatible. HLA matching is not routinely performed. When accepting donor lungs, it is important to rule out infectious processes and malignancy. In addition, the partial pressure of oxygen (Po_2) at 100% oxygen and 5 cm H_2O of positive end-expiratory pressure (PEEP) should exceed 350 mm Hg. The donor chest x-ray must show clear lung fields, and bronchoscopy is routinely performed. Because the lung graft can maintain a low level of aerobic metabolism by utilizing oxygen that diffuses from the alveoli to endothelial and parenchymal cells, the lungs are removed from the donor by clamping the trachea after a full volume of ventilation, maintaining them in an inflated state. The lung is generally the most fragile organ in brain-dead patients and is the least likely organ to be suitable for transplantation. Shortage of donor organs has expanded the indications for single-lung transplantation and has led to the development of living-related lobar transplantation.

Single-lung transplantations have traditionally been performed through a posterolateral thoracotomy, although there is an increasing trend toward the use of muscle-sparing thoracotomies, anterior thoracotomies, and sternotomies to minimize postoperative discomfort. Usually the lung receiving less blood, as determined by nuclear perfusion scan, is replaced. Double-lung transplantations have traditionally been performed through a clamshell incision (bilateral thoracosternotomy) with division of both internal mammary arteries. However, recently several groups have moved to bilateral anterior thoracotomy without sternal division to minimize wound complications. Cardiopulmonary bypass (CPB) is used routinely for patients with pulmonary vascular disease and in 10% to 20% of the time for bilateral lung transplantations, particularly when the first lung that was implanted does not show immediate function. In single-lung transplantations, CPB is used for poor right ventricular function, hemodynamic instability, hypoxemia, and worsening hypercarbia.

Complications in the early postoperative period usually involve the bronchial anastomosis, generally as a result of ischemia of the donor segment of bronchus. Superficial patches of necrosis usually heal without clinical sequelae, but necrosis at the suture line may lead to disruption of the airway. This may manifest as an air leak, sepsis associated with mediastinal infection, or bronchopulmonary fistula. Complete dehiscence and bronchopulmonary fistula require immediate surgical correction or retransplantation, but partial dehiscence can be treated with gentle mechanical débridement and drainage. Long term, bronchial ischemia leads to airway stenosis, which can often be managed by repeated dilatation and placement of an endobronchial stent. During the first 72 hours posttransplantation, pulmonary edema can develop, ranging from mild, transient hypoxemia to acute severe respiratory distress requiring prolonged mechanical ventilation, inhaled nitric oxide, and even extracorporeal membrane oxygenation. Early acute respiratory distress syndrome (ARDS), also known as primary graft failure, is associated with mortality rates as high as 60%, and emergency retransplantation does not result in an improvement in survival, unlike primary nonfunction following liver transplantation.

Because the lung has direct exposure to airborne pathogens, it is more susceptible to various bacterial, viral, and fungal infections, and lung transplant recipients have a rate of infection several times higher than that of other organ recipients. *Pseudomonas aeruginosa* and other gram-negative organisms are most often isolated, but CMV pneumonitis and invasive aspergillus infection are also of particular concern in lung transplant recipients. Airway infections and acute rejection both present with fevers, leukocytosis, dyspnea, increased secretions, and infiltrates or pleural effusions on chest radiographs. Bronchoscopy with transbronchial biopsies and bronchoalveolar lavage for microbiologic cultures are essential to differentiate these conditions. Acute rejection episodes usually respond well to pulse treatment with steroids. Alternative regimens include OKT3 or antithymocyte globulin.

The primary cause of late mortality and morbidity after lung transplantation is bronchiolitis obliterans. More than one third of all lung transplant recipients develop this fibroproliferative process of the small airways, leading to luminal obstruction and airflow limitation. Clinically, patients present with a sudden and persistent drop FEV_1. Acute rejection is the most important risk factor in the development of bronchiolitis obliterans. Infectious episodes, particularly resulting from CMV, and ischemia-reperfusion injury also contribute to the development of obliterative bronchiolitis.

KEY CONCEPTS

▲ Interleukin (IL)-1 is produced by macrophages and is the main pyogenic cytokine.

▲ The main complication of calcineurin inhibitor immunosuppression is nephrotoxicity.

▲ Indirect presentation refers to presentation of alloantigens by antigen-presenting cells (APCs) of the recipient; direct presentation refers to presenting of alloantigens by donor APCs.

▲ The first-line treatment for posttransplantation lymphoproliferative disorder (PTLD) is reduction of immunosuppression.

▲ Cross-matching is done by combining donor lymphocytes with recipient serum.

SUGGESTED READINGS

Becker YT, Becker BN, Pirsch JD, et al. Rituximab as treatment for refractory kidney transplant rejection. *Am J Transplant* 2004;4: 996–1001.

Brinkmann V, Cyster JG, Hla T. FTY720: sphingosine 1-phosphate receptor-1 in the control of lymphocyte egress and endothelial barrier function. *Am J Transplant* 2004;4:1019–1025.

Ganne V, Siddiqi N, Kamaplath B, et al. Humanized anti-CD20 monoclonal antibody (rituximab) treatment for post-transplant lymphoproliferative disorder. *Clin Transplant* 2003;17:417–422.

Pace KT, Dyer SJ, Phan V, et al. Laparoscopic vs open donor nephrectomy: a cost-utility analysis. *Surg Endosc* 2003;17:134–142.

Robertson RP. Islet transplantation as a treatment for diabetes—a work in progress. *N Engl J Med* 2004;350:694–705.

Tedesco-silva H, Mourad G, Kahan BD, et al. FTY720, a novel immunomodulator: efficacy and safety results from the first phase 2A study in de novo renal transplantation. *Transplantation* 2004; 77(12):1826–1833.

Yopp AC, Fu S, Honig SM, et al. FTY720-enhanced T Cell homing is dependent on CCR2, CCR5, CCR7, and CXCR4: evidence for distinct chemokine compartments. *J Immunol* 2004;173:855–865.

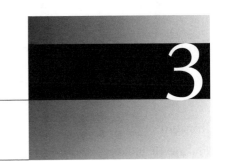

Surgical Infectious Diseases

3

Bradley G. Leshnower   **Thomas G. Gleason**

In 1867, Joseph Lister dramatically changed the practice of surgery after publishing *On the Antiseptic Principle in the Practice of Surgery*. Use of antiseptic techniques immediately impacted morbidity and mortality, reducing postoperative infections from 90% to 10%. Surgical infectious diseases include infections that require surgical intervention and infections that result from surgical intervention. An understanding of host defenses, microbiology, antimicrobial therapies, and proper antiseptic technique is required of all practicing surgeons.

HOST DEFENSE MECHANISMS

Barriers

The body has many natural barriers that serve important roles in preventing infection. The *skin* is the first line of defense against infectious diseases. Skin functions as a mechanical barrier against microbial invasion and provides an unfavorable environment for microbial growth with its acidic pH (5 to 6) and relative lack of water. The skin's constant epithelial cell proliferation allows daily cell turnover and sloughing of both dead cells and resident flora.

Throughout the epithelial surface of the respiratory tract lies a mucous blanket that contains immunoglobulin (Ig) A. The *mucociliary mechanism* captures inhaled particulates within the superficial mucous blanket that rests on the ciliated respiratory epithelium from the larynx to the terminal bronchioles. The mucus is rolled steadily toward the mouth by the motion of the cilia. The regularly beating cilia convey particles and alveolar macrophages embedded in the mucous blanket from the distal airways toward the pharynx, where they are expelled by coughing. This process efficiently clears particles by the mucociliary mechanism every 14 minutes. Secretory IgA, produced by lymphoid tissue throughout the respiratory tract, offers additional protection to the host by preventing bacterial adherence to the respiratory epithelium.

The *acidic pH* of gastric secretions prevents the growth of most bacteria in the stomach keeping it essentially sterile.

The introduction of antacids into the stomach compromises this natural barrier, and the stomach becomes vulnerable to bacterial and fungal colonization or both. Aspiration in the setting of gastric pH neutralization poses an increased risk of developing pneumonia.

The small and large intestines are colonized with abundant bacterial flora, and there is an increasing gradient in the concentration of bacteria proceeding from the small to the large bowel. *Peristalsis* and *a normal motility pattern* keep the bacterial population of the small bowel constant. Bacterial content increases significantly in the colon.

The urinary tract is normally sterile except at the urethral orifice. Urine also contains IgA, which prevents bacterial adherence to the urothelium. The most important natural defense of the bladder in males is the long urethra that is distant from and thus protected from contamination by bacteria present in and around the anus. The incidence of urinary tract infections is increased in women because the urethra is short and in proximity to the fecal stream.

Microbial Flora

Microbes themselves contribute to host defense, particularly in the gastrointestinal tract. The gut, which is sterile *in utero*, is initially exposed to microbes during birth and during the initial feedings. Thereafter, the gastrointestinal tract becomes colonized. The composition of the resident flora changes as the host diet changes. The normal microflora of the gastrointestinal tract add to host defense by occupying potential epithelial binding sites, thereby limiting penetration of pathologic microbials. This is known as *colonization resistance* or *tropism*. The resident microflora also function as a physical mucobacterial barrier, which is constantly maintained by rapid cell turnover, the shedding of enterocytes, mucus production, and bacterial growth. The presence of microflora in the gastrointestinal tract also promotes the development of gut-associated lymphoid tissue.

The distal small intestine and colon harbor the largest concentrations of microorganisms in the gastrointestinal tract. Bacterial anaerobes (*Bacteroides fragilis* and *Fusobacterium* species) outnumber aerobes (*Escherichia coli* and *Enterococcus faecalis*) in the colon by a ratio of 300:1. The total concentration of bacteria in stool is 10^{12} cfug^{-1}, which represents approximately 30% of the dry weight of feces.

Immunology

Phagocytic leukocytes, in concert with the cellular and humoral immune systems, constitute the host's most formidable defense mechanism against infection. Phagocytes in the circulating blood are monocytes and granulocytes (neutrophils, eosinophils, and basophils). Macrophages are differentiated monocytes that reside in all living tissues of the body but are heavily concentrated in the lungs, liver, and spleen. These noncirculating cells are referred to as the reticuloendothelial system. Macrophages, monocytes, and granulocytes initiate the eradication of bacteria and fungi by ingesting these pathogens in a process known as *phagocytosis*. This is the single most important process in the control of infection. Although phagocytes can eliminate microbes independently, they play a more important role in the host's immune response by serving as antigen-presenting cells (APCs) to T lymphocytes. Circulating phagocytes migrate to areas of inflammation by following a gradient of chemoattractant molecules in a highly efficient process known as *chemotaxis*. At the site of inflammation, opsonization facilitates phagocytic recognition of the pathogenic species. *Opsonization* is the process by which opsonins (immunoglobulins and complement) that are bound to the surface of microbes interact with receptors on the phagocyte and promote ingestion. Disorders in opsonization result in a failure to clear the offending microbe and place the host at a high risk for bacterial infection, especially from encapsulated bacteria. Opsonization and subsequent phagocytosis are the host's primary method of eliminating extracellular pathogens.

Microbes that live inside cells (primarily viruses) are cleared by the host's cellular immune system. Cellular immunity consists of an afferent limb, which is responsible for recognizing foreign antigen, and an efferent limb, which destroys the infected cell. Upon induction of an immune response, macrophages process and then present antigen on their cell surfaces in conjunction with major histocompatibility complex (MHC) molecules (see Chapter 2). The antigen–MHC complex binds to T lymphocytes, which express the CD4 molecule and are known as *helper T cells*. Helper T cells interact with the antigen-presenting macrophages and proliferate into a subpopulation of T-cell clones that recognize the specific antigen(s) and amplify the immune response. These cells produce specific lymphokines that promote B-cell differentiation into antibody-generating plasma cells and stimulate the effector arm of the immune response. *Effector cells* consist of monocytes, macrophages, granulocytes, and T cells, which express the CD8 molecule. Cytotoxic CD8 T cells can kill virally infected cells by direct contact. Although the contributions of the cytotoxic T cells are significant, the majority of antigen elimination is handled by the monocytes, macrophages, and

granulocytes. In this manner a small number of sensitized T lymphocytes can respond to a microbial invasion, stimulate a large immune response, and eliminate infection from the host.

Humoral responses to infection are dependent upon immunoglobulins and complement. *Immunoglobulins* are directed primarily against extracellular pathogens. They protect the host from infection by (i) neutralizing viruses and bacterial toxins, (ii) inhibiting microbial attachment to host cells, (iii) opsonizing pathogens for elimination by phagocytes, and (iv) activating the complement cascade. Five classes of immunoglobulins are produced by B-cell-derived plasma cells: IgG, IgA, IgM, IgD, and IgE. IgM, IgG, and IgA are most directly involved in microbial defense. IgM is the first immunoglobulin produced in the initial response to antigen and is a potent activator of complement. IgG is transported across the placenta from mother to fetus and protects the newborn until the fourth month of life. IgG is the predominant immunoglobulin produced and circulated during anamnestic responses. IgA is a monomer in the circulating blood and combines with a secretory component and an amino acid chain (J chain) to form the polymeric secretory IgA (S-IgA). S-IgA acts as a first line of defense against pathogens by preventing bacterial adherence to the mucosal epithelium of the respiratory, gastrointestinal, and genitourinary tracts. IgA deficiency is the most common of the immunoglobulin deficiencies. Patients with IgA deficiency can present with recurrent mucosal infections resulting in bronchitis, allergies, or gastrointestinal malabsorption.

The *complement* system is a nonspecific defense system designed to allow for an immediate response to invading organisms. It is an efficient and self-regulated cascade that requires the binding of only a few molecules of antibody to activate large amounts of complement. The proteins that constitute the complement system are inactive by themselves, but interaction with antigen–antibody complexes or microbial cell surfaces activates these substances and initiates a cascade of reactions that ultimately results in cell lysis. The complement cascade can be activated through two separate pathways, which converge into a common final pathway (Fig. 3-1). The classical pathway is activated by the binding of complement protein C1q to an antigen–antibody complex that initiates a series of reactions resulting in the cleavage of the C3 protein. The alternative pathway can be activated by circulating microbes, polysaccharide molecules, or endotoxin and also results in the cleavage of C3. The activation of C3 amplifies the immune response and facilitates (i) the formation of the membrane attack complex (C5-C9), (ii) opsonization, (iii) further activation of the complement cascade, and (iv) mast cell degranulation. The membrane attack complex disrupts the target cell membrane and causes cell death.

Most microbial elimination is carried out by the phagocytic leukocytes. These effector cells are attracted to the area of inflammation by chemokines released during mast cell degranulation and engulf the opsonized pathogens. Patients with recurrent infections should be screened for complement deficiencies. The most serious is C3 deficiency, which results in recurrent infections with gram-negative and encapsulated organisms.

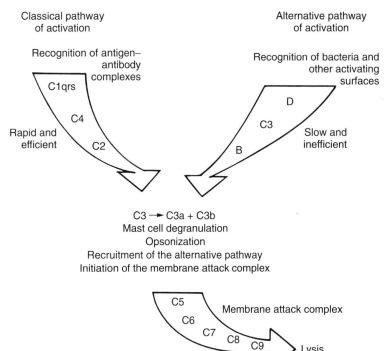

Figure 3-1 Pathways of complement activation. (From Paul W. The immune system: an introduction. In: Paul W, ed. *Fundamental immunology*. New York: Raven Press, 1984:3–22, with permission.)

SURGICAL MICROBIOLOGY AND PATHOGENICITY

Viruses

Viruses are obligate intracellular pathogens composed of a central core of genetic material [deoxyribonucleic acid (DNA) or ribonucleic acid (RNA)] surrounded by a protein coat (the capsid), which protects the nucleic acid and serves as a vehicle of transmission from one cell to another. Some viruses have an outer membrane (the envelope) comprising lipids that are acquired from the host's nuclear membrane. Viruses do not contain any cell machinery and therefore depend entirely upon the host cell to provide the energy and the biosynthetic organelles for viral replication. As the virus replicates, the process continues until the host cell lyses or the virus buds off to infect another cell. Viruses cause disease by cell lysis or by interfering with normal cell machinery to cause cellular dysfunction. One concern during viral infection is the associated risk of bacterial superinfection. This may occur in part because of the impaired phagocytic capacity of virally infected macrophages or polymorphonuclear leukocytes (PMNLs) rendering the host more vulnerable to bacterial infection. Viral infections can cause congenital malformations (TORCH viruses), chromosomal damage (herpes), altered immune function [human immunodeficiency virus (HIV)], and increased cellular proliferation and oncogenesis [human T-cell lymphotropic virus 1 (HTLV-I)]. Viruses have been implicated in surgical diseases such as appendicitis (enterovirus), ulcerative colitis [cytomegalovirus (CMV)], and intussusception (adenovirus). Viral illnesses rarely require surgical intervention. One notable exception is hepatitis B or C virus infection causing cirrhosis and end-stage liver disease, which may ultimately require liver transplantation (see Chapter 15).

Bacteria

Bacteria generate their own energy and contain all of the biosynthetic machinery necessary for self-replication. Their structure includes a single circular molecule of DNA, ribosomes, a cytoplasmic membrane, and a cell wall. Some bacteria carry plasmids, which are autonomously replicating strands of DNA that may carry genes conferring resistance to antibiotics. Bacteria are prokaryotes and have no nuclear membrane. They have three general shapes: rods, spheres, and spirals. Differences in cell-wall structure determine whether bacteria are gram-positive or gram-negative (Fig. 3-2).

The initial step in bacterial pathogenicity is adherence to an epithelial surface. Once attached to the host, bacteria cause disease by invading tissues, producing toxins, or inciting pathologic immune responses. *Streptococcus pneumoniae* is an example of a bacterial species that invades tissue. Other bacteria produce toxins that can be subdivided into two classes: *exotoxins* and *endotoxins*. Protein exotoxins cause hemolysis of red blood cells, white blood cell death, necrosis of tissues, degradation of intercellular substances, and clotting of plasma. Important surgical diseases resulting from bacterial exotoxins include necrotizing fasciitis caused by *Clostridium perfringens* and toxic megacolon caused by *Clostridium difficile*. Endotoxins are macromolecular complexes of phospholipids, polysaccharide, and protein, which form the outer layer of the cell wall of gram-negative bacteria. *Lipopolysaccharide* (LPS or endotoxin) is composed of a "core" polysaccharide region and a unique "O-antigen" polysaccharide region, which are covalently bound to the "lipid A" lipid region (Fig. 3-3). The toxic properties of LPS rest largely with the lipid A moiety of the molecule. LPS induces fever by direct action on the hypothalamus and by stimulating the release of pyrogens like interleukin (IL)-1, IL-6, and tumor necrosis factor

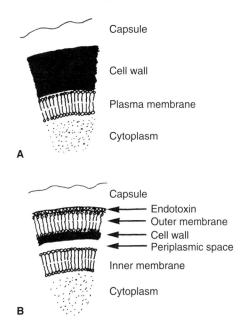

A

B

Figure 3-2   The wall of the gram-positive organism **(A)** contains a much larger cell wall, whereas the gram-negative bacteria **(B)** has both an inner and an outer membrane around the relatively thin cell wall. (From Fry DE. Surgical infections. In: O'Leary JP, ed. *The Physiologic basis of surgery*, 2nd ed. Philadelphia: Williams & Wilkins, 1996:185, with permission.)

(TNF). It can cause septic shock by activating the complement system, thereby causing the release of vasoactive substances such as prostaglandins, collagenases, and serotonin and inducing disseminated intravascular coagulation, platelet aggregation, and thrombocytopenia.

Fungi

Fungi are primitive eukaryotes that contain DNA in their nucleus and organelles capable of biosynthesis and energy generation in their cytoplasm. External to their plasma membrane lies a rigid cell wall that protects the cell from osmotic rupture. Most medically important fungi are molds. *Molds* are multicellular fungi that form long filaments called hyphae and reproduce by forming spores. *Yeasts* are unicellular fungi that reproduce by budding. Many fungi are dimorphic and grow as either form depending on their environment. An immunocompetent

host rarely develops fungal infections. However, there are three main mechanisms by which fungi can gain access to human tissues and cause disease: (i) inhalation; (ii) inoculation of the subcutaneous tissues; and (iii) colonization of mucosal surfaces. Histoplasmosis, blastomycosis, and coccidioidomycosis are examples of fungal diseases caused by inhalation of spores into the lung. Inoculation of the subcutaneous tissues by spores occurs in sporotrichosis. In this uncommon occupational disease, gardeners who injure their skin with contaminated thorns or branches present with nodules and ulcers on their hands and feet that may require surgical drainage. Fungal colonization of mucosal surfaces in a healthy, immunocompetent host rarely causes infection. However, in the immunocompromised patient, opportunistic infections such as esophageal candidiasis or pulmonary aspergillosis can occur. Fungal disease must always be considered when treating infections in immunocompromised groups such as patients with diabetes or patients who have undergone transplantation. Other risk factors for the development of fungal disease include prolonged hospitalization, intravenous cannulae, prolonged or broad-spectrum antibiotic administration, hyperalimentation, immunosuppressive drugs, burns, trauma, and malnutrition.

ANTIMICROBIAL THERAPY

Proper selection of antimicrobial therapy requires the knowledge of: (i) the most common pathogens causing the specific infection; (ii) the mechanism of action of the selected agent; (iii) the mechanisms of resistance to the selected agent; (iv) potential side effects of the selected agent; and, finally, (v) sensitivity patterns of the most common microbes in the environment (e.g., hospital) in which the antimicrobial agents are being prescribed. The following text is a brief overview of the most common classes of antimicrobials. Table 3-1 offers a comprehensive list of antimicrobial agents and their spectrum of activity against common bacterial pathogens.

Inhibitors of Cell Wall Synthesis

The majority of antimicrobial agents that inhibit cell wall synthesis share a common structural element, a *β*-lactam ring. The *β-lactam ring* binds to division-plate proteins on

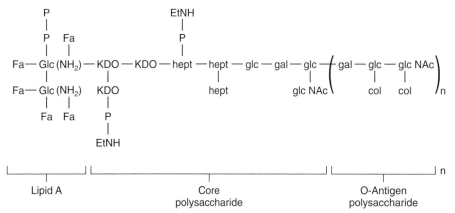

Figure 3-3   The chemical structure of lipopolysaccharide (endotoxin) includes lipid A, the O-antigen side chain, and the core polysaccharide. Lipid A is the toxic moiety of endotoxin and interacts with various cells to induce the septic response.

TABLE 3-1

GENERAL SPECTRUM OF ACTIVITY OF COMMONLY USED ANTIMICROBIAL AGENTS

Antimicrobial Agent	Microorganism						
	Gram-positive			Gram-negative		Anaerobic	
	Streptococci	Staphylococci	Enterococci	Enterics	Pseudomonas	Cocci	Bacteroides
Penicillins							
Penicillin	3	1	1	0	0	2	1
Ampicillin	2	1	3	1	0	2	1
Carboxypenicillin	1	1	1	3	2	1	1
Ureidopenicillin	2	2	2	3	3	1	2
Ampicillin +β-lactamase Inhibitor	2	2	3	2	1	2	2
Carboxypenicillin +β-lactamase Inhibitor	2	2	2	3	2	2	3
Cephalosporins							
First generation	2	3	0	1	0	2	0
Second generation[a]	1	2	0	2	1	1	2
Third generation[a]	0	0	0	3	3	1	1
Monobactams	0	0	0	3	2	0	0
Carbapenems	3	3	0	3	3	2	3
Aminoglycosides	0	1	1	3	3	0	0
Vancomycin	3	3	3	0	0	3	0
Erythromycin	2	2	2	0	0	2	0
Quinolones[a]	2	1	1	3	2	1	0
Tetracyclines	2	1	1	1	0	1	2
Chloramphenicol	2	2	1	1	0	2	2
Clindamycin	2	1	2	0	0	2	3
Metronidazole	0	0	0	0	0	1	3
Trimethoprim-sulfamethoxazole	2	1	0	3	2	1	0

Note: Higher numbers correspond to higher sensitivity of the organism to the antibiotic.
[a] Different specific agents within the same gereral class vary markedly with respect to spectrum of activity.
From Dunn DL, Rotstein OD. Diagnosis, prevention, and treatment of infection in surgical patients. In: Greenfield LJ, Mulholland MW, Oldham KT et al., eds. *Surgery: scientific principles and practice*, 3rd ed. Philadelphia: Lippincott Williams & Wilkins, 2001:187, with permission.

the bacteria and inhibits cell-wall peptidoglycan synthesis, thereby inducing autolytic bacteriolysis. Side chains of the β-lactam ring distinguish the agents of this class from one another and are responsible for the variance in their activity. The major mechanism of resistance against this class of antibiotics is bacterial production of the enzyme β-*lactamase*, which disrupts the β-lactam ring.

Penicillin G, the prototypical β-lactam, has excellent bactericidal activity against most gram-positive and anaerobic organisms. The broad-spectrum penicillins (e.g., ampicillin and piperacillin) add coverage against gram-negative organisms. The most common adverse effect of the penicillins is the development of an allergic reaction that can range from a benign rash to, on rare occasions, anaphylactic shock.

The cephalosporins are also broad-spectrum β-lactams, which are classified by generation according to their antimicrobial activity. First-generation cephalosporins have strong gram-positive, modest gram-negative, and poor anaerobic coverage. Second-generation cephalosporins have increased gram-negative and anaerobic activity but weaker gram-positive activity. Third-generation cephalosporins target gram-negative enteric organisms, and fourth-generation

cephalosporins have extended activity against *Pseudomonas* species. Despite their broad spectrum of activity, all cephalosporins are ineffective against enterococcal infections.

Other synthetic β-lactams include imipenem and meropenem, which offer the broadest range of activity (gram-positive, gram-negative, and anaerobic) of all antibiotics. Aztreonam provides good selective gram-negative and pseudomonal coverage. Vancomycin does not contain a β-lactam ring in its structure, but it inhibits cell wall synthesis by preventing glycopeptide polymerization. It is effective against the majority of gram-positive organisms and is the treatment of choice for infections caused by methicillin- or oxacillin-resistant *Staphylococcus aureus* and *Staphylococcus epidermidis*.

Inhibitors of Ribosomal Protein Synthesis

Aminoglycosides, macrolides, tetracyclines, and *chloramphenicol* inhibit bacterial protein synthesis by interfering with ribosomal activity. All of these agents are considered *bacteriostatic* except for the aminoglycosides, which are *bactericidal*. The *aminoglycosides* bind irreversibly to the 30S subunit of bacterial ribosomes and are especially active against aerobic gram-negative bacilli, *Pseudomonas* species and *S. aureus*. They are ineffective against anaerobes. The most common mechanism of resistance is plasmid-induced modification of the aminoglycoside, which decreases its ability to penetrate the bacteria and reduces its binding affinity for the ribosome. Other less common mechanisms include modified bacterial enzymes, which reduce aminoglycoside transport into the bacteria and the evolution of bacteria deficient in aminoglycoside binding sites. The two most common adverse effects of the aminoglycosides are nephrotoxicity and ototoxicity.

The *macrolides* (erythromycin and clindamycin) bind to the 50S ribosomal subunit to prevent protein synthesis. This class of agents has a broad spectrum of activity against gram-positive bacteria. Erythromycin is commonly combined with neomycin orally to prepare the bowel for surgery. Clindamycin is also effective against anaerobes. Resistance to this class of agents is usually caused by decreased permeability of the cell wall or alteration of the ribosomal subunit.

Tetracyclines bind to the 30S ribosomal subunit and have a broad spectrum of activity against gram-positive and gram-negative aerobes and anaerobes. Gonococci, meningococci, pneumococci, and *Haemophilus influenzae* are highly susceptible to the tetracyclines, and they are the treatment of choice for chlamydia, syphilis, and Lyme disease. The predominant mechanism of resistance manifests as decreased transport of the drug into the bacteria. Adverse reactions include nausea, vomiting, esophageal ulcerations, vertigo (minocycline), and permanent discoloration of the teeth in children (tetracycline).

Chloramphenicol is a very effective broad-spectrum bactericidal agent, but its use is limited to critically ill patients or for infections caused by highly resistant organisms because of its potential to cause bone marrow suppression and irreversible aplastic anemia. Like the macrolides, chloramphenicol binds to the 50S ribosomal subunit and is active against virtually all gram-positive and gram-negative bacteria, spirochetes, rickettsiae, chlamydiae, and mycoplasmas. The notable exceptions are methicillin-resistant *S. aureus*, *Pseudomonas aeruginosa*, *Serratia marcescens* and many of the *Enterobacter* species. Resistance to chloramphenicol can occur and results from alteration of the bacterial cell membrane permeability.

Inhibitors of Folic Acid Synthesis

Sulfonamides and *trimethoprim* are bacteriostatic antimicrobial agents that inhibit bacterial DNA replication by interfering with the folic acid synthetic pathway. *Sulfonamides* are structurally similar to paraaminobenzoic acid (PABA), and are readily incorporated into the folic acid biosynthetic pathway. *Trimethoprim* inhibits dihydrofolate reductase, a vital enzyme in the pathway. These agents work synergistically to inhibit the production of folic acid. Without folic acid, bacteria are unable to synthesize the purine bases which, along with the pyrimidines, are necessary to form the backbone of DNA strands (humans get folic acid through their diet, and therefore host purine synthesis is unaffected). Bacteria are unable to replicate, and the pathogen is eliminated. A sulfonamide and trimethoprim are typically administered together and are commonly used

for the treatment of acute and chronic urinary tract infections. They are effective prophylactics against *Pneumocystis carinii* infection in immunocompromised patients. Adverse reactions are usually caused by the sulfonamide portion of the molecule and include nausea, vomiting, diarrhea, rash, acute hemolytic anemia, aplastic anemia, agranulocytosis, and thrombocytopenia. Organisms develop resistance by overproduction of PABA or decreased affinity for the sulfonamide.

Inhibitors of DNA Synthesis

The *fluoroquinolones* inhibit DNA synthesis by binding to DNA helicase proteins, which are vital to unwinding of the double helix during replication. These agents have a broad spectrum of activity against both gram-positive and gram-negative pathogens including *Pseudomonas* species and methicillin-resistant *S. aureus*. They are ineffective against anaerobes. The mechanisms of resistance are decreased bacterial permeability and alteration of the target DNA helicase proteins. The most common reported adverse effects of fluoroquinolones are nausea, vomiting, and abdominal discomfort. Fluoroquinolones are frequently used in the treatment of respiratory, gastrointestinal, and genitourinary infections because of their broad spectrum of activity and their ability to achieve high serum drug levels with oral administration.

Metronidazole's mechanism of action is poorly understood, but it is believed to cause DNA strand breakage and fatal DNA helicase destabilization. It is the most effective antimicrobial agent against anaerobes, including all *Bacteroides* species. Because of its rapid oral absorption and low cost, metronidazole is the treatment of choice for *C. difficile* enterocolitis. Adverse effects include nausea and diarrhea, and its disulfiram-like properties when mixed with alcohol result in severe abdominal cramping, flushing, and vomiting. Despite its frequent use, resistance to metronidazole by anaerobes is extremely rare.

Antifungal Therapy

Amphotericin B and fluconazole are the two most commonly prescribed antifungal agents in surgical patients. Amphotericin B has a broad spectrum of activity against fungi and can be used for the majority of fungal infections. It is a polyene macrolide that binds to fungal membrane sterols to cause cell lysis, and it is considered the definitive treatment for all systemic fungal infections. Amphotericin B is a potent drug, but it is also toxic and its side effects can limit use. Frequent adverse effects at the onset of therapy include fever, chills, nausea, vomiting, and hypotension. Nephrotoxicity is the most common serious side effect associated with use of amphotericin B and develops in up to 80% of patients. Amphotericin B can also cause a reversible normocytic anemia, thrombocytopenia, leukopenia, severe electrolyte disturbances, and thrombophlebitis at the injection site. Resistance to amphotericin B is very rare.

Fluconazole is a safer alternative to amphotericin B in the treatment of many fungal diseases. Its mechanism of action is the disruption of fungal membrane sterol synthesis. Fluconazole is most commonly used for infections caused by *Candida* species. It is highly effective in the treatment of mucosal candidiasis and candiduria, and it is administered as life-long maintenance therapy (after induction therapy with amphotericin B) for HIV-infected patients with cryptococcal meningitis. Life-threatening infections caused by any of these fungi usually require treatment with amphotericin B. Nausea, vomiting, and diarrhea are the most commonly reported side effects of fluconazole.

SURGICAL PROPHYLAXIS

Surgical wound infections are the most common nosocomial infections among surgical patients. Up to 5% of all patients undergoing an operation develop wound infections, which result in prolonged hospitalizations, increased costs, and significant morbidity. The majority of wound infections can be attributed to endogenous contamination from the host's resident microflora (e.g., skin and gastrointestinal tract) or exogenous contamination from a break in sterile technique. Careful maintenance of sterile technique can be overlooked during prolonged operations. Endogenous contamination of the surgical site is a persistent threat starting from the time of incision until the sterile incision re-epithelializes. Proper preparation of the surgical site begins with hair removal using clippers just before the procedure. Shaving the surgical site the night before surgery actually increases the infection rate by 100%. Shaving promotes bacterial growth in the razor nicks on the skin. The operative site should be scrubbed with a germicidal detergent and then painted with an antimicrobial solution of iodine, povidone-iodine, or chlorhexidine. Both iodine and chlorhexidine are bactericidal, but chlorhexidine may provide a longer period of bactericidal activity after its application. This preparation significantly reduces the quantity of skin microflora present at the time of the incision. If the respiratory, gastrointestinal, or genitourinary tracts are entered during the procedure, a separate set of instruments should be used and then removed from the field after the "dirty" portion of the procedure is complete. These easily applied principles can have a dramatic impact on reducing the incidence of wound infections from endogenous contamination.

Preoperative intravenous antibiotic administration has proved to reduce the risk of postoperative wound infection in clean-contaminated and contaminated cases (See Table 3-2). Patients who are undergoing "clean case" surgery do not require prophylactic antibiotics because the infection rate is low (1.5%) and not significantly lowered by prophylaxis. Conversely, when prosthetic materials are implanted in clean cases, especially during cardiac surgery through a median sternotomy, and for all neurosurgical procedures, prophylactic antibiotics do significantly reduce the rate of infection. The optimal time of antibiotic administration is 30 minutes prior to skin incision or at the induction of anesthesia, so that therapeutic blood levels are achieved at skin incision. Prolonged operations may require an additional dose; however, postoperative dosing does not significantly alter the rate of infection and may lead to the development of resistant organisms and an increased risk of adverse reactions.

Cefazolin, a first-generation broad-spectrum cephalosporin, is used as the prophylactic agent for the majority of

TABLE 3-2

WOUND INFECTION STRATIFICATION SCHEME

Class I/clean: An uninfected operative wound in which no inflammation is encountered and the respiratory, alimentary, genital, or uninfected urinary tract is not entered. In addition, clean wounds are primarily closed and, if necessary, drained with closed drainage. Operative incisional wounds that follow nonpenetrating (blunt) trauma should be included in this category if they meet the criteria.

Class II/clean-contaminated: An operative wound in which the respiratory, alimentary, genital, or urinary tracts are entered under controlled conditions and without unusual contamination. specifically, operations involving the biliary tract, appendix, vagina, and oropharynx are included in this category, provided no evidence of infection or major break in technique is encountered.

Class III/contaminated: Open, fresh, accidental wounds. In addition, operations with major breaks in sterile technique (e.g., open cardiac massage) or gross spillage from the gastrointestinal tract, and incisions in which acute, nonpurulent inflammation is encountered are included in this category.

Class IV/dirty-infected: Old traumatic wounds with retained devitalized tissue and those that involve existing clinical infection or perforated viscera. This definition suggests that the organisms causing postoperative infection were present in the operative field before the operation.

Note: As one progresses from Class I to Class IV, the probability of a wound infection increases.
Adapted from Mangram AJ, Horan TC, Pearson ML, et al., and the Hospital Infection Control Practices Advisory Committee. Guidelines for prevention surgical site infection—1999. *Infect Control Hosp Epidemiol* 1999;20:247, with permission.

surgical procedures. If gram-negative organisms and anaerobes are anticipated in the operative site (e.g., during bowel surgery), the second-generation cephalosporins cefotetan or cefoxitin may be superior. For patients allergic to cephalosporins, vancomycin is a good alternative, but it lacks activity against gram-negative and anaerobic organisms. Certain operative sites have higher risks of infections and require additional prophylaxis. Historically, patients undergoing colorectal surgery have benefited from mechanical cleansing of the bowel and oral administration of erythromycin and neomycin in order to reduce the bacterial concentration within the colon. This practice has been shown to reduce the wound infection rate in colorectal surgery. Recently, there are new data suggesting that mechanical bowel preparation may not significantly alter wound infection rate, although this remains controversial.

Halsted identified a number of surgical principles that reduce wound infection rates. These include the obliteration of dead space, the removal of devitalized tissue, wound closure without tension, complete hemostasis, the use of nonabsorbable suture, and adequate blood supply to the wound. The presence of hematomas, seromas, and dead tissue supply sufficient adjuvant and media for bacterial growth. Although drains were originally designed to evacuate hematomas and reduce the risk of infection, open drains (e.g., Penrose) have been shown to increase infection rates by serving as an entry portal for bacteria. Closed suction drains (e.g., Jackson-Pratt bulb suction) enable the drain tip to remain sterile and have proved effective in reducing infection rates in certain settings. Generally, the presence of any foreign body, including drains, increases the risk of infection; therefore, drains should be used only when the accumulation of blood or fluid is anticipated.

Immunotherapy is rarely used to prevent surgical infections, but it is very successful in preventing tetanus. The tetanus toxin is produced by the organism *Clostridium tetani* and inhibits neurotransmitter release leading to spastic paralysis. After a full course of active immunization (full childhood series or three doses in adults), passive immunization with a booster injection of the toxoid protects adults for as long as 10 years. Patients with dirty wounds should receive a booster injection of the toxoid if their last booster was more than five years before the current event. It is imperative to ask all patients with wounds about their tetanus immunization history. Patients with unclear or incomplete immunization histories and those who have never received immunization should receive the tetanus immunoglobulin and toxoid booster at the same time in different injection sites.

SPECIFIC INFECTIONS

Intraabdominal Infections

Peritonitis is a surgical disease that can be rapidly fatal if untreated. *Primary peritonitis* occurs in patients with impaired host defenses. *Secondary peritonitis* results from contamination of the peritoneal cavity by a perforated viscus or external trauma. *Tertiary peritonitis* is the result of a change in the host microbial flora following antibiotic treatment of secondary peritonitis so that microbes of normally low virulence become pathogenic. Prosthetic-device–associated peritonitis occurs in patients with indwelling intraperitoneal prosthetic devices such as peritoneal dialysis catheters or ventriculoperitoneal shunts.

The induction of secondary peritonitis requires the presence of both bacteria and an adjuvant like blood, stool, or debris. The host response to microbial invasion of the peritoneal cavity occurs by three different mechanisms: phagocytosis, clearance, and sequestration. Following a bacterial inoculation of the peritoneal cavity, bacteria undergo *phagocytosis* by resident macrophages. These activated macrophages release cytokines that attract additional phagocytic leukocytes (e.g., PMNLs) to assist in engulfing the invading organisms and eliminating them from the peritoneal cavity. The resident macrophages represent the host's first line of defense. *Clearance* occurs via translymphatic absorption of bacteria, fluid, and other particles through specialized structures in the peritoneal mesothelium on the underside of the diaphragm. The bacteria transit through stomata located between mesothelial cells into lymph vessels that drain into the thoracic duct. The bacteria gain access to the bloodstream when the thoracic duct empties into the left subclavian vein. Clearance of the peritoneal cavity is a highly efficient process that results in bacteremia within minutes of bacterial invasion into the peritoneal cavity. Pathogens that escape phagocytosis and clearance undergo *sequestration*. It is hypothesized that once the mesothelial cells of the peritoneal cavity recognize

infection or injury, they produce an inflammatory exudate rich in opsonins and fibrinogen. This exudative fluid forms fibrin polymers, which, along with the omentum and other mobile viscera, wall off contaminated enteric contents, seal perforations, and prevent further bacterial seeding of the peritoneal cavity. If the inflammatory fluid and fibrin deposition completely isolate bacteria from the host's phagocytic cells, a cavity is created that promotes bacterial proliferation and results in the formation of an *abscess*. An average of four to five isolates usually occur in patients with intraabdominal infections, and 80% to 90% of specimens contain both aerobic, and anaerobic bacteria. Commonly encountered aerobic isolates include gram-negative bacilli (*E. coli*, *Enterobacter* species, and *Klebsiella* species), gram-positive cocci (streptococci, staphylococci and enterococci), and the *Bacteroides* species (especially *B. fragilis*). *Clostridium* species and the anaerobic cocci are the other common anaerobes isolated.

Antibiotic therapy should be initiated as soon as the diagnosis of peritonitis is established. Initial therapy is empiric and must cover a wide spectrum of microorganisms. If the likelihood of resistant gram-negative rod infection is small, then ampicillin/sulbactam or a second-generation cephalosporin is a good initial option. If the perforated viscus is in the lower rather than upper gastrointestinal tract, anaerobic coverage should be included. Surgical intervention for peritonitis is aimed at identifying and controlling the source of the infection, evacuating pus and enteric contents, and preventing sepsis. Antibiotics should be tailored according to the results of intraoperative cultures and should be continued postoperatively. General guidelines for the discontinuation of antibiotics include: (i) when the patient is hemodynamically stable; well-appearing and afebrile for 48 hours; (ii) when the leukocyte count has normalized for 48 hours; and (iii) the band count is less than 3%.

Postoperative Pneumonia

Postoperative pneumonia is the most common infection in surgical intensive care units (ICUs). Pneumonia is the leading cause of mortality in ICUs and is the result of compromised host defenses. Postoperative pneumonia can be classified into three categories: ventilator-associated pneumonia, nonventilator-associated pneumonia, and aspiration-associated pneumonia. Ventilator-associated pneumonia (VAP) is defined as the development of a pulmonary infection 48 hours after the initiation of mechanical ventilation. Endotracheal intubation allows the microflora of the oropharynx direct access to the tracheobronchial tree, eliminates the host's natural defense mechanism of coughing, and disrupts the competency of the glottis. The mortality rate of VAP is 40% to 70%.

Nonventilator-associated pneumonia begins with the development of atelectasis from reduced tidal volumes. Decreased tidal volumes in the postoperative patient are secondary to the lingering effects of general anesthesia, postoperative pain and splinting, and reduced respiratory drive from narcotics. The collapse of airways in atelectatic lung segments impairs the mucociliary mechanism and prevents clearance of bacteria. This leads to local bacterial proliferation in an enclosed space, which can progress into lobar pneumonia.

The development of aspiration-associated pneumonia may or may not be preceded by an obvious aspiration event. Gross aspiration, commonly caused by an altered sensorium and a distended stomach, causes a chemical pneumonitis that places the lung at high risk of bacterial infection. Microaspiration causes pneumonia in a more subtle manner.

In healthy patients, microaspiration of normal oropharyngeal flora is typically a benign event, which stimulates the cough reflex and results in expectoration of the aspirated microbes. Postoperative patients have an impaired cough reflex, and the composition of their oropharyngeal flora is altered by gastric acid–reducing medications. These medications alkalinize the normally acidic milieu of the stomach, which results in gastric proliferation of intestinal bacteria and retrograde colonization of the oropharynx. In this circumstance microaspiration poses an increased risk of pneumonia as each occult event exposes the tracheobronchial tree to more virulent gram-negative enteric pathogens.

Restoration of the normal host defenses is the key to preventing postoperative pneumonia. This includes early extubation, ambulation, coughing, deep breathing, incentive spirometry, and postural chest physiotherapy. Aggressive suctioning of the airways helps manage secretions and prevents mucous plugging in both ventilated and nonventilated patients. Aspiration precautions include gastric decompression and an upright position during oral intake. Treatment of postoperative pneumonia consists of the maintenance of the pulmonary toilet by the methods described in the preceding text, and broad-spectrum or culture-directed antibiotics.

Necrotizing Soft Tissue Infections

Necrotizing fasciitis is the most serious of all soft tissue infections and is associated with a mortality rate of 40% or higher. Diagnosing these infections can be challenging, and a high index of suspicion is critical because the classic signs of a wound infection are often absent. The infection is always introduced through a break in the skin (e.g., incision, perineal decubitus ulcer, or enterostomy). Signs of a necrotizing soft tissue infection include skin discoloration or necrosis; subcutaneous crepitus; blebs; or a thin, grayish foul-smelling drainage. Often, the overlying skin may have a relatively normal appearance, masking significant infection of the underlying tissues. The presence of gas on x-ray or computerized tomographic (CT) scans of the involved soft tissue may aid in the diagnosis. However, the absence of gas does not rule out the diagnosis. A failure to respond to conventional nonoperative therapy, rapid progression of any clinical signs of soft tissue infection, or a significant change in the patient's hemodynamic status may be the earliest signs of a necrotizing soft tissue infection necessitating urgent operative intervention.

Primary operative therapy of necrotizing fasciitis is radical débridement of all infected and necrotic tissue so that margins several centimeters into grossly normal, healthy tissue are achieved. Amputation of extremities may be required to gain control of this infection. Wounds are packed loosely open with gauze that is changed frequently. Reexploration should be planned within 24 hours. These infections tend to be polymicrobial and synergistic in nature, and both aerobic and anaerobic organisms are usually present. Empiric broad-spectrum antibiotic therapy should be initiated immediately with high doses of penicillin G included in the regimen as coverage against *Clostridium* species. Gram-staining and culture data sent from intraoperative specimens can aid in subsequent direction of the postoperative antibiotic regimen.

Gram-negative Bacterial Sepsis

Gram-negative bacterial sepsis is one of the most lethal disease processes that can occur in the surgical population. Factors that predispose patients to this disease include old age, disability, malnutrition, immunosuppression, prior or concurrent antimicrobial administration, renal insufficiency, diabetes mellitus, congestive heart failure, malignancy, and respiratory or urinary tract intubation. Many different organisms can cause this devastating septic cascade, but *E. coli* is the most common. Fever, arterial hypoxemia, abnormal metabolism, activation of the complement and coagulation cascades, decreased systemic vascular resistance, increased cardiac output, and hypotension are features of this disease. Gram-negative sepsis can lead to multisystem organ dysfunction. The mechanisms by which gram-negative infections produce these detrimental physiologic host responses are not fully understood.

It is widely agreed that the lipid A moiety of LPS of the bacterial cell wall is responsible for much of the toxicity in gram-negative sepsis. LPS is a potent immunogen that activates macrophages, stimulates B-cell proliferation, and causes antibody production. The activated macrophages secrete various cytokines including TNF-α, IL-1, IL-6, and interferon (IFN)-γ. Il-1 is known to stimulate B- and T-cell proliferation, which results in amplification of immune responses. In experimental models of gram-negative sepsis, the administration of large quantities of TNF-α mimics the devastating physiologic effects of LPS (fever, leukopenia, hypotension, and death). However, small quantities of TNF-α administered in these same models have been shown to enhance survival. This suggests that the level of the host immune system response may be important in the pathophysiology of the disease. At low levels, the immune response to endotoxin (LPS) may be beneficial; however, at higher levels the immune response becomes detrimental to the host, ultimately resulting in septic physiology, multiorgan dysfunction, and death.

Blood cultures confirm the diagnosis, but gram-negative sepsis is usually suspected when septic physiology is recognized, especially in the setting of a known source of infection. Empiric antibiotic administration initiated early in the course of the disease is beneficial, but the mortality rate of this disease despite antibiotic therapy remains 20% to 30%.

Catheter and Prosthetic Device Infections

Many patients require long-term indwelling intravenous catheters for chemotherapy or parenteral hyperalimentation. Infection is a major problem with such devices. The most common pathogenic organisms involved are *S. aureus* and *S. epidermidis*. These bacteria produce a biofilm that facilitates adherence to the catheters and prevents antimicrobial penetration. Fungal and gram-negative organisms also infect indwelling catheters, especially in immunocompromised patients who have been receiving long-term antibiotic therapy. Optimal treatment of these types of infections consists of device removal and initiation of an appropriate antimicrobial agent. In patients receiving long-term hyperalimentation without alternative intravenous access sites, the catheter may be left in place and the patient treated with a prolonged course of antibiotic therapy. However, sepsis, bacteremia, or fungemia necessitates catheter removal regardless of the circumstances.

Urinary Tract Infections

Urinary tract infections (UTIs) are the most common cause of gram-negative bacterial sepsis in hospitalized patients. The presence of a bacterial level of 10^5 cfu/mL of urine in a patient is diagnostic of a UTI. Many antimicrobial agents concentrate in the urine, facilitating very efficient therapies. Culture and sensitivity reports should be obtained and follow-up specimens should be sent to the laboratory to confirm eradication. More than 80% of UTIs are caused by *E. coli*; other common pathogens include *Klebsiella*, *Proteus*, *Pseudomonas*, and *Enterobacter* species.

Human Immunodeficiency Virus in the Surgical Patient

The *HIV* epidemic over the last 25 years has created new infectious diseases challenges for the surgeon. This blood-borne virus is transmitted by exposure to infected blood or body fluids. The virus infects CD4 lymphocytes and releases RNA and the enzyme *reverse transcriptase*. This enzyme, using the host cell machinery, produces multiple copies of viral DNA (cDNA) from the template RNA. This cDNA incorporates itself into the host's chromosomes and new virions are produced. Viral synthesis continues until the capacity of the cell has been exceeded and the T lymphocyte ruptures, releasing multiple copies of the virus into the blood to infect other host CD4 lymphocytes. This ultimately results in depletion of host CD4 cells and immunosuppression. When the CD4 count drops to lower than 200 or the patient manifests an indicator condition/infection (e.g., *P. carinii* pneumonia, toxoplasmosis, and cryptosporidiosis) then the patient is considered to have *acquired immunodeficiency syndrome (AIDS)*.

Patients with AIDS often present with abdominal pain that requires the attention of a surgeon. Because of their immunocompromised state, these patients are susceptible to a variety of opportunistic infections, but more often they have uncommon presentations of common diseases. Acute appendicitis may present as fever, right lower quadrant pain, with a normal white blood cell count. In addition to a fecalith, appendicitis may be incited by obstruction of the appendiceal orifice by Kaposi sarcoma or a CMV infection leading to acute appendicitis. Gastrointestinal tract obstruction may be caused by Kaposi sarcoma, mycobacterial infection, and lymphoma. Gastrointestinal symptoms are common in patients with AIDS and usually have nonsurgical etiologies. However, there is an increased incidence of gastrointestinal tract perforations in patients with AIDS, which are often masked by a relative lack of peritoneal signs. CMV infection is the most frequent cause, typically occurring in the terminal ileum and colon. CMV-induced perforation of the gastrointestinal tract has a poor prognosis and is a marker of advanced-stage AIDS. These patients have a high probability of death from peritonitis or other AIDS-related illnesses. When treating patients with HIV or AIDS, surgeons must be vigilant in recognizing both unusual presentations of common diseases and rare presentations of opportunistic infections not seen in immunocompetent hosts.

KEY POINTS

▲ The toxic properties of gram-negative bacterial endotoxin rests in the lipid A moiety of the lipopolysaccharide (LPS) molecule. The endotoxin stimulates the hypothalamus to produce fever and stimulates macrophages to release tumor necrosis factor alpha (TNF-α, which can result in septic shock).

▲ Necrotizing fasciitis is a polymicrobial infection requiring radical operative débridement and a broad-spectrum antibiotic regimen, which includes high-dose penicillin as coverage for *Clostridium* species.

▲ Bacterial inoculation of the peritoneal cavity results in (i) *phagocytosis* of bacteria by macrophages, (ii) *clearance* of bacteria via translymphatic absorption, and (iii) *sequestration* of the remaining intraperitoneal bacteria by a inflammatory exudates.

▲ The most common cause of a wound infection in a clean case is a break in sterile technique.

▲ β-Lactams and vancomycin inhibit cell wall synthesis, whereas tetracyclines, aminoglycosides, macrolides, and chloramphenicol bind to ribosomes and inhibit ribonucleic acid (RNA) transcription. Fluoroquinolones inhibit deoxyribonucleic acid (DNA) helicase.

SUGGESTED READINGS

Dellinger EP. Surgical infections and choices of antibiotics. In: Townsend CM Jr, Beauchamp RD, Evers BM et al., eds. *Sabiston textbook of surgery*, 16th ed. Philadelphia: WB Saunders, 2001:171–188.

Dunn DL, Rotstein OD. Diagnosis, prevention, and treatment of infection in surgical patients. In: Greenfield LJ, Mulholland MW, Oldham KT et al., eds. *Surgery: scientific principles and practice*, 3rd ed. Philadelphia: Lippincott Williams & Wilkins, 2001:178–202.

Fry DE. Surgical problems in the immunosuppressed patient. In: Townsend CM Jr, Beauchamp RD, Evers BM et al., eds. *Sabiston textbook of surgery*, 16th ed. Philadelphia: WB Saunders, 2001:189–197.

Fry DE. Surgical infection. In: O'Leary JP, ed. *The physiologic basis of surgery*, 3rd ed. Philadelphia: Lippincott Williams & Wilkins, 2002:212–258.

Howard RJ, Simmons RL. *Surgical infectious diseases*, 3rd ed. Norwalk: Appleton & Lange, 1998.

Tumor Biology

4

Susan B. Kesmodel   Jeffrey A. Drebin

Cancer is a significant public health problem that affects patients of all ages, socioeconomic groups, races, and ethnicities. It remains the second leading cause of death in the United States. In 2005 alone, more than 1.3 million new cases of cancer are expected with estimated deaths of over 500,000. Recent data on cancer incidence and mortality in the United States demonstrate that the three most common cancers in men are prostate, lung and bronchus, and colorectal, whereas in women the three most common cancers are breast, lung and bronchus, and colorectal. In both genders, cancer of the lung and bronchus is the leading cause of death (Fig. 4-1). Although the incidence of many types of cancers has increased in recent years, advances in our understanding of cancer biology may lead to improvements in diagnosis, therapy, and prevention.

Carcinogenesis is a complex and varied process that is influenced by genetic, environmental, and host factors. Recent advances in molecular biology have resulted in a more complete understanding of this process and have led to the identification of new targets for cancer therapy. It is now clear that malignant transformation results from the accumulation of genetic defects within a cell, which eventually release the cell from normal cellular mechanisms that control growth and development. It appears that malignant transformation is a multistep process that requires between five and ten genetic alterations for a cell to develop the cancer phenotype. The process of multistep carcinogenesis has been particularly well characterized for colon cancer (Fig. 4-2).

Significant geographic disparity in cancer incidence is found, confirming the importance of environmental factors in cancer development. Examples of this include the high incidence of hepatocellular carcinoma in Southeast Asia owing to the prevalence of hepatitis B infection in this region, the incidence of gastric carcinoma in Japan influenced by dietary factors, and the incidence of thyroid cancer in the areas surrounding Chernobyl resulting from radiation exposure.

Once a cell has acquired the genetic defects that lead to malignant transformation, a series of tumor and host interactions predominate that promote tumor growth, invasion, and metastasis. During this time tumor cells continue to accumulate genetic alterations that support growth and favor an invasive phenotype. This leads to a heterogeneous population of cells with different metastatic potentials. Some of the changes include upregulation of growth factor receptors, upregulation of proangiogenic factors, and changes in cell-surface adhesion molecules.

This chapter focuses on three main areas of tumor biology. The first section focuses on the genetic, environmental, and host factors that influence malignant transformation. The second section reviews the cancer phenotype, including tumor growth characteristics, the tumor microenvironment, and factors necessary to develop an invasive and metastatic phenotype. Finally, treatment modalities for cancer are reviewed including standard surgical, chemotherapeutic, and radiation therapies, as well as immunotherapy, gene therapy, and molecular therapies.

MALIGNANT TRANSFORMATION

Malignant transformation results from the accumulation of genetic defects within a cell, which release the cell from normal mechanisms that regulate cell growth, differentiation, and cell death. Numerous genetic, environmental, and host factors contribute to this process.

Genetic Factors

Oncogenes
Oncogenes are altered forms of normal cellular genes known as protooncogenes and are involved in multiple steps in cell growth and differentiation. Identification of these genes and an understanding of how they are involved in carcinogenesis were made possible by the identification of viral oncogenes. In 1909, Rous demonstrated that transplanted sarcomas in chickens could be induced by a cell-free agent. This agent was identified as a retrovirus containing a transduced part of a normal cellular gene known as *src*. It was found that the *src* gene was mutated when compared to the normal cellular gene, leading to a constitutively activated protein that had transforming capacity. This was the first demonstration of how an alteration in a normal cellular gene could result in a gene with transforming activity.

Several mechanisms for the activation of oncogenes have been identified including point mutation, chromosomal translocation, and gene amplification. Examples of

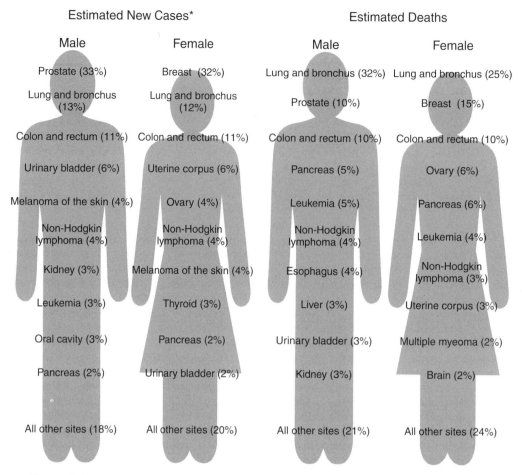

Figure 4-1 Ten leading cancer types for the estimated new cancer cases and deaths by sex, United States 2004. (From Jemal A, Tiwari RC, Murray T, et al. Cancer Statistics, 2004. *CA Cancer J Clin*, 2004;54:8–29, with permission.)

oncogenes that are activated by point mutation are the *ras* oncogenes. Activated (mutant) *ras* genes are found in a significant fraction of colon, pancreas, and lung cancers. The *ras* oncogenes encode guanosine triphosphate (GTP) binding (G) proteins that are involved in signal transduction. A single-point mutation difference has been identified between the oncogene and protooncogene leading to a protein product with transforming activity. A second mechanism of oncogene activation is chromosomal translocation. The most well-known example of this is the Philadelphia chromosome in chronic myelogenous leukemia. A translocation of the *c-abl* protooncogene from chromosome 9 to chromosome 22 leads to a fusion protein Bcr/abl. This new

fusion protein has enhanced tyrosine kinase activity that plays a critical role in the development of leukemia. An additional mechanism by which oncogenes are activated is through amplification, which leads to increased gene expression. An example of an oncogene that is activated by amplification is the *N-myc* oncogene in neuroblastoma. Amplification of this gene has been shown to correlate with tumor progression, recurrence, and resistance to chemotherapy.

Numerous oncogenes have been identified that are involved in various steps in cell growth, differentiation, and signal transduction (Table 4-1). These oncogenes can be classified according to their cellular location and mechanism

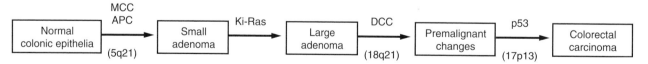

Figure 4-2 The multistep pathway to colorectal cancer. The accumulation of five to ten mutations in several tumor suppressor genes or oncogenes over a lifetime results in cancer. In some cases, an inherited mutation adenomatous polyposis coli produces thousands of adenomas, which results in cancer at a younger age. MCC, mutated in colorectal cancer; APC, adenomatous polyposis coli; Ki-ras, the Kirsten *ras* oncogene; DCC, deleted in colorectal cancer; *p53*, the *p53* gene. (From Leach SD, Pearson AS, Beauchamp RD. Tumor biology. In: Greenfield LJ, Mulholland MW, Oldham KT et al., eds. *Surgery: scientific principles and practice*, 3rd ed. Philadelphia: Lippincott Williams & Wilkins, 2001:471, with permission.)

TABLE 4-1
ONCOGENES

Oncogene	Lesion	Neoplasm	Protooncogene
Growth factors			
v-sis		Glioma/fibrosarcoma	B-chain PDGF
int 2	Proviral insertion	Mammary carcinoma	Member of FGF family
KS3	DNA transfection	Kaposi sarcoma	Member of FGF family
HST	DNA transfection	Stomach carcinoma	Member of FGF family
int-l	Proviral insertion	Mammary carcinoma	Possible growth factor
Receptors lacking protein kinase activity			
mas	DNA transfection	Mammary carcinoma	Angiotensin receptor
Tyrosine kinases: integral membrane proteins, growth factor receptors			
EGFR	Amplification	Squamous cell carcinoma	Protein kinase (tyr) EGFR
v-fms		Sarcoma	Protein kinase (tyr) CSF-1R
v-kit		Sarcoma	Protein kinase (tyr) stem cell factor R
v-ros		Sarcoma	Protein kinase (tyr)
MET	Rearrangement	MNNG-treated human osteocarcinoma cell line	Protein kinase (tyr) HGF/SFR
TRK	Rearrangement	Colon carcinoma	Protein kinase (tyr) NGFR
NEU	Point mutation	Neuroblastoma	Protein kinase (tyr)
	Amplification	Carcinoma of breast	
RET	Rearrangement	Carcinoma of thyroid MEN 2A, MEN 2B	Protein kinase (tyr) GDNFR
Tyrosine kinases: membrane associated			
scr		Colon carcinoma	Protein kinase (tyr)
v-yes		Sarcoma	Protein kinase (tyr)
v-fgr		Sarcoma	Protein kinase (tyr)
v-fps		Sarcoma	Protein kinase (tyr)
v-fes		Sarcoma	Protein kinase (tyr)
Bcr/abl	Chromosome translocation	Chronic myelogenous leukemia	Protein kinase (tyr)
Membrane-associated G proteins			
H-RAS	Point mutation	Colon, lung, pancreatic carcinoma	GTPase
K-RAS	Point mutation	Acute myelogenous leukemia thyroid carcinoma, melanoma	GTPase
N-RAS	Point mutation	Carcinoma, melanoma	GTPase
gsp	Point mutation	Carcinoma of thyroid	$G_6\alpha$
gip	Point mutation	Ovarian, adrenal carcinoma	$G_1\alpha$
GEF family of proteins			
Dbl	Rearrangement	Diffuse B-cell lymphoma	GEF for Rho and Cdc42Hs
Ost		Osteosarcomas	GEF for RhoA and Cdc42Hs
Tiam-1	Metastatic and oncogenic	T lymphoma	GEF for Rac and Cdc42Hs
Vay	Rearrangement	Hematopoietic cells	GEF for Ras?
Lbc	Oncogenic	Myeloid leukemias	GEF for Rho
Serine/threonine kinases: cytoplasmic			
v-mos		Sarcoma	Protein kinase (ser/thr)
v-raf		Sarcoma	Protein kinase (ser/thr)
pim-1	Proviral insertion	T-cell lymphoma	Protein kinase (ser/thr)
Cytoplasmic regulators			
v-crk			SH-2/SH-3 adaptor
Nuclear protein family			
v-myc		Carcinoma myelocytomatosis	Transcription factor
N-MYC	Gene amplification	Neuroblastoma, lung carcinoma	Transcription factor
L-MYC	Gene amplification	Carcinoma of lung	Transcription factor
v-myb		Myeloblastosis	Transcription factor
v-fos		Osteosarcoma	Transcription factor API
v-jun		Sarcoma	Transcription factor API
v-ski		Carcinoma	Transcription factor
v-rel		Lymphatic leukemia	Mutant NFκB
v-ets		Myeloblastosis	Transcription factor
v-erbA		Erythroblastosis	Mutant thioredoxine receptor

EGFR, epidermal growth factor receptor; DNA, deoxyribonucleic acid; PDGF, platelet-derived growth factor; CSF-1R, macrophage colony-stimulating factor-1 receptor; FGF, fibroblast growth factor; GEF, guanine nucleotide exchange factor; GDNR, glial derived neurotropic factor receptor; HGF/SFR, hepatic growth factor/scatter factor receptor; NGF, nerve growth factor.
From Park M. Oncogenes. In: Volgelstein B, Kinzler KW, eds. *The genetic basis of human cancer*, 2nd ed. New York: McGraw-Hill, 2002:181, with permission.

of action into growth factors, growth factor receptors, membrane-associated tyrosine kinases and G proteins, cytoplasmic serine and threonine kinases, cytoplasmic hormone receptors, and nuclear factors. A significant number of oncogenes are growth factor receptors with tyrosine kinase activity. Ligand-independent activation of these receptors, often caused by truncation of the extracellular binding domain, has been identified. This leads to a growth factor receptor that is constitutively active. Examples of oncogene products that are growth factor receptors with tyrosine kinase activity include the epidermal growth factor receptor (EGFR), RET, and NEU.

Tumor-Suppressor Genes

In contrast to oncogenes in which mutations to normal cellular genes lead to gain of function, mutations in tumor-suppressor genes result in loss of function. Tumor-suppressor genes are therefore considered recessive genes in cancer, since a single normal copy of the gene is sufficient for normal cellular function and loss of both copies of the gene is required to contribute to the cancer phenotype. Similar to oncogenes, tumor-suppressor genes are involved in many of the processes that regulate cell growth and differentiation. In addition, tumor-suppressor genes have been identified that play important roles in cell adhesion, programmed cell death, and the maintenance of genomic integrity.

The theory of the existence of tumor-suppressor genes came from two concurrent lines of research. In the first, it was found that growth of tumor cells could be suppressed following the fusion of malignant cells with normal cells. However, when these cells were cultured for extended periods, many reverted back to the malignant state and it was found that the cells that reverted to the malignant state had lost specific chromosomes. The second line of research was epidemiologic studies that were performed by Knudson in patients with retinoblastoma. Knudson found that in certain families there was an autosomal dominant inheritance of retinoblastoma and that in these families, onset of the disease was earlier and often bilateral and multifocal. From this information, Knudson generated the two-hit hypothesis, in which he suggested that in order for the malignant phenotype to occur, both copies of the gene had to be lost. In those families with autosomal dominant retinoblastoma, a germ-line mutation in a gene was present, and, therefore, a single additional somatic mutation was necessary to generate the cancer phenotype. In patients with a germ-line mutation, loss of heterozygosity at the chromosomal allele for the tumor-suppressor gene resulted in the cancer phenotype. In the sporadic form of the disease, however, two somatic mutations were necessary.

Tumor-suppressor genes can be categorized into two broad groups, which Volgelstein and Kinzler have termed gatekeepers and caretakers. Gatekeepers are tumor-suppressor genes that directly regulate cell growth and death. Examples of gatekeepers include the adenomatous polyposis coli (*APC*) gene in familial adenomatous polyposis and the retinoblastoma (*Rb*) gene, as described in preceding text. Conversely, caretaker tumor-suppressor genes are generally involved in the maintenance of genomic stability. Mutations to these genes lead to the accumulation of mutations in other genes, thereby resulting in the activation of oncogenes or loss of gatekeeper tumor-suppressor genes.

Examples of caretaker tumor-suppressor genes include mismatch repair genes in hereditary nonpolyposis colon cancer (HNPCC) and nucleotide excision repair genes in xeroderma pigmentosum (XP).

The original studies by Knudson in patients with retinoblastoma led to the recognition that inheritance of germ-line mutations in certain genes predisposes to development of specific cancer phenotypes. Numerous familial cancer syndromes have since been identified that result from germ-line mutations in tumor-suppressor genes (Table 4-2). Many of these inherited familial cancer syndromes are reviewed in detail elsewhere in this textbook.

Environmental Factors

Multiple environmental factors have been shown to influence cancer development in humans. These include exogenous factors (physical, chemical, viral, and dietary carcinogens) as well as endogenous factors (hormone levels and immune system status).

Physical Carcinogens

Radiation, either in the form of ionizing radiation or ultraviolet (UV) light, is the most important physical carcinogen that has been identified in the environment. The potential for ionizing radiation to induce carcinogenesis was recognized soon after the discovery of x-rays, with skin cancers developing in irradiated areas and with leukemia developing in radiation workers. Numerous studies have subsequently shown that ionizing radiation is a "universal carcinogen," which can induce carcinogenesis in most species at any age and which penetrates tissues in a random fashion.

Although numerous mechanisms have been proposed for the mutagenic effects of ionizing radiation, it appears that induction of double-stranded DNA breaks (DSBs) is the primary lesion. Patients with ataxia-telangiectasia (A-T), an inherited cancer syndrome, are extremely sensitive to the effects of ionizing radiation. These patients often develop fatal complications after conventional radiation doses, and are prone to developing lymphoreticular malignancies at a young age. The genetic defect in A-T is in a protein that senses DSBs. The defect in this protein prevents phosphorylation of important molecules that are involved in cell cycle arrest. The result is lack of DNA repair prior to initiation of the next cell cycle and propagation of genetic defects.

Striking examples of the impact of ionizing radiation on cancer rates and genetic mutation can be seen in epidemiologic studies of populations that have been exposed to large doses of radiation, including inhabitants of the areas surrounding Chernobyl and survivors of the atomic bombs in Hiroshima and Nagasaki. Studies of children born in Belarus following the Chernobyl accident demonstrate an increased frequency of germ-line mutations that is directly related to the amount of parental radiation exposure. Ionizing radiation has also been shown to be a risk factor in the development of several other malignancies including papillary thyroid cancer, sarcoma, breast cancer, and lymphoma.

In addition to the mutagenic effects of ionizing radiation, UV light has also been implicated in carcinogenesis, contributing to the development nonmelanocytic skin cancers. UVA, UVB, and UVC light have all been shown to induce

TABLE 4-2

GERM LINE AND SOMATIC MUTATIONS IN TUMOR-SUPPRESSOR GENES AND FUNCTIONS OF THE TUMOR-SUPPRESSOR PROTEINS

Gene	Associated Inherited Cancer Syndrome	Cancers with Somatic Mutations	Presumed Function of Protein
RB1	Familial retinoblastoma	Retinoblastoma, osteosarcoma, SCLC, breast, prostate, bladder, pancreas, esophageal, others	Transcriptional regulator; E2F binding
TP53	Li–Fraumeni syndrome	Approx. 50% of all cancers (rare in some types, such as prostate carcinoma and neuroblastoma)	Transcription factor; regulates cell cycle and apoptosis
p16/INK4A	Familial melanoma, familial pancreatic carcinoma	25%–30% of many different cancer types (e.g., breast, lung, pancreatic, bladder)	Cyclin-dependent kinase inhibitor (i.e., cdk4 and cdk6)
p14^{Arf}(p19^{Arf})	Familial melanoma?	Approx. 15% of many different cancer types	Regulates Mdm-2 protein stability and hence p53 stability; alternative reading frame of p16/INK4A gene
APC	FAP (Familial adenomatous polyposis coli), Gardner syndrome, Turcot syndrome	Colorectal, desmoid tumors	Regulates levels of β-catenin protein in the cytsol; binding to microtubules
WT-1	WAGR, Denys–Drash syndrome	Wilms tumor	Transcription factor
NF-1	Neurofibromatosis type 1	Melanoma, neuroblastoma	p21 ras-GTPase
NF-2	Neurofibromatosis type 2	Schwannoma, meningioma, ependymoma	Juxtamembrane link to cytoskeleton
VHL	von Hippel–Lindau syndrome	Renal (clear cell type), hemangioblastoma	Regulator of protein stability (e.g., HIFα)
BRCA1	Inherited breast and ovarian cancer	Ovarian (approx. 10%), rare in breast cancer	DNA repair; complexes with Rad 51 and BRCA2; transcriptional regulation
BRCA2	Inherited breast (both female and male), pancreatic cancer, others?	Rare mutations in pancreatic, others?	DNA repair; complexes with Rad 51 and BRCA1
MEN-1	Multiple endocrine neoplasia type 1	Parathyroid adenoma, pituitary adenoma, endocrine tumors of the pancreas	Not known
PTCH	Gorlin syndrome, hereditary basal-cell carcinoma syndrome	Basal-cell skin carcinoma, medulloblastoma	Transmembrane receptor for sonic hedgehog factor; negative regulator of smoothened protein
PTEN/MMAC1	Cowden syndrome; sporadic cases of juvenile polyposis syndrome	Glioma, breast, prostate, follicular thyroid, carcinoma, and head and neck squamous carcinoma	Phosphoinositide 3-phosphatase; protein tyrosine phosphatase
DPC4	Familial juvenile polyposis syndrome	Pancreatic (approx. 50%), 10%–15% of colorectal cancers, rare in others	Transcriptional factor in TGF-β signaling pathway
E-CAD	Familial diffuse-type gastric cancer	Gastric (diffuse type), lobular breast carcinoma, rare in other types (e.g., ovarian)	Cell–cell adhesion molecule
LKB1/STK1	Peutz–Jeghers syndrome	Rare in colorectal, not known in others	Serine/threonine protein kinase
EXT1	Hereditary multiple exostoses	Not known	Glycosyltransferase; heparan sulfate chain elongation
EXT2	Hereditary multiple exostoses	Not known	Glycosyltransferase; heparan sulfate chain elongation
TSC1	Tuberous sclerosis	Not known	Not known; cytoplasmic vesicle localization
TSC2	Tuberous sclerosis	Not known	Putative GTPase-activating protein F or Rap1 and rab5; golgi localization
MSH2, MLH1, PMS1, PMS2, MSH6	Hereditary nonpolyposis colorectal cancer	Colorectal, gastric, endometrial cancer	DNA mismatch repair

FAP, familial adenomatous polyposis coli; WAGR, Wilms' tumor-aniridia-genitourinary anomalies-mental retardation; SCLC, small cell lung cancer; GTP, guanosine triphosphates; DNA, deoxyribonucleic acid.
From Fearon ER. Tumor-suppressor genes. In: Volgelstein B, Kinzler KW, eds. *The genetic basis of human cancer*, 2nd ed. New York: McGraw-Hill, 2002:199, with permission.

DNA damage by generating pyrimidine photoproducts. Support for an association between UV light and skin cancer comes from studies of patients with XP. Patients with XP have a defect in nucleotide excision repair (NER) genes that prevents excision of UV-induced pyrimidine dimers. Patients with XP have a significantly increased incidence of UV-induced skin cancers.

Chemical Carcinogens

Numerous chemical carcinogens have been identified, with tobacco being the most prevalent. Although evidence of the carcinogenicity of tobacco has existed for more than 50 years, a reduction in tobacco use in men has only been seen in the last 20 years, and, tobacco use continues to increase in women. Tobacco consumption has clearly been shown to be a risk for lung cancer, with approximately 90% of lung cancers in men and 75% to 80% in women attributed to its use. The duration and amount of tobacco use have been shown to affect the lifetime risk of developing lung cancer, and cessation of smoking results in a considerable decrease in mortality from lung cancer. Numerous carcinogens are present in tobacco smoke, so it is difficult to determine the relative carcinogenicity of each of these agents. However, important carcinogens that are present in smoke include polycyclic aromatic hydrocarbons, nitrosamine 4-(N-nitrosomethyl-amino)-1-(3-pyridyl)-1-butanone, and free radicals. Other malignancies that are causally associated with tobacco use include cancers of the oropharynx, esophagus, pancreas, kidney, and bladder.

Occupational chemical exposures have also been shown to be carcinogenic including exposure to asbestos, benzene, and aromatic amines. The association between pleural mesothelioma and asbestos exposure has been demonstrated following both occupational and household exposure. Recent estimates predict that mortality from mesothelioma will be approximately 250,000 in the next 35 years. Although the use of asbestos in developed countries has decreased considerably, there continues to be a significant use of this material in developing countries.

Dietary Carcinogens

Dietary constituents and nutrition have also been implicated in carcinogenesis. Alcohol consumption has been shown to be associated with multiple cancers, including those of the oropharynx, esophagus, and liver. This increased cancer risk is directly related to the amount of alcohol intake. Aflatoxins are produced by *Aspergillus parasiticum* and *Aspergillus flavus*, and are found as contaminants in food. These toxins are most prevalent in Southeast Asia and sub-Saharan Africa, and have been shown to induce hepatocellular carcinoma in several animal species. High salt intake, generally resulting from the consumption of salted foods, is associated with an increased risk of nasopharyngeal cancer and gastric cancer. In gastric cancer, high doses of salt may disrupt the protective mucin layer in the stomach, thereby exposing the underlying epithelial cells to damage. This leads to increased epithelial proliferation in the stomach, which increases the potential for mutation. In addition, salted foods are often also smoked, which increases their carcinogenicity. More recently, heterocyclic amines (HCAs) have been identified in meat and other proteinaceous foods that have been exposed to open flames. HCAs are known carcinogens that can induce cancers of the breast, colon, prostate, skin, lymphoid tissue, and liver. Methods to decrease production of HCAs include avoiding open flame cooking or covering meat that will be cooked on an open flame. Finally, nitrosamines, which are present in foods as preservatives or generated in the stomach from nitrites, have been found to be associated with cancers of the esophagus, stomach, bladder, and colon.

In addition to the carcinogenic effects of dietary constituents, the amount and type of food consumed also influence the development of cancer. Diets high in animal fats are associated with an increased risk of breast cancer and colon cancer. Obesity increases the risk for endometrial, kidney, gallbladder, and esophageal cancers, and patients with diets deficient in fruits and vegetables have been shown to be at increased risk for developing cancers of the upper digestive tract, stomach, and lung. Conversely, diets rich in antioxidant vitamins may be associated with decreased cancer risk, although this remains controversial.

Viral Carcinogens

Transforming retroviruses in animals were first identified by Rous in 1909 while he was studying the cause of a chicken sarcoma, as noted previously. Subsequent research has led to the identification of numerous acutely transforming retroviruses that contain oncogenes derived from normal cellular genes, as well as nontransforming retroviruses that lead to malignant transformation by insertional mutagenesis and activation of protooncogenes.

In contrast to retroviruses, DNA tumor viruses induce tumorigenesis by two mechanisms. First, because DNA tumor viruses are small, they are dependent on the host cell for replication. Virally encoded nonstructural proteins stimulate cells to enter the S phase, providing an environment that is conducive to viral replication. Therefore, DNA viruses interfere with normal cell cycle control. Second, viral oncoproteins are transcribed that bind to and inhibit the function of cellular proteins. In many cases these viral oncoproteins affect the function of tumor suppressor genes products such as p53 and pRb, which play critical roles in cell cycle control and programmed cell death.

Although a causal role for viruses in human cancer was initially rejected, several human cancers have since been shown to be induced by viral pathogens and several candidate human tumor viruses exist. Viral carcinogenesis in humans generally results from infection with either nontransforming retroviruses [human lymphotrophic virus 1 (HTLV-1) and human immunodeficiency virus (HIV)] or DNA tumor viruses [hepatitis B virus (HBV), Epstein-Barr virus (EBV), human herpesvirus 8 (HHV-8), human papilloma virus (HPV), and polyomavirus], although the flavivirus hepatitis C virus (HCV) has also been implicated in hepatocellular carcinoma. Approximately 15% of all human cancers are virally induced. The majority of these are virally induced cervical and hepatocellular carcinomas, which are seen with increased frequency in developing countries where the incidence of HPV, HBV, and HCV infection is high. Table 4-3 lists the properties of accepted and potential human tumor viruses. These viruses have different tissue tropism, require a long latent period from infection to tumor induction, and are dependent on host–virus interactions and environmental factors. Therefore, in each host, there is significant variability in response to viral infection and the potential for carcinogenesis.

Host Factors

Hormonal Balance

Several human cancers can be categorized as hormonally induced tumors, including breast, endometrial, ovarian, testicular, prostate, thyroid, and osteosarcoma. These tumors share a common mechanism of carcinogenesis in which elevated or unopposed hormone levels induce cellular proliferation, thereby increasing the frequency of additional random genetic mutations and eventually leading to the development of a malignant phenotype. These hormones may be endogenous, such as increased

TABLE 4-3
PROPERTIES OF ACCEPTED AND POTENTIAL HUMAN TUMOR VIRUSES

Characteristic	HBV	EBV	HPV	HTLV-I	HCV	HHV-8 (KSHV)	SV40	MCV
Genome								
Nucleic acid	dsDNA[a]	dsDNA	dsDNA	ssRNA → dsDNA	ssRNA	dsDNA	dsDNA	dsDNA
Size (kb/kbp)	3.2	172	8	9.0	9.4	165	5.2	190
No. genes	4	≈90	8–10	6	9	≈90	6	≈180
Cell tropism	Hepatocytes, white blood cells	Oropharyngeal epithelial cells, B cells	Squamous epithelial cells (mucosal, cutaneous)	T cells	Hepatocytes	Vascular endothelial cells, lymphocytes	Kidney epithelial cells, others	Epidermal cells
Unique biology	May cause chronic infection and inflammation	Immortalizes B cells	Highly species and tissue specific, replication dependent on cell differentiation	Immortalizes T cells, encodes trans-acting factor	High rate of chronic infection and inflammation	Contains many cellular genes	Stimulates cell DNA synthesis	Species and tissue specific
Prevalence of infection	Chronic infections common—Asia, Africa	Common	Common	Common—Japan, Caribbean	Common	Not ubiquitous	—	—
Transmission	Vertical, parenteral, horizontal, venereal	Saliva	Venereal, skin abrasions	Breast milk, parenteral, venereal	Parenteral, horizontal	Horizontal, venereal	Urine?	Contact, venereal
Human diseases	Hepatitis, cirrhosis	IM, oral hairy leukoplakia	Skin warts, EV, genital warts, LP	HAM/TSP	Hepatitis, cirrhosis	—	—	—
Human cancers	HCC	BL,[b] NPC,[c] HD, lymphomas	Cervical, skin, oropharynx	ATL	HCC	KS, PEL, Castleman disease	Brain, bone, mesothelioma	MC
Transforming genes	HBx?	LMP-1	E6, E7	Tax?	NS3?	—	Large T-antigen, small t-antigen	—
Viral genome integrated in human tumors	Usually		Usually	Yes (provirus)	No	—	—	No

HBV, hepatitis B virus; EBV, Epstien–Barr virus; HPV, human papilloma virus; HTLV-1, human lymphotrophic virus-1; HCV, Hepatitis C virus; HHV-8, human herpes virus-8; SV40, simian virus 40; MCV, molluscum contagiosum virus; EV, echo virus; HD, Hodgkin disease; IM, infectious mononucleosis; KS, Kaposi sarcoma; LP, laryngeal papillomas; MC, molluscum contagiosum; PEL, primary effusion lymphoma; HAM/TSP, HTLV-1 associated myelopathy/tropical spartic paraparesis; BL, Burkitt lymphoma; NPC, nasopharyngeal carcinoma.

[a] Partially double-stranded (ds) and partially single-stranded (ss) in virion.
[b] Equatorial Africa = endemic; elsewhere = sporadic.
[c] Southeast Asia = common.
From Butel JS. Viral carcinogenesis: revelation of molecular mechanisms and etiology of human disease. *Carcinogenesis* 2000;21:415, with permission.

estrogen production in postmenopausal, obese women or may be exogenous, such as estrogen replacement therapy or sequential oral contraceptives.

Breast cancer and prostate cancer, the two most common malignancies in women and men in the United States, are generally hormonally dependent tumors. The role of estrogens in breast cancer has been established from epidemiologic and experimental studies. These studies have identified numerous risk factors for breast cancer that result in increased exposure to estrogen including early menarche, late menopause, obesity, alcohol consumption, and hormone replacement therapy. Epidemiologic studies have demonstrated that postmenopausal women who develop breast cancer have mean estradiol serum concentrations that are 15% higher than unaffected women. In addition, hormone replacement therapy in postmenopausal women has been shown to increase the risk of breast cancer. In the case of prostate cancer, higher levels of testosterone have been shown to increase the risk of developing prostate cancer.

Currently chemoprevention cancer therapies that target the production or action of endogenously circulating hormones are being utilized. The effectiveness of tamoxifen in reducing the risk of breast cancer in high risk patients has been demonstrated, and a trial to evaluate the efficacy of finasteride in reducing the incidence of prostate cancer is underway. Although the actual genes that contribute to the development of hormonally induced tumors are still unknown, several candidate genes have been identified that are involved in the production and transport of hormones. Identification of these genes may lead to new targets for cancer prevention therapies.

Immune System

The increased incidence of malignancies in patients following bone marrow or solid organ transplantation, as well as in patients with inherited or acquired immune deficiency syndrome (AIDS), suggests a role for the immune system in prevention of some malignancies. Many of the malignancies seen in immunocompromised individuals appeared to be virally induced.

Following bone marrow or solid organ transplantation there is a significant increase in a small number of malignancies. Several of these conditions appear to be virally induced malignancy that may respond to decreases in immunosuppressive therapy. Posttransplantation lymphoproliferative disorders and Hodgkin disease are related to EBV infection in the majority of cases. In addition, HHV-8 also appears to be a causative agent in the development of Kaposi sarcoma in patients following solid organ transplantation, with an incidence up to 500 times that of the general population. Although there is also an increased incidence of other solid tumors in patients following transplantation including skin cancer, oropharyngeal cancer, and bone cancer, the pathogenesis of these cancers, as well as the role of the immune system in preventing them, remains elusive.

Patients with HIV and AIDS have a significantly increased risk of developing several malignancies. In fact, three malignant conditions are now considered AIDS-defining illnesses in patients with HIV: Kaposi sarcoma, aggressive non-Hodgkin lymphomas (NHLs), and invasive cervical cancer. Viruses have been implicated in the pathogenesis of all three of these malignancies. HHV-8 has been shown to be a causative agent for all forms of Kaposi sarcoma. The majority of large B-cell and primary central nervous system lymphomas in HIV-infected patients are associated with EBV infection. In addition, persistent HPV infection is found in a greater number of HIV-infected women, which may account for the increased incidence of invasive cervical cancer in this population.

TUMOR PHENOTYPE

Although many genetic, environmental, and host factors influence the process of malignant transformation, not all cells that are exposed to these insults will become transformed. The majority of transforming events are lethal, and of the remaining cells that survive, many will undergo terminal differentiation or apoptosis. Tumors develop from a single transformed cell leading to a clonal population. These progeny inherit the same genetic alterations and growth characteristics of the parent cell. Transformed cells demonstrate many phenotypic, biochemical, and immunologic characteristics that are altered from normal cells (Fig. 4-3). These characteristics include changes in cell surface receptors and antigens, disordered cytoskeletal arrangements, nuclear and cellular polymorphism, karyotypic changes, and increased antigenicity.

Growth Characteristics

The growth of many tumors has been described by the idealized Gompertzian growth model, in which tumor growth proceeds exponentially with a shortening of the doubling time as the tumor enlarges. However, because exponential growth in tumors occurs only when nutrient availability is optimal, this growth generally occurs only in the early phases of tumor development. As tumors enlarge, they eventually outstrip their blood supply and source of nutrients. Therefore, tumors actually demonstrate a deceleration of growth in the latter stages of development (Fig. 4-4).

By the time a tumor becomes clinically apparent (1 cm in greatest dimension), it will have already undergone approximately 30 doublings to reach that size. To reach a lethal size of 1 kg, only 10 additional doublings are required. Therefore, the time during which a tumor is clinically detectable represents only a small fraction of the tumor's actual growth and history (Fig. 4-5).

The rate of tumor growth depends of three factors: tumor growth fraction, duration of the cell cycle, and the balance between cell proliferation and loss. The tumor growth fraction is the proportion of cells in a tumor mass that is cycling at a given time. Because tumors comprise heterogeneous cell populations, most of which are not dividing, the majority of cells are not part of the growth fraction. This growth fraction ranges from 4% to 24% for many solid tumors and varies during the duration of tumor development. A maximum growth fraction of 37% may be reached during early, exponential tumor growth.

The duration of the cell cycle and the balance between cell proliferation and loss are also important determinants of rate of tumor growth. The duration of the cell cycle is similar for most tumors, ranging from 2 to 4.5 days. However, it is the fate of cells completing the cell cycle that is significant. At the end of the cell cycle, cells may proceed through the cell cycle again, undergo programmed cell

[handwritten margin notes: "Effect of Hormone on Breast CA" and "HIV and Cancer"]

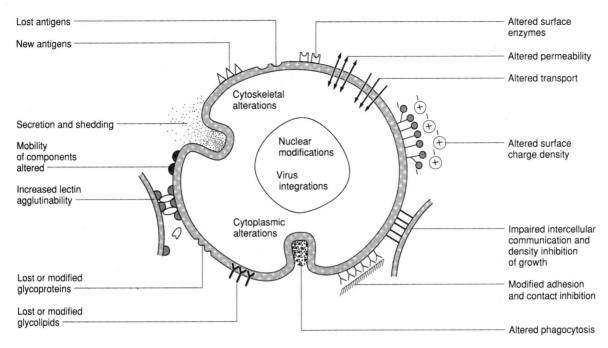

Figure 4-3   Alterations of cell structure and function that have been noted with neoplastic transformation. (From Ellis LM, Jones Jr DV, Chiao PJ, et al. Tumor biology. In: Greenfield LJ, Mulholland MW, Oldham KT et al., eds. *Surgery: scientific principles and practice*, 2nd ed. Philadelphia: Lippincott-Raven Publishers, 1997:465, with permission.)

death, enter a reversible quiescent phase, or reach a state of terminal differentiation. In neoplastic tissues, an imbalance between continued proliferation and cell loss or terminal differentiation occurs leading to a net positive balance and continued tumor growth.

Tumor Antigens

For many years it was thought that tumors did not generate antitumor immune responses and that manipulation of the immune system was not a viable approach to cancer therapy. However, in patients with melanoma, the identification of tumor-infiltrating lymphocytes (TILs) that demonstrated specific antitumor immune responses against autologous and allogeneic melanoma cells established the presence of tumor antigens that could be targeted by the cellular immune system. Numerous types of tumor antigens have been identified, which can be grouped into several categories: (i) antigens that are expressed in both normal and neoplastic cells derived from the same tissue but that elicit a host immune response only when expressed on tumor cells; (ii) antigens that are expressed only in immune-privileged areas of the testis and on certain neoplastic cells; (iii) antigens that are derived from the overexpression of certain genes or from gene mutations; (iv) antigens that are generated from oncoviral proteins; and (v) antigens that are

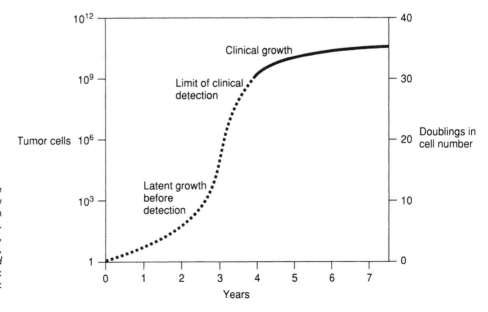

Figure 4-4   Theoretic growth curve for human tumors. Growth rates slow as tumors approach lethal mass. (From Ellis LM, Jones Jr DV, Chiao PJ, et al. Tumor biology. In: Greenfield LJ, Mulholland MW, Oldham KT et al., eds. *Surgery: scientific principles and practice*, 2nd ed. Philadelphia: Lippincott-Raven Publishers, 1997: 467, with permission.)

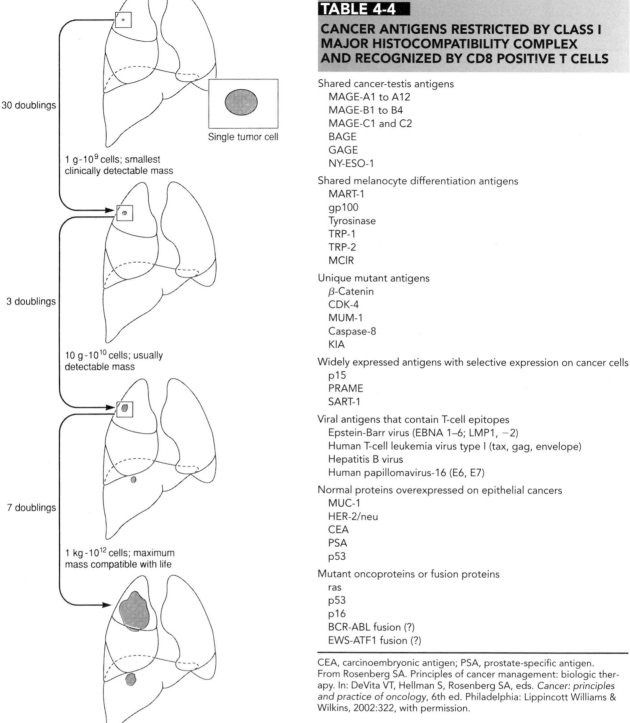

30 doublings

1 g - 10^9 cells; smallest clinically detectable mass

Single tumor cell

3 doublings

10 g - 10^{10} cells; usually detectable mass

7 doublings

1 kg - 10^{12} cells; maximum mass compatible with life

Figure 4-5 Growth of a solid tumor from a single transformed cell into a lethal tumor mass. (From Ellis LM, Jones Jr DV, Chiao PJ, et al. Tumor biology. In: Greenfield LJ, Mulholland MW, Oldham KT et al., eds. *Surgery: scientific principles and practice*, 2nd ed. Philadelphia: Lippincott-Raven Publishers, 1997:466, with permission.)

TABLE 4-4

CANCER ANTIGENS RESTRICTED BY CLASS I MAJOR HISTOCOMPATIBILITY COMPLEX AND RECOGNIZED BY CD8 POSITIVE T CELLS

Shared cancer-testis antigens
    MAGE-A1 to A12
    MAGE-B1 to B4
    MAGE-C1 and C2
    BAGE
    GAGE
    NY-ESO-1

Shared melanocyte differentiation antigens
    MART-1
    gp100
    Tyrosinase
    TRP-1
    TRP-2
    MCIR

Unique mutant antigens
    β-Catenin
    CDK-4
    MUM-1
    Caspase-8
    KIA

Widely expressed antigens with selective expression on cancer cells
    p15
    PRAME
    SART-1

Viral antigens that contain T-cell epitopes
    Epstein-Barr virus (EBNA 1–6; LMP1, −2)
    Human T-cell leukemia virus type I (tax, gag, envelope)
    Hepatitis B virus
    Human papillomavirus-16 (E6, E7)

Normal proteins overexpressed on epithelial cancers
    MUC-1
    HER-2/neu
    CEA
    PSA
    p53

Mutant oncoproteins or fusion proteins
    ras
    p53
    p16
    BCR-ABL fusion (?)
    EWS-ATF1 fusion (?)

CEA, carcinoembryonic antigen; PSA, prostate-specific antigen.
From Rosenberg SA. Principles of cancer management: biologic therapy. In: DeVita VT, Hellman S, Rosenberg SA, eds. *Cancer: principles and practice of oncology*, 6th ed. Philadelphia: Lippincott Williams & Wilkins, 2002:322, with permission.

---

oncofetal proteins that are overexpressed in neoplastic tissues (Tables 4-4 and 4-5). Immunotherapy strategies that target these specific tumor antigens are being developed in an effort to generate high levels of specific antitumor reactivity.

There are numerous examples of these different tumor antigens. MART-1/MelanA is a tumor antigen that is expressed on both normal melanocytes and melanoma cells, and it is the most common antitumor reactivity found in patients with melanoma. The *MAGE* gene family, comprising at least 12 genes, is an example of genes that are expressed only in the testis and on neoplastic cells. The proteins produced by the expression of these genes have been identified as tumor antigens in patients with melanoma, as well as in patients with breast, prostate, esophageal, lung, and colon carcinoma. Some genes, such as the *HER2/neu*

TABLE 4-5

CANCER ANTIGENS RESTRICTED BY CLASS II MAJOR HISTOCOMPATIBILITY COMPLEX AND RECOGNIZED BY CD4-POSITIVE TUMOR-INFILTRATING LYMPHOCYTES

Antigens	HLA Restrictions	Peptides
Tyrosine	HLA-DR4	QNILLSNAPLGPQFP (56–70)
	HLA-DR4	SYLQDSDPDSFQD (448–462)
	HLA-DR15	FILHHAFVDSIFEQWLQRHRP (386–406)
	HLA-DR4	EIWRDIDFAHE (193–203)
gp100	HLA-DR4	WNRQLYPEWTEAQRLD (44–59)
MAGE-3	HLA-DR11	TSYVKVLHHMVKISG (281–295)
	HLA-DR13	AELVHFLLLKYRAR (114–127)
	HLA-DR13	FLLLKYRAREPVTKAE (119–134)
TPI	HLA-DR1	GELIGILNAAKVPAD (23–37)
LDFP	HLA-DR1	PVIWRRAPA (312–323)
	HLA-DR1	WRRAPAPGA (315–323)
CDC27	HLA-DR4	FSWAMDLDPKGA (760–771)

From Rosenberg SA. Principles of cancer management: biologic therapy. In: DeVita VT, Hellman S, Rosenberg SA, eds. *Cancer: principles and practice of oncology*, 6th ed. Philadelphia: Lippincott Williams & Wilkins, 2002:323, with permission.

gene, which is overexpressed in breast cancer, and the *p53* gene, which is mutated in more than 50% of human malignancies, have been shown to generate antitumor immune responses. Oncoviral proteins, such as the E6 and E7 proteins generated by HPV, act as tumor antigens. Finally, examples of oncofetal proteins that act as tumor antigens are carcinoembryonic antigen (CEA) in colon cancer and α-fetoprotein (AFP) in hepatocellular carcinoma.

Tumor Microenvironment

The tumor microenvironment plays an important role in the development of the tumor phenotype. In this microenvironment there are complex interactions between tumor cells, stromal cells, endothelial cells, and the extracellular matrix (ECM) that drive tumor growth, invasion, and metastasis. These interactions result in changes in the production and response to growth factors, lead to decreased apoptosis, and stimulate angiogenesis.

Growth Factors and Apoptosis

The uncontrolled cellular proliferation that is seen in tumors results from a combination of activation of growth stimulatory signals, evasion of growth inhibitory and differentiation signals, and avoidance of apoptosis. Tumor cells develop autonomous growth-signaling mechanisms that circumvent normal growth controls. Many oncogene products have been identified that are involved in growth-signaling pathways including growth factors, growth factor receptors, or intracellular mitogenic signal transduction molecules. These oncogenes induce cellular proliferation by autonomous production of growth factors with autocrine stimulation, overexpression of growth factor receptors, expression of constitutively active growth factor receptors, and deregulation of intracellular, mitogenic, signal

transduction pathways. One example of this is the HER2/neu growth factor receptor that is overexpressed in breast cancer and ovarian cancer and that has been shown to be associated with recurrence and poor outcomes.

In addition to growth stimulatory signals, tumor cells develop mechanisms that block growth inhibitory and differentiation signals. The most commonly affected growth inhibitory pathway is the pRb pathway, which controls the majority of cellular antiproliferative signals. When pRb is in a hypophosphorylated state, cell progression from G1 to S phase is blocked by interaction of pRb with the E2F transcription factor. This prevents cellular proliferation. The pRb pathway may be affected in multiple ways including direct mutation of the *Rb* gene, sequestering of pRb by viral oncoproteins, mutations or alterations in the expression of cyclin-dependent kinases that phosphorylate and inhibit pRb, and decreased production of transforming growth factor β (TGF-β) or TGF-β receptors that block phosphorylation of pRb. In addition, cells may downregulate cell surface receptors such as integrins that produce growth inhibitory signals, favoring cell proliferation.

Although normal tissue growth is controlled through balanced cell proliferation and attrition, tumor cells develop mechanisms to evade apoptosis in response to intracellular and extracellular abnormalities such as DNA damage, activation of oncogenes, and hypoxia. These mechanisms include increased expression of antiapoptotic proteins, such as members of the Bcl-2 family, and mutations in genes involved in the apoptotic pathway, such as *p53*. The *p53* tumor-suppressor gene is involved in apoptosis through upregulation of proapoptotic proteins in response to DNA damage. This gene is mutated in more than 50% of all human malignancies and is one of the most common ways in which tumor cells develop resistance to apoptosis.

Angiogenesis

The importance of angiogenesis in tumor growth and metastasis was recognized more than 30 years ago, on the basis of the observation that the delivery of nutrients and growth factors to sustain tumor growth and development requires proximity to blood vessels. Therefore, without neovascularization, tumors fail to grow beyond a small size or to metastasize. Numerous endogenous proangiogenic and antiangiogenic factors have been identified, and it is the balance between these factors that is thought to be important in controlling angiogenesis (Tables 4-6 and 4-7). At some point during tumor development, an "angiogenic switch" occurs, which tips the balance in favor of proangiogenic factors. This may result from an increase in proangiogenic factors such as vascular endothelial growth factor (VEGF) or basic fibroblast growth factor (bFGF), or from a decrease in antiangiogenic factors such as thrombospondin-1 (TSP-1). The end result is neovascularization leading to tumor growth and metastasis.

Because of the importance of angiogenesis in tumor progression and the numerous angiogenic targets that have been identified, antiangiogenic cancer therapies are currently under investigation. These agents function by either inhibiting proangiogenic factors (e.g., anti-VEGF antibodies) or increasing antiangiogenic factors (e.g., angiostatin and endostatin). Multiple clinical trials investigating a variety of these antiangiogenic agents are ongoing (Table 4-8).

TABLE 4-6

PROANGIOGENIC GROWTH FACTORS

Factor	Properties	Receptor	Study
Vascular endothelial growth factor—vascular permeability factor	Endothelial mitogen, survival factor, and permeability inducer produced by many types of tumor cells	Flk-1/KDR (VEGFR-2), Flt-1 (VEGFR-1) (both present on activated endothelium)	Veikkola et al. (2000)
Placental growth factor	Weak endothelial mitogen	Flt-1 (VEGFR-1)	Veikkola et al. (2000)
Basic fibroblast growth factor (bFGF/FGF-2)	Endothelial mitogen, angiogenesis inducer, and survival factor; inducer of Flk-1 expression	FGF-R1–4	Baird and Klagsbrun, (1991) Gimenez-Gallego and Cuevas (1994)
Acidic fibroblast growth factor (aFGF/FGF-1)	Endothelial mitogen and angiogenesis inducer	FGF-R1–4	Baird and Klagsbrun, (1991) Gimenez-Gallego and Cuevas (1994)
Fibroblast growth factor 3 (FGF-3/*int*-2)	Endothelial mitogen and angiogenesis inducer	FGF-R1–4	Baird and Klagsbrun, (1991) Gimenez-Gallego and Cuevas (1991)
Fibroblast growth factor 4 (FGF-4/*hst*/K-FGF)	Endothelial mitogen and angiogenesis inducer	FGF-R1–4	Baird and Klagsbrun, Gimenez-Gallego and Cuevas (1991)
Transforming growth factor-α (TGF-α)	Endothelial mitogen and angiogenesis inducer; inducer of vascular endothelial growth factor expression	Epidermal growth factor-R	Schmitt and Soares (1999)
Epidermal growth factor (EGF)	Weak endothelial mitogen; inducer of vascular endothelial growth factor expression	Epidermal growth factor-R	Mooradian and Diglio (1990)
Hepatocyte growth factor/scatter factor (HGF/SF)	Endothelial mitogen, motogen, and angiogenesis inducer	c-Met	Lamszus et al. (1999)
Transforming growth factor-β (TGF-β)	*In vivo*—acting angiogenesis inducer; endothelial growth inhibitor; inducer of vascular endothelial growth factor expression	Transforming growth factor-β–RI, II, III	Pepper (1997)
Tumor necrosis factor-α (TNF-α)	*In vivo*—acting angiogenesis inducer; endothelial mitogen (low concentrations) or inhibitor (at high concentrations); inducer of vascular endothelial growth factor expression	TNF-R55	Yoshida et al. (1997)
Platelet-derived growth factor	Mitogen and motility factor for endothelial cells and fibroblasts; *in vivo*—acting angiogenesis inducer	Platelet-derived growth factor-R	Kuwabara et al. (1995)
Granulocyte colony-stimulating factor	*In vivo*—acting angiogenesis-inducing factor with some mitogenic and motogenic activity for endothelial cells	Granulocyte colony-stimulating factor	Bussolino et al. (1991)
Interleukin-8	*In vivo*—acting, possibly indirect angiogenesis inducer	Interleukin-8R presence on endothelial cells remains uncertain	Desbaillets et al. (1997)
Pleiotropin	Angiogenesis-inducing pleiotropic growth factor	Proteoglycan	Choudhuri et al. (1997)
Thymidine phosphorylase (TP)–platelet-derived endothelial cell growth factor (PD-ECGF)	*In vivo*—acting angiogenesis factor	Unknown	Takahashi et al. (1996)
Angiogenin	*In vivo*—acting angiogenesis inducer with RNAse activity	170-kD angiogenin receptor	Hartmann et al. (1999)
Proliferin	35-kD a angiogenesis-inducing protein in mouse	Unknown	Jackson et al. (1994)

From Fidler IJ, Kerbel RS, Ellis LM. Biology of cancer: angiogenesis. In: DeVita VT, Hellman S, Rosenberg SA, eds. *Cancer: principles and practice of oncology*, 6th ed. Philadelphia: Lippincott Williams & Wilkins, 2002:139, with permission.

TABLE 4-7

SOME ENDOGENOUS INHIBITORS OF ANGIOGENESIS

Name	Description	Study
Thrombospondin-1 and internal fragments of thrombospondin-1	Large, modular (180-kD) extracellular matrix protein	Tolsma et al. (1993)
Angiostatin	38-kD a fragment of plasminogen involving either kringle domains 1–3 or smaller kringle 5 fragments	O'Reilly et al. (1994)
Endostatin	20-kD a zinc-binding fragment of type XVIII collagen	O'Reilly et al. (1997)
Vasostatin	NH_2 terminal fragment (amino acids 1–80) of calreticulin	Pike et al. (1998)
Vascular endothelial growth factor inhibitor	174-amino acid protein with 20%–30% homology to tumor necrosis factor superfamily	Zhai et al. (1999)
Fragment of platelet factor-4	N-terminal fragment of platelet factor-4	Gupta et al. (1995)
Derivative of prolactin	16-kD fragment of prolactin	Clapp et al. (1993)
Restin	NC10 domain of human collagen XV	Ramchandran et al. (1999)
Proliferin-related protein	Protein related to the proangiogenic molecule proliferin	Jackson et al. (1994)
SPARC cleavage product	Fragments of secreted protein, acidic and rich in cysteine	Vasquez (1999)
Osteopontin cleavage product	Thrombin-generated fragment containing an RGD sequence	Sage (1999)
Interferon-α-β	Well-known antiviral proteins, may downregulate angiogenic factor expression	Ezekowitz et al. (1992)
METH-1 and METH-2	Proteins containing metalloprotease and thrombospondin domains, and disintegrin domains in NH_2 termini	Vasquez (1999), Sage (1999)
Angiopoietin-2	Antagonist of angiopoietin-I that binds to Tie-2 receptor	Davis and Yankopoulos (1999), Maisonpierre et al. (1997)
Antithrombin III fragment	A fragment missing the carboxy-terminal loop of antithrombin III (a member of the serpin family)	O'Reilly et al. (1999)
Interferon-inducible protein-10	Up-regulated by IFN-γ and whose mechanism of antiangiogenic effect is unknown	Moore et al. (1998)

From Fidler IJ, Kerbel RS, Ellis LM. Biology of cancer: angiogenesis. In: DeVita VT, Hellman S, Rosenberg SA, eds. *Cancer: principles and practice of oncology*, 6th ed. Philadelphia: Lippincott Williams & Wilkins, 2002:141, with permission.

TABLE 4-8

INHIBITORS OF ANGIOGENESIS IN VARIOUS STAGES OF CLINICAL TRIALS IN CANCER

Agent	Sponsor	Mechanism	Location
Phase 1			
SU6668	Sugen	Inhibition of receptor signaling	South San Francisco, CA
Angiostatin	EntreMed	Inhibition of endothelial proliferation	Rockville, MD
Endostatin	EntreMed	Inhibition of endothelial proliferation	Rockville, MD
Combretastatin	Oxigene	Stimulation of endothelial apoptosis	Watertown, MA
ZD6474	AstraZeneca	Inhibition of VEGFR-2	Wilmington, DE
Phase 2			
CAI	National Cancer Institute	Inhibition of calcium influx	Bethesda, MD
COL-3	Collagenex	Inhibition of matrix metalloproteinases	Newtown, PA
Squalamine	Geneara	Inhibition of sodium/hydrogen ion exchange	Plymouth Meeting, PA
TNP-470	TAP Pharmaceutical Products, Inc	Inhibition of endothelial proliferation	Lake Forest, IL
Interleukin-12	Wyeth	Inhibition of interferon-γ	Madison, NJ
Prinomastat	Pfizer	Inhibition of matrix metalloproteinases	New York, NY
Phase 3			
Bevacizumab	Genentech	Inhibition of VEGF	South San Francisco, CA
IMC-ICII	ImClone	Inhibition of VEGFR-2	New York, NY
Marimastat	British Biotech	Inhibition of matrix metalloproteinases	Oxford, UK
SU5416	Sugen	Inhibition of VEGFR-2	South San Francisco, CA

VEGF, vascular endothelial growth factor; VEGFR, vascular endothelial growth factor receptor.
From Folkman J. Role of angiogenesis in tumor growth and metastasis. *Semin Oncol* 2002;29:16, with permission.

Invasion and Metastasis

Tumors consist of heterogeneous populations of cells that vary in their growth rates, production of growth factors, stimulation of angiogenesis, and receptor expression. In addition, these heterogeneous cell populations have different propensities to metastasize. Although angiogenesis functions as a key component of tumor growth by providing oxygen and nutrients for continued cellular proliferation, it is also an important factor in invasion and metastasis, providing the route for tumor cells to escape their local environment and settle at distant sites. The hallmark of the invasive phenotype is the ability to disrupt and traverse the basement membrane. In order to develop this phenotype, several additional characteristics must be acquired by tumor cells that result in changes in cell–cell adhesions, changes in cell–ECM interactions, and disruption of the ECM.

Several classes of cell surface proteins are involved in cell–cell adhesions and cell–ECM interactions including the cell adhesion molecules (CAMs) of the cadherin, immunoglobulin, and integrin superfamilies. Changes in cell surface expression of these receptors enable tumor cells to invade the stromal compartment and to eventually metastasize. One important cell surface receptor, the function of which is lost in numerous epithelial cancers is epithelial cadherin (E-cadherin). E-Cadherin is a transmembrane glycoprotein that mediates homotypic cell–cell adhesions and functions through cytoplasmic interaction with B-catenin to produce antigrowth signals that suppress invasion and metastasis. Several mechanisms are involved in disrupting the function of E-cadherin, including mutational inactivation of the E-cadherin or B-catenin genes, transcriptional repression by hypermethylation, and proteolytic modification of the extracellular domain. It is of interest to note that a germ-line mutation in E-cadherin has been linked to an inherited gastric cancer syndrome.

In addition to changes in cell–cell adhesions, changes in the interaction between tumor cells and ECM are also necessary for tumor invasion and metastasis. Integrins play an important role in this process as tumor cells encounter changing microenvironments during invasion and metastasis. The changing integrin profile on the surface of a tumor cell may favor invasion into the degraded ECM in some cases, whereas a completely different set of integrin receptors may be required for extravasation to produce metastases.

In addition to changes in CAMs, acquisition of the invasive phenotype requires activation of extracellular proteases that degrade the ECM and disrupt basement membranes. Matrix metalloproteinases (MMPs) make up one family of proteases that plays a key role in matrix degradation, thereby allowing for tumor cell motility. These proteases exert their effects in several ways including the degradation of cell surface adhesion molecules such as E-cadherin or CD44, which is a cell–matrix adhesion molecule, or by degradation of structural proteins within basement membranes. This process of ECM degradation requires a balance between prodegradative factors and inhibitors of degradation to provide the optimal environment for tumor cell migration.

Once tumor cells have developed the invasive phenotype, intravasation into vascular or lymph vessels is possible and may result in regional or distant metastases. Although a significant number of tumor cells may enter the circulation, only a small fraction (<0.1%) will survive to produce metastatic disease, since there are many sequential steps that tumor cells must follow and barriers to metastasis that are encountered (Fig. 4-6). There are two theories as to the organ distribution of metastases for various malignancies. The first is the "seed" and "soil" hypothesis proposed by Paget in 1889. On the basis of the organ distribution of specific metastases, Paget concluded that metastatic disease does not occur by chance and that specific tumors metastasize to specific organs where the microenvironment is favorable and compatible. A second hypothesis for the distribution of metastatic disease was proposed by J. Ewing who attributed the distribution mainly to mechanical and anatomic factors such as the structure of the vascular system. There is support for both of these theories. For example, colorectal cancer generally metastasizes to the regional lymph nodes first and then to the liver, as a result of the draining lymphatics and venous drainage of the colon. In the case of ocular melanoma, however, metastases are generally found in the liver with not a clear lymphatic or hematogenous relationship.

TREATMENT MODALITIES

Historically, surgical resection was the only effective treatment for cancer cure. Therefore, surgeons developed and performed radical surgical procedures in an effort to completely eradicate disease (Table 4-9). However, a more complete understanding of the biology of cancer and patterns of metastasis, the realization that micrometastatic disease may still be present after surgical resection, and advances in surgical technique have shifted the focus of cancer treatment away from radical surgical resection in favor of multimodality therapy, including less extensive surgery in combination with chemotherapy, radiation therapy, immunotherapy, and newer modalities such as gene therapy. Combining these therapeutic modalities has decreased the morbidity and mortality associated with radical surgical procedures while maintaining similar overall survival and has improved the quality of life for cancer patients.

Principles of Surgical Oncology

Surgical oncologists play an important role in the management of cancer patients. This role includes surgical interventions for staging, cancer prevention, definitive resection, treatment of metastatic disease, and palliation. In addition, it is necessary for surgical oncologist to have an understanding of tumor biology and the use of multimodality therapy for cancer treatment to plan appropriate surgical procedures based on the extent of disease and the clinical status of the patient.

The role of surgical oncologists in the diagnosis and staging of malignancies has decreased with the development of sensitive cross-sectional imaging techniques, nuclear imaging modalities, and minimally invasive diagnostic techniques such as core biopsy. For example, core biopsy of breast masses and soft tissue tumors has taken the place of operative incisional or excisional biopsy, except in cases where nondiagnostic results are obtained using needle biopsy techniques. There are multiple genetic and medical conditions that have a high incidence of cancer

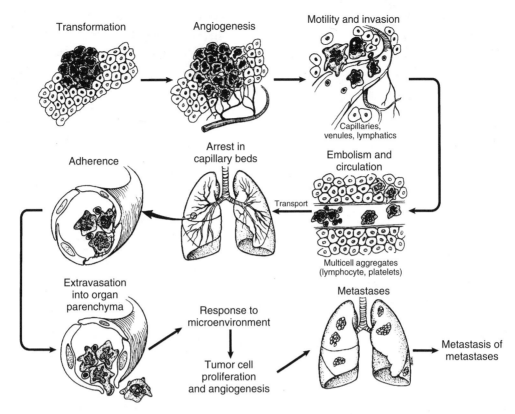

Figure 4-6 The pathogenesis of cancer metastasis. To produce metastases, tumor cells must detach from the primary tumor, invade the extracellular membrane and enter the circulation, survive in the circulation to arrest in the capillary bed, adhere to subendothelial basement membrane, gain entrance into the organ parenchyma, respond to paracrine growth factors, proliferate and induce angiogenesis, and evade host defenses. The pathogenesis of metastasis is, therefore, complex and consists of multiple sequential, selective, and interdependent steps the outcome of which depends on the interaction of tumor cells with homeostatic factors. (From Stetler-Stevenson WG. Invasion and metastases. In: DeVita VT, Hellman S, Rosenberg SA, eds. *Cancer: principles and practice of oncology*, 7th ed. Philadelphia: Lippincott Williams & Wilkins, 2005:117, with permission.)

development in which the surgical oncologist may play a role in cancer prevention by resection of nonvital organs. Examples of these conditions include familial adenomatous polyposis coli and ulcerative colitis, which often require total colectomy, and familial breast cancer syndromes, which in some cases may be managed with prophylactic mastectomy. Additional conditions in which surgeons play a role in cancer prevention are listed in Table 4-10.

The principal role of surgical oncologists remains surgical resection for primary cancers. In addition to providing local control, surgery allows for confirmation of histologic diagnosis, staging of tumors (which may be necessary to guide postoperative adjuvant therapy), and tumor debulking (cytoreductive surgery) prior to the initiation of other treatment modalities. There are numerous cases in which surgical resection may be the only necessary intervention. Examples include wide local excision for low-risk patients with thin melanoma, partial colectomy for patients with stages I and II colon cancer, and total thyroidectomy for patients with papillary thyroid carcinoma. In other cases, surgical resection may reveal metastasis to regional lymph nodes, which may necessitate the use of adjuvant chemotherapy, as in patients with stage III colon cancer. The key for surgical oncologists is to thoroughly evaluate patients preoperatively to determine the extent of local and metastatic disease and to understand the role for and efficacy of other treatment modalities for various malignancies.

In addition to surgical resection for primary cancers, cancer patients may also be candidates for surgery for resection of metastatic disease, for palliation, or in for surgical emergencies. Hepatic resection for isolated colorectal liver metastases has been shown to significantly improve 5-year survival, and the resection of pulmonary sarcoma metastases has been shown to lead to cure rates of up to 30%. Surgical oncologists may also be able to provide palliation through surgery by relief of chronic intestinal obstruction or by the removal of large tumors causing significant discomfort. In addition, cancer patients may require surgical intervention for surgical emergencies including obstruction, hemorrhage, or perforation.

Numerous advances in technology and surgical technique have been made in the field of surgical oncology and have resulted in a changing role for the surgical oncologist in the management of cancer patients. These advances include the use of diagnostic laparoscopy, intraoperative ultrasonography, and regional therapies for metastatic disease. One of the most notable developments in the last decade is sentinel mapping and lymphadenectomy for patients with breast cancer and melanoma. In the case of

TABLE 4-9

**SELECTED HISTORICAL MILESTONES
IN SURGICAL ONCOLOGY**

Year	Surgeon	Event
1809	Ephraim McDowell	Elective abdominal surgery (excised ovarian tumor)
1846	John Collins Warren	Use of ether anesthesia (excised submaxillary gland)
1867	Joseph Lister	Introduction of antisepsis
1860–1890	Albert Theodore Billroth	First gastrectomy, laryngectomy, and esophagectomy
1878	Richard von Volkmann	Excision of cancerous rectum
1880s	Theodore Kocher	Development of thyroid surgery
1890	William Stewart Halsted	Radical mastectomy
1896	G. T. Beatson	Oophorectomy for breast cancer
1904	Hugh H. Young	Radical prostatectomy
1906	Ernest Wertheim	Radical hysterectomy
1908	W. Ernest Miles	Abdomenoperineal resection for rectal cancer
1912	E. Martin	Cordotomy for the treatment of pain
1910–1930	Harvey Cushing	Development of surgery for brain tumors
1913	Franz Torek	Successful resection of cancer of the thoracic esophagus
1927	G. Divis	Successful resection of pulmonary metastases
1933	Evarts Graham	Pneumonectomy
1935	A. O. Whipple	Pancreaticoduodenectomy
1945	Charles B. Huggins	Adrenalectomy for prostate cancer
1958	Bernard Fisher	Organization of NSABP to conduct prospective randomized trials

NSABP, National Surgical Adjuvant Breast and Bowel Project.
From Rosenberg SA. Principles of cancer management: surgical oncology. In: DeVita VT, Hellman S, Rosenberg SA, eds. *Cancer: principles and practice of oncology*, 6th ed. Philadelphia: Lippincott Williams & Wilkins, 2002:254, with permission.

TABLE 4-10

**CONDITIONS IN WHICH PROPHYLACTIC
SURGERY CAN PREVENT CANCER**

Underlying Condition	Associated Cancer	Prophylactic Surgery
Cryptorchidism	Testicular	Orchiopexy
Polyposis coli	Colon	Colectomy
Familial colon cancer	Colon	Colectomy
Ulcerative colitis	Colon	Colectomy
Multiple endocrine neoplasia types 2 and 3	Medullary cancer of the thyroid	Thyroidectomy
Familial breast cancer	Breast	Mastectomy
Familial ovarian cancer	Ovary	Oophorectomy

From Rosenberg SA. Principles of cancer management: surgical oncology. In: DeVita VT, Hellman S, Rosenberg SA, eds. *Cancer: principles and practice of oncology*, 6th ed. Philadelphia: Lippincott Williams & Wilkins, 2002:259, with permission.

the number of sphincter-sparing procedures that can be performed, thereby eliminating the need for a permanent ostomy and improving quality of life considerably. In the case of patients with large breast cancers, neoadjuvant therapy may increase the frequency of successful breast conservation therapy.

Principles of Chemotherapy

The use of chemotherapeutic agents in the clinical setting as the primary treatment for cancer began in the 1940s, when it was noted that exposure to alkylating agents led to significant myelosuppression. The subsequent use of these agents in patients with lymphoid and hematologic malignancies produced dramatic tumor regression, even in advanced cases. Complete cancer cures using chemotherapy alone were first noted in the 1960s, when combination chemotherapy was used to treat childhood leukemias and Hodgkin disease. The successful treatment of these lymphoid and hematologic malignancies led to the application of chemotherapy to the treatment of patients with solid tumors with variable success. Chemotherapy, with surgical resection and radiation therapy, has become one of the three major modalities currently used to treat cancer.

Chemotherapeutic agents target those tumor cells that are actively proliferating. Because most cells within a solid tumor are quiescent, however, only a small proportion of tumor cells will be susceptible to a chemotherapeutic agent at any given time. In addition, although tumors start out as a clonal proliferation of cells, mutations during tumor growth lead to subpopulations of tumor cells that may be variably sensitive to different chemotherapeutic agents. There are numerous mechanisms for the development of drug resistance. One inherent mechanism is the multidrug resistance gene, which encodes a membrane glycoprotein that extrudes various chemotherapeutic agents from the cell.

Because solid tumors contain so many cells (10^{10} to 10^{12}), even under perfect conditions, with a 100% tumor growth fraction and no inherent or acquired drug resistance, elimination of greater that 99.9999% of a tumor

melanoma, this minimally invasive staging technique has replaced the sporadic use of elective lymph node dissection and has allowed for more complete staging in this group of patients. For breast cancer patients, this procedure has decreased the need for axillary lymph node dissection (ALND) in the considerable number of node-negative patients with stages I and II disease, thereby avoiding the morbidity associated with that procedure. Several regional therapies have also been developed for the treatment of colorectal liver metastases including hepatic arterial infusion pumps and radiofrequency ablation.

The use of neoadjuvant therapy has also changed the surgical approach to several malignancies by increasing the number of patients who are candidates for surgical resection and by decreasing the extent of surgical procedures. For example, in the case of rectal cancer, the use of preoperative chemotherapy and radiation therapy has increased (a 5-log kill), although leading to a complete clinical remission, will still leave enough viable tumor cells to generate a recurrence. Because chemotherapeutic agents are not selective for neoplastic cells, normal proliferating cells will also be adversely affected by these agents. The normal cells that are most affected are those with the highest growth rates and turnover, namely the gut mucosa, hair follicles, and bone marrow.

Most chemotherapeutic agents have a dose-response curve and known toxicities. These agents are dosed to maximize tumor cell kill while taking into account the clinical status of the patient, prior response to agents, and development of toxicities. The interval between doses is determined by the amount of time necessary for recovery of normal tissues that are also affected by these agents. Myelosuppression is the most common side effect of chemotherapeutic agents. For the majority of drugs a nadir is reached 2 weeks after administration with an additional 2 weeks required for full recovery. Multidrug treatment regimens using drugs with different actions and toxicity profiles are generally used to maximize cancer cell death while limiting toxicities. In addition, these multidrug regimens may target tumor cells with different resistance profiles. Table 4-11 lists some common chemotherapeutic agents, the tumors in which they have efficacy, and their dose-limiting toxicities.

The timing for delivery of chemotherapeutic agents varies according to the clinical situation and the goals of treatment. Chemotherapy administered to patients as the primary treatment for metastatic disease is known as induction or primary chemotherapy. The goal of this treatment is generally not cure, but to control tumor growth and to improve quality of life. Chemotherapy delivered following another treatment modality such as local surgical resection or radiation therapy is known as adjuvant chemotherapy. The goal of adjuvant chemotherapy is to target micrometastatic disease in patients with a high risk of tumor recurrence following another treatment modality. For example, postoperative adjuvant therapy in patients with stage III colon cancer using 5-fluorouracil and leucovorin has been shown to improve 5-year survival rates. When chemotherapeutic agents are used as the primary modality for cancer cure or prior to administration of a different treatment modality, this is known as neoadjuvant therapy. Prior to local surgical resection, the goal of neoadjuvant therapy is generally to decrease tumor size preoperatively to allow for a less extensive surgical resection. In addition, the efficacy of a particular chemotherapeutic regimen may be determined by response of the primary tumor and may lend support for continued use of a regimen postoperatively to treat additional micrometastases. Table 4-12 lists numerous malignancies in which neoadjuvant therapy plays an important role.

Although the majority of chemotherapeutic agents are administered systemically by intravenous infusion, several regional infusion strategies have been developed. These regional approaches allow for increased doses of a drug to be administered while limiting systemic toxicities. Hepatic arterial infusion therapy for the treatment of colorectal liver metastases has been evaluated in numerous studies, and while response rates are significantly higher that systemic chemotherapy, the overall survival benefit has been marginal. Another example is the use of regional infusion therapy for metastatic melanoma isolated to the extremities. Isolated limb perfusion using melphalan and moderate hyperthermia in this clinical situation has been shown to produce complete response rates of up to 50% to 90%.

Principles of Radiation Therapy

Ionizing radiation is one of the primary treatment modalities for cancer. The energy that is absorbed by tissues that are irradiated leads to ionization of various molecules that have direct and indirect effects on the cell, leading to cell death. The direct effects of ionizing radiation occur through induction of double-stranded DNA breaks, which prevent cell replication. Indirect effects are seen through the generation of free radical species that further damage DNA and other intracellular molecules.

The two principal methods by which radiation is delivered to patients are brachytherapy and teletherapy. With brachytherapy, the source of radiation is placed within or adjacent to the target tissue. This is accomplished by the use of catheters that are loaded with different radioactive isotopes. Concentrated doses of radiation will be delivered immediately surrounding the catheters, as the dose delivered is inversely proportional to the distance squared from the source of the radiation. Therefore, normal tissues will be significantly spared. Examples of brachytherapy include the use of intrauterine devices for cervical cancer and the placement of brachytherapy catheters in the tumor bed following the removal of sarcomas to improve local control. With teletherapy, the source of radiation is outside the patient and is delivered as a high-energy electromagnetic beam. Delivery of radiation by this method can be modified by the use of filters and collimators to focus the radiation source on the target tissue while maximally sparing surrounding tissues.

Tumor cells are variably sensitive to the effects of ionizing radiation according to their oxygen status and stage in the cell cycle (Fig. 4-7). Those tumor cells that are well-oxygenated will be more susceptible to the effects of ionizing radiation, since the generation of oxygen free radicals is one of the ways in which ionizing radiation produces it effects. Pharmacologic modifiers have been used to increase the sensitivity of cells to ionizing radiation. Nitroimidazole compounds can substitute for oxygen and sensitize hypoxic cells, and halogenated pyrimidines when incorporated into DNA increase the sensitivity of cells to radiation. Hyperbaric oxygen treatment has also been used to increase the sensitivity of tumor cells. In addition to varying susceptibilities based on oxygen status, it has also been shown that those cells that are in the mitotic phase of the cell cycle are most susceptible to the effects of ionizing radiation.

Radiation survival curves are used to describe the sensitivity of cells to ionizing radiation (Fig. 4-8). These curves have a shallow initial slope, which represents the ability of a particular cell to recover from sublethal doses of radiation. Clinical doses of radiation are generally along the steeper slope of the radiation survival curve. Ionizing radiation is usually delivered in a series of smaller doses known as fractionation. This method of delivery has two main advantages over delivery of larger single or multiple doses. First, normal tissues have time to recover from sublethal doses of radiation and can repopulate. Second,

TABLE 4-11
PRIMARY CHEMOTHERAPY

Drug	Indication	Toxicities
Alkylating agents: transfer alkyl groups to nucleic acids and other biologically important molecules		
Busulfan	Chronic myelogenous leukemia, myeloproliferative disorders	Myelosuppression, pulmonary fibrosis, gonadal dysfunction, marrow failure
Chlorambucil	Chronic lymphocytic leukemia, Waldenström macroglobulinemia	Myelosuppression, gonadal dysfunction, secondary leukemia
Cyclophosphamide	Hematologic malignancies, Hodgkin disease, non-Hodgkin lymphomas, carcinomas of the breast and ovary, sarcomas, small cell lung cancer, pediatric malignancies	Leukopenia, cystitis, nausea and vomiting, alopecia, cardiac necrosis, gonadal dysfunction, SIADH
Ifosfamide	Carcinomas of the breast, ovaries, lung, testicles; lymphomas; sarcomas	Myelosuppression, cystitis, nephrotoxicity, hepatotoxicity, lethargy and confusion
Dacarbazine	Hodgkin disease, non-Hodgkin lymphomas, melanoma, sarcomas	Nausea and vomiting, flu-like syndrome, myelosuppression, hepatotoxicity
Cisplatin	Carcinomas of the ovary, testis, cervix, head and neck, bladder, lung (small and non–small cell), esophagus; lymphomas	Nausea and vomiting, nephrotoxicity, neurotoxicity, hearing loss, electrolyte imbalance
Carboplatin	Carcinoma of the ovary; bone marrow transplantation	Myelosuppression, nausea and vomiting
Melphalan	Multiple myeloma, ovarian cancer	Myelosuppression, anorexia, nausea and vomiting
Mechlorethamine	Lymphomas, Hodgkin disease	Myelosuppression, secondary leukemia, severe vesicant, nausea and vomiting, alopecia, rash, gonadal dysfunction, neurotoxicity
Nitrosoureas (Carmustine, BCNU; lomustine, CCNU)	Lymphomas, Hodgkin disease, brain cancer, bone marrow transplantation	Myelosuppression, secondary leukemia, hepatotoxicity, pulmonary fibrosis, nausea and vomiting, nephrotoxicity, confusion
Streptozocin	Neuroendocrine tumors	Nephrotoxicity, nausea and vomiting, myelosuppression, hepatotoxicity, hypoglycemia
Procarbazine	Hodgkin disease, lymphomas, brain cancer	Myelosuppression, monoamine oxidase inhibition, nausea and vomiting, lethargy, myalgias, arthralgias, neurotoxicity, dermatitis
Mitomycin C	Carcinomas of the breast, lung, gastrointestinal tract, cervix, bladder	Myelosuppression, severe vesicant, weakness, anorexia, hemolytic anemia, renal insufficiency, nausea and vomiting
Antimetabolites: interfere with nucleic acid synthesis and are cell cycle specific		
Cytosine arabinoside	Acute myelogenous leukemia, leptomeningeal carcinomatosis, lymphomas	Myelosuppression, ischemic bowel, stomatitis, nausea and vomiting, hepatotoxicity, cerebellar toxicity
5-Fluorouracil	Carcinomas of the breast, cervix, head and neck, gastrointestinal tract; nonmelanoma skin cancer	Mucositis, diarrhea, myelosuppression, dermatitis, hepatotoxicity (intraarterial therapy), nausea and vomiting
Floxuridine	Hepatic arterial therapy	Mucositis, biliary sclerosis, nausea and vomiting, abdominal pain
6-Mercaptopurine	Acute lymphoblastic leukemia	Myelosuppression, cholestasis, rash, anorexia, nausea and vomiting
Methotrexate	Carcinomas of the breast, head and neck, esophagus; choriocarcinoma; leptomeningeal carcinomatosis; osteogenic sarcoma	Myelosuppression, stomatitis, diarrhea, intestinal bleeding and perforation, arachnoiditis, hepatic dysfunction, cirrhosis, radiation recall, pneumonitis, renal dysfunction
Gemcitabine (Difluorodeoxycytidine)	Experimental	Myelosuppression, weakness
Pentostatin	Hairy cell leukemia, T-cell lymphomas	Nephrotoxicity, risk of severe infections without neutropenia, lethargy, hepatotoxicity, mild myelosuppression
Fludarabine	B-cell chronic lymphocytic leukemia	Myelosuppression, tumor lysis syndrome, weakness, neurotoxicity, edema, pneumonitis, nausea and vomiting, anorexia, gastrointestinal bleeding, stomatitis, diarrhea

SIADH, syndrome of inappropriate antidiuretic hormone secretion.
From Ellis LM, Jones Jr DV, Chiao PJ, et al. Tumor biology. In: Greenfield LJ, Mulholland MW, Oldham KT et al., eds. *Surgery: scientific principles and practice*, 2nd ed. Philadelphia: Lippincott-Raven Publishers, 1997:501, with permission.

TABLE 4-12
PRIMARY CHEMOTHERAPY

Neoplasms in which chemotherapy is the primary therapeutic modality for localized tumors

Large cell lymphoma
Lymphoblastic lymphoma
Burkitt and non-Burkitt, undifferentiated lymphoma
Childhood and some adult stages of Hodgkin disease
Wilms tumor
Embryonal rhabdomyosarcoma
Small cell lung cancer
Central nervous system lymphomas

Neoplasms in which primary chemotherapy can allow less mutilating surgery

Anal carcinoma
Bladder carcinoma
Breast cancer
Esophageal cancer
Laryngeal cancer
Osteogenic sarcoma
Soft tissue sarcoma

Neoplasms in which clinical trials indicate an expanding role for primary chemotherapy in the future

Nonsmall cell lung cancer
Bladder cancer
Breast cancer
Cervical cancer
Esophageal cancer
Gastric cancer
Nasopharyngeal cancer
Other cancers of the head and neck region
Pancreatic cancer
Prostate cancer

From Chu E, DeVita Jr VT. Principles of cancer management: Chemotherapy. In: DeVita VT, Hellman S, Rosenberg SA, eds. *Cancer: principles and practice of oncology*, 6th ed. Philadelphia: Lippincott Williams & Wilkins, 2002:292, with permission.

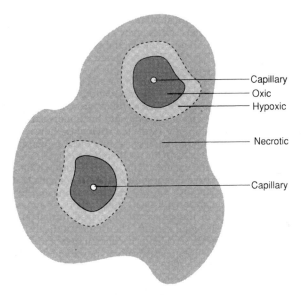

Figure 4-7 Tumors contain regions that are anoxic, hypoxic, and well-oxygenated and that vary in distance from capillaries. The response to ionizing radiation varies with the degree of tissue oxygenation. (From Ellis LM, Jones Jr DV, Chiao PJ, et al. Tumor biology. In: Greenfield LJ, Mulholland MW, Oldham KT et al., eds. *Surgery: scientific principles and practice*, 2nd ed. Philadelphia: Lippincott-Raven Publishers, 1997:493, with permission.)

Active immunotherapy approaches include those in which a host antitumor immune response is elicited following the delivery of either nonspecific or specific stimulants of the immune system. Examples of nonspecific stimulants include viable or nonviable microorganisms such as bacille

because only a proportion of tumor cells will be sensitive to ionizing radiation at a given time, fractionation allows for reoxygenation of hypoxic areas of the tumor following the death of those cells that were initially susceptible.

Radiation therapy may be used as the primary treatment for some tumors or may be used in combination with surgical resection to provide local tumor control. Radiation therapy has been used in management of soft tissue sarcomas of the extremities, delivered either preoperatively or postoperatively as external beam radiation or using brachytherapy. The use of radiation therapy following the resection of large soft tissue sarcomas with positive margins has also been shown to improve local control. Radiation therapy is frequently used as the primary modality for early stage head and neck cancers or may be used in the adjuvant setting following surgical resection to improve local control.

Immunotherapy

The goal of immunotherapy is to generate antitumor immune responses by stimulating or bolstering the host immune system. Both active and passive immunotherapy approaches have been utilized for cancer therapy.

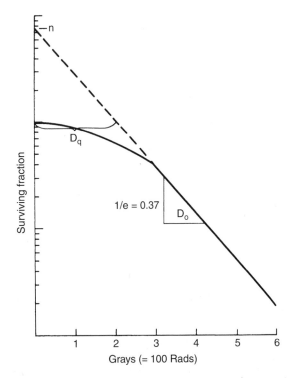

Figure 4-8 Idealized radiation survival curve. D_o, dose required to reduce the survival fraction to 37% on the exponential curve; D_q, the quasi-threshold dose; $1/e$, dose energy divided by dose loss. (From Hellman S. Principles of cancer management: radiation therapy. In: DeVita VT, Hellman S, Rosenberg SA, eds. *Cancer: principles and practice of oncology*, 6th ed. Philadelphia: Lippincott Williams & Wilkins, 2002:272, with permission.)

Calmette-Guérin (BCG), levamisole, and cytokines. Some clinical efficacy has been demonstrated with use of BCG for melanoma metastases and superficial bladder cancer; levamisole, when used in concert with 5-fluorouracil, to decrease colon cancer recurrence and improve survival; and interferons when used for hematologic malignancies and certain epithelial carcinomas. It was the use of the cytokine, interleukin-2 (IL-2), however, in patients with metastatic melanoma, renal cell carcinoma, and non-Hodgkin lymphoma that first demonstrated that manipulation of the immune system could lead to regression of bulky solid tumors and metastatic disease. In these initial studies, systemic delivery of IL-2 led to observed responses in 15% to 20% of patients with durable complete responses in approximately one half of those patients. Specific active immunotherapy strategies using vaccines derived from tumor cell preparations or antigen-presenting cells (APCs) have also been utilized.

Passive immunotherapy strategies include the delivery of agents that already possess antitumor activity such as monoclonal antibodies and immune cells. The two most widely studied passive immunotherapy strategies are those that have utilized nonspecific lymphokine-activated killer (LAK) cells and specific TILs.

Several important discoveries and developments have been critical to continued progress in the field of immunotherapy. The first of these was the initial identification and isolation of T-cell growth factor (TCGF), now known as IL-2, which could be utilized for the *in vitro* expansion of lymphocytes. It was found that the incubation of lymphocytes with IL-2 led to the development of nonspecific cytotoxic cells which were called LAK cells. Preclinical animal models using IL-2 and LAK cell therapy demonstrated improved efficacy when both agents were used. In addition, a direct relationship was noted between clinical outcomes and the number of LAK cells delivered and dose of IL-2 administered. Subsequent clinical trials using IL-2 therapy in combination with LAK cells in patients with metastatic melanoma and renal cell carcinoma resulted in higher objective responses in 15% to 30% of patients.

A second important discovery was the identification of TILs that had specific antitumor activity, and techniques were developed to isolate these lymphocytes from solid tumors and to expand them *in vitro*. The identification of TILs was a clear indication that the immune system did play a role in fighting cancer and that there were specific tumor antigens that could be recognized and targeted by the immune system. This finding led to the identification of numerous tumor antigens that are recognized by the cellular immune system and provide potential targets for immunotherapeutic strategies. Subsequent preclinical studies using TILs demonstrated that they possessed antitumor activity without the presence of IL-2, and that similar to LAK cells, there was a direct relationship between outcomes and the number of TILs and dose of IL-2 delivered. Overall, TILs were found to be 50 to 100 times as effective as LAK cells. In clinical trials combining TILs and IL-2 therapy in patients with metastatic melanoma, objective responses were observed in 35% to 40% of patients.

Finally, the development of methods to genetically manipulate lymphocytes, tumor cells, and APCs *in vitro* to enhance their *in vivo* antitumor activity or their ability to stimulate the immune system, has had a considerable impact on immunotherapy. Genetic manipulation of these cells has included insertion of genes that express cytokines, costimulatory molecules, and tumor antigens. The importance of APCs in stimulating the immune system has been recognized, and, therefore, attempts have been made to use these cells for cancer vaccines. APCs have been pulsed with tumor antigens, tumor lysates, tumor peptides, or transduced with recombinant viruses *in vitro* to generate specific antitumor immune responses *in vivo*.

Gene Therapy

The introduction of cancer gene therapy more than a decade ago was greeted with considerable optimism that this would provide a novel therapy for cancer. Although numerous preclinical studies and clinical trials have been initiated since that time with variable results, multiple limitations still exist in the field. Increasing knowledge of the molecular basis of malignant transformation, however, and a more complete understanding of tumor biology, including the tumor microenvironment and host–tumor interactions, have led to the identification of an increasing number of potential targets for cancer gene therapy. Therefore, there is continued interest and growth in the field in an effort to develop new therapies for cancer.

Successful gene therapy strategies require delivery vectors that are safe, efficient, and selective. Both nonviral and viral vectors have been developed and utilized. Examples of nonviral gene delivery methods include the injection of naked DNA and DNA complexed to cationic carriers. The advantages of nonviral gene delivery methods are that they are less immunogenic than viral vectors and can be produced in higher titers *in vitro*. Viral vectors that have been used frequently in cancer gene therapy include delivery vectors using adenovirus, retrovirus, herpes simplex virus, and adeno-associated virus. These viral vectors vary in their size, DNA carrying capacity, ability to transduce dividing and nondividing cells, potential for long-term gene expression, and in the titers that can be generated *in vitro* (Table 4-13). The advantages of viral vectors are that they have higher transduction efficiencies as compared to nonviral vectors and that some have the potential for long-term gene expression.

Gene therapy strategies that have been evaluated for the treatment of cancer are generally divided into five main categories: mutation compensation, molecular chemotherapy, immunopotentiation, antiangiogenic therapy, and viral-mediated oncolysis. Mutation compensation gene therapy approaches attempt to correct the genetic alterations that occur during malignant transformation by restoring the function or expression of tumor-suppressor genes or by inactivating oncogenes. Two strategies that have been the focus of research in this area are restoration of *p53* function and targeting the *HER-2/Neu* growth factor receptor gene. The goal of molecular chemotherapy is to produce high local concentrations of cytotoxic metabolites, and thereby circumvent the dose-limiting toxicities of systemic chemotherapy. This is accomplished by transducing cells with a converting enzyme that leads to the conversion of an inactive prodrug to a cytotoxic metabolite. The two most frequently utilized enzyme-prodrug combinations are HSV thymidine kinase with ganciclovir and *Escherichia coli* cytosine deaminase with 5-fluorocytosine. Immunopotentiation gene therapy strategies attempt to enhance antitumor immune responses. Numerous approaches have been evaluated including

TABLE 4-13
GENE THERAPY VECTORS

Vector	Genome	Maximum Insert Size	Efficiency of Transduction	Requires Replication for Transduction	Location of Vector Genome in Host	Expression	Immunogenicity	Advantages	Disadvantages	Clinical Trials
Viral vectors										
Adeno-associated virus	Single-stranded DNA	4.5 kb	Moderate	No	In the absence of rep protein: episomal or randomly integrated into host genome in the presence of rep protein: preferential site-specific integration into chromosome 19	Stable	No	Stable expression, nonimmunogenic	Small transgene capacity	Cystic fibrosis, Canavan disease
Adenovirus	Double-stranded DNA	8 kb	High	No	Episomal	Transient	Yes	High transduction efficiency	Immunogenicity leads to elimination of transduced cells and loss of transgene expression	More than 65 trials in a wide range of applications
Guted adenovirus	Double-stranded DNA	37 kb	High	No	Episomal	Variable, depending on immunogenicity of transgene	Low	High transduction efficiency, low immunogenicity compared with earlier adenoviral vectors	Elimination of transduced cells after expression of immunogenic construct	No
Retrovirus	Single-stranded RNA	7 kb	Moderate	Yes	Random integration into host genome	Stable	No	Integration, long-term expression	Requirement for cell division, labile in vivo, insertional mutagenesis	More than 150 trials in a wide variety of applications, especially for ex vivo manipulation of hematopoietic cells
Lentivirus	Single-stranded RNA	8.8 kb	High	No	Random integration into host genome	Stable	No	Ability to infect nondividing and quiescent cells, integration, long-term expression	Biosafety issues regarding parental virus, insertional mutagenesis	No
Herpes simplex	Double-stranded DNA	30 kb	Moderate	No	Episomal	Transient	No	Neuronal tropism, ability to establish latency, large transgene capacity	Transient transgene expression, viral toxicity in some cell types	One trial for treatment of malignant glioma
Poxviruses	Double-stranded DNA	25 kb	Moderate	No	Cytoplasm	Transient	Yes	Large transgene capacity, wide tropism	Immunogenicity	Cancer immunotherapy and vaccination
Nonviral vectors										
Liposomes	DNA or RNA	50 kb	Low	No	Episomal	Transient	No	Large transgene capacity, nonimmunogenic, ease of manufacture	Low transduction efficiency and transient expression	More than 70 trials in a wide range of applications
Naked DNA	DNA	50 kb	Low	No	Episomal	Transient	No	Large transgene capacity, nonimmunogenic, ease of manufacture	Low transduction efficiency	Several trials in various applications including myocardial angiogenesis, cancer, and hemophilia A
DNA–protein conjugate	DNA	48 kb	Low	No	Episomal	Transient	No	Large transgene capacity, nonimmunogenic, ability to target specific cell types through surface receptors	Low transduction efficiency, degradation within lysosomes	Few

From Beseth BD, Cameron RB, Mulé JJ. Human gene therapy. In: Greenfield LJ, Mulholland MW, Oldham KT et al., eds. *Surgery: scientific principles and practice*, 3rd ed. Philadelphia: Lippincott Williams & Wilkins, 2001:497, with permission.

delivery of cytokines, development of tumor vaccines based on tumor antigens, upregulation of costimulatory molecules, and inhibition of immunosuppressive molecules. Antiangiogenic gene therapy strategies have focused on blocking proangiogenic factors or increasing inhibitors of angiogenesis. One approach that has been evaluated in several preclinical studies is targeting the proangiogenic cytokine vascular endothelial growth factor. Finally, viral-mediated oncolysis uses the pathologic replication of viruses within cells to produce cell death. The most widely studied tumor oncolytic virus in ONYX-015, which preferentially replicates in and leads to cytotoxicity in *p53*-deficient tumor cells.

Each of these gene therapy approaches has been evaluated in multiple preclinical studies and clinical trials, for numerous malignancies, targeting local, regional, and metastatic disease. Although preclinical studies have produced promising results, only limited responses have been observed in clinical trials. For example, delivery of WT *p53* by intratumoral injection in animal models for colon cancer and prostate cancer resulted in clinically significant tumor growth inhibition, and in several animals led to tumor eradication. In a similar phase I trial conducted at The University of Texas MD Anderson Cancer Center in patients with recurrent head and neck squamous cell carcinoma (HNSCC), although *p53* transduction and intratumoral expression were demonstrated, only two partial responses were observed in 17 patients. In an example of regional therapy, intraperitoneal and intrapleural animal models of malignant mesothelioma were generated using a human mesothelioma cell line transduced *in vitro* with an AV vector containing the HSV-tk gene. Following the administration of author to define ganciclovir (GCV), macroscopic tumor was eliminated in 90% of animals and microscopic tumor in 80% of animals. In a phase I trial of AV-mediated intrapleural HSV-tk/GCV therapy for malignant mesothelioma, while gene transfer was observed in approximately 50% of patients, there were no significant clinical responses and only 20% of patients demonstrated stabilization of disease. Although the reasons for the limited efficacy observed in clinical trials have not been clearly identified, some of the contributing factors are low transduction efficiencies, antiviral immune responses, and targeting of only single genetic defects.

In addition to using gene therapy as a single modality, combination gene therapy approaches, as well as gene therapy in concert with radiation therapy and chemotherapy have been evaluated with improved efficacy in many cases. Enhanced antitumor immune responses have been demonstrated in preclinical models by delivery of multiple cytokines or upregulation of costimulatory molecules in combination with cytokine delivery. Molecular chemotherapy and immunopotentiation gene therapy strategies using HSV-tk/GCV with IL-2, IL-12, or granulocyte macrophage colony-stimulating factor (GM-CSF) have been combined in several preclinical studies for the treatment of peritoneal carcinomatosis and for colon and lung cancer metastases. In these studies, improved animal survival was demonstrated using combination therapy when compared to a single gene therapy approach. In addition, improved efficacy has been demonstrated in preclinical studies and in clinical trials when gene therapy approaches are combined with standard treatment modalities. Radiosensitization has

been demonstrated *in vitro* following the transduction of colon cancer and prostate cancer cells in vitro with WT *p53*. Furthermore, in a phase II trial for recurrent HNSCC, the combination of standard cytotoxic chemotherapeutic agents with intratumoral administration of ONYX-015 resulted in 8 complete and 11 partial responses in 30 patients.

Molecular Diagnostics and Therapeutics

As our understanding of the specific genetic alterations that are necessary for malignant transformation has increased, potential new targets for cancer therapy are being identified that are directed at these changes in gene expression and in protein expression and function. Identification of these targets has been facilitated by the development of new technologies that allow for rapid transcription and molecular profiling of individual cancers. Gene expression and protein microarrays are examples of these emerging technologies, which when used in concert can provide a significant amount of information about genetic alterations within cancer cells, as well as the functional state of these genetic changes. The identification of genetic and epigenetic alterations in cancer cells, as well as changes in protein expression and function, may lead to the detection of new molecular markers for malignancies, may improve the classification of cancers beyond what is currently possible by histopathologic methods, may allow oncologists to tailor therapy to a particular tumor, and may provide important information for prognosis.

The use of molecular diagnostics to identify genetic mutations in cancer cells has led to the development of molecular inhibitors that target specific genetic alterations and modulate signaling pathways in cancer cells. The first successful example of targeted molecular therapy was the development of the tyrosine kinase inhibitor imatinib mesylate (Gleevec) for the treatment of patients with chronic myeloid leukemia (CML) and gastrointestinal stromal tumors (GISTs). The principal genetic defect in 95% of patients with CML is a reciprocal translocation between chromosomes 9 and 22, which leads to a *bcr-abl* fusion gene and a resultant fusion protein that functions as a constitutively active tyrosine kinase. In the case of GISTs, the majority of tumors have a gain-of-function mutation in the *c-kit* protooncogene, which leads to a constitutively active tyrosine kinase receptor. In the initial clinical trials in patients with CML, up to 95% of chronic-phase patients who failed interferon therapy had a clinical response to imatinib mesylate and approximately one half of these patients also had a molecular remission. The use of imatinib mesylate has also revolutionized the treatment of patients with metastatic GISTs, and the efficacy of this agent is currently being evaluated as adjuvant therapy in patients following primary resection.

Since the success of imatinib mesylate, several additional molecular therapies have been developed and are currently in clinical trials. The overexpression of epidermal growth factor receptors (EGFRs) in numerous cancers has led to the development of agents that target these receptors. Overexpression of the HER2/neu receptor in 25% to 30% of patients with breast cancer leads to an aggressive form of the disease. Trastuzumab (Herceptin), a monoclonal antibody against the HER2/neu receptor, has proved effective as a single agent in these patients, and in combination with chemotherapy has been shown to slow disease progression and improve overall survival. The reversible EGFR kinase inhibitor gefitinib (Iressa) is currently being evaluated in patients with glioblastoma multiforme in which the overexpression of EGFR genes is common and in patients with non–small cell lung cancer in which the expression or overexpression of EGFR may correlate with aggressive tumor behavior and poor prognosis.

CONCLUSIONS

Cancer remains a significant public health problem. More than 50% of patients with malignancies still succumb to metastatic disease that cannot be controlled by standard treatment modalities. Although advances in molecular biology have markedly increased our understanding of malignant transformation and the cancer phenotype, they have also highlighted the complexity and heterogeneity of carcinogenesis that make prevention and treatment so difficult. Surgery, chemotherapy, and radiation therapy continue to be the standard treatment modalities; however, molecular diagnostic techniques and targeted molecular therapies will likely play an increasing role in cancer detection and treatment in the future as therapies are tailored for specific genetic alterations in individual patients. Researchers continue to increase our understanding of tumor biology and produce novel therapies for malignancies, with the ultimate goal of improving quality of life and outcomes for cancer patients.

KEY POINTS

▲ Malignant transformation results from the accumulation of genetic defects within a cell, frequently involving mutations to oncogenes and tumor-suppressor genes. Genetic, environmental, and host factors are involved in this process. Generally between four and seven genetic alterations are necessary for a cell to become transformed.

▲ The tumor microenvironment plays an important role in tumor growth and development supporting cell–cell and cell–matrix interactions that drive growth, invasion, and metastasis. These interactions result in changes in the production and response to growth factors, lead to decreased apoptosis, and stimulate angiogenesis.

▲ Angiogenesis is critical to tumor growth, invasion, and metastasis in delivering of nutrients that sustain cell growth, as well as providing an egress for cancer cells from the local tumor microenvironment resulting in disseminated disease.

▲ Multimodality therapy using a combination of surgery, chemotherapy, and radiation therapy remains the standard of care for cancer patients.

▲ Targeted molecular therapy will likely become an important treatment modality for cancer in the future as specific genetic defects in various malignancies are identified and treatment is tailored for individual tumors.

SUGGESTED READINGS

Baird A, Klagsbrun M. The fibroblast growth factor family. *Cancer Cells* 1991;3:239.

Bussolino F, Ziche M, Wang JM, et al. In vitro and in vivo activation of endothelial cells by colony-stimulating factors. *J Clin Invest* 1991;87:986.

Choudhuri R, Zhang HT, Donnini S, et al. An angiogenic role for the neurokines midkine and pleiotrophin in tumorigenesis. *Cancer Res* 1997;57:1814.

Clapp C, Martial JA, Guzman RC, et al. The 16-kilodalton N-terminal fragment of human prolactin is a potent inhibitor of angiogenesis. *Endocrinology* 1993;133:1292.

Davis S, Yancopoulos GD. The angiopoietins: Yin and Yang in angiogenesis. *Curr Topics Microbiol Immunol* 1999;237:173.

Desbaillets I, Diserens AC, Tribolet N, et al. Upregulation of interleukin 8 by oxygen-deprived cells in glioblastoma suggests a role in leukocyte activation, chemotaxis, and angiogenesis. *J Exp Med* 1997;186:1201.

DeVita VT, Hellman S, Rosenberg SA, eds. *Cancer: principles and practice of oncology*, 6th ed. Philadelphia: Lippincott Williams & Wilkins, 2002.

Espina V, Mehta AI, Winters ME, et al. Protein microarrays: molecular profiling technologies for clinical specimens. *Proteomics* 2003;3:2091–2100.

Ezekowitz RAB, Mulliken JB, Folkman J. Interferon alpha-2a therapy for life-threatening hemangiomas of infancy. *N Engl J Med* 1992;326:1456-1463.

Gimenez-Gallego G, Cuevas P. Fibroblast growth factors, proteins with a broad spectrum of biological activities. *Neurol Res* 1994;16:313.

Greenfield LJ, Mulholland MW, Oldham KT et al., eds. *Surgery: scientific principles and practice*, 2nd ed. Philadelphia: Lippincott-Raven Publishers, 1997.

Greenfield LJ, Mulholland MW, Oldham KT et al., eds. *Surgery: scientific principles and practice*, 3rd ed. Philadelphia: Lippincott Williams & Wilkins, 2001.

Gupta SK, Hassel T, Singh JP. A potent inhibitor of endothelial cell proliferation is generated by proteolytic cleavage of the chemokine platelet factor 4. *Proc Natl Acad Sci USA* 1995;92:7799.

Hanahan D, Weinberg RA. The hallmarks of cancer. *Cell* 2000;100:57–70.

Hartmann A, Kunz M, Kostlin S, et al. Hypoxia-induced up-regulation of angiogenin in human malignant melanoma. *Cancer Res* 1999;59:1578.

Hughes RM. Strategies for cancer gene therapy. *J Surg Oncol* 2004;85:28–35.

Jackson D, Volpert OV, Bouck N, et al. Stimulation and inhibition of angiogenesis by placental proliferin and proliferin-related protein. *Science* 1994;266:1581.

Kuwabara K, Ogawa S, Matsumoto M, et al. Hypoxia-mediated induction of acidic/basic fibroblast growth factor and platelet-derived growth factor in mononuclear phagocytes stimulates growth of hypoxic endothelial cells. *Proc Natl Acad Sci USA* 1995;92:4606.

Lamszus K, Laterra J, Westphal M, et al. Scatter factor/hepatocyte growth factor (SF/HGF) content and function in human gliomas. *Int J Dev Neurosci* 1999;17:517.

Luo J, Isaacs WB, Trent JM, et al. Looking beyond morphology: cancer gene expression profiling using DNA microarrays. *Cancer Invest* 2003;21:937–949.

Maisonpierre PC, Suri C, Jones PF, et al. Angiopoietin-2, a natural antagonist for Tie2 that disrupts in vivo angiogenesis. *Science* 1997;277:55.

Mooradian DL, Diglio CA. Effects of epidermal growth factor and transforming growth factor-β1 on rat heart endothelial cell anchorage-dependent and independent growth. *Exp Cell Res* 1990;186:122.

Moore BB, Arenberg DA, Addison CL, et al. Tumor angiogenesis is regulated by CXC chemokines. *J Lab Clin Med* 1998;132:97.

O'Reilly MS, Boehm T, Shing Y, et al. Endostatin: an endogenous inhibitor of angiogenesis and tumor growth. *Cell* 1997;88:277.

O'Reilly MS, Holmgren L, Shing Y, et al. Angiostatin: a novel angiogenesis inhibitor that mediates the suppression of metastases by a Lewis lung carcinoma. *Cell* 1994;79:315.

O'Reilly MS, Pirie-Shepherd S, Lane WE, Folkman J. Antiangiogenic activity of the cleaved conformation of the Serpin antithrombin III. *Science* 1999;285:1926.

Pepper MS. Transforming growth factor-beta: vasculogenesis, angiogenesis, and vessel wall integrity. *Cytokine Growth Factor Rev* 1997;8:21.

Pike SE, Yao L, Jones KD, et al. Vasostatin, a calretriculin fragment, inhibits angiogenesis and suppresses tumor growth. *J Exp Med* 1998;188:2349.

Ramchandran R, Dhanabal M, Volk R, et al. Antiangiogenic activity of restin, NC10 domain of human collagen XV: comparison to endostatin. *Biochem Biophys Res Commun* 1999;255:735.

Rosenberg SA. Progress in human tumour immunology and immunotherapy. *Nature* 2001;411:380–384.

Sage EH. Pieces of eight: bioactive fragments of extracellular proteins as regulators of angiogenesis. *Trends Biol Sci* 1999;7:182.

Schmitt FC, Soares R. TGF-α and angiogenesis. *Am J Surg Pathol* 1999; 23:358.

Takahashi Y, Bucana CD, Liu W, et al. Platelet derived endothelial cell growth factor in human colon cancer angiogenesis: role of infiltrating cells. *J Natl Cancer Inst* 1996;88:1146.

Tolsma SS, Volpert OV, Good DJ, et al. Peptides derived from two separate domains of the matrix protein thrombospondin-1 have anti-angiogenic activity. *J Cell Biol* 1993;122:497.

Vasquez F, Hastings G, Ortega MA, et al. METH-1, a human ortholog of ADAMTS-1, and METH-2 are members of a new family of proteins with angioinhibitory activity. *J Biol Chem* 1999;274:23349.

Veikkola T, Karkkainen M, Claesson-Welsh L, et al. Regulation of angiogenesis via vascular endothelial growth factor receptors. *Cancer Res* 2000;60:203.

Volgelstetin B, Kinzler KW, eds. *The genetic basis of human cancer*, 2nd ed. New York: McGraw-Hill, 2002.

Yoshida S, Ono M, Shono T, et al. Involvement of interleukin-8 , vascular endothelial growth factor, and basic fibroblast growth factor in tumor necrosis factor alpha-dependent angiogenesis. *Mol Cell Biol* 1997;17:4015.

Zhai Y, Ni J, Jiang GW, et al. VEGI, a novel cytokine of the tumor necrosis factor family, is an angiogenesis inhibitor that suppresses the growth of colon carcinomas in vivo. *FASEB J* 1999;13:181.

Melanoma, Sarcoma, Lymphoma, and the Spleen

5

Robert J. Canter   Mark B. Faries   Francis R. Spitz

This chapter contains a diverse set of topics, each important in its own right to the general surgeon. The first three sections deal with malignancies. Melanoma and sarcoma are diseases for which surgery is the primary treatment and the only potentially curative intervention. Surgery is also the best palliative modality for these diseases. Surgical treatment for lymphoma is unusual and is becoming even less common as medical treatments advance. However, surgeons are frequently involved in obtaining tissue for diagnosis and treating gastrointestinal lymphomas. The final section deals with the spleen in lymphoma and other hematologic malignancies, diseases in which this organ is frequently involved.

MELANOMA

The incidence of *melanoma* continues to increase worldwide, particularly in the United States. Since 1971 the incidence of this cancer has increased by 83% (Fig. 5-1). The incidence is now 4 to 26 cases of melanoma per 100,000 population, with the highest rates in the southern United States. In the year 2000, the lifetime risk of developing melanoma was estimated to be 1 in 90. Over the last 30 years, melanoma has also become more localized to the primary site, with 81% of melanomas localized in 1990 versus 73% in 1960. During this same period, the average thickness of melanomas has decreased from 3 mm to less than 1 mm, a trend that may reflect increased surveillance for primary lesions.

Differential Diagnosis of the Pigmented Lesion

The most common initial presentation of a patient is for evaluation of a *pigmented lesion*. The vast majority of such lesions are benign, but differentiation between benign and malignant is not always clear. The differential diagnosis of a pigmented lesion is extensive (Table 5-1). *Congenital nevi*

develop in approximately 1% of children before or shortly after birth. Risk of progression to melanoma correlates with size. Small lesions (0 to 1.5 cm in diameter) have little or no increased risk, whereas lesions exceeding 20 cm in diameter have as high as a 30% lifetime risk of developing into melanoma. *Acquired nevi* appear after the first few months of life and can be divided into junctional nevi, compound nevi, and intradermal nevi, among others.

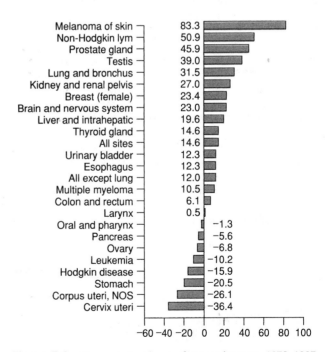

Figure 5-1 Change in incidence of cancer by type, 1973–1987. (From Chang AE, Johnson TM, Rees RS. Cutaneous neoplasms. In: Greenfield LJ, Mulholland MW, Oldham KT et al., eds. *Surgery: scientific principles and practice*, 2nd ed. Philadelphia: Lippincott-Raven Publishers, 1997:2232, with permission.)

TABLE 5-1

PIGMENTED LESION, DIFFERENTIAL DIAGNOSIS

Melanocytic	Nonmelanocytic
Congenital nevus	Hemangioma
Acquired nevus	Kaposi sarcoma
Atypical nevus	Pyogenic granuloma
Melanosis of the genitalia	Dermatofibroma
Blue nevus	Angiokeratoma
Solar lentigo	

Junctional nevi are macular and generally have smooth, regular borders. They appear in childhood and adolescence and consist of a proliferation of melanocytes limited by the basement membrane. *Compound nevi* occur when melanocytes penetrate the basement membrane and are located in nests within the dermis. *Intradermal nevi* are entirely within the dermis and are clinically evident as dome-shaped, or nodular, and less pigmented.

History and Physical Examination

Patients undergoing evaluation of pigmented lesions should be evaluated for *risk factors* for melanoma. Elements of the history should include any family history of melanoma, as this is indicative of increased risk. Specific mutations have been identified in melanoma in four distinct genes. These mutations, located on chromosomes 1, 6, 7, and 9, are believed to play a role in developing melanoma. A genetic predisposition to melanoma is seen in families with familial atypical mole and melanoma syndrome. This disorder was formerly known as the *dysplastic nevus syndrome*.

An additional risk factor is a history of previous melanomas. Such patients have a ninefold increased risk for developing a second primary melanoma when compared to a population without a history of previous melanomas.

Another predisposing factor is previous exposure to environmental risk factors such as ultraviolet radiation. An increased risk of melanoma has been found with even one blistering sunburn. The increased exposure of the population to radiation from decreased ozone shielding of ultraviolet solar radiation and the increased use of tanning booths has been thought to contribute to the increasing rates of melanoma and other skin cancers.

In addition, compared to the black population, whites have an approximately 20-fold increased risk of developing melanoma. Finally, during history taking, the history of the lesion itself should be elicited. Lesions that have recently developed or changed should arouse more suspicion than long-standing nevi that have not changed. Changes in size, shape, or color and any history of itching or bleeding are worrisome for malignant transformation.

Patients who are undergoing evaluation for a pigmented lesion should have all areas of their skin examined for evidence of other lesions. Patients with a large number of benign nevi are at increased risk of developing melanoma.

Individual lesions should be examined for several characteristics. These include the so-called *ABCDEs*: *asymmetry*, irregular *borders*, variegated *color*, large *diameter*, and *elevated* surface. When examining the color of a lesion, shades of red, pink, white, blue, black, or brown mixed together are suspicious. Lesions with diameters greater than 6 mm are also associated with malignancy. Although the presence of these characteristics may be suggestive of malignancy, their absence does not rule out melanoma.

Classification of Melanomas

Suspicious lesions should be *biopsied*. The incision should be oriented so that it can be incorporated into a subsequent wide local excision. Minimal margins of normal tissue should be obtained when biopsying a pigmented lesion, since the majority of such lesions will be benign. Punch or incisional biopsies should be avoided, as an area of increased thickness or malignancy may be missed in the sampling. With large lesions in critical locations (such as above joints or near facial structures), an incisional biopsy may be the only practical option. Shave biopsies may also be used, but it may be difficult to accurately determine the thickness of a lesion that has been removed by shaving.

Melanomas can be classified into four main types according to their appearance and clinical behavior. *Superficial spreading melanoma* is the most common type. It is found in 70% of cases and often arises from preexisting nevi. Superficial spreading melanomas are initially characterized by the radial growth phase. Then, over variable periods of time, vertical growth develops within the lesion, often seen clinically as a raised papule.

Nodular melanoma is the second most common type and accounts for 15% to 30% of cases and lacks a radial growth phase. These tumors are characterized by a vertical growth phase without radial growth and are more aggressive than the superficial spreading type. Clinically, the lesions tend to be darker and more uniform and are more prevalent in men. Five percent of nodular melanomas lack pigment, which is associated with a higher rate of metastatic spread.

Lentigo maligna melanomas constitute 4% to 10% of cases and have a tendency to develop in older patients in sun-exposed areas of the body such as the face. They are relatively more common in women and tend to be large at diagnosis, often greater than 3 cm in diameter. These lesions also characteristically develop over many years from a precursor macular brown nevus, the so-called *Hutchinson freckle*. In addition, this type of melanoma tends to be less aggressive and is, therefore, associated with a better prognosis.

Acral lentiginous melanomas are relatively uncommon. They make up only 2% to 8% of melanomas in white patients, but 35% to 60% of melanomas in patients with dark skin. Typically these lesions occur on the palms or soles. This class of melanoma is the most aggressive and has the highest risk of metastasis.

Although most melanomas develop on the skin, it is important to remember that melanoma may be found in noncutaneous sites. Ocular melanoma is the most common noncutaneous melanoma. Treatment typically requires enucleation, although radiotherapy and photocoagulation have been employed in an attempt to reduce ocular morbidity with apparently similar results. Primary melanoma may also occur in the mucous membranes of the genitalia, the anus, the oropharynx, and the gastrointestinal tract, among other locations.

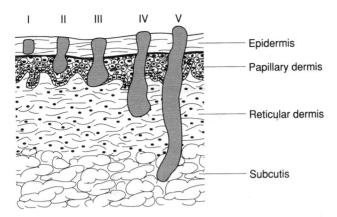

Figure 5-2 Clark levels of invasion. (From Chang AE, Johnson TM, Rees RS. Cutaneous neoplasms. In: Greenfield LJ, Mulholland MW, Oldham KT et al., eds. *Surgery: scientific principles and practice*, 2nd ed. Philadelphia: Lippincott-Raven Publishers, 1997:2233, with permission.)

Staging

The *staging system* for melanomas was developed by the American Joint Committee on Cancer (AJCC) and is based on the level or depth of invasion of the primary tumor (based on the systems of *Clark* and *Breslow,* respectively), involvement of regional lymph nodes, in-transit sites, and distant metastases. Figure 5-2 outlines Clark classification and Tables 5-2 and 5-3 describe the most current staging system by the AJCC.

Revisions to the staging system were published in 2002, reflecting a systematic multiregression analysis of over

TABLE 5-2

AMERICAN JOINT COMMITTEE ON CANCER (AJCC) 2002 TNM CLASSIFICATION FOR MELANOMA

Tumor (T) classification

T1a, b	Primary melanoma ≤1 mm
T2a, b	Primary melanoma 1.01 to 2.0 mm
T3a, b	Primary melanoma 2.01 to 4.0 mm
T4a, b	Primary melanoma >4 mm thick

a, without ulceration; *b,* with ulceration.

Node (N) classification

N1a, b	One positive lymph node
N2a, b, c	Two to three positive lymph nodes
N3	Four or more positive lymph nodes, or matted lymph nodes, or in-transit metastasis with metastatic node(s)

a, micrometastases diagnosed after sentinel or elective lymphadenectomy; *b,* macrometastases diagnosed on clinical examination or when nodal metastasis exhibits gross extracapsular extension; *c,* in-transit met(s)/satellite lesion(s) without metastatic nodes.

Metastasis (M) classification

M1a	Distant skin, subcutaneous, or lymph node metastases with normal LDH level
M1b	Lung metastases with normal LDH level
M1c	All other visceral metastases with normal LDH level or any distant metastases with elevated LDH level

LDH, lactate dehydrogenase.

TABLE 5-3

AMERICAN JOINT COMMITTEE ON CANCER 2002 PATHOLOGIC STAGING CLASSIFICATION FOR MELANOMA

IA	T1a, N0, M0
IB	T1b, N0, M0
	T2a, N0, M0
IIA	T2b, N0, M0
	T3a, N0, M0
IIB	T3b, N0, M0
	T4a, N0, M0
IIC	T4b, N0, M0
IIIA	Any Ta, N1a, M0
	Any Ta, N2a, M0
IIIB	Any Tb, N1a, M0
	Any Tb, N2a, M0
	Any Ta, N1b, M0
	Any Ta, N2b, M0
	Any T, N2c, M0
IIIC	Any Tb, N1b, M0
	Any Tb, N2b, M0
	Any Ta, N3, M0
	Any Tb, N3, M0
IV	Any T, Any N, M1a
	Any T, Any N, M1b
	Any T, Any N, M1c

17,000 patients that correlated histopathologic risk factors with long-term survival. *Tumor thickness* emerged as the most reproducible and powerful predictor of survival, as opposed to Clark level of invasion, and thickness cutoffs were modified to less than or equal to 1 mm, 1.01 to 2 mm, 2.01 to 4 mm, and greater than 4 mm because these values more accurately segregate patients into survival groups and are easier to remember. *Ulceration* also emerged as a key prognostic feature in this analysis and was, therefore, incorporated into the new staging system. For regional, so-called N disease, the key changes to the new staging system were the consideration of in-transit metastases as equivalent to nodal disease, the elimination of nodal size as a factor, the incorporation of number of positive nodes as a prognostic factor, and the distinction between microscopic and macroscopic nodal metastases. Finally, the data demonstrated that the prognosis of distant metastases could be separated according to site, with distant skin, subcutaneous, and lymph node metastases being more favorable than lung metastases, which in turn were more favorable than other visceral organ metastases. In addition, it was recognized that an elevated *lactate dehydrogenase* (LDH) level represents an unfavorable prognostic factor in patients with disseminated melanoma.

Surgical Treatment of Melanoma

The cornerstone of treatment of melanoma remains wide local excision. Width of margins is dictated by the thickness of the primary tumor, and several studies have led to decreasing margin requirements. One study done by the World Health Organization (WHO) randomized 612 patients with melanomas less than 2 mm in thickness to undergo excision with 1- or 2-cm margins. There were four local recurrences, all of which occurred in patients with melanomas 1 to 2 mm in thickness that were excised with a 1-cm margin. However, there were no statistically significant differences in disease-free or overall survival between the 1-cm and 2-cm margin groups. A subsequent study randomized 486 patients with intermediate thickness melanoma (1 to 4 mm) to either a 2-cm or 4-cm margin. There were no statistically significant differences between the two groups in terms of local recurrence or overall survival. The wide-margin group required skin grafting for closure more frequently than did the narrow-margin group. The results of this study were updated in 1996 to include 742 patients, and again no statistically significant recurrence or survival differences were observed at that time. The Swedish Melanoma Study Group trial included 769 patients randomized to either 2-cm or 5-cm margins for melanomas 0.8 to 2.0 mm thick. No differences in local or regional recurrence or overall survival were seen during a median follow-up of 5.8 years. In 1998, The University of Texas MD Anderson Cancer Center reported the results of a retrospective analysis of 278 patients with thick (greater than 4 mm) melanomas. Again, no relation was found between margin width (greater than or less than 2 cm) and disease-free or overall survival.

As a result, overall reasonable *guidelines for resection margin* are 1 cm for melanomas less than 1 mm thick and 2-cm margins for intermediate (1 to 4 mm) thickness melanomas. For thick melanomas, there is a paucity of data examining optimal margins, but local recurrence rates of 10% to 20% suggest wider margins should be attained when possible. Ensuring adequate resection margins in melanomas occurring on the digits generally requires amputation of the digit. The proximal phalanges can often be preserved, frequently with distal or subungual melanomas. An important goal with resection of melanomas of the hands and feet should be the preservation of a functional limb. For the lower extremity, this entails weight bearing, which is dependent on the heel and ball of the plantar surface.

Most excision sites can be closed primarily, provided adequate skin flaps are raised on either side of the site. In the event that primary closure is not possible, a split-thickness skin graft is favored for most areas, since this is technically easier to perform, can cover a larger area, and has a higher rate of engraftment. An important exception is the face, where for cosmetic and occasionally functional reasons, a full-thickness skin graft should be used.

Regional lymph nodes are often the first site of melanoma metastasis. If lymph nodes are the only site of tumor spread, their surgical resection may be curative. However, patients with metastatic spread to lymph nodes have markedly decreased survival and are therefore candidates for further, more aggressive treatment. Morbidity associated with lymph node dissections makes elective removal of draining basins somewhat controversial, and a substantial effort has been made to determine which patients may benefit from *elective lymph node dissection* (ELND). In patients with thin (less than 1 mm) melanomas, primary wide local excision results in an approximate 95% cure rate, so elective lymph node dissection would appear unnecessary. Conversely, in patients with thick (greater

than 4 mm) melanoma, even if there is no clinical evidence of nodal disease, approximately 60% of patients will have lymphatic spread in a resected lymph node basin. However, 70% will have distant disease and will not benefit from a lymph node dissection, except for control of clinically evident regional disease. Vigorous debate has persisted over the role of ELND for patients with intermediate (1 to 4 mm) melanomas. Although there is extensive literature examining this topic with proponents both for and against the procedure, the importance of ELND in the care of patients with melanoma has diminished greatly in recent years with the advent and widespread acceptance of *sentinel lymph node biopsy* as the regional staging procedure of choice.

In patients who undergo *therapeutic lymph node dissection* for clinically evident metastases, an effort should be made to perform a thorough lymphadenectomy. In the axilla, this includes level III nodes medial to the pectoralis minor. In the inguinal region, this includes all superficial femoral nodes (Fig. 5-3). These nodes fill the triangle between the sartorius laterally, the adductor muscles medially, and the inguinal ligament superiorly. The femoral vein is the deep margin of this group, and removal of the group requires ligation of the saphenous vein. The inguinal ligament may need to be incised to enable adequate exposure of the basin. Most authors agree that dissection of the deeper iliac and obturator nodes is indicated in only the following

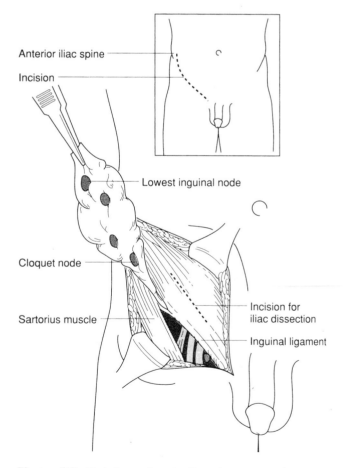

Figure 5-3 Technique of groin dissection. (From Chang AE, Johnson TM, Rees RS. Cutaneous neoplasms. In: Greenfield LJ, Mulholland MW, Oldham KT et al., eds. *Surgery: scientific principles and practice,* 2nd ed. Philadelphia: Lippincott-Raven Publishers, 1997:2240, with permission.)

circumstances: the nodes appear to be clinically involved, there are three or more positive nodes in the superficial group, or a Cloquet node is involved (which is felt to be indicative of deeper lymphatic spread).

For primary melanomas of the head and neck, lymphatic drainage patterns have been mapped and dictate appropriate areas for dissection. Parotid, submandibular, submental, jugular, and posterior triangle lymph nodes drain areas anterior to the ear and superior to the mouth. Anterior lesions inferior to the mouth drain to cervical nodes and posterior lesions drain to occipital, postauricular, posterior triangle, and jugular nodes. A radical neck dissection is generally performed for clinically apparent disease, and a less aggressive, modified dissection is done as part of an elective node dissection.

Complications of lymph node dissections include infection in 5% to 19% of patients, seroma or lymphocele in 2% to 23%, and lymphedema in 2% to 27%. Incidence of infection can be reduced by perioperative antibiotic therapy and limb elevation. Over the long-term, patients should be careful to protect the involved limb from insults such as trauma, burns, needle sticks (iatrogenic or accidental), and blood pressure measurements. Development of limb edema may be indicative of lymphatic recurrence. Lymphedema can be treated with limb elevation, application of compression stockings, or gentle diuresis. Severe cases of lymphedema may be treated surgically, although success has been limited. Surgical treatment generally includes excision of subcutaneous tissues or microsurgical insertion of lymphatics into local veins using a needle and single securing suture.

The development of *sentinel lymph node biopsy* has had a dramatic impact on the staging of patients with melanoma. This technique, described by Morton in 1992, involves the selective removal of the specific lymph node or nodes that first receive drainage from the primary tumor. Identification of the sentinel node is accomplished by injection of the primary tumor site with tracers shortly before the exploration, generally a vital blue dye and a radiocolloid.

Multiple, well-controlled studies have demonstrated that this technique leads to identification of the sentinel node in 93% to 100% of cases. The accuracy of the procedure in evaluating the status of a lymphatic basin is excellent, with false-negative rates of 1% to 4%. The procedure allows identification of patients with subclinical spread to regional lymphatics, as defined by metastatic spread to the sentinel lymph node. These patients then have established stage III disease and should form the population most likely to benefit from complete regional node dissections. At the same time, unnecessary dissections are avoided, and patients without nodal involvement are spared the morbidity association with a formal regional lymphadenectomy, which can be significant.

Adjuvant Therapy for Lymphatic Spread

Radiation therapy may be used as an adjunct to surgery for locoregional control. Patients with involvement of multiple regional lymph nodes or extracapsular spread should be considered for radiotherapy. When used alone in clinically node-negative patients or with surgery in node-positive patients, an 85% local control rate is achieved. It should be remembered, however, that the risk of complications after a combination of surgical resection of the lymphatic basin and radiation to the basin is several-fold greater than with either modality alone.

In-transit metastases are sites of tumor growth in subcutaneous tissues along the lymphatic drainage pathway between the primary tumor and the regional lymph node basin. There is a 2% to 3% incidence of these metastases. Because they are an indication of tumor spread, in-transit metastases are associated with a poorer prognosis. In addition, the prognosis worsens with an increased number of in-transit metastases. In two of three patients with in-transit metastases, the regional lymph nodes are also involved.

Treatment includes excision and lymph node dissection. If the extent or location of disease renders the patient unresectable, radiation therapy may provide effective palliation. More recently, isolated limb perfusion has been used with good results in achieving local control. This technique involves vascular isolation of the limb and circulation of high doses of heated chemotherapeutic and biologic agents. The most commonly used chemotherapeutic agent is melphalan. This has been combined with tumor necrosis factor α (TNF-α) and/or interferon γ (IFN-γ). Complete local response rates for melphalan alone are approximately 60% to 70%, and complete local responses as high as 100% have been reported for combinations of melphalan, TNF-α, and IFN-γ. Intralesional injection of nonspecific immunostimulatory agents such as BCG has also been used with some response. Systemic chemotherapy is a poor option and should be used only as a last resort.

Distant Metastases

Initial evaluation of patients with melanoma should include a history and physical examination, chest x-ray, and liver function tests including determination of LDH level. If *distant disease* is suspected, computerized tomographic (CT) scans of the head, chest, abdomen, and pelvis should be obtained because melanoma spreads most commonly to lung, liver, brain, and bone, in decreasing order of frequency. Cardiac, adrenal, pancreatic, visceral, and renal metastases are less commonly encountered. Brain metastases can lead to hemorrhage in 33% to 55% of cases, and strong consideration should be given to their resection, particularly given that a percentage of patients with solitary brain metastases who undergo resection and radiation therapy survive for more than 5 years. As a rule, however, distant metastases portend a poor prognosis. Median survival after diagnosis is 11 months for lung metastases and 2 to 6 months for liver, brain, or bone metastases.

Treatment of systemic melanoma has not met with much success to date. In patients who are asymptomatic and in poor medical condition, observation alone is often warranted. Surgical resection of metastases can often provide effective palliation of symptoms and lead to a median survival of 16 to 23 months. Radiation therapy may also provide some benefit, particularly with hyperfractionated dosing. Although several chemotherapy regimens have achieved some response rates, success in improving survival has been more difficult to achieve. Combination regimens including dacarbazine (DTIC), carmustine (BCNU), and tamoxifen have resulted in response rates of up to 46% and complete responses in up to 11% of patients.

Biologic therapies have also been tried with limited success. Cytokine therapy with IL-2 results in a 10% to 20%

response rate, and some of these responses are dramatic. Numerous types of vaccines have also been used or are currently undergoing clinical trials. Infusion of monoclonal antibodies directed against melanoma-specific markers is also being evaluated, as are vaccines using dendritic cells pulsed with melanoma-associated tumor antigens.

Treatment of Local Recurrences

Overall there is an approximately 3% rate of local recurrence. *Recurrence* is defined as regrowth of tumor within 5 cm of the primary resection site. It occurs more frequently in patients with thick (greater than 4 mm) primary tumors (13%); ulcerated tumors (11.5%); and in lesions of the foot, hand, scalp, and face (5% to 12%). Initial local recurrences of low-risk tumors are treated with wide excision. Conversely, multiple recurrences or recurrences from the high-risk tumor categories noted in the preceding text should be treated with excision and consideration of isolated limb perfusion. Radiation therapy should be used when isolated limb perfusion is not possible. Local recurrence signals a poor prognosis, with a 3-year median survival and a 20% 10-year survival.

Prognosis

Multiple factors influence the prognosis of melanoma. These include location, gender, thickness, Clark level, ulceration, growth pattern, age, regression, and tumor-infiltrating lymphocytes. Melanomas of the trunk have a worse prognosis than those of the extremities. Primary tumors of the leg carry a worse prognosis than that of the arm, and prognosis for scalp melanoma is worse than those for other locations of the head and neck. Disease in women is associated with a better prognosis than in men, due to which women may have a higher incidence of extremity melanomas and fewer ulcerated lesions. Matched for stage, however, survival is similar.

Thickness of the primary melanoma (Breslow scale) has been found to be the most powerful predictor of prognosis. Provided a representative biopsy is available, it is relatively simple for a pathologist to obtain this measurement, even with limited experience. The scale is divided into increments of thickness. Tumor thickness is inversely correlated with survival (Fig. 5-4).

The other common measure of depth of invasion, the Clark level, has also been shown to be highly predictive of prognosis. This measurement provides an indicator of biologic invasiveness, but its determination requires an experienced pathologist for optimal accuracy.

Ulceration is another important prognostic factor. In stage I and stage II lesions with ulceration, there is a 50% 5-year survival, whereas survival for similar, nonulcerated lesions is 75%. In stage III lesions, ulceration decreases 3-year survival from 61% to 29%.

The growth pattern of melanoma is also predictive of survival. Acral lentiginous melanoma is associated with a worse prognosis than superficial spreading and nodular melanoma. Superficial spreading melanomas are less aggressive than nodular melanomas. Of the four histologic types of melanoma, lentigo maligna melanoma carries the best prognosis; even lesions exceeding 3 mm in thickness are association with an 80% 10-year survival.

Presence of nodal or distant metastases is a strong predictor of a poor outcome. Patients with clinically positive

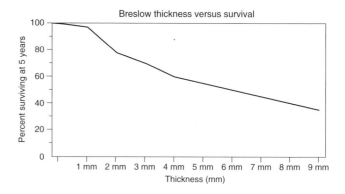

Figure 5-4 There is a linear relationship between increasing melanoma tumor thickness at diagnosis and decreasing survival.

nodes have a 12% 10-year survival; those with occult positive nodes found during ELND have a 48% 10-year survival, whereas those who are node negative have a 64% 10-year survival.

There exists an inverse correlation between age and survival. Older patients generally present with thicker melanomas and do accordingly worse, although, for unexplained reasons, the incidence of lymph node metastases in this patient population is reduced. Regression of lesions is a poor prognostic indicator, whereas tumor-infiltrating lymphocytes are associated with increased survival. Multifactorial analyses have consistently underscored the importance of thickness and ulceration as key independent prognostic factors in patients with melanoma, whereas other, smaller studies have shown location of the primary tumor, gender, mitotic rate, and the presence of vertical growth phase to also influence prognosis.

SOFT TISSUE SARCOMA

Sarcomas are tumors derived from mesenchymal cells. The term *sarcoma* comes from the Greek *sar*, meaning flesh. For clinical purposes, a basic division exists between extremity and truncal sarcomas. Extremity sarcomas represent approximately one half of adult sarcomas, whereas truncal sarcomas represent 40%. About one half of truncal sarcomas occur in the retroperitoneum.

Sarcomas have an age-adjusted incidence of 2 per 100,000 and represent about 1% of adult malignancies and approximately 15% of pediatric malignancies. In the United States there are approximately 8,000 cases per year, and cases are divided equally between men and women.

Etiology

Several genetic syndromes are associated with the development of sarcomas. Gardner syndrome is associated with the formation of multiple desmoid tumors. Li–Fraumeni syndrome, a familial cancer syndrome that is associated with an increased risk of soft tissue sarcomas, osteosarcomas, breast cancer, acute leukemia, brain tumors, adrenocortical carcinomas, and gonadal germ-cell tumors, is linked to a mutation in the p53 tumor suppressor gene. Neurofibromatosis I, or von Recklinghausen disease, is an autosomal dominant disorder characterized by multiple neurofibromas and café-au-lait spots. Sarcomas have also been associated with amplification of the MDM2 gene, whose product interacts with p53.

Environmental factors have also been linked to the occurrence of sarcomas. It has been speculated that herbicides may play a role in some cases as well as previous radiation exposure. There is generally a considerable delay of 10 years or more between radiation exposure and onset of disease. Stewart-Treves syndrome is defined as the development of an angiosarcoma associated with lymphedema, classically in breast cancer patients following removal of the tumor and axillary lymph node dissection.

Extremity Sarcomas

The clinical evaluation and treatment of sarcomas is dictated in part by their location. Extremity soft tissue sarcomas will be considered first followed by retroperitoneal sarcomas.

Diagnosis

Diagnosis begins with a comprehensive history and physical examination. During the early course of disease, clinical manifestations are infrequent, and a mass is the most common presenting complaint. Frequently, a trivial traumatic event may initially draw attention to the area, although there is probably no causal relation between a history of trauma and the development of a sarcoma.

When a suspicious mass is discovered, a biopsy is indicated. In centers in which there is significant experience with sarcomas, a core-needle biopsy may be performed as a first step. Care should be taken to insert the needle through areas that would be incorporated into a definitive resection. However, in most centers, an open biopsy is the most reliable means of obtaining a diagnosis. Lesions 3 cm or smaller can be completely excised, whereas an incisional biopsy is often appropriate for lesions 3 cm or larger. It is critical that the dissection is planned, including the skin incision, so that the biopsy tract can be excised completely in the final resection. Therefore, incisional biopsies on extremities are performed through longitudinal skin incisions.

Staging

Once a tissue specimen has been obtained, the pathologist can determine the histologic type of sarcoma. These include liposarcoma, fibrosarcoma, fibroxanthoma, leiomyosarcoma, rhabdomyosarcoma, lymphangiosarcoma, synovial sarcoma, and malignant neurilemoma. These categories are based on the appearance of the tumors and their presumed sites of origin. The most common soft tissue sarcomas in adults are malignant fibrous histiocytomas and liposarcomas, whereas rhabdomyosarcomas and fibrosarcomas are the most prevalent types in the pediatric population. There is only a 65% concordance among different pathologists in assigning type. Pathologic grade is a much more significant prognostic parameter and is more reproducible between pathologists. It is based on differentiation of cells, cellularity of the specimen, amount of stroma, vascularity, degree of necrosis, and number of mitoses per high power field.

Radiologic imaging studies provide invaluable information prior to the definitive resection of sarcomas. The goal of these studies is to define the extent of the tumor so that a resection can be planned and patients can be informed of probable outcomes. The most commonly used imaging modalities for evaluation of soft tissue sarcomas are computerized tomography and magnetic resonance imaging (MRI) with or without magnetic resonance angiography (MRA). Although CT scanning is less expensive and easier to obtain, MRI provides better resolution of soft tissues. In addition, the relationship of tumors to blood vessels can be more accurately determined by MRA. Bone scanning is sensitive for bony involvement but is not sufficiently specific to distinguish tumor extension from reactive inflammation. Angiography was previously employed in select cases of retroperitoneal or extremity sarcomas to delineate vascular anatomy, but it is rarely required with current cross-sectional imaging modalities. Because sarcomas commonly spread to the lungs via the hematogenous route, a CT scan of the chest is also indicated to rule out metastatic disease.

The combination of histologic and radiographic information can then be used to stage the patient's disease. Multiple staging systems have been developed. These systems are based on the histologic grade of the tumor, its size, and the presence of metastases in regional lymph nodes or distant sites. The AJCC produced a revised staging system in 1997. Histopathologic grade is divided into well differentiated (G1), moderately differentiated (G2), and poorly differentiated (G3). Tumors less than or equal to 5 cm in greatest dimension (T1) are separated from tumors that are greater than 5 cm (T2). The size classification is further subdivided into superficial and deep tumors noted with the suffixes a and b, respectively. Stage IV disease is defined as the presence of regional lymph node metastases (N1) or distant metastases (M1) (Table 5-4).

TABLE 5-4

AMERICAN JOINT COMMITTEE ON CANCER (AJCC) SARCOMA STAGING SYSTEM

G	Histologic grade of malignancy	
	G1	Well differentiated
	G2	Moderately differentiated
	G3	Poorly differentiated

T	Primary tumor	
	T1	Tumor ≤5 cm
	T2	Tumor >5 cm

a, tumor superficial to the fascia; b, tumor deep to the fascia, also includes retroperitoneal, mediastinal, and pelvic sarcomas.

N	Regional lymph nodes	
	N0	Absent regional lymph node involvement
	N1	Present regional lymph node involvement

M	Distant metastasis	
	M0	Absent distant metastasis
	M1	Present distant metastasis

Pathologic staging classification

I	G1, T1a-b, N0, M0
	G1, T2a-b, N0, M0
II	G2-3, T1a-b, N0, M0
	G2-3, T2a, N0, M0
III	G2-3, T2b, N0, M0
IV	Any G, Any T, N1, M0
	Any G, Any T, N0, M1

This staging system has been found to correlate well with rates of local recurrence, disease-free survival, and overall survival. Five-year survival is only 10% if metastatic disease is present (Fig. 5-5).

Surgical Treatment

Resection is the mainstay of treatment, although other modalities are useful as adjuvants. Sarcomas are characterized by a pseudocapsule. This cannot be used as a plane of dissection, as microscopic disease extends beyond the pseudocapsule and will uniformly lead to local recurrence. Local recurrence rates decreased dramatically when this was recognized, and radical resection was performed with excision of entire muscle groups. However, significant morbidity is associated with this approach because it can lead to significant impairment of limb function or even amputation. In addition, in patients who eventually succumb to distant disease, the increased morbidity of radical resection seems unnecessary. Therefore, recent focus has been placed on preservation of limbs and limb function by limiting resection.

Limb preservation has been increased by acceptance of a 2-cm resection margin in the setting of low-grade sarcomas that are less than 5 cm in diameter (Fig. 5-6). In the case of high-grade sarcomas, limb function can be preserved through a combination of limited resection and adjuvant radiotherapy. Equivalent disease-free and overall survival rates have been reported with limb-sparing procedures in conjunction with radiotherapy, compared to amputation.

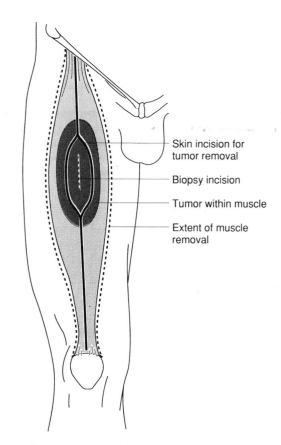

Figure 5-6 Plan for sarcoma resection showing longitudinal biopsy incision and wide excision border, sparing limb function. (From Sondak VK. Sarcomas of bone and soft tissue. In: Greenfield LJ, Mulholland MW, Oldham KT et al., eds. *Surgery: scientific principles and practice*, 2nd ed. Philadelphia: Lippincott-Raven Publishers, 1997:2257, with permission.)

Adjuvant Therapy

Radiotherapy can be administered before, after, or during surgery and is indicated in patients with tumors greater than 5 cm in diameter or close resection margins. The therapy may be given as beam radiation or in the form of brachytherapy. There have been no studies directly comparing these methods of administration, and no marked difference in local control has been noted with each method measured separately. Each technique offers some advantages and disadvantages, which may guide the physician's choice of modality. Preoperative radiotherapy has the advantages of requiring a smaller field of radiation exposure as well as a lower dose than postoperative radiation owing to relative hypoxia at the resection site. However, preoperative radiation has been demonstrated to have a significantly higher wound complication rate than postoperative radiation without a significant benefit in terms of local recurrence or survival. Therefore, preoperative radiotherapy is generally reserved for patients whose tumors are initially considered too large to resect with acceptable morbidity.

Brachytherapy is a relatively new technique in which radioactive isotopes are placed in proximity to the tumor for a period of 5 to 6 days. Although this technique is associated with rates of wound complications similar to that of postoperative external beam radiotherapy (provided therapy is delayed at least 5 days after surgery), it has the advantages of less radiation scatter and a much shorter

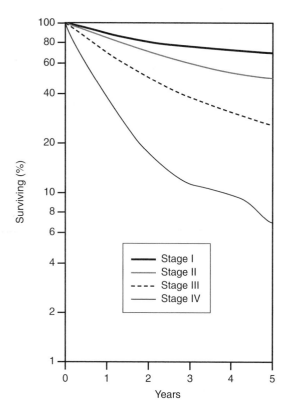

Figure 5-5 Sarcoma survival by stage of disease. (From Sondak VK. Sarcomas of bone and soft tissue. In: Greenfield LJ, Mulholland MW, Oldham KT et al., eds. *Surgery: scientific principles and practice*, 2nd ed. Philadelphia: Lippincott-Raven Publishers, 1997:2250, with permission.)

duration of therapy. Brachytherapy is indicated only in the setting of high-grade lesions, whereas external beam radiation is indicated for low-grade lesions.

Adjuvant systemic *chemotherapy* has also been used in patients with sarcoma. Trials of postoperative chemotherapy have generally demonstrated no survival benefit. A recent meta-analysis of data from previous trials revealed statistically significant improvements in local recurrence-free and disease-free survival rates in patients who received doxorubicin-containing postoperative chemotherapy. However, the same analysis did not show any improvement in overall survival, and postoperative chemotherapy cannot be considered standard therapy.

Preoperative or neoadjuvant chemotherapy has also had fairly poor results with doxorubicin-based regimens, resulting in 3% to 27% response rates. Preliminary studies using combinations of doxorubicin and ifosfamide have shown some improvement in response rates. Approaches using chemotherapy alone as adjuvant treatment have been largely abandoned in favor of protocols that combine multiple modalities.

Sequential or concurrent use of chemotherapy and radiation therapy has demonstrated promising short-term results, with improvements in local control, disease-free survival, and overall survival. However, these results will require longer follow-up and confirmation before combined modality therapy can move beyond the investigational stage.

Finally, localized therapy in the form of *isolated limb perfusion* (ILP) with chemotherapeutic agents such as melphalan in combination with TNF-α and IFN-γ or both can be used in cases where local control or limb salvage is particularly challenging. Toxicity in the perfused limb is generally not severe and is often related to necrosis of the tumor. Systemic toxicity can be severe if there is a leak of perfusate into the systemic circulation.

This technique provides only regional therapy, so its application is limited to certain specific situations. These include locally advanced disease that would otherwise require amputation for local control. ILP has demonstrated limb salvage rates of greater than 80%. In addition, ILP may be used in patients with stage IV disease that is advanced at the site of origin. ILP may preserve the function of the affected limb and quality of life over the anticipated short period of survival of these patients.

Sarcomas spread by a hematogenous route. Therefore, regional lymph node involvement is unusual, and elective lymph node dissection is not indicated. One possible exception is in the case of epithelioid sarcomas in which metastases to regional lymph nodes are found in approximately 20% of cases. Nodal metastases are also seen in 10% of rhabdomyosarcomas and 5% of malignant fibrous histiocytomas.

Local recurrence of sarcoma is associated with a poor prognosis. However, it has not been determined if there exists a causal relationship to decreased survival. The site of recurrence may be a source for further metastasis, but the fact that even amputation of the recurrent site does not improve survival suggests that distant disease may already be present at the time of the local recurrence. Local recurrences should be treated by excision. Considerations for preservation of limb function are analogous to those in primary resections, and radiotherapy should also be considered.

Even if the site has been irradiated previously, brachytherapy or intraoperative radiotherapy may be options for additional treatment. Finally, chemotherapy should be considered for patients with local recurrences of high-grade tumors. Approximately two thirds of patients who undergo resections for local recurrences will experience long-term survival.

Patients who die from their disease generally succumb to distant metastases. The tumors with higher histologic grade and those exceeding 5 cm in greatest dimension have a greater propensity to metastasize. Longer intervals from the treatment of the primary tumor to the occurrence of metastatic disease are associated with a better prognosis. The lungs are the most common site of metastasis. Pulmonary lesions should be resected, provided the patient can tolerate the operation and has adequate pulmonary reserve. Survival at 5 years in patients with completely resected pulmonary metastases is 15% to 30%.

Retroperitoneal Sarcoma

Retroperitoneal sarcomas are considerably less common than extremity sarcomas, making up only 15% to 25% of all cases. However, these tumors carry a much worse prognosis, because approximately 60% are high grade, and given a relative lack of clinical signs during the early stages of disease, they are frequently not diagnosed until they have reached a relatively advanced stage. The progress in patient outcomes and quality of life, which has been evident in the treatment of extremity sarcoma, has unfortunately not been mirrored in retroperitoneal sarcomas.

Diagnosis

Most patients present with an abdominal mass (80%) and frequently with lower extremity neurologic symptoms (42%) or pain (37%). Most tumors are greater than 10 cm in diameter at the time of presentation and the most common histologic types are liposarcoma (41%), leiomyosarcoma (27%), and malignant fibrous histiocytoma (7%).

Evaluation of a suspected retroperitoneal sarcoma should include CT scanning to evaluate the local extent of disease and the presence of hepatic metastases. It is important in this anatomic region to distinguish sarcoma from lymphoma and germ-cell tumors, both of which are amenable to chemotherapy. This can be accomplished with a CT scan or ultrasound-guided fine-needle aspirate, or if that is inadequate, a guided core biopsy. If lymphoma or germ-cell tumor is not part of the differential diagnosis, biopsy is performed only if neoadjuvant therapy is considered because of concerns of seeding the needle tract with malignant tumor cells. An abdominal/pelvic MRI and/or MRA may be necessary to delineate involvement of adjacent vasculature. Metastatic workup should include a CT scan of the chest.

Treatment

Chemotherapy has not been shown to be effective for these tumors and use of radiation is limited because of toxicity to adjacent structures; consequently, surgery offers the only effective treatment. Complete gross resection is possible in more than 75% of initial presentations and frequently requires resection of neighboring organs. Patients who have unresectable tumors on the basis of radiologic studies may be candidates for neoadjuvant chemoradiation in an

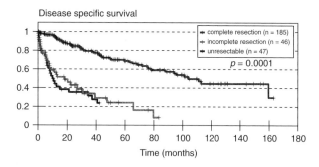

Figure 5-7 Incomplete resection provides no survival benefit. (From Lewis JJ, Leung D, Woodruff JM, et al. Retroperitoneal soft-tissue sarcoma: analysis of 500 patients treated and followed at a single institution. *Ann Surg* 1998;228(3):355–365, with permission.)

attempt to decrease tumor size to the point where resection is possible. However, resection should be attempted only if a complete resection is anticipated because incomplete resection has not been shown to offer any benefit in survival (Fig. 5-7).

Approximately 25% of patients with complete gross resections will nevertheless have positive microscopic margins. Patients who have high-grade sarcomas fare significantly worse than those with low-grade tumors (median survival 33 months vs. 149 months). Approximately one half of the patients who experience local recurrences will have disease that is grossly resectable. Resection is the only effective treatment for such a recurrence. Distant disease most frequently occurs in the liver (44%), lung (38%), or both (18%). If the distant disease is isolated, it should be considered for resection, since long-term survival is possible following metastasectomy. Overall, however, patients with metastatic disease have only a 10-month median survival.

Because early recognition of metastases while resection is still possible, offers patients the only hope of cure, patients with no evidence of disease should be followed closely for signs of recurrence. This follow-up should include history taking and physical examination every 3 months for the first 2 years, with a chest radiograph every 6 months. Any radiographic abnormalities should be further evaluated with a CT scan of the chest. The site of the primary tumor should be evaluated with MRI every 6 months for the first 2 years, particularly if the primary tumor was in a deep location. After the first 2 years, patients should undergo a history and physical examination every 6 months for the next 3 years.

LYMPHOMA

Surgeons are often asked to participate in the care of patients with lymphoma for specific reasons: diagnosis, intravenous access, or to treat complications of the disease. Hematologic malignancies are the most common malignancies in children younger than 15 years and constitute 6% to 8% of adult cancers.

Lymph Node Biopsy

One of the most common reasons for surgical consultation for patients with lymphoma is to obtain tissue for diagnosis. The importance of tissue architecture in pathologic classification and the need for a considerable amount of

tissue for special studies leads to the need for surgical biopsy rather than fine-needle aspirate or core biopsy. One exception is for evaluation of recurrence when a needle biopsy may be sufficient. Generally, the largest node is removed because this provides the greatest chance for a positive result and the greatest amount of tissue for study. Although ease of removal is a consideration for choosing the biopsy site, cervical or axillary nodes are generally preferred over inguinal nodes, as nodal enlargement caused by reactive inflammation is less likely.

Hodgkin Lymphoma

Patients with Hodgkin lymphoma typically present in young adulthood with nontender lymphadenopathy. Cervical lymph node basins are the most commonly involved sites at presentation, followed by those in the axillary, inguinal, mediastinal, and retroperitoneal basins. Patients may report the presence of other symptoms such as fever (greater than 38°C), night sweats, or weight loss of more than 10% of body weight over a 6-month period. These are the so-called *B symptoms* and have staging and prognostic significance, as discussed in subsequent text.

In addition to a complete history focusing on duration of lymph node enlargement as well as recent injury to sites drained by that lymphatic basin, the evaluation of patients referred for lymph node biopsy should include a physical examination, with detailed evaluation of all accessible lymphatic tissue. This includes palpation of all superficial lymph node basins, oropharyngeal examination with evaluation of tonsils, and abdominal palpation for hepatic or splenic enlargement. Laboratory studies should include a complete blood count with differential and peripheral blood smear examination.

Staging in Hodgkin disease is based on the extent of disease and the presence or absence of the symptoms. Stage I disease is limited to a single lymph node region or single extralymphatic site. Stage II is characterized by involvement of two or more lymph node regions on the same side of the diaphragm or one extralymphatic site with only adjacent lymph nodes involved. In stage III disease, lymph nodes on both sides of the diaphragm or the spleen (denoted with an *S*) are involved, and stage IV consists of diffuse or disseminated involvement of one or more extralymphatic sites with or without associated lymph node involvement. The absence of constitutional symptoms is denoted with an *A*, whereas their presence is denoted with a *B*. Staging workup includes tests for liver function and chest radiographs. CT scans have also become routine to evaluate the presence of mediastinal or retroperitoneal lymphadenopathy. Bone marrow biopsies provide additional information regarding the extent of disease, although their overall impact on disease management has been questioned.

The cornerstones of treatment of Hodgkin lymphoma are radiation therapy for stage I and IIA disease, and chemotherapy in combination with radiation for patients with stage IIB disease and greater.

The *staging laparotomy* has historically played an important role in the evaluation of patients with Hodgkin disease. The goal of this procedure is to provide a thorough evaluation of the abdomen and retroperitoneum for the presence of disease, and thereby distinguish between low-stage and advanced lymphoma. The procedure entails a midline

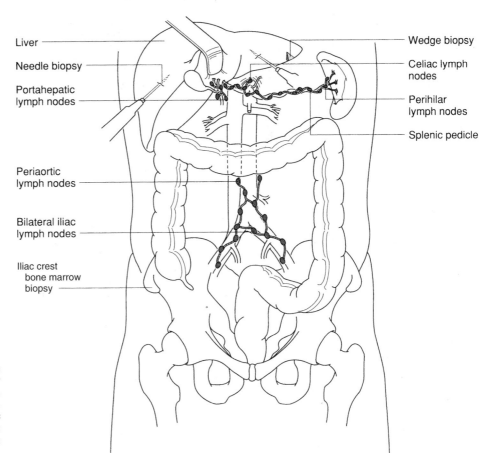

Figure 5-8 Biopsy sites during staging laparotomy. (From Meyer AA. Spleen. In: Greenfield LJ, Mulholland MW, Oldham KT et al., eds. *Surgery: scientific principles and practice*, 2nd ed. Philadelphia: Lippincott-Raven Publishers, 1997: 1275, with permission.)

laparotomy and palpation of the liver, small bowel, colon, and mesentery. Intraoperative ultrasonography may be used as an adjunct to palpation for evaluation of deeper areas within solid organs. Splenectomy and wedge biopsies of the liver are also performed with additional core needle biopsies of deeper hepatic tissue. Each major nodal group is then dissected. Nodes associated with the hepatic artery and celiac axis are removed via an incision in the gastrohepatic ligament, and nodes from the porta hepatis are sampled as well. Finally, the aorta is exposed inferior to the transverse mesocolon and nodes are removed along the inferior mesenteric artery. If there are any nodes that are suspicious based on evaluation at laparotomy or preoperative lymphangiography, these should also be removed with concomitant oophoropexy in anticipation of radiation to the pelvis (Fig. 5-8).

Improved radiographic imaging has led to a significantly reduced need for staging laparotomies to choose a therapeutic approach (Fig. 5-9). Patients with early stage disease and favorable histology almost always have disease limited to supradiaphragmatic nodal tissue and can be treated safely with mantle radiation therapy only. In addition, improved efficacy and safety of chemotherapy have led to its more liberal administration in cases of suspected advanced Hodgkin disease, with laparotomy for pathologic confirmation deemed unnecessary. However, staging laparotomy is still indicated in select cases where negative results would obviate the need for chemotherapy. Hodgkin disease may also be staged laparoscopically. Use of this technique decreases postoperative ileus and length of hospitalization, which may increase the use of operative staging.

Non-Hodgkin Lymphoma

Non-Hodgkin lymphoma is increasing in incidence in the United States and now represents approximately 7% of malignancies. Some of this increase can be attributed to increasing numbers and life expectancies of patients with acquired immunodeficiency syndrome (AIDS). Patients typically present with lymphadenopathy. On histologic

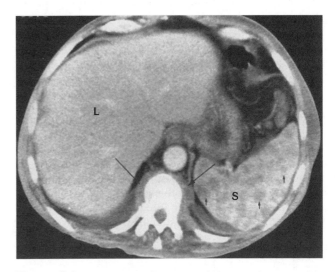

Figure 5-9 Computerized tomographic scan demonstrating involvement of both the spleen and paraaortic lymph nodes. L, liver; S, spleen. (From Brant WE. Pancreas and spleen. In: Brant WE, Helms CA, eds. *Fundamentals of diagnostic radiology*, 2nd ed. Philadelphia: Lippincott Williams & Wilkins, 1998:710, with permission.)

evaluation the tumors are classified as diffuse versus follicular, small cell versus large cell, and cleaved versus noncleaved nuclear morphology. Most cases are of B-cell origin (80%). With use of histopathologic information, non-Hodgkin lymphomas are classified as low-, intermediate-, or high grade according to their prognosis.

Surgeons are typically called upon to obtain tissue for diagnosis. The use of a staging laparotomy is extremely limited in patients with non-Hodgkin lymphoma because this disease generally does not progress in the orderly manner seen in Hodgkin lymphoma and patients therefore typically present with advanced disease.

Gastrointestinal Lymphoma

The *stomach* is the most common site of extranodal non-Hodgkin lymphoma in the United States. Gastric lymphoma is the second most common tumor of the stomach, representing 2% to 7% of primary gastric malignancies. Patients typically present with abdominal pain (71% to 85%), weight loss (11% to 68%), nausea or vomiting (14% to 28%), bleeding (7% to 23%), or, rarely, perforation (0% to 6%).

Patients will usually undergo endoscopic evaluation, which has become increasingly effective in diagnosing lymphoma. The sensitivity of endoscopy is reported to be 92% to 100%. However, the technique is not completely specific, as 25% of cases of gastric lymphoma are diagnosed only as cancer, and not lymphoma, before operation.

There are several systems for staging gastrointestinal lymphomas. The Ann Arbor system uses the suffix *E* to identify lymphomas that originate in extranodal tissue. The TNM staging system is also used. Tumor stage is based on level of invasion, nodal stage is based on the presence and location of lymph nodes positive for tumor, and metastasis stage is based on the presence of distant metastasis (Table 5-5).

This system correlates well with patient survival but does not take into account tumor grade. A third system proposed as a result of a workshop in 1994 presents a system for pathologic classification that incorporates tumor grade. Prognosis correlates with both stage and grade and correlates more closely when both variables are considered.

Treatment for gastric lymphomas is highly variable. Numerous studies have demonstrated that surgery alone is an effective therapy for early (stage I$_E$ or II$_E$) stage disease. However, other studies have demonstrated no additional benefit to surgery in patients treated with chemotherapy and radiation therapy. One difficulty in evaluating these results is that there are no prospective randomized trials of surgical versus nonsurgical treatment. Single-modality treatment with surgery, radiation, or chemotherapy is appropriate for early stage disease, and multimodality treatment including chemotherapy is indicated for more advanced (stage II$_E$ or stage I, high grade) disease. Most centers employ surgical treatment in patients with early stage disease as well as in patients with advanced stages of disease who present with bleeding or obstruction.

Gastric Mucosa–Associated Lymphoma Tissue

Gastric mucosa–associated lymphoid tissue (MALT) lymphoma is a collection of lymphoid tissue in the stomach

TABLE 5-5
PRIMARY GASTRIC LYMPHOMA STAGING: TNM

Tumor stage (depth of invasion)
T1: lamina propria or submucosa
T2: muscularis propria
T3: subserosa
T4: serosa (adjacent structures free)
T5: adjacent structures

Metastasis stage
M0: no metastases
M1: distant metastases

Nodal stage
N0: node negative
N1: perigastric nodes
N2: perigastric nodes >3 cm from stomach or along hepatic, left gastric, splenic or celiac arteries
N3: hepatoduodenal, paraaortic, or distant abdominal nodes
N4: nodes beyond N3

Stage	Tumor	Nodes	Metastasis	5-yr survival
I	T1	N0,N1	M0	100%
II	T1	N2	M0	88.9%
	T2,T3	N0,N1,N2	M0	
III	T4,T5	Any N	M0	52.1%
	Any T	N3,N4	M0	
IV	Any T	Any N	M1	25%

that resembles mucosa-associated lymphoid tissue rather than nodal lymphoid tissue. It is believed to be a precursor of gastric lymphoma and is associated with *Helicobacter pylori* infection. Proliferation of malignant, monoclonal B cells is stimulated by IL-2 released by nonneoplastic T cells in response to the infection. Treatment with antibiotics to eliminate the infection is highly effective in cases of low-grade MALT lymphoma. Patients who fail to respond completely to antibiotic therapy should undergo surgical resection and possibly chemotherapy based on the pathology of the surgical specimen.

Other Gastrointestinal Lymphomas

Lymphomas of the small bowel are less common in the United States but are the most common extranodal lymphoma in the Middle East. These tumors have a higher incidence in patients who suffer from celiac disease and are typically located in the proximal jejunum. These tumors can present with obstruction, intussusception, or bleeding and are multiple in 20% of cases. Appropriate treatment is limited resection followed by chemotherapy. Radiation therapy can be considered as an additional modality, but its utility is limited by radiation enteritis. Survival at 5 years is approximately 40%.

Colonic lymphomas are rare, although they are the most common noncarcinomatous tumors of the large bowel. Occasionally, systemic non-Hodgkin lymphoma can lead to diffuse lymphomatous polyposis. Treatment of these tumors also consists of local resection of involved bowel with adjuvant therapy dictated by the stage and grade of the disease. Overall survival at 5 years after complete resection is 50%.

SPLEEN

Surgical intervention is frequently required in the care of patients with splenic complications of hematologic disorders or trauma. This section will consider the normal anatomy and function of the spleen and discuss the surgical care of patients with abnormalities manifested in the spleen as a result of systemic disease.

Anatomy and Normal Function

The spleen arises from embryologic mesoderm along the left side of the dorsal mesogastrium and attains a weight of 100 to 150 g in the normal adult. It is a solid, purplish organ located in the left upper quadrant that measures approximately 12 × 7 × 4 cm and stretches from the eighth to the eleventh rib. Its blood supply arises from the splenic artery off the celiac trunk and from the short gastric arteries. It is surrounded by a fibroelastic capsule of 1 to 2 mm in thickness. Humans lack any significant smooth muscle in the capsule and are, therefore, not able to produce autotransfusion in response to circulating catecholamines, as is the case of other mammals. The spleen is attached by so-called *ligaments* of connective tissue to surrounding structures. These include the gastrosplenic ligament containing the short gastric arteries as well as the avascular splenorenal, splenophrenic, and splenocolic ligaments.

The parenchyma of the spleen is divided into the red and white pulps, which are the sites of filtration of senescent or abnormal red blood cells and other unwanted elements from the blood and generation of effective lymphoid immune responses, respectively. Blood is carried into the spleen from the hilum via trabecular arteries, which branch to form the central arterioles. Central arterioles are surrounded by white pulp over much of their course and empty either into the red pulp from open-ended penicillary arterioles or into venules through a closed circulation without being directly exposed to the red pulp. After entering venous sinusoids, blood drains into trabecular veins and exits via the splenic vein (Fig. 5-10).

The red pulp is composed of sponge-like areas of tissue known as the *cords of Billroth*. They contain a large number of macrophages that function to remove aged or defective red blood cells. They also remove inclusions from cells such as Heinz or Howell-Jolly bodies. In autoimmune hemolytic anemia, these macrophages recognize and destroy red blood cells coated with autoantibodies. Bacteria, cellular debris, and other abnormal debris are also filtered in the red pulp.

The spleen is one of the secondary lymphoid organs. The majority of splenic lymphoid activity occurs in the white pulp. One particularly important lymphoid function performed by the spleen is the generation of primary antibody responses. It is well suited to this function, as serum and any foreign antigens contained within it are skimmed from trabecular and central arteries and pass through the white pulp and sinusoids where they may be taken up, processed, and presented by macrophages or dendritic cells. This generally takes place in the T-cell dominated periarterial sheaths. Lymphocyte responses are generated in lymphoid nodules that are composed primarily of B cells and follicular dendritic cells and are spaced out along the artery. If an antigen is presented by antigen-presenting cells (APCs) and recognized by lymphocytes, a germinal center containing proliferating lymphocytes forms within the follicle. The spleen is central to the development of new antibody responses characterized by the production of immunoglobulin (Ig)M.

The spleen has other functions including production of monocytes and lymphocytes and storage of 30% to 40% of the body's platelets. It serves as a site of hematopoiesis during early development and in some pathologic conditions.

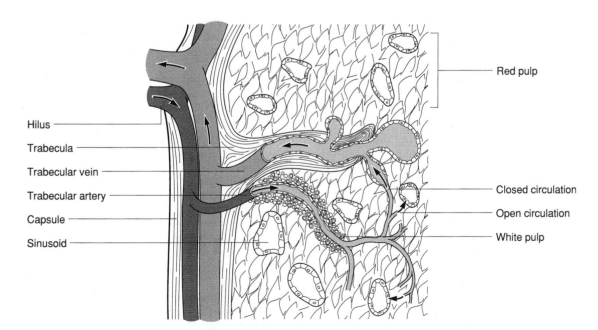

Figure 5-10 The splenic microcirculation is shown with depictions of both open and closed circulation. (From Meyer AA. Spleen. In: Greenfield LJ, Mulholland MW, Oldham KT et al., eds. *Surgery: scientific principles and practice*, 2nd ed. Philadelphia: Lippincott-Raven Publishers, 1997:1265, with permission.)

Splenomegaly

Surgical consultation is frequently sought for splenomegaly. The differential diagnosis includes infectious, hematologic, neoplastic (both hematologic and nonhematologic), congestive, inflammatory, and infiltrative processes.

Malaria is the most common *infectious* cause for splenic enlargement in tropical regions of the world, whereas splenomegaly caused by mononucleosis is more prevalent in the developed world. In addition, AIDS, viral hepatitis, cytomegalovirus, tuberculosis, hepatic echinococcosis, and congenital syphilis may lead to splenomegaly.

Hematologic disorders are among the most common causes of splenic enlargement. These include disorders of red blood cells such as spherocytosis, early sickle cell disease, thalassemia major, paroxysmal nocturnal hemoglobinuria, hemoglobinopathies, and autoimmune hemolytic anemia. Generally in these disorders the spleen is congested because of an attempt to clear abnormal erythrocytes from the circulation. In advanced stages of sickle cell disease, the spleen eventually undergoes autoinfarction owing to occlusion of its vasculature by distorted red blood cells.

Myeloproliferative disorders are characterized by overproduction of one or more hematologic cell lines. These syndromes include polycythemia vera, myelogenous leukemia, and idiopathic thrombocytosis. Myeloproliferative disorders are often accompanied by replacement of bone marrow with fibrous tissue, or myelofibrosis, leading to extramedullary hematopoiesis. This combined with infiltration of the spleen with abnormal blood components can result in massive splenomegaly.

Hematologic neoplasms such as lymphomas and leukemias are also responsible for a significant proportion of enlarged spleens. Hairy cell leukemia is commonly associated with pancytopenia and splenomegaly, and select cases respond well to splenectomy as primary treatment.

Although rare, *extrasplenic* tumors such as melanoma and lung and breast malignancies may metastasize to the spleen. Generally, involvement of the spleen occurs when the primary tumor becomes widely metastatic. In addition, nonhematologic primary tumors such as sarcomas, hemangiomas, and hamartomas may arise in the spleen.

Congestion within the portal venous system, which may be due to primary hepatic disease, thrombosis of the hepatic, portal, or splenic veins, or right ventricular dysfunction, can result in splenomegaly. Pancreatitis is the most common cause of *splenic vein thrombosis*. This condition frequently results in gastric varices and can be treated with splenectomy. The likelihood of functional hypersplenism increases with the duration of congestion and splenomegaly.

Inflammatory or *autoimmune conditions* may result in reactive hyperplasia of the spleen and splenomegaly. This is seen in a variety of disorders including infectious mononucleosis, autoimmune hemolytic anemia, and systemic lupus erythematosus. Rheumatoid arthritis, when accompanied by splenomegaly and neutropenia, is known as *Felty syndrome*. This condition is associated with antibodies against granulocytes and responds well to splenectomy.

Splenomegaly may also result from *infiltration with extracellular or intracellular material*. Sarcoidosis and amyloidosis are examples of disorders in which extracellular accumulation occurs. Several enzymatic defects that result in abnormal storage or degradation products such as gangliosides and mucopolysaccharides can lead to their accumulation in the reticuloendothelial system and consequently enlargement of the liver, spleen, and lymph nodes. Gaucher disease (β-glucocerebrosidase deficiency) and Niemann-Pick disease (sphingomyelinase deficiency) are examples of such disorders.

Splenectomy

Splenectomy is indicated as treatment for severe symptoms of splenomegaly and hypersplenism, as a diagnostic procedure, and in some cases of splenic trauma, as discussed in more detail in Section III (Trauma section) of this book. Splenectomy may be indicated in some cases to relieve the effects of increased splenic size alone. In such cases, the massive size of the spleen causes symptoms such as shortness of breath, early satiety, and weight loss secondary to displacement of neighboring structures including the stomach or diaphragm.

In other cases, the spleen may need to be removed owing to clinical consequences of its function, as in the case of *hypersplenism*. Although hypersplenism may be associated with splenomegaly, the syndrome is currently defined on the basis of its functional consequences rather than according to organ size. The clinical picture is one of deficiency and increased turnover in one or more hematologic cell lines with increased or normal cellularity of the bone marrow. Hypersplenism may in rare cases be a primary disorder, but it is generally secondary to another systemic abnormality. In such cases of secondary hypersplenism, the spleen functions normally but abnormalities in blood components lead to excessive destruction or sequestration in the spleen.

Some *hematologic diseases* respond well to splenectomy. *Hereditary spherocytosis*, the most common symptomatic familial hemolytic anemia, is characterized by defective erythrocyte membranes owing to a deficiency in *spectrin*. The red blood cells are relatively fragile and are therefore destroyed after only a few passes through the splenic cords, resulting in anemia, jaundice, intractable leg ulcers, and an increased incidence of gallstones. Splenectomy should be delayed until after the age of 3 years in order to reduce the incidence of infectious complications. Although the red blood cell defect persists after splenectomy, symptoms are typically completely relieved. Cholecystectomy should be performed at the time of splenectomy in patients who have developed pigment gallstones before the procedure. *Hereditary elliptocytosis* is a similar, though less severe, disorder of red blood cell membranes. Splenectomy may be indicated in these patients depending on the severity of associated symptoms. *Thalassemia major* and *sickle cell disease* are red blood cell disorders characterized by abnormal hemoglobin and increased red blood cell destruction. Splenectomy is generally not indicated in these disorders, but it may decrease transfusion requirements in some cases of thalassemia and may be useful in certain cases of splenic sequestration in sickle cell disease.

Autoimmune hemolytic anemia is characterized by autoantibodies to red blood cells, which develop after exposure to certain drugs during the course of a collagen vascular disease or infection, or in up to 50% of cases without an identifiable cause. Penicillin, quinidine, hydralazine, and methyldopa are the drugs most commonly implicated in inducing autoimmune hemolysis. Antibodies are classified as *warm* or *cold*, depending on the temperature at which they bind optimally to red blood cells. Cold antibodies are typically of the IgM isotype, and warm antibodies are usually IgG. Some patients experience only a self-limited acute episode of the disease. Corticosteroids induce a remission in approximately 75% of cases and are the first-line treatment for patients who have more severe forms of the disease. Approximately two thirds of these patients will have a relapse after steroid withdrawal. Splenectomy is indicated only for patients with warm antibodies in whom steroids have failed or are contraindicated. Removal of the spleen is therapeutic in about 80% of these patients. Other medical therapies such as azathioprine or cyclophosphamide have been used in patients for whom steroids and splenectomy have failed.

Hematologic disorders may also result in increased *platelet destruction,* and splenectomy is often an effective treatment. *Idiopathic thrombocytopenic purpura* (ITP) is characterized by IgG antibodies directed at platelets. The spleen contributes both to the production of these antibodies and to the sequestration of antibody-bound platelets. Clinical manifestations of the disease include thrombocytopenia with platelet counts generally lower than 50,000, prolonged bleeding times with fairly normal clotting times, and normal to hyperplastic megakaryocytes. *The spleen is generally not enlarged.* Bleeding from the gums or gastrointestinal tract may occur and women, who make up 75% of patients, often experience excessive menstrual bleeding. Although acute ITP is frequently self-limited, particularly in children, patients may require treatment. Steroids are the first-line treatment in this disorder. Patients who do not respond within the first 6 to 8 weeks of treatment, or who relapse after withdrawal of steroids, should undergo splenectomy. Approximately 75% to 85% of these patients will attain a permanent response with increased platelet counts or normalization of bleeding diathesis even if the platelet count does not fully return to normal. Persistence of symptoms may indicate the presence of an accessory spleen. Technetium scanning is a sensitive method of detecting accessory spleens, which should be removed if they are found. Intracranial hemorrhage resulting from ITP is an indication for emergent splenectomy.

TTP is defined by a pentad of clinical features: fever, thrombocytopenic purpura, hemolytic anemia, neurologic manifestations, and renal dysfunction. Arteriolar damage results in activation or destruction of multiple blood components, resulting in anemia, thrombocytopenia, and thrombosis. Cerebral hemorrhage and renal failure are the most frequent causes of death in these patients. Plasmapheresis and transfusion with fresh-frozen plasma has proved to be the most effective treatment. Splenectomy is indicated in cases refractory to plasmapheresis. Steroids and dextran may also provide some benefit. Most patients can achieve remission with one or more of these therapies.

Technical Considerations of Splenectomy

The spleen is generally approached through a midline or left subcostal incision. The former is used in trauma cases. The ligamentous attachments of the spleen are taken down to mobilize the spleen. These normally avascular attachments may develop collateral vessels in myeloid metaplasia

and secondary hypersplenism. The short gastric vessels are doubly ligated, but care must be taken to preserve gastric circulation. The hilar vessels are then dissected and ligated. During elective splenectomies, the hilar dissection may be completed before mobilization of ligamentous attachments. Initial ligation of the splenic artery serves to decrease the size of the spleen and facilitate complete mobilization. The pancreatic tail is in proximity to the splenic hilum, so careful dissection is required to avoid damaging the pancreas during the hilar dissection. In patients undergoing splenectomy to treat hematologic disease, a careful search should be made for accessory spleens in the peritoneal cavity, as their presence frequently causes postoperative recurrent hypersplenism.

There is controversy regarding preoperative embolization as a method of reducing splenic size and intraoperative blood loss. Data supporting the use of this technique have failed to clearly demonstrate a benefit to date, and the technique is not utilized at our institution.

Many patients undergoing splenectomy in the context of hematologic disorders have had numerous previous blood transfusions and may therefore have developed antibodies to blood products. This makes cross-matching of banked blood difficult, and ample time must be allowed to complete the task before surgery.

Gastric decompression should be accomplished both intraoperatively and postoperatively until bowel function has returned. This prevents gastric distention, which may hinder intraoperative exposure and place strain on short gastric ligatures.

Laparoscopic Splenectomy

Improvements in video technology and laparoscopic instruments as well as increased surgical experience with laparoscopic techniques have resulted in the performance of considerably more laparoscopic splenectomies. The procedure is typically performed with the patient in either a lithotomy or a right lateral decubitus position. Port placement is variable but typically includes a 10-mm umbilical camera port and three to five other ports for placement of instruments and retractors. Initially, the short gastric vessels are exposed, ligated or cauterized, and divided. The splenic hilum is then dissected, and the splenic artery and vein are isolated and divided individually using an endoscopic stapling device. The spleen can then be removed either by enlarging one of the port-site incisions to allow for removal or by morcellation within a plastic retrieval bag placed into the peritoneal cavity.

The indications for laparoscopic splenectomy are the same as those for open splenectomy, although several relative contraindications for using the laparoscopic approach exist. Trauma patients are not appropriate candidates, because unstable patients cannot tolerate the operative time required to perform the technique, and stable patients are generally treated with nonoperative therapy or splenorrhaphy. Massive splenomegaly is a relative but not absolute contraindication, as similar results of cases involving smaller spleens have been reported.

In general, the operative times have been found to be longer and the operative costs higher with the laparoscopic approach. The blood loss, transfusion requirements, and complication rates are generally similar. The postoperative ileus and length of hospital stay are significantly decreased, leading to an overall cost comparable to that of the open technique.

Complications of Splenectomy

Splenectomy, both when it is elective and when it is performed for isolated trauma, is generally well tolerated. Mean operative blood loss is between 250 and 400 mL in most series, and transfusions are required in about 10% to 15% of patients. An incidence of subphrenic abscess as high as 3.4% has been reported in some trauma series. However, when patients with isolated splenic injuries, or patients undergoing elective splenectomy, are considered alone, the rate is well below 1%. Leukocytosis and thrombocytosis are frequently observed in the postsplenectomy patient. These elevations generally occur 1 to 2 days after surgery and may persist for several weeks. These laboratory abnormalities generally are not clinically significant, but antiplatelet agents such as aspirin should be considered if the platelet count increases to greater than 1×10^6 per millimeter cubed. Delayed complications may also arise from splenectomy. These include pseudoaneurysm formation of the splenic artery and pancreatic fistula or pseudocyst formation resulting from iatrogenic injury to the pancreas.

Patients who have undergone a splenectomy are more susceptible to infections than the general population. Although this increase has been reported as high as 200 to 600 times the normal risk, this translates into an estimated incidence of less than 0.2%. The risk is somewhat higher in the pediatric population, with an estimated incidence of 0.6%. The disease process leading to splenectomy appears to affect risk, with posttraumatic splenectomy engendering the least risk. The first 2 years after splenectomy are the most dangerous in both the adult and pediatric populations, but some increased risk continues throughout the patient's life.

Encapsulated bacteria are the most frequent infectious agents responsible for *overwhelming postsplenectomy sepsis* (OPSS). *Pneumococcus* is the most common organism, accounting for between 50% and 90% of cases. *Haemophilus influenzae*, another significant agent, accounts for 32% of OPSS deaths. *Neisseria meningitidis* is the third important encapsulated organism. The clinical course of OPSS is frequently fulminant. Patients may develop fever and mild symptoms of infection, followed rapidly by severe sepsis and death. Progression from good health to death may occur in less than 24 hours. Treatment of patients who may be developing OPSS must be early and aggressive. Empiric antibiotic therapy is instituted with drugs tailored to treat resistance patterns of pneumococci prevalent in the respective area.

Vaccines exist for the three encapsulated organisms noted previously. Because the spleen plays an important role in the development of new immune responses, the vaccine should be given at least 2 weeks before splenectomy. In emergent cases, such as trauma, in which preoperative administration of vaccines is not feasible, the vaccines must be given postoperatively. Consensus has not been reached regarding the optimal timing for postsplenectomy vaccination. Some investigators advocate early vaccination, whereas others find that it should be delayed until the patient is in positive nitrogen balance.

Pediatric patients are frequently treated with prophylactic antibiotics following splenectomy because they are at a higher risk of developing OPSS. Prophylactic antibiotics have traditionally consisted of penicillin or amoxicillin, but changing bacterial resistance patterns has made this recommendation less uniform. Patients located in areas of high resistance to penicillin should receive trimethoprim-sulfamethoxazole or possibly amoxicillin/clavulanic acid. There is also no uniform recommendation with regard to the duration of prophylactic antibiotic therapy. Some authors suggest that treatment may be stopped at the age of 6 years, whereas others advocate the continuation of therapy until the age of 18. Some authors also recommend treating adult patients with prophylactic antibiotics for the first 2 years following splenectomy while the patient is considered to be at highest risk.

KEY CONCEPTS

▲ Tumor thickness and ulceration in that order are the most important pathologic factors in predicting risk of disease progression and death in patients with melanoma.

▲ The accepted resection margins for thin (less than 1 mm) and intermediate (1 to 4 mm) thickness melanomas are 1 cm and 2 cm, respectively. Insufficient data exist regarding thick (greater than 4 mm) melanomas, but margins should be as wide as possible without compromising cosmetic or functional results.

▲ Elective lymph node dissection for melanoma has been largely replaced by sentinel lymph node biopsy for staging regional lymph nodes. Therapeutic lymph node dissection is important for patients with a positive sentinel lymph node.

▲ With suspicious large masses on an extremity, incisional biopsies should be performed through longitudinal skin incisions so that the biopsy tract can be excised completely in the final resection.

▲ Pathologic grade is the most significant prognostic parameter, and the most reproducible between pathologists, for soft tissue sarcoma.

▲ Radiation therapy has been shown to affect only local recurrence rates, not overall survival, in patients with extremity sarcoma. Chemotherapy given in a neoadjuvant setting may help down stage patients to enable complete resection, but it has not been shown to improve overall survival.

▲ Retroperitoneal sarcoma carries a worse prognosis than extremity sarcoma because a large percentage of these tumors are high grade and because they are frequently not diagnosed until they have reached a relatively advanced stage.

▲ Non-Hodgkin lymphoma is increasing in incidence in the United States in large part because of the increasing prevalence of acquired immunodeficiency syndrome (AIDS).

▲ Hereditary spherocytosis, a type of familial hemolytic anemia, is characterized by defective erythrocyte membranes resulting from a deficiency in spectrin. Splenectomy is typically curative.

▲ Idiopathic thrombocytopenic purpura (ITP) is characterized by immunoglobulin (Ig)G antibodies directed at platelets. The spleen is generally not enlarged. Steroids are the first-line therapy for this disorder, but splenectomy is indicated for those in whom steroids fail or are contraindicated.

SUGGESTED READINGS

Aisenberg AC. Coherent view of non-Hodgkin's lymphoma. *J Clin Oncol* 1995;13:2656–2675.

Balch CM, Soong SJ, Gershenwald JE. Prognostic factors analysis of 17,600 melanoma patients: validation of the American Joint Committee on Cancer melanoma staging system. *J Clin Oncol* 2001; 19:3622–3634.

Lewis JJ, Brennan MF. Soft tissue sarcomas. In: *Current problems in surgery*. Chicago: Yearbook Medical Publishers, 1996.

McClelland RN. *The spleen. Selected readings in general surgery*, Vol 24, No 8. Texas: University of Texas, Southwestern Medical Center at Dallas, 1997.

Tsao H, Atkins MB, Sober AJ. Medical progress: management of cutaneous melanoma. *N Engl J Med* 2004;351:998–1012.

Wound Healing

6

Stephen M. Bauer   Omaida C. Velazquez

INTRODUCTION

Tissue injury is often followed by resolution, regeneration, or repair. Resolution is the removal of dead cellular material and debris by macrophage-mediated phagocytosis that leaves the tissue's original architecture intact. In regeneration, lost tissue is replaced by the proliferation of cells, of the same type, that reconstruct the normal architecture. Finally, repair is the process through which lost tissue is replaced by a fibrous scar that is produced from the granulation of tissue.

TYPES OF WOUND HEALING

Wound healing occurs by different processes, which depend on the type of injury and whether the wound margins are in approximation. The classic three wound healing processes are primary, secondary, and tertiary intention. Healing by primary intention occurs when a sharp instrument, such as a scalpel, is used to make the wound where the wound margins are closely approximated with sutures or staples shortly after the wound was incurred. Within 48 hours rapid reepithelialization occurs, followed by the deposition and cross-linking of the collagen matrix.

Healing by secondary intention occurs when there is severe disruption to the tissue by a large defect in which the margins cannot be approximated. Often, these wounds occur after wide débridement of infected tissue. Alternatively, surgically created sharp wounds can be left unapproximated and allowed to close by secondary intention because of concerns about contamination and infection. This type of healing is characterized by prolonged periods of healing repair. The wound bed fills with granulation tissue, which is characterized by ingrowth of capillaries, fibroblasts, and extracellular matrix, and the margins subsequently close by contraction. An advantage of this process is that it allows large contaminated wounds to heal while also minimizing the risk of abscess formation. However, this process results in a large, often unsightly, scar and longer healing times. In addition, the combination of contractures and a large scar, especially around a joint, can affect mobility.

Healing by tertiary intention occurs when a large or contaminated defect is closed several days later, usually after a period of local wound care results in significant decontamination of the wound. The initial formation of granulation tissue at the wound base offers significant protection against infection in a contaminated wound, where infection is less likely to occur when bacterial counts are less than 10^5 organisms per gram of tissue. Healing by tertiary intention provides faster wound closure, less contraction, and smaller scar formation than if the wound is allowed to close by secondary intention.

STAGES OF WOUND HEALING

Wound healing involves a continuum of processes and for academic purposes is divided into four stages based on the (i) time after wounding, (ii) predominant cell type, and (iii) predominant biologic activities occurring within the wound. Following injury to the tissue, the stages of wound healing are the (i) coagulation phase, (ii) inflammatory phase, (iii) proliferative phase, and (iv) remodeling phase.

Coagulation Phase

Following tissue injury, the first stage is the coagulation phase, which occurs from the time of injury to one hour after injury. This phase is dominated by the platelet. The major events of this phase are control of hemorrhage and the initial release of cytokines to initiate the repair process. In uninjured tissue the endothelial cell acts to inhibit thrombosis, but damage to the endothelium exposes subendothelial collagen to circulating factor VII and platelets. Exposure of factor VII to tissue factor that is expressed on cells in the extravascular tissue initiates the extrinsic coagulation cascade that culminates in the production of fibrin.

Platelets become activated when exposed to subendothelial collagen. Platelets are anucleate cells of myeloid lineage derived from megakaryocytes. Platelets contain two cytoplasmic granules: alpha and dense. Alpha granules contain platelet-specific proteins such as transforming growth factor β (TGF-β), platelet-derived growth factor (PDGF), and platelet factor 4. The dense granules contain serotonin, calcium, adenosine diphosphate, histamine, and epinephrine (Table 6-1).

TABLE 6-1

CONTENT OF PLATELET AND GRANULES

Alpha Granules	Dense Granules
PDGF	Serotonin, adenosine diphosphate
TGF-β	Calcium, histamine
Platelet factor 4	Epinephrine

PDGF, platelet-derived growth factor; TGF-β transforming growth factor β.

Upon activation, platelets undergo three very important reactions: adhesion, secretion, and aggregation. Platelets adhere to the damaged endothelium via von Willebrand factor, which is produced by endothelial cells via their glycoprotein Ib receptor. Soon after adhesion, platelets secrete the contents of their granules to further promote thrombosis. Platelet aggregation, distinct from adhesion, occurs when platelets adhere to one another to form the initial platelet plug via fibrinogen bridging to the platelet receptor glycoprotein IIb/IIIa. Adenosine diphosphate (ADP), thromboxane A$_2$, and thrombin are three very important stimuli for aggregation. Further fibrin formation will stabilize this plug to a clot. This clot is the initial extracellular matrix formed in the healing wound and acts as scaffolding for the subsequent stages to build upon.

Activated platelets increase the release of arachidonic acid from the membrane by phospholipase, which then proceeds through the cyclooxygenase pathway to produce thromboxane A$_2$, a potent vasoconstrictor and platelet aggregant. The subsequent vasoconstriction helps to control hemorrhage and to decrease flow, thereby aiding in the formation of the platelet plug. Aspirin irreversibly inhibits cyclooxygenase activity. Since platelets lack a nucleus and are incapable of synthesizing more enzymes, this results in inactivation of thromboxane A$_2$ for the life of the platelet. With further activation of the intrinsic coagulation cascade and the increase in production of fibrin the platelet plug is stabilized.

In addition to the early control of hemorrhage, the platelet plug initiates the wound healing process by releasing two very important cytokines, PDGF and TGF-β. Cytokines are the basis of cell–cell communication regulating cellular proliferation, migration, and protein synthesis, and are an area of intense research. Cytokines may act in an endocrine function, where they are released by a cell and circulate in the bloodstream to reach the target cell; in a paracrine manner, where they are secreted by a cell and affect an adjacent target cell; and in an autocrine manner, where the secreting cell is the target cell. Some cytokines also act in an intracrine manner where they are produced in a cell and act within the cell. The cytokine nomenclature is complex and can be misleading. Many cytokines were initially named according to their cell of origin, such as PDGF, or according to their first observed action, such as epidermal growth factor (EGF) and TGF-β. Many cytokines have since been found to be synthesized by many cell types and have more than one function. Cytokines play an integral role in the wound healing processes.

During the coagulation phase, the initial cytokines that are released orchestrate the following phases. First released is PDGF, a heterodimer protein consisting of an α chain and a β chain. PDGF is synthesized by the megakaryocyte and packaged into the platelet alpha granules. PDGF is secreted during the platelet-secretion reaction and supplemented by production from endothelial cells, fibroblasts, and macrophages. PDGF actions are mediated by tyrosine kinase receptors on the target cell. It is chemotactic for neutrophils, fibroblasts, and smooth muscle cells and also stimulates production of fibronectin and hyaluronic acid from fibroblasts and activates macrophages, important for the inflammatory stage. TGF-β is then released and is the predominant cytokine in the wound. It is produced by platelets, fibroblasts, smooth muscle cells, endothelial cells, keratinocytes, lymphocytes, and macrophages. TGF-β is a chemotractant for neutrophils, T cells, and fibroblasts. TGF-β also activates monocytes and is a potent inducer of extracellular matrix production, and it stimulates fibroblasts to produce collagen I, II, and V. TGF-β decreases matrix degradation by inhibiting gene expression of proteases and promoting synthesis of protease inhibitors. As a result, there is a net increase in collagen deposition by the fibroblast that is necessary for the healing wound. However, there has been recent evidence demonstrating that excessive TGF-β plays a role in the pathophysiology of hypertrophic scarring and fibrosis.

Inflammatory Phase

The inflammatory phase is characterized by the migration of leukocytes into the wound, occurring from 1 hour to 4 days post injury. The major events that characterize this phase include decontamination, cytokine manufacturing, and neovascularization. After the initial vasoconstriction to control hemorrhage and promote formation of a stable clot, the vessels at the site of injury dilate and become more permeable. These processes are mediated via histamine (derived from platelet decarboxylation of l-histidine), endothelial cell–derived prostacyclin (PGI2), nitric oxide (endothelium-derived relaxing factor), and bradykinin. Clinically, the results are hyperemia, edema, warmth, and pain, or the classic findings of rubor, tumor, calor, and dolor, respectively.

The predominant cells during the inflammatory phase are leukocytes, initially the neutrophil, followed by the monocyte. The neutrophil is a granulocyte derived from the myeloid lineage in the bone marrow. It is a migratory, phagocytic cell that circulates in the blood and homes to injured tissue by cytokine gradients. Neutrophils enter the wounded tissue by means of coordinated interaction of endothelial adhesion molecules and integrins on the neutrophil. Initially, the expression of selectins on the endothelial cell surface binds loosely to neutrophils causing them to roll along the endothelial surface. Examples are P-selectin found in the Weibel-Palade bodies of endothelial cells, L-selectin, and E-selectin. L-Selectin specifically binds to sialylated Lewis X on the neutrophil. Induction of leukocyte integrins increases affinity to intercellular adhesion molecule 1 (ICAM-1) on the endothelial cell, largely through the β2-integrin-ICAM-1 complexes, and traps the neutrophil. The neutrophil then undergoes transmigration through the capillary wall into the injured tissue, a process known as diapedesis. Leukocyte diapedesis,

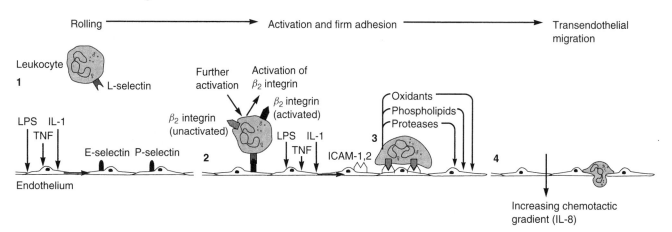

Figure 6-1 The process of leukocyte recruitment into areas of inflammation. At first, the cell exhibits a rolling type of motion due to loose adhesion between L-selectin and E-selectin. Progressive activation results in the expression of more adhesion molecules, firmer connections between the leukocyte and endothelial cell surface, and, finally, transendothelial leukocyte migration. (From Colletti LM, Kunkel SL, Strieter RM. Cytokines. In: Greenfield LJ, Mulholland MW, Oldham KT et al., eds. *Surgery: scientific principles and practice*, 2nd ed. Philadelphia: Lippincott-Raven Publishers, 1997:117, with permission.)

as well as increased vascular permeability, occurs predominantly in the venules, where blood flow is slow and nonpulsatile (Fig. 6-1).

After diapedesis, the function of the neutrophil is to engulf foreign material, remove necrotic debris, and destroy infiltrating bacteria. Neutrophils contain three types of cytoplasmic granules: primary (azurophilic) granules, secondary (specific) granules, and tertiary granules. Most importantly, the azurophilic granules contain the enzyme myeloperoxidase, bactericidal factors, and proteases. The secondary granules contain the components of the nicotinamide adenine dinucleotide phosphate (NADPH) oxidase system. Upon engulfing of bacteria the phagosome fuses with the secondary granule where the NADPH oxidase system produces superoxide and peroxide (H_2O_2). The phagosome then fuses with the azurophil granule, which releases myeloperoxidase. This catalyzes the formation of a more lethal agent that kills bacteria by oxidizing proteins and disrupting the cell wall. This NADPH oxidase mechanism is extremely important, as patients with a defect in this system develop chronic granulomatous disease. In this disorder, neutrophils can phagocytose bacteria but are unable to kill them, thereby leading to chronic infections.

Macrophages appear in the wound within 5 hours after injury and peak at 72 hours, replacing the neutrophil as the predominant cell type. Macrophages are monocytes that differentiate once at the site of injury. Monocytes are bone marrow–derived granulocytes that remain in circulation until called upon by injured tissue, whereby, through mechanisms similar to that of the neutrophil, they migrate to the site of injury. Unlike the neutrophil, the role of the macrophagerole is more than tissue débridement and bacterial killing. Macrophages replace the platelet as a source of cytokines to orchestrate the healing process.

Neovascularization

Vital to the healing process is the formation of new capillary beds to replace the ones disrupted during the injury. These new capillaries then supply oxygen and nutrients to the healing tissue. Neovascularization is the process by

which these new capillary beds form at the wound base, and this process begins during the inflammatory phase of wound healing. Platelets, neutrophils, and monocytes are all sources of angiogenic factors that stimulate neovascularization, and their release is stimulated by the local hypoxia of the wound bed.

Neovascularization occurs by two processes: angiogenesis and vasculogenesis. Angiogenesis is the process by which new vessels are formed from the sprouting of endothelial cells from preexisting vessels. Resident endothelial cells of the microvascular beds first release proteinases, most importantly the matrix metalloproteinases (MMPs), to digest the basement membrane and extracellular matrix. The cells then migrate into the avascular tissue following an angiogenic cytokine gradient and by using components of the extracellular matrix, fibronectin and degraded collagen, via their integrin receptors, as their migration scaffolding. These cells then lay their basement membrane and form primitive tubules that will later mature into capillary networks.

Neovascularization also occurs by the process of vasculogenesis. Initially believed to occur only during fetal development, there is recent evidence that this process occurs in the adult. Vasculogenesis is the *de novo* formation of blood vessels from bone marrow–derived precursor cells. During fetal vasculature development, primitive cells known as hemangioblasts of mesodermal origin form blood islands. These blood islands are spatially oriented in a specific way, whereas, cells programmed to differentiate into endothelial cells, known as angioblasts, are located at the periphery of the blood islands. Cells destined for the hematopoietic lineage, known as hematopoietic stem cells (HSCs), are located in the center of the blood islands.

The adult bone marrow contains a reservoir of adult stem cells known as multipotent adult progenitor cells (MAPCs). These cells have been shown to have the ability to differentiate into many adult tissue types when placed in the proper cytokine milieu. During vasculogenesis MAPCs differentiate to endothelial progenitor cells (EPCs) in the bone marrow. EPCs then exit the marrow and enter the peripheral circulation where they traffic to sites of vasculogenesis. The extent of their involvement in physiologic neovascularization is a matter of ongoing intense research efforts.

The cells involved in healing tissue express angiogenic and vasculogenic cytokines. Many families of cytokines have been implicated including fibroblast growth factor (FGF), EGF, insulin-like growth factor (IGF), PDGF, and vascular endothelial growth factor (VEGF), to name a few. The platelet begins the process with the release of PDGF. It is becoming increasingly more recognized that the monocyte/macrophage and the resident fibroblasts secrete potent angiogenic/vasculogenic cytokines. The most potent of these cytokines is the VEGF family. This family consists of five members: VEGF-A, VEGF-B, VEGF-C, VEGF-D, and PLGF (placenta-like growth factor). These five growth factors work through three tyrosine kinase receptors: VEGFR-1, VEGFR-2, and VEGFR-3. Of these, the most important is VEGF-A, which binds avidly to VEGFR-2 on endothelial cells and EPCs to exert its potential angiogenic and vasculogenic (also mediated by VEGFR-1) effects, respectively. The other members of the VEGF family have been found to have some effects on neovascularization, but not as potent as that of VEGF-A. Of note, the VEGF-C–VEGFR-3 ligand receptor complex is a potent mediator in lymphangiogenesis.

Proliferative Phase

The proliferative phase of wound healing is characterized by the production of collagen tissue. This phase occurs from day 3 to day 21 post injury. With the removal of the proinflammatory stimuli, such as foreign bodies and bacteria, and with the onset of neovascularization, the inflammatory phase subsides giving way to the initiation of fibroblast migration into the injured tissue. Fibroblast migration begins at day 3, and by day 5 it is the dominant cell type. Numerous cytokines mediate fibroblast migration into the wound, most importantly PDGF and TGF-β. TGF-β is a potent mitogenic stimulus for fibroblasts as well as promotor of collagen synthesis. The fibroblast will transform the early wound matrix into a mature scar.

The early wound matrix is rich in ground substance. Ground substance is composed of proteoglycans. Proteoglycans are negatively charged macromolecules composed of glycosaminoglycan (GAG) subunits attached by covalent bonds via serine residues. These subunits form a bottlebrush-like structure that occupies a large amount of space in the extracellular matrix. These large molecules absorb a large amount of water and cytokines. The negatively charged, hydrophilic molecules bind the chemotactic cytokines, thereby allowing the formation of the chemotactic gradients for the migration of cells. Hyaluronic acid is one such GAG. Hyaluronic acid is a large, nonsulfated molecule that maintains a fluid environment to allow for easy cell migration, proliferation, and matrix synthesis. Hyaluronic acid appears only transiently in the early phases of wound healing in the adult but in the fetus it persists and may play a role in the regenerative response seen in fetal wound healing.

The extracellular matrix will change from a loose array of GAGs and fibronectin to a strong, multilayered structure of cross-linking collagen, or a scar, by the process of fibroplasia. A scar is defined as a disordered collection of collagen that replaces the native tissue lost by the injury.

Collagen, most notably type I collagen, is an insoluble fiber with high tensile strength. It is the dominant structural component of the final scar and succeeds fibrin as the predominant and final component of extracellular matrix. There have been 19 forms of collagen that were identified. The first five are described briefly. Type I collagen is the predominant type in the body, makes up most connective tissue, and is the predominant type in scar tissue. Type II collagen makes up cartilage. Type III is associated with type I, and its concentrations are high in the initial phase of healing and in the developing fetus. Type IV collagen makes up basement membranes. Type V is found in the cornea and maintains transparency (Table 6-2).

Collagen Synthesis

As mentioned in the preceding text, collagen is an insoluble fiber with high tensile strength and collagen type I is the most abundant collagen type within scar tissue. Collagen is synthesized by the fibroblast.

Collagen is composed of three polypeptide chains, which form a triple helix. The polypeptides contain a high frequency of glycine, proline, and lysine amino acids. Glycine is a small amino acid that allows the collagen to form its triple helix structure by fitting within the helix and forming the intermolecular hydrogen bonds to hold the helix together. Posttranslational modification hydroxylates 40% of the proline residues and 14% of the lysine residues. Specifically, proline and lysine get hydroxylated to 4-hydroxyproline and 5-hydroxylysine by prolyl hydrolase and lysyl hydrolase, respectively. These modified amino acids afford the collagen molecule its high tensile strength and stability.

If hydroxylation of these amino acids does not occur, the ensuing collagen undergoes degradation in both the intracellular and extracellular environments. Both hydrolase enzymes rely on the cosubstrate ascorbate (vitamin C) to maintain the iron atom of the active enzymatic site in the reduced state. Molecular oxygen acts as the donor of the oxygen atom in this reaction. Hypoxia and vitamin C deficiency decrease the activity of these hydrolase enzymes and result in the subsequent failure of hydroxylation of the proline and lysine residues.

The triple helix collagen molecule is formed as a procollagen molecule containing extra amino acid residues at the carboxy and amino terminals. This procollagen molecule is soluble in the cell cytoplasm and does not interact with other procollagen molecules until it is secreted into the extracellular matrix, where there is digestion of the propeptides on either end by extracellular procollagen peptidases. After digestion the triple helix is known as tropocollagen, which undergoes spontaneous terminal and lateral elongation by the formation of cross-links with other tropocollagen bundles and is insoluble. The sequential

TABLE 6-2

COLLAGEN DISTRIBUTION

Type I	All connective tissue, 90% of body collagen
Type II	Cartilage, vitreous humor
Type III	Fetal tissues, healing wound, blood vessels, cornea
Type IV	Basement membranes
Type V	Cornea

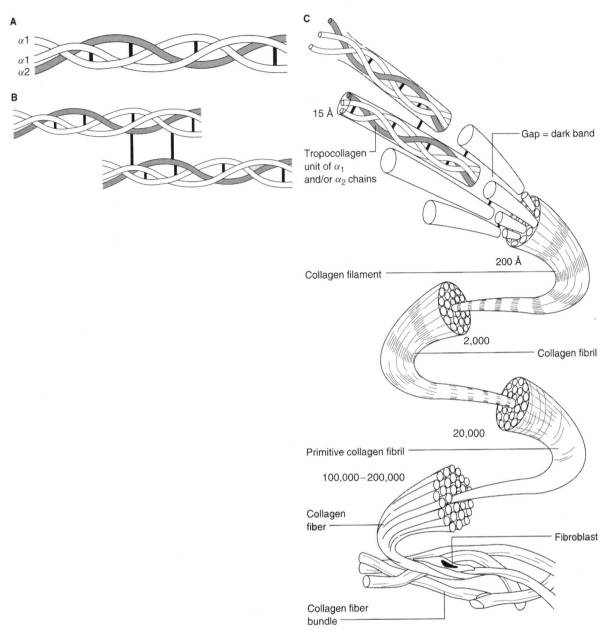

Figure 6-2   A: Type I collagen showing triple helix and intramolecular cross-links. **B:** Intermolecular cross-links provide tensile strength. **C:** Assembly of collagen fibrils, fibers, and fiber bundles. (From Fine NA, Mustoe TA. Wound healing. In: Greenfield LJ, Mulholland MW, Oldham KT et al., eds. *Surgery: scientific principles and practice*, 3rd ed. Philadelphia: Lippincott Williams & Wilkins, 2001, with permission.)

assembly of tropocollagen leads to the production of filaments, fibrils, and fibers (Fig. 6-2).

The strength of collagen is derived from its extensive intramolecular and intermolecular bonds. The three α chains of the procollagen molecule are held together by extensive hydrogen bonding between the glycine residues. The hydroxylation of the proline and lysine residues confers ionic bonds. In addition, there is covalent bonding between two hydroxyl lysine residues and one lysine residue. Lysine oxidase, to be distinguished from lysine hydroxylase, is a copper-containing enzyme that forms the intramolecular cross-linking between two lysine residues (Table 6-3). The significance of lysine oxidase enzyme was the rationale for the clinical trials of D-penicillamine, a copper-binding agent, in scleroderma to inhibit the excessive collagen formation

that leads to fibrosis. The overall strength of the final molecule is caused by the cooperative interaction of numerous relatively weak bonds. Collagen synthesis and accumulation occur by day 3 to day 5 and reach a maximum level by 2 to 3 weeks.

There is much similarity between the early fibrin matrix and the final collagen matrix of the scar. Both proteins appear in the extracellular matrix in an inactive form, fibrinogen and procollagen, where they then undergo enzymatic cleavage by thrombin and procollagen peptidase, respectively. The molecules then undergo extensive intramolecular and intermolecular cross-linking to achieve strength. In addition, both require an activated cell for the protein's successful assembly, the platelet and the fibroblast for fibrin and collagen, respectively.

TABLE 6-3

ENZYMES INVOLVED IN COLLAGEN PRODUCTION

Prolyl hydroxylase	Hydroxylation of proline residues
Lysyl hydroxylase	Hydroxylation of lysine residues
N- and C-terminal propeptidases	Cleavage of terminal propeptides
Lysine oxidase	Linkage of lysine residues

Deficiencies in the collagen pathway also have severe clinical outcomes. Vitamin C deficiency causes scurvy, which is caused by a dysfunction of the enzymes required for the hydroxylation of proline and lysine, prolyl and lysyl hydroxylase. Scurvy is characterized by poor wound healing, fragile gums, and skin lesions.

Remodeling Phase

The final phase of the healing wound is the remodeling phase, which begins around day 21, where collagen synthesis comes into equilibrium with collagen breakdown with no collagen accumulation. This phase is significant for strengthening the collagen matrix and the subsequent scar. At 6 weeks postinjury the wound is at 50% of its final tensile strength. For normal wound healing, collagen must be degraded as well as produced.

The digestion of the extracellular matrix is accomplished with MMPs, which are divided into four subclasses based on substrate specificity. The interstitial collagenases, MMP 1, 8, and 13, will initially cleave the collagen and then the gelatinases, MMP 2 and 9, will further digest these breakdown products. The MMPs are secreted as an inactive form, or as a zymogen, and are activated by other proteases such as plasmin. Tissue inhibitors of MMPs, known as TIMPs, downregulate MMP activity.

During the remodeling phase, disorganized fibers are degraded and replaced with more organized bundles. These new collagen fibers will be placed in the direction of the tensile forces and will have an increased amount of molecular bonds. Clinically, as one observes the wound base, the proliferative and remodeling phases replace the beefy, friable granulation tissue with the light, strong scar tissue.

With wound healing by secondary intention, wound contraction and reepithelialization are two vital processes. Wound contraction is the contraction of the normal tissue around the scar to decrease the cross-sectional area of the open wound. Because human skin is loosely connected to fascia and the underlying muscle, wound contraction can decrease the area by 30% to 90%. This process is mediated by the actin filaments of fibroblasts, which contact the extracellular matrix via fibronexi. Specifically, the cell type responsible for wound contraction is the myofibroblast, a more differentiated fibroblast that expresses α smooth muscle actin and develops the contractile properties of the smooth muscle cell. TGF-β has been shown to promote the differentiation of fibroblast to myofibroblasts.

An important distinction exists between wound contraction and scar contracture. Contractures are pathologic conditions caused by increased fibrosis and wound contraction. Contractures involving limbs, especially the joints, can lead to decreased range of motion. Contractures can also be unsightly.

Figure 6-3 summarizes the stages of wound healing, their timing in the healing process, the primary event, the dominant cell type, and the dominant cytokines.

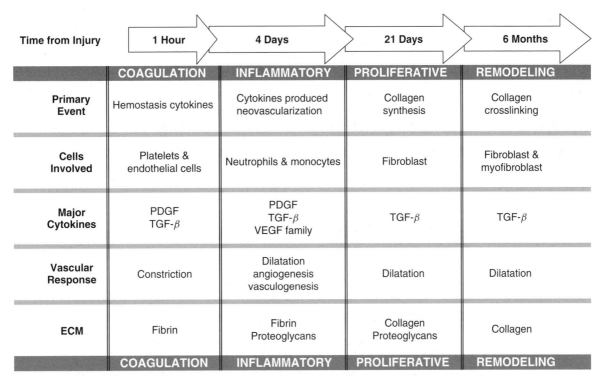

Time from Injury	1 Hour	4 Days	21 Days	6 Months
	COAGULATION	**INFLAMMATORY**	**PROLIFERATIVE**	**REMODELING**
Primary Event	Hemostasis cytokines	Cytokines produced neovascularization	Collagen synthesis	Collagen crosslinking
Cells Involved	Platelets & endothelial cells	Neutrophils & monocytes	Fibroblast	Fibroblast & myofibroblast
Major Cytokines	PDGF TGF-β	PDGF TGF-β VEGF family	TGF-β	TGF-β
Vascular Response	Constriction	Dilatation angiogenesis vasculogenesis	Dilatation	Dilatation
ECM	Fibrin	Fibrin Proteoglycans	Collagen Proteoglycans	Collagen
	COAGULATION	**INFLAMMATORY**	**PROLIFERATIVE**	**REMODELING**

Figure 6-3 Phases of wound healing. Time after injury, primary event, dominant cell type, cytokines, and vascular response are depicted. ECM, extracellular matrix.

PATHOLOGIC WOUND HEALING

Chronic Nonhealing Wounds

Chronic wounds remain a costly and debilitating health problem leading to amputations, infections, and increased mortality. As detailed in the preceding text, normal wound healing is a well-organized response to injury that is characterized by diverse cellular activities. Multiple cytokines and growth factors contribute to the timely and successful repair of wounds. Despite the numerous advances in wound healing research, the treatment of chronic nonhealing wounds still presents a challenge.

A chronic wound is one that fails to heal because an underlying pathologic condition disrupts the phases of well-organized healing. Chronic wounds may result from a variety of factors usually associated with comorbidities of the host including diabetes mellitus, venous stasis, and arterial disease.

In patients with diabetes the cause of chronic wounds is secondary to neuropathy, arterial insufficiency, and leukocyte abnormality. The pathophysiology of the venous stasis ulcer begins with the insufficiency of the venous valves in the lower extremity causing blood to pool in the veins, and the increase in hydrostatic pressure causes a transudate with ensuing edema. The continuous pressure on the capillary beds causes the gap junctions between the endothelial cells to widen, thereby allowing exudates high in fibrinogen to extravasate into the extravascular space. The polymerization of fibrin around the vessels forms a sleeve around the capillary and acts as a diffusion barrier for oxygen and other nutrients. This sleeve also sequesters cytokines culminating in the "brawny edema" used to describe the clinical appearance. The decrease in oxygen and nutrients then leads to tissue breakdown, ulceration, and infection.

These conditions all culminate with the local environment of the wound having one or more of the following factors that have been found to impair healing. First is the propensity of chronic wounds to become colonized with bacteria and sometimes fungi. A level greater or equal to 10^6 organisms per gram of tissue is associated with impaired healing. Secondly, the extravasation of macromolecules, such as fibrinogen and α_2-macroglobulin, "trap" growth factors and cytokines important for healing. For example, TGF-β binds to the perivascular cuffs formed by these macromolecules and is no longer biologically active. The study of fluid from acute wounds demonstrates a proliferative effect on fibroblasts, keratinocytes, and endothelial cells. However, the fluid of chronic wounds blocks cellular proliferation and angiogenesis. In addition, the fluid of chronic wounds has been found to have increased levels of MMPs that break down extracellular matrix proteins and growth factors. Lastly, prolonged hypoxia correlates with the inability to heal.

The first step in treating chronic wounds is sharp débridement to healthy, well-vascularized tissue. The intent of débridement is for the surgeon to remove necrotic debris, foci of infection, edema with its harmful proteinases, and to reestablish the dynamic processes of normal wound healing, essentially transforming a chronic wound into an acute one. In the setting of arterial insufficiency, it is important to return the delivery of oxygen and nutrients before any wound healing can take place; this is often accomplished via revascularization surgical procedures.

Several recombinant growth factors have been tested for their ability to accelerate healing. Positive results have been demonstrated with EGF, keratinocyte growth factor-2, fibroblast growth factor, and PDGF. Only PDGF is approved by the U.S. Food and Drug Administration (FDA). Topical PDGF, or becaplermin topical gel, is a homodimeric protein produced by recombinant DNA technology. The biologic activity of becaplermin is similar to that of endogenous PDGF, specifically, the recruitment and the proliferation of cells involved in wound repair.

Extensive studies have demonstrated that becaplermin is an effective adjunctive measure for the healing of chronic wounds when used in conjunction with standard wound healing therapies. Specifically these practices include the provision of a moist environment free of debris and necrotic tissue, control of infection, and optimal weight displacement from the affected area. Becaplermin is safe and easy to use, being applied once daily. However, response rates are only 30% at best and wounds require excellent vascularization and a healthy bed of granulation tissue as a prerequisite for effectiveness. There is ongoing research in applying platelet gels on chronic wounds as a source of stimulatory cytokines.

There is work being done on agents to decrease the amount of proteinases found in chronic wounds. Vacuum-assisted closure (VAC) is a new device for wound treatment that uses negative pressure. The method has proved successful on chronic wounds of many etiologies. Pressure is exerted on the wound with foam and then covered with an airtight, occlusive dressing. Negative pressure is applied through vacuum suction, which removes third space fluid adjacent to the wound thereby decreasing the pressure on the small neovessels and improving blood supply, as well as removing proteinases and bacteria.

Other areas of research include gene therapy and stem cell therapy. With gene therapy, a viral vector carrying a plasmid DNA encoding a desirable cytokine can be injected into the wound bed and temporarily increase the local expression of a prohealing cytokine. For instance, the gene encoding VEGF has been reported to enhance healing and angiogenesis in ischemic ulcers, but effects are limited by induction of immature and leaky capillaries by VEGF. More recently, the rationale of stem cell therapy is to locally inject multipotent adult progenitor cells found in the adult bone marrow to replace the senescent fibroblasts, endothelial cells, and keratinocytes found in the chronic wound.

In chronic wounds resulting from trauma, especially in patients without comorbidities to explain the cause, the physician must be alerted to the possibility of retained foreign body or onset of malignancy. Squamous cell carcinoma may form in such a wound and clinically mimic a chronic wound. This is termed Marjolin ulcer. A high index of suspicion should lead one to biopsy such a wound.

Hypertrophic Scars and Keloids

Hypertrophic scarring and keloid disease are the result of abnormal healing responses to cutaneous injury, which lead to disfiguring and dysfunctional scarring. In predisposed individuals, an exuberant healing process may occur after cutaneous injury resulting in the accumulation of abundant extracellular matrix. Clinically this is seen as a raised, inflexible scar. Hypertrophic scars are defined as raised scars that remain within the boundaries of the original injury, regress spontaneously, and rarely recur after surgical excision. They mostly occur in patients with a dark-skinned complexion.

Keloids, unlike hypertrophic scars, are defined as lesions that extend beyond the boundaries of the original injury, behave like a benign tumor, continue to grow over time, do not regress spontaneously, commonly recur after excision, and are present for a minimum of 1 year. Keloid disease is a familial condition occurring in all races, but more commonly in dark-skinned individuals.

Recent evidence suggests two basic mechanisms involved in the pathophysiology of keloid disease, a continuous state of inflammation and excessive accumulation of extracellular matrix. Clinically, keloids are described as having a reddish border at the edge of the expanding or inflammatory zone. Histologic studies of the inflammatory zone at the peripheral border of the expanding keloid reveal abundant vessel density and multiple foci of inflammatory cells. This persistent inflammatory response is a source of cytokines, such as TGF-β, IGF-1, PDGF, interleukins, and EGF, which all promote angiogenesis and fibroplasia, thereby leading to abundant production of extracellular matrix and synthesis beyond the margins of the original lesion. Recently, IGF-1 has been shown to act in a paracrine fashion between keratinocytes and fibroblasts to promote production of extracellular matrix. It has been shown that blocking the IGF-1 receptor attenuates the proliferation of keloid-derived fibroblasts.

The local overexpression of TGF-β has been implicated in promoting overproduction of extracellular matrix and supporting keloid formation. Scarless fetal wound healing occurs in the relative absence of TGF-β, and the addition of this cytokine induces scar formation. Systemic administration of TGF-β can induce fibroproliferative disorders, such as cirrhosis, pulmonary fibrosis, and scleroderma. Therapies to treat keloid disease may focus on blocking the production or actions of TGF-β in the wound.

Keloids have been treated with many modalities with varying success rates. The most successful treatment is prevention. In patients prone to keloid formation, incisions should be avoided unless absolutely necessary. In patients with keloids, silicone sheeting and/or pressure should be tried first. If there is no response, intralesional steroid injections can be tried. Other modalities are being investigated. Verapamil, a calcium channel antagonist, inhibits the synthesis and secretion of extracellular matrix molecules and increases collagenase. Intralesional verapamil injection after keloid excision had moderate results. Single-fraction radiotherapy following excision was found to decrease recurrence. The pyrimidine analog 5-fluorouracil is a potent inhibitor of TGF-β-induced collagen synthesis. Intralesional 5-fluorouracil injections have shown some promise: greater than 50% improvement in the lesions and no patient had complete failure. However, long-term follow-up for recurrence is needed. Other modalities currently being tested in the basic science laboratories include inhibiting the effects of growth factors and cytokines in the wound, such as IGF-1 as mentioned previously.

Adverse Effects of Immunosuppression on Wound Healing

With the advent and success of organ transplantation and prolonged survival of organ transplant recipients, wound healing in the immunosuppressed patient has become very important clinically. Patients who undergo transplantation are treated with multiple immunosuppressive agents and the most commonly used drugs are corticosteroids. Corticosteroids interfere with prostaglandin synthesis, leukocyte migration, and cytokine production by the macrophage (all important steps during the inflammatory phase to ward off infection and to continue the healing process). Steroids may also inhibit fibroblast function and collagen synthesis. Patients taking steroids chronically develop thin and fragile skin. Vitamin A, in oral doses of 25,000 U per day, can overcome the antihealing effects of steroids. The effect may be mediated through TGF-β, which is decreased by steroids but returned to normal levels by vitamin A. Once the inflammatory phase of wound healing has occurred, the effects of steroids on healing are less. However, steroids still cause abnormal collagen remodeling, even when administered after the inflammatory phase.

Effects of Human Immunodeficiency Virus on Wound Healing

Acquired immunodeficiency syndrome (AIDS) manifests with a very diverse array of symptoms. Interestingly, a direct relationship between leukocyte count and healing has not been reported. The wound complications from AIDS are secondary to other manifestations of the disease, such as infection or Kaposi sarcoma.

Effects of Nutrition on Wound Healing

Optimal nutrition is paramount to proper wound healing. Ignoring of the nutritional status may compromise the patient's ability to heal and subsequently prolong the stages of wound healing. Glucose provides the energy needed for wound healing, angiogenesis, and the deposition of extracellular matrix. Fatty acids are essential for cell structure. Protein calorie intake must be maintained throughout the healing process; if stopped even for 24 hours, collagen synthesis ceases and wound dehiscence may occur. High exudative losses from wounds can result in an enormous protein deficit and an increased requirement for protein and caloric intake.

Vitamins and minerals are also extremely important. Vitamin C deficiency is the etiology of scurvy. In this disease, scars can break open even many years after full healing. The acute healing process is impaired with scurvy. In the United States, approximately 20% of the inner city population seen in the trauma bay is vitamin C deficient. After trauma, one gram per day of vitamin C replacement is recommended. Zinc deficiency also delays wound healing. The mechanism for this is thought to be secondary to decreases in production of inflammatory cytokines and decreased neutrophil migration to the injured site.

Effects of Oxygen on Wound Healing

In addition to adequate nutrition, wounds require adequate oxygenation. Oxygen is needed for the hydroxylation of the proline and lysine residues and also for bacterial killing. An increase in tissue oxygen tension can be effective in healing some chronic or infected wounds, as is seen in clinical benefits of hyperbaric therapy. Hyperbaric therapy can also enhance angiogenesis by mechanisms related to nitric oxide synthase induction.

KEY POINTS

▲ Four phases of wound healing are the coagulation phase, inflammatory phase, proliferative phase, and re-modeling phase.

▲ The key cell in wound healing is the monocyte, which becomes the macrophage when it enters the tissue from the blood. The neutrophil only débrides and kills bacteria, the wound will go on to heal in the absence of neutrophils.

▲ Aspirin irreversibly inhibits cyclooxygenase and therefore thromboxane A_2 synthesis. The thromboxane A_2 synthesis is inactive for the life of the platelet.

▲ Hypoxia and vitamin C deficiency decrease activity of the hydrolase enzymes. Failure of hydroxylation of the proline and lysine residues results in unstable collagen molecules, more prone to degradation.

▲ Marjolin ulcer is squamous cell carcinoma that forms in a wound and can mimic a chronic wound.

▲ Keloids, unlike hypertrophic scars, are defined as lesions that extend beyond the boundaries of the original injury, behave like a benign tumor, continue to grow over time, do not regress spontaneously, commonly recur after excision, and are present for a minimum of 1 year.

▲ Oral vitamin A can overcome the antihealing effects of corticosteroids.

SUGGESTED READINGS

Falanga V. The chronic wound: impaired healing and solutions in the context of wound bed preparation. *Blood Cells Mol Dis* 2004;32: 88–94.

Fine NA, Mustoe TA. Wound healing. In: Greenfield LJ, Mullholland MW, Oldham KT et al., eds. *Surgery: scientific principles and practice,* 3rd ed. Philadelphia: Lippincott Williams & Wilkins, 2001.

Harry L, Paleolog EM. From the cradle to the clinic: VEGF in developmental, physiological, and pathological angiogenesis. *Birth Defects Res* 2003;69:363–374.

Le A, Zhang Q, Wu Y, et al. Elevated vascular endothelial growth factor in keloids: relevance to tissue fibrosis. *Cells Tissues Organs* 2004;176:87–94.

Nanda S, Negi Reddy BS. Intralesional 5-fluorouracil as a treatment modality of keloids. *Dermatol Surg* 2004;30:54–57.

Anesthesia

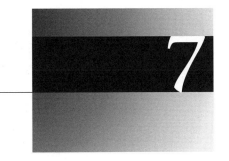

William J. Vernick   C. William Hanson III

Anesthesia, perhaps more so than any other specialty, has its roots in the United States. William T.G. Morton, on October 16, 1846, gave the first public demonstration of general anesthesia at the Massachusetts General Hospital. From this initial display, the discipline of anesthesiology was born. It is imperative that surgeons be familiar with the basic concepts of operative anesthesia. To function most effectively in the operating room, surgeons and anesthesiologists must work together as a team. Information pertaining to sudden or large amounts of blood loss, adequacy of relaxation, and forewarning before clamping or unclamping of vessels should be conveyed to the anesthesiologist. The anesthesiologist, in turn, has a responsibility to inform the surgeon of important physiologic information, such as hemodynamic stability.

The principles of operative anesthesia include the five As: amnesia, analgesia, anxiolysis, akinesia, and areflexia. Akinesia ensures a quiet surgical field, allows the surgeon to function efficiently, and prevents mishaps associated with patient movement. Areflexia implies attenuation or abolishment of the hemodynamic responses associated with surgery.

PREOPERATIVE ASSESSMENT

An anesthetist begins with the preoperative assessment, which consists of a history, a physical examination, and a review of pertinent patient data. The goal of the preoperative assessment is to summarize the patient's health status and to help formulate an anesthetic plan. The evaluation may take place on the day of surgery, in the patient's hospital room the night before surgery, or in a physician's office or preoperative evaluation center days to weeks before an elective procedure. The obvious advantage of an evaluation one or more days before surgery is that it allows further studies to be performed, if indicated, and interventions to take place so that the patient may be "optimized." In today's medical environment that is focused on efficiency and cost savings, usually the first time the anesthesiologist meets the patient is on the day of surgery. In order to maximize time and resources, the surgeon should know what information to acquire preoperatively, so that the anesthesiologist's assessment can be made quickly and easily.

Assessment of cardiac and pulmonary function is crucial, as many perioperative complications involve these organ systems. However, evaluation of all organ systems is important, as they all may affect perioperative care. A level of functional status should be obtained, which can be expressed in metabolic equivalents (METs). Perioperative cardiac morbidity is increased in those unable to achieve 4 METS. Examples of four MET activities include: climbing stairs, walking up a hill, or running a short distance (Table 7-1).

The assessment of cardiac risk has been aided by the American College of Cardiology/American Heart Association (ACC/AHA), which published a series of guidelines regarding perioperative care. They define surgical procedures as high risk if they are associated with a greater than 5% incidence of perioperative cardiac complications. High risk procedures include aortic or major vascular surgery, emergent major operations, and long procedures with significant blood loss or fluid shifts. Examples of intermediate risk surgery (incidence of cardiac complications of 1% to 5%) are intrathoracic, intraperitoneal, and orthopedic procedures (Table 7-2). Clinical predictors of cardiac risk that are independent of the surgical procedure

TABLE 7-1

ESTIMATED ENERGY REQUIREMENT FOR VARIOUS ACTIVITIES

1 MET	Can you take care of yourself? Eat, dress, or use the toilet? Walk indoors around the house? Walk a block or two on level ground at 2–3 mph or 3.2–4.8 km/h? Do light work around the house like dusting or washing dishes?
4 METs	Climb a flight of stairs or walk up a hill? Walk on level ground at 4 mph or 6.4 km/h? Run a short distance? Do heavy work around the house such as scrubbing floors or lifting or moving heavy furniture? Participate in moderate recreational activities like golf, bowling, dancing, doubles tennis, or throwing a baseball or football?
>10 METs	Participate in strenuous sports like swimming, singles tennis, football, basketball, or skiing?

MET, metabolic equivalent.
From Eagle K, Brundage B, Chaitman B, et al. Guidelines for perioperative cardiovascular evaluation of the noncardiac surgical patient. A report of the American Heart Association/American College of Cardiology Task Force on Assignment of Diagnostic and Therapeutic Cardiovascular Procedures. *Circulation* 1996;93:1278, with permission.

TABLE 7-2

CARDIAC RISK[a] STRATIFICATION FOR NONCARDIAC SURGICAL PROCEDURES

Risk Level	Procedure
High (Reported cardiac risk often >5%)	• Emergent major operations, particularly in older individuals • Aortic and other major vascular • Peripheral vascular • Anticipated prolonged surgical procedures associated with large fluid shifts and/or blood loss
Intermediate (Reported cardiac risk generally <5%)	• Carotid endarterectomy • Head and neck • Intraperitoneal and intrathoracic • Orthopedic • Prostate
Low[b] (Reported cardiac risk generally <1%)	• Endoscopic procedures • Superficial procedures • Cataract • Breast

[a] Combined incidence of cardiac death and nonfatal myocardial infarction.
[b] Do not generally require further preoperative cardiac testing.
From Eagle K, Brundage B, Chaitman B, et al. Guidelines for perioperative cardiovascular evaluation of the noncardiac surgical patient. A report of the American Heart Association/American College of Cardiology Task Force on Assignment of Diagnostic and Therapeutic Cardiovascular Procedures. *Circulation* 1996;93:1278, with permission.

TABLE 7-3

CLINICAL PREDICTORS OF INCREASED PERIOPERATIVE CARDIOVASCULAR RISK (MYOCARDIAL INFARCTION, CONGESTIVE HEART FAILURE, DEATH)

Major	Unstable coronary syndromes • Recent myocardial infarction[a] with evidence of important ischemic risk by clinical symptoms or noninvasive study • Unstable or severe[b] angina (Canadian Class III or IV)[c] Decompensated congestive heart failure Significant dysrhythmias • High-grade atrioventricular block • Symptomatic ventricular arrhythmias in the presence of underlying heart disease • Supraventricular dysrhythmias with uncontrolled ventricular rate Severe valvular disease
Intermediate	Mild angina pectoris (Canadian Class I or II) Prior myocardial infarction by history or pathologic Q waves Compensated or prior congestive heart failure Diabetes mellitus
Minor	Advanced age Abnormal electrocardiogram (left ventricular hypertrophy, left bundle branch block, ST-T abnormalities) Rhythm other than sinus (e.g., atrial fibrillation) Low functional capacity (e.g., inability to climb one flight of stairs with a bag of groceries) History of stroke Uncontrolled systemic hypertension

[a] The American College of Cardiology National Database Library defines recent myocardial infarction (MI) as greater than 7 days but less than or equal to 1 month (30 days).
[b] May include "stable" angina in patients who are unusually sedentary.
[c] Campeau L. Grading of angina pectoris. *Circulation* 1976;54:522.
From Eagle K, Brundage B, Chaitman B, et al. Guidelines for perioperative cardiovascular evaluation of the noncardiac surgical patient. A report of the American Heart Association/American College of Cardiology Task Force on Assignment of Diagnostic and Therapeutic Cardiovascular Procedures. *Circulation* 1996;93:1278, with permission.

have also been defined. Examples of major clinical risk factors include unstable angina or acute myocardial infarction (MI) (within 1 week), recent MI (7 days to 1 month), severe valvular abnormalities, or decompensated congestive heart failure (CHF). Examples of intermediate clinical risk factors include a history of MI greater than 1 month before surgery, compensated heart failure, or diabetes mellitus (Table 7-3).

The evaluation of the pulmonary system includes an inquiry for reactive airway disease, chronic obstructive pulmonary disease, tobacco use, and recent upper respiratory tract infections. Patients should be strongly encouraged to refrain from tobacco use before surgery. Twenty-four hours of smoking abstinence will reduce carboxyhemoglobin levels, although an improvement in mucociliary transport takes several weeks of smoking cessation in order to occur. The value of preoperative pulmonary function tests (PFTs) remains very controversial, except in the case of lung resection. Any patient with a forced expiratory volume in 1 second (FEV_1) of less than 70%-predicted may be at increased risk of pulmonary complications. However, clinical findings may be more predictive than spirometry. PFTs may be useful to determine if recent interventions have optimized a patient's lung function.

The patient's current medications need to be reviewed during the preoperative assessment. In general, most cardiovascular drugs should be continued up to the day of surgery. Diuretics tend to cause hypovolemia and hypokalemia. β-Blockers may blunt sympathetic nervous system (SNS) responses. There have been reports of intractable vasodilation in patients receiving angiotensin-converting enzyme (ACE) inhibitors. Recent use of antiplatelet drugs and

anticoagulants such as heparins and warfarin could increase intraoperative blood loss and potentially contraindicate neuraxial anesthetic techniques. Use of oral hypoglycemics or insulin therapy necessitates an intraoperative plan for glucose control and monitoring. Monoamine oxidase inhibitors (MAOIs) may cause significant hypertension when used in combination with indirect acting sympathomimetic drugs such as ephedrine or life-threatening hyperthermia and hypertension when combined with meperidine.

A physical examination with special emphasis on the vital signs, airway, heart, lungs, and central nervous system (CNS) is performed. Signs of hypovolemia should be sought, especially in patients who have required colonic preparation prior to surgery. Particular attention should be placed on the airway evaluation in order to predict the degree of difficulty with intubation and mask ventilation. Laboratory data should be ordered on the basis of findings on history and physical examination, with consideration given to the planned procedure. The haphazard ordering of laboratory tests is expensive and is rarely of any utility. A general guideline for ordering laboratory studies is provided in Table 7-4.

The decision to obtain preoperative cardiac evaluation studies is aided by the ACC/AHA guidelines and depends

---

TABLE 7-4

RECOMMENDED LABORATORY TESTING SYSTEM UTILIZED AT THE JOHNS HOPKINS HOSPITAL

Electrocardiogram

Age 50 yr or older
Significant cardiocirculatory disease
Diabetes mellitus (age 40 yr or older)
Renal disease
Other major metabolic disease
Procedure level 5[a]

Chest x-ray

Asthma or COPD that is debilitating or with change of symptoms
    or acute episode within last 6 mo
Cardiothoracic procedure
Procedure level 4

Serum chemistries

Renal disease
Adrenal or thyroid disorders
Diuretic therapy
Chemotherapy
Procedure level 5

Urinalysis

Diabetes mellitus
Renal disease
Genitourologic procedure
Recent genitourinary infection
Metabolic disorder involving renal function
Procedure level 3

Complete blood count

Hematologic disorder
Vascular procedure
Chemotherapy
Procedure level 4

Coagulation studies

Anticoagulation therapy
Vascular procedure
Procedure level 5

Pregnancy testing

Patients for whom pregnancy might complicate the surgery
Patients of uncertain status by history

COPD, chronic obstructive pulmonary disease.
[a] Five surgical categories are defined, with a higher category denoting increasing invasiveness. Blood loss and estimated risk are also taken into account in this system. Procedure level 4, defined as highly invasive procedures with blood loss less than 1500 mL and major risk to patients independent of anesthesia, includes major orthopedic surgery, reconstruction of the gastrointestinal tract, and vascular repair without an intensive care unit (ICU) stay. Procedure level 5 is similar to level 4 but includes a usual postoperative ICU stay with invasive monitoring. From Pasternal LR. Screening patients: strategies and studies. In: McGoldrick K, ed. *Ambulatory anesthesiology: a problem-oriented approach.* Baltimore: Williams & Wilkins, 1995:15, with permission.

---

on the urgency of the surgery, the patient's clinical risk predictors, the risk of the surgery itself, the patient's functional status, and the results of previous cardiac evaluations or interventions (Fig. 7-1). It is important to keep in mind that these are only guidelines and cases need to be individualized.

Recently, much attention has focused on the use of perioperative β-blockade. Two large randomized trials have demonstrated improved outcomes for high risk vascular patients who were treated perioperatively with β-blockers. One study showed a decrease in perioperative cardiac complications and the other demonstrated improved 6-month survival. β-Blockers should be started ideally at least 1 week prior to surgery, with a target resting heart rate of 50 to 60 beats per minute. However, they may be titrated intravenously intraoperatively either as a bolus or infusion and then begun postoperatively. Class I evidence supports the use of perioperative β-blockade in patients who have required β-blockers for angina or hypertension in the past or in patients found to have inducible ischemia on preoperative testing and who undergo vascular surgery. Class II evidence supports the use of β-blockers in patients found to have untreated hypertension (HTN), coronary artery disease (CAD), or major risk factors for CAD.

The role of a consultant in the perioperative assessment is important but is often misunderstood. The consultant should define the patient's medical conditions in terms of severity and interpret the results of previous studies as they pertain to their field of expertise. In addition, recommendations on the necessity of further evaluations should be made. Finally, the consultant should make recommendations on how to optimize the patient's medical status preoperatively. The consultant's role is not to provide "medical clearance" for surgery. The decision to proceed with surgery should be made by the surgeon and the anesthesiologist, with assistance from the consultant.

The anesthesiologist must determine the patient's risk for gastric aspiration during induction as well as emergence of anesthesia. Aspiration occurs in these settings because of a decreased level of consciousness and loss of airway reflexes. If the airway is not protected intraoperatively with an endotracheal tube (ETT), the patient may be at risk for aspiration, even during maintenance of anesthesia. Situations that increase the risk of aspiration include gastrointestinal dysfunction, increased intraabdominal pressure, the use of opioids, and recent gastrointestinal intake. Current recommendations for preoperative fasting in adults are clear liquids up to 2 hours preoperatively, light solid foods up to 6 hours preoperatively, and heavy meals up to 8 hours preoperatively. If a patient is at increased risk for aspiration, a rapid sequence induction is often necessary, and heavy sedation should not be administered without an ETT to protect the airway.

On the basis of the patient's state of health, a physical status (PS status) is assigned (Table 7-5). Physical status is a means of classifying patients according to their overall condition and does not take the planned procedure into account. The PS status is typically used to help anesthesiologists communicate with each other to quickly summarize a patient's overall health status. An elevated PS status has been shown to correlate with increased perioperative mortality.

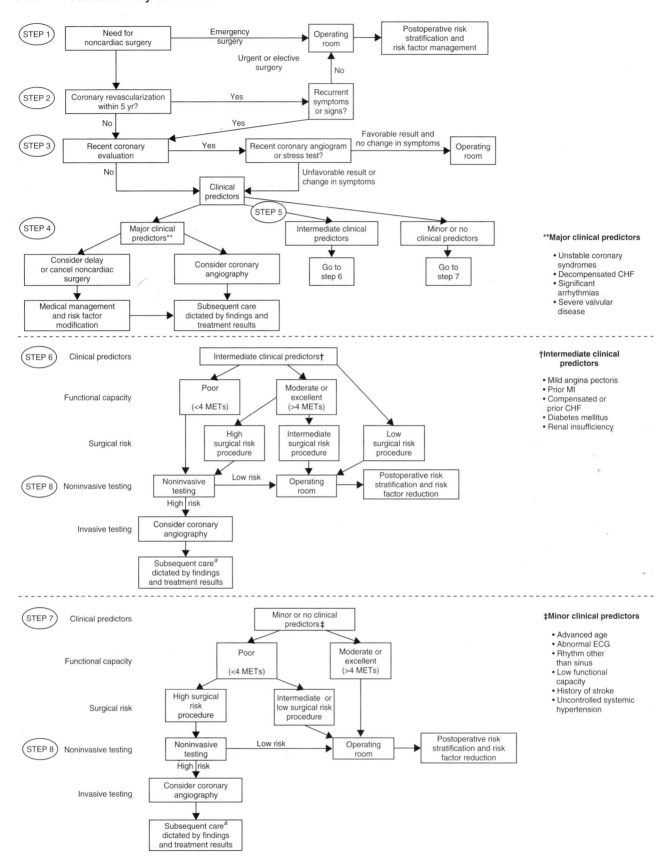

Figure 7-1 Stepwise approach to preoperative cardiac assessment. Steps are discussed in text. [a] Subsequent care may include cancellation or delay of surgery, coronary revascularization followed by noncardiac surgery, or intensified care. CHF, congestive heart failure; ECG, electrocardiogram; MET, metabolic equivalent; MI, myocardial infarction. [From Eagle KA, Berger PB, Calkins H, et al. American College of Cardiology/American Heart Association Task Force on Practice Guidelines (Committee to Update the 1996 Guidelines on Perioperative Cardiovascular Evaluation for Noncardiac Surgery). *Circulation* 2002;105:1257–1267, with permission.]

TABLE 7-5

THE PHYSICAL STATUS CLASSIFICATION OF THE AMERICAN SOCIETY OF ANESTHESIOLOGISTS

Physical Status	Definition
PS-1	Healthy patient (free of systemic disease)
PS-2	Patient with mild systemic disease that results in no functional limitations
PS-3	Patient with moderate to severe systemic disease that results in some functional limitation
PS-4	Patient with severe systemic disease that is a constant threat to life and is incapacitating
PS-5	Moribund patient who is not expected to live beyond 24 h, with or without surgery
PS-6	Brain-dead patient for organ harvest
E	Any patient in whom an emergency operation is required; e.g., a healthy patient undergoing an emergency procedure is classified as PS-IE

PS, physical status; E, emergency.

ANESTHETIC TECHNIQUES

On the basis of the proposed surgery, the patient's condition and preference, the surgeon's needs, and the anesthesiologist's judgment, an anesthetic technique is chosen. General anesthesia, regional anesthesia, and monitored anesthesia care (MAC) represent the various options. General *anesthesia* implies a loss of consciousness. This is achieved by either inhaled or intravenous anesthetic agents. Inhaled anesthetics can be delivered via an ETT, a laryngeal mask airway (LMA), or a face mask. The volatile agents can be inspired either via spontaneous, negative pressure ventilation, or via mechanical, positive pressure ventilation. *Regional anesthesia* involves injecting medications, most commonly local anesthetics, to prevent nerve transmission of surgical stimuli. Epidural, spinal, and caudal anesthesia, collectively known as *neuraxial blockade*, work by acting at the spinal cord and spinal nerves. A *peripheral nerve block* is achieved by infiltration of a nerve or nerves to anesthetize a given sensory distribution. Peripheral nerve blocks are an attractive option for patients with poor cardiac or pulmonary reserve, as hemodynamic and respiratory perturbations are minimized. *Monitored anesthesia care* involves the administration of sedation and analgesics for patient comfort. This technique often relies on the surgeon to infiltrate the operative site with a local anesthetic.

MONITORING

Certain tools have become standard intraoperative monitors for almost all anesthetics in modern operating rooms. They include the pulse oximeter, noninvasive blood pressure monitor, electrocardiogram, temperature monitor, and a means of assessing adequacy of ventilation, usually with an end-tidal carbon dioxide (CO_2) monitor.

All operating rooms employ end-tidal capnometry to measures the level of CO_2 in the circuit. The presence of sustained CO_2 in exhaled gas is the gold standard for successful endotracheal intubation, although the presence of end-tidal CO_2 cannot rule out an endobronchial intubation. Capnometry serves as a noninvasive measure of systemic partial pressure of CO_2, albeit an inaccurate one. It is, however, very sensitive in detecting changes in dead space ventilation. With normal lungs, end-tidal CO_2 is approximately 5 to 6 mm Hg below that of arterial CO_2. This gap results from dead space ventilation and normal intrapulmonary right-to-left shunting. An increase in the gap suggests that an increase in dead space ventilation has occurred. An extreme example of this occurs during cardiac arrest or a pulmonary embolism, as the end-tidal CO_2 concentration acutely and profoundly decreases. An obstruction to expiration such as bronchospasm can be detected by a delayed upstroke of the end-tidal CO_2 tracing.

Mass spectrometry is used to measure the exhaled concentration of oxygen, nitrogen, nitrous oxide, and inhalational anesthetics, permitting a real-time correlation between exhaled concentration of gases and anesthetic levels. There are various ventilator monitors and alarms built into most modern anesthesia machines. Low oxygen concentration alarms are universal. A low pressure alarm will signal decreased airway pressure and allow the detection of a circuit disconnection. A kink in the circuit, main stem bronchus intubation, patient respiratory effort, and bronchospasm will often set off the high pressure alarm. Spirometry allows the measurement of minute ventilation and tidal volumes.

An intra-arterial catheter may be inserted for "beat to beat" blood pressure monitoring or frequent blood gas and electrolyte monitoring. Cannulation of a central vein may be chosen to provide large bore venous access, for administration of vasoactive or caustic medications, or for central venous pressure (CVP) monitoring. The CVP may be used as a surrogate of left ventricular end-diastolic pressure (LVEDP) in order to monitor intravascular volume. The absolute CVP value is often difficult to interpret, especially in the setting of positive pressure ventilation. However, the trend may give valuable information.

Traditionally, pulmonary artery catheters (PACs) are placed in situations where the CVP is not a reliable indicator of LVEDP. Conditions where the pulmonary artery occlusion pressure (PAOP) is a more accurate measure of LVEDP than CVP include abnormalities of the tricuspid valve, the right ventricle, the pulmonary vasculature, or the pericardium. The use of PAOP as an indicator of left ventricular end-diastolic volume (LVEDV) relies on the assumption that there is a predictable relationship among the PAOP, the left atrial pressure (LAP), the LVEDP, and the LVEDV. Mitral valve disease, aortic insufficiency, positive pressure ventilation, positive end-expiratory pressure, catheter position in the lung, and alterations in left ventricular compliance can all confound the relationship between PAOP and LVEDV. Many studies have shown a poor relationship between PAOP and echocardiographic measurements of LVEDV.

The PAC can provide other important information. Pulmonary artery pressures can be measured as well as cardiac output. Newer catheters have the ability to measure mixed venous saturations ($S\bar{v}O_2$) and provide continuous cardiac output measurements. Fluid therapy can be titrated to cardiac output and stroke volume. Systemic vascular resistance can be calculated by using CVP and cardiac output. Although most studies have failed to show any improvement in perioperative morbidity or mortality with the use of PACs, it must be kept in mind that most of these studies have either been retrospective, nonblinded, or underpowered. In addition, the PAC is a monitor, not an intervention. Therefore, its value depends on what the physician does with the information obtained from it, making its utility difficult to prove in a study.

Cutaneous application of a peripheral nerve stimulator allows an objective assessment of the level of neuromuscular blockade when paralytic agents are used. A sequence of four electrical stimuli (train-of-four) of 50 to 60 mA is applied at a frequency of 2 Hz over a peripheral nerve. This is meant to simulate nerve conduction. Typically, the ulnar nerve, which innervates the adductor pollicis muscle, is stimulated, and thumb opposition is monitored for effect. When nondepolarizing drugs (pancuronium, cisatracurium) are used, the train-of-four demonstrates "fade," with the last twitch amplitude smaller than the first. This is analogous to the "fatigue" seen with myasthenic patients.

A number of specialized neurologic monitors may be employed during procedures in which the integrity of the CNS may be compromised. Electroencephalographic (EEG) monitoring may be used for carotid endarterectomies and during some cardiac surgical procedures. Somatosensory evoked potentials are useful for monitoring the spinal cord and its vascular supply, such as in thoracic aneurysmectomy or scoliosis repair. Monitoring may be done by the anesthesiologist or more typically by a dedicated neurophysiology technician.

Recently, newer technologies for assessment of the depth of anesthesia have been developed. The method that has gained the most popularity in clinical practice is the *BIS index*. It integrates bispectral analyses of EEG findings with more traditional spectral and burst suppression analyses to monitor the effects of many, although not all, hypnotic intravenous and inhalational agents on the EEG. The BIS index has been shown to correlate well with the loss of consciousness caused by these agents and therefore has the potential to reduce the incidence of intraoperative recall. However, it has many limitations. For example, it is a poor predictor of movement under anesthesia. It also correlates poorly with loss of consciousness induced by ketamine, nitrous oxide, and high dose opioids.

Transesophageal echocardiography (TEE) is currently used primarily in the cardiac surgical suites. TEE permits real-time evaluation of left ventricular wall motion, end-diastolic volume, and valvular function. It is used to detect air embolism, aortic dissection, valve malfunction, endocarditis, and MI.

INHALATIONAL AGENTS

The primary effector site of anesthetic gases is the CNS, with the lungs providing a conduit for delivery of gas to the CNS. The standard measure of potency for inhaled anesthetics is defined as the *minimum alveolar concentration* (MAC) of a given gas at 1 atmosphere that produces immobility in 50% of subjects exposed to a noxious stimulus.

The inhalational agents in common use today include the volatile anesthetics isoflurane, sevoflurane, and desflurane, as well as the gas nitrous oxide. Each has its own unique set of properties. It is the partial pressure of an inhaled anesthetic in the brain that results in anesthesia. Therefore, the more soluble the agent that is in the blood, the slower its rise in partial pressure, and the slower the onset of anesthesia. Increased solubility of inhaled anesthetics in tissues leads to an increased uptake in the muscle and fat, which prolongs awakening once administration of the agent has been discontinued. All volatile anesthetics cause dose-dependent cardiac depression; decreases in systemic, pulmonary, and venous vascular resistance; respiratory depression; bronchodilation; decreases in cerebral metabolic rate ($CMRo_2$); and increases in intracranial pressure (ICP). When choosing an inhaled anesthetic, one must consider an agent's side-effect profile, its potential for airway irritation, and its degree of metabolism in the body.

Desflurane is the most insoluble agent in the blood, thereby allowing a very quick onset and offset of anesthesia. Both its pungent odor and its propensity to induce airway irritation and laryngospasm make desflurane unsuitable for masked inductions. Catecholamine surges may occur from rapid increases in inspired concentrations. Desflurane is the least metabolized of all volatile anesthetics. *Sevoflurane* is a nonpungent agent and is therefore ideal for mask inductions. Its blood solubility falls between those of isoflurane and desflurane. Sevoflurane is metabolized in the liver with the production of fluoride ions. *Isoflurane* is the oldest of the three inhaled anesthetics discussed herein. It is more pungent then sevoflurane and undergoes minimal metabolism.

Nitrous oxide is a colorless, odorless gas. It has a very low solubility in blood and the lowest tissue solubility of the volatile anesthetic agents. It has a very low potency, which results in its use only as an adjuvant anesthetic at relatively high inspired concentrations. Its major shortcoming is a tendency to diffuse into closed air-containing spaces. It is, therefore, contraindicated in the presence of a pneumothorax, small bowel obstruction, air embolism, and middle ear surgery. Nitrous oxide will activate the SNS and increase $CMRo_2$. The use of nitrous oxide has been associated with an increased incidence of postoperative nausea.

INTRAVENOUS ANESTHETICS

These are a group of unrelated medications that are administered parenterally to provide hypnosis. Most work by activation of γ-aminobutyric acid (GABA) pathways. These include barbiturates, propofol, etomidate, ketamine, and benzodiazepines. Traditionally these medications have been used for the induction of anesthesia because of their rapid onset, which results from high lipid solubility. High lipid solubility allows these agents to traverse cell membranes rapidly, including the blood–brain barrier. The high lipid solubility also leads to a rapid offset because of extensive redistribution out of the brain into the blood and then into peripheral tissues. Extensive hepatic metabolism also leads to a relatively short half-life for these drugs. During prolonged infusions, the drugs begin to accumulate in peripheral tissues, such as muscle and fat, which prolongs awakening once the infusion is discontinued. In these situations, the offset of the drug is dependent more on metabolism and clearance than on redistribution. Other than ketamine, these drugs possess no analgesic properties.

Barbiturates

Sodium thiopental is the most commonly used barbiturate. Thiopental causes profound respiratory depression when administered as a bolus. It also causes peripheral vasodilation and myocardial depression. The dose should be decreased in the presence of decreased protein binding states (chronic renal failure and cirrhosis) and in patients with decreased central blood volume (elderly and patients with hypovolemia) as the free drug concentration in plasma will be higher in these situations. A beneficial effect of barbiturates is a reduction of cerebral metabolism and oxygen consumption. Barbiturates may provide cerebral protection in the face of focal ischemia but not in the event of global ischemic episodes like cardiac arrest. A contraindication to barbiturate administration is acute intermittent porphyria, as an attack may be precipitated.

Profolol

Propofol is rapidly and extensively metabolized in the liver. Its metabolism and rapid redistribution provide a very short elimination half-life. Propofol causes even larger decreases in vascular tone and cardiac contractility than thiopental. Like thiopental, propofol will decrease $CMRO_2$, cerebral blood flow (CBF), and ICP. Continuous infusions of propofol can be used in combination with other agents, such as opioids, for total intravenous anesthesia (TIVA). In addition, propofol has antiemetic properties.

Etomidate

Etomidate is an imidazole-containing compound. Etomidate is well suited for the induction of anesthesia in patients with compromised hemodynamics, as it causes minimal cardiorespiratory depression. Subcortical inhibition may lead to occasional myoclonic activity during induction. It can suppress adrenal hormone synthesis even after a single dose for up to 5 to 6 hours. The significance of this suppression in the short term is unknown. However, the use of long-term infusions in critically ill patients has been associated with increased mortality, presumably from adrenal suppression.

Ketamine

Ketamine is a phenylcyclidine derivative that induces a dissociative state of anesthesia by inhibition of thalamocortical pathways and activation of the limbic system. Ketamine's CNS effects are mediated via inhibition of N-methyl-D-aspartate (NMDA) receptors. Unlike other agents, ketamine stimulates the SNS, causing an increase in heart rate, blood pressure, and cardiac output. Ketamine has negligible effects on ventilatory drive and induces bronchodilation. It possesses potent analgesic properties. Cerebral blood flow and oxygen consumption are increased with the administration of ketamine. Because of this, it is undesirable in patients with head injury and/or elevations in intracranial pressure. Its stimulation of the SNS makes ketamine relatively contraindicated in the presence of CAD or uncontrolled hypertension. Emergence dysphoria and hallucinations are common following ketamine-based anesthesia. Benzodiazepines can be used to decrease these complications.

Benzodiazepines

Benzodiazepines are used primarily as anxiolytics. However, they may also be used for anesthetic induction and in combination with other agents for total intravenous anesthesia. Midazolam, because of its short duration of action, is the predominant benzodiazepine encountered in anesthetic practice. Midazolam has profound amnestic properties. Benzodiazepines have no analgesic properties and are, therefore, often combined with opioids. Flumazenil is a specific benzodiazepine antagonist. Bolus administration of flumazenil may cause seizure activity in patients on chronic benzodiazepine therapy.

Opioids

Opioids are not sedative-hypnotics and have minimal amnestic properties. They interact with opioid receptors in the CNS and mediate effects on pain, mood, respiration, circulation, and bowel and bladder function. The liver is the site of most opioid metabolism.

In general, opioids are not associated with a decrease in cardiac contractility. Blood pressure may, however, fall as a result of vagally mediated bradycardia and blunting of the SNS. There is a direct dose-dependent depression of ventilation with opioid administration. Opioids have a prominent effect on the gastrointestinal tract, as peristalsis is slowed and gastric emptying is delayed. Nausea and vomiting, as well as constipation and urinary retention, are common side effects of opioids.

Morphine and meperidine have been associated with histamine release. Both are known to have active renally excreted metabolites, which will accumulate in patients with renal failure. Meperidine has a metabolite that can induce seizures. Fentanyl has minimal cardiovascular effects, no active metabolites, and a short half-life.

MUSCLE RELAXANTS

Neuromuscular blocking agents are used to facilitate intubation as well as to enhance surgical exposure, to ensure immobility, and to enable a patient to be anesthetized with lower concentrations of inhalational agents. The degree of paralysis can be objectively assessed with a peripheral nerve stimulator.

The two major classes of neuromuscular blocking agents include depolarizing and nondepolarizing agents. The only depolarizing agent used in the United States today is *succinylcholine*. Succinylcholine binds to nicotinic acetylcholine receptors at the neuromuscular junction (NMJ), causing an initial depolarization that leads to a diffuse non-coordinated muscle contraction referred to as a fasciculation. A stylized picture of the NMJ is found in Figure 7-2. Succinylcholine remains bound to the acetylcholine receptor and flaccid paralysis follows. It eventually dissociates from the receptor and diffuses into the bloodstream, where it is metabolized by plasma pseudocholinesterase. The major advantages of succinylcholine are its rapid onset, provision of reliable intubating conditions in 60 seconds, and an ultrashort duration of action of 3 to 5 minutes.

Succinylcholine, however, is associated with various adverse side effects (Table 7-6). Succinylcholine can cause the

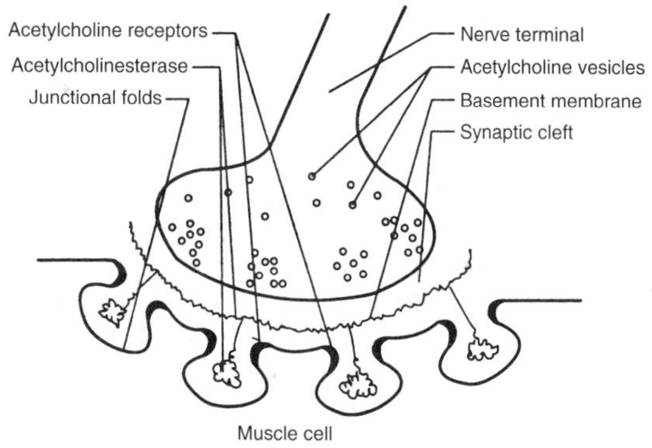

Figure 7-2 The neuromuscular junction. (From Bevan DR, Donati F. Muscle relaxants. In: Barash PG, Cullen BF, Stoelting RK, eds. *Clinical anesthesia*, 4th ed. Philadelphia: Lippincott Williams & Wilkins, 2001, with permission.)

release of potassium from muscle, with a rise of 0.5 to 1 mEq per L, owing to its depolarizing effects at the acetylcholine receptor. In susceptible patients, life-threatening hyperkalemia may ensue. Those at risk include patients with extensive burns, massive tissue injuries, neurologic injuries (spinal cord injuries or hemiparesis), and neuromuscular disorders [muscular dystrophy or amyotrophic lateral sclerosis (ALS)]. The common pathway appears to be the loss of neurologic innervation of the NMJ or defective muscle membranes. In either case, there is a subsequent diffusion of nicotinic receptors from the NMJ to the rest of the muscle membrane. Patients may be at risk for severe hyperkalemia with succinylcholine as soon as 24 to 48 hours after the acute injury and stay at risk for months to years later. In 1994 the FDA issued a warning to avoid the routine use of succinylcholine in pediatric patients, as many children may have subclinical myopathies predisposing them to hyperkalemia. Relative contraindications to succinylcholine include its use in patients with intracranial hypertension or open orbital injuries because of a sudden but brief increase in intracranial or intraocular pressure.

Nondepolarizing neuromuscular blocking (NDNMB) agents do not activate the acetylcholine receptor. Their mechanism of action is through the competitive inhibition of acetylcholine binding at the NMJ. The elimination of

most NDNMBs is via hepatic and renal mechanisms. For the most part, *vecuronium* is excreted nonenzymatically by way of the biliary system, although some is metabolized in the liver and some is excreted unchanged in the urine. *Pancuronium* is excreted mostly unchanged in the urine with some hepatic extraction. *Mivacurium* and *cisatracurium* are metabolized enzymatically in the plasma. The choice of a particular agent usually depends on the desired length of paralysis and the presence of any hepatic or renal disease (Table 7-7). The paralysis induced by NDNMB agents can be reversed with acetylcholinesterase inhibitors (*neostigmine* and *edrophonium*). Their mechanism of action is via inhibition of acetylcholine breakdown at the NMJ. This leads to a rise in intrasynaptic levels of acetylcholine, causing a shift in the competitive binding at the NMJ between the paralytic and acetylcholine. Reversal with acetylcholinesterase inhibitors will increase acetylcholine levels at muscarinic receptors as well, resulting in a diffuse vagal response. To counteract this, anticholinergics such as glycopyrrolate or atropine are administered with the acetylcholinesterase inhibitors.

LOCAL ANESTHETICS

Local anesthetics can be classified as either amides (*lidocaine* and *bupivacaine*) or esters (*procaine*) on the basis of their intermediate linkage structure. Plasma cholinesterase is responsible for the metabolism of the ester family of agents, whereas local anesthetics with an amide linkage undergo hepatic metabolism. Esters have a higher incidence of "true" allergic reactions based on a cross-sensitivity to paraaminobenzoic acid (PABA), which is a product of ester metabolism.

Local anesthetics act on the sodium channels of nerve membranes. They bind to specific receptors within the inner portion of the sodium channel and stabilize the channel in the inactivated state, thereby terminating the initiation and conduction of action potentials.

Local anesthetics may be used topically, subcutaneously, and in a wide variety of perineural locations for major nerve blocks. The choice of agent is based on the location to be blocked, the desired duration of action, and the toxicity. The addition of epinephrine to a local anesthetic causes vasoconstriction in that region. This will prolong an agent's duration of action, limit systemic absorption and toxicity, and may serve as a marker for intravascular injection by inducing tachycardia. Local anesthetics are weak bases; therefore, alkalinization of a local anesthetic solution with bicarbonate will speed onset, as it increases the percentage of local anesthetic present in the nonionized form. It is the nonionized form of these weak bases that penetrates nerve cell membranes.

Lidocaine is perhaps the most commonly used local anesthetic, having a wide margin of safety and a moderate duration of action. The maximum dose of lidocaine for infiltration is 5 mg per kg, and 7 mg per kg if epinephrine is added.

Bupivacaine is an amide agent that provides excellent sensory and motor blockade and lasts approximately twice as long as lidocaine. The maximum dose for infiltration is 3 mg per kg. Ropivacaine is a relatively new amide agent. It shares a similar pharmacokinetic profile with bupivacaine. The major advantage of ropivacaine over bupivacaine is decreased cardiac toxicity.

The major concern regarding the use of local anesthetics is cardiovascular and CNS toxicity. CNS symptoms tend to

---

TABLE 7-6

ADVERSE EFFECTS OF SUCCINYLCHOLINE

1. It is a known trigger for malignant hyperthermia.
2. A prolonged duration of action is seen in patients with atypical pseudocholinesterase or severe liver disease.
3. Increases in intragastric, intraocular, and intracranial pressures follow its administration.
4. Arrhythmias including bradycardia, junctional arrhythmias, and ventricular dysrhythmias may occur because of vagotonic effects.
5. Although usually mild (a rise of 0.5–1.0 mEq/dL is typical) and transient, hyperkalemia follows succinylcholine administration. This effect can be profound in patients with burns, upper and lower motor neuron injuries or disease, and after significant trauma. The hyperkalemic response is most pronounced beginning 24 h after a burn or injury and lasts 6 mo. In predisposed patients, the precipitous rise in potassium level may cause cardiac arrest.
6. Because of the potential for undiagnosed muscular dystrophy, succinylcholine is relatively contraindicated in children.

TABLE 7-7
MUSCLE RELAXANTS

Agent	Intubating Dose (mg/kg)	Duration	Clearance	Autonomic Effects	Of Note
Depolarizing:					
Succinylcholine	1.5–2.0	3–5 min	Enzymatic	+ vagatonic	↑ K, arrhythmias
Nondepolarizing:					
Pancuronium	0.08–0.10	90 min	Renal	Vagolytic	Tachycardia
Cisatracurium	0.20	60 min	Enzymatic	—	Organ-independent elimination
Vecuronium	0.10	60 min	Renal, hepatic	—	Cardiovascularly inert
Rocuronium	0.6–1.0	60 min	Hepatic	—	Rapid onset of intubating conditions
Rapacuronium	1.0–1.5	20 min	Hepatic	—	Histamine release; renally excreted active metabolite

precede cardiovascular symptoms. The first signs of neurologic toxicity may be a metallic taste in the mouth, circumoral tingling, or tinnitus. CNS depression may be followed by excitation in the form of tonic-clonic seizures. Local anesthetic–induced seizures may be terminated with barbiturates or benzodiazepines.

Larger doses of local anesthetics are needed to produce cardiovascular toxicity than are needed to produce convulsions. Lidocaine toxicity typically produces bradycardia and vasodilation. Bupivacaine can cause significantly more cardiac toxicity then the other local anesthetics. Although it suppresses cardiac contractility to the same degree as lidocaine does, it can have profound effects on cardiac conduction. Bupivacaine binds avidly to cardiac sodium channels and dissociates very slowly. The first sign of bupivacaine toxicity may be a ventricular dysrhythmia or cardiovascular collapse. Treatment often involves cardiopulmonary resuscitation (CPR) and may require temporary cardiopulmonary bypass.

Toxicity is frequently said to occur at a given dose for a given weight. However, it is more complicated than this. Toxicity is primarily related to the plasma concentration. The accidental injection of a small amount of lidocaine into the vertebral artery may cause a seizure, whereas subcutaneous infiltration of large amounts of lidocaine has minimal side effects. Systemic blood levels vary as a function of the rate of absorption from a particular injection site. Drugs injected for intercostal nerve blocks are absorbed much more rapidly than drugs infiltrated subcutaneously. Therefore, the intercostal nerve block will result in a higher peak plasma concentration and a higher risk for toxicity.

MAINTENANCE OF ANESTHESIA

During surgery the anesthesiologist is responsible for maintaining optimal operating conditions for the surgeon while maintaining optimal physiologic conditions for the patient. The surgical stress response, combined with the anesthetic-induced decrease in sympathetic tone, as well as the cardiorespiratory depressant effects of the anesthetic drugs, can often make this challenging. Superimposed on these challenges is the presence of any intrinsic disease state. Fluid deficits from either preoperative fasting or from bowel preparations must be replaced. Isotonic crystalloids are typically used for maintenance fluids, administered at dosages of approximately 2 mL/kg/h. Blood loss is replaced with either crystalloid or colloids until transfusion becomes

necessary. Often large fluid volumes are administered to replenish the intravascular volume because of fluid sequestration in the interstitial spaces from capillary leaks. "Third space losses" from large abdominal procedures can require crystalloid dosages of up to 10 mL/kg/h for replacement.

REGIONAL ANESTHESIA

The major regional modalities include epidural and spinal anesthesia as well as peripheral nerve blocks. Regional blockade may be used as the sole form of anesthesia or as an adjunct to general anesthesia. Regional anesthesia can provide analgesia into the postoperative period, especially when catheters are left in place. Studies have shown that surgery performed under neuraxial anesthesia leads to higher rates of graft viability following peripheral revascularization, decreased intraoperative blood loss, and lower rates of deep venous thrombosis for hip surgery.

Epidural anesthesia is achieved by the administration of local anesthetic into the epidural space. A needle is used to traverse the skin, subcutaneous tissue, supraspinous ligament, interspinous ligament, and ligamentum flavum, after which the epidural space is reached. Typically, a catheter is threaded into the epidural space for subsequent use. Placement of a spinal needle is similar to that of an epidural; however, the epidural space is traversed and the subarachnoid space entered, which is heralded by return of cerebrospinal fluid (CSF). A much finer needle is typically useed for spinal anesthesia, and it is less common to place an indwelling catheter. As the spinal cord terminates at the L1-2 level in adults, the spinal needle is introduced at least one interspace below this during induction of spinal anesthesia.

The systemic implications of neuraxial anesthesia may be considerable. In addition to their sensory and motor effects, local anesthetics create a chemical sympathectomy in the affected body region that results in vasodilation. When the block is proximal to the high thoracic cardiac accelerator fibers, bradycardia can also ensue. The combination of bradycardia and peripheral pooling of blood can cause profound hypotension. Mental status changes from impaired cerebral blood flow may occur. Treatment of hypotension includes fluid administration, vasoconstrictors, and inotropic agents. Occasionally anticholinergics are required for severe bradycardia. The vasodilation associated with neuraxial techniques may be particularly harmful in hypovolemic patients as well as in those with stenotic valvular heart disease, severe coronary artery disease, or hypertrophic obstructive cardiomyopathies. Although neuraxial techniques have been employed safely in these settings, a degree of caution must be used and a thorough assessment of the risk-to-benefit ratio examined when considering the use of general versus regional anesthetic techniques. In addition, the consequences of treating this pharmacologic sympathectomy must be considered.

A "total spinal" implies a regional block that spreads throughout the entire spinal cord. The block may inhibit the muscles of respiration, requiring temporary positive pressure ventilation. However, apnea often resolves with the restoration of a normal blood pressure. A postdural puncture headache (PDPH) may occur following spinal anesthesia or after inadvertent dural puncture with attempted epidural placement. PDPH is the result of CSF leakage, which leads to sagging of the brain in the cranial vault which applies traction to the pain-sensitive dural fibers. These headaches are exacerbated by the erect position and ameliorated by assumption of a supine position. PDPH can occur anywhere but are usually occipital or frontal in location. Visual and auditory disturbances can occasionally occur. Treatment of PDPH includes bed rest, IV hydration, caffeine, and if these conservative measures fail, an epidural blood patch. An epidural blood patch involves the sterile placement of 10 to 20 mL of blood into the epidural space. It affords relief in 1 to 24 hours for 85% to 90% of patients with PDPH.

The most feared neurologic complication of neuraxial anesthesia is an *epidural hematoma*. Fortunately, the incidence is 1 per 150,000. The most common presenting symptoms are backache and lower extremity weakness or numbness. The risk of hematoma formation is not limited to the placement of a spinal or epidural but also is present upon removal of catheters. Hematoma formation is more likely in the setting of coagulopathy or platelet dysfunction, either from medications or intrinsic disease. Aspirin therapy and nonsteroidal antiinflammatory drugs (NSAIDs), either alone or in combination, do not increase the risk of hematoma formation. However, antiplatelet drugs such as ticlopidine and clopidine do increase the risk. The current American Society of Regional Anesthesia guidelines recommend discontinuing ticlopidine for 14 days and clopidine for 7 days prior to performing neuraxial anesthesia. One is referred to these guidelines for further information regarding the timing and use of the heparins, warfarin, fibrinolytics, and GP IIb/IIIa inhibitors in the setting of regional anesthesia. If there is a suspicion for a hematoma, emergent magnetic resonance imaging (MRI) is indicated, followed by surgical decompression. The chance for recovery is decreased considerably if surgery occurs more than 8 hours after the event.

Commonly used peripheral nerve blocks include those of the brachial plexus, the sciatic and femoral nerves, the intercostal nerves, the ilioinguinal nerve, and the nerves of the ankle. Advantages of peripheral nerve blocks over neuraxial blockade include greater hemodynamic stability and less risk of serious neurologic injury. Complications of peripheral nerve block include hematoma, block failure, intravascular injection, and, rarely, infection or nerve damage. Intercostal or interscalene nerve blocks may cause pneumothorax, which may result in respiratory decompensation. An interscalene block can also cause phrenic nerve paralysis. Additional relative contraindications to regional nerve blocks include sepsis, skin infection in the area of proposed needle placement, and preexistent neurologic deficit/neuropathy. Finally, patients with increased ICP are at risk for brain herniation after a spinal or an inadvertent dural puncture with an epidural needle, owing to a sudden loss of CSF.

MALIGNANT HYPERTHERMIA

Malignant hyperthermia (MH) is an extremely rare complication of anesthesia. It has an incidence of 1 per 12,000 anesthetics in children and 1 per 40,000 anesthetics in adults. Susceptible patients have a genetic predisposition. Known triggers of malignant hyperthermia include all volatile agents as well as succinylcholine. The pathophysiology of malignant hyperthermia is the inability of the sarcoplasmic reticulum to reaccumulate calcium in skeletal muscle, which causes sustained muscle contractions.

MH is a clinical diagnosis. The first sign frequently is an elevation in the end-tidal CO_2 level. Other findings include tachycardia, dysrhythmias, skeletal muscle rigidity, and, eventually, an elevated body temperature. Laboratory abnormalities include a combined metabolic and respiratory acidosis, hyperkalemia, and extremely high levels of creatine kinase.

Therapy includes immediate discontinuation of volatile anesthetics, hyperventilation with 100% oxygen, conclusion of surgery as quickly as possible, maintenance of urine output to protect the kidneys from myoglobin, and active cooling measures. *Dantrolene* is the drug of choice for treatment of MH. It acts by interfering with the release of calcium from the sarcoplasmic reticulum.

KEY POINTS

▲ All inhaled anesthetics cause a dose-dependent decrease in systemic and venous resistance, decrease in cardiac contractility, decrease in ventilatory drive, decrease in cerebral metabolic drive, and increase in intracranial pressure (ICP) and cerebral blood flow.

▲ Nitrous oxide will expand closed air spaces and should be avoided in cases where a bowel obstruction or a pneumothorax is present, as well as in cases involving middle ear surgery.

▲ Severe hyperkalemia may be seen after the administration of succinylcholine to patients with extensive burns. The risk of hyperkalemia may occur as soon as 24 to 48

hours and may last for months. Patients with damaged muscle membranes or with denervated muscle are also at risk, and the risk may persist for years after the initial injury.

▲ The risk of a spinal hematoma is increased in the setting of coagulopathy either from intrinsic disease or anticoagulation. The risk is also increased in the setting of thrombocytopenia or platelet dysfunction from platelet inhibitors other than aspirin.

▲ The early signs of malignant hyperthermia (MH) are an increase in carbon dioxide production, tachycardia, hypertension, and a metabolic acidosis.

SUGGESTED READINGS

American Society of Regional Anesthesia and Pain Medicine (US). C2002. Available at: http://www.asra.com/items_of_interest/consensus_statement.html. Accessed June, 2004.

Barash PG, Cullen BF, Stoelting RK, eds. *Clinical anesthesia*, 4th ed. Philadelphia: Lippincott Williams & Wilkins, 2000.

Eagle KA, Berger PB, Calkins H, et al. ACC/AHA guideline update for perioperative cardiovascular evaluation for non-cardiac surgery-executive summary. *Anesth Analg* 2002;94:1052–1064.

Miller RD, ed. *Anesthesia*, 5th ed. Philadelphia: Churchill Livingstone, 2000.

Morgan GE, Mikhail MS, eds. *Clinical anesthesiology*, 3rd ed. New York: McGraw-Hill, 2002.

Hernias

Ibrahim Abdullah   Jon B. Morris

8

Hernia, which in Latin means "rupture" in the abdominal wall, is a protrusion of abdominal cavity contents beyond their inherent domain. In the United States, approximately one million hernia operations are performed each year. A large part of any general surgical practice is devoted to the diagnosis and treatment of hernias and their complications. As such, it is important for the surgeon to fully understand the types of hernias that can occur, their natural history, the pertinent regional anatomy, and the treatment options available.

DEFINITIONS AND TERMS

Several terms are used to describe hernias and the status of the herniated organs. A *reducible* hernia is one in which the herniated contents can be returned to their anatomic position manually; they may, however, spontaneously herniate again after the manual control is removed. A hernia is called *incarcerated* if its contents cannot be returned to their normal position in a nonsurgical manner. This type of hernia is often associated with complications and *may* require urgent or emergent treatment. In cases of chronic hernias, adhesions may cause a hernia to become incarcerated. In such cases an elective repair may offer less risk than an emergent repair. At the other extreme, an incarcerated hollow viscus may become obstructed while any incarcerated organ may have its blood supply compromised, resulting in a dangerous *strangulated* hernia. Such hernias undoubtedly require emergent repair. When part of the hernia sac is composed of the herniating organ, this is known as a *sliding* hernia. A *Richter* hernia occurs when less than the full circumference of the bowel wall becomes entrapped in a hernia defect, rendering possible ischemia but no obstruction (Fig. 8-1). A *Littre* hernia is a *Richter* hernia in which there is herniation of a Meckel diverticulum. *Incisional* hernias develop through a surgical incision in the abdominal wall.

PATHOPHYSIOLOGY OF HERNIA DEVELOPMENT

Hernias may develop in any of the structures surrounding or supporting the abdominal cavity. They are particularly prone to develop at naturally weak points of the abdominal wall. Congenital maldevelopment of an abdominal support structure coupled with physical stresses play a significant role.

Inguinal hernias, by far the most common, and, in particular, indirect inguinal hernias occur because of an unobliterated processus vaginalis, the peritoneal connection between the abdominal cavity and the scrotum. In women, the canal of Nuck is an analogous embryologic remnant related to the migration of the gubernaculum of the round ligament to the labium majus. It must be understood that although necessary, a patent processus vaginalis alone does not necessarily lead to an indirect inguinal hernia, as autopsy results have demonstrated that 20% of individuals without any clinical evidence of a hernia have had a patent processus vaginalis.

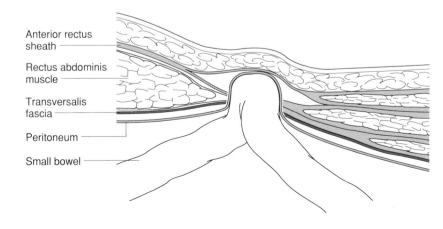

Anterior rectus sheath

Rectus abdominis muscle

Transversalis fascia

Peritoneum

Small bowel

Figure 8-1 Richter hernia of the small bowel. (From Richards AT, Quinn TH, Fitzgibbons RJ. Abdominal wall hernias. In: Greenfield LJ, Mulholland M, Oldham KT et al., eds. *Surgery: scientific principles and practice*, 3rd ed. Philadelphia: Lippincott Williams & Wilkins, 2001:1200, with permission.)

Other factors of note include integrity of fascial tissue in terms of collagen strength as well as factors that increase intraabdominal pressure such as morbid obesity, chronic pulmonary disease, constipation, pregnancy, and urinary obstruction. Overexpression of matrix metalloproteinasis involved in extracelullar matrix synthesis and degradation has also been implicated in predisposing individuals to hernia formation. Individuals with Marfan syndrome, a well-known disease associated with a collagen disorder, have a known prediliction to developing hernias. Although much more research may be needed, certain studies have demonstrated the development of inguinal hernias in young rats and mice that were fed a diet of flowering sweet peas. The active agent in the pea, β-aminoproprionitirile, is known to prevent collagen maturation.

TABLE 8-1

LAYERS OF THE ANTERIOR ABDOMINAL WALL

Skin	Superficial
Subcutaneous fat	
Scarpa fascia	
External oblique muscle	
Internal oblique muscle	
Transversus abdominus muscle	
Transversalis (endoabdominal) fascia	
Properitoneal fat	
Peritoneum	Deep

GROIN HERNIAS

Abdominal hernias may occur at any location that supports intrabdominal contents, with abdominal wall hernias being by far the most predominant. Among abdominal wall hernias, groin hernias represent approximately 90% of cases. Among groin hernias, indirect hernias are the predominant type, followed by direct hernias and femoral hernias, respectively. Consequently, a thorough understanding of the groin hernia is important for all surgeons.

Anatomy of the Lower Abdominal Wall

The lower abdominal wall is made up of three musculoaponeurotic layers covered by subcutaneous fat and skin (Fig. 8-2 and Table 8-1). The *external oblique muscle* arises from the lower eight ribs interdigitating with the serratus anterior and the latissimus dorsi, with its fibers running in an inferomedial direction. The aponeurosis contributes to the anterior rectus sheath before inserting into the linea alba in the midline. The portion of the external oblique aponeurosis that stretches between the anterior superior iliac spine and the pubic tubercle is somewhat thickened and folds back onto itself, forming the *inguinal (Poupart) ligament*. Medially, the inguinal ligament reflects back onto the pectin pubis as the *lacunar ligament*. Just superior to the medial part of the inguinal ligament is a triangular opening in the external oblique aponeurosis known as the *superficial inguinal ring*, through which the spermatic cord in men, or the round ligament in women, exits the inguinal canal (Fig. 8-3).

The *internal oblique muscle* is the middle layer of the abdominal wall musculature. Its fibers course in a superomedial direction at approximately right angles to the external oblique fibers. It serves as the superior border of the inguinal canal.

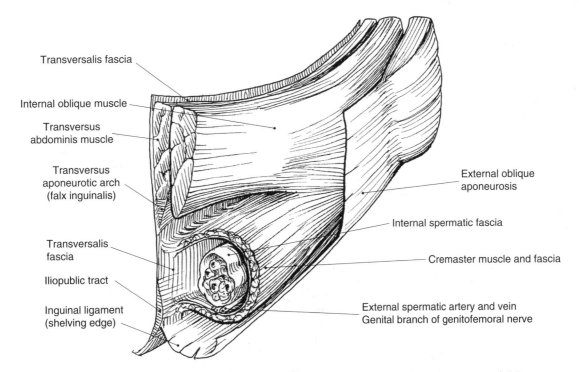

Figure 8-2 Anterior view of the inguinal canal as seen from medial to lateral. (From Wind GG. *Applied laparascopic anatomy.* Baltimore: Williams & Wilkins, 1997, with permission.)

Labels on figure:
- Transversalis fascia
- Internal oblique muscle
- Transversus abdominis muscle
- Transversus aponeurotic arch (falx inguinalis)
- Transversalis fascia
- Iliopublic tract
- Inguinal ligament (shelving edge)
- External oblique aponeurosis
- Internal spermatic fascia
- Cremaster muscle and fascia
- External spermatic artery and vein
- Genital branch of genitofemoral nerve

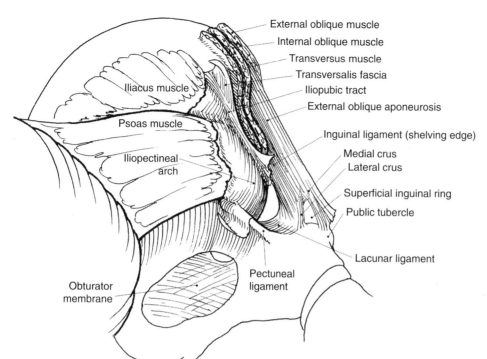

Figure 8-3 Posterior view of the inguinal canal with the spermatic cord removed. (From Wind GG. *Applied laparascopic anatomy.* Baltimore: Williams & Wilkins, 1997, with permission.)

The medial aspect of the internal oblique aponeurosis joins the aponeurosis of the transversus abdominis in 5% to 10% of individuals to form the *conjoined* tendon. The aponeurosis of the internal oblique muscle contributes to both the anterior and posterior rectus sheaths above the arcuate line. The arcuate line defines the inferior margin of the posterior rectus sheath. In contrast, below the arcuate line, the aponeurosis of the internal oblique muscle contributes solely to the anterior rectus sheath.

The *transversus abdominis* forms the innermost muscular layer of the abdominal wall. The transversus abdominis courses transversely, medially contributing to the rectus sheath. Above the arcuate line, the aponeurosis contributes to the posterior rectus sheath along with the internal oblique; below the arcuate line, it joins the internal and external oblique to form the anterior rectus sheath. The inferior edge of the transversus abdominis aponeurosis inserts onto *Cooper* ligament, which is formed of periosteum and fascial condensations along the posterior aspect of the superior pubic ramus.

The *deep inguinal ring* is a defect in the transversalis fascia approximately halfway between the anterior superior iliac spine and the pubic tubercle, through which the spermatic cord and round ligament exit the abdominal cavity and enter the inguinal canal.

The *inguinal canal* courses from the deep inguinal ring to the superficial inguinal ring (Fig. 8-2). The transversalis fascia forms the posterior border or floor of the inguinal canal. The external oblique fascia forms the anterior border of the canal. The arching fibers of the internal oblique and transversus abdominis muscles (*falx inguinalis*) form the superior border, whereas the inguinal and lacunar ligaments form the inferior border of the canal.

Hesselbach triangle defines a region of the abdominal wall through which a direct inguinal hernia protrudes. The triangle is bounded by the inferior epigastric artery laterally, the inguinal ligament inferiorly, and the rectus sheath medially (Fig. 8-4).

The *spermatic cord* passes through the deep inguinal ring with the vas deferens, testicular vessels, and the usually obliterated processus vaginalis (Table 8-2). The transversalis fascia extends onto the cord, forming the internal spermatic fascia as the cord passes through the deep inguinal ring. The internal oblique muscle extends fibers onto the

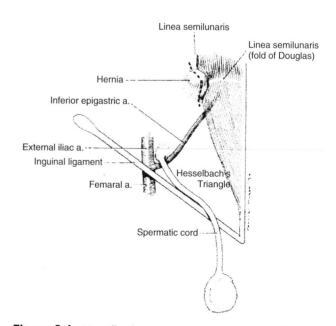

Figure 8-4 Hesselbach triangle. (From Skandalakis JE, Skandalakis LJ, et al. Anatomy of the hernial rings. In: Nyhus LM, Baker RJ, eds. *Mastery of surgery,* 4th ed. Philadelphia: Lippincott Williams & Wilkins, 2001:1884, with permission.)

TABLE 8-2
RELATION OF ABDOMINAL WALL LAYERS TO SPERMATIC CORD LAYERS

Abdominal Wall	Spermatic Cord
External oblique	External spermatic fascia
Internal oblique	Cremaster muscle
Transversalis fascia	Internal spermatic fascia
Peritoneum	Processus vaginalis

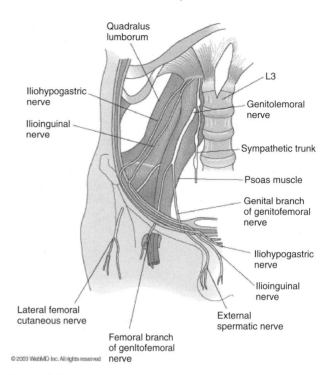

Figure 8-5 Nerves of the inguinal region. [From ACSSurgery.com (Fig. 3 from Chapter 22, Section 3).]

cord as the cremaster muscle, whereas the external oblique muscle fascia adds the external spermatic fascia at the superficial inguinal ring. The cremaster muscle forms an extension of the internal oblique muscle onto the cord. The external spermatic fascia is likewise derived from the external oblique muscle fascia at the superficial inguinal ring.

The *iliopubic tract* is a thickening of the endoabdominal fascia where the transversalis fascia and the iliopsoas fascia meet. It courses from the anterior superior iliac spine to the superior pubic ramus and pubic tubercle. It is located deep to and slightly superior to the inguinal ligament forming the inferior margin of the deep inguinal ring. Medially, it forms the anterior and medial walls of the femoral canal (Figs. 8-2 and 8-3).

The *femoral canal* is a potential space deep to the inguinal ligament that can allow potential herniation. It is bounded laterally by the external iliac vein, superoanteriorly by the inguinal ligament, posteriorly by Cooper ligament, and medially by the lacunar ligament (Fig. 8-3).

An understanding of the sensory-motor neural anatomy is important in the surgical treatment of a groin hernia. The *iliohypogastric nerve* and *ilioinguinal nerves* originate from the L1 nerve root. The ilioinguinal nerve runs superior to the spermatic cord through the superficial inguinal ring to innervate the scrotum or labium majus canal. The genital branch of the *genitofemoral* nerve arises from the L1 and L2 nerve roots and enters the inguinal canal inferior to the deep inguinal ring. It provides motor innervation for the cremaster muscle and sensory innervation to the scrotum and medial thigh (Fig. 8-5).

Indirect Inguinal Hernias

Indirect inguinal hernias are protrusions through the deep internal ring that pass lateral to the inferior epigastric vessels. They arise because of a patent processus vaginalis and may course completely into the scrotum after passing through the superficial inguinal ring. The indirect sac is present within the cremaster muscle and is located on the anteromedial aspect of the cord. These are the most common abdominal wall hernias in both men and women, although men are more likely than women to develop these hernias.

Direct Inguinal Hernias

Direct inguinal hernias arise medial to the inferior epigastric vessels and occur secondary to a weakening of the transversalis fasica in Hesselbach triangle. This type of hernia also occurs predominantly in men and incarceration is rare given the wide neck. If a sliding component is present, especially on the left side, it may contain the sigmoid colon or bladder.

Femoral Hernias

Femoral hernias develop secondary to a peritoneal outpouching through the femoral ring. The borders of a femoral hernia include the femoral vessels laterally, the inguinal ligament superiorly, the lacunar ligament medially, and Cooper ligament inferiorly. These hernias are much more common in elderly women than men and given the narrow neck, are prone to incarceration and strangulation.

Clinical Presentation

The diagnosis of a groin hernia is primarily made by history and physical examination. Symptoms often occur after extended periods of standing. Most patients initially notice a lump in the groin. The lump may or may not be associated with pain and it may be intermittent or persistent. A sensation of pulling or tearing may radiate to the scrotum. If a segment of bowel becomes entrapped in the hernia sac, symptoms of bowel obstruction may ensue—nausea, vomiting, distention, constipation, diarrhea, and abdominal pain. Erythema over the sac portends an ominous scenario—that of possible bowel strangulation. Possible systemic manifestations of a strangulated hernia include fever, tachycardia, hypotension, and peritoneal irritation.

On physical examination, if possible, the patient should initially be made to stand. The inguinal region is visually inspected for a lump with and without the patient performing a Valsalva maneuver. In men, the examination finger is invaginated into the scrotum and taken up to the superficial inguinal ring. While palpating the superficial inguinal ring, the examiner may ask the patient to perform a Valsalva maneuver, which in turn may elicit a "tap" against the finger—suggesting an indirect hernia. With the examination finger in this position, the integrity of the floor of the inguinal canal can also be assessed. Of note, clinical assessment of inguinal hernias may be challenging in women. The small external ring does not easily admit the examining finger; however the round ligament may be thickened and palpable as it courses toward the labia. In women a strong clinical history (i.e., recurrent, red, tender, and reducible bulge) is sufficient to support inguinal exploration in which case 75% of the time an indirect hernia may be encountered. In either men or women, if the patient does not show signs of strangulation, an attempt to manually reduce the hernia may be made. It is best, however, to perform an operative herniorraphy for acutely incarcerated hernias and imperative for strangulated hernias.

Investigations

In addition to the physical examination, imaging studies may also aid in the diagnosis of an abdominal hernia. This may be especially relevant when dealing with hernias that often are challenging to diagnose physically, such as the femoral hernia. In such situations, ultrasonography or computerized tomography may be performed. These may demonstrate loops of bowel in nonanatomic locations. It must be noted that a negative study does not exclude the presence of a hernia. Imaging may also help discern possibilities in the differential diagnosis of a hernia such as inguinal adenopathy, undescended testis, spermatocele, varicocele, hydrocele, lipoma, or testicular cancer.

Treatment

The goal of a groin hernia repair is restoration of all herniated structures to their previous anatomic position behind and deep to the transversalis fascia. Effective anesthesia is tailored to specific patient needs in consultation with an anesthesiologist and can include a local field block of the iliohypogastric and ilioinguinal nerve, general, epidural, or spinal anesthesia.

With the patient positioned supine, an incision is made approximately 2 cm above and parallel to the inguinal ligament. In the case of a femoral hernia, an infrainguinal approach is an option. Dissection is carried until the external oblique aponeurosis is encountered. An incision is made parallel to its fibers to expose the inguinal canal. Care must be taken not to injure the iliohypogastric and ilioinguinal nerves. The spermatic cord is then mobilized. The hernia sac is exposed by dividing the cremaster muscle longitudinally. The sac usually lies along the anteromedial aspect of the spermatic cord. The sac is dissected free of the cord and displaced into the peritoneal cavity or divided and ligated near the internal ring. If the sac extends into the scrotum, no attempt should be made to retrieve the sac distal to the pubic tubercle. Instead, the sac should be divided at the pubic tubercle and the distal end left open or marsupialized to prevent hydrocele and to minimize cord trauma.

In addition to restoring the herniated structures to their anatomic position, the floor of inguinal canal needs to be reinforced, especially in adults. This has classically been achieved by one of four methods: the Bassini repair, the Shouldice repair, the McVay repair, and the mesh (Lichtenstein, plug patch, or laparoscopic) repair.

In the *Bassini* repair, the aponeurosis of the transversus abdominus muscle is approximated to the shelving edge of the inguinal ligament below (Fig. 8-6). If there is believed to be too much tension in the repair, a relaxing incision can be made in the aponeurosis of the rectus muscle. Recurrence rates vary from 5% to 20%, depending on the size of the initial hernia.

In the *Shouldice* repair, the transversalis fascia is divided from the internal ring to the pubic tubercle. The fascia is then imbricated to itself and the inguinal ligament with two suture lines (Fig. 8-7). As with the Bassini repair, relaxing incisions may be necessary. Recurrence rates are much lower at 0.6%.

In the *McVay* or *Cooper ligament repair* (Fig. 8-8), the floor of the inguinal canal is excised and reconstructed by initially approximating the transversus abdominis aponeurosis and transversalis fascia to Cooper ligament medially from the pubic tubercle to the femoral vein. The reapproximation lateral to this point is then transitioned to the femoral sheath and inguinal ligament. This repair essentially closes off the femoral canal and can be used in femoral hernia repairs as well. A relaxing incision is often required in this procedure as well.

In the *Lichtenstein* repair, the floor of the inguinal canal is reconstructed with prosthetic mesh (Fig. 8-9). The mesh

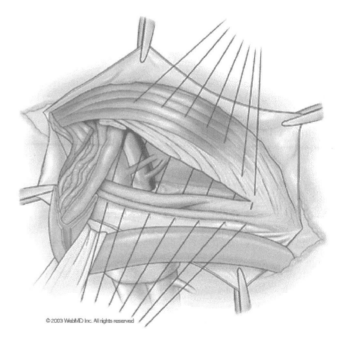

Figure 8-6 The Bassini inguinal hernia repair. [From ACSSurgery.com (Fig. 5b from Chapter 22, Section 3).]

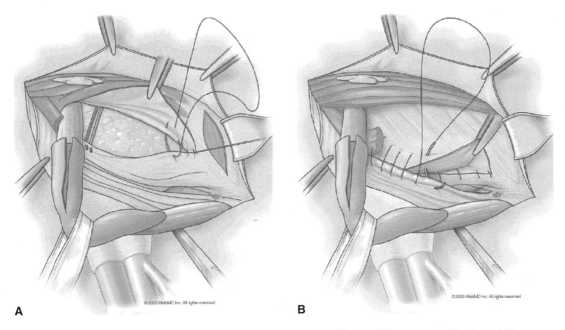

A   **B**

Figure 8-7   The Shouldice inguinal hernia repair. Fig. 10-7 [From ACSSurgery.com (Fig. 6a and 6b from Chapter 22, Section 3).]

affords a tension-free repair of the floor and has come into wide use. It lies posterior to the spermatic cord and is sutured to the inguinal ligament inferiorly and transversus abdominis aponeurosis or internal oblique aponeurosis superiorly. The mesh is split laterally to allow room for the cord to exit the deep inguinal ring.

In a variation of the Lichtenstein repair, often referred to as the "plug-and-patch" repair, a method popularized by Rutkow, a mesh plug is placed within the deep ring adjacent to the spermatic cord to help minimize the aperture of the deep inguinal ring (Fig. 8-10). In addition, a mesh is placed over the floor of the inguinal canal with

minimal or no suture fixation, thereby reducing postoperative disability.

In addition to the anterior approach, a posterior, or preperitoneal approach can be used (Fig. 8-11A). This type of repair is often used for femoral or recurrent hernias. In this approach, an incision is made 2 to 3 cm superior and parallel to the inguinal ligament while staying superior to the deep inguinal ring. Upon approaching the rectus sheath, the anterior sheath is incised and the rectus

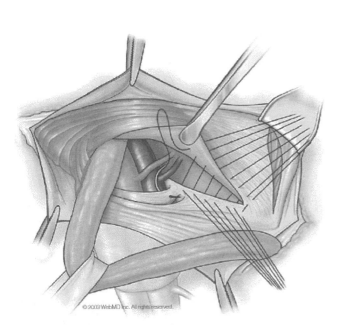

Figure 8-8   The McVay or Cooper ligament repair. [From AC-SSurgery.com (Fig. 7 from Chapter 22, Section 3).]

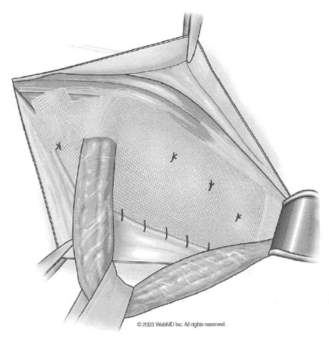

Figure 8-9   The placement of mesh to create a tension-free repair of an inguinal hernia was initially popularized by Lichtenstein. [From ACSSurgery.com (Fig. 9 from Chapter 22, Section 3).]

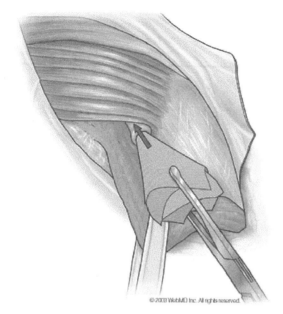

Figure 8-10 The placement of a mesh plug used in a "plug and patch" repair to help minimize the aperture of the deep inguinal ring. [From ACSSurgery.com (Fig. 10 from Chapter 22, Section 3).]

abdominus muscle is retracted medially. The exposed transversalis fascia is then incised to gain access to the properitoneal space. The peritoneum is then bluntly separated from the abdominal wall inferiorly, exposing the internal surface of the inguinal region. After reducing the hernia by gentle traction, the sac is amputated and the hernia defect is either repaired by approximating the transversus abdominis aponeurosis to Cooper ligament medially

followed by the iliopubic tract laterally or by suturing a prosthetic mesh to the inner abdominal wall.

The laparoscopic approach to the groin hernia is also an option (Fig. 8-11B). Two popular techniques exist: the transabdominal preperitoneal (TAPP) repair and the totally extraperitoneal (TEP) approach. Both techniques involve placement of a mesh patch over the deep ring and the floor of the inguinal canal—similar to the open preperitoneal procedure. The main difference between the TAPP and TEP approaches is the manner in which access to the preperitoneal spce is achieved. TAPP repair uses intraperitoneal trocars and involves creation of a peritoneal flap over the posterior inguinal area. The TEP approach provides access to the preperitoneal space without entering the peritoneal cavity.

In the TAPP herniorrhaphy, pneumoperitoneum is created to aid in the visualization of the inguinal region and critical landmarks: the spermatic vessels, the obliterated umbilical artery, the inferior epigastric vessels, and the external iliac vessels. The peritoneum is divided transversely superior to the deep inguinal ring, and upper and lower flaps are created using blunt dissection. Prosthetic mesh is then placed in the preperitoneal space to cover the entire inguinal and femoral region. Medial to the inferior epigastric vessels, the mesh is secured to Cooper ligament, the lacunar ligament, the posterior rectus musculature, and the transversus abdominis aponeurotic arch. Laterally, the mesh is secured to the lateral extension of the transversus aponeurotic arch and the superior edge of the iliopubic tract. Care must be taken not to place staples below the lateral iliopubic tract to avoid injuring the genitofemoral nerve and the lateral femoral cutaneous nerve. Care must also be taken not to place staples inferior to the deep inguinal ring so as to avoid injury to the ductus deferens,

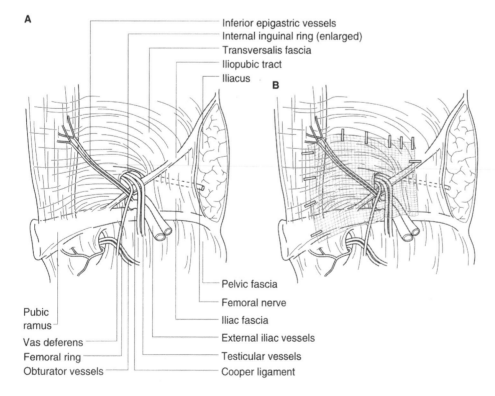

A

- Inferior epigastric vessels
- Internal inguinal ring (enlarged)
- Transversalis fascia
- Iliopubic tract
- Iliacus

B

- Pelvic fascia
- Femoral nerve
- Iliac fascia
- External iliac vessels
- Testicular vessels
- Cooper ligament

Pubic ramus
Vas deferens
Femoral ring
Obturator vessels

Figure 8-11 Internal anatomy of a right groin hernia **(A)** and placement of mesh during a laparoscopic repair **(B)**. (From Knol JA, Eckhauser FE. Inguinal anatomy and abdominal wall hernias. In: Greenfield LJ, Mulholland M, Oldham KT et al., eds. *Surgery: scientific principles and practice*, 2nd ed. Philadelphia: Lippincott-Raven Publishers, 1997:1226, with permission.)

spermatic vessels, external iliac vessels, and the femoral nerve. Finally the cut edges of the peritoneum are reapproximated to prevent the mesh from coming into contact with bowel.

In the TEP approach, a skin incision is made in the periumbilical region and dissection is carried to the level of the rectus sheath. The rectus sheath is entered and a pneumatic balloon is placed along the anterior surface of the posterior rectus sheath and advanced to the space of Retzius. The balloon is inflated and additional trocars can then be placed without traversing the peritoneum. A sheet of prosthetic mesh large enough to cover the entire region is then placed in the preperitoneal space and held in place by the peritoneum upon deflation of the preperitoneal space.

Much debate has centered over the use of laparoscopic techniques for hernia repair. Proponents contend that the laparoscopic techniques afford excellent visualization, minimal pain, and rapid return to work and normal activities. Furthermore, they contend that a laparoscopic approach facilitates repair of recurrent hernias in that it allows one to avoid scar tissue and potentially distorted anatomy, thereby minimizing risk of injuring critical structures. In addition, in cases of bilateral groin hernias, proponents emphasize the ability to accomplish both repairs in the same setting. Critics contend that laparoscopic techniques require the use of general anesthesia, higher operative costs, and violation of the peritoneal cavity (TAPP) and associated comorbidities. A recent prospective 2-year study of 2,164 Veterans Administration patients comparing the laparoscopic mesh approach versus the open anterior mesh approach for inguinal hernia repairs has demonstrated a higher recurrence rate for the laparoscopic mesh repair (10.1% vs. 4.9%). However, recurrence rates for repair of recurrences using either technique were similar.

Complications

As with any operation, bleeding, infection, and recurrence must be described as possible complications. However, testicular atrophy and residual neuralgia represent serious complications unique to inguinal hernia repair.

Testicular atrophy occurs as a consequence of ischemic orchitis. Ischemic orchitis occurs secondary to thrombosis of the delicate veins of the pampiniform plexus. Primary arterial ischemia to the testicle is rare because of the rich blood supply to the testicle (the testicular artery from the aorta, the artery of the ductus deferens from the superior vesical artery, and the cremasteric artery from the inferior epigastric artery). Pathology evaluation shows significant venous congestion. Thrombosis is likely attributed to traumatic handling of the cord during dissection. Clinical manifestations include cord and testicular hardening, pain, and retraction, and often do not become apparent until 2 to 5 days after repair. The process may last 6 to 12 weeks, either resulting in complete resolution or testicular atrophy. Two common modalities used to aid diagnosis are Doppler flow studies or nuclear medicine scans. Orchiectomy is usually not necessary and care is supportive henceforth. Orchiectomy is indicated for intractable pain or lack of flow to the testicle. Furthermore,

antibodies can develop to the atrophic testicle, which may render risk of infertility, in which case, orchiectomy is reasonable.

Neuralgia may result from surgical trauma to the sensory nerves in the groin or secondary to nearby inflammatory and fibrotic responses. Neuralgias may develop either early or late postoperatively. A special case of residual neuralgia is a neuroma. This results from a proliferation of nerve fibers outside the neurilemma of a partially or completely divided nerve. Pain associated with a neuroma is variable and may depend on changes in position. Hyperesthesia may be present, and tapping at the site may produce severe shooting pain. Deafferentiation chronic pain differs from pain associated with a neuroma in that it is burning, permanent, and with intermittent paroxysmal exacerbations. Onset in such cases is delayed for about a week after injury and tapping produces no exquisite pain.

Management of neuralgia is difficult and may involve local antesthetic blocks, or in the case of the genitofemoral nerve, block of L1 and L2 paravertebrally. Analgesics, antidepressants, anxiolytics, transcutaneous electrical stimulation, acupuncture, and steroid injections have also been used. When all else fails, surgical neurolysis can be performed.

ANTERIOR AND POSTERIOR ABDOMINAL WALL HERNIAS

Anterior abdominal wall hernias as a group are less common than inguinal hernias, but given the risk of bowel strangulation, it is important to accurately diagnose these hernias and treat them accordingly.

Umbilical hernias are more commonly congenital in origin but may be acquired in adults. The umbilicus forms a site of potential weakness where the round ligament, urachus, and obliterated umbilical arteries converge. In adults, umbilical hernias do not regress spontaneously as in children and occur secondary to conditions leading to increased intraabdominal pressure and straining. Incarceration and strangulation are unusual, but repair is nevertheless warranted if the patient's condition permits. Repair of an umbilical hernia is typically initiated with a periumbilical curvilinear incision. The hernia sac is identified and isolated by blunt dissection. The hernia and its contents are reduced and the fascial edges are reapproximated transversely.

Epigastric hernias occur in the linea alba superior to the umbilicus. They may result from congenital variations in the decussation patterns of the linea alba and can lead to weak areas in the epigastrum. With repetitive stresses or persistent elevation in intraabdominal pressure, defects can develop in areas of weakness. Epigastric hernias occur more commonly in men and approximately 20% of these hernias are multiple, with 80% located slightly off the midline. Small defects can be repaired primarily. Larger or multiple defects may require repair with a prosthetic mesh. Recurrence occurs in 5% to 10% of patients.

Spigelian hernias are rare spontaneous hernias of the abdominal wall. The hernia protrudes through a weakness in the Spigelian fascia (Fig. 8-12), where the transversus

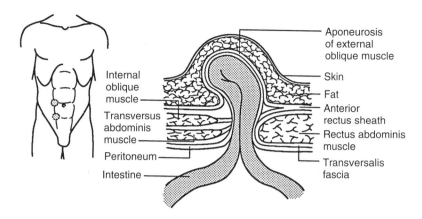

Figure 8-12 A Spigelian hernia occurs through the linea semilunaris. (From Richards AT, Quinn TH, Fitzgibbons RJ. Abdominal wall hernias. In: Greenfield LJ, Mulholland M, Oldham KT et al., eds. *Surgery: scientific principles and practice*, 3rd ed. Philadelphia: Lippincott Williams & Wilkins, 2001: 1218, with permission.)

abdominis aponeurosis joins the edge of the rectus sheath from the semilunar line. Most of these occur where the Spigelian fasica crosses the arcuate line in the lower abdomen. Given the high likelihood of incarceration or strangulation of a Spigelian hernia, repair is indicated when these herniations are identified.

As mentioned in the preceding text, *incisional* hernias develop through a surgical incision in the abdominal wall. These most commonly involve vertical incisions of the anterior abdominal wall, but may occur from incisions in the lumbar and perineal regions. Incidence varies from 0.5% to 13.9% of patients who undergo abdominal surgery. Factors contributing to the development of incisional hernias include poor postoperative wound healing, use of steroids, wound infections, and poor technique. Increased intraabdominal pressure, increased age, nutritional depletion, male gender, and jaundice also increase the risk for developing incisional hernias. Small incisional hernias, those less than 3 to 4 cm in greatest dimension, can be closed primarily, provided the underlying causes are addressed, for example, wound infection. Larger hernias with significant prolapse of abdominal contents for extended periods may lead to respiratory compromise following reduction of the hernia. In such situations, surgeons may use progressive pneumoperitoneum to increase the intraabdominal volume prior to repair. For large incisional hernias, relaxing incisions may be needed along the lateral aspects of the anterior rectus sheath. These allow the medial aspect of the anterior sheath to close the midline. For even larger hernias, prosthetic Marlex mesh may be used to allow for a tension-free repair. The mesh should have significant overlap with the fascia (4 to 8 cm) to allow for secure repair. Furthermore, nonabsorbable sutures should be used. Certain risks associated with mesh placement include infection and possible erosion of mesh into the bowel. To minimize such risks, omentum or peritoneum may be placed between the mesh and the bowel. Recent use of Alloderm, an intact biologic tissue matrix, has shown promising potential in minimizing the previously described risks associated with prosthetic mesh. Furthermore, fluid collections, as sources of the infection, can be minimized with closed suction drains. The recurrence rate for incisional hernias is 30% to 50%. With mesh, the recurrence rate is as low as 10%. An alternative to the open repair is laparoscopic repair. It resembles open repair in that mesh is inserted to cover the defect in the abdominal wall fascia and

avoids the extensive dissection associated with open repairs. Several preliminary studies suggest that laparascopic repair may be highly promising. A randomized trial of 60 patients by Carbajo and colleagues comparing laparoscopic incisional hernia repair to open repair has shown significantly shorter hospital stays and fewer postoperative complications for the laparoscopic group as compared to the open group. A retrospective study of 105 patients by Park and colleagues has likewise shown similar results.

Lumbar hernias arise in the lumbar region through the posterior abdominal wall either spontaneously or from previous nephrectomy incisions. These hernias occur through one of two sites (Fig. 8-13). The superior lumbar triangle, also called Grynfelt triangle, is the most common site of origin. The inferior lumbar triangle, also called Petit triangle, is less commonly involved. The common clinical presentation is usually a mass in the flank that may or may not be associated with pain. Lumbar hernias progress in size over time and have a 10% incidence of incarceration and strangulation; therefore, they should be repaired when found. They may be repaired primarily or with mesh.

Diastasis recti refers to a condition in which there is attenuation of the linea alba. It is primarily of aesthetic concern and not usually a surgical problem. This condition typically occurs in infancy, although it may occur during pregnancy. Usually there is no treatment for infants as the defect corrects while the infant continues to grow. For pregnant women, abdominal exercises may help strengthen the abdominal musculature and help close the defect. Rarely, an umbilical hernia associated with a diastasis recti may need surgical correction.

PELVIC HERNIAS

Pelvic hernias comprise a rare group that form protrusions through muscles that make up the pelvic floor. There are essentially three types: the *obturator* hernia, the *sciatic* hernia, and the *perineal* hernia.

Obturator hernias are acquired defects through the obturator canal and course along the tract taken by the obturator neurovascular bundle as it exits the pelvis. These occur primarily in elderly women and are associated with radicular pain extending down the medial thigh with abduction or internal rotation of the knee. This is

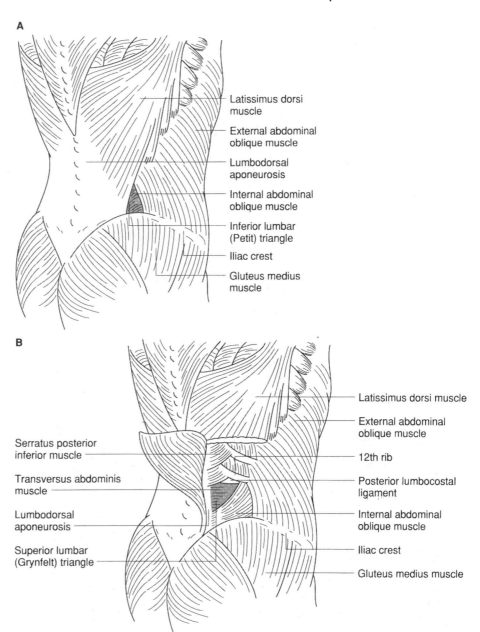

Figure 8-13 A hernia in the lumbar region can occur through the **(A)** inferior lumbar triangle and the **(B)** superior lumbar triangle. (From Knol JA, Eckhauser FE. Inguinal anatomy and abdominal wall hernias. In: Greenfield LJ, Mulholland M, Oldham KT et al., eds. *Surgery: scientific principles and practice*, 2nd ed. Philadelphia: Lippincott-Raven Publishers, 1997:1210, with permission.)

known as the classic *Howship-Romberg* sign, although it is present in less than one half of patients with an obturator hernia. The most common presentation is crampy abdominal pain and small bowel obstruction. On physical examination, a mass may be felt on vaginal or rectal examination. Given the high mortality associated with an obturator hernia, accurate diagnosis and prompt treatment is vital.

Obturator hernias are treated operatively via a transabdominal approach. Any nonviable bowel is resected and the hernia sac is removed. An attempt should be made to close the fascial defect primarily, and if this is not possible then a prosthetic mesh may be used. Recurrences are rare.

Sciatic hernias are rare defects that occur through the greater or lesser sciatic foramina. Patients present with a gradually enlarging mass in the infragluteal region. Sciatic nerve compression may result along with symptoms of bowel obstruction and ischemia. A computerized tomographic (CT) scan or ultrasonography may be necessary to aid in the diagnosis. Sciatic hernias can be repaired via either the transabdominal and transgluteal approach, with the transabdominal approach preferred for signs of bowel obstruction or strangulation. In addition prosthetitc mesh may be required.

Perineal hernias occur through a defect in the levator sling in the pelvic floor. These hernias are typically the result of multiple pregnancies or surgery of the pelvic floor. They appear as a bulge just lateral to midline perineal raphe and are frequently asymptomatic and reducible. Depending on their location, they may be associated with pain on sitting or a variety of urinary complaints, namely dysuria. Strangulation and incarceration are rare. Diagnosis can be made by careful history and physical examination, particularly the vaginal and rectal examinations. These hernias may be repaired directly via a transabdominal aproach with or without a mesh.

KEY POINTS

▲ A Richter hernia occurs when less than the full circumference of the bowel wall becomes entrapped in a hernia defect.

▲ A Littre hernia is a Richter hernia in which there is herniation of a Meckel diverticulum.

▲ Borders of the inguinal canal include the aponeurosis of the external oblique anteriorly, the transversalis fascia posteriorly, the aponeurosis of the internal oblique superiorly, and the inguinal ligament inferiorly.

▲ Borders of a femoral hernia include the femoral vessels laterally, the inguinal ligament superiorly, the lacunar ligament medially, and Cooper ligament inferiorly.

▲ Open techniques include the Bassini repair, the Shouldice repair, the McVay repair, the tension-free mesh Lichtenstein repair, and the Rutkow plug and patch repair.

SUGGESTED READINGS

American College of Surgeons. ACS Surgery: Principles & Practices. Available at: www.acssurgery.com/cgi-bin/publiccgi.pl. Accessed April 28, 2005.

Cameron JL. *Current surgical therapy*, 7th ed. Philadelphia: Mosby, 2001.

Carbajo MA, Martin del Olmo JC, Blanco JI, et al. Laparoscopic treatment vs open surgery in the solution of major incisional and abdominal wall hernias with mesh. *Surg Endosc* 1999;13:250–252.

Corson JD, Williamson RCN, eds. *Surgery*. Philadelphia: Mosby International Ltd, 2001.

Fitzgibbons RJ, Greenburg AG, eds. *Nyhus & Condon's hernia*. Philadelphia: Lippincott Williams & Wilkins, 2002.

Greenfield LJ, Mulholland M, Oldham KT et al., eds. *Surgery: scientific principles and practice*, 3rd ed. Philadelphia: Lippincott Williams & Wilkins, 2001.

Jansen PL, Mertens PR, Klinge U, et al. The biology of hernia formation. *Surgery* 2004;136:1–4.

Neumayer L, Giobbie-Hurder A, Jonasson O, et al. Open mesh versus laparoscopic mesh repair of inguinal hernia. *N Engl J Med* 2004;350: 1819–1827.

Nyhus LM, Baker RJ, eds. *Mastery of surgery*, 4th ed. Philadelphia: Lippincott Williams & Wilkins, 2001.

Park A, Birch DW, Lovrics P. Laparoscopic and open incisional hernia repair: a comparison study. *Surgery* 1998;124:816.

Townsend CM, Beauchamp RD, Evers BM et al., eds. *Sabiston textbook of surgery*, 16th ed. Philadelphia: WB Saunders, 2001.

Wind GG. *Applied laparascopic anatomy*. Baltimore: Williams & Wilkins, 1997.

Statistics and Epidemiology

Laura Kruper   Seema S. Sonnad

FUNDAMENTALS OF STUDY DESIGN

Understanding both study design and analytic methods is essential to interpreting medical literature or performing clinical studies. This chapter will cover study design, basic statistics, and the fundamentals of economic analysis.

Epidemiology is often defined as the study of the distribution of health and disease in groups of people, as well as the study of factors influencing this distribution. There are two basic categories of epidemiologic studies: descriptive and analytic. *Descriptive studies* observe and describe the health and factors influencing health in selected groups of people. This information serves as a context for developing hypotheses, designing further studies, and interpreting results. Then, *analytic studies* allow inferences about causality, using formal hypothesis testing.

DESCRIPTIVE STUDIES

Descriptive studies include case reports, case series, and surveillance. The *case report* is a detailed clinical description of a single patient, often used to document a rare or uncommon presentation of a disease and its management. No statistical analyses can be performed on the sample of one and observations cannot be generalized to other subjects. Case reports may suggest hypotheses for further study.

The individual case report can be expanded to a *case series*, which is a clinical description of a group of patients with a specific disease or condition. It usually provides descriptions of diagnoses as well as of the interventions and outcomes. Routine surveillance programs often use accumulating case reports to suggest an outbreak of an epidemic or the emergence of a new disease. Like case reports, case series cannot prove causation but can be used for hypothesis generation. Because there is no comparison or control group, statistical analyses cannot be performed.

ANALYTIC STUDIES

Analytic studies allow quantitative analysis of relationships between health outcomes and causal factors. Design options for analytic studies fall into two broad categories: observational and intervention (experimental). Analytic studies typically include testing specific hypotheses.

Observational Studies

Observational studies include case–control and cohort studies. In a *case–control study*, patients with a given disease of interest are paired with subjects without the disease, who serve as the control group (Fig. 9-1). Participants are usually either interviewed or their medical records are reviewed regarding one or more exposures of interest to determine if there is an association between a prior exposure and subsequent development of a disease. A comparison is made between the proportions of the exposure of interest in each of the two groups to determine if the proportions are different. Many risk factors and exposures can be studied simultaneously in a case–control study. These studies are particularly well suited to investigations of rare diseases or of diseases that take a long time to develop. Otherwise, many subjects would need to be followed for a very long time to generate a sufficient number of diseased individuals to produce accurate results. An example of a simple case–control design is a study in which the last 100 cases of thyroid cancer seen at one institution are matched with 100 normal controls. If an investigator wishes to determine whether prior radiation is a risk factor for the development of thyroid cancer, prior radiation exposures would be determined for all subjects to determine whether patients with thyroid cancer were exposed to more radiation when compared to the controls.

Case–control studies often require a relatively small sample size and often may be completed quickly and economically. One of the major disadvantages is the potential for bias. Because subjects are interviewed about past exposures, subjects may selectively recall past events, which introduces *recall bias*. *Interviewer bias* occurs when an interviewer, aware

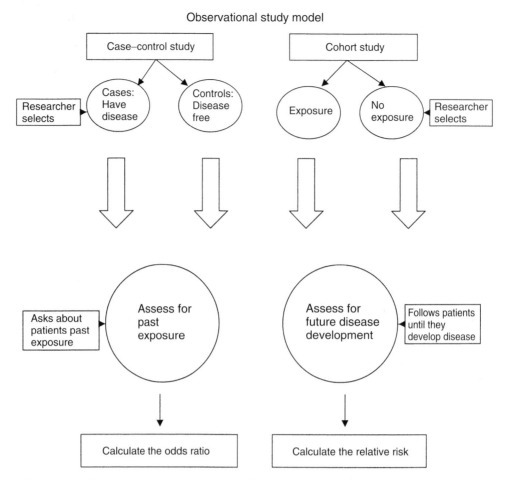

Figure 9-1 Schematic representation of the difference between a case–control and a cohort study.

of exposure of interest, interviews the case subjects more thoroughly than the controls. *Selection bias* occurs when the presence or absence of the exposure influences which particular diseased or nondiseased individuals are entered into the study; subjects are selected according to their exposure status.

In case–control studies, the association between exposure and disease is reported as an odds ratio (OR). The OR is defined as the odds of developing disease in the exposed group relative to the odds in the unexposed group. Examination of a 2×2 contingency table shows the odds of exposure for those with disease would be a/c and the odds of exposure for those without disease would be b/d (Fig. 9-2). The OR would then be: $a/c \div b/d$ or ad/bc.

In a cohort study, subjects are classified on the basis of the presence or absence of an exposure and then followed for a given period to determine which individuals develop a certain disease. One advantage of a cohort study is that multiple outcomes can be studied, such as the development of lung cancer, stroke, and cardiac disease in a cohort of smokers. These studies are well suited to investigate the risks of rare exposures, including rare occupational exposures such as working in a vinyl chloride factory. Cohort studies provide information on the temporal relationship between exposure and disease, important in proving causality. Some of the disadvantages of cohort studies are the expense involved, the long time

needed for follow-up, and the potential for patient withdrawal and loss to follow-up.

The association of the risk factor (exposure) and disease in a cohort study is reported as the *relative risk*, or risk ratio (RR), which is $a/(a + b) \div c/(c + d)$ (Fig. 9-3). The RR is the risk of disease in the exposed population divided by the risk of disease in the unexposed population. If the relative risk is greater than 1, then the factor under investigation increases risk; if less than 1, it reduces risk. In case–control studies, because subjects are selected on the basis of disease status, it is not possible to determine the rate of development of disease; therefore, a relative risk cannot be determined. However, if the disease in a case–control is rare, the odds ratio can estimate the RR. By looking again at Figure 9-2, in a rare condition, a and c are very small compared to b and d. If one then conducted a prospective cohort study, the RR would be $a/(a + b) \div c/(c + d)$, but since a and c are very small $(a + b) \approx b$ and $(c + d) \approx d$. The equation then becomes: $a/b \div c/d$, which equals the OR ad/bc.

Intervention Studies

Intervention studies (experimental studies or clinical trials) can be thought of as a type of prospective cohort study, since subjects are identified on the basis of their exposure status and followed to determine whether they develop disease. The main difference between this study design and

	Outcome +	Outcome −
Exposure +	a	b
Exposure −	c	d
	a/c Odds of being exposed in cases	b/d Odds of being exposed in controls

a = the subjects who have disease and the exposure of interest

b = the subjects who have the exposure of interest and no disease

c = the subjects who have not been exposed but have disease

d = the subjects who do not have the exposure of interest or disease. Note that $a + c$ equals all the patients with disease (the cases); $b + d$ equals the total number of patients without disease (the controls).

Figure 9-2   Sample calculation of the odds ratio from a case–control study using a 2 × 2 table.

Odds ratio = $OR = (a/c)/(b/d) = ad/bc$

an observational study design is that the investigator assigns the exposure status of each participant. In a randomized control trial (RCT), subjects are allocated to treatment group on the basis of some chance mechanism. This ensures that unrecognized risk factors, or confounders, are allocated equally between the two groups, and minimizes bias. As with a cohort study, an intervention study can be expensive and be subject to large losses of follow-up. These types of studies are often considered to provide the most reliable evidence. This type of design, however, is not always possible owing to reasons of ethics and feasibility.

DESCRIPTIVE STATISTICS

After data collection is complete, the first step in looking at data is to describe the material in a concise, comprehensible way. One of the goals is then to collapse the data into summaries that can be used to evaluate relationships among sets of numbers or compare sets of numbers from different sources. This section will review basic methods frequently used for presenting and summarizing data.

Statistics involves computations performed on variables. Variables are classified into different types, and these

	Outcome +	Outcome −	
Exposure +	a	b	a/(a + b) Risk rate of developing outcome in exposed
Exposure −	c	d	c/(c + d) Risk rate of developing outcome in unexposed

Figure 9-3   Calculation of the relative risk of a cohort study.

Given a, b, c, and d as previously defined in the example for case–control studies, the relative risk of disease development given exposure may be represented as follows:
Relative Risk = $RR = a/(a + c)/b/(b + d)$.

types determine the analytical methods used to interpret the data. Any variable can be categorized as either discrete or continuous. *Discrete* data can take on only certain values within a given range, increasing in steps, such as the number of patients operated upon in one month: 34, 35, 36, etc. *Continuous* variables have no such limitation and can assume all possible values along a continuum within a specified range. Most clinical parameters are continuous, including blood pressure, height, weight, and cholesterol level.

Categorical, or *nominal*, data are used for named categories that may be represented by numbers, but have no implied order. A *binary* variable is a special type of categorical variable, one that only has two outcomes or levels. Examples include gender (male/female) and disease outcome (disease/no disease).

Ordinal data can also be used for named categories represented by numbers, but unlike categorical data, these variables can be placed into a meaningful order. Common examples are responses recorded as poor/satisfactory/good, which exhibit an underlying order, but without the requirement that the differences between categories be equal. Interval data can also be placed in a meaningful order with consistent intervals between data points. The intervals are based on an accepted convention, but the zero point is arbitrary. An example of interval data is the reading on a thermometer, where the zero point has a different meaning for Fahrenheit and Celsius temperatures. Ratio data is like interval data but the zero point is fixed, such as blood pressure and body weight, where the zero points are well defined.

Frequency Tables

Describing the data is crucial because the analytical methods used for interpretation depend on the type of information presented. It is also important to present the data in a manner that communicates information in the most efficient format. Frequency tables present counts of defined subgroups of numbers. A hypothetical example might look at diagnosed breast cancers and count how often cancer is diagnosed as stage I, II, II, or IV (Table 9-1). For example, of 872 diagnosed cancers, 589 might be stage I, representing 67.5%. For stage II, 153 might be diagnosed, representing 17.5%. A frequency is the number of times that a value occurs in a given data set, so for stage II in our hypothetical data set, the frequency is 153. The *relative* frequency is the proportion of all observations in the data set with that value; therefore, for stage II, the relative frequency would be 0.175. By adding the relative frequency for one value at a time, one can obtain the *cumulative* frequency. For stage II, this would be 0.85 (0.675 for stage I added to 0.175 for stage II).

Histograms

The purpose of a graphic display is to give a quick overall impression of the data. Histograms and bar graphs are often used to display grouped data. Bar graphs are preferable when groups are characterized by nonnumeric attributes, such as nonsmoker/light smoker/heavy smoker. When groups are characterized by numeric attributes, such as systolic blood pressure or body mass index (BMI), histograms are preferred. The *y* axis represents frequency and the *x* axis is typically marked in equal units by most statistical software programs. Histograms are analogous to frequencies tables, but provide more information, such as whether the data follows a normal distribution or is skewed (Fig. 9-4).

Tables are a convenient way to present numeric information, but it is also valuable to provide a summary of the important characteristics of the collected data. An important parameter used to describe a sample is a measure of central tendency. The measures most commonly used are the mean, median, and mode (Fig. 9-5A). The *mean* (often referred to as the average) of a data set is the sum of all the values of observations divided by the number of observations. The mean of a distribution is sensitive to extreme values, or outliers. When they are present, it may be more appropriate to use the median to describe the center of the data. When observations are arranged in order, the *median* (or the 50th percentile) is the midpoint, with half of the observations below the median, and half above. If the number of observations is odd, then the median is the middle observation. If the number is even, the median will be the average of the middle pair of observations. The median is relatively insensitive to extreme values within the distribution. The mode of a distribution is the observation or value that occurs with the greatest frequency. Some distributions may be bimodal or multimodal, with two or more values occurring with equal frequency.

TABLE 9-1

FREQUENCIES, RELATIVE FREQUENCIES, AND CUMULATIVE FREQUENCIES OF CANCER STAGING DISTRIBUTION

Cancer Stage	Frequency	Cumulative Frequency	Percentage	Relative Frequency (proportion)
I	589	0.675	67.5%	0.675
II	153	0.85	17.5%	0.175
III	87	0.949	10.0%	0.10
IV	43	1.0	5.0%	0.05

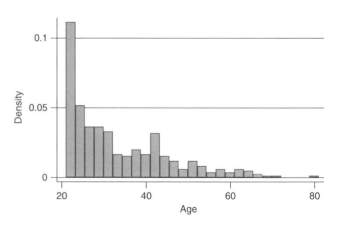

Figure 9-4 Representative histogram from hypothetical data of age distribution in sample population. The data are not normally distributed; they are skewed to the right, with a long tail on the right.

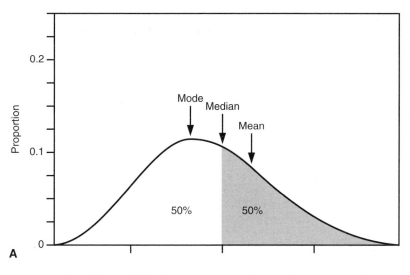

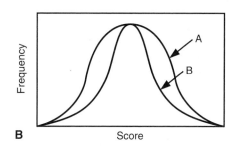

Figure 9-5 **A:** Representation of the mode, median, and mean of a normal distribution. **B:** Example of two normal distributions in which the mode, median, and mean are similar but the variances differ.

Complete description of a data set should also include a measure of spread or variability. In Figure 9-5B, the two distributions have the same median, mode, and mean yet the curves look different because of differences in variability of the two sets of data. Three measures of variability are the range, variance, and standard deviation (SD). The range is calculated by subtracting the lowest observed value from the highest. The most common measures of variability are the variance and its related function, the SD. Both of these parameters are used to describe the spread of individual observations around the center when the center is expressed as a mean. The variance is computed by calculating the difference between each observation (obs) and the mean. These differences are squared and all of the calculated quantities are then added together. This total sum is then divided by the number of observations minus one, or $n - 1$. The term $n - 1$ is used in the denominator to adjust for the fact that in studies we are typically looking at samples, rather than at the entire population. The mean of the sample is used as an estimate of the mean of the underlying population. If data are available from the entire population, then n can be used instead of $n - 1$. The SD is the square root of the variance. The SD can be thought of as the average distance of observations from the mean. The SD is greatly affected by large outliers, as is the mean.

For distributions that are roughly symmetric and unimodal, the mean and standard deviation alone can sufficiently describe the normal distribution. Such distributions follow a bell-shaped curve and are referred to as Gaussian or normal. One useful property of the normal distribution is that 95% of the individual observations in such distributions lie within 2 standard deviations (± 2 SD) of the mean. Asymmetrical data are referred to as skewed. In biologic studies, data are often skewed right because many measurements involve variables that have natural lower boundaries but no definitive upper boundaries. An example is length of hospital stay, for which the lower boundary can be no shorter than one day but can be as long as several hundred days. Skewness shows up as a distribution with a long tail on the right.

ANALYTICAL METHODS

Statistics involves making inferences about occurrences and relationships by using data from relatively limited samples. Biostatistics is the branch of applied statistics that applies statistical methods to medical and biologic questions. Analysis of epidemiologic studies involves determining associations between exposure and disease observed in a sample result from true associations in the underlying population or from chance, bias, or confounding. This section will review the various methods used in assessing the degree to which observations of associations are caused by real relationships rather than chance.

To understand why the role of chance as an alternative explanation is important in determining associations, it is important to understand the concept of inference. Inference involves using a subset or sample to make assumptions about the population as a whole. One of the investigator's goals is to select a sample representative of the entire source population. A sampling method that yields a random sample of the source population is the best way to ensure this. When there is error in the way individuals are sampled from the source population, then bias is introduced, and the inference could be imprecise or inaccurate. However, the likelihood that an incorrect inference will be made about the true characteristics of the population based on the representative sample decreases as the size of the sample increases.

HYPOTHESIS TESTING

Investigators are concerned about whether the results of a study occur by chance or are due to a true difference. Hypothesis testing involves conducting a test of statistical significance and determining the degree to which sampling variability, or chance, could explain the observed results. Two hypotheses are tested; the null hypothesis states that there is no association between exposure and disease. The alternative hypothesis states the opposite, that there is some relation between exposure and disease. Once these two hypotheses have been identified, a test of statistical significance can be performed. These types of tests lead to probability statements or what is known as a p value. The p value is the likelihood of obtaining a result at least as extreme as that observed in the study by chance alone. In medical research, the p value by convention is set at 0.05. This means that at most there is a 5% chance of observing an association as large as that found in the study by chance.

Although a result may be statistically significant, with a p value less than 0.05, it must be remembered that statistical significance does not mean clinical significance. For example, a new drug may be tested and found to lower a person's cholesterol level by 1 mg, with a statistically significant result. However, in a clinical sense, a reduction of 1 mg in a person's cholesterol does not mean much, especially when there are costs and potential side effects to taking a medication.

A measure related to the p value, also evaluating the role of chance, is the confidence interval (CI). The CI represents a range of values that we are fairly confident will contain the true magnitude of effect. Conceptually, if a study were to be repeated an infinite number of times, and a 95% confidence interval was obtained for each one, 95% of such intervals would contain the true value being estimated. Like a p value, the CI can provide information about statistical significance at a specified level. For example, if the null value (relative risk = 1 or difference = 0) is included in a 95% CI, then the corresponding p value is greater than 0.05, by definition. But the added information that a CI provides is a measure of true magnitude of the relative risk associated with a particular exposure. The width of the CI indicates the amount of variability in the estimate. A wider CI indicates a less accurate result. With a narrower CI, the precision of the estimate is greater. The p value and CI are complementary and together provide the most information about the role of chance.

STATISTICAL TESTS

Although hypothesis tests share a similar underlying concept, the selection of a particular statistical test depends on the data characteristics and the specific hypothesis being evaluated. To go into great detail about the different tests is beyond the scope of this book; however, there are certain tests that appear frequently in the literature and some of these will be discussed herein.

t Test

A t test evaluates the observed difference between the mean values of the study groups to determine statistical significance. If the variance of the underlying population is known, or if the sample size is large enough, the normal distribution is used to determine the test statistic. However, usually the variance of a population is not known and a t distribution is used. Once a t test is performed, a t statistic is obtained and converted into a p value with the use of a t table. t Tests are used for continuous data, which as mentioned previously, represents clinical measurements such as height, blood pressure, or cholesterol level.

A *paired t test* is used and is similar to a t test but is most often used in studies that look at pre- and posttreatment effects, with patients serving as their own controls. An

example would be the effects of an antihypertensive drug, comparing the mean value of a patient's blood pressure level before the new therapy, compared to his/her level after the therapy. A t statistic would be calculated with accompanying p value to determine if the difference in observed effect was statistically significant.

Analysis of variance (ANOVA) is used when comparisons are being made among the means of 3 or more groups. It provides an overall test of equality of several means, but does not specify which group or means differ. If one were to test three different diets and their effects on cholesterol levels, a significant ANOVA result would only indicate that the means of the three groups were not the same, but one would need to perform additional tests to determine which diet group had a different mean level in cholesterol.

Chi-Square Test

For discrete data that do not follow a normal distribution, a chi-square test is a simple and common method to determine whether the differences in proportions between study groups are statistically significant. The chi-square test is analogous to the t test for comparing means between two study groups, except that proportions are being compared instead of means. This test compares the expected proportion of individuals with a certain outcome against the proportion that is actually observed. Expected values are determined based on the assumption that the null hypothesis is true: there is no difference in the proportions between the two groups.

Usually a 2×2 table is used to present the observed data. One can also use what is called an $r \times c$ contingency table, which contains counts of observations in r rows and c columns, representing the various levels of disease and exposure. An example of an $r \times c$ table would have disease status represented as a binary outcome (yes/no) in columns and exposure status as categories in rows. Examples of categorical exposure status are age categories (ages 20–29, 30–39, etc.) or smoking level [never, light smoker (less than 1 pack per day), heavy smoker (greater than 1 pack per day)]. One then constructs another 2×2 table, or $r \times c$ table, of expected frequencies based on exposure rates in the study and the total number of cases in the study. The larger the chi-square value, the more likely the difference between the observed and expected frequencies is not due to chance. To determine whether the results are significant, the chi-square result can be found in a chi-square table with associated p value.

When the data to be evaluated are paired, such as in a matched case–control study, a *McNemar test* is used, which is a variant of the chi-square test. Another chi-square variant is the *Fisher exact test*, which is used when sample sizes are small. The Fisher exact test must be used when any one of the expected frequencies from the chi-square analysis is less than 5, which can be seen in a study if there are very few "events" or cases of disease.

When data do not follow a normal distribution or cannot be defined by certain parameters, such as the mean and standard deviation, nonparametric statistical tests are used. Examples of nonparametric tests are the *signed-rank* test, *Wilcoxon Rank-Sum* and *Kruskal Wallis*. These tests are used frequently when data are subjective, such as determining whether an arm looks less red, redder, or the same after application of an anti-inflammatory cream. Nonparametric tests have less power than do the parametric alternatives because they make no assumption about the shape or distribution of the data, and some of the information is ignored. For example, the precise distance between two data points is ignored, instead only the relative order is used when the data are ranked. Because parametric tests do not ignore aspects of the data, they are more powerful and should be used whenever possible.

SAMPLE SIZE AND POWER

In addition to chance, the size of a study influences the p value: the larger the sample size, the greater the probability of a statistically significant result. Conversely, a large effect may not achieve statistical significance because if the sample size is too small, the variability may be substantial. Often the number of subjects available for a study is limited, so the relevant factor to determine in this case is the power of the study, given the sample size, to detect a statistically significant difference. For both sample size and power calculations, the underlying assumption is that the null hypothesis is not true and that the alternative hypothesis (that there is a true difference) is true. This is in contrast to hypothesis testing, where the underlying assumption is that the null hypothesis is true.

To begin, we define the null hypothesis and the alternative. One way to begin is to determine the smallest effect worth detecting. For example, in a case–control study of smoking as risk factor for stroke, one might be interested in detecting a relative risk of 2.0 or more: in other words, individuals who smoke have at least a 100% increase in risk of stroke compared with those who do not smoke. The null hypothesis could be written as H_0: RR = 1, with the alternative hypothesis written as H_1: RR $\geq$ 2.0. If the result of our statistical test is significant, we reject the null hypothesis and conclude that the alternative hypothesis is true (in this case that the RR is greater than or equal to 2, that there is an increased risk of stroke with smoking). If it is not significant, we do not reject the null hypothesis.

However, in rejecting or not rejecting the null hypothesis, two types of errors can occur. The first type of error, type I error, occurs when the null hypothesis is rejected when it is actually true. The probability of making a type I error, represented by Greek letter alpha (α), is equal to the p value. In a study where the p value is 0.05, the α level would also be equal to 0.05, which would indicate that the probability of incorrectly rejecting the null hypothesis would be 1 in 20. In other words, if a study were to be repeated an infinite number of times, 5% of the time, the results of the study would be accepted as real when in reality the difference was due to chance.

A type II error is made when there truly is a difference between two study groups—the alternative hypothesis is true—and one fails to reject the null hypothesis, or makes the conclusion that there is no difference. The likelihood of making a type II error is represented by the Greek letter beta (β). The power of a study is the probability of being able to conclude that there is a statistical difference between two study groups, if one truly exists, and is calculated by $1 - \beta$. If β is set at 0.20, the power of the study would be $1 - 0.20$, or 0.80, which would mean 80% power to detect a differ-

ence of a certain magnitude if one truly exists, or a 20% chance of making a type II error. Both types of error should be minimized when designing a study, however, because these two errors are interrelated—as the probability of making a type I error decreases, the probability of making a type II error increases, and vice versa.

To determine the necessary sample size for a proposed study, one needs to specify the values for the probabilities of type I (α) and type II (β) errors, the magnitude of the desired effect (or detectable difference) and the proportion of the baseline population that either has the disease of interest (cohort studies or RCTs) or is exposed to the factor under study. Traditionally, the α level is set at 0.05 and $1 - \beta$ is either 0.80 or 0.90. The estimate of the baseline proportion is usually determined from published studies. Prior studies can also be used to estimate the detectable difference, or if there are no estimates, the value could represent what is believed to be the smallest, clinically meaningful effect size by the investigators. There are multiple formulas that can be used to determine sample size; the formula used depends on the research question, the study design, and the type of data to be collected.

Sample Size

Ideally, the sample size required to draw meaningful conclusions from the data should be predetermined by the investigators, and the study performed using that sample size. However, more often than not, studies are constrained by budget demands, time limits, or low disease rates (few cases) making it almost impossible to obtain enough subjects. In these situations, it is helpful to determine the power of a study given the fixed sample size and various estimated magnitudes of effect. In these power calculations, it becomes apparent that if a sample size is small, a study has adequate power (defined as 80% or higher) only if the postulated magnitude of effect is large. Basically, the power of a study is dependent on both the sample size and the magnitude of the effect, so for a study to have adequate power, if one value is small, the other will need to be large. Sometimes there is a true difference between two groups (not due to chance). Because the study was underpowered, however, the difference (or magnitude of effect) was too small to be detected. In other words, the study might have had enough power only to detect a very large difference, such as a 100% reduction in risk from a new therapy, and usually such large effects are not seen in studies.

Meta-analysis is a quantitative method by which multiple comparable studies are combined to obtain an overall estimate of effect. This type of systematic review is used to gain statistical power when individual studies are underpowered, mostly because of small sample sizes. Often, a pooled risk estimate is obtained that is statistically significant. Meta-analyses are also used to identify needs for future studies and determine future sample sizes.

DIAGNOSTIC TESTS

In clinical practice, diagnostic tests are often used to guide patient management. A patient with a constellation of signs and symptoms is the basis of any diagnostic process. Diagnostic tests are most often used to classify patients

	Disease +	Disease −
Test +	True Positive (TP)	False Positive (FP)
Test −	False Negative (FN)	True Negative (TN)

Sensitivity = TP/(TP + FN) = the percentage of patients with a positive test result who truly have disease = true positive rate (rate—not number!)

Specificity = TN/(FP + TN) = the percentage of patients with a negative test result who do not have disease = true negative rate (rate—not number!)

Prevalence = (TP + FN)/ (TP + FP + FN + FN)

Positive predictive value (PPV) = TP/(TP + FP) = patients with true disease and a positive test result/all those with a positive test result

Negative predictive value (NPV) = TN/(FN + TN) = patients without disease who have a negative test result/all subjects with a negative test result

Figure 9-6 A 2 × 2 table used in the calculation of the test operating characteristics of a hypothetical diagnostic test.

according to some binary outcome variable, such as disease status (yes/no). Diagnostic tests can also classify patients according to categorical outcome variables, such as low, intermediate, and high probability in cases of suspected pulmonary emboli. Physicians are required to interpret the results of these tests. Some examples of diagnostic tests are mammograms, as a screening tool for breast cancer, or laboratory procedures, such as an elevated white blood cell count for signs of infection.

The *sensitivity* of a test is the ability of a test to detect disease when it is present, or the probability of having a positive test given that the patient has disease. Sensitivity is often referred to as the *true-positive rate*. The *specificity* of a test is the ability of a test to identify patients without disease, or the probability of having a negative test given that the patient does not have disease. Specificity is often referred to as the *true-negative rate*. There are two types of error that occur during diagnostic testing. One is incorrectly classifying a patient with disease as disease-free, otherwise known as a *false-negative test*. The other type of error is a *false-positive test*, or classifying a patient who is not diseased as having disease. Sensitivity and specificity are characteristics of the test and remain constant.

The basis for statistics concerning diagnostic test results is the 2 × 2 contingency table (Fig. 9-6). To complete the 2 × 2 table, one needs to know three proportions: the sensitivity (true-positive rate), which is calculated by TP/(TP + FN), the specificity (false-negative rate), which is calculated by TN/(FP + TN), and the prevalence of the disease in the sample represented, TP + FN/(TP + FP + FN + TN). *Prevalence* is the proportion of individuals in a population who have the disease at a specific instant. For diagnostic tests, prevalence is often referred to as the *prior probability*.

To complete a 2 × 2 table, we will use an example of a sample population of 1,000 individuals (Fig. 9-7). The prevalence of peptic ulcer disease (PUD) is 0.25. This means that 250 individuals will be in the disease column and 750 in the no disease column. The sensitivity of a new laboratory test to determine PUD is 60%, so of 250 patients in the disease column, 150 will have true-positive results

	Disease +	Disease −
Test +	150	150
Test −	100	600
	250	750

Sensitivity = 60%, specificity = 80%, prevalence = 25%

If prevalence = 25%, of 1000 people, 250 have disease, 750 no disease

If sensitivity = 60%, then 150 (250 × 0.6) in D+/T+ cell; 100 in D+/T− cell

If specificity = 80%, then 600 (750 × 0.8) in D−/T− cell; 600 in D−/T+ cell

PPV = TP/(TP + FP) = 150/(150 + 150) = 0.50

Figure 9-7 Example of diagnostic test in sample population.

and the remaining 100 will have false-negative results. The specificity of the test is 80%, so of 750 patients in the no-disease column, 600 will have true-negative results and 150 will have false-positive results.

Usually a physician wants to know the probability of a patient having disease, once the test is positive. The *positive predictive value* (PPV) is the most clinically relevant probability calculated from a 2×2 table. It is the probability that a patient has the disease, given that the test result is positive, and it is often referred to as *posterior probability* or *post-test probability*. Because the positive predictive value is dependent on the prevalence of disease in a population, the pretest probability exerts a major influence on the diagnostic process. When the prevalence of a disease is low, even use of a test with high sensitivity and specificity will result in a low positive predictive value. Unlike sensitivity and specificity, which remain constant and are characteristics of the test, positive predictive value will change depending on prevalence. To finish with the example in the preceding text, the positive predictive value would be TP/(TP + FP), or $150/(150 + 150) = 0.50$. This means that the probability of a patient having PUD, without any other information, would be 25% in this sample population. But, if the new laboratory test is positive for a patient, then the probability has increased to 50%. To show how the PPV is dependent on prevalence, if we lower the prevalence to 10%, then the new PPV would be 0.25 (TP = 60 FP = 180, PPV = $60/(60 + 180) = 0.25$).

The validity of a diagnostic test depends on how well the test does what it is supposed to do: correctly categorize individuals who have disease as positive and those without disease as negative. Sensitivity and specificity are two measures of the validity of a diagnostic test. One way to determine the validity of a test is to compare it to a *gold standard*, a test that has been used and is accepted in the field. To do so, one administers the standard at the same time as the newer diagnostic test. It must be noted, however, that most "gold standard" tests are not 100% accurate.

Often a physician's decision to perform a given medical intervention is based on the determination that the benefit of the intervention outweighs the risk of providing the therapy. The decision-making process can be represented schematically (Fig. 9-8). The treatment threshold X represents the probability of disease at which a physician could choose either to treat or to observe. Below this threshold, the probability of disease is sufficiently low that a physician will decide not to provide intervention. Beyond the treatment threshold, the probability of disease is sufficiently high that intervention is warranted. Diagnostic testing serves the purpose of moving a physician either farther to the right or to the left on Figure 9-8 so that there is less ambiguity in the decision-making process. In the example just noted, when the prevalence of PUD was 25%, one

might not be certain about whether to start treatment for PUD, but with a positive test, the patient now has a post-test probability of 50%, which might lend more weight toward treatment. The treatment threshold is physician dependent and varies on factors such as physician experience, availability of diagnostic testing, and disease severity.

CLINICAL ECONOMICS

Clinical economics is applied to provide information concerning more efficient uses of resources, considering both costs and outcomes. Because medical resources are limited, choices must be made among alternatives involving trade-offs. As new or existing therapies are evaluated, there are certain factors to consider, with the initial emphasis on efficacy: that a health care intervention achieves its stated goal in controlled settings. A second factor to address is effectiveness, that a therapy does more good than harm in usual circumstances. The third stage of assessment involves both the effectiveness and the resources involved in providing a given intervention. There are three primary types of economic analysis: cost-identification, cost-effectiveness, and cost-benefit.

Cost Identification

Cost identification, or *cost minimization*, simply defines the cost of alternative modes of therapy, for example, the costs of medical management versus surgical intervention. The goal of this type of analysis is used to identify the least expensive therapy. The underlying assumption with cost identification is that the outcomes of the various strategies are considered equal. This type of analysis is often used to determine the financial burden of disease, but does not evaluate what health outcomes are achieved for the resources provided.

Cost-Effectiveness Analysis

Both cost and effect are incorporated in cost-effectiveness analysis. The net cost is measured as well as the outcome, which is reported either as a conventional clinical outcome (such as years of life saved) or as a combined result of several different outcomes. Disparate outcomes can be compared with one another by combining these outcomes into a common scale. This is accomplished most frequently by means of utility analysis. Individuals (patients, general public, and experts in the field) are asked to compare the relative values of a range of outcomes, such as disability, pain, side effects, or death. By using a variety of techniques—such as standard gamble references, time tradeoff, and rank and scale—the values of different outcomes can be combined into a single utility score. A utility score is a quantitative measure of an individual's preference for a given state of health. Cost-utility analysis may be considered as a form of cost-effectiveness analysis.

Frequently used in cost-effectiveness analysis is measurement of outcomes in quality-adjusted life-years (QALYs). By using QALYs, the years of life gained through an intervention are weighed against the quality of those years. For example, a year of life with bladder dysfunction might be equivalent to 0.6 years of life in perfect health, equaling

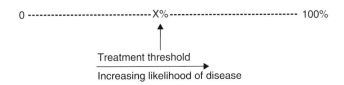

Figure 9-8   Decision to treat based on the results of a test.

0.6 QALYs. The results of such analyses are reported in cost per unit of outcome. No therapy, however, can be evaluated in isolation; it must be compared to at least one other service so that an incremental cost-effectiveness ratio can be obtained.

Cost-Benefit Analysis

In *cost-benefit analysis*, clinical outcomes are converted into dollar amounts. Benefits are converted by either measuring a patient's wages or income as a measure of worth or by determining the patient's "willingness-to-pay" for a certain outcome. This kind of conversion is controversial at times, since it requires several value judgments. Therefore, analysts prefer to measure outcomes in utilities or QALYs, even though there remains skepticism regarding the techniques surrounding those measurements. Ultimately, with cost-benefit analysis, one can make an explicit decision about whether the cost of an intervention is worth the benefit by measuring both in dollar amounts and obtaining a net monetary benefit that includes costs and outcomes in the same units.

KEY POINTS

▲ The *median* of a distribution is the value that equals the 50th percentile. The *mean* is the arithmetic average of the distribution. The *mode* is the value of the distribution that occurs most frequently.

▲ A confidence interval that includes "1" indicates that the result is not significant.

▲ *t* Tests and analysis of variance (*ANOVA*) are used to analyze data sets that contain continuous variables. *t* Tests compare the means between two groups, whereas ANOVA is used to compare the means of more than two groups. The *Chi square* test is used to analyze categorical data or compare proportions.

▲ *Sensitivity* = TP/(TP + FN), the percentage of patients with a positive test result who truly have disease. *Specificity* = TN/(FP + TN), the percentage of patients with a negative test result who do not have disease. *Positive predictive value* (PPV) = TP/(TP + FP), patients with true disease and a positive test result/all those with a positive test result.

SUGGESTED READINGS

Clarke JR. A scientific approach to surgical reasoning: diagnostic accuracy—sensitivity, specificity, prevalence and predictive value. *Theor Surg* 1990;5:129–132.

Detsky AS, Naglie IG. A clinician's guide to cost-effectiveness analysis. *Ann Intern Med* 1990;113(2):147–154.

Eisenberg J. Clinical economics: a guide to the economic analysis of clinical practices. *JAMA* 1989;262(20):2879–2886.

Hennekens CH, Buring JE. In: Mayrent SL, ed. *Epidemiology in medicine*. Philadelphia: JB. Lippincott, 1987.

Rosner B. *Fundamentals of biostatistics*, 5th ed. Pacific Grove: Duxbury Press, 2000.

Sonnad S. Describing data: statistical and graphical methods. *Radiology* 2002;225:622–628.

Woodward M. *Epidemiology: study design and data analysis*. Boca Raton: Chapman & Hall/CRC, 1999.

Pediatric Surgery

10

Michael J. Morowitz   Michael L. Nance

Pediatric surgeons care for children with a broad range of conditions, including congenital anomalies, cancer, and trauma. During past decades, advances in critical care, anesthesia, and nutrition have allowed for dramatic improvements in the survival of infants and children requiring surgery. In recent years, additional incremental advances in survival have been achieved through pharmacologic (e.g., surfactant and nitric oxide) and technologic (e.g., extracorporeal membrane oxygenation) improvements. The discipline of pediatric surgery has welcomed refinements in surgical technique for common surgical diseases and has also adopted novel treatment strategies such as fetal intervention. This chapter provides a review of major topics in pediatric surgery.

DISORDERS OF THE RESPIRATORY SYSTEM

Congenital Diaphragmatic Hernia

During normal fetal development, the pleuroperitoneal canal maintains continuity between the pleural and coelomic cavities until formation of the diaphragm is complete midway through the first trimester. The last portion of the canal to close is a posterolateral communication between the transverse septum and pleuroperitoneal membranes. Incomplete development at this location results in a defect known as a Bochdalek hernia. This defect is most commonly observed on the left (90%) and its most severe forms result in complete agenesis of the affected hemidiaphragm. Diaphragmatic hernias through the foramen of Morgagni (anterior parasternal defects) represent less than 5% of all congenital diaphragmatic hernias (CDHs) and typically result in fewer physiologic derangements at birth. Congenital diaphragmatic hernias occur in 1 in 4,000 live births.

The presence of a diaphragmatic hernia allows the abdominal viscera to migrate into the ipsilateral thorax with several developmental consequences (Fig. 10-1). As a result of displacement of abdominal contents into the chest, the abdominal cavity is undeveloped. This loss of domain can be problematic at the time of diaphragm repair with reduction of the herniated viscera. More important is that herniation of the abdominal contents into the chest and mechanical compression of local structures result in hypoplasia of the ipsilateral lung or, in more severe cases, hypoplasia of both

lungs. Histologic examination of lungs in affected neonates demonstrates decreased bronchial and pulmonary artery branching, as would normally be seen in a fetus of 14 weeks of gestation. As a consequence of the pulmonary hypoplasia, inadequate alveolar gas exchange and pulmonary hypertension develop. Prognosis is largely determined by the degree of pulmonary hypoplasia and pulmonary hypertension.

Increasingly, newborns with CDH are diagnosed by prenatal ultrasonography as early as 15 weeks of gestation. Sonographic findings include polyhydramnios, herniated abdominal viscera, abnormal anatomy of the upper abdomen, and mediastinal shift due to mass effect on the ipsilateral side. Ultrafast magnetic resonance imaging (MRI) of the fetus may provide additional anatomic information of clinical value. Correlation between prenatal imaging and outcome has proven unreliable; however, a decreased ratio of lung volume-to-head circumference and evidence of herniation of the liver into the chest are both associated with a poor outcome. At delivery, affected infants characteristically demonstrate a scaphoid abdomen. Postnatal diagnosis is confirmed with a plain chest radiograph demonstrating the typical findings of intrathoracic intestine, absent diaphragmatic silhouette, and contralateral mediastinal shift. Up to

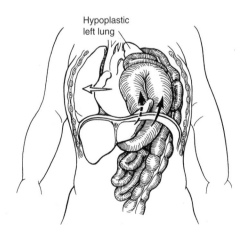

Figure 10-1 Left-sided congenital diaphragmatic hernia with migration of stomach (*solid black arrow*), liver (*dashed black arrow*), and intestines into the left hemithorax. The mediastinum is shifted right, and a hypoplastic left lung is seen at the apex of the left chest. (From Baker RJ, Fischer JE. *Mastery of surgery*, 4th ed. Philadelphia: Lippincott Williams & Wilkins, 2001:699, with permission.)

25% of infants with diaphragmatic hernia will have associated anomalies, most notably severe cardiac defects.

Emergent surgical repair of CDH is no longer advocated. The immediate priority in treating newborns with CDH is resuscitation and stabilization of cardiac and pulmonary function. Infants typically will demonstrate hypoxia, hypercarbia, and metabolic acidosis, as well as persistent pulmonary hypertension resulting in right-to-left shunting across the foramen ovale and ductus arteriosus. Respiratory support in CDH should consist of supplemental oxygen as needed and gentle mechanical ventilation. Aggressive or prolonged manual ventilation ("bagging") should be avoided to prevent distention of the bowel and further compromise of gas exchange. A major treatment goal should be to avoid barotrauma from hyperventilation and high inspiratory pressures. Infants with CDH who fail to respond to conventional mechanical ventilatory support may require interventions such as oscillatory ventilation or extracorporeal membrane oxygenation (ECMO). The efficacy of ECMO support in this setting has been debated. Infants may be maintained on these circuits until pulmonary hypertension and lung compliance (and function) are improved. The duration of ECMO therapy in CDH patients is typically from 1 to 3 weeks. More recently, "gentilation" or permissive hypercapnia strategies have been advocated. Early experience with this approach appears favorable. Although efficacious in respiratory failure from other causes, nitric oxide and surfactant administration have no proven survival benefit in newborns with CDH.

There is no current consensus regarding the optimal timing of surgical repair of CDH. The spectrum of surgical approaches includes early repair with or without bypass, delayed repair on bypass after pulmonary function is improved, and delayed repair after the infant is successfully weaned from the bypass circuit. For the newborn that requires ECMO support, one must balance the risk of bleeding with repair while anticoagulated against the benefit of full respiratory support afforded by ECMO. A standard approach is to proceed with surgery in stable infants who have progressed to a point where consideration of extubation is reasonable. Open repair of the diaphragmatic hernia is usually performed via an abdominal approach through a subcostal incision. After herniated abdominal viscera are carefully reduced, the diaphragmatic defect is exposed. When possible, the defect is closed primarily with nonabsorbable suture. Frequently, large defects with poorly defined tissue margins are closed with prosthetic patches anchored to the diaphragmatic remnant or thoracic cage. The successful application of minimally invasive techniques to CDH repair has been reported but is not widely practiced. Reported survival rates for infants with congenital diaphragmatic hernia range from 60% to greater than 90%.

Congenital Pulmonary Cystic Diseases

Congenital lobar emphysema (CLE), pulmonary sequestration, congenital cystic adenomatoid malformation (CCAM), and bronchogenic cysts are congenital lesions of the thorax that share similar embryologic and clinical features.

Congenital lobar emphysema is a rare condition characterized by hyperexpansion of one or more lobes of the lung. Inspired air is trapped in the affected lobes, which progressively overexpand and cannot deflate. Atelectasis of adjacent pulmonary tissue results, and eventually mediastinal shift ensues with compromise of the contralateral lung. CLE occurs most frequently in the upper lobes of the lung, due to either extrinsic airway compression or intrinsic obstruction from aberrant airway development. Extrinsic compression may be the result of associated cardiovascular anomalies.

CCAMs are cystic or hybrid solid/cystic lesions that communicate with the normal tracheobronchial tree. Proliferation of the terminal airway yields cystic structures lined with respiratory epithelium capable of producing mucus. Either single isolated cysts or collections of multiple associated cysts may be observed. The left lower lobe is most frequently affected, but CCAMs may occur in other lobes as well.

Pulmonary sequestrations are anomalous collections of lung parenchymal tissue with abnormal communications to the pulmonary artery and/or tracheobronchial tree. Sequestration may be extralobar or intralobar and usually occurs in the left lower chest. Extralobar sequestration, often found in cases of CDH, is a collection of nonventilated lung tissue with a systemic blood supply usually located immediately superior to the left diaphragm. Intralobar sequestration is most commonly found within the left lower lobe parenchyma. Again, there is no major connection to the tracheobronchial tree and the arterial supply is systemic, often arising from the abdominal aorta. Venous drainage may be systemic or pulmonary.

Bronchogenic cysts consist of immature bronchial tissue that does not communicate with the tracheobronchial tree and that does not possess a unique blood supply. Hilar and carinal bronchogenic cysts are thought to represent clusters of epithelial cells that become separated from the tracheobronchial tree and lung buds. These cells do not undergo further differentiation into alveolar units, as seen in sequestration. These cysts generally become extrapulmonary masses lined with ciliated columnar epithelium and surrounded by a fibrous tissue wall.

These congenital cystic lesions of the chest frequently become superinfected. Each may also result in respiratory distress by compression of adjacent bronchi and lung tissue. Bronchogenic cysts and extralobar sequestrations often remain asymptomatic. Congenital lobar emphysema usually causes severe air-trapping and respiratory distress within the first few days of life. A plain chest radiograph is the initial study of choice to evaluate all of the lesions described in the preceding text. Further imaging with computerized tomography, ultrasonography, or MRI is useful when necessary to delineate cystic from solid components or to identify an aberrant systemic artery. A barium esophagram is indicated in patients with dysphagia to search for a communication with the gastrointestinal tract.

Congenital cystic thoracic lesions should be resected to avoid the pulmonary complications described above. Asymptomatic lesions should be excised to eliminate the risk of superinfection or, rarely, malignant degeneration. Lobectomy is generally required for management of CCAMs and intralobar sequestration. In congenital lobar emphysema, positive pressure ventilation after intubation may be poorly tolerated and, therefore, the surgeon should be present during induction of anesthesia. Lobectomy is tolerated quite well in children, who frequently undergo such robust growth and expansion of the remaining lung tissue postoperatively that total lung volume returns to normal.

DISORDERS OF THE ESOPHAGUS

Esophageal Atresia and Tracheoesophageal Fistula

The survival of the newborn with tracheoesophageal fistula (TEF) and esophageal atresia has markedly improved over the last 100 years. Although newborns with this problem uniformly died a century ago, the majority of infants with this problem today survive because of improvements in surgical technique, perioperative care, and nutrition.

The precise etiology of this malformation is uncertain but is related to the common embryologic origin of the esophagus and trachea. Under normal circumstances, these foregut structures divide into separate tubes by 36 days of gestation. Incomplete separation of these structures is likely what results in a variety of malformations. The most common anatomic variant (85%) includes a blind-ending upper esophageal pouch and fistula between the distal esophagus and trachea (Fig. 10-2). Other congenital anomalies are commonly associated with esophageal atresia and represent the most important factor determining survival. These anomalies often present as a constellation of malformations known as the VACTERRL association (vertebral, anorectal, cardiac, tracheoesophageal, renal, radial, and limb deformities). Nearly 20% of affected newborns will demonstrate some form of congenital heart disease, and up to 10% demonstrate imperforate anus.

Infants with esophageal atresia present difficulties with feeding and managing secretions. Abdominal distention may be present owing to passage of inspired air into the stomach via the fistula. Because the esophagus ends in a blind pouch, attempts to place a tube into the stomach are unsuccessful. Reflux of gastric secretions into the lungs and a resultant chemical pneumonitis may cause respiratory distress, and this can be exacerbated by atelectasis secondary to gastric distention and diaphragmatic elevation.

Diagnosis is often made with a plain film demonstrating a coiled nasogastric tube within an air-filled esophageal pouch (Fig. 10-2). Contrast imaging is rarely required, although it can confirm the diagnosis and document the presence of an upper pouch fistula. Radiographic evidence of air in the stomach confirms the presence of a fistula between the trachea and the lower esophagus. In stable infants, preoperative bronchoscopy allows confirmation of the presence of a single fistula and the absence of a second more proximal fistula. In addition, echocardiography should be performed prior to repair to exclude the presence of cardiac defects and to determine the location of the aortic arch. Isolated TEF without atresia ("H-type" fistula) is difficult to diagnose; this typically presents later at several months of life with a history of recurrent respiratory problems. This type of fistula can often be demonstrated by a specialized "pullback" upper gastrointestinal series.

Treatment priorities after confirmation of diagnosis include aspiration precautions with upright positioning and catheter decompression of the upper esophagus. Primary surgical repair should be attempted once the patient is stabilized unless concomitant anomalies preclude such an approach. Primary repair is delayed in unstable infants, who may receive an initial gastrostomy for decompression and feeding, and who may also require ligation of the fistula to prevent recurrent soilage of the lungs.

For infants with a proximal atresia and distal fistula, the goal of treatment is to restore continuity in a single procedure. Surgical repair includes division of the TEF and an esophagoesophagostomy. A right posterolateral, extrapleural thoracotomy is used, unless a right-sided aortic arch is present. The distal esophageal fistula usually lies immediately beneath the azygous vein. The fistula is divided, taking care not to remove any tracheal wall. The proximal and distal esophageal ends are carefully mobilized such that a tension-free anastomosis may be performed. Complications of anastomotic leak and stricture can be seen in up to 20% of patients. Overall survival for patients with esophageal atresia is close to 90%. In the absence of associated anomalies, survival approaches 100%.

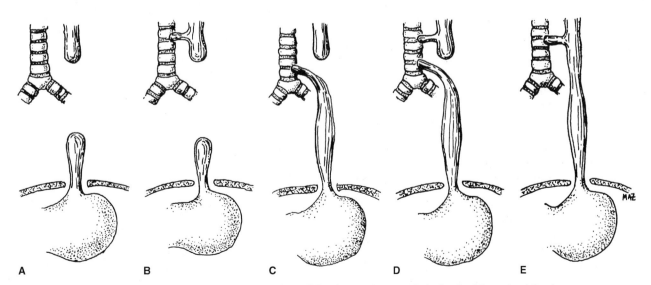

A   B   C   D   E

Figure 10-2 Variants of tracheoesophageal fistula. **A:** Atresia without fistula, (**B**) proximal fistula and distal pouch, (**C**) proximal pouch and distal fistula (*most common*), (**D**) atresia with both proximal and distal fistulas, and (**E**) fistula without atresia (H-type fistula). (From Doherty GM, Lowney JK, Mason JE, et al. *The Washington manual of surgery*, 3rd ed. Lippincott Williams & Wilkins, 2002:642, with permission.)

Pure esophageal atresia without tracheoesophageal fistula is often characterized by a long gap between the proximal and distal esophagus. These infants are managed by placing a gastrostomy for nutrition, establishing proximal pouch suction drainage to prevent aspiration, and dilatation of the proximal pouch by bougienage. After 3 to 6 weeks of dilatations, the esophageal gap frequently narrows sufficiently to allow primary repair. TEFs without atresia can frequently be ligated via a right cervical incision.

Corrosive Injury of the Esophagus

Corrosive esophageal injury from caustic ingestion occurs in adults who attempt suicide and in young children who accidentally swallow caustic substances. Mild burns from bleach and detergents may produce no symptoms, whereas alkali and acid ingestion typically cause severe mucosal damage, ulceration, and, potentially, perforation. The most destructive injury pattern is the liquefactive necrosis caused by alkali ingestion, which may result in full-thickness injury. Acids typically cause coagulation necrosis, which tends not to penetrate as deeply as alkali injuries.

Patients with suspected corrosive injuries from caustic ingestion should be hospitalized for stabilization and thorough evaluation of the injury. Patients should be monitored closely for evidence of airway compromise. After an adequate airway is ensured, the initial diagnostic evaluation should include an esophagogram with dilute barium to rule out a perforation and urgent esophagogastroscopy to evaluate the extent of disease. First- and second-degree burns are characterized by mucosal erythema and ulceration, respectively, whereas third-degree burns involve deep ulceration and severe edema that may narrow the esophageal lumen. Patients with mild injury may be discharged after a brief period of observation. Patients with moderate-to-severe esophageal injury should be placed on bowel rest and receive broad-spectrum intravenous antibiotics to reduce the risk of pneumonitis from aspiration. A gastrostomy tube is usually placed for nutritional support. Those with clinical evidence of peritonitis from full-thickness necrosis must undergo surgical exploration and may require esophagogastrectomy. When stable, patients may be discharged on antibiotics with plans for repeat endoscopy after 3 weeks. Nearly all patients with significant burns will develop esophageal strictures requiring chronic esophageal dilatations beginning at 6 weeks after injury until a patent lumen results. Repeated retrograde bougie dilatation via a large gastrostomy is safer than chronic balloon dilatation. Unyielding strictures may require esophageal resection and replacement with a gastric conduit or colon interposition. Additional potential late sequelae of corrosive injuries include hiatal hernia and malignant degeneration.

DISORDERS OF THE GASTROINTESTINAL TRACT

Hypertrophic Pyloric Stenosis

Hypertrophic pyloric stenosis refers to the progressive concentric hypertrophy of pyloric smooth muscle with resultant luminal narrowing and subsequent gastric outlet obstruction. The etiology of the disorder is unknown, but may be related to the loss of nitric oxide–mediated relaxation of muscle fibers. The incidence is highest in first-born male children, and the incidence is significantly increased among children of an affected parent. Overall, about 1 in 250 to 1,000 live births are affected.

Classically, an infant with pyloric stenosis presents at 4 to 6 weeks of age with nonbilious projectile vomiting, which occurs within minutes of feeding. The infant appears generally well and feeds enthusiastically until late in the course of the disease. The pathognomonic finding on physical examination is the firm, palpable pyloric "olive" in the epigastrium or right upper quadrant. Visible gastric peristaltic waves may also be present. Laboratory evaluation may reveal a hypokalemic, hypochloremic metabolic acidosis caused by persistent loss of gastric contents. Fluid resuscitation and electrolyte repletion should be complete prior to surgical repair. The diagnosis of pyloric stenosis can be made confidently with an appropriate history and physical examination. When further imaging is required, both ultrasonography and upper gastrointestinal series provide sensitive and specific means of diagnosis.

The treatment for hypertrophic pyloric stenosis is a surgical pyloromyotomy following adequate fluid and electrolyte resuscitation (Fig. 10-3). Traditionally a Ramstedt-Friedet pyloromyotomy is performed after delivering the pylorus into a right upper quadrant incision. A single longitudinal incision in the hypertrophied muscle is made, dividing the circular muscle of the stomach onto the pylorus. When this

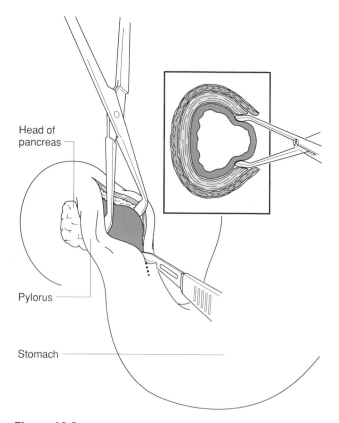

Figure 10-3   Ramstedt pyloromyotomy for hypertrophic pyloric stenosis. A longitudinal incision of the gastric wall allows the submucosa to herniate into the myotomy site. (From Greenfield L, Mulholland MW, Zelenock GB, et al. *Surgery: scientific principles and practice*, 3rd ed. Philadelphia: Lippincott Williams & Wilkins, 2001:2008, with permission.)

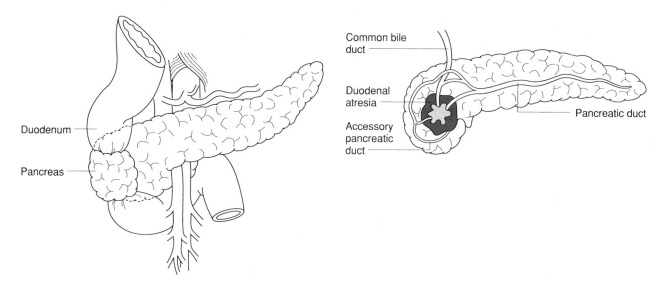

Figure 10-4 In annular pancreas, circumferential pancreatic tissue is always associated with duodenal obstruction or atresia. (From Greenfield L, Mulholland MW, Zelenock GB, et al. *Surgery: scientific principles and practice*, 3rd ed. Philadelphia: Lippincott Williams & Wilkins, 2001:1979, with permission.)

incision is done properly, the gastric submucosa should bulge into the myotomy site. In recent years, this procedure has been performed increasingly via a laparoscopic approach. Both procedures are generally well tolerated. Infants may resume feeding several hours postoperatively and typically are discharged to home the following day. Postoperative complications are uncommon, and are related to either an inadequate pyloromyotomy or inadvertent duodenotomy.

Congenital Obstruction of the Duodenum

Congenital duodenal obstruction is a rare condition that may result from a pure duodenal atresia, an intraluminal web, or an annular pancreas. Roughly 1 per 10,000 to 40,000 infants is affected, nearly one third of whom also have trisomy 21. In 90% of cases, the site of obstruction is distal to the ampulla of Vater. Complete atresia and intraluminal stenotic webs are observed with similar frequency. Annular pancreas results when the normal migration of embryonic pancreatic diverticula is interrupted. Persistent circumferential pancreatic tissue compresses the duodenal lumen (Fig. 10-4). Annular pancreas is always associated with duodenal obstruction and a patent accessory pancreatic duct.

Prenatal ultrasonography in affected infants often reveals polyhydramnios. Feeding intolerance and bilious vomiting without abdominal distention within the first 48 hours of life are typical. The classic x-ray finding in duodenal atresia is the double bubble, representing distention of both the stomach and the duodenal bulb in the absence of distal bowel gas (Fig. 10-5). An upper gastrointestinal series is helpful if the diagnosis remains uncertain. A routine karyotype and echocardiogram should be obtained in all infants born with duodenal obstruction because of a high incidence of trisomy 21 and congenital heart disease. It is important to differentiate this clinical picture from that of the newborn with malrotation and volvulus.

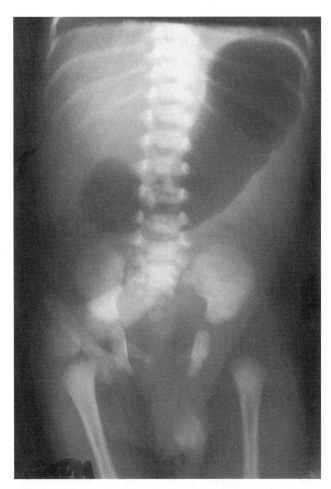

Figure 10-5 When the duodenum is obstructed, a plain film of the abdomen typically demonstrates the "double bubble," which represents distension of both the stomach and proximal duodenum in the absence of distal intestinal air. (From Baker RJ, Fischer JE. *Mastery of surgery*, 4th ed. Philadelphia: Lippincott Williams & Wilkins, 2001:976, with permission.)

Surgical correction of congenital duodenal obstruction should be performed urgently, after adequate preoperative assessment and resuscitation. Bypassing the obstruction provides the simplest approach to restoring intestinal continuity without sacrificing bowel length and without injuring the pancreas or ampulla of Vater. The preferred approach to correcting both duodenal atresia and annular pancreas is to perform a duodenoduodenostomy. Duodenal webs are excised via a longitudinal duodenotomy and subsequent transverse closure, or may be bypassed by duodenoduodenostomy. Several weeks may be required before enteral feeding is tolerated after correction of congenital duodenal obstruction, but long-term outcome is excellent in the absence of comorbidities.

Intestinal Atresia

Congenital atresia of the jejunum or ileum is believed to result from segmental interruption of mesenteric blood flow during fetal development. This disruption in blood supply may be idiopathic, or may result from intrauterine volvulus, malrotation, or intussusception. The jejunum and ileum are affected equally, and the atresia is nearly always complete. Up to 20% of affected infants present with multiple atresias. The incidence of associated congenital anomalies is relatively low (less than 10%).

Prenatal ultrasonography may detect intestinal distention and polyhydramnios. Neonates present with bilious vomiting, abdominal distention, and failure to pass meconium. Plain radiographs of the abdomen demonstrate proximal intestinal distention and a collapsed colon. Confirmatory barium enema demonstrating a normal colon is useful.

The goal of surgical therapy for intestinal atresia is to reestablish intestinal continuity while preserving bowel length. Affected segments of bowel are resected, and one or more primary anastomoses are performed. Any size discrepancy observed between proximal and distal lumens may be reduced by tapering the proximal end. A careful evaluation of the bowel is necessary to exclude the presence of multiple atresias. Transient postoperative dysfunction of the gut is common, but overall survival after surgery for uncomplicated intestinal atresia approaches 100%.

Malrotation

Malrotation refers to a spectrum of conditions in which improper midgut rotation during embryologic development leads to abnormal intestinal anatomy at birth. Autopsy studies have suggested that rotational abnormalities occur as frequently as in 1% of the population, but the observed incidence is much lower because most patients are asymptomatic. More than one half of cases present in the first month of life, and the majority are discovered by 1 year of age. However, older children and adults may also present later in life with either symptomatic or incidentally discovered malrotation. Surgical correction is always recommended to avoid possible midgut volvulus, and subsequent vascular occlusion of the narrowed mesenteric pedicle.

Normal growth of the midgut is a complex and dynamic process characterized by three stages: herniation of the midgut loop into the umbilical cord with a 270-degree rotation, reduction back into the abdominal cavity, and fixation to the posterior body wall. The normal rotation process includes fixation of the duodenojejunal junction at the ligament of Treitz to the left of the aorta and fixation of the cecum in the right iliac fossa.

Interruption of normal positioning of the intestines may lead to three common anomalies, which fall under the category of malrotation. In nonrotation, the 270-degree turn is not observed, and the colon resides in the left abdomen and the small intestine is seen on the right. The duodenojejunal junction is fixed caudally and to the right of the midline. The midline cecum is fixed via peritoneal attachments (Ladd bands) that cross anterior and lateral to the duodenum and may cause obstruction. Midgut volvulus is a significant risk. With incomplete rotation, the normal rotational arc ceases at or near 180 degrees, usually with the colon on the left and the small intestine on the right. Risk of midgut volvulus and duodenal obstruction remains high. In congenital mesocolic hernia, nonrotation of the midgut is associated with a failure of fixation of the intestine to the posterior body wall. This may occur on either the left or the right, with resultant entrapment of the small bowel behind the colon and possible strangulation.

Malrotation may present with either duodenal obstruction or midgut volvulus, or both. Ladd peritoneal bands fixing the cecum to the right abdominal wall may cause extrinsic compression of the duodenum, feeding intolerance, and bilious emesis. With midgut volvulus, compromised blood flow threatens the intestines in the distribution of the superior mesenteric vessels. Transmural necrosis and fulminant sepsis may be life-threatening. Prompt diagnosis and intervention are critical for survival. Plain films may appear normal or demonstrate duodenal obstruction, and they may not distinguish the condition from duodenal atresia. An upper gastrointestinal series will typically demonstrate a distal duodenal obstruction due to the volvulus.

Neonates diagnosed with malrotation or internal hernia should be taken emergently to the operating room. The corrective procedure for such infants is the Ladd procedure (Fig. 10-6). Correction of malrotation involves reduction of the midgut volvulus, division of Ladd bands, broadening of the mesentery, and appendectomy. Nonviable bowel is resected while attempting to preserve maximal intestinal length. Upon completion, the small bowel will reside in the right abdomen and the cecum in the left upper quadrant. The abnormally located appendix is removed. The Ladd procedure minimizes but does not completely eliminate the risk for future volvulus.

Meconium Ileus

Meconium ileus refers to the characteristic obstruction of the terminal ileum observed in neonates with cystic fibrosis. Cystic fibrosis is seen in 1 in 2,500 live births, and up to 20% of these infants will present with meconium ileus. The molecular defect in cystic fibrosis is a deoxyribonucleic acid (DNA) point mutation that leads to impermeability of the chloride ion in epithelial tissues. Decreased chloride permeability in the airways leads to abnormally viscous secretions that are poorly cleared and engender recurrent pulmonary infections. Similarly, pancreatic exocrine secretions are highly viscous and inadequate, and pancreatic exocrine insufficiency ensues.

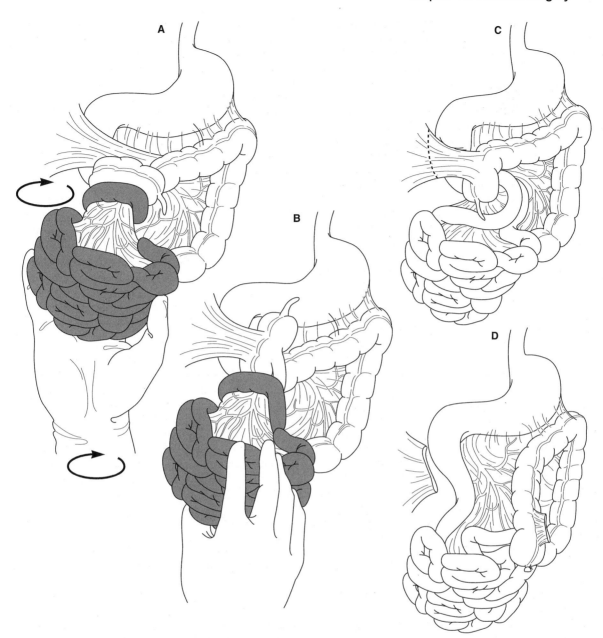

Figure 10-6 Ladd procedure. **A,B:** Counterclockwise detorsion of midgut volvulus. **C,D:** Division of peritoneal attachments (Ladd bands) of cecum to abdominal cavity. (From Greenfield L, Mulholland MW, Zelenock GB, et al. *Surgery: scientific principles and practice*, 3rd ed. Philadelphia: Lippincott Williams & Wilkins, 2001:1998, with permission.)

The lack of pancreatic proteinases results in meconium ileus, characterized by unusually thick, protein-laden meconium that characteristically obstructs the terminal ileum. The colon is small and unused but otherwise normal.

Infants develop signs of small bowel obstruction in the first day of life. Bilious emesis and abdominal distention are common, and thickened loops of distended intestine may be palpable. Plain abdominal radiographs will demonstrate multiple distended intestinal loops and may demonstrate the "soap-bubble" sign, termed for the ground-glass appearance of meconium mixed with air in the bowel. A contrast enema should be obtained to demonstrate a small unused colon and reflux into the terminal ileum. Meconium ileus usually occurs in the absence of associated congenital anomalies. However, up to 50% of cases are complicated by

in utero complications such as proximal volvulus, atresia, or intestinal perforation. When perforation occurs, sterile meconium peritonitis may yield a calcified pseudocyst. The pseudocyst may be detectable on prenatal ultrasonography or palpable on examination at birth.

Repeated contrast enemas with water soluble contrast relieve the distal small bowel obstruction in up to 70% of cases of meconium ileus. Care must be taken to avoid dehydration associated with the contrast enemas. When medical management fails, laparotomy is indicated. External massage and direct transmural irrigation may be attempted, but frequently an enterotomy and subsequent primary closure is required for evacuation. In complicated meconium ileus, an intrauterine complication, atresia, or perforation may result in segmental bowel necrosis necessitating resection.

Mortality rates approaching 30% following treatment for meconium ileus reflect the severity of associated pulmonary disease, both in the neonatal period and later in life.

Necrotizing Enterocolitis

Necrotizing enterocolitis (NEC) is a poorly understood condition characterized by intestinal injury during the newborn period. The extent of this injury may range from mucosal ischemia to transmural necrosis. The etiology of the disease is unknown but it is exclusively a disease of critically ill newborns. Thus, prematurity, hypoxia, hypotension, sepsis, and maternal drug use have all been associated. It is unclear whether mucosal ischemia in NEC results from a discrete vascular insult or a period of prolonged focal hypoperfusion. Evidence exists to support both concepts. Inconclusive epidemiologic data have also been published that link NEC to various infectious agents, for example, *Clostridium difficile*. A likely hypothesis is that NEC represents a final common pathway of intestinal damage resulting from nonspecific causes in uniquely susceptible neonates. NEC is the most common surgical emergency in neonates in North America.

The overall incidence of the disease is estimated to be 1 per 500 to 1,000 live births. Most newborns with NEC weigh less than 2,500 g at birth, and present during the first 2 weeks of life with bilious emesis and hematochezia. Symptoms typically follow the initiation of enteral feedings. Nonspecific findings such as abdominal distention and diarrhea are common, whereas a fixed abdominal mass and abdominal wall erythema suggest intestinal perforation. Lethargy and other signs of hypoperfusion occur late. The classic finding on plain films is pneumatosis intestinalis, indicating the invasion of the bowel wall by gas-forming organisms. Portal venous air and pneumoperitoneum are radiographic signs that transmural necrosis has developed. Serial abdominal radiographs should be obtained in suspected cases of NEC to detect pneumatosis or other complications. A primary goal of clinical management is to distinguish between reversible mucosal injury and frank necrosis necessitating surgical intervention.

Up to 90% of infants with NEC are managed conservatively and do not require surgical intervention. Nasogastric decompression, broad-spectrum antibiotics, and close monitoring for progression of the disease are mandatory. Under these circumstances, most infants will experience significant improvement within a period of days. A typical course of antibiotics is 2 weeks. Total parenteral nutrition is delivered via a central venous catheter until enteral feedings are tolerated.

Most surgeons reserve operative intervention in NEC for those neonates with evidence of intestinal perforation or refractory sepsis. Generally, infants who progress to surgery do so within the first 48 hours of diagnosis. A fixed abdominal mass, abdominal wall erythema, and portal venous air are relative indications for surgery. At laparotomy, nonviable bowel is resected with exteriorization of proximal and distal ends. Preservation of marginal areas of intestine with subsequent operative reexploration is common. When possible, maximal bowel length and the ileocecal valve should be preserved. In affected neonates weighing less than 1,000 g, some have advocated placement of a peritoneal drain at bedside. In this micropreemie population, survival

is 60% with drainage alone. Half of survivors will later require surgery for complications of NEC that can be performed when the patient is stable.

In general, outcomes for infants with NEC are roughly similar to long-term outcomes for other premature infants. Overall survival after both operative and nonoperative management for NEC exceeds 60%. Survival rates have improved significantly in recent decades because of improvements in critical care for neonates and aggressive early treatment for presumed NEC. Complications after surgery for NEC are common and include intestinal leak, fistula formation, and nonviable stomas. An important late complication of NEC is stricture formation, which occurs commonly in infants with advanced clinical disease, regardless of whether they receive nonoperative or operative therapy. The colon is the site of stricture formation in 70% of cases, and surgery is indicated when these are symptomatic.

Meckel Diverticulum

A Meckel diverticulum is a remnant of the embryonic yolk stalk (omphalomesenteric duct). This stalk connects the developing midgut with the embryonic yolk sac and normally closes by the seventh gestational week. Failure of the normal closure of the yolk sac results in a true diverticulum of the ileum. Meckel diverticula are invariably found on the antimesenteric border of the terminal ileum, usually within 2 feet of the ileocecal valve. The blood supply is derived from persistent vitelline vessels from the superior mesenteric artery. In up to 25% of patients, the diverticulum is fixed to the anterior abdominal wall via a fibrous band at the umbilicus. The incidence of Meckel diverticulum is estimated to be 2% in the general population, although only approximately 2% of total cases are symptomatic. Heterotopic gastric mucosa is present within the diverticulum in 50% of cases, and another 5% of diverticula contain pancreatic tissue.

A symptomatic Meckel diverticulum may present with bleeding, obstruction, or perforation. Because ectopic gastric mucosa may bleed, Meckel diverticulum represents the most common cause of hematochezia in children. Such cases should be evaluated with technetium pertechnetate nuclear scans, since this isotope has a high affinity for gastric mucosa and can demonstrate the presence of a bleeding diverticulum in at least 80% of patients. Negative scans should be repeated if clinical suspicion is high. A Meckel diverticulum may become inflamed or necrotic and present with right lower quadrant pain similar to that of appendicitis. In addition, patients may present with small bowel obstruction, either from intussusception with the diverticulum as the lead point or volvulus around an attachment to the abdominal wall. A symptomatic Meckel diverticulum should be surgically resected, either by wedge resection and transverse ileal closure or by segmental ileal resection. The management of asymptomatic diverticula is controversial. In general, incidentally discovered diverticula are removed in children but left *in situ* in adults.

Hirschsprung Disease

Hirschsprung disease is characterized by the absence of ganglion cells in the myenteric plexus of the intestinal wall. Hirschsprung disease is observed in 1 per 5,000 live births, with male infants affected four times as frequently as female infants. During normal fetal development, ganglion cells derived from the neural crest migrate into the intestine in a cephalad to caudal direction. Dysregulation of this process is poorly understood but can result in aganglionic segments of bowel extending proximally from the rectum for a variable distance. In 85% of cases disease is limited to the rectum and sigmoid colon. Aganglionic segments of bowel demonstrate abnormal peristalsis and fail to relax. A defect in nitric oxide–mediated muscle relaxation may be responsible for clinical features of the disease. Most cases are sporadic, but a familial pattern of disease does exist. Female gender, total colonic aganglionosis, and a mutation of the *RET* protooncogene are strongly associated with familial disease. Up to 15% of affected children also have trisomy 21.

Affected infants develop a functional large bowel obstruction from a failure of relaxation of the diseased segment. Abdominal distention, bilious emesis, and failure to pass meconium in the first 24 hours of life are characteristic findings. Rectal examination reveals normal external anatomy and rules out anorectal anomalies. Presentation may be more subacute with failure to thrive in newborns or constipation in older children as the principal findings. Up to 30% of patients will present with enterocolitis. Fever and diarrhea are seen early, and rapid progression to sepsis and intestinal perforation can occur within 24 hours if untreated. Hirschsprung enterocolitis still carries a significant mortality rate, underscoring the need for early and aggressive treatment with fluid resuscitation, intravenous antibiotics, rectal irrigation, and a diverting colostomy in severe cases.

Infants with clinical signs of a large bowel obstruction should be studied with plain films and a contrast enema (Fig. 10-7). The classic finding on barium enema of a transition zone of aganglionosis is a reliable indicator of the presence of Hirschsprung disease. However, definitive diagnosis in all patients should be made with rectal biopsy. In the newborn period, suction rectal biopsy may be performed at the bedside. Histopathologic evaluation reveals the absence of ganglion cells in all intramural plexuses, increased staining of a cholinesterase dye, and the presence of hypertrophied nerve bundles. A deficiency of nitric oxide synthetase may also be observed.

The cornerstone of treatment for Hirschsprung disease is an endorectal pull-through procedure allowing anastomosis of ganglionated bowel to the anus. In recent years, the surgical management of Hirschsprung disease has evolved substantially. Traditionally, a three-stage management approach was employed involving colostomy, pull-through, and a subsequent colostomy takedown. Currently, three distinct single-stage pull-through procedures are regularly used, and long-term success has been reported with each. The Swenson procedure was the initial pull-through described for Hirschsprung disease and consists of colon resection, extensive rectal dissection, and colorectal anastomosis. In the Duhamel-Martin procedure, the aganglionic rectal stump is left *in situ* and a pull-through with colorectal anastomosis is performed with substantially less rectal dissection. The Soave-Boley procedure involves resection of aganglionic bowel and mucosal proctectomy, followed by coloanal anastomosis via endorectal pull-through. Complications after each procedure include enterocolitis, constipation, and anastomotic stricture. Mortality in Hirschsprung disease is rare in the absence of severe enterocolitis. These procedures

have been performed laparoscopically with good success. Recently, surgeons have reported performing one-stage pull-through procedures via a transanal approach, both with and without laparoscopic assistance.

Imperforate Anus

Imperforate anus occurs when the normal descent of the urorectal septum is disrupted or incomplete, resulting in a spectrum of anorectal and cloacal anomalies. The level to which the urorectal septum descends determines whether the urinary tract effectively separates from hindgut structures. "High" lesions are those in which the rectum fails to descend below the striated muscle complex including the levator ani, and "low" lesions are those in which the rectum at least partially descends below this point. The incidence is 1 per 5,000 births, with a slight male predominance.

Low lesions in male and female patients are associated with a fistula from the rectum to the perineum. Because the rectum has descended below the levator ani, surgical correction of the anomaly can be accomplished via a perineal or limited posterior approach and affected children can be expected to be continent postoperatively. Correction of high imperforate anus is more extensive. In male patients, the rectum typically ends as a fistula into the genitourinary tract. In female patients, high imperforate anus is rare but may be part of a cloacal anomaly with severe derangement of development of the abdominal wall and pelvic structures. Up to 70% of infants with imperforate anus, particularly those with high lesions, have anomalies of the VACTERRL association. A tethered spinal cord may be observed in the presence of a high imperforate anus and sacral dysplasia.

The diagnosis of imperforate anus is typically apparent on physical examination. Accurate classification of the anatomic defects as high or low lesions requires further assessment. Leakage of mucus or meconium along the perineum suggests a low imperforate anus and draining fistula in the male. The classic diagnostic study for neonates is the Wangensteen-Rice invertogram, in which a pelvic x-ray of an infant held upside down demonstrates the position of the air-filled rectum relative to the perineum. A retrograde urethrogram with contrast may demonstrate the urinary fistula of high imperforate anus of the male. Most lesions in the female are low, and careful evaluation of the perineum, fourchette, and vestibule of the vagina will locate the fistula. Ultrasonography and MRI allow further evaluation of pelvic anatomy and, specifically, the striated muscle complex.

Affected infants with a high imperforate lesion require a colostomy in the newborn period with definitive corrective anorectoplasty as early as 6 weeks of age. Goals for definitive surgical therapy include closure of the rectourinary fistula and placement of the rectum into the striated muscle complex. The commonly employed approach to this procedure is the posterior sagittal anorectoplasty devised by Pena and DeVries. With use of this approach, the levator ani and external sphincter complex are divided posteriorly in the midline, allowing the rectum to be delivered after satisfactory mobilization. The muscle complexes are then reconstructed and sutured to the rectum. The colostomy may be reversed 4 to 6 weeks later. Serious complications are uncommon. Low malformations are repaired during

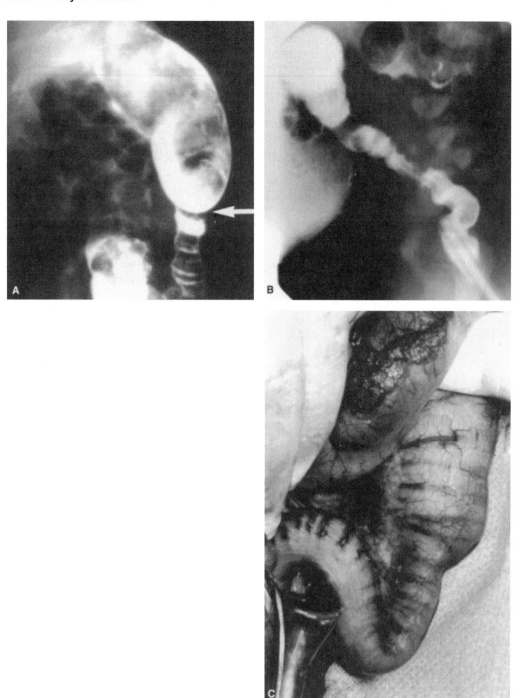

Figure 10-7   A,B: Contrast enema and **(C)** intraoperative photograph in Hirschsprung disease demonstrating a classic rectosigmoid transition zone. (From Greenfield L, Mulholland MW, Zelenock GB, et al. *Surgery: scientific principles and practice*, 3rd ed. Philadelphia: Lippincott Williams & Wilkins, 2001:2001, with permission.)

the newborn period with relatively simple perineal procedures. These do not require a diverting colostomy.

Following repair of low imperforate anus, affected infants enjoy good results regarding fecal incontinence. Generally, those with high lesions have poorer functional results. Long-term functional outcomes are variable, but about one half of patients can be expected to require only a minimal bowel regimen and to live without accidental soilage. The remainder of patients may be challenging to manage and may require major lifestyle adjustments.

Mortality for imperforate anus is related to the severity of associated anomalies.

Intussusception

Intussusception refers to the pathologic invagination of a proximal segment of intestine (*intussusceptum*) into an adjacent distal segment (*intussuscipiens*). The most commonly observed intussusception is ileocolic, in which a portion of the terminal ileum passes across the ileocecal valve into the colon. In 95% of cases, the intussusception is idiopathic without an intrinsic anatomic abnormality. The peak incidence of idiopathic intussusception is between 3 months and 3 years of age. Hyperplastic lymphoid nodules (Peyer patches) may serve as "lead points" in these cases. Children presenting at later ages are more likely to have a pathologic lead point. Other conditions predisposing to intussusception include Meckel diverticulum, bowel polyps and neoplasms, and cystic fibrosis with inspissated feces. Regardless of etiology, prolonged intussusception may lead to ischemia of the proximal bowel and progress to gangrene and perforation.

The reported incidence of intussusception ranges between 1 per 250 to 1,000 children. Reproducible seasonal peaks in midsummer and midwinter suggest an infectious (viral) etiology, but this has not been definitively proven. The typical presentation involves the onset of colicky abdominal pain in an otherwise healthy child. Asymptomatic intervals between bouts of pain are common early, whereas bilious vomiting and abdominal distention may be late findings. Focal mucosal ischemia yields heme-positive stool in over 90% of cases. Classic findings include bloody mucoid stools ("currant jelly stools") and a palpable sausage-shaped right lower quadrant mass. Plain films may demonstrate a paucity of air in the right lower quadrant but are usually nondiagnostic. Ultrasonography can reliably demonstrate the presence of intussusception, but it is rarely used because it does not offer a therapeutic option.

All children with a suspected intussusception should be evaluated with a contrast enema (air, water soluble, or barium). The classic finding of intussusception on contrast enema is the coiled-spring sign, in which the ileum is folded onto itself within the cecum. Reduction of intussusception can be achieved radiologically in 80% to 90% of children, although success rates diminish as the duration of symptoms extends beyond 24 hours. Successful reduction must be documented by confirming the free flow of contrast into the terminal ileum. Risk of bowel perforation is relatively low with a carefully performed contrast enema. However, antibiotics are generally administered prior to attempts at reduction to prevent infectious complications associated with manipulation of ischemic bowel. After successful reduction of a symptomatic intussusception, patients must be admitted to the hospital for intravenous fluid resuscitation and close observation as the most common time for recurrence is the first 24 hours after reduction.

Laparotomy is required in cases of failed enema reduction of an intussusception or for affected infants with signs of peritonitis. Via a right lower quadrant incision, the intussusception should be reduced by gently massaging distally to proximally rather than forcefully pulling apart. Bowel resection and primary end-to-end anastomosis is performed if gangrene or a suspicious mass is observed, or when the bowel cannot be manually reduced. Appendectomy is routinely performed during surgical reduction of intussusception. Recurrence of idiopathic intussusception is roughly 5% after both operative or enema reduction, and this can usually be managed with a repeat enema.

Appendicitis

Appendicitis is a common clinical problem caused by obstruction of the lumen of the appendix. In children, luminal obstruction most commonly results from lymphoid hyperplasia within the submucosal follicles of the appendix in the setting of viral infection or dehydration. Less common causes of pediatric appendiceal obstruction include fecaliths, pinworm infection, and carcinoid tumors.

Early and accurate diagnosis of appendicitis in children can be challenging. History and physical examination are extremely useful in distinguishing appendicitis from other conditions that may present in a similar fashion. About one half of patients present with the classic history of periumbilical pain that eventually migrates and localizes to the right lower quadrant. The pain perceived in early appendicitis is dull because visceral organs have autonomic innervation only and do not possess somatic pain fibers. With progressive local inflammation near the appendix, irritation of the pain fibers of the visceral peritoneum produces localized right lower quadrant pain. Alternatively, atypical abdominal pain in appendicitis may include pain that begins in the right lower quadrant or pain that remains vague and periumbilical. Nearly all patients report abdominal pain and anorexia, and most will also describe nausea. Fever is uncommon in the absence of perforation.

With a thorough physical examination of the patient with appendicitis, one can readily detect parietal peritoneal inflammation and the presence of somatic pain. Right lower quadrant pain on light palpation is usually present and may be associated with guarding. Physical signs associated with acute appendicitis include pain in the right lower quadrant with palpation of the left side of the abdomen (Rovsing sign), pain on internal rotation of the hip (obturator sign), and pain on extension of the hip (iliopsoas sign). Unusual anatomic variations in the location of the appendix may affect the constellation of presenting symptoms. Because of delay in diagnosis is common, the rate of perforation in acute appendicitis during childhood is significantly increased and may approach 50%.

Laboratory and radiologic investigation is unnecessary when the history and physical examination strongly suggest the presence of appendicitis. However, further tests can be helpful with indeterminate cases. Most patients will present with a leukocytosis and left shift. Conventional radiographs occasionally demonstrate the presence of an appendicolith but do not routinely contribute to the diagnosis of appendicitis. Both ultrasonography and computerized tomography have been demonstrated to be sensitive and specific means of diagnosing appendicitis. Various studies have shown ultrasonography to be 80% to 92% sensitive and 86% to 98% specific for appendicitis, but this modality is highly user-dependent. Sonographic findings of appendicitis include increased wall thickness, luminal distension, and lack of compressibility. Computerized tomography has a published sensitivity ranging from 87% to 100% and specificity from 83% to 97%. Computerized tomographic (CT) findings of appendicitis include inflammatory streaking of surrounding fat and a thick-walled, distended appendix that does not fill with contrast. Various investigators have studied specific diagnostic algorithms with ultrasonography and/or computerized tomography for children suspected of having appendicitis, but no consensus has emerged. A practical approach to managing appendicitis during childhood is to avoid radiographic imaging when the diagnosis is unequivocal, and to use ultrasonography as a first-line imaging modality over computerized tomography if the prerequisite expertise exists.

Patients with appendicitis should undergo surgical removal of the inflamed appendix after initiation of broad-spectrum antibiotic therapy and fluid resuscitation. Open appendectomy is performed via a limited right lower quadrant incision at the point of maximal tenderness or at the McBurney point. After delivery of the cecum and appendix into the wound, the appendiceal artery is ligated and the appendix is removed. The appendiceal stump is cauterized and inverted to prevent mucocele formation. In recent years, many surgeons have expressed a preference for the minimally invasive laparoscopic appendectomy. In clinically stable patients with perforated appendicitis, an acceptable alternative to emergency surgery is nonoperative management with intravenous antibiotics for 2 weeks, percutaneous drainage of an abscess if present, and an interval appendectomy performed 6 to 12 weeks later.

DISORDERS OF THE BILIARY TRACT

Biliary Atresia

Biliary atresia is a rare disease affecting 1 per 15,000 infants, in which the extrahepatic biliary ducts are replaced with dense fibrous tissue. Most patients exhibit a form of the disease in which the entire biliary tract, including the gallbladder, is obliterated. The pathogenesis of biliary atresia remains poorly understood. However, clinical and experimental data suggest that it results from an obliterative inflammatory process similar to sclerosing cholangitis in adults rather than a true atresia or failure of ductal recanalization during embryogenesis. Progression of bile duct proliferation, cholestasis, and portal fibrosis leads to liver parenchymal injury and cirrhosis. Early intervention to establish bile drainage is important for long-term hepatic function. When surgical intervention is late or inadequate, cirrhosis and liver failure invariably result. Diagnosis of biliary atresia is often delayed because of the overwhelming prevalence of routine physiologic jaundice as the source of jaundice in the newborn and the relative infrequency of a true obstructive lesion.

Affected neonates are commonly anicteric full-term infants who develop progressive neonatal jaundice during the first several weeks of life. Most infants become jaundiced by 1 month of age, with associated acholic stools and dark urine. Aside from jaundice and perhaps hepatosplenomegaly, physical examination is unremarkable. Radionuclide imaging of the hepatobiliary tree with technetium-99m-iminodiacetic acid (99mTc-IDA) provides a highly sensitive and specific method for diagnosis. Such imaging reveals normal efficient uptake but no excretion of the radioisotope into the duodenum. An abdominal ultrasonographic examination should also be obtained to document anatomic evidence of an absent or diminutive extrahepatic biliary tree. Diagnosis is confirmed by intraoperative cholangiogram and percutaneous or open biopsy demonstrating bile duct proliferation and hepatic fibrosis.

First developed in Japan in the 1950s and subsequently adopted in North America, the Kasai portoenterostomy is the recommended procedure for the initial management of infants with proven biliary atresia. This procedure is performed via a right upper quadrant incision. Diagnosis should be confirmed by open liver biopsy if not performed preoperatively and an intraoperative cholangiogram via the gallbladder if possible. Evaluation of the hepatoduodenal ligament reveals a nonpatent fibrous cord replacing the common bile duct. This cord is transected distal to the cystic duct, and dissection is carried out into the porta hepatis to the bifurcation of the portal vein. The ductal remnant is transected at the level of the hepatic parenchyma. Mobilization of a short retrocolic Roux-en-Y jejunal conduit allows the creation of a single-layer anastomosis between the jejunum and the transected ducts at the liver hilum. The level of transection is determined by frozen section examination of the proximal ducts.

The overall failure rate after portoenterostomy is between 40% and 60% at 5 years, and survival is inversely related to age at the time of operation. Whereas 75% of infants operated on before 60 days of age will ultimately develop bile flow, infants operated on at 120 days of age have little chance of regaining bile flow. Cholangitis occurs as a late complication in up to 50% of patients, necessitating intravenous antibiotics and fluid resuscitation. Cessation of bile flow may be associated with cholangitis, and this may respond to a brief steroid taper. Nearly all patients with biliary atresia have some degree of residual liver injury after portoenterostomy. Some develop fat malnutrition and fat-soluble vitamin deficiency, which is treated with medium chain fat triglycerides. Others will develop progressive fibrosis and portal hypertension despite a successful portoenterostomy. Two thirds of biliary atresia patients ultimately require hepatic transplantation.

Choledochal Cysts

Choledochal cysts are congenital malformations of the bile duct that cause cystic dilatation. A classification system for choledochal cysts was described in 1959 and remains in use today (Fig. 10-8). Most observed choledochal cysts are type I cysts, characterized by fusiform dilation of the entire common bile duct with minimal proximal disease. These cysts are generally large, and may extend from the porta hepatis into the pelvis to displace adjacent viscera. The distal aspect of the common bile duct is narrow and predisposes affected infants to obstructive jaundice. Type II cysts are true diverticula of the common bile duct. The type III cyst is defined as a choledochocele, a local dilation of the distal common bile duct. Type IV disease is defined as multiple cysts, and type V anomalies (Caroli disease) are rare cystic malformations of the intrahepatic ducts. Any variation or combination of these anomalies may be observed.

The incidence of choledochal cysts is highest in Japan and among females. Infants may be diagnosed as a result of prenatal ultrasonographic screening. Otherwise, most infants and older children present with obstructive jaundice, or less commonly with extrinsic compression of adjacent viscera by a palpable mass. The classic presentation in older children of recurrent abdominal pain, jaundice, and a palpable right upper quadrant mass is infrequently observed. Both ultrasonography and hepatobiliary iminodiacetic acid (HIDA) scan should be obtained for definitive diagnosis. Percutaneous cholangiography, magnetic resonance cholangiopancreatography, or endoscopic retrograde cholangiopancreatography (ERCP) are recommended to further define aberrant anatomy.

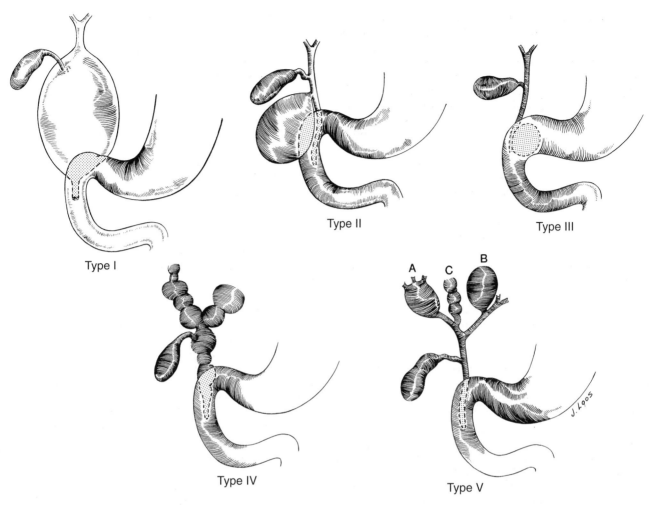

Figure 10-8 Common types of choledochal cysts (types I–V), as described in the text. Fusiform dilatation of the common bile duct, type I, represents the most common variant. (From Baker RJ, Fischer JE. *Mastery of surgery*, 4th ed. Philadelphia: Lippincott Williams & Wilkins, 2001:1207, with permission.)

Treatment of choledochal cysts is always surgical. Operative procedures should include a cholangiogram via the gallbladder and a subsequent cholecystectomy. Cyst enterostomy and internal drainage procedures were routinely performed for type I choledochal cysts until the 1970s. These procedures have been abandoned owing to a high rate of failure and the recognition that residual unexcised cysts have a risk of malignant degeneration. Currently, standard management for type I cysts includes primary transmural cyst excision and reconstruction with a Roux-en-Y hepaticojejunostomy. Recurrent cholangitis, stricture or stone formation, and pancreatitis are potential complications after choledochal cyst excisions.

DEFORMITIES OF THE CHEST WALL AND ABDOMINAL WALL

Pectus Excavatum

Pectus excavatum (funnel chest) is a deformity of the chest wall characterized by a variable posterior curve in the body of the sternum (Fig. 10-9). The incidence of pectus excavatum is between 1 and 8 cases per 1,000 children. Both pectus

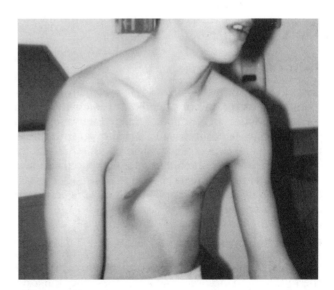

Figure 10-9 Pectus excavatum. Typical appearance of an adolescent boy with funnel chest depression deformity of the chest wall. (From Greenfield L, Mulholland MW, Zelenock GB, et al. *Surgery: scientific principles and practice*, 3rd ed. Philadelphia: Lippincott Williams & Wilkins, 2001:1939, with permission.)

excavatum and pectus carinatum (see below) are believed to result from disordered regulation of cartilaginous growth in costal cartilages rather than a bony rib or sternal abnormality. In pectus excavatum, a posterior displacement of the sternum begins superiorly at the manubrium and extends to the xiphoid. The funnel-shaped depression is associated with a dorsal bend in costal cartilages. The deformity is generally present at birth but progresses to a variable degree during childhood, and may become most prominent during adolescence after periods of rapid somatic growth. Concurrent scoliosis is commonly observed. Most affected children are asymptomatic without evidence of cardiopulmonary compromise, although patients with Marfan syndrome and concomitant pectus excavatum tend to have respiratory impairment. A negative self-perception is often generated through insensitive peer–peer interactions.

The indications for repairing pectus excavatum are to improve cosmetic appearance and psychosocial development. In recent years, surgical management of this deformity has changed dramatically. The classic surgical repair for pectus excavatum is performed via an inframammary transverse incision. Liberal anterior displacement of the sternum is possible after resection of the deformed costal cartilages, anterior osteotomy, and sternal fracture. Preservation of the perichondrium is important for regeneration of new cartilage. The corrected sternal position is maintained by inserting a stainless steel strut that lies under the sternum and overlaps the ribs. This strut is removed surgically at a later date once healing is complete. In 1997, the Nuss procedure, a minimally invasive technique for pectus excavatum repair, was introduced. In this procedure, the sternum is elevated without cartilage resection or sternal osteotomy. A stainless steel bar is custom contoured and placed below the sternum, where it is supported by the adjacent rib cage. This procedure allows the cartilage to remodel while the bar supports the sternum. Typically, the supporting bar is removed at 2 years. Cosmetic and functional outcomes after both of these procedures are excellent with a low rate of recurrence. In rare cases, a postoperative asphyxiating thoracic dystrophy may occur after the open procedure.

Pectus Carinatum

Pectus carinatum (pigeon breast) is considerably less common than pectus excavatum. Unlike the concavity seen in pectus excavatum, an elevation of the sternum is seen with the carinatum deformity, again a result of a cartilaginous abnormality rather than a bony deformity. Techniques for surgical repair are similar to those for open pectus excavatum repair, although the metal strut may not be necessary to maintain the corrected sternal position. Long-term outcomes are excellent.

Poland Syndrome

Poland syndrome refers to a rare constellation of unilateral chest wall anomalies, vertebral anomalies, and upper extremity deformities. Findings include a deficiency of the pectoralis major and minor muscles; absence of the serratus anterior and external oblique muscles; ipsilateral syndactyly of the hand; ipsilateral hypoplasia of the breast; deformity of the costal cartilages. These skeletal defects are

not symptomatic. Surgical repair of the chest wall deformities in Poland syndrome is similar to the repair for pectus excavatum and pectus carinum. Including a prosthetic mesh may provide additional protection to vulnerable intrathoracic structures. In the female, a mammary implant is required after puberty to compensate for hypoplasia of the ipsilateral breast.

Gastroschisis and Omphalocele

During normal fetal development, the complete abdominal wall is formed by four distinct embryologic folds—the cephalic, caudal, and right and left lateral folds. Each of the folds migrates toward the anterior central portion of the coelomic cavity, where they join and form a large umbilical ring. The umbilical ring envelops the two umbilical arteries, the umbilical vein, and the yolk sac (omphalomesenteric duct). This group of structures together, covered by a layer of amnion, comprises the umbilical cord. During the first trimester, the intestinal tract temporarily resides within the proximal cord, where it undergoes rapid growth and rotation and then gradually returns to the abdominal cavity. With contraction of the umbilical ring, the formation of the abdominal wall is complete.

Incomplete central migration of the lateral embryologic folds is thought to result in *omphalocele*. Prenatal ultrasonography currently identifies many such defects and leads to appropriate genetic evaluation and counseling. The incidence of omphalocele is estimated to be 1 per 6,000 to 10,000 births. Postnatally, an omphalocele is diagnosed by inspection, revealing a mass of bowel and solid viscera in the central abdomen covered by a translucent sac composed of amniotic membrane and peritoneum (Fig. 10-10). The umbilical cord is attached to the sac. Small defects allow herniation of a small length of intestine, whereas large defects result in massive herniation of much of the abdominal contents including solid organs and an underdeveloped abdominal cavity (loss of domain). The intestine is malrotated but otherwise normal because its overlying sac

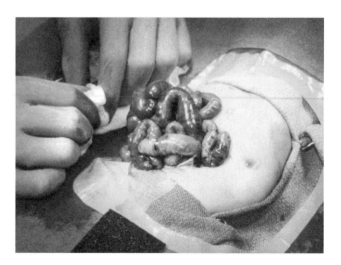

Figure 10-10 In omphalocele, relatively normal appearing bowel protrudes from an undeveloped abdominal cavity through a large central defect in the abdominal wall. (From Greenfield L, Mulholland MW, Zelenock GB, et al. *Surgery: scientific principles and practice*, 3rd ed. Philadelphia: Lippincott Williams & Wilkins, 2001:1969, with permission.)

prevents exposure to amniotic fluid. Roughly two thirds of infants with omphalocele have associated congenital anomalies, notably cardiac and chromosomal anomalies. Infants with large defects may have significant pulmonary hypoplasia.

Gastroschisis is also an embryologic failure of abdominal wall formation and is characterized by a full-thickness defect and herniation of intestines without an overlying protective sac. This defect always lies to the right of the umbilicus. Prenatal ultrasonography is also effective in diagnosing gastroschisis, which occurs with an incidence of 1 per 3,000 to 8,000 live births. Experimental evidence supports the hypothesis that gastroschisis results from an intrauterine rupture of a hernia of the umbilical cord after complete development of the abdominal wall. Chemical irritation of the unprotected intestine by substances in the amniotic fluid result in the appearance of edematous and matted bowel covered by a gelatinous exudate. The intestine is malrotated and often dysfunctional owing to extensive inflammation. Unlike omphalocele, associated anomalies (with the exception of intestinal atresia) are uncommon in gastroschisis.

The priorities in management of both omphalocele and gastroschisis are resuscitation of the infant and protection of the bowel. Nasogastric tube decompression prevents aspiration and reduces bowel distention. Note that the omphalocele sac or the herniated viscera in gastroschisis are initially wrapped with moist gauze and covered with a plastic drape to prevent hypothermia and avoid contamination. Broad-spectrum intravenous antibiotics and maintenance fluids should be started immediately, and infants are transported in a warm incubator to the intensive care unit. A thorough examination for associated congenital anomalies should be carried out prior to operative repair. Nonoperative conservative approaches to managing omphalocele are indicated in the presence of severe associated anomalies that are life-threatening or preclude a conventional surgical repair of the defect. In gastroschisis, fluid requirements are high because of the large, exposed surface of inflamed intestine.

Immediate primary repair of the abdominal wall defect after reduction of herniated viscera is successful for 60% to 70% of infants with omphalocele and gastroschisis. However, excessive intra-abdominal pressure after closure may compromise venous return and respiratory function, and should be avoided. For larger omphaloceles, a gradual reduction is performed either by wrapping of the omphalocele or creation of a temporary silo. For gastroschisis, prefabricated silos are now available, which can be placed in the neonatal intensive care unit without the need for anesthesia. Serial reductions are then performed at bedside until the bowel is completely reduced into the abdomen and definitive closure may be scheduled. At the time of abdominal closure, the bowel should be inspected for possible associated atresias. Nutritional support with total parenteral nutrition is indicated for infants with gastroschisis or giant omphalocele until enteral feedings can be tolerated. Infants with gastroschisis are at particular risk for developing necrotizing enterocolitis, and thus feedings should be increased judiciously.

The mortality rate of infants with omphalocele is 20% to 30% and largely reflects the severity of associated anomalies rather than the omphalocele itself. Survival of infants with gastroschisis exceeds 90% because of the absence of associated congenital anomalies. Long-term complications include malabsorption from transmural intestinal inflammation and hepatotoxicity from total parenteral nutrition.

Umbilical Hernia

Congenital umbilical hernias represent the most common abdominal wall defects in infants and children. The incidence of umbilical hernias is 5% to 10% in white children and may be as high as 25% to 50% in black children. Prematurity is a significant risk factor. These hernias result when incomplete closure of the umbilical ring after birth leaves a central defect in the linea alba. Abdominal contents protruding through the defect are covered only by skin and subcutaneous tissue, and, therefore, umbilical hernias are easily recognized. Most will close spontaneously by 4 years of age, and small hernias tend to close earlier than large hernias. Incarceration is rarely seen in a pediatric umbilical hernia.

Because most congenital umbilical hernias close spontaneously, surgical repair is generally not performed until the patient is 4 years of age. Defects that fail to close by this time should be repaired. The repair is performed through a small curved infraumbilical incision that allows primary closure of the fascial defect with an acceptable cosmetic result.

Inguinal Hernia and Hydrocele

Inguinal hernias occur in 1% to 3% of all children. Nearly all inguinal hernias in childhood are indirect inguinal hernias and represent incomplete obliteration of the processus vaginalis. During normal fetal development, the testicle descends into the scrotum during the third trimester. The processus vaginalis is an extension of peritoneum that is drawn with the testicle into the scrotum until birth, at which time it forms a serous covering around the testicle known as the tunica vaginalis. Incomplete obliteration of this space near the time of birth results in an indirect inguinal hernia, with or without an associated hydrocele (Fig. 10-11). The origin of an indirect hernia is always lateral to the inferior epigastric vessels, and the hernia extends caudally with the spermatic cord within the cremasteric fascia. It may lie completely within the inguinal canal, or it may protrude down to the level of the testicle. Because development of the inferior vena cava can delay the normal descent of the right testicle, right-sided inguinal hernias are more common in children than left-sided hernias.

Inguinal hernias are six times more common in males than females, and are twice as common in premature infants. Affected infants typically present with an intermittent unilateral bulge in the groin, scrotum, or labia. The mass is usually noted at times of increased intraabdominal pressure (e.g., crying) and reduces spontaneously or with gentle external pressure. Even when the hernia cannot be demonstrated at the time of clinical examination, an appropriate clinical history is adequate for confidently making the diagnosis. Incarcerated inguinal hernias do not reduce spontaneously but can usually be reduced with gentle bimanual pressure. Incarcerated hernias may result in intestinal obstruction if left untreated. Further progression will result in strangulation of hernia contents and bowel

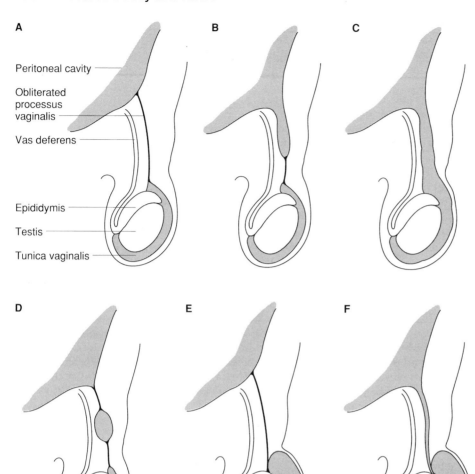

A

Peritoneal cavity

Obliterated processus vaginalis

Vas deferens

Epididymis

Testis

Tunica vaginalis

B

C

D

E

F

Figure 10-11 Schematic representation of the anatomic variations observed with varying degrees of obliteration of the processus vaginalis. **A:** Normal; obliterated processus vaginalis. **B:** Proximal hernia sac; distal obliterated processus. **C:** Hernia sac extending into scrotum; no obliteration. **D:** Proximal and distal obliteration with hydrocele of the cord. **E:** Hydrocele of the scrotum; obliterated processus. **F:** Patent processus with communicating hydrocele. (From Greenfield L, Mulholland MW, Zelenock GB, et al. *Surgery: scientific principles and practice*, 3rd ed. Philadelphia: Lippincott Williams & Wilkins, 2001:1972, with permission.)

necrosis. An incarcerated hernia must be distinguished from an acute hydrocele.

Because of the high risk of incarceration, all pediatric inguinal hernias should be surgically repaired. These hernias will not resolve spontaneously. Otherwise healthy full-term infants with reducible hernias undergo elective repair in an outpatient unit. A critical distinction between modern hernia surgery in adults and children is that mesh prostheses are not used under normal circumstances in children. The principal technical consideration in pediatric hernia repair is high ligation of the hernia sac at the level of its origin at the internal inguinal ring. The operation is performed through a small incision in a skin crease in the groin over the external internal ring. The hernia sac (located medially) and cord structures (located laterally) are delivered into the wound, and care must be taken in all cases to identify and preserve the vas deferens and the testicular blood supply. On occasion, large, chronic hernias during childhood or adolescence may result in a dilated internal ring necessitating fascial repair or mesh plug insertion. Because roughly one sixth of patients have bilateral hernias, infants younger than 2 years usually undergo routine exploration of the contralateral side. Laparoscopy performed via the hernia sac or transabdominally can be

utilized to exclude a contralateral hernia. Incarcerated hernias should be reduced if possible and repaired electively within 24 hours. Nonreducible incarcerated hernias should be repaired promptly with concomitant fluid resuscitation. Recurrent inguinal hernias in children are rare (1%).

Scrotal hydrocele is a collection of fluid within the tunica vaginalis of the scrotum. A communicating hydrocele is in continuity with a patent processus vaginalis and is characterized by intermittent accumulation of peritoneal fluid within the tunica vaginalis. The anatomic defect in communicating hydrocele is identical to that of indirect inguinal hernia, and so treatment is the same. A noncommunicating hydrocele is an accumulation of fluid in the tunica vaginalis in the presence of an obliterated processus vaginalis. This entity tends to resolve spontaneously by 1 year of age. Classically, diagnosis is by transillumination of the simple fluid collection, but this technique is not reliable in the presence of a hernia because fluid-filled bowel may transilluminate. A careful history from a parent is most helpful in diagnosis. Repair of communicating hydroceles or unresolving noncommunicating hydroceles should be performed via the inguinal approach such that an associated hernia may be repaired.

NEOPLASTIC DISEASE

Cancer is the second leading cause of death in children. However, in recent years, a more detailed understanding of tumor biology and progress in cancer diagnosis and treatment has yielded improved long-term survival of children with cancer.

Wilms Tumor

Wilms tumor (nephroblastoma) is an embryonal renal malignancy with high cure rates. Most cases occur between 1 and 5 years of age. The incidence is 7 per 1 million children, and is highest among black children. Conditions associated with Wilms tumor include aniridia, Beckwith-Wiedemann syndrome, and urinary tract malformations. Mutations in the tumor suppressor genes WT1 and WT2 have been described which contribute partially to the development of Wilms tumors. In addition, a familiar form of the disease has been described that is associated with chromosomal 11p deletion.

Most Wilms tumors are unilateral and unifocal. About 7% of tumors are multifocal within a single kidney and another 7% of patients have bilateral disease. The tumors are generally friable and easily ruptured. When spontaneous hemorrhage has occurred, it is not uncommon to see a characteristic pattern of "egg-shell" or linear calcification on plain films. This radiographic pattern is to be distinguished from the stippled calcifications seen in neuroblastoma. On histopathologic evaluation Wilms tumors demonstrate a triphasic pattern of blastemic, stromal, and epithelial cells. Rarely an anaplastic histologic appearance is observed and designated as "unfavorable histology." Anaplastic tumors carry a significantly worsened prognosis.

Most Wilms tumors present as large but asymptomatic abdominal masses. Occasionally patients will present with acute onset pain from a spontaneously ruptured tumor. Suspected Wilms patients should undergo either conventional excretory or CT urography to study both the affected and contralateral kidney. Duplex ultrasonography should be performed to study the mass and to identify intracaval tumor extension, hepatic metastases, and enlarged regional lymph nodes. Finally, plain chest radiographs are obtained to identify pulmonary metastases. Treatment of pulmonary nodules seen on CT scanning but not on plain films remains controversial. Final tumor staging is assigned after surgical staging and pathologic review.

All patients undergo unilateral nephroureterectomy with local lymph node dissection via a generous transverse abdominal incision. Palpation and inspection of both the contralateral kidney and the liver is important, and early ligation of the renal vein is recommended to prevent tumor embolization. Wilms tumors are staged according to the extent of disease observed at surgery. Stage I and II tumors represent fully resected abdominal tumors, whereas stages III and IV refer, respectively, to incompletely resected tumors or metastatic disease (Table 10-1).

Postoperative therapy is determined by tumor histopathology and the clinical stage of the patient. All patients receive a course of chemotherapy with actinomycin D and vincristine, with longer and more intensive regimens with adriamycin reserved for advanced disease. External beam radiation to the primary tumor bed is recommended for all patients with

TABLE 10-1
STAGING CRITERIA FOR WILMS TUMOR

Wilms Tumor Staging System[a]		4-Year Survival Rate (%)
Stage 1	Tumor limited to kidney and completely excised; surface intact with no evidence of rupture	97
Stage 2	Tumor extends beyond kidney but completely excised; infiltration through the renal capsule, or extension into vessels outside the kidney substance, or local open biopsy or spillage confined to the flank; no residual tumor	95
Stage 3	Residual nonhematogenous tumor	91
Stage 4	Hematogenous metastases to lung, liver, bone, brain, etc.	78
Stage 5	Bilateral renal involvement at diagnosis	Same as for higher stage unilateral

[a] Survival based on outcome for patients with favorable histologic-types in the National Wilms Tumor Study-3.
From Greenfield L, Mulholland MW, Zelenock GB, et al. *Surgery: scientific principles and practice*, 3rd ed. Philadelphia: Lippincott Williams & Wilkins, 2001:2063, with permission.

advanced disease as well as localized disease with unfavorable histologic findings. Isolated pulmonary or hepatic metastases should be resected.

Outcomes for patients with Wilms tumor are generally excellent with current treatment protocols. Patients with locally confined disease and favorable histologic findings can achieve cure rates as high as 97%, whereas even stage IV patients with distant metastasis experience survival rates close to 80%. Long-term follow-up is required for all patients with Wilms tumor because of the risk of developing a second malignancy.

Neuroblastoma

Neuroblastoma is a childhood tumor derived from primitive neural crest cells. It is the third most common tumor of childhood. The median age at diagnosis is 2 years, and the incidence is 10 per 1 million children. Neuroblastoma may occur anywhere along the normal path of embryonic descent of sympathetic ganglia. The adrenal glands are the most frequent site of disease, but tumors may also arise from cervical, posterior mediastinal, retroperitoneal, or pelvic sites. Unlike Wilms tumors, neuroblastomas represent a heterogeneous class of tumors, and long-term outcomes vary significantly among patients according to the biologic and clinical features of their disease. Although outcomes are excellent for patients with resectable tumors, survival rates for patients with advanced disease remain poor.

Much effort has been devoted to characterizing the extensive genetic changes observed in neuroblastoma cells. Neuroblastoma was the first human tumor for which the presence of an oncogene was demonstrated to be clinically significant. It has been clearly demonstrated that an increased number of copies of the *NMYC* oncogene within tumor cells is associated with rapid tumor progression and a poor prognosis. Although the function and mechanism of this oncogene remain unknown, all neuroblastoma tumors are evaluated for *NMYC* amplification so that treatment plans may be determined accordingly. Deletion of chromosome 1p also appears to be a clinically significant cytogenetic abnormality that correlates with adverse outcomes in neuroblastoma.

Clinical presentation of neuroblastoma varies with site of origin, age at diagnosis, and the biologic aggressiveness of the tumor. Most patients present with asymptomatic abdominal masses, and, unlike Wilms tumors, these tumors may cross the midline. Cervical tumors may present as lateral neck masses associated with a Horner syndrome, owing to tumor replacement of the cervical sympathetic ganglia. Thoracic tumors may be associated with opsoclonus-myoclonus, a paraneoplastic syndrome characterized by polymyoclonia, opsoclonus, and cerebellar ataxia. Pelvic tumors may cause bladder and bowel symptoms resulting from direct compression of tumor on local organs.

In all cases, the goal of diagnostic evaluation is to determine the location of the primary tumor and characterize any metastatic disease. Cross-sectional imaging with CT scanning or MRI should be obtained to evaluate the neck, chest, abdomen, and pelvis. Radiolabeled metaiodobenzylguanidine (MIBG) is a norepinephrine derivative that localizes to neuroblastoma and can be used to accurately assess sites of disease. Bone marrow is assessed routinely by aspiration and biopsy. Timed collection and measurement of urinary catecholamines and their derivatives may aid with diagnosis and provide a tumor marker for evaluating therapeutic response. Serum levels of neuron-specific enolase, which correlates with advanced disease, are measured. Finally, histologic confirmation of neuroblastoma is required, either by direct tumor biopsy or identification of tumor cells in bone marrow specimens. For unresectable tumors, a generous biopsy should be obtained for histopathologic evaluation and determination of the status of the *NMYC* oncogene.

A complete diagnostic evaluation allows patients to be stratified as low risk, intermediate risk, or high risk, according to clinical stage, age at diagnosis, and *NMYC* status (Table 10-2). Low-risk patients generally undergo surgical resection and do not need further treatment. A transverse incision is used, which allows for tumor excision and lymphadenectomy. Intermediate-risk tumors are often

TABLE 10-2

RISK STATUS DETERMINANTS IN NEUROBLASTOMA

	Low Risk	High Risk
Age	<1 yr (especially <6 mo)	>1 yr at diagnosis
Stage	1, 2A, 2B, 4S	3, 4
NMYC amplification	<3 copies	>3 copies
Cytogenetics	No 1p abnormality	1p deletion
Neuron-specific enolase	≤100 ng/mL	≥100 ng/mL

From Greenfield L, Mulholland MW, Zelenock GB, et al. *Surgery: scientific principles and practice*, 3rd ed. Philadelphia: Lippincott Williams & Wilkins, 2001:2059, with permission.

resected, whereas initial surgery in high-risk disease consists of biopsy, surgical staging, and establishment of vascular access. Both of these latter groups of patients receive several courses of multiagent chemotherapy and may then qualify for a "second-look" attempt at resection. Regimens incorporating bone marrow transplantation have also been evaluated for patients with advanced disease.

Outcomes vary widely between low- and high-risk neuroblastoma patients. Survival rates for patients with localized resectable disease are excellent. However, outcomes in high-risk neuroblastoma remain poor. Despite aggressive experimental protocols, survival for older children with metastatic disease is only 20% at 2 years. Novel therapies for high-risk neuroblastoma are clearly needed and remain under active investigation.

Rhabdomyosarcoma

Rhabdomyosarcoma is a soft tissue sarcoma of childhood. Derived from primitive fetal mesenchymal tissue, this tumor always displays characteristics of striated muscle. The incidence is roughly 4 cases per million children, and is highest among white children. Peak incidence occurs during infancy and again during adolescence. Rhabdomyosarcoma can be associated with the Li-Fraumeni syndrome, a familial cancer syndrome characterized by a defective p53 gene, or with congenital anomalies of the genitourinary and cardiac systems. Of the four described histopathologic subtypes, the most common childhood form of the disease is the more favorable embryonal rhabdomyosarcoma. The less common variants are the alveolar, botryoid, and pleomorphic subtypes.

Rhabdomyosarcoma occurs most frequently in the head and neck region, extremities, and genitourinary tract, although it may also be found in the trunk. Presentation varies with site of tumor origin. Head and neck lesions may present with local swelling or infections of the ear or sinuses. Genitourinary lesions may present with hematuria or a suprapubic mass. Lesions of the extremities can be either painless or painful, depending upon the presence of local bony invasion. Patients should be evaluated thoroughly for metastatic disease with both cross-sectional imaging and positron emission tomographic (PET) scanning. Following radiologic evaluation and bone marrow biopsy, tissue diagnosis should be confirmed with an incisional or core needle biopsy. Rhabdomyosarcoma has a propensity to grow aggressively into local surrounding structures and to metastasize widely to distant sites.

The multidisciplinary approach to the treatment of rhabdomyosarcoma involves surgical resection, chemotherapy, and radiotherapy after complete staging according the TNM staging system for rhabdomyosarcoma. Histologic tumor grade and the presence of metastases are the most important determinants of postoperative therapy.

Wide local excision with negative margins is the goal of treatment for localized tumors. Radical and debilitating resections (i.e., amputation or cystectomy) are avoided when possible. Radiation therapy is added to surgical resection for all high-grade tumors, all tumors greater than 5 cm in diameter, and all incomplete resections. Most patients with advanced disease receive chemotherapy as well. Overall survival at 5 years is 60%. Prognosis for the embryonal tumor subtype (80%) is significantly more favorable than for the alveolar histology.

Teratoma

Teratomas are germ cell tumors containing elements of all three embryonic germ layers: endoderm, mesoderm, and ectoderm. They may be benign or malignant. Teratomas commonly contain tissue that is foreign to the location of the tumor, such as skin, teeth, or neural tissue. They may occur anywhere in the body but are found frequently in midline structures. Sacrococcygeal teratoma represents the most common teratoma of neonates and the most common extragonadal teratoma overall. The ovary is the most common site of teratomas in adolescents. These tumors generally present by exerting a mass effect on local structures, or with torsion or rupture in the case of ovarian teratomas.

Serum levels of human chorionic gonadotropin, α-fetoprotein, and lactate dehydrogenase isoenzyme 1 may be elevated and followed serially as tumor markers.

Sacrococcygeal teratomas present as large masses protruding from the space between the anus and coccyx. Prenatal diagnosis can accurately identify many teratomas. The mass can be as small as a few centimeters in diameter or as large as the infant. The differential diagnosis includes myelomeningocele, neural tumor, or lipoma. Complete resection of the tumor should be performed promptly after diagnosis, as there is a risk of malignant degeneration with advancing age. Resection of the coccyx should be included for sacrococcygeal teratomas to reduce the risk of local recurrence. Hypothermia and hemorrhage can be significant complications, particularly in newborns with massive tumors. Aggressive chemotherapy is indicated for malignant tumors. Fetuses with evidence of hydrops and a large sacrococcygeal tumor have poor outcomes.

PEDIATRIC TRAUMA

Trauma represents the largest threat to the lives of American children. Each year 20,000 children die from accidental injuries. This number exceeds the total number of pediatric deaths from *all other diseases* combined. In addition to this unsettling number of traumatic deaths, another 100,000 children sustain injuries causing permanent disabilities each year. Both the financial and psychosocial costs of pediatric trauma are substantial. Optimizing the care of the pediatric trauma patient requires understanding common patterns of injury and considering unique physiologic and anatomic characteristics of children.

More than 80% to 90% of traumatic injuries during childhood result from blunt trauma. The most common mechanisms of blunt injuries are falls and motor vehicle crashes in which children are passengers or pedestrians. Falls are common among infants and toddlers, whereas school-aged children are more likely to be struck by a car while riding a bicycle or walking. During adolescence, high-speed motor vehicle crashes and penetrating injuries are more common. Different anatomic injury patterns result from these different mechanisms of injury. Head injuries are frequently seen after falls, whereas chest and abdominal injuries typically accompany penetrating injuries or injuries

caused by motor vehicles. Motor vehicle crashes claim the highest number of pediatric trauma deaths, but actual case-fatality rates are highest in drowning, penetrating wounds, and child abuse. An estimated 20,000 children each year are injured by firearms, often within the home after discharge of a weapon by somebody known to the child. Finally, health care providers must always consider and are obligated to report the possibility of child abuse, a significant public health problem in the United States.

Evaluation of the trauma patient begins with a primary survey conducted in a manner similar to that of adult patients, that is, by evaluation of airway, breathing, and circulation (the ABCs) with immobilization of the cervical spine. Optimal airway protection of the awake patient is provided in the sniffing position, with the face moved superiorly and anteriorly. When endotracheal intubation is indicated, an uncuffed endotracheal tube should be used in younger children to avoid airway edema and subglottic stenosis. One should consider the short length of the pediatric trachea (only 5 cm in infants) to avoid mainstem bronchial intubation. If needed, a surgical airway in children is best provided via needle cricothyroidotomy with subsequent conversion to tracheostomy in the operating room.

In evaluating hemodynamic stability in children, tachycardia is the first indicator of hypovolemia. Because injured children possess an ability to maintain blood pressure by constricting small- and medium-sized arteries, hypotension may not be observed until 40% of the blood volume has been lost. Because the blood volume of a child is relatively small (80 mL per kg or 800 mL in a healthy 10-kg infant), a seemingly small blood loss can have dramatic physiologic consequences. Volume resuscitation begins after prompt establishment of intravenous access. Preferred sites for venous access are the greater saphenous vein at the ankle, cephalic vein at the antecubital fossa, and the external jugular vein. When peripheral lines cannot be successfully inserted and the patient is in shock, intraosseous infusion of fluid and drugs is appropriate (for patients younger than 6 years of age). Fluid resuscitation should begin with an initial bolus of 20 mL per kg of lactated Ringer solution, and this may be repeated for persistent hypotension. Hypotension that does not respond to these two initial boluses should be managed with transfusion of red blood cells (10 mL per kg) and evaluation for surgical bleeding. Hypothermia, which may potentiate the adverse effects of shock and metabolic acidosis, should be aggressively corrected. Thin skin, lack of subcutaneous fat, and large ratio of surface area-to-total body weight all predispose the injured child to hypothermia. Overhead warmers and warming of all infused products should be priorities.

Following the primary survey and initial volume resuscitation, a rapid but systematic physical examination is performed to identify injuries. Multisystem injury is more common in children than adults because of the proximity of organs and the lack of body fat and elastic connective tissue. Standard laboratory studies, including blood typing and cross-matching, are performed during the secondary survey as indicated. Vital signs should be monitored continuously. Plain radiographs of the cervical spine, chest, and pelvis are often obtained as clinically indicated. The CT scan is still the imaging study of choice for the pediatric abdomen but ultrasonography in the trauma bay may be of some benefit.

Head injury, usually the result of a fall or motor vehicle crash, is the most common cause of death after pediatric trauma. A thin skull, weaker supporting musculature of the cervical spine, and relatively larger size of the head predispose the injured child to head injuries. Aggressively treating hypoxia, hypotension, and intracranial hypertension is critical to prevent secondary brain injury and to maximize the chance for long-term recovery from central nervous system injury. This may require placement of an intraventricular monitor for measuring intracranial pressure or craniotomy for clot evacuation. In general, children surviving serious head injuries possess a better prognosis than adults with similar injuries. Nevertheless, up to 30% of children with serious head injuries do not survive.

Thoracic injuries occur in up to 30% of injured children, and the associated mortality rate can be as high as 25% in children younger than 5 years of age. The immature rib cage in children is particularly compliant and allows kinetic energy to be directly transmitted to underlying structures. Rib fractures are, therefore, relatively uncommon in children, but their presence implies a significant force and should increase suspicion for a major thoracic injury. Pulmonary contusion is the most common thoracic injury. Because the mediastinum in children is unusually mobile, a tension pneumothorax can cause severe hypotension if rapid mediastinal shift obstructs vena caval return to the heart. Both blunt and penetrating thoracic injuries rarely require operative intervention.

Serious abdominal injuries occur in up to 25% of patients with multisystem trauma. A nasogastric tube should be inserted early to facilitate abdominal examination and to avoid aspiration of gastric contents. Diagnostic peritoneal lavage historically has served as a rapid and sensitive test to detect significant intraabdominal hemorrhage, but currently is used only in highly selected circumstances. CT scan of the abdomen is the preferred radiographic means of evaluating patients with blunt abdominal trauma. Injuries to the spleen and liver represent approximately 75% of pediatric abdominal injuries. Decades of experience have validated the safety and efficacy of a nonoperative approach to nearly all cases of hepatic and splenic injury. These patients should be monitored in an intensive care unit with serial abdominal examinations and hematocrit determinations. Indications for laparotomy after blunt trauma are refractory hypotension and ongoing transfusion. A similar management approach is gaining popularity for renal and pancreatic injuries as well.

Orthopedic trauma in children is common. Pediatric pelvic fractures can be life-threatening, particularly those with bilateral anterior and posterior fractures. Extremity fractures range from those that heal spontaneously to long-bone fractures involving the epiphysis that have long-term implications for growth and development. Fractures at the level of the knee and elbow may be associated with accompanying vascular injuries. Such injuries should be monitored with frequent neurovascular examinations to detect a possible compartment syndrome.

Most deaths following pediatric trauma are preventable. To date, injury prevention programs have successfully implemented strategies to encourage use of seatbelts, bicycle helmets, smoke detectors, and window guards. Comprehensive injury prevention programs represent a realistic opportunity to successfully address this major health problem for children today.

EXTRACORPOREAL MEMBRANE OXYGENATION (ECMO)

ECMO has been utilized for support of pediatric patients with pulmonary failure of various reversible causes. The use of ECMO involves the cannulation of the internal jugular vein and common carotid artery (veno-arterial) for full cardiopulmonary support or placement of an internal jugular double lumen cannula (veno-venous) if the heart is functioning adequately. The most common indications for ECMO cannulation in the newborn are: meconium aspiration syndrome, CDH, and persistent pulmonary hypertension of the newborn. Survival rates vary by indication and range from 54% to 94%. Success in the application of ECMO in the pediatric population has not been as good as in the newborn. Appropriate patient selection is critical. ECHO and head ultrasonography are performed prior to cannulation to exclude a cardiac source of hypoxia and to confirm the absence of intracranial hemorrhage prior to the systemic heparinization necessary for the ECMO circuit.

PRENATAL DIAGNOSIS AND FETAL SURGERY

Prenatal imaging and diagnosis of congenital anomalies has improved dramatically in recent years because of refinements in duplex ultrasonography and the advent of ultrafast fetal MRI. Commonly diagnosed conditions include abdominal wall defects, bowel obstruction, diaphragmatic hernia, lung lesions, obstructive uropathy, myelomeningocele, twin–twin transfusion syndromes, and sacrococcygeal teratoma. Prenatal evaluation of these conditions has increased the understanding of the pathophysiology and natural history of these lesions. In some cases, imaging studies can alter the management plan for the fetus, for example, by influencing the timing of delivery or by leading to termination of the pregnancy. Although most correctable anomalies are treated after delivery, some conditions may be amenable to surgical intervention *in utero*.

Fetal surgery has been employed to treat several life-threatening congenital anomalies. Congenital diaphragmatic hernia with severe associated pulmonary hypoplasia has been treated both by open *in utero* repair and by temporary tracheal occlusion to promote pulmonary development. Large space-occupying cystic lung lesions such as CCAM, which prevent normal lung growth and result in pulmonary hypoplasia, can be resected or occasionally drained by percutaneous thoracoamniotic shunting. Massive sacrococcygeal teratomas with associated high-output cardiac failure have been resected to prevent intrauterine demise. Percutaneous decompression of bilateral hydronephrosis due to urethral obstruction can be performed to prevent associated renal failure. Lastly, fetal repair of myelomeningocele can potentially minimize postnatal neurologic sequelae of the disease. At present, all of these procedures are performed only at a small number of highly specialized centers worldwide. The safety and efficacy of these and other fetal procedures remain under study, and further experience is needed to build a consensus regarding indications for fetal surgery.

KEY POINTS

▲ The prognosis for infants with congenital diaphragmatic hernia is determined by the extent of pulmonary hypoplasia and the presence of associated malformations.

▲ Congenital cystic adenomatoid malformation (CCAM) and sequestration both represent abnormal collections of lung tissue, but only sequestration commonly possesses a systemic arterial supply and venous drainage.

▲ The most common type (85%) of tracheoesophageal fistula, type C, is characterized by esophageal atresia and distal transesophageal fistula (TEF) and should be repaired in stable infants via an extrapleural right thoracotomy.

▲ Infants diagnosed with intestinal malrotation should undergo an emergent laparotomy and Ladd procedure to prevent the development of midgut volvulus.

▲ Duodenal obstruction of the newborn is frequently associated with trisomy 21 and should be managed if technically possible with duodenoduodenostomy.

▲ Up to 90% of infants with necrotizing enterocolitis are managed conservatively and do not require surgical intervention.

▲ Multiple procedures have been demonstrated to be successful in the surgical treatment of Hirschsprung disease, and each of these feature resection of distal aganglionic rectum and a low rectal anastomosis to normally innervated pulled-through proximal intestine.

▲ Reduction of intussusception can be achieved nonoperatively with contrast enema in 80% to 90% of children, although success rates diminish as the duration of symptoms extends beyond 24 hours.

▲ A type I choledochal cyst, characterized by fusiform dilation of the common bile duct, is the most common choledochal cyst and is optimally treated by total transmural excision with Roux-en-Y hepaticojejunostomy.

▲ Severe congenital anomalies are commonly associated with omphalocele but are uncommon in gastroschisis; transmural inflammatory damage to the intestines is common in gastroschisis but uncommon in omphalocele.

▲ Inguinal hernias during childhood are indirect hernias in which the peritoneum protrudes through the internal inguinal ring via a patent processus vaginalis.

▲ Outcomes for patients with Wilms tumor are generally excellent with current treatment protocols; outcomes for patients with advanced neuroblastoma remain poor.

▲ Blunt injuries to the spleen and liver during childhood should be managed conservatively in the absence of refractory hypotension or ongoing transfusion requirements.

SUGGESTED READINGS

Adzick NS, Nance ML. Medical progress: pediatric surgery. *N Engl J Med* 2000;342:1651–1657, 1726–1732.

Baker RJ, Fischer JE, eds. *Mastery of surgery*, 4th ed. Philadelphia: Lippincott Williams & Wilkins, 2001.

Blackbourne LH, Fleischer KJ, Binns O et al., eds. *Advanced surgical recall*, 1st ed. Baltimore: Williams & Wilkins, 1997.

Greenfield LJ, Mulholland MW, Oldham KT, et al. *Surgery: scientific principles and practice*, 2nd ed. Philadelphia: Lippincott-Raven Publishers, 1997.

Hernanz-Schulman M. Infantile hypertrophic pyloric stenosis. *Radiology* 2003;227:319–331.

Paulson EK, Kalady MF, Pappas TN. Suspected appendicitis. *N Engl J Med* 2003;348:236–242.

Rothrock SG, Pagane J. Acute appendicitis in children: emergency department diagnosis and management. *Ann Emerg Med* 2000;36:39–51.

Schwartz S, Shires GT, Spencer FC, eds. *Principles of surgery*, 6th ed. New York: McGraw-Hill, 1994.

The Esophagus

Richard J. Myung   John C. Kucharczuk

ANATOMY

Between the fourth and fifth weeks of gestation, the esophagus develops from the embryonic foregut, comprising endoderm and mesoderm from separation of the tracheal bud by the tracheoesophageal septum or ridge. Similar to other segments of the gastrointestinal tract, the esophagus is a tube composed of mucosa, muscularis mucosa, submucosa, and an inner circular and an outer longitudinal muscularis layer. The esophagus lacks a true serosal layer.

The esophagus can be broken down into three regional parts: the cervical, intrathoracic, and intraabdominal. The esophagus begins in the distal oropharynx, approximately 15 cm from the incisors, at the level of the sixth cervical vertebra. The striated muscles of the proximal esophagus are located just inferior to the cricopharyngeus muscle, which is a continuation of the inferior pharyngeal constrictor. This region has distinct clinical significance, because the posterior space between the cricopharyngeus and thyropharyngeus fibers in the inferior oropharynx is an area of potential weakness known as the Killian triangle. This area is a common site from which a Zenker diverticulum or an iatrogenic perforation occurs. The remaining two thirds of the esophagus continues as smooth muscle to its termination at the cardia of the stomach. The termination of the esophageal mucosa here forms the Z-line or squamocolumnar junction.

Anatomically, the esophagus has three areas of narrowing: the upper esophageal sphincter (UES), the bronchoaortic constriction at the level of T4 (approximately 24 to 26 cm from the incisors), and the diaphragmatic hiatus at the level of T10. The cervical esophagus lies left of the midline allowing for adequate access via a left cervical incision. The thoracic esophagus lies right of the midline and can be best approached through a right thoracotomy. The remaining distal esophagus returns to left of the midline and is approached by a left thoracotomy or thoracoabdominal incision. (Figure 11-1 outlines the pertinent topography of the esophagus.) In proximity to the esophagus, the thoracic duct enters the chest to the right of the distal esophagus, crosses midline at the level of T5 as it passes posterior to the aorta, and empties into the left subclavian vein.

The vascular supply of the esophagus occurs in a segmental distribution according to its embryologic origin from the branchial arch arteries or the celiac artery. The cervical distribution occurs mainly through the inferior thyroid artery, a branch of the thyrocervical trunk. Blood then drains via the inferior thyroid vein. The thoracic portion of the esophagus receives its blood supply from the bronchial arteries and from branches arising directly off the descending aorta. The venous drainage of this portion drains via the azygos-hemiazygos system and intercostal veins. The remaining intraabdominal portion of the esophagus receives its blood supply from the left gastric and inferior phrenic arteries. Drainage occurs via the left gastric vein. The left gastric vein, as an extension of the portal venous system, allows for the formation of esophageal varices in patients with portal hypertension. (Figure 11-2 details the segmental arterial blood supply.)

Lymphatic drainage also occurs in a segmental fashion. The cervical esophagus drains to the internal jugular, paratracheal, and deep cervical lymph nodes. The midthoracic esophagus drains into the subcarinal and pulmonary ligament nodes. The lower one third of the esophagus drains into the paraesophageal and celiac nodes. In many cases, owing to the rich network of submucosal lymphatics in the esophagus, tumor has been found at distant sites several centimeters from the primary lesion. As a consequence of the segmental distribution of the esophagus, the direction of blood and lymphatic drainage varies with anatomic position relative to the level of the tracheal bifurcation in the chest. In general, blood and lymphatic drainage flows cephalad along the esophagus superior to the level of the tracheal bifurcation, while flow inferior the tracheal bifurcation is oriented caudad. the blood and lymphatic drainage superior to the tracheal bifurcation returns cephalad, whereas drainage inferior to the bifurcation flows caudad.

Esophageal motility is coordinated by both sympathetic and parasympathetic innervation. Most important, the left and right vagus nerves course along the esophagus, with the left vagus rotating anteriorly and the right vagus posteriorly as they enter the abdomen. The vagus nerve and its recurrent laryngeal branches supply sympathetic innervation to the striated portion of the esophagus and the UES to coordinate the initiation of esophageal peristalsis. The remainder of the esophagus receives parasympathetic innervation from the vagus nerve and an intrinsic autonomic nerve plexus located in the submucosa of the esophageal wall.

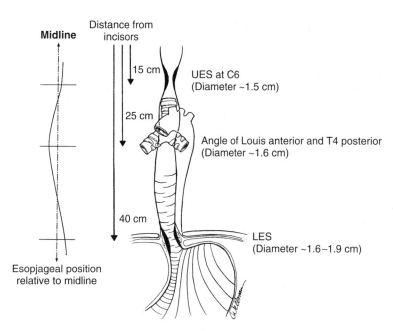

Figure 11-1 Topography of the esophagus with pertinent clinical endoscopic measurements in adults. LES, lower esphageal sphincter; UES, upper esophageal sphincter. (From Nyhus LM, Baker RJ, Fischer JE, eds. *Mastery of surgery*, 3rd ed. Boston: Little, Brown and Company, 1996:722, with permission.)

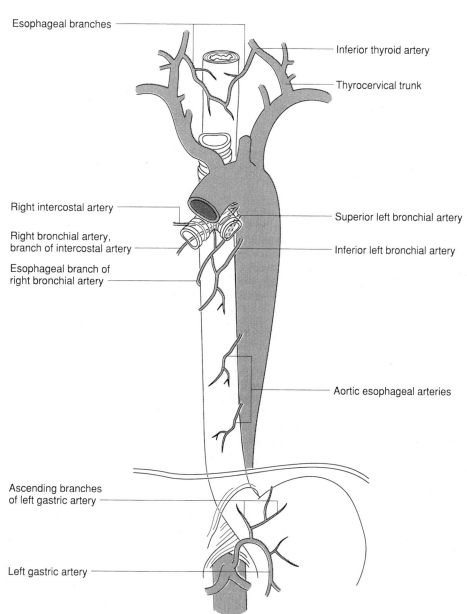

Figure 11-2 Arterial blood supply of the esophagus. (From Greenfield LJ. *Surgery: scientific principles and practice*, 1st ed. Lippincott-Raven, 1996:597, with permission.)

ESOPHAGEAL PHYSIOLOGY

The primary function of the esophagus is to provide a conduit by which food is propelled to the stomach and to prevent its regurgitation from the stomach. The physiology of swallowing will be discussed in greater detail in Chapter 16, "Nutrition, Digestion, and Absorption." The basics are discussed herein for review. During the swallowing phase, as food enters the esophagus, the cricopharyngeus muscle or UES reaches twice its normal resting pressure of 30 mm Hg and initiates a primary peristaltic wave in the upper esophagus. Smooth muscle activation continues the peristaltic wave in the remainder of the esophagus, allowing food to overcome the pressure gradient of approximately 10 mm Hg from the chest into the abdomen. Further relaxation of the lower esophageal sphincter (LES) allows food to easily enter the stomach. Secondary peristaltic waves continue to clear the esophagus of food. Loss of coordination of these events leads to the swallowing disorders discussed in subsequent text.

EVALUATION OF THE ESOPHAGUS

Functional and structural abnormalities of the esophagus can be evaluated with several modalities. In most cases, a combination of tests is required to form an accurate diagnosis.

Endoscopy is a valuable tool for both the diagnosis and treatment of a wide range of esophageal diseases. It is generally indicated in any patient complaining of dysphagia, even in the presence of normal radiographic studies. Endoscopy has a high degree of sensitivity and specificity for both structural and functional lesions, especially lesions confined to the mucosa. When combined with endoscopic ultrasonography (EUS), endoscopy has 90% sensitivity in predicting tumor and node status in esophageal cancer. However, its diagnostic strength must be weighed against the rare risks of both aspiration and perforation.

Imaging of the esophagus can be performed by the use of computerized tomographic scanning (CT) or magnetic resonance imaging (MRI). Cross-sectional imaging with these modalities is particularly useful for evaluating esophageal tumor invasion into surrounding structures. CT or MRI may also be used to detect lymphadenopathy or localize metastatic disease.

A barium swallow provides both structural and functional information. Aspiration is documented by residual contrast in the larynx after swallowing. Esophageal peristalsis can be documented by the presence of a stripping wave after a swallowed bolus of contrast. The addition of motion-recording techniques greatly facilitates the evaluation of function.

Esophageal manometry allows precise measurement of the contractility and resting pressures of various portions of the esophagus. The test is indicated in any patient with a suspected motor abnormality when barium swallow or endoscopy does not show a clear structural defect. A manometric study consists of four parts: the assessment of the LES, measurement of LES relaxation, esophageal body manometry, and assessment of the UES. Manometry is most widely used in conjunction with pH monitoring in the diagnosis of gastroesophageal reflux disease. A normal manometric test would include (i) a resting basal LES pressure of 10 to 45 mm Hg with complete relaxation during the average of ten wet swallows (swallows performed with the administration of a small water bolus), (ii) peristaltic wave progression at a rate of 2 to 8 cm per second, and (iii) distal wave amplitudes of 30 to 180 mm Hg. An abnormal LES is suggested by a low basal pressure less than 6 mm Hg, an average length exposed to the positive-pressure abdomen less than 1 cm, and an overall sphincter length of less than 2 cm.

Twenty-four hour pH monitoring is performed by placement of a pH probe 5 cm superior to the manometrically determined LES. Monitoring of pH is not a test for reflux but rather an indication of the severity and duration of acid exposure to the esophagus. However, reflux symptoms correlate well with an esophageal pH of less than 4.0. The test is indicated in patients with reflux-like symptoms who have failed to respond to a 12-week course of acid-suppression therapy and as a work-up for all patients being considered for an antireflux procedure.

The Bernstein test is discussed primarily for historical interest. The test represents a provocative maneuver by administering 0.1 N HCl at 15 cm superior to the LES to reproduce reflux symptoms. A positive test suggests mucosal sensitivity to acid but does not diagnose the presence or absence of reflux or esophagitis.

MOTILITY DISORDERS

An esophageal dysmotility evaluation is indicated in patients presenting with either dysphagia or chest pain in whom other primary cardiac, thoracic, or esophageal disorders (i.e., stenosis, malignancy) have been ruled out. There are four basic categories of primary motor disorders of the esophagus, which include: inadequate relaxation of the LES (achalasia), uncoordinated contractions (diffuse esophageal spasm), hypercontractions (nutcracker esophagus and hypertensive LES), and hypocontraction (ineffective esophageal motility). Regardless of the type of disorder, the etiology of most primary motility disorders remains unknown. However, neuromuscular impairment resulting from cerebrovascular ischemia, myasthenia gravis, Parkinson disease, motor neuron disease, multiple sclerosis, collagen vascular diseases, and polymyositis has been implicated.

Inadequate relaxation of the LES is best characterized by *achalasia*. Achalasia is characterized by peristalsis of the esophageal body against an incompletely relaxed LES. Possible etiologies of achalasia include viral (varicella-zoster) and parasitic (*Trypanosoma cruzi*, Chagas disease) infections, which may be responsible in neuronal degeneration of the myenteric plexus. Preferential regression of the nitric oxide–producing inhibitory neurons results in incomplete relaxation of the LES. Patients often present with progressive dysphagia, chest pain, weight loss, and occasionally regurgitation. If regurgitation occurs, it is usually associated with meals and may accompany respiratory symptoms from aspiration. In addition, these patients also suffer from pneumonitis, bronchiectasis, hemoptysis, and esophagitis. Late-stage achalasia causes dilation of the esophagus resulting in an air–fluid level and a characteristic *bird's beak* appearance on barium esophagram as show in Figure 11-3. Manometric findings include incomplete relaxation of the LES to less than 8 mm Hg and low amplitude contractions of less than 40 mm Hg of the esophageal body after swallowing

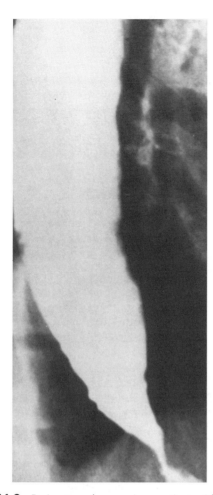

Figure 11-3 Barium esophagram in a patient with achalasia demonstrating a persistent "bird's beak" taper at the gastroesophageal junction. (From Bell RH, Rikkers LF, Mulholland MW. *Digestive tract surgery: a text and atlas*. Philadelphia: Lippincott-Raven, 1996:34, with permission.)

(Fig. 11-4). This condition is considered premalignant, with the occurrence of squamous cell carcinoma occurring in 1% to 10% of patients over 15 to 25 years.

Treatment has traditionally been a conservative attempt to lower resting LES pressures with the use of calcium channel blockers, nitrates, repetitive balloon dilatations, or injection of botulinum toxin. Surgical therapy was previously reserved for the 30% of patients who failed conservative treatment. However, recent prospective trials comparing laparoscopic myotomy with botulinum toxin injection have demonstrated improved results after surgery, with approximately 90% of patients symptom-free at 2 years, compared to 34% in the botulinum toxin injection group. Because of this, many surgeons are beginning to advocate early surgery for these patients because of the improved outcomes and the difficulty of performing a myotomy after repeated dilatations and injections. In most cases, myotomy can be performed using an extended Heller myotomy via a laparoscopic approach with the addition of an antireflux procedure such as a Nissen fundoplication. In cases involving proximal motility disorders or patients with progressive disease despite a laparoscopic myotomy, a right thoracoscopy can be performed for a complete esophagocardiomyotomy. In both approaches, the myotomy involves division of both the longitudinal and circular muscle layers without injury

to the underlying mucosa. Alleviation of dysphagia, regurgitation, and chest pain can be expected in 80% to 90% of patients at 5 years. Reflux can be expected in 15% to 25% of patients who do not undergo an antireflux procedure.

Uncoordinated esophageal contraction is best characterized by *diffuse esophageal spasm* (DES). DES is primarily a disorder of the esophageal body, which results in manometric abnormalities of frequent (occurring in greater than 10% of wet swallows), simultaneous esophageal contractions of high amplitude (greater than 30 mm Hg), with normal relaxation of the LES. Unlike achalasia, the LES in these patients is frequently normal, and consequently these patients do not experience symptoms of reflux. The etiology of DES is unknown but it is frequently associated with irritable bowel syndrome and stress. Patients often present with angina-like chest pain or dysphagia and often undergo a normal cardiac evaluation. DES often resembles a "cork screw" esophagus on barium esophagram as shown in Figure 11-5. This disease has no malignant potential. Treatment is usually conservative with the use of calcium channel blockers and long-acting nitrates to help attenuate the esophageal contractions. Surgery is recommended for only the most severe cases, which are refractory to conservative management.

Esophageal hypercontraction or "nutcracker esophagus" is the most common motility disorder observed in patients with noncardiac chest pain. Manometric amplitudes of the esophageal body two standard deviations (SDs) greater than normal (peaks of greater than 180 mm Hg) characterize this disorder. Similar to patients with DES, patients often present with crushing chest pain occurring frequently at rest. Again, the mainstay of treatment is conservative management with the use of calcium channel blockers and nitrates.

Hypertensive LES is characterized by elevated resting LES pressures or exaggerated contraction of the LES after relaxation, with normal LES relaxation and esophageal peristalsis. Patients commonly present with dysphagia and chest pain, but it remains unclear how attributable their symptoms are to these findings. LES myotomy is reserved for patients who do not respond to repeated dilatations.

The last group includes *esophageal hypocontraction*, best described in patients with scleroderma. Manometric evidence of contractions less than 30 mm Hg and moderately reduced resting LES pressures affects up to 80% of these patients, but can affect patients with other collagen vascular diseases as well.

ESOPHAGEAL DIVERTICULA

Esophageal diverticula often result from disorders of esophageal motility and can be separated into two broad categories: traction and pulsion diverticula. *Pulsion diverticula* arise from elevated intraluminal pressures that force mucosa and submucosa through the esophageal wall. *Traction diverticula* result from an adjacent inflammatory process that pulls the entire esophageal wall as a "true diverticulum" toward it. *Parabronchial diverticula* are characterized as traction diverticula associated with mediastinal granulomatous disease such as histoplasmosis or tuberculosis.

A *Zenker diverticulum* is a false diverticulum arising from the area of weakness inferior to the oblique fibers of the thyropharyngeus and the horizontal fibers of the cricopharyngeus or UES, as illustrated in Figure 11-6. The incidence has

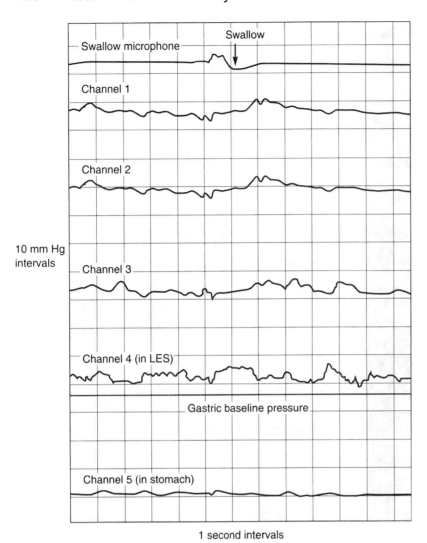

Figure 11-4 Manometric tracing of achalasia; nonrelaxation of the lower esophageal sphincter (LES) and absent peristalsis. (From Crookes PF, Demeester TR. Esophageal anatomy and physiology, and gastroesophageal reflux. In: Greenfield LJ, Mulholland M, Oldham KT et al., eds. *Surgery: scientific principles and practice*, 2nd ed. Lippincott-Raven Publishers, 1997:676, with permission)

been reported to occur in 0.1% of 20,000 routine barium esophagrams, usually occurring in elderly white men. Patients often complain of symptoms associated with cervical dysphagia, regurgitation of undigested food, recurrent aspiration, gastrointestinal reflux, and halitosis. Surgical treatment includes cervical esophagomyotomy with resection of the diverticulum, or diverticulopexy with cricopharyngeal myotomy. Recently, endoscopic cricopharyngomyotomy has been described, although the indications for this approach are still unclear.

Epiphrenic or subdiaphragmatic diverticula are pulsion diverticula that result secondary to motor dysfunction or mechanical obstruction within 10 cm of the distal esophagus, as illustrated in Figure 11-7. Generally, patients with diverticula greater than 3 cm or moderate-to-severe symptoms should undergo surgery. Surgical intervention includes resection of the diverticulum and a long esophagomyotomy, with or without an antireflux procedure.

ESOPHAGEAL PERFORATION

The absence of serosa predisposes the esophagus to rupture at lower pressures than other parts of the alimentary tract. Clinical and radiographic manifestations are determined by esophageal anatomy: lower esophageal rupture

drains into the left thoracic cavity, whereas rupture of the midesophagus will drain into the right thoracic cavity. Clinical presentation may include a pleural effusion, pneumothorax, pneumomediastinum, atelectasis, subcutaneous emphysema, chest pain, dysphagia, tachycardia, tachypnea, and fever. Patients may also present with a *Hamman sign*, a mediastinal crunch caused by mediastinal emphysema that is appreciated during auscultation of the chest on physical examination. Esophageal perforation is caused by spontaneous rupture in approximately 15% of cases, traumatic rupture in 20%, and iatrogenic rupture in 60%.

Iatrogenic perforation is commonly caused by esophagoscopy with or without sclerotherapy, variceal ligation, pneumatic dilatation, bougienage, laser therapy, endotracheal intubation, and nasogastric tubes. Most iatrogenic injuries occur at the level of the cricopharyngeal constrictor at Killian triangle. Any patient reporting chest pain or fever after instrumentation of the esophagus should be evaluated for a perforation. Other less frequent causes include foreign body ingestion, trauma, and operative injury.

Spontaneous rupture can occur from increased pressure against a closed glottis. *Boerhaave syndrome* classically presents with a *Mackler triad*: vomiting, lower thoracic pain, and subcutaneous emphysema. Perforations are localized to the left lateral wall, just superior to the diaphragm. In the *Mallory-Weiss syndrome*, increased pressure causes mucosal

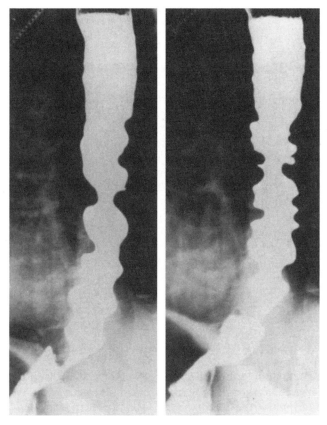

Figure 11-5 Barium esophagram demonstrating tertiary contractions of the circular muscle "corkscrew" characteristic of diffuse esophageal spasm. (From Bell RH, Rikkers LF, Mulholland MW. *Digestive tract surgery: a text and atlas.* Philadelphia: Lippincott-Raven, 1996:38, with permission.)

laceration on the gastric side of the gastroesophageal junction, commonly presenting with bleeding. Patients with the Mallory-Weiss syndrome present with esophageal injury but do not have esophageal perforation.

Early diagnosis of esophageal perforation can dramatically reduce the morbidity and mortality associated with this disease. Radiographic studies include chest x-ray to identify pneumomediastinum, which may be present in up to 40% of patients with perforation, although normal radiographic findings do not rule out perforation. A water soluble contrast esophagram followed by a dilute barium esophagram will diagnose approximately 60% of cervical

perforations and up to 90% of mediastinal perforations. Serial barium esophagrams may be required if the initial esophagram is negative and the clinical suspicion remains high. Perforations can also be diagnosed with esophagoscopy; esophagoscopy has high sensitivity for perforations caused by external trauma. Computerized tomographic (CT) scans may suggest perforation with the presence of extraluminal air, esophageal thickening, or fluid collections. Pleural fluid collected by thoracentesis is suggestive of perforation with a pH less than 6.0, the presence of food particles, or elevated salivary amylase.

Treatment options include both conservative and surgical management, depending on the time from injury to diagnosis and the degree of injury. Surgical management should be the treatment of choice for patients presenting with sepsis, shock, respiratory failure, pneumothorax, pneumoperitoneum, and extensive mediastinal emphysema or abscess. Well-contained cervical perforations are treated with cervical incision and drainage alone. More distal perforations can be managed with several options, including primary repair with or without reinforcement and drainage. Patients with severe gastrointestinal reflux should receive an antireflux procedure at the time of repair. Regardless of type of primary repair or time to presentation, the lowest mortality rates are achieved in patients managed operatively, ranging from 0 to 31% and averaging 12%. Therefore, primary repair remains the treatment of choice for patients without extensive esophageal necrosis or esophageal malignancy regardless of the time to presentation.

In cases of severe necrosis or an underlying esophageal carcinoma, an esophagectomy is required. The use of a transhiatal approach or a staged transthoracic approach is debatable depending on the time to presentation and the extent of necrosis or spillage. The mortality rate in these cases averages 17%. Severe contamination with delay in diagnosis can best be managed with exclusion and diversion or use of a T-tube for creation of a controlled fistula. However, these other surgical therapies are associated with a higher mortality rate of 24%. Overall, the highest mortality (37%) occurs in patients receiving drainage alone.

Nonoperative management is reserved for stable patients. These patients often present early with well-contained perforations and minimal mediastinal or pleural contamination. Other criteria suggested for the selection of nonoperative candidates include drainage into the esophageal lumen on

Figure 11-6 Formation of a Zenker diverticulum **(A)**. Herniation of the pharyngeal mucosa and submucosa occurs at the point of transition (*arrow*) between the oblique fibers of the thyropharyngeus muscle and the more horizontal fibers of the cricopharyngeus muscle **(B and C)**. As the diverticulum enlarges, it dissects toward the left side and downward into the superior mediastinum in the prevertebral space, forming a false diverticulum. (From Bell RH, Rikkers LF, Mulholland MW. *Digestive tract surgery: a text and atlas.* Philadelphia: Lippincott-Raven, 1996:33, with permission.)

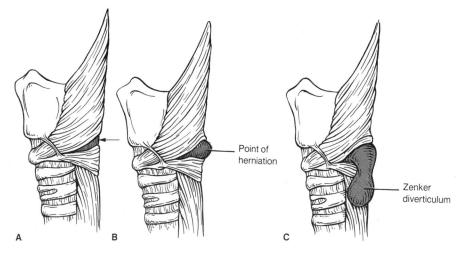

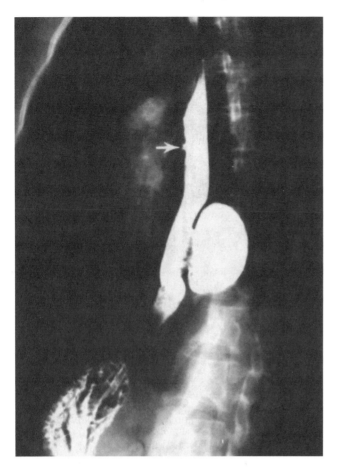

Figure 11-7 Esophagram of a patient with a large epiphrenic pulsion diverticulum and a small midesophageal traction diverticulum (*arrow*). (From Sabiston DC Jr. *Textbook of surgery: the biological basis of modern surgical practice*, 15th ed. Philadelphia: WB Saunders, 1997:731, with permission.)

contrast imaging, injury outside of the abdomen, perforation not involving neoplastic tissue, injury not proximal to an obstruction, and the immediate availability of contrast imaging and an experienced thoracic surgeon. Management includes the use of broad-spectrum antibiotics, nothing by mouth for up to 72 hours, drainage of collections by thoracostomy tubes or image-guided catheters, and total parenteral nutrition. Although endoscopically placed stents have been described, their indication for use remains ill-defined and reserved for patients who cannot otherwise tolerate surgery. Nonoperative management is most successful in patients with perforations recognized early following instrumentation. The mortality rate has been reported to be extremely low in highly select groups, with an overall average of 18%.

Despite prompt diagnosis and treatment, mortality from esophageal perforation still remains high. The etiology clearly determines outcome, with spontaneous perforations associated with a mortality of 36%, iatrogenic perforations 19%, and traumatic perforations 7%. In addition, cervical perforations are associated with the lowest mortality of 6%, whereas thoracic and abdominal perforations are associated with mortality rates of 27% and 21%, respectively. The most critical determinant remains the time of injury to treatment. Patients treated less than 24 hours after the time of injury have a mortality

rate of approximately 10% to 15% and those diagnosed later have rates upward of 50%.

CAUSTIC INJURY

The incidence of caustic injury to the esophagus has a bimodal distribution, with its peak occurring at ages younger than 5 years followed by a secondary peak later in adolescence and young adulthood. The latter group usually swallows greater quantities as a result of deliberate suicide attempts. The most common ingested chemicals include alkali (65%), acid (16%), and bleach. Alkali, an odorless and tasteless liquid, usually causes the most damage via liquefaction necrosis to surrounding tissues. Acid usually causes upper airway injury because of gagging, although results in less injury owing to coagulation necrosis. Bleaches are esophageal irritants and pose no serious esophageal injury.

Patients present with mouth and chest pain, hypersalivation, dysphagia, bleeding, and vomiting. Assessment of mucosal injury is performed by esophagoscopy within the first 24 hours after presentation. Because of the risk of perforation, the endoscope should not be passed beyond the proximal lesion. Treatment consists of broad-spectrum antibiotics and corticosteroids. Emetics are contraindicated. Early surgical intervention is reserved for patients with extensive hemorrhage or necrosis, burns beyond the pylorus, and peritonitis. If gastric necrosis is present, a transhiatal esophagogastrectomy with end-cervical esophagostomy, mediastinal drainage, and feeding jejunostomy is performed. Gastrointestinal continuity is restored at a later date with colonic interposition.

After the acute phase of injury is complete, surgical management is directed toward the prevention of strictures. Mucosal injuries require 20 to 30 days to heal, and strictures will develop in 20% of patients. In patients who go on to develop esophageal stricture post injury, 60% of strictures occur in 1 month and 80% within 2 months. Beyond 8 months, it is unlikely a stricture will develop in the absence of symptoms. Satisfactory treatment is usually obtained by early, repeated bougie dilatation. Surgical intervention is reserved for complete stenosis, fistula, mediastinitis, and inability to maintain a sizable lumen. Esophageal resection with gastric, colonic, or jejunal interposition is the procedure of choice unless severe periesophagitis precludes safe dissection of the esophagus. Strictures are at risk to undergo malignant degeneration and therefore endoscopic surveillance is recommended.

FOREIGN BODIES

Foreign body ingestion occurs frequently in the pediatric population. Generally, ingested foreign bodies lodge in regions of anatomic narrowing, as previously noted. Foreign bodies are usually easily diagnosed with chest x-ray, dilute barium esophagram, or flexible endoscopy. Objects can usually be removed with flexible endoscopy. Sharp foreign bodies should always be removed because of a 15% to 30% risk of perforation at the ileocecal valve. Surgical removal is indicated for sharp objects, for objects that cannot be removed endoscopically, or for blunt objects that have not advanced within 3 days.

BENIGN ESOPHAGEAL LESIONS

Benign neoplasms of the esophagus are extremely rare and account for 0.5% of all esophageal masses. These tumors are usually divided into intraluminal and extraluminal subgroups. Most intramural lesions are *leiomyomas* comprising 60% of benign lesions. The incidence of this lesion is approximately 5% in autopsy series, with a peak between the third and fifth decades of life, although rarely do they become symptomatic. Approximately 80% of these lesions occur in the distal two thirds of the esophagus and are multiple in 10% of patients. Those leiomyomas arising in the distal esophagus are derived from smooth muscle, which originates in the muscularis propria.

Leiomyomas are slow-growing tumors, and patients with these lesions present with a long history of generalized upper gastrointestinal symptoms of regurgitation, belching, dysphagia, and pain. Hiatal hernia is the most common coexisting diagnosis, which predisposes the patient to reflux esophagitis and subsequent ulceration. Diagnosis is usually made by barium esophagram, which shows a smooth concave defect with sharp borders (Fig. 11-8). Endoscopy with EUS also reveals a lesion with normal overlying mucosa and a freely movable mass with narrowing but not complete obstruction of the lumen. Biopsy is contraindicated, since mucosal interruption will complicate subsequent surgical excision.

Treatment for leiomyomas must be tailored to the lesion's tumor size, location, and morphology as well as the clinical condition of the patient. Treatment for asymptomatic leiomyomas remains controversial. The majority of small lesions can be followed with expectant management and surveillance, with routine radiography and endoscopy. Indications for surgical removal include unremitting symptoms, tumor size greater than 3 cm in diameter, progressive increase in tumor size, mucosal ulceration, and confirmation of histopathologic diagnosis. The procedure is performed via thoracotomy or thoracoscopy with a longitudinal esophageal myotomy, enucleation of the mass, and reapproximation of the myotomy. With this approach, mortality is approximately 0.5% to 1%, with more than 90% of patients remaining symptom-free at 5 years. Complications, although rare, include esophageal leak, cardiopulmonary complications, chyle leak, and chronic thoracotomy pain. Recurrence is extremely rare. Esophageal resection is usually required with larger lesions greater than 8 cm or with annular lesions.

Benign mucosal polyps are also extremely rare. These lesions typically arise in older men and are localized to the cervical esophagus, where they are frequently attached to the cricoid cartilage. Polyps tend to lengthen progressively by pedicles over time owing to peristaltic contractions. Polyps that cannot be removed endoscopically can be removed surgically, usually by a lateral esophagostomy and resection of the mucosal base.

Hemangiomas account for 2% to 3% of benign lesions and typically present with upper gastrointestinal bleeding. Laser coagulation via endoscopy usually provides an effective treatment with excision reserved for recurrent bleeding.

Esophageal duplication cysts are a variation of a foregut cyst. They are lined with various types of epithelium and can occur anywhere along the length of the thoracic esophagus. Enteric and bronchogenic cysts are the most common and are of foregut origin. They usually present in childhood, are located on the right side in 60% of cases, and are associated with vertebral and spinal cord abnormalities. Over time, cysts have a tendency to ulcerate, bleed, and become infected. Surgical excision is generally recommended.

Schatzki ring is a submucosal band encircling the esophagus at the squamocolumnar junction. Symptoms of dysphagia generally arise during the ingestion of food. The treatment of choice is dilatation alone, with the majority of patients responding to the first dilatation. The natural history of these lesions remains unknown.

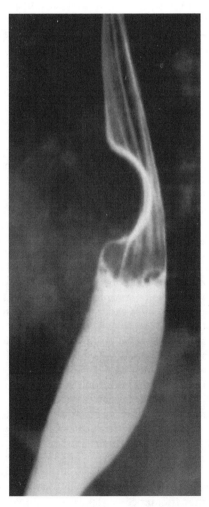

Figure 11-8 Barium esophagram showing a leiomyoma. (From Orringer MB. Tumors, injuries, and Miscellaneous conditions of the esophagus. In: Greenfield LJ, Mulholland MW, Oldham KT et al., eds. *Surgery: scientific principles and practice*, 3rd ed. Philadelphia: Lippincott Williams & Wilkins, 2001:694.)

MALIGNANT ESOPHAGEAL NEOPLASMS

The prevalence of esophageal carcinoma varies worldwide, primarily because of the influence of local dietary and environmental factors. In high-risk areas such as China and Iran, the incidence can be as high as 180 per 100,000 men. In the United States, the highest prevalence occurs in men; the incidence is 6 per 100,000 men annually (13 per 100,000 black men). Approximately 13,900 new cases are diagnosed and 13,000 deaths occur per year.

These numbers represent a 15% to 20% increase over the last decade.

Histologically, 90% of esophageal cancers can be divided into either squamous cell carcinoma (SCCA) or adenocarcinoma. The other 10% usually comprise rare melanomas, leiomyosarcomas, carcinoids, and lymphomas. Of interest, over the last 20 years, the incidence of SCCA has decreased dramatically, for unknown reasons, whereas adenocarcinoma has increased 450% in white men and 50% in black men. Approximately three fourths of adenocarcinomas arise in the distal two thirds of the esophagus, whereas SCCA arises more commonly in the middle and lower thirds of the esophagus. The etiology of the various carcinomas varies significantly. Common etiologies of both types of cancer include smoking tobacco (both quantity and duration of smoking), carcinogens including *N*-nitrosamines, and a prior history of radiotherapy to the mediastinum. Unlike adenocarcinoma, SCCA is implicated with chronic irritation associated with alcohol, achalasia, chronic esophagitis, diverticula, caustic injury, extremely hot fluids, and possibly human papillomavirus (HPV). SCCA has also been linked to rare deficiency syndromes such as *Plummer-Vinson* (dysphagia, iron-deficiency anemia, atrophic oral mucosa, spoon-shaped fingers with brittle nails, and esophageal webs) as well as genetic syndromes such as nonepidermolytic palmoplantar keratoderma (autosomal dominant hyperkeratosis of palms and soles, thickening of oral mucosa, and 95% risk of SSCA by the age of 70). Unlike adenocarcinoma, SCCA has a strong predilection for low socioeconomic class.

The incidence of adenocarcinoma has increased considerably in Western countries, such as the United States and those in Europe, for unclear reasons. Patients with reflux symptoms have an eightfold increased risk of adenocarcinoma of the esophagus. The most important reason is likely linked to gastroesophageal reflux and the development of Barrett columnar cell metaplasia in 5% to 8% of these patients. Patients with Barrett esophagus are at a high risk for adenocarcinoma, with an annual rate of neoplastic transformation estimated at 0.5% per year. In addition, Barrett esophagus is present in 80% of patients with adenocarcinoma of the distal esophagus. Obesity is also a risk factor for adenocarcinoma.

Screening has not been advocated, except in high-risk patients such as those with Barrett esophagus, because of the high cost and low prevalence of the disease. In these patients, endoscopy is recommended every 3 to 5 years and more frequently in the presence of low-grade dysplasia. Patients treated with proton-pump inhibitors may often experience reversal of the metaplasia to normal squamous mucosa. Whether this reduces the overall risk of cancer in these patients remains unknown. High-grade dysplasia is an indication for esophagectomy. Without treatment, up to one half of patients with high-grade dysplasia will develop adenocarcinoma within 3 years.

Patients with esophageal cancer usually present with dysphagia, odynophagia, anorexia, and weight loss. Lymphadenopathy (Virchow node), hepatomegaly, or pleural effusions are highly suggestive of distant disease. Diagnosis can usually be confirmed with esophagoscopy. Other studies during the workup should include a chest radiograph, barium esophagram, and CT scan or MRI for metastatic disease. Endoscopic ultrasonography has 90% accuracy in determining T stage in 80% to 90% of patients and N stage in 70% to 80% of patients. Endoscopic ultrasonographic–guided fine needle aspiration has also been used to increase staging accuracy. Positron emission tomography can be used to detect metastatic disease and has been shown to detect distant disease in 15% of patients thought to have localized cancers. Although extremely accurate, thoracoscopic and laparoscopic staging has largely been replaced by less invasive methods.

Tumors are classified according to the 2002 American Joint Committee on Cancer (AJCC) Tumor-Node-Metastasis (TNM) system (Table 11-1). Overall survival depends on stage, with approximately 50% of patients presenting with distant metastases. Unfortunately, these patients have a survival rate of less than 1 year. Among the other patients undergoing treatment, overall 5-year survival rates exceed 95% for stage 0, 50% to 80% for stage I, 30% to 40% for stage IIA, 10% to 30% for stage IIB, and 10% to 15% for stage III. In addition, lymphatic micrometastases, advanced age, large tumor burden, dysphagia, and weight loss greater than 10% of body mass confer a poor outcome.

Surgery remains the mainstay of treatment for localized esophageal carcinoma. Tumors of the middle third of the esophagus are approached via a right thoracotomy combined with an abdominal incision and an intrathoracic anastomosis: the *Ivor-Lewis procedure* (Fig. 11-9). Resection can also be accomplished by a cervical anastomosis with use of the three-field technique, the *McKeown procedure*. Tumors of the lower third of the esophagus are best approached via a transhiatal approach or a left thoracoabdominal incision (Fig. 11-10). Minimally invasive esophagectomy has also been described, although its role remains to be defined. Regardless of the approach, the procedure involves resection of the esophagus with anastomosis to an interposed colon, stomach, or jejunum. Stomach reconstruction involves division of the short gastrics, left gastric, left gastroepiploic, and right gastric arteries, with the sole blood supply via the right gastroepiploic artery.

The advantages and disadvantages among approaches are debatable. The transhiatal approach does not permit a formal lymph node dissection because of the limited exposure of the mediastinal lymph node compartment. However, the transhiatal approach avoids the morbidity associated with a thoracotomy and its subsequent cardiopulmonary sequelae. In addition, a cervical anastomotic leak complicating a transhiatal esophagectomy is easier to control than an intrathoracic leak that may complicate an anastomosis within the chest. Comparable survival results have been reported with either transthoracic or transhiatal procedures, with an overall mortality rate of 5%, perioperative morbidity rates of 26% to 41%, and 5-year survival rates approaching 15% to 24%.

The use of other modalities as an alternative or adjunct to surgery remains controversial. Radiotherapy alone (doses of 5,000 to 6,800 cGy) yields 5-year survival rates similar to that of surgery without the perioperative morbidity and mortality associated with surgery. However, radiotherapy is not as effective at providing long-term relief from dysphagia and odynophagia, and it is associated with a higher incidence of devastating local complications such as the formation of esophageal-tracheal fistulas. In addition, preoperative neoadjuvant radiotherapy (doses of 2,000 to 4,000 cGy) has failed to demonstrate any survival advantage.

TABLE 11-1

TNM STAGING CLASSIFICATION FOR CANCER OF THE ESOPHAGUS

TNM DEFINITIONS

Primary tumor (T)

TX	Primary tumor cannot be assessed (cytologically positive tumor not evident endoscopically or radiographically)
T0	No evidence of primary tumor (e.g., after treatment with radiation and chemotherapy)
Tis	Carcinoma in situ
T1	Tumor invades lamina propria or submucosa, but not beyond it
T2	Tumor invades muscularis propria
T3	Tumor invades adventitia
T4	Tumor invades adjacent structures (e.g., aorta, tracheobronchial tree, vertebral bodies, and pericardium)

Regional lymph node involvement (N)

NX	Regional nodes cannot be assessed
N0	No regional node metastasis
N1	Regional node metastasis

Distant metastasis (M)

MX	Presence of distant metastasis cannot be assessed
M0	No distant metastasis
M1	**Distant metastasis**

Tumors of the lower thoracic esophagus
   M1a Metastasis in celiac lymph nodes
   M1b Other distant metastasis
Tumors of the midthoracic esophagus
   M1a Not applicable
   M1b Nonregional lymph nodes and/or other distant metastasis
Tumors of the upper thoracic esophagus
   M1a Metastasis in cervical nodes
   M1b Other distant metastasis

STAGE GROUPING

Stage 0	Tis N0 M0
Stage I	T1 N0 M0
Stage IIA	T2 N0 M0
	T3 N0 M0
Stage IIB	T1 N1 M0
	T2 N1 M0
Stage III	T3 N1 M0
	T4 any N M0
Stage IV	Any T any N M1
Stage IVA	Any T any N M1a
Stage IVB	Any T any N M1b

From Fleming ID, Cooper JS, Henson DE et al., eds. *American Joint Commission on Cancer staging handbook.* From the AJCC staging manual, 5th ed. Philadelphia: Lippincott Williams & Wilkins, 1998:65–69, with permission.

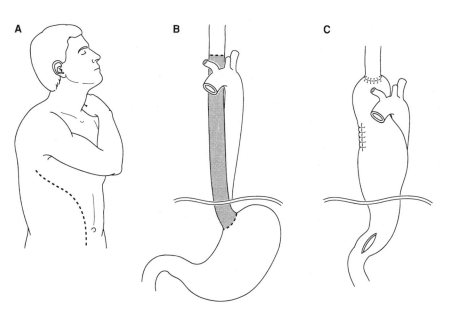

Figure 11-9 Standard Ivor-Lewis esophagogastrectomy for lesions of the lower and middle third of the thoracic esophagus. **A:** The continuous thoracoabdominal incision and the separate thoracic and abdominal incisions that may be used. **B:** Portion of the esophagus to be resected (*shaded area*). **C:** Completed reconstruction with high intrathoracic esophagogastroanastomosis and gastric drainage procedure. (From Ellis FH, Jr. Treatment of carcinoma of the esophagus and cardia. *Mayo Clin Proc* 1960;35:653, with permission.)

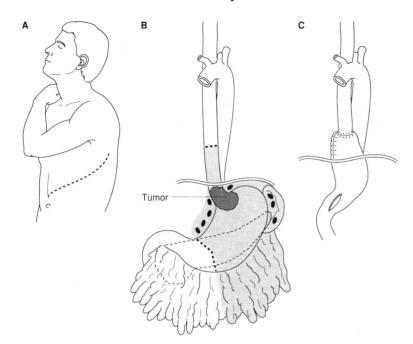

Tumor

Figure 11-10 Standard thoracoabdominal esophagogastrectomy for lesions of the distal esophagus and cardia. **A:** Incision. **B:** Margins of resection (*shaded area*). **C:** Completed reconstruction with intrathoracic esophagogastroanastomosis and either pyloromyotomy or pyloroplasty to prevent postvagotomy pylorospasm. (From Ellis FH, Jr. Treatment of carcinoma of the esophagus and cardia. *Mayo Clin Proc* 1960;35:653, with permission.)

Large randomized multi-institutional trials involving neoadjuvant chemotherapy (cisplatin and fluorouracil) demonstrate conflicting results. Although one study showed no survival benefit, another resulted in a 2-year survival benefit of 43% compared to 34% in those receiving surgery alone. Overall, any benefit obtained following preoperative chemotherapy seems to be small if at all present.

Furthermore, several large randomized trials testing preoperative chemoradiotherapy resulted in similar controversial results. Only one study demonstrated a favorable 3-year survival advantage in those patients treated with cisplatin and fluorouracil followed by 4,000 cGy of radiation. The remaining studies failed to demonstrate any survival advantage. Postoperative chemoradiotherapy is reserved for patients with incomplete resections. Chemotherapy with radiotherapy without surgery has been shown to offer a long-term survival benefit of 26%, similar to surgery alone.

Treatment for advanced esophageal cancer includes palliative measures aimed at improving dysphagia, preventing obstruction, and improving overall quality of life. Chemotherapy is the main treatment of choice aimed at the palliation of dysphagia and obstruction. Patients receiving chemotherapy can have response rates of upward of 50%. Recently, encouraging results have been obtained with the use of endoscopically placed coated stents. Stents offer immediate relief from symptoms of obstruction. In addition, palliative stents have also dramatically changed the management of esophageal-airway fistulas. The development of an esophageal-airway fistula can be a life-threatening complication and usually presents with cough, aspiration, or pneumonia. Endoscopic stents can successfully seal these fistulas. Unfortunately, esophageal cancer remains an overwhelmingly aggressive tumor and any benefit from palliative measures is usually short-lived.

KEY POINTS

▲ Laparoscopic myotomy is the procedure of choice for inadequate relaxation of the lower esophageal sphincter (LES); achalasia.

▲ Early endoscopy and repeated dilatations are indicated for caustic injuries to the esophagus.

▲ Early recognition (less than 24 hours) and primary repair of esophageal perforations improve mortality.

▲ Esophagectomy is the treatment of choice for local esophageal cancer; there is yet no clear role for adjuvant or neoadjuvant chemoradiation in esophageal cancer.

SUGGESTED READINGS

Brinster CJ, Singhal S, Lee L, et al. Evolving options in the management of esophageal perforation. *Ann Thorac Surg* 2004;77(4):1475–1483.

Enzinger PC, Mayer RJ. Esophageal cancer. *N Engl J Med* 2003;349: 2241–2252.

Lee LS, Singhal S, Brinster CJ, et al. Current management of esophageal leiomyoma. *J Am Coll Surg* 2004;198:136–146.

Richter JE. Oesophageal motility disorders. *Lancet* 2001;358:823–828.

The Stomach

12

Jagajan Karmacharya   *Jon B. Morris*

ANATOMY

The stomach and duodenum are derived from the caudal portion of the embryonic foregut as a dilation during the fifth week of gestation. Morphologic development is completed by the sixth to seventh week of gestation. The primitive stomach is invested within the ventral mesentery and the dorsal mesentery. In postnatal life, the ventral mesentery is represented as the lesser omentum, consisting of the falciform ligament, and the gastrohepatic and hepatoduodenal mesenteries. The greater omentum (former dorsal mesentery) forms the gastrosplenic and gastrophrenic ligaments. Rotation of the gut causes the left vagal trunk to lie in its anterior portion, whereas the right trunk lies farther posterior in relation to the stomach wall. The stomach lies most commonly between the tenth thoracic and the third lumbar vertebral segments, fixed at these points by the gastroesophageal junction proximally and the retroperitoneal junction distally.

The stomach is divided into four parts, serving as guidelines in planning surgical resection (Fig. 12-1). The *cardia* is located immediately distal to the gastroesophageal junction while the *fundus* is the portion above the gastroesophageal junction. The *body* (corpus) is the central portion of the stomach, marked distally by the *angularis incisura*, a crease on the lesser curvature, just proximal to the terminal nerves of Latarjet (terminal posterior branches of the vagus to the antrum). The distal thickened segment of the stomach is the *pylorus*, often identified by palpation and presence of the *vein of Mayo*. Finally, the *antrum* is the inferior portion of the stomach just proximal to the pyloric sphincter.

Anteriorly, the stomach comes in contact with the left hemidiaphragm, the left lobe of the liver, the anterior portion of the right lobe of the liver, and the parietal surface of the abdominal wall. On its posterior surface, the topographic relations of the stomach are as follows: left diaphragm; left kidney; left adrenal gland; neck, tail, and body of pancreas; aorta; celiac trunk; and periaortic nerve plexus. Nestled in the concavity of the spleen is the left lateral portion of the stomach. The transverse colon and its mesentery lie caudad to the greater curvature.

An abundant network of extramural and intramural vascular collaterals exists in the stomach. The blood supply of the stomach is primarily derived from branches of the celiac trunk, as detailed below. The *left gastric artery*, the first branch

of the celiac trunk, and the *right gastric artery*, a branch of the hepatic artery, supply the lesser curvature. Branches of the *splenic artery*—the *short gastric arteries*, and the *left gastroepiploic*—supply the greater curvature. The greater curvature is also supplied by the *right gastroepiploic artery*, a branch of the gastroduodenal artery. The venous drainage parallels the arterial supply (Fig. 12-2). The left gastric vein is also known as the coronary vein.

Lymph nodes drain from the proximal lesser curvature into the superior gastric lymph nodes surrounding the left gastric artery and from the distal lesser curvature portion to the suprapyloric lymph nodes. Pancreaticosplenic nodes and subpyloric and omental nodes drain the proximal and the antral portions of the greater curve, respectively. Ultimately, all of the lymph nodes drain via the base of the celiac axis. Metastatic disease can bypass and present beyond the primary nodes owing to extensive intramural and extramural communications.

Two vagal trunks emerge through the esophageal hiatus of the diaphragm. The left trunk is on the anterior surface of the esophagus and the right is posterior, between the esophagus and the aorta. The anterior vagus nerve gives off the hepatic branch and then courses along the lesser curvature. This nerve provides vagal innervation to the anterior gastric wall (Fig. 12-3). The posterior vagus nerve branches into

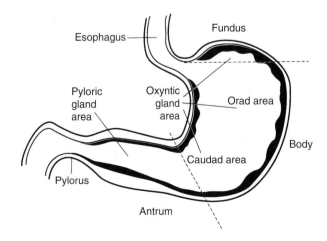

Figure 12-1 The stomach is anatomically divided into four parts with different anatomic functions. (From Johnson LR. Secretion. In: Johnson LR, ed. *Essential medical physiology.* New York: JB Lippincott, 1992:482, with permission.)

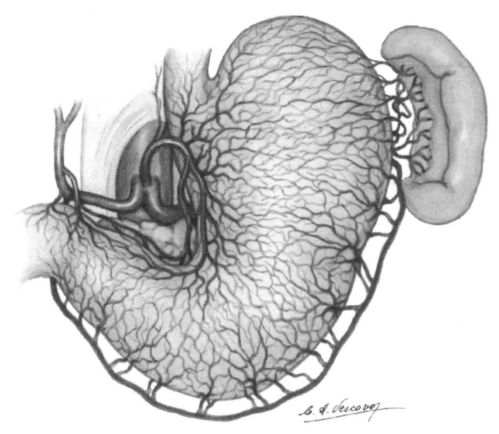

Figure 12-2   The stomach is an extremely vascular organ with blood supply from the left and right gastroepiploic arteries, left and right gastric arteries, and the short splenic vessels. (From Etala E. *Atlas of gastrointestinal surgery*. Philadelphia: Lippincott-Raven, 1997:879, with permission.)

the celiac division and the posterior division, which supplies the posterior gastric wall. A high branch also known as the *criminal nerve of Grassi* should be identified during truncal vagotomy.

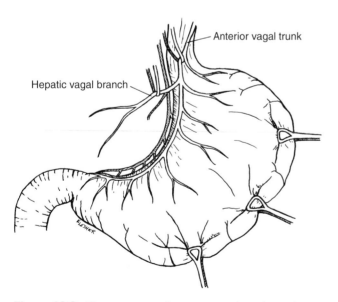

Figure 12-3   The vagus nerve forms two vagal trunks on the anterior and posterior surfaces of the stomach. The anterior vagal trunk gives off the hepatic vagal branch. (From Sawers JL. Selective vagotomy and pyloroplasty. In: Nyhus LM, Baker RJ, eds. *Mastery of surgery*, 2nd ed. Philadelphia: Little, Brown and Company, 1992:674, with permission.)

Mostly afferent, the vagal trunks transmit information to the central nervous system. Ten percent of the vagal fibers are motor or secretory efferents. Parasympathetic fibers originate in the dorsal nucleus of the medulla. They synapse in the myenteric and submucosal plexus and secondary neurons that directly innervate the gastric smooth and epithelial cells. Pain from the stomach and the duodenum are sensed through the afferent fibers of the sympathetic system. These fibers are derived from spinal segments T5 through T10, entering gray rami communicantes to the prevertebral ganglia. Presynaptic nerves then pass through the greater splanchnic nerve to the celiac plexus. Postsynaptic fibers from the celiac plexus innervate the stomach.

Gastric mucosa is lined by simple columnar cells with three types of specialized gastric glands: cardiac, oxyntic, and antral. Cardiac glands occupy the narrow transition zone between stratified squamous epithelium of the esophagus and simple columnar cells of the stomach. The functional importance of the cardiac gland, other than the secretion of mucus, is not completely understood. The fundus and body of the stomach contain the tubular oxyntic glands in which the acid-secreting parietal cells are prominent (Fig. 12-4). Oxyntic glands also contain chief cells that synthesize pepsinogen. The gland is divided into three regions: (i) isthmus, containing surface mucosal cells and a few parietal cells; (ii) neck, containing a high concentration of parietal cells and few mucosal cells; and (iii) base, containing chief cells, few parietal cells, scattered mucosal cells, and undifferentiated cells. The parietal cell has a unique canalicular structure that extends from the basal

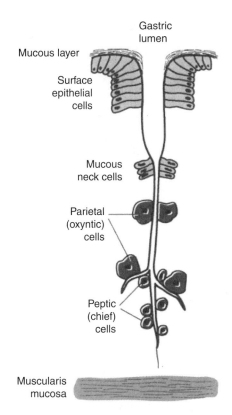

Figure 12-4 The oxyntic gland is divided into three regions: (i) the surface, containing mucosal cells; (ii) the neck, containing mainly parietal cells and a few mucosal cells; (iii) and the base, containing mainly chief cells. (From Johnson LR. Secretion. In: Johnson LR, ed. *Essential medical physiology.* New York: JB Lippincott, 1992:482, with permission.)

cytoplasm to the gastric lumen. This canalicular system becomes prominent and conspicuous on stimulation. The canaliculi is lined by microvilli. Parietal cells have high oxidative rates, as reflected by an increased number of mitochondria during stimulation. Antral glands are located in the distal stomach, or antrum, as well as in the pyloric channel. Gastrin-secreting cells are a distinctive feature of this gland and can be identified morphologically by numerous dense granules containing this hormone. Upon stimulation, gastrin diffuses through the basal membrane and into the bloodstream. Endocrine cells are generally found in all three regions.

PHYSIOLOGY

The complex physiologic function of the stomach is linked with its overall role in digestion and is discussed in detail in Chapter 16, "Nutrition, Digestion, and Absorption." We briefly summarize herein the elements of gastric physiology most pertinent to the gastric disease processes that are subsequently discussed in this chapter.

Gastric acid is a known contributor to the pathogenesis of peptic ulcer disease. Under normal circumstances, the stimulation of acid secretion occurs in three phases: cephalic, gastric, and intestinal. The basal acid secretion is 2 to 5 mEq per hour in a fasting state and is determined by the ambient histamine secretion plus the vagal tone. The *cephalic phase* is mediated by the vagus nerve, and it begins

with the thought, sight, and smell of food. Cholinergic stimulation is by direct action on gastrin cells. Binding of acetylcholine and related cholinergic agonists to muscarinic receptors results in mobilization of intracellular calcium via protein phosphorylation, resulting in hydrogen ion secretion. The maximum output in a normal person is 10 mEq per hour during the cephalic phase. Entry of food marks the beginning of the *gastric phase*. The most important stimulants are the presence of partially hydrolyzed food and gastric distention. Small peptide fragments and amino acids, particularly tryptophan and phenylalanine, stimulate the release of gastrin. This acid regulatory peptide is derived from its prehormone (preprogastrin). Local cholinergic intramural reflexes increase sensitization of parietal cells to the effects of gastrin. Stimulation of gastrin receptors (situated in the basolateral membrane) result in acid secretion. Gastrin, like histamine and acetylcholine, acts via the membrane-bound parietal cell proton pump or the hydrogen ion pump. (Fig. 12-5). Entry of gastric contents into the intestine marks the *intestinal phase*. The hormones enterooxyntin, secretin, somatostatin, peptide YY, gastric inhibitory peptide, and neurotensin have been proposed as the mediators during this phase of gastric-acid secretion.

The stomach also serves to store, mix, and triturate (reduction of size) ingested food. Postprandial gastric distention, texture, volume, and osmolality of meals influence gastric peristalsis. The most important factor is vagally controlled distention known as "receptive relaxation," which allows the accommodation of food in the proximal stomach. This function is lost in patients who have undergone truncal vagotomy.

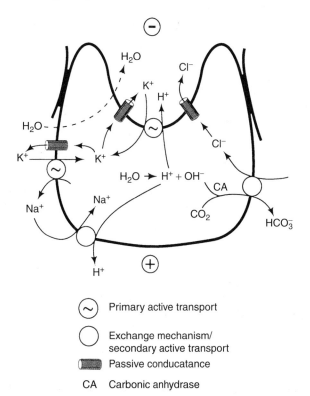

○~ Primary active transport

○ Exchange mechanism/ secondary active transport

▭ Passive conducatance

CA Carbonic anhydrase

Figure 12-5 The gastric parietal cell produces hydrochloric acid and creates and acidic intraluminal gastric environment. (From Johnson LR. Secretion. In: Johnson LR, ed. *Essential medical physiology.* New York: JB Lippincott, 1992:485, with permission.)

After every meal, approximately 1,000 mL of gastric juice is secreted by the stomach. Important components are mucus, HCO_3, pepsinogen, and intrinsic factor. *Mucus*, produced by the parietal and oxyntic glands, is 95% water combined with high molecular weight glycoproteins. Mucus is extremely important in lubrication and protection of the gastric mucosa from the locally acidic milieu. This mucoid gel forms a layer on the gastric mucosal surface known as the "unstirred layer." HCO_3 ions formed as a byproduct of acid secretion are trapped in this layer, and maintain neutrality over the gastric mucosa, despite the low luminal pH. The combination of HCO_3 and the unstirred layer of mucoid gel acts as a mechanical barrier to the effects of acid. *Pepsinogen* is synthesized by chief cells and is stored as visible granules. Its precursor zymogen is activated by falling pH level, resulting in cleavage of a polypeptide fragment to active enzyme pepsin. Pepsin catalyzes hydrolysis of peptide bonds containing phenylalanine, tyrosine, and leucine. The most important stimulus for pepsin secretion is stimulation of muscarinic receptors of the M1 type (cholinergic). The major function of pepsin is to initiate protein digestion, and pepsin functions optimally at a pH of 2.0 and is irreversibly denatured at a pH of 7.0 or greater. Finally, a mucoprotein, *intrinsic factor*, is secreted by parietal cells of the gastric mucosa. This factor is necessary for the absorption of cobalamin (vitamin B_{12}) from the terminal ileum. Histamine, acetylcholine, and gastrin stimulate intrinsic factor secretion. Atrophy of the parietal cells results in a deficiency of intrinsic factor and pernicious anemia. This deficiency can be corrected by parenteral administration of vitamin B_{12}. Total gastrectomy results in the permanent dependency of parenteral vitamin B_{12} administration.

PEPTIC ULCER DISEASE

Pathophysiology of Peptic Ulcer Disease

Current theory underlying the pathogenesis of peptic ulcer disease (PUD) involves the disequilibrium of acid secretion and mucosal defense (Table 12-1). The dictum "no acid, no ulcer" still holds true. Environmental factors such as smoking and use of alcohol and nonsteroidal antiinflammatory drugs (NSAIDs) have all been implicated in ulcerogenesis (Table 12-2). Cigarette smoking is a major risk factor. Smoking has been shown to impair ulcer healing, increase the rate of recurrence, and decrease effective medical therapy, thereby resulting in the need for surgical inter-

TABLE 12-1

FACTORS MODULATING GASTRIC MUCOSAL PROTECTION

Stimulation	Inhibition
cAMP	NSAID
Prostaglandins	α-Adrenergic agonists
Cholinomimetics	Bile acids
CCK	Acetazolamide
Glucagon	Ethanol

cAMP, cyclic adenosine monophosphate; CCK, cholecystokinin; NSAID, nonsteroidal antiinflammatory drug.

TABLE 12-2

POSTULATED PATHOGENETIC FACTORS IN PATIENTS WITH DUODENAL ULCERS

Acid secretion

Increased acid secretory capacity
Increased basal secretion
Increased pentagastrin-stimulated output
Increased meal response
Abnormal gastric emptying

Environment

Cigarette smoking
Nonsteroidal antiinflammatory drug
Helicobacter infection

Mucosal defense

Decreased duodenal HCO_3 production
Decreased gastric mucosal prostaglandin production

From Mulholland MW. Duodenal ulcer. In: Greenfield LJ, Mulholland MW, Oldham KT et al., eds. *Surgery: scientific principles and practice*, 2nd ed. Philadelphia: Lippincott-Raven, 1997:759, with permission.

vention. The suggested mechanisms include altered mucosal blood flow, increased bile reflux, decreased mucosal prostaglandin (PGE_2) production, and increased acid stimulation. All of these are key factors that affect patients who continue to smoke. Clearly, counseling regarding cessation of smoking is mandatory. Widespread belief that dietary factors cause ulcers is not generally supported by the scientific evidence. Alcohol in moderation is not harmful, but there is evidence to indicate that alcohol consumption in excess impairs ulcer healing. The use of NSAIDs can result in a variety of duodenal and gastric lesions, leading to hemorrhage, superficial erosions, and deep ulcerations. The U.S. Food and Drug Administration (FDA) estimates the rate of NSAID-induced ulcers to be 2% to 4% per patient-year. The mechanism involves systemic suppression of PGE_2 production and loss of mucosal protection. All NSAIDs pose the risk of peptic ulceration, and all patients should therefore use NSAIDs with caution. Concurrent use of NSAIDs with alcohol and tobacco increases the rate of ulceration. A large body of evidence now supports the view that infection with the bacterium *Helicobacter pylori* causes peptic ulceration. Warren and Marshall were the first to demonstrate a spiral urease-producing, gram-negative organism that caused antral gastritis and peptic ulceration. They subsequently demonstrated that eradication of the organism resulted in healing of the ulcer. Evidence supporting the pathogenesis of *H. pylori* in duodenal ulcer disease is summarized in Table 12-3.

Clinical Features and Treatment

Many patients report epigastric pain. This burning, stabbing, gnawing pain is worse in the morning and is commonly relieved by eating or taking antacids. Pain referred to the back may signal perforation or penetration into the head of the pancreas. Physical examination is typically nonspecific in uncomplicated cases. The differential diagnosis includes nonspecific dyspepsia, gastric neoplasia, cholelithiasis, pancreatitis, and pancreatic neoplasia. Diagnostic evaluation

TABLE 12-3

SUPPORT FOR THE ROLE OF *HELICOBACTER PYLORI* IN ULCER DISEASE

1. *Helicobacter pylori*–positive patients almost always demonstrate antral gastritis, characterized by nonerosive mucosal inflammation.
2. *H. pylori* binds only to gastric epithelium.
3. Eradication of *H. pylori* results in resolution of gastritis with antimicrobials, and recurrence is associated with reinfection.
4. Intragastric administration of isolated organism in animal models and in two humans resulted in lesions of chronic superficial gastritis.

From Mulholland MW. Duodenal ulcer. In: Greenfield LJ, Mulholland MW, Oldham KT et al., eds. *Surgery: scientific principles and practice*, 2nd ed. Philadelphia: Lippincott-Raven, 1997:768, with permission.

typically involves either a barium contrast study or endoscopy. Acid secretory studies are no longer used routinely.

Of all dyspeptic patients referred for endoscopy, 13% have duodenal ulcers, 10% have gastric ulcers, 2% have gastric cancer, and up to 15% have esophagitis. Duodenal ulcers have a typical appearance with sharp edges and a clean smooth base. Recent hemorrhage is characterized by an eschar or exudate. Ulcers are usually surrounded by a local inflammatory response. Histolopathologic evaluation of duodenal ulcers demonstrates gastric metaplasia in the surrounding tissue, infiltration with chronic and acute inflammatory cells, and fibrosis. Radiographic signs of an acute ulcer usually are seen in profile or en face, with erosion of the normal smooth outline. Changes associated with chronicity and scarring can be evident with distortion of the duodenal bulb or pseudodiverticulum formation. Despite the predilection for higher acid secretion in those with duodenal ulcer, circulating serum gastrin levels are typically normal (50 to 100 pg per mL), and measuring gastrin levels is only helpful if *Zollinger–Ellison syndrome* is suspected.

Diagnosis and eradication of *H. pylori* infection is paramount to successful therapy. Presence of the organism can be determined by endoscopic or nonendoscopic methods. Serology is a reliable marker of initial infection, because most people harboring the organism will develop circulating antibodies. However, this is unreliable in documenting clearance as patients can retain serologic positivity for a prolonged period of time, even after the eradication of the bacteria. The urea breath test is a more reliable, nonendoscopic measure of infection. It relies on the principle that labeled urea is converted into ammonia and labeled carbon dioxide by the *H. pylori* urease in the stomach. The carbon dioxide is then absorbed through the stomach wall and can be detected upon expiration. Endoscopic diagnosis relies on the ability to detect *H. pylori* within endoscopic biopsies of the gastric mucosa or the prescence of urease.

Medical therapy is directed toward both the healing of the ulcer with reduction of acid secretion and definitive cure with eradication of *H. pylori*. Powerful antisecretory drugs include histamine antagonists (cimetidine and ranitidine) and proton pump inhibitors (omeprazole). *Histamine receptor antagonists* bind competitively to parietal cell histamine receptors, producing reversible inhibition of

acid secretion. Peak plasma concentrations are generally reached within 1 to 3 hours after oral administration. Renal failure significantly alters plasma clearance of these drugs. Six weeks of treatment with histamine receptor antagonists will heal a duodenal ulcer in 80% of patients. If the medication is stopped, however, half of the patients may present with recurrent ulceration within the year. This can be avoided by long-term, single-dose bedtime administration of a histamine antagonist. *Proton pump inhibitors* (omeprazole) in therapeutic doses cause near-complete inhibition of acid secretion. These drugs act specifically in the gastric mucosa, binding to the parietal cell membrane–associated H^+/K^+ ATPase. Several studies have demonstrated the superiority of proton pump inhibitors over histamine antagonists given higher healing rates (80% within 2 weeks) and a reduction in associated epigastric pain. However, ulcer recurrence is common after the cessation of treatment with proton pump inhibitors as well. Long-term maintenance on omeprazole is not recommended, as effects of sustained hypergastrinemia are not known. If long-term maintenance is necessary, an attractive option is *sucralfate*, an aluminum salt of sulfated sucrose. This polymer acts by providing a protective coat over the gastric and duodenal mucosa, which binds bile acids and inhibits pepsin while stimulating mucus, prostaglandin, and HCO_3 secretion. Side effects are minimal, and there is virtually negligible systemic absorption. It is also the drug of choice for ulcer therapy during pregnancy. When administered at a dose of 1 g four times a day, ulcer healing is achieved within 4 weeks in 80% of patients. *Misoprostol*, a prostaglandin analog, should be avoided during pregnancy because of its abortifacient properties. Three fourths of patients treated with misoprostal achieve healing in 4 weeks. The major side effect of misoprostol in nonpregnant patients is diarrhea. *Antacids* should be used as supplements to the antisecretory drugs mentioned previously.

Eradication of *H. pylori* infection eliminates recurrent ulceration, unless recurrent ulceration is caused by reinfection (10% of cases). Various therapeutic combinations exist and treatment with bismuth subsalicylate, metronidazole, tetracycline, and omeprazole has the highest cure rate (94% to 98%), but compliance is difficult to achieve. Less expensive alternatives consist of clarithromycin and metronidazole or amoxicillin with omeprazole for 1 week. An equally effective regimen involves the combination of antibiotics with a histamine receptor antagonist for 2 weeks. It is generally accepted that acid-suppressive therapy continue for 6 weeks after eradication of *H. pylori*.

Surgical treatment for duodenal ulcer disease is indicated if medical treatment fails or if the patient presents with the classical complications of peptic ulcer disease such as hemorrhage, perforation, or obstruction. Widely used procedures include (i) *truncal vagotomy with drainage*, (ii) *truncal vagotomy and antrectomy*, and (iii) *highly selective vagotomy*. Truncal vagotomy must be combined with a drainage procedure, as denervation will result in impaired pyloric coordination and gastric emptying as first described by Dragstedt. The method of drainage usually selected is a *pyloroplasty*. Heineke-Mikulicz pyloroplasty is most commonly performed, as it offers the advantage of preserving continuity of the duodenal loop, hence the integrity of the hormonal milieu (Fig. 12-6). If the duodenum is scarred, then another option involves the creation of a posterior

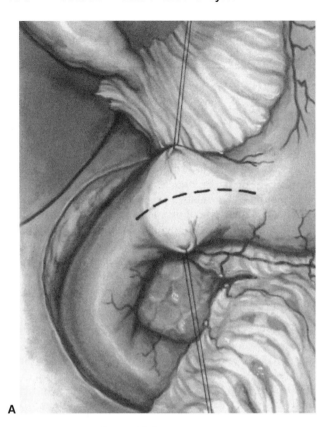

A

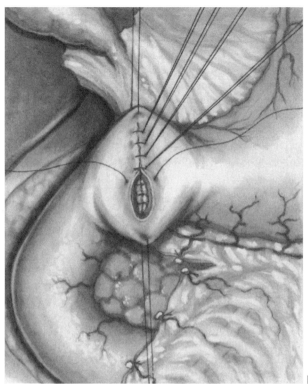

B

Figure 12-6   The Heineke-Mikulicz pyloroplasty enlarges the gastric outlet by closing a longitudinal pyloric incision **(A)** in a transverse fashion **(B)**. (From Etala E. *Atlas of gastrointestinal surgery.* Philadelphia: Lippincott-Raven, 1997:1085, with permission.)

gastrojejunostomy. Complete acid reduction is achieved by truncal vagotomy combined with resection of gastric antrum. This entails a 50% resection of the distal stomach, and the remnant is anastomosed to the duodenum (Billroth I resection) or to the proximal jejunum (Billroth II resection) (Fig. 12-7). The morbidity rate of this operation is higher owing to the combination of partial gastric resection with vagotomy. Highly selective vagotomy involves resection of the nerve fibers to the acid-secreting fundic mucosa while preserving the fibers to the antrum and the pylorus, thereby preserving gastric emptying. The denervation of the nerve fibers begins at the distal 5 to 7 cm of the esophagus and extends along the lesser curvature to 5 cm of the proximal pylorus (Fig. 12-8).

Complications of Ulcer Surgery

The physiologic consequences of truncal vagotomy are listed in Table 12-4. All forms of vagotomy cause postoperative hypergastrinemia owing to decreased luminal acid, loss of inhibitory feedback, and loss of vagal inhibition. In most cases chronic hypergastrinemia is caused by gastrin-cell hyperplasia. Antrectomy combined with truncal vagotomy causes greater reduction in acid secretion than vagotomy alone. Vagotomy alters gastric emptying, as vagus-mediated receptive relaxation is lost. Truncal vagotomy affects the motor activity of both the proximal and the distal stomach. Liquids are emptied at a faster rate because of alteration in gastroduodenal gastric pressure gradient for any given volume. Decreased gastric emptying can be improved when combined with pyloroplasty. Conversely, highly selective

vagotomy preserves mixing and triturating capacity of solid food, and emptying of solids is near normal.

Early complications of peptic ulcer surgery include duodenal stump leakage after a Billroth II resection, gastric retention, and hemorrhage. Later complications are recurrent ulcer, gastrojejunocolic and gastrocolic fistula, dumping syndrome, alkaline gastritis, anemia, postvagotomy diarrhea, chronic gastroparesis, and afferent loop syndrome. Recurrence rate of ulceration after a proximal vagotomy is 10%, and the rate is slightly lower when a truncal vagotomy is combined with pyloroplasty. There is a significant decrease in ulceration when truncal vagotomy is combined with antrectomy. Ulcers almost always develop on the intestinal side of the anastomosis. Patients classically complain of pain that is improved by eating or by antacids. In some patients, the pain is referred to the shoulder. Complications such as hemorrhage or perforation can also occur. The treatment for these complications are similar to that of the original ulcer. Patients presenting with severe diarrhea, weight loss, and a history of abdominal pain preceding the onset of diarrhea is characteristic of gastrocolic fistula. Low protein level and fluid electrolyte imbalance are typical. Barium enema is the investigation of choice. Once the patient's fluid and electrolytes are corrected, the fistula is excised and bowel continuity restored.

Dumping syndrome is characterized by gastrointestinal (GI) and vasomotor symptoms. It occurs to some extent in most patients with impaired gastric emptying but becomes a problem in about 2% when truncal vagotomy is combined with antrectomy. It is believed to result from symptoms, but definitive treatment involves prevention of reflux by creating a Roux-en-Y gastrojejunostomy with a 50- to 60-cm efferent jejunal limb. Iron deficiency anemia develops in one third of the patients after partial gastric resection owing to failure of organic iron absorption. Ferrous sulfate or ferrous gluconate, the inorganic form of iron, is normally absorbed and can be used to overcome this form of iron deficiency.

Gastric Ulcer

The peak incidence of gastric ulceration occurs in patients 40 to 60 years of age. Ninety-five percent of the ulcers are located along the lesser curvature. Signs and symptoms are similar to those of duodenal ulcer. Gastric ulcers are divided into four different types. Type I ulcers are usually found along the lesser curvature. Antral gastritis is always present, and in most cases, *H. pylori* infection is present. Type II ulcers are usually prepyloric and occur in association with duodenal ulcers. Type III ulcers occur in the antrum as a result of NSAID use. Type IV ulcers occur high on the lesser curvature and are similar in pathophysiology to type I ulcers (Fig. 12-9). Patients present with a history of epigastric pain are often relieved by food or antacids. The pain associated with gastric ulceration may appear soon after eating but at other times is aggravated by eating. Endoscopy should be performed to rule out a malignant gastric ulcer. Benign ulcers are characterized by flat edges, as opposed to malignant ulcers which are classically rolled. At least six biopsies from the margins should be obtained at the time of initial endoscopic examination to differentiate benign from malignant ulcers. An upper GI series can also demonstrate a gastric ulcer. Radiographic characteristics of a malignant ulcer include a prominent rim of radiolucency around the ulcer (meniscus sign) and a large ulcer size (more than 2 cm). The principal complications of gastric ulcer disease include bleeding, obstruction, and perforation. Etiology of gastric ulceration is often similar to that of duodenal ulcers, but patients with gastric ulcerations are rarely acid hypersecretors and pathogenesis lies mostly in loss of mucosal defense. The medical treatment is the same as for duodenal ulcers. Endoscopic evaluation is recommended at 2 to 3 months, particularly if the ulcer was greater than 2 cm, and *H. pylori* eradication should be confirmed after a course of medical management. Surgical treatment for primary, nonmalignant gastric ulcer is rarely indicated. Today, most surgical procedures are reserved for treatment of nonhealing gastric ulcers as well as for complications of ulcer disease such as bleeding, perforation, or obstruction. Truncal vagotomy combined with a drainage procedure or truncal vagotomy and Billroth I including the ulcer may suffice. The operation should be tailored with regard to the position of the ulcer.

Upper Gastrointestinal Hemorrhage

The most common causes of upper GI bleeding requiring hospital admission include peptic ulceration, esophageal or gastric bleeding from portal hypertension, and gastritis. An upper GI bleed is defined as bleeding that originates proximal to the ligament of Treitz and is usually bright red or dark. The presence of coffee-ground emesis indicates that blood has been in the stomach long enough for hemoglobin to convert to methemoglobin. Melena (passage

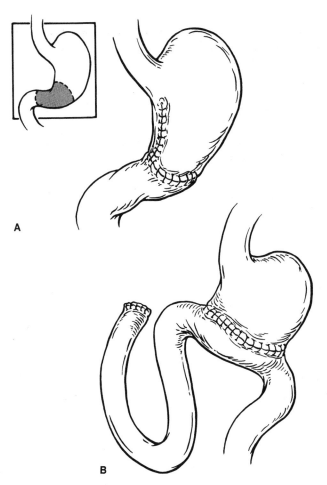

Figure 12-7 The anatomic differences between an antrectomy with a **(A)** Billroth I reconstruction and a **(B)** Billroth II resection. (From Mulholland MW. Peptic ulcer disease. In: Bell RH, Rikkers LF, Mulholland MW, eds. *Digestive tract surgery: a text and atlas.* Philadelphia: Lippincott-Raven, 1996:180, with permission.)

sudden osmotic load of ingested food in the small bowel. Symptoms include palpitations, sweating, weakness, dyspnea, flushing, nausea, abdominal cramps, belching, vomiting, diarrhea, and occasionally syncope. These symptoms classically occur shortly after a meal. In severe cases, patients may lie down for 30 to 40 minutes to achieve relief. A dietary regimen of low carbohydrates, with meals high in fat and protein content, as well as fluid restriction is sucessful in most patients and symptoms improve with time. Subcutaneous injection of a somatostatin analog (octreotide, at 50 to 100 μg) before a meal, may reduce symptoms of dumping in some patients. Although its mechanism of action is uncertain, it may act by reducing splanchnic blood flow, inhibiting release of vasoactive peptides, decreasing peak plasma insulin, and slowing intestinal transit time.

Alkaline reflux gastritis consists of postprandial epigastric pain, bile reflux, and histologic evidence of gastritis. The epigastric pain must be differentiated from recurrent ulceration, biliary and pancreatic conditions, afferent loop obstruction, and esophagitis. Endoscopic examination may show bile reflux and a patchy nonulcerative edematous mucosa. A more quantitative study may be obtained by using nuclear scans. Dietary and drug therapies improve

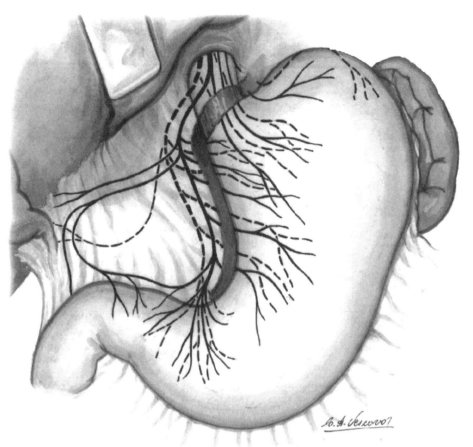

Figure 12-8 Unlike the truncal vagotomy, the proximal gastric vagotomy selectively denervates the lesser curvature of the stomach but spares the nerves to the pylorus and antrum. (From Etala E. *Atlas of gastrointestinal surgery*. Philadelphia: Lippincott-Raven Publishers, 1997:1047, with permission.)

of black tarry stools) is a nonspecific sign that, in general, poorly indicates the rate of bleeding and represents blood that has been in the intestine. The black color is due to *hematin*, the product of heme oxidation by bacterial and intestinal enzymes. *Hematochezia*, or the passage of

bright-red blood per rectum, due to upper GI bleeding is very unusual but, when present, may indicate massive upper GI bleeding.

Patients presenting with a history of hematemesis or melena of less than 12 hours require hospital admission. Patients should be questioned about predisposing factors for upper GI bleeding including NSAID use and other bleeding tendencies. A large nasogastric tube should be placed to check for intragastric blood, and a positive lavage result can confirm an upper GI source of bleeding. A negative lavage may occur in 20% of bleeding duodenal ulcers. Once the patient is stabilized and blood volume is restored, endoscopy should be performed within 24 hours. In 80% of the cases, the source of bleeding can be identified and treated endoscopically. Rarely it is necessary to use angiographic techniques to embolize a bleeding vessel.

A persistently hypotensive patient who requires more then 4 units of blood or 1 unit every 8 hours usually has a poor prognosis and surgical treatment may be indicated. In the operating room, a duodenotomy or gastroduodenostomy is performed to expose the bleeding ulcer. The bleeding vessel is controlled by three sutures, and a truncal vagotomy is then performed in the elderly or in those patients with poor operative risk. In patients who are better able to tolerate surgical intervention, a selective vagotomy is an alternative choice once bleeding is controlled. It is important to note that if a truncal vagotomy is performed, a pyloroplasty must accompany the operation in order to facilitate gastric emptying, as the denervated pylorus will no longer allow spontaneous emptying of the stomach.

TABLE 12-4

PHYSIOLOGIC ALTERATIONS CAUSED BY TRUNCAL VAGOTOMY

Gastric effects

Decreased basal acid output
Reduced cholinergic input to parietal cells
Decreased stimulated maximal acid output
Diminished sensitivity to histamine gastrin
Decreased meal-induced acid secretion
Increased fasting and postprandial gastrin
Gastrin cell hyperplasia
Accelerated liquid emptying
Altered emptying of solids

Nongastric effects

Decreased pancreatic exocrine secretion
Decreased pancreatic enzymes and HCO_3
Decreased postprandial bile flow
Increased gallbladder volumes
Diminished release of vagally mediated peptide hormones

From Mulholland MW. Duodenal ulcer. In: Greenfield LJ, Mulholland MW, Oldham KT et al., eds. *Surgery: scientific principles and practice*, 2nd ed. Philadelphia: Lippincott-Raven, 1997:768, with permission.

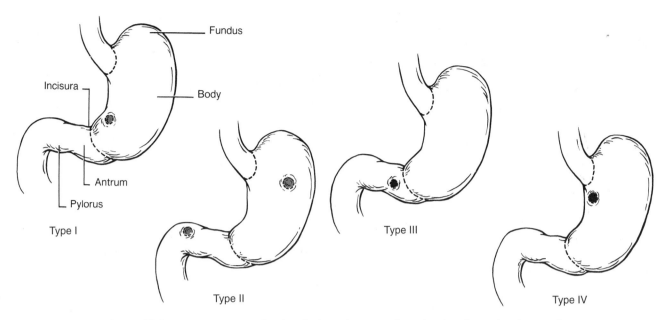

Figure 12-9 Gastric ulcers can be classified into four types based on location and pathogenesis. (From Mulholland MW. Peptic ulcer disease. In: Bell RH, Rikkers LF, Mulholland MW, eds. *Digestive tract surgery: a text and atlas.* Philadelphia: Lippincott-Raven, 1996:190, with permission.)

Rebleeding from peptic ulcer disease occurs in about 25% of patients treated medically and is more common in patients with gastric ulcers. Rebleeding has been associated with a 30% mortality rate, and to reduce this patients should undergo early surgical intervention. Those at a higher risk of rebleeding include patients older than 60 years, those that initially presented with hematemesis, those with a visible vessel actively bleeding during endoscopy, and those with a hemoglobin level lower than 8 g per dL upon admission. These patients usually rebleed within the first 48 hours of hospital admission and will generally benefit from early surgical intervention. The use of histamine blockers or proton pump inhibitors reduces the risk of rebleeding over time but does not alter the outcome of acute, active bleeding.

Perforated Peptic Ulcer

The most common site of perforation for peptic ulcer is the anterior gastric or duodenal wall. Erosions of ulcers through the anterior wall tend to present as perforation rather than bleeding because of the absence of major blood vessels on this surface. So-called "kissing ulcers" or posterior bleeding ulcers complicating an anterior perforation are rare and carry a high mortality rate. Following gastric perforation, patients present with sudden onset of severe upper abdominal pain, typically several hours after a meal. Pain may be referred to the shoulder or to the back. History of peptic ulcer disease is not a consistent finding. Classically, patients are severely distressed, lying still with knees drawn up, and taking shallow breaths. There may be temporary improvement of symptoms with the onset of bacterial peritonitis, as initial chemical peritonitis is diluted by peritoneal fluid. Patients are usually afebrile upon presentation with boardlike rigidity of the abdomen. The continual loss of air from the perforation can result in tympany and abdominal distention. Peristaltic sounds are usually reduced or absent. However, patients can present with abdominal pain without any classic physical findings. The incidence of this masked presentation is higher in hospitalized patients who are being treated for other unrelated causes or on steroids. Significance of pain often goes unnoticed, resulting in delay of appropriate treatment. A reasonable initial approach is to obtain an abdominal radiograph or upright chest film, which will demonstrate free intraperitoneal air. Duodenal leaks can track down the paracolic gutter and cause signs and symptoms that may be confused with appendicitis or colonic diverticulitis. Subclinical perforations can also be sealed off by the omentum or liver and present as a subdiaphragmatic or subphrenic abscess. Laboratory findings usually will show a mild leukocytosis (12,000 per μL) in the early stages, which can rise during the course of illness. Serum amylase levels are usually mildly elevated. If the diagnosis remains unclear, an abdominal computerized tomographic (CT) scan, which is very sensitive for free intraperitoneal air, can be obtained, or 400 mL of air may be insufflated into the stomach via a nasogastric tube to demonstrate the perforation. Treatment is dictated by the overall condition of the patient. Fluid resuscitation and intravenous antibiotics should be started. A nasogastric tube should be passed and abdominal films acquired. The surgical method of repair involves sealing the perforation with an omental patch (Graham Steell patch). One should start medical therapy for peptic ulcer. Surgical treatment of ulcer disease with a truncal vagotomy or pyloroplasty is rarely necessary today. However, perforation in the presence of pyloric obstruction is best treated by pyloroplasty or a gastroenterostomy. Antrectomy combined with truncal vagotomy is another option. Nonoperative treatment with fluids and antibiotics is occasionally indicated but is associated with higher rates of peritoneal and subphrenic abscess. A conservative approach does not necessarily carry a higher mortality rate and has been shown to be effective if the risk of operative intervention is high. An increased mortality rate is associated with a delay in treatment, in the presence of other systemic illnesses and in the elderly.

Pyloric Oruction

Pyloric obstruction from peptic ulcer disease is less common than peptic perforation. Duodenal ulcers cause obstruction more frequently than do gastric ulcers. Most patients have a long history of peptic ulcer disease and up to one third have had some treatment for a previous obstruction or perforation. Anorexia and vomiting of undigested food without biliary staining is the usual presentation. Weight loss is seen if the patient has delayed seeking medical attention and malignant ulcers are present. A succussion splash can be elicited in some patients from gastric dilation and retained gastric contents, but a visible peristaltic wave in the abdominal wall is rare in adults. The usual laboratory studies reveal a metabolic alkalosis with hypochloremia, hypokalemia, hyponatremia, and increased HCO_3. Tetany has been reported in severe cases of alkalosis owing to prolonged vomiting. Prerenal azotemia may result. A large nasogastric tube should be passed into the stomach and gastric contents lavaged. Medical therapy consists of decompression of the stomach, which allows resolution of pyloric edema and muscular spasm. In most circumstances improvement is seen within 72 hours of conservative management. Endoscopic evaluation is favored over an upper GI series because biopsy specimens can be obtained to exclude malignancy. Early surgical intervention is indicated if medical therapy and decompression for 1 week do not relieve the obstruction. Endoscopic-guided balloon dilatation can relieve symptoms in most patients. The surgical treatment of choice in cases of chronic or recurrent obstruction is usually a truncal vagotomy and drainage procedure.

Stress Ulcers

Stress gastritis is defined by ulcers or frank gastric ulceration occurr after major physiologic shock resulting from sepsis, severe burn involving more than 35% of body surface area (Curling ulcer), or trauma. Stress gastritis can also occur as a result of central nervous system disease (Cushing disease). The pathogenesis is mainly decreased mucosal resistance as an effect of ischemia, decreased production of prostanoids, and thinning of the mucous layer, which becomes vulnerable to acid, pepsin, and lysosomal enzymes. Ulcers associated with central nervous system pathology (Cushing disease) are generally associated with increased gastrin levels and increased gastric acid secretion. Most stress ulcers occur in acid-secreting portion of the stomach, and bleeding ulcers are more common than perforation. Perforation is more common, however, in a Cushing ulcer. The ulcers are shallow and discrete with little inflammation and edema. The condition becomes clinically prominent 4 to 5 days after the onset of the initial illness. Prophylaxis with a histamine receptor antagonist can decrease the incidence and avert bleeding. Antacids given hourly by a nasogastric tube can also be effective as long as the gastric pH level remains higher than 3.5. Sucralfate can also be used as a prophylactic drug and is as effective as antacids or histamine receptor antagonists. Initial therapy involves resuscitation and treatment of the underlying condition. Hemorrhagic shock should be corrected with whole blood replacement, and antimicrobial therapy should be started to combat sepsis while any abscess or undrained collection is drained. Medical management of gastric bleeding can be achieved by gastric lavage. This can control bleeding 80% of the time, but infusion of a vasoconstricting agent by selective angiographic catheterization may sometimes be needed. Despite aggressive medical therapy a definitive surgical procedure is unavoidable in some patients. The possible choices include vagotomy and pyloroplasty, vagotomy and antrectomy, vagotomy and subtotal gastrectomy, and total gastrectomy. There is no evidence supporting the superiority of one procedure over the other. There is a trend toward vagotomy and pyloroplasty with suture ligation to control bleeding points. The mortality rate is high (30% to 60%) in patients with acute hemorrhagic stress ulcers requiring surgical intervention.

GASTROESOPHAGEAL REFLUX DISEASE

Gastroesophageal reflux disease (GERD) is the most common GI disorder in the western hemisphere. The prevalence is approximately 5%. Symptoms are principally heartburn and regurgitation. The findings range from normal endoscopic and manometric findings to severe esophagitis, strictures, Barrett metaplasia, and deformities of the cardia from a defective lower esophageal sphincter (LES). The maintenance of the high pressure zone in the LES, which helps prevent reflux, has been attributed to the intrinsic musculature at the lower esophagus, the sling fibers of the stomach, the diaphragmatic crura, and abdominal pressure. Antireflux surgery has been designed to restore the defective LES. The indications for surgery are (i) persistent symptoms despite optimal medical management for 4 weeks or more, (ii) complications from the disease, or (iii) manometric evidence of a defective LES, as well as the presence of a low pH in the esophagus during a 24-hour pH test. Typical preoperative evaluation includes endoscopy, manometry, pH monitoring, and esophagogram. Thorough pre-operative evaluation will identify those patients who will most likely benefit from antireflux surgery. Multivariate analyses indicate excellent (97%) outcome in patients with typical symptoms, a documented response to acid suppression, and the presence of an abnormal 24-hour pH score.

The operation should be tailored to the pathophysiologic data that are available. Patients with early disease with normal esophageal length and normal body motility should be treated with a laparoscopic or transabdominal *Nissen fundoplication*. If the patient is severely obese, a transthoracic approach can be made. If the peristaltic amplitude is below 20 mm Hg in the distal one third of the esophagus, a *Belsey fundoplication* is a better choice. If the esophagus is shortened because of chronic disease or the site of previous surgery, a *Colles gastroplasty* with a partial wrap is a reasonable option. In the presence of complications of GERD, such as high grade esophageal dysplasia, undilatable esophageal stricture, or esophageal carcinoma, a total esophagectomy should be performed. The essential principles of the fundoplication are identification and preservation of the vagus nerve and the anterior hepatic branch, dissection of the esophagus, crural apposition, mobilization and division of the short gastric vessels, and lastly, creation of a loose wrap enveloping the anterior and posterior wall of the fundus around the esophagus.

SURGICAL TREATMENT FOR MORBID OBESITY

The surgical treatment of morbid obesity has become more frequent in the United States, owing to the increasing incidence of morbid obesity nationwide. Over the last 40 years, the incidence of morbid obesity has increased from 13% to 35%, thus becoming a very serious national health problem.

Obesity is defined as having a body mass index (BMI) greater than 30 kg per m^2. Patients with severe obesity have a BMI greater then 35 kg per m^2, and patients classified as morbidly obese have a BMI greater than 40 kg per m^2. Complications related to obesity include obstructive sleep apnea, hypertension, and coronary artery disease. Bariatric surgery is recommended for patients who are severely obese with obesity related complications, as well as in the morbidly obese, according to the BMI criteria outlined above. Patients who are likely candidates for bariatric surgery have failed medically supervised weight reduction, have no active history of alcohol or other substance abuse, have acceptable medical risks for surgery, and who have realistic outcomes and are capable of long-term commitment.

The most commonly offered operations in the United States are *vertical banded gastroplasty* (VBG) and *roux-en-Y gastric bypass*. The VBG is a restrictive procedure that involves the creation of a small reservoir or pouch with a vertical staple line. This new pouch empties into the residual stomach via a narrow outlet banded with mesh. The advantage of this procedure is that it avoids a GI anastomosis and preserves gastroduodenal continuity. The primary disadvantages include (i) pouch stretching with enlargement over time, (ii) staple line dehiscence, (iii) gastric outlet obstruction, and (iv) intraluminal band migration. This procedure may also be associated with severe GERD. The treatment for this complication of VGB is conversion to gastric bypass. Because it provides many patients with more significant weight loss than does the VGB, the *gastric bypass* (either laparascopic or laparotomic) has largely replaced VBG and is the treatment of choice in most centers. This procedure involves the creation of a small gastric pouch and a gastrojejunostomy with a roux-en-Y limb of jejunum to facilitate emptying. Although weight loss is significantly better in comparison to the VBG, there is a higher incidence of stomal ulcer, stomal stenosis, gallstones and vitamin B_{12} deficiency. Finally, laparascopic techniques, including the recent development of adjustable gastric bands, are gaining popularity in bariatric surgery as the risks and benefits of these techniques become better defined in this emerging field.

GASTRIC CANCER

The incidence of gastric cancer in the United States is decreasing, but the reason for this decline is not known. The factors that play a key role in the pathogenesis of gastric carcinogenesis include diet, exogenous chemicals, intragastric synthesis of carcinogens, genetic factors, infectious agents, and antral gastritis. Dietary factors probably play an important role in countries such as Japan and other nations where the incidence of gastric cancer is high. Studies of individuals emigrating from endemic areas to Europe or the United States show a lower incidence of gastric cancer after migration. Dietary nitrites and their derivatives such as nitrosamines have been shown to induce gastric cancer under experimental conditions, but specific dietary factors have yet to be identified in humans. *H. pylori* has recently been classified as a carcinogen by the World Health Organization (WHO). *H. pylori* infection also causes atrophic gastritis, which is a recognized precursor to gastric adenocarcinoma. However, it is not known if eradication of *H. pylori* infection will prevent gastric cancer. Patients with longstanding pernicious anemia characterized by fundic mucosal atrophy, hypochlorhydria, hypergastrinemia, and loss of parietal and chief cells are at increased risk (twice that of age-matched controls) of developing gastric cancer. The other premalignant lesion that has a distinct risk of leading to gastric malignancy is an adenomatous polyp. Ten percent to 20% of patients with polyps greater then 2 cm in diameter develop gastric cancer.

Gastric cancers usually are adenocarcinomas. The morphologic types include ulcerating carcinoma, polypoid carcinoma, superficial spreading carcinoma, and linitis plastica. In *ulcerating carcinoma*, a deeply penetrating malignant ulcer involves the entire gastric wall. *Polypoid carcinoma* is defined as a large intraluminal tumor with late metastasis. *Superficial spreading* carcinoma is an early gastric cancer that is often confined to the superficial layers of the gastric wall. Unlike other subtypes, only one third of these present with metastatic disease. *Linitis plastica* is a spreading tumor involving all the layers of the gastric wall. The stomach loses its pliability early because of malignant infiltration, and metastasis occurs early. Most commonly, patients present with advanced disease. Gastric cancer can also be classified as inflammatory, glandular (intestinal), and diffuse (stromal). Tumors eliciting an inflammatory response are generally found to have a better prognosis. Gastric cancer is predominately found in the antrum along the lesser curvature. This is also a common location for benign gastric ulcers. Ulcers along the greater curvature and the cardia have a higher incidence of malignancy than do ulcers along the lesser curvature.

Patients with gastric cancer frequently present with new onset of discomfort on top of a history of chronic dyspeptic symptoms. Anorexia develops early with concurrent weight loss. Vomiting is associated with pyloric obstruction, whereas involvement of the cardia is associated with dysphagia. A mass can be palpated in some patients. Occult blood can be detected in the stool of 50% of patients, but frank anemia is present in fewer individuals. Physical signs of dissemination include a palpable *Virchow node* in the left supraclavicular space, indicating metastasis along the thoracic duct, and intraperitoneal spread may involve the ovaries (*Krukenberg tumors*) or other intraperitoneal organs. "Drop" metastases present on the rectum can occasionally be palpated as a *Blumer shelf* on rectal examination. Distant metastasis can involve the liver, lungs, brain, or bone. Carcinoembryonic antigen level is usually elevated in metastatic disease. The initial diagnostic procedure of choice is an upper endoscopy. Polyps or ulcers that are suspicious for cancer should be biopsied. An upper gastrointestinal series (UGI) can be diagnostic in most instances, but the false-negative rate can be as high as 20%.

Surgical resection is the only curative treatment, but only one half of resectable tumors are potentially curable because of micrometastasis. The location of the tumor dictates the extent of resection necessary. Antral tumors necessitate a distal gastrectomy with a proximal resection margin of approximately 6 cm from the tumor and 3 to 4 cm from the duodenum, along with an *en bloc* resection of the omentum, the subpyloric lymph nodes, and the left gastric artery and lymph nodes. Bowel continuity is then reestablished, preferably using a Billroth II procedure. Proximal tumors usually require a total gastrectomy, whereas tumors of the cardia require an esophagogastrectomy and splenectomy. Antral tumors with extragastric spread or pyloric obstruction may require a palliative gastrectomy. If a gastrectomy is impossible, then a palliative gastrojejunostomy for bypass is the procedure of choice. Adjuvant chemotherapy and/or radiation therapy have not proven efficacious. The overall 5-year survival rate for gastric cancer in the United States is 12%.

KEY POINTS

▲ Bleeding peptic ulcers that have failed endoscopic interventions should be controlled by the three suture technique and truncal vagotomy or selective vagotomy. Any stomach denervation should have a pyloroplasty to facilitate gastric emptying.

▲ The essential principles of the fundoplication are identification and preservation of the vagus nerve proper and the anterior hepatic branch of the vagus nerve, dissection of the esophagus, crural apposition, mobilization and division of the short gastric vessels, and, lastly, creation of a loose wrap enveloping the anterior and posterior wall of the fundus around the esophagus.

▲ Obesity is defined as having a body mass index (BMI) of greater than 30 kg per m². Patients with severe obesity have a BMI greater then 35 kg per m², and patients classified as morbidly obese have a BMI greater than 40 kg per m².

▲ The indications for antireflux surgery are persistent symptoms despite optimal medical management for 4 weeks or more, complications from the disease, manometric evidence of a defective lower esophageal sphincter (LES), and 24-hour pH test demonstrating gastroesophageal reflux disease (GERD).

▲ The majority of gastric cancer patients have micrometastasis at the time of presentation. Physical signs of dissemination include a palpable *Virchow node* in the left supraclavicular space, or palpable peritoneal deposits on rectal examination, known as a *Blumer shelf*.

SUGGESTED READINGS

Baker RJ, Fisher JE, eds. *Mastery of surgery*, 4th ed. Philadelphia: Lippincott Williams & Wilkins, 2001.

Cameron JL, ed. *Current surgical therapy*, 8th ed. St. Louis: Mosby, 2004.

Mulholland MW. Duodenal ulcer. *Surgery: scientific principles and practice*, 2nd ed. Philadelphia: Lippincott-Raven Publishers, 1997.

Mulholland MW. Gastric anatomy and physiology. In: Greenfield LJ, Mulholland MW, Oldham KT et al., eds. *Surgery: scientific principles and practice*, 3rd ed. Philadelphia: Lippincott Williams & Wilkins, 2001.

Small Bowel

13

Jin Hee Ra   *Steven E. Raper*

OVERVIEW

The small bowel is a highly specialized, hollow viscus, approximately 8 m in length, the major function of which is vital to nutrition. In addition, the small bowel has many endocrine and immunologic functions as well as a complex nervous system. This chapter describes the anatomy and physiology of the small bowel in addition to the pathologic processes affecting this organ. Gastrointestinal (GI) hormones, nutrition, immunology, and motility are discussed in Chapter 16, "Nutrition, Digestion, and Absorption." Embryology and pediatric small bowel diseases are discussed in Chapter 10, "Pediatric Surgery."

ANATOMY AND PHYSIOLOGY

The small bowel is a highly specialized organ, the anatomy of which is very important to its function. The small bowel is divided into three sections: the *duodenum* (approximately 40 cm in length), the *jejunum* (approximately 200 cm), and the *ileum* (approximately 300 cm). The jejunum and ileum are covered by visceral peritoneum and are tethered to the posterior abdominal wall by mesentery. The duodenum, a retroperitoneal organ, is divided into four parts. The first portion, also called the duodenal bulb, is superior to the pancreatic head and anterior to the gastroduodenal artery (Fig. 13-1). Ninety percent of duodenal ulcers occur in the bulb. The first portion of the duodenum is the only intraperitoneal section of the duodenum, and it derives its blood supply from the supraduodenal branch of the hepatic artery and the gastroduodenal artery. The second portion of the duodenum is attached to the head of the pancreas and is retroperitoneal; this portion is where the major ampulla of Vater and minor ampulla of Santorini enter the duodenum. Additional features of the duodenum include plicae circulares (transverse folds or folds of Kerckring). The third portion is also retroperitoneal and is attached to the uncinate process of the pancreas. It is located between the superior mesenteric artery (SMA) and the aorta. The blood supply for the second and third portion of the duodenum extends from the anterosuperior and posterosuperior pancreaticoduodenal branches of the gastroduodenal artery and the anteroinferior and posteroinferior pancreaticoduodenal branches of the SMA. The fourth, ascending, portion of the duodenum receives its blood supply from the first jejunal branch of the SMA. The *ligament of Treitz* is a suspensory fold of peritoneum derived from the right crus of diaphragm, and it is the anatomic landmark by which surgeons differentiate the duodenum from the jejunum.

The small bowel may be differentiated from the remainder of the intestine both grossly and radiographically by the *valvulae conniventes*, circular folds of mucosa and submucosa that markedly increase the absorptive surface area. Characteristics of the small bowel that allow differentiation of the jejunum from the ileum include larger circumference and mesenteric vascular anatomy. The mesenteric vessels of the jejunum form only one or two arterial arcades and send out long vasa recta. The jejunal mesentery contains less fat and appears thinner than the ileal mesentery. It usually occupies the mid- to upper abdomen to the left of midline. In contrast, the ileum has fewer plicae, is smaller in diameter, has a thicker mesentery, and has short vasa recta with multiple arterial arcades. It is usually located in the lower abdomen to the right of midline (i.e., right lower quadrant). Embryologically, the jejunum and ileum are derived predominantly from the midgut and as such are vascularized by the SMA. The superior mesenteric vein (SMV) constitutes the venous drainage and runs parallel to the arterial supply. Abundant lymphatic tissue, such as the Peyer patches of the ileal wall, allows the small bowel to play a major role in immunologic function. Furthermore, the pronounced lymphatic drainage of the small bowel also allows for fat absorption, which is integral to the small bowel's role in digestion.

Histologically, the bowel consists of four layers: the mucosa, the submucosa, the muscularis, and serosa. The innermost layer, the *mucosa* lines the lumen of the bowel and is made up of many villi and crypts, which provide the small bowel with a massive surface area important in its role of secretion and absorption (Figs. 13-2 and 13-3). Small bowel mucosa can be subdivided into three layers: the muscularis mucosa, lamina propria, and the epithelium. The outermost layer, the muscularis mucosa, is a thin layer of muscle separating the mucosa from the submucosa. The middle mucosal layer, the lamina propria, is a continuous layer of connective tissue between the muscularis mucosa and epithelium and serves as a supportive base for the villi and a protective barrier from microorganisms. Immune cells reside in this layer. The epithelium constitutes the innermost layer of mucosa. The major functions of the epithelial lining of the villi and crypts of

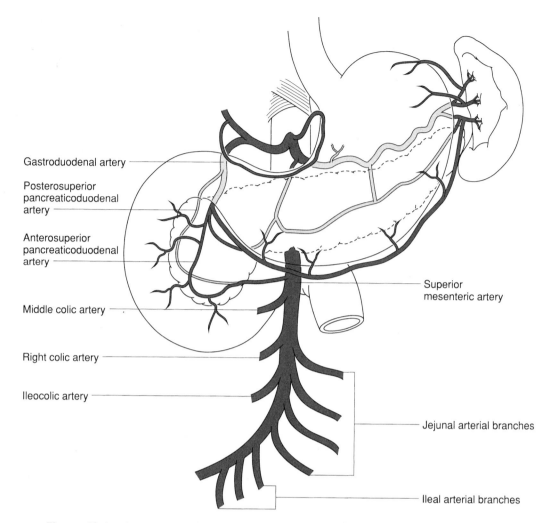

Gastroduodenal artery

Posterosuperior pancreaticoduodenal artery

Anterosuperior pancreaticoduodenal artery

Middle colic artery

Right colic artery

Ileocolic artery

Superior mesenteric artery

Jejunal arterial branches

Ileal arterial branches

Figure 13-1   The arterial blood distribution of the celiac artery, superior mesenteric artery, and their branches. (From Greenfield LJ, Mulholland MW, Oldham KT et al., eds. *Surgery: scientific principles and practice*, 3rd ed. Philadelphia: Lippincott Williams & Wilkins, 2001:1693, with permission.)

Lieberkühn are digestion, absorption, cell renewal, and secretion of hormones. The *submucosa* is the supportive layer of fibroelastic connective tissue, which consists of the blood supply, lymphatics, and nerves. Finally, the *muscular layer* is composed of two muscle layers: the inner circular and the outer longitudinal. These muscles have specialized

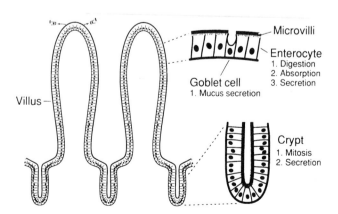

Villus

Microvilli

Enterocyte
1. Digestion
2. Absorption
3. Secretion

Goblet cell
1. Mucus secretion

Crypt
1. Mitosis
2. Secretion

Figure 13-2   Two sectioned villi and a crypt from the small intestinal mucosa. (From Johnson LR. *Essential medical physiology.* New York: Raven Press, 1992:508, with permission.)

gaps in the muscle-cell membrane allowing the bowel to function as an electrical syncytium. Sandwiched between the layers is a group of ganglion cells from the myenteric (Auerbach) plexus. The *serosa* is the outermost layer and is composed of flattened mesothelial cells and consists of the visceral peritoneum.

Innervation of the small bowel comes from both sympathetic and parasympathetic nervous systems. The three sympathetic ganglia are located around the base of the SMA, which affect the blood vessel motility and to a lesser extent gut secretion and motility. Pain is also mediated through the general visceral afferent fibers of the sympathetic nervous system. Parasympathetic fibers come from the vagus nerve and predominantly affect gut secretion and motility. The most common disorder of motility is ileus, a temporary loss of peristalsis caused by gastroenteritis, medication, or surgery.

Postoperative ileus is the most common form of ileus and may result from unbalanced autonomic stimulation to the gut after surgery. The basal motility pattern, or migrating motor complex (MMC), is disturbed for approximately 24 hours after laparotomy owing in part to the anesthetic technique. Bowel resection temporarily blocks the MMC and peristalsis at the site of resection; however,

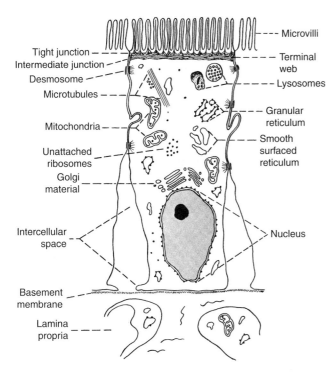

Figure 13-3 An intestinal epithelial cell. (From Trier JS, Rubin CE. Electron microscopy of the small intestine: a review. *Gastroenterology* 1965;49:574, with permission.)

motility usually quickly returns to normal. Generally, small bowel function returns within hours of manipulation but return of stomach and colon function requires 48 to 72 hours. Return of bowel function may not necessarily be clinically apparent, as a recent prospective randomized control trial found that many patients may be discharged on a clear liquid diet even before the resumption of flatus or stool.

DISEASES OF THE SMALL BOWEL

Obstruction

Small bowel obstruction (SBO) is one of the most common diseases affecting the small bowel. There are many causes of small bowel obstruction (Table 13-1). The three most common causes of mechanical obstruction include adhesive disease, tumors, and hernias. Sixty percent of SBOs are secondary to adhesive disease, which has increased in incidence as a result of the increase in elective abdominal surgery. Hernias are the most common cause of SBO in patients with no history of prior abdominal surgery (Fig. 13-4). Lower abdominal and pelvic operations (appendectomy and female adnexal procedures) appear to be associated with a higher incidence of adhesive obstruction than are upper abdominal procedures. The incidence of small bowel obstruction due to hernia or inflammatory bowel diseases (IBDs) is higher in young adults. The small bowel may be partially or completely obstructed. With either type of obstruction, all or part of the bowel wall may be incarcerated or strangulated.

Clinical Manifestations

Patients usually present with nausea, vomiting, crampy abdominal pain, distention, obstipation, and high pitched or absent bowel sounds (Table 13-2). The pain may be intermittent and associated with episodes of intense pain and bowel sounds, the so-called "peristaltic rush." Clinically relevant signs and symptoms include fever (if bowel is strangulated or obstruction is caused by IBD), tachycardia (if the patient is hypovolemic, or if bowel is strangulated), and peritonitis if bowel is ischemic or perforated. Four classic findings of gangrenous bowel include leukocytosis, tachycardia, localized pain or tenderness, and fever. It is optimal

TABLE 13-1

CLASSIFICATION OF ADULT MECHANICAL INSTESTINAL OBSTRUCTIONS

Intraluminal	Intramural	Extrinsic
Foreign bodies	Congenital	Adhesions
Barium inspissation (colon)	Atresia, stricture, or stenosis	Congenital
Bezoar	Web	Ladd or Meckel bands
Inspissated feces	Intestinal duplication	Postoperative
Gallstone	Meckel diverticulum	Postinflammatory
Meconium (cystic fibrosis)	Inflammatory process	Hernias
Parasites	Crohn disease	External
Other (e.g., swallowed objects, enteroliths)	Diverticulitis	Internal
Intussusception	Chronic intestinal ischemia or	Volvulus
Polypoid, exophytic lesions	postischemic stricture	External mass effect
	Radiation enteritis	Abscess
	Medication induced (nonsteroidal	Annular pancreas
	antiinflammatory drugs, potassium	Carcinomatosis
	chloride tablets)	Endometriosis
	Neoplasms	Pregnancy
	Primary bowel (malignant or benign)	Pancreatic pseudocyst
	Secondary (metastases, especially	
	melanoma)	
	Traumatic	
	Intramural hematoma of duodenum	

From Greenfield LJ, Mulholland MW, Oldham KT et al., eds. *Surgery: scientific principles and practice*, 3rd ed. Philadelphia: Lippincott Williams & Wilkins, 2001:800, with permission.

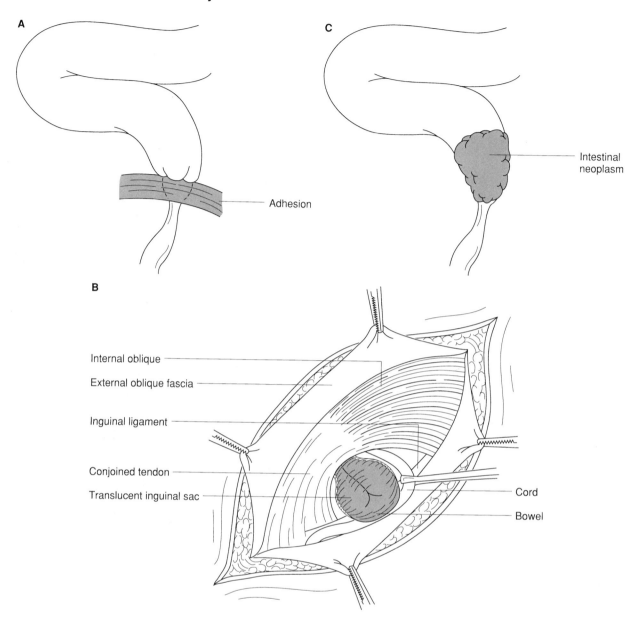

Figure 13-4 Schematic illustration of different forms of simple mechanical obstruction. Simple obstruction is most often caused by adhesion **(A)**, groin hernia **(B)**, or neoplasm **(C)**. The hernia can act as a tourniquet, causing a closed-loop obstruction and strangulation. (From Greenfield LJ, Mulholland MW, Oldham KT et al., eds. *Surgery: scientific principles and practice*, 3rd ed. Philadelphia: Lippincott Williams & Wilkins, 2001:799, with permission.)

not to allow a patient under observation to progress to these signs. Laboratory values may be normal in patients with SBO. However, leukocytosis may be present if bowel is strangulated, or if inflammation or infection occurs. Hypokalemic, hypochloremic metabolic alkalosis secondary to vomiting or metabolic acidosis may also be observed. The hematocrit may be falsely elevated because of hemoconcentration resulting from volume depletion. The presence of anemia may indicate underlying malignancy. Abnormal laboratory values of lactate dehydrogenase (LDH), phosphorus, amylase, alkaline phosphatase, ammonia, or creatine phosphokinase (CPK) have not been particularly helpful in determining strangulation of bowel. In contrast, elevated serum lactate levels have been 90% sensitive and 87% specific for the presence of bowel ischemia.

Diagnosis

If there is clinical suspicion for SBO, an obstruction series (upright chest and abdominal radiographs and supine abdominal radiograph) should be obtained. In SBO, there are classically dilated loops of bowel—often in a step ladder–like appearance—with air-fluid levels and a paucity of or no gas past the point of the obstruction. Small bowel may be differentiated from colon by the presence of plicae circulares versus haustral markings. Plain radiographs are only 50% to 60% correct in making the diagnosis.

Computerized tomographic scan of the abdomen and pelvis with intravenous and oral contrast has become a common and important diagnostic tool in differentiating the many causes of SBO. CT imaging can detect the specific location of the lesion (by visualization of a transition point and discrepancy in the caliber of the proximal and

TABLE 13-2

SYMPTOMS AND SIGNS OF BOWEL OBSTRUCTIONS

Symptom or Sign	Proximal Small Bowel (Open Loop)	Distal Small Bowel (Open Loop)	Small Bowel (Closed Loop)	Colon and Rectum
Pain	Colicky, often relieved by vomiting	Intermittent, sometimes constant	Progressive, intermittent or constant, worsens quickly	Continuous
Vomiting	Frequent, bilious, large volume	Low volume, low frequency, becomes feculent with time	May be prominent (reflex)	Intermittent, not prominent; feculent when present
Tenderness	Epigastric or periumbilical, usually mild unless strangulation present	Diffuse and progressive	Diffuse and progressive	Diffuse
Distention	Absent	Moderate to marked	Often absent	Marked
Obstipation	May not be present	Present	May not be present	Present

From Greenfield LJ, Mulholland M, Oldham KT et al., eds. *Surgery: Scientific Principles and Practice*, 2nd ed. Philadelphia: Lippincott-Raven, 1997:819, with permission.

distal small bowel) as well as differentiate the cause and signs of bowel infarction or perforation. Studies support the use of computerized tomography, as it is approximately 95% sensitive and specific in making the correct diagnosis. Furthermore, data suggest that two groups of patients benefit from CT scan: those with SBO and a history of abdominal malignancy and those with simple adhesive disease. For example, if a patient has a history of malignancy, a CT scan may help determine whether treatment should be surgical or conservative, while a CT scan without evidence of tumor or obstructing mass can suggest adhesive disease as the underlying etiology of the SBO. CT findings that require immediate surgical intervention include closed loop obstruction and strangulation. Strangulation is characterized by thickening of the bowel wall, *pneumatosis intestinalis*, ascites, or mesenteric hematoma. Closed loop obstruction findings include a C- or U-shaped section of bowel with dilation of the loop and proximal bowel and decompression of the distal bowel. There is also a fixed-to-radial distribution of dilated loops with stretched proximal mesentery.

Barium upper GI series with small bowel follow-through (SBFT) may also be employed in the evaluation of small bowel obstruction, and is greater than 80% accurate in diagnosing obstruction in subacute cases. Following the introduction of oral contrast into the bowel, serial abdominal films are taken over time to follow the contrast's passage through the bowel. This is helpful in differentiating adynamic ileus from mechanical obstruction. Ileus is characterized by overall delay in contrast transit time, whereas a discrete transition point will be noted in cases of mechanical obstruction. Considerable judgment is necessary to determine when a barium study is needed, as intraoperative enterolysis of obstructed bowel full of barium adds significant technical challenge to the operation.

Enteroclysis, a less frequently used study, involves the placement of a nasal–small bowel tube past the ligament of Treitz. Diluted barium (sometimes air and contrast) is then injected into the tube at a constant rate and radiographs are taken. This procedure is more sensitive and specific than an upper GI SBFT because the injection of air and contrast allows for better evaluation of the mucosa, and allows for better determination of bowel distensibility. This test is particularly useful in the diagnosis of small bowel tumors or the demonstration of mucosal signs of inflammatory bowel disease.

Treatment

The initial management should include intravascular volume resuscitation, electrolyte correction, and the placement of a nasogastric tube and urinary catheter. Intravascular volume is often depleted, the extent of which can be underestimated owing to sequestration of large amounts of fluid in the bowel lumen. Multiple factors contribute to the intraluminal fluid accumulation in patients with SBO. Reabsorption of fluid and increased secretion are caused by increased intraluminal pressure, release of vasoactive agents such as vasoactive intestinal peptide and prostaglandins, and digestion of intestinal contents, leading to increased osmolarity and further retention of fluid. Although it initially increases, blood flow is compromised and strangulation begins when intraluminal pressure exceeds intramural capillary and venous pressure. Intravenous antibiotics are generally not necessary unless surgery is undertaken and bowel resection is anticipated. In patients with partial SBO, treatment initially is nonoperative. If there is no or minimal improvement in 3 to 5 days, parenteral nutrition should be started. Timing of surgery in such cases is usually individualized. If the patient's signs and symptoms worsen at any time, surgery should be performed. Patients who initially resolve a partial SBO but then recur generally are best served by surgical exploration. Patients with complete SBO are at high risk of strangulation, which is a surgical emergency. The risks of nonoperative therapy in complete SBO are compounded by the fact that only 60% to 70% of patients with strangulation will manifest the expected signs and symptoms. In general, once the decision to operate on small bowel obstruction has been made, there is little to gain by waiting. In some circumstances, a delay in operative management of between 6 and 8 hours may be warranted for resuscitation purposes or to stabilize a comorbid condition, such as diabetic ketoacidosis or acute myocardial infarction. Most operations, however, should be performed without delay.

Surgical treatment may include lysis of adhesions (LOAs), resection of nonviable bowel with anastomosis, or intestinal bypass. If the small bowel is greatly distended with fluid and air, it is susceptible to inadvertent enterotomy and can make abdominal wall closure difficult. A small enterotomy can be made and a small catheter placed to decompress the bowel. Milking a large volume of intestinal contents into the stomach is not advisable as pulmonary aspiration may result. Bowel viability must be determined and can be performed intraoperatively by using one of several methods. Fluorescein angiography is performed by intravenous injection followed by black light (Wood lamp) examination of the bowel. There are two main fluorescein patterns. Homogeneous hyperfluorescence with a fine granular or reticular pattern suggests normal bowel perfusion, whereas patchy fluorescence or nonfluorescence suggest nonviable bowel. The limiting feature of this method is that it is subject to interpretation. Black light examination must be undertaken within 2 to 3 minutes of revascularization/ treatment of obstruction. The method is approximately 80% sensitive. Doppler ultrasonography may also be used but is examiner dependent. Obvious nonviable bowel should be resected and a "second look" laparotomy planned in 24 to 48 hours from the initial exploration to assess the presence of further nonviability. The decision to perform a "second look" should be made at the first operation, and the decision should be firm. Resection should be limited in patients with Crohn disease and radiation enteritis in an attempt to preserve as much bowel as possible.

Patients with SBO should be evaluated for hernias, especially if there is no history of prior abdominal surgery. Hernias may be external or internal. Common external hernias are inguinal, femoral, and incisional. Internal hernias include those related to inadequate closure of mesenteric defects created by prior operations, congenital mesenteric defects, and obturator foramen hernias.

A bowel obstruction in a patient with known malignancy requires special consideration. Recent studies have suggested that between 20% and 80% of SBOs in patients with a known history of abdominal cancer but without documented recurrence are caused by adhesive disease and should be treated accordingly. However, if obstruction is caused by tumor, operative management should be carefully considered secondary to the high rate of morbidity and mortality postoperatively. It is generally accepted to attempt a trial of conservative medical management. Most patients with malignancy deserve one serious attempt at nonsurgical resolution of bowel obstruction.

Prevention

Once formed, adhesions are likely to recur. Surgical techniques to decrease the formation of adhesions may include the use of sharp scalpel dissection, avoidance of tissue ischemia, minimal use of foreign material, and avoidance of bowel manipulation with rough instruments or sponges. A variety of topical agents are available which allegedly decrease adhesion rate, but their efficacy remains in question.

Prognosis

Approximately 10% of patients after LOA will have recurrence of SBO and the incidence increases with each subsequent LOA. Plication of the small bowel may be considered in patients with multiple adhesive obstructions to promote the formation of adhesion of the bowel in a nonobstructive arrangement. Strangulated bowel is associated with increased morbidity and mortality. There is a 0.5% mortality rate with SBO. The following diseases are less common but important causes of SBO and they will be discussed separately.

Gallstone Ileus

The development of a cholecystoduodenal fistula with distal propagation of a gallstone is an uncommon but fascinating cause of SBO associated with considerable morbidity and mortality. It occurs more frequently in the elderly, in patients with severe concomitant disease, and in patients with gallstones 2 to 5 cm in diameter. Classical findings include intestinal obstruction (greater than 70%), pneumobilia (greater than 50%), an aberrantly located gallstone usually in the right lower quadrant (greater than 30%), or a change in position of a gallstone from previous studies. The pathophysiology of the disease begins with cystic duct obstruction, cholecystitis, biliary-enteric fistula, stone erosion into the small bowel, distal migration and ends with obstruction of the gallstone at a narrowing, usually the ileocecal valve. Surgical intervention generally includes laparotomy and removal of the stone. If the clinical situation permits, cholecystectomy is performed, but this procedure is usually delayed until a second operation. The biliary-enteric fistula usually closes by itself. Rarely, if the patient is a prohibitive surgical candidate, lithotripsy may be attempted.

Intussusception

In adults, intussusception is caused by small bowel pathology approximately 80% of the time. The leading edge or intussusceptum is usually an intraluminal lesion (Fig. 13-5).

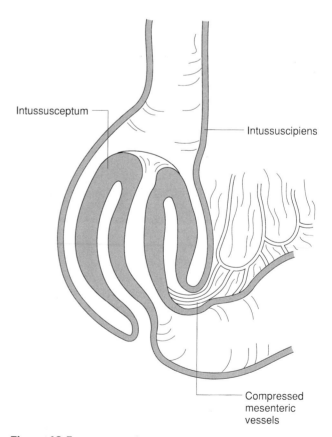

Figure 13-5 Anatomy of intussusception. The intussusceptum is the segment if bowel that invaginates into the intussuscipiens. (From Greenfield LJ, Mulholland MW, Oldham KT et al., eds. *Surgery: scientific principles and practice*, 3rd ed. Philadelphia: Lippincott Williams & Wilkins, 2001:808, with permission.)

The patient may present with crampy abdominal pain, nausea, vomiting, and heme-positive stools. Unlike the pediatric population, hydrostatic reduction by barium enema is not recommended in adults. The diagnosis is now usually made by computerized tomography. The CT finding most indicative of intussusception is an intraluminal soft tissue mass with high attenuation peripherally and low attenuation centrally, known as the "target sign." Surgical exploration is warranted in all but the most unusual circumstances as up to 40% of intussuscepta are caused by malignant tumors.

Volvulus

Volvulus is the twisting of a loop of bowel around the axis of a long narrow mesentery, often associated with malrotation or internal herniation (Fig. 13-6). Volvulus accounts for approximately 4% of SBOs. The incidence is equal in men and women. Clinical presentation is usually acute abdominal pain and distention, nausea, and bilious vomiting. Leukocytosis is the only common laboratory abnormality. Diagnosis is often made by plain films, barium GI studies, or CT scanning, and should be sought during exploration for bowel obstruction. Treatment begins with fluid resuscitation and intravenous antibiotics and is followed by exploratory laparotomy. If the bowel appears viable, then a simple enterolysis and Ladd procedure (counterclockwise reduction of the volvulus, splitting of Ladd bands/adhesions, and appendectomy) is adequate. If the bowel appears nonviable, then a Ladd procedure and bowel resection is required followed by a second-look laparotomy.

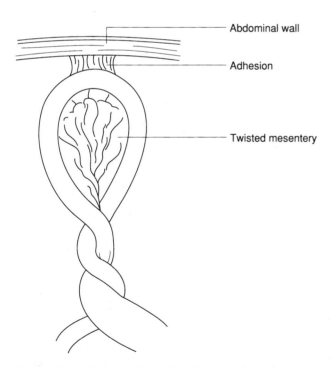

- Abdominal wall
- Adhesion
- Twisted mesentery

Figure 13-6 Schematic illustration of a closed-loop obstruction. The small intestine twists around its mesentery, compromising inflow and outflow of luminal contents from the loop. In addition, the vascular supply to the loop may be compromised because of the twisting of the mesentery. The risk of strangulation is high. (From Greenfield LJ, Mulholland MW, Oldham KT et al., eds. *Surgery: scientific principles and practice*, 3rd ed. Philadelphia: Lippincott Williams & Wilkins, 2001:801, with permission.)

INFLAMMATORY DISEASES

Crohn Disease

Crohn disease, or *regional enteritis,* is a chronic granulomatous disease of unknown cause. Any part of the GI system from the mouth to the anus can be affected, although the terminal ileum is most commonly affected (approximately 70% to 90% of cases). The incidence is approximately 5 per 100,000 in the general population. It has a bimodal distribution, affecting people in the second and third decades of life, and there is a small increase in incidence in the sixth decade. There is a slight female predominance and a familial association has been demonstrated. The disease more commonly affects smokers, people who reside in industrial areas, and is more frequent in Ashkenazi Jews. The disease is characterized by periods of remissions and exacerbations.

Etiology

Although the cause of Crohn disease remains unknown, there are several theories. Autoimmune, infectious, and genetic factors have all been proposed as likely possibilities. Humoral and cell-mediated immune reactions against gut cells have been found in patients with Crohn disease, which suggests autoimmunity, although there has been no direct correlation between this and the development of Crohn disease. There has been speculation as to whether certain organisms such as atypical mycobacterium or viruses could be the cause. However, clinical trials in which treatment for these microbes was administered failed to demonstrate any improvement in the disease process. Genetic factors may also contribute to the development of Crohn disease; however, research is still ongoing. Other possible contributing factors such as environment, psychosomatic origin, smoking history, and diet have yet to be conclusively proven.

Pathology

Macroscopically, the small bowel is characterized by grayish pink to purplish serosa with areas of thick grayish-white exudates or fibrosis. The affected bowel is usually thick, firm, and rubbery. The portion of the bowel proximal to the involved segment is usually dilated because of the obstruction of diseased bowel. There is also "fat creeping" of the mesenteric fat over the antimesenteric portion of the bowel. There may be bowel perforation, abscess formation, or an entero-enteric fistula found at the time of surgical exploration. Microscopically, there is segmental, transmural involvement of the affected bowel with varying amounts of fibrosis and ulceration. There is linear ulceration with mucosal and submucosal edema surrounding the ulcer creating a "cobblestone" appearance. The edema can be sufficiently extensive to cause obstruction. The lesions are segmental, meaning that normal bowel is located in between areas of diseased bowel, also known as "skip lesions." Sixty percent to 70% of patients may have areas of discrete noncaseating granulomas with Langerhans giant cells. The autoimmune hypothesis is supported by the finding of gut lamina propria with a two- to threefold increase in lymphocytes.

Clinical Manifestations

Crohn disease is characterized by symptomatic periods of crampy to dull aching abdominal pain (most common)

TABLE 13-3

HISTOPATHOLOGIC DIFFERENTIATION OF CROHN COLITIS AND ULCERATIVE COLITIS

Crohn Colitis	Ulcerative Colitis
Macroscopic	
Transmural involvement	Disease confined to mucosa except in toxic dilation
Segmental disease, fistulae	Rectum always involved
Thickened wall with "creeping fat"	Normal thickness of bowel wal
Occasional pseudopolyps	Pseudopolyps
Small bowel may be involved	Small bowel not involved (except as backwash ileitis)
Perianal disease common	Perianal disease less common
Microscopic	
Transmural inflammation and fibrosis	Inflammation of mucosa and submucosa
Crypt abscesses less common	Crypt abscesses common
Cobblestoning	Pseudopolyps
Narrow, deeply penetrating ulcers	Shallow, wide ulcers
Fissures, fistulae	
Granuloma common	Granuloma rare
Mucus secretion increased	Mucus secretion decreased

From Greenfield LJ, Mulholland MW, Oldham KT et al., eds. *Surgery: scientific principles and practice*, 2nd ed. Philadelphia: Lippincott-Raven Publishers, 1997:835, with permission.

and diarrhea (second most common), interspersed with periods of remission. The onset is usually insidious, and during the natural course of the disease, intervals of remission become progressively shorter while symptomatic periods become longer and more severe. Bloody diarrhea is less frequent in patients with Crohn disease when compared to patients with ulcerative colitis (Table 13-3). There usually is no mucus or pus in the stools. Frank lower GI bleeding is unusual. Other symptoms that are less commonly encountered include fever (one third of patients), weight loss, malaise (greater than one half of patients), and malnutrition. Extraintestinal manifestations such as arthralgias, iritis, uveitis, erythema nodosum, pyoderma gangrenosum, arthritis, hepatitis, and pericholangitis occur in approximately 30% patients. Patients with Crohn disease have multiple complications often requiring surgical intervention, which include obstruction and perforation, and the development of fistulae, abscesses, and perianal disease (fistula, fissure, stricture, and abscess in approximately 25% of patients). Obstruction occurs secondary to the chronic inflammation causing fibrosis and progressive narrowing of the bowel lumen. Fistulae occur to adjacent organs such as bladder, vagina, adjacent bowel segments, and skin. Although toxic megacolon has also been described in patients with Crohn disease, this diagnosis most commonly suggests ulcerative colitis. The incidence of colonic malignancy, although less common in patients with Crohn disease than in patients with ulcerative colitis, is approximately six times greater than in the general population. Perianal disease has been known to precede intestinal disease by months to years; therefore, patients with recurrent perianal disease should be evaluated for Crohn disease.

Diagnosis

Evaluation for Crohn disease is usually performed with endoscopy and biopsy (colonoscopy for distal ileal and colonic involvement, esophagogastroduodenoscopy for upper tract involvement) as well as radiographic studies [computerized tomography/magnetic resonance imaging (MRI), upper GI and SBFT, and barium or Gastrografin enema]. Stool cultures should also be obtained to rule out infectious enteritis. Endoscopic findings include granular, discrete, aphthous ulcerations surrounded by normal tissue and mucosa with cobblestone-like appearance. Discontinuous segments of diseased bowel are classic signs of Crohn disease. Radiographic findings include cobblestone-like appearance of mucosa (linear ulcers, transverse sinuses, and clefts), diffuse narrowing of bowel lumen (narrowed terminal ileum known as Kantor string sign), and asymmetric involvement of bowel wall with a nodular contour. Fistulae and abscesses may also be present.

Nutritional Considerations

Protein calorie malnutrition may occur in 80% to 90% of patients with Crohn disease. Although multiple factors contribute to the malnutrition, abdominal pain, anorexia, nausea, and emesis are the most common. The cytokines interleukin-1 (IL-1) and tumor necrosis factor (TNF) may contribute to cachexia. Total parenteral, total enteral nutrition, or elemental diets may also be used as needed for nutritional derangements. Nutritional therapy as primary treatment for Crohn disease is no longer used as a result of negative controlled trials. However, several important indications for nutritional therapy remain, such as correction of preexisting malnutrition and maintenance of remission. In general, enteral formulas are preferred over parenteral nutrition, as they are more effective, easier to administer, cost less, and have fewer complications. Studies have shown that "resting" the bowel from its absorptive function in and of itself is no longer a valid indication for total parenteral nutrition (TPN).

Medical Treatment

Crohn disease is chronic and incurable. The main goal of therapy is, therefore, symptomatic relief and control of inflammation until such time that a complication requires surgical therapy. Antiinflammatory and immunosuppressive medications that are commonly used for flares of Crohn disease include steroids (intravenous or oral), and sulfasalazine. Other immunosuppressive agents such as azathioprine, 6-mercaptopurine, methotrexate, and cyclosporine have been shown to be effective as maintenance therapies. Antibiotics are also prescribed during acute exacerbations and anal disease, typically metronidazole.

Surgical Treatment

Eventually, most patients diagnosed with Crohn disease will require surgical intervention. Overtreatment with immunosuppression or other medical therapy in hopes of preventing a surgical procedure should not be allowed to compromise patient care. The most common indication for surgery is an acute Crohn flare not responding to therapy or occurring in a patient who cannot tolerate the side-effects of medical treatment. Additional indications for surgical intervention are obstruction, perforation, abscess and fistula formation, perianal disease, and malignancy.

The goal of surgery is to eradicate the acute problem while limiting resection to the grossly involved segment of bowel. Many patients with the Crohn disease will undergo more than one resection during their lifetime and multiple indiscriminate resections may lead to short bowel syndrome, which has been reported variably between 2% and 13%.

Obstruction

Another frequent indication for surgical intervention is obstruction. Partial obstruction is often treated conservatively with nasogastric tube placement, bowel rest, fluid hydration, and electrolyte correction. Complete obstruction and partial obstruction that does not resolve require operative treatment. Again, minimal resection is recommended. Healthy bowel should be resected only if it separates the diseased segments by 5 cm or less. If a healthy intervening segment is greater than 5 cm, it should be salvaged; if a short stricture is the cause of obstruction, than stricturoplasty can be performed. This is done by making a longitudinal incision through the stricture and closing it in a transverse fashion. Bypass with exclusion procedures may also be used but is usually reserved for those patients at high risk (for short gut syndrome and further complications) and the elderly. Most small bowel adenocarcinomas in patients with Crohn disease arise in the bypassed, anatomically excluded bowel segments.

Fistulae

The second most common indication for surgery is fistula formation. Enterocutaneous fistulae are common in Crohn patients and can originate spontaneously or from prior bowel anastomoses or external drainage of an intraabdominal abscess. Simple fistulae (those not complicated by sepsis or other complications) can be treated conservatively (with bowel rest and TPN). Those patients whose conditions fail medical management or who have fistulae that are complicated should be surgically treated. For enterocutaneous fistulae, affected bowel should be resected and the fistula tract in the abdominal wall débrided. Also, the bowel should be separated from the abdominal wall by omentum. Entero-enteric fistulae may be left alone if asymptomatic; however if large segments are bypassed, significant malabsorption and fluid loss may mandate surgery. For entero-vesical and entero-adnexal fistulae, the affected bowel and fistula tract should be resected and the defect in the organ closed.

Acute ileitis is a self-limited disease of the terminal ileum of unknown etiology, although infectious causes have been suggested (*Yersinia* species and *Campylobacter* species). Inflammation of this segment may give a clinical picture similar to appendicitis. The ileum may appear beefy red, with edema, a thickened mesentery, and enlarged lymph nodes. The intent of surgical intervention is to resect affected bowel and to perform an appendectomy even in the absence of appendicitis. If the cecum is also involved, a limited ileocolic resection may be indicated as unresected inflamed bowel may lead to fistula formation.

Prognosis

There is no cure. Recurrences increase in frequency and severity over the years. The most common site of recurrence is the small bowel, usually proximal to the prior site of resection. Many patients will undergo multiple procedures. The disease does gradually recede with increasing age.

DIVERTICULAR DISEASE

Meckel Diverticulum

A Meckel diverticulum is the most common true diverticulum of the GI tract. Although common in the pediatric population, such diverticula should enter into the differential diagnosis in adults as well. The overall incidence is thought to be approximately 2%, and only a small percentage of these become symptomatic. Hemorrhage and inflammation mimicking acute appendicitis are the most common clinical presentations. All symptomatic Meckel diverticula should be resected, including segmental ileal resection if necessary, to eliminate the base where ectopic tissue such as gastric mucosa may be found. Although resection of an incidental asymptomatic Meckel diverticulum can be debated, many surgeons resect lesions greater than 2 cm at the base, in individuals younger than 40 years of age, or for suspicion of ectopic tissue.

Duodenal Diverticula

Duodenal diverticula are the most common acquired or false diverticula in the small bowel (second most common site next to the colon). The true incidence is unknown but may be as high as 10% to 20% of the general population. Duodenal diverticula are more common in women and in individuals older than 50 years of age. Greater than 95% of these defects are asymptomatic and less than 5% require any surgical intervention. More than 60% of these diverticula are found in the periampullary region projecting from the medial wall.

Clinical Manifestations

Patients may present with obstruction, perforation, or bleeding into the small bowel. Periampullary diverticula may also be responsible for recurrent pancreatitis, cholangitis, and recurrent common bile duct (CBD) stones even after cholecystectomy, secondary to mechanical distortion of the CBD.

Treatment

The main goal is to control the complications. The most common and effective treatment is to perform a diverticulectomy. A *Kocher maneuver* (dissecting the lateral peritoneal attachments of the duodenum to allow access to the pancreas, duodenum, and other retroperitoneal structures) is performed, and a duodenotomy is made. The diverticulum is then excised, followed by closure of the defect in a transverse fashion to avoid narrowing the lumen.

Jejunoileal Diverticula

Most jejunoileal diverticula are acquired pulsion pseudodiverticula associated with increasing age. They are frequently a marker for an underlying dysmotility syndrome. Like colonic diverticula, most are located on the mesenteric aspect of the bowel, at locations where blood vessels perforate the muscularis propria. They may be multiple and are usually asymptomatic but can be complicated by infection, obstruction, and perforation. Associated bacterial overgrowth occasionally leads to malabsorption. Enteroclysis (small bowel enema) is the study of choice for making the diagnosis. Complications of diverticulitis, obstruction, or perforation are treated similarly to those associated with colonic diverticular disease. Jejunoileal diverticula render patients at increased risk for lymphoma.

VASCULAR DISEASE

Acute Mesenteric Ischemia

Acute mesenteric ischemia may result from (i) SMA embolization (cardiac origin), (ii) SMA thrombosis (underlying atherosclerotic disease), (iii) nonocclusive mesenteric ischemia (low cardiac output state), and (iv) acute mesenteric venous thrombosis (dehydration and infection). Rarely, visceral ischemia may result from an aortic dissection if the visceral vessels are disconnected from the true lumen.

Clinical Manifestations

Patients usually present with abdominal pain out of proportion to physical findings. The pain is usually periumbilical with symptoms of nausea, vomiting, and bloody diarrhea. Laboratory studies may reveal leukocytosis, hyperkalemia, metabolic acidosis, or elevations levels of lactate levels, LDH, alanine aminotransferase (ALT), aspartate aminotransferase (AST), or CPK. Changes in the mucosa can be detected under light microscopy within minutes of the onset of ischemia; these changes later develop into hemorrhagic necrosis, edema of the bowel wall, sloughing of the mucosa, and finally hemorrhage into the lumen. The insult to the mucosa causes it to be permeable to the luminal bacterial flora leading to peritonitis, bacteremia, and septicemia.

Diagnosis

Clinical diagnosis is difficult because the symptoms are vague, it occurs infrequently, and patients frequently have other comorbidities. If the diagnosis is delayed, especially beyond 24 hours, the disease is associated with high mortality. Traditionally, consideration of visceral ischemia in patients with acute abdominal pain mandated visceral arteriography. Other diagnostic modalities now being used with increasing frequency are CT angiography and magnetic resonance arteriography/venography. These studies can also assist in differentiating between the four main causes of ischemia. SMA embolism is characterized by emboli at the origin of the middle colic artery distal to the first few jejunal branches. SMA thrombus is characterized by thrombus at the origin of the SMA proximal to the jejunal branches. Nonocclusive ischemia is characterized by segmental mesenteric vasospasm involving the branches of the SMA (Fig. 13-1).

Treatment

The treatment varies with the cause of bowel ischemia. For SMA embolus, operative management is required, and the preoperative arteriogram will assist with appropriate planning of therapy. Through a midline incision, the root of the SMA is exposed. A transverse arteriotomy is performed, and a balloon catheter is passed distally and proximally to remove the thrombus/embolus. Assessment of intestinal reperfusion is required after revascularization.

Several diagnostic tools may be utilized to estimate bowel viability. These include intraoperative intravenous fluorescein injection with Wood light inspection of the bowel and Doppler assessment of pulsatile flow in the vascular arcades. A second-look procedure is necessary approximately 24 hours postrevascularization to establish viability of bowel segments deemed marginal at the first operation. For SMA thrombus, a bypass graft is often needed to reestablish flow to the affected bowel. There are advantages to placing the proximal graft in the supraceliac portion of the intraabdominal aorta, as the vessel tends to be less calcified and there are fewer tendencies for the graft to kink. Vein grafts are preferred to prosthetic grafts because of the risk of bacterial seeding. For nonocclusive mesenteric ischemia, treatment is usually nonoperative, and the cause of the low flow state is corrected with appropriate volume resuscitation, vasopressors, or cardiac support as is clinically indicated. In general, restoration of adequate cardiac index will alleviate the symptoms. Vasodilating agents such as papaverine and tolazoline may be used at the time of arteriography. Surgical resection should be performed should medical management fail.

Chronic Mesenteric Ischemia

Chronic mesenteric ischemia is usually caused by atherosclerotic disease of the SMA and celiac arteries. Other etiologies include fibromuscular dysplasia, radiation enteritis, autoimmune arteritides, and external compression. The atherosclerotic process usually begins with plaque formation, which occurs at the origin of the visceral arteries. The chronicity of the disease allows for the development of collateral circulation, an important characteristic of the disease. The common collateral circuits are the communication between the celiac artery and the gastroduodenal artery, the SMA and the pancreatic branches, as well as the SMA and the inferior mesenteric artery (IMA) through the meandering mesenteric artery (most important), the marginal artery of Drummond (Fig. 13-7), and the left colic and middle colic arteries. The meandering mesenteric artery is present only in occlusive disease. It is more tortuous, shorter in length, and more medial than the marginal artery of Drummond.

Diagnosis

Patients classically complain of postprandial abdominal pain starting approximately 20 minutes to 1 hour after a meal. Many patients have a pre-existing history of atherosclerotic disease. The intensity of pain correlates with the amount of food ingested; chronic mesenteric ischemia has, therefore, also been referred to as "intestinal angina." Patients may also complain of weight loss secondary to "food fear," as fear of associated pain may result in decreased food intake. Patients are usually cachectic, with a midabdominal bruit, and have other clinical signs of atherosclerotic disease such as the absence of palpable lower extremity pulses, as well as carotid, femoral, and/or abdominal aortic bruits. The gold standard study is arteriography, which may reveal occlusion or stenosis of the celiac axis, the SMA, and any collateral vessels. Chronic mesenteric ischemia rarely occurs with a single arterial occlusion. Duplex ultrasonography has also been used for screening for mesenteric ischemia. Occult blood in the stool is unusual in chronic mesenteric ischemia; therefore,

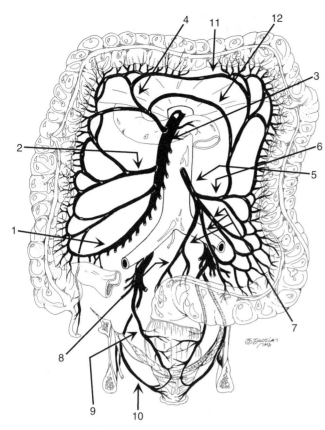

Figure 13-7 The arterial blood supply to the colon: *(1)* ileocolic artery, *(2)* right colic artery, *(3)* superior mesenteric artery, *(4)* middle colic artery, *(5)* inferior mesenteric artery, *(6)* left colic artery, *(7)* sigmoidal artery, *(8)* superior hemorrhoidal artery, *(9)* middle hemorrhoidal artery, *(10)* Inferior hemorrhoidal artery, *(11)* marginal artery of Drummond, *(12)* meandering artery of Gonzalez. (From Blackbourne LH, ed. *Surgical recall*, 2nd ed. Philadelphia: Lippincott Williams & Wilkins, 1998:274, with permission.)

if occult blood is found, another diagnosis such as acute ischemia or malignancy must be sought.

Treatment

To prevent bowel infarction, revascularization is indicated in all symptomatic patients. Bypass procedures are preferred over endarterectomy techniques because an intimal flap inadvertently created during endarterectomy may cause early thrombosis of the artery. Although the supraceliac and infrarenal aorta, as well as the iliac arteries may all provide adequate inflow into the new bypass graft, placement of a supraceliac aortic graft in an antegrade fashion leads results in superior outcomes. Venous and prosthetic grafts have equally good outcomes, but there is a decreased risk of persistent bacterial infection with autogenous grafts. Endovascular techniques, such as percutaneous balloon angioplasty and stent placement, are still under investigation for safety and efficacy in the treatment of mesenteric ischemia.

SMALL BOWEL NEOPLASMS

Several hypotheses exist that attempt to explain the extremely low incidence of primary small bowel neoplasms. The increased transit time of the small bowel may decrease contact of carcinogens with the mucosa, or the highly developed immune system of the small bowel mucosa may eliminate premalignant transformed cells. Additional theories describe a protective effect of the basic pH of the bowel contents, as well as the absence of bacteria that can convert certain products into carcinogens and the presence of mucosal enzymes that eliminate carcinogens. Small bowel neoplasms are usually asymptomatic but can present with obstruction, diarrhea, abdominal distention, obstipation, cramping, or anemia secondary to bleeding. Benign tumors include hamartomas, adenomas, hemangiomas, fibromas, lipomas, and leiomyomas. Malignant tumors include adenocarcinomas, lymphomas, and leiomyosarcomas. Malignant and benign neoplasms occur with equal frequency, but malignant tumors are more likely to produce symptoms.

Benign Neoplasms

The majority of benign small bowel tumors are asymptomatic and found incidentally at autopsy. The diagnosis is often delayed or missed. Benign small bowel tumors are of epithelial or connective tissue origin. Histologic benign tumors include adenomas (most common and found usually at autopsy), leiomyomas (most common benign tumor to cause symptoms), and lipomas. These neoplasms are usually slow growing but may grow enough to cause intraluminal obstruction. They may also be polypoid and cause intussusception or may twist axially causing hemorrhage. Diagnosis is often made secondary to suspicion because of the infrequency and vague symptoms associated with this disease. The physical examination is usually not revealing. Diagnostic studies used include upper endoscopy, SBFT, and enteroclysis. Enteroclysis is superior to SBFT in detecting small filling defects in the mucosa and determining changes in the mucosal pattern; it is approximately 90% accurate. Capsule enteroscopy for diagnosis is being evaluated, but it is not currently able to allow biopsy of identified lesions. Surgical intervention is indicated because of the possibility of cancer and the risks of subsequent mechanical complications. Surgery usually consists of segmental resection and primary anastomosis, though small lesions may be excised by enterotomy.

Adenoma

There are two types of true adenomas—villous adenomas and Brunner gland adenomas. Approximately 20% are located in the duodenum, 30% in the jejunum, and 50% are found in the ileum. Most occur singly and are asymptomatic. *Villous adenomas* are rare and most commonly are found in the duodenum. They can be quite large (larger than 5 cm) and have a 30% to 50% malignancy potential. *Brunner gland adenomas* are located in the duodenum and are caused by the hyperplastic proliferation of the normal exocrine glands located in the submucosa. Diagnosis is usually made by endoscopy and biopsy. These tumors have no malignant potential; therefore, conservative local resection should be attempted.

Leiomyoma

Leiomyomas are the most common symptomatic benign lesion. Histologically, these are smooth muscle tumors and are most commonly located in the jejunum. Leiomyomas can occur singly or multiply, with equal male and female incidence. They can grow to a large size intramurally or extramurally. If they grow large enough, they can outgrow their blood supply, thereby causing tumor necrosis and bleeding. The most common indication for operative intervention is bleeding. Angiography may be useful for diagnosis and even temporary control of hemorrhage.

Lipoma

Lipomas are most commonly found intramurally or in the submucosa of the ileum. They are usually single and small and may cause obstruction by becoming the lead point of an intussusception. Bleeding can also occur from ulceration of the overlying mucosa. They have no malignant potential. Surgical excision is the usual treatment.

Hamartoma

Hamartomas commonly occur as part of the Peutz–Jeghers syndrome, an autosomal dominant inherited syndrome of mucocutaneous melanotic pigmentation and GI polyps. The polyps are not true polyps and are therefore not premalignant; however, patients diagnosed with Peutz–Jeghers are at increased risk of other GI malignancies. Classically, patients have small, 1 to 2 mm brown-black spots located in a circumoral region of the face, buccal mucosa, palms and soles, lips, digits, and the perianal area. The hamartomas are most frequently located in the jejunum and ileum. Approximately 50% of patients also have a concomitant lesion in the colon or rectum and about 25% may have gastric polyps as well. If the colonic, rectal, or gastric polyps are found to be hamartomas, then the small bowel should also be investigated for polyps. Patients may complain of colicky abdominal pain secondary to intermittent intussusception, obstruction, or bleeding. Surgical treatment is primarily indicated for obstruction or persistent hemorrhage. Bowel resection should be limited to the affected portion.

Hemangiomas

Hemangiomas are developmental malformations of proliferating submucosal blood vessels and account for 3% to 4% of all benign small bowel tumors. They are most common in the jejunum but can occur anywhere in the GI tract. Most patients with hemangiomas are asymptomatic with the onset of GI bleeding, usually the only indication of their existence. Diagnostic studies most useful in diagnosis are angiography and Technetium-99m-labeled red blood cell scan, although diagnosis is usually difficult. If the lesion can be localized, conservative resection is recommended. However, if the lesion cannot be localized, then intraoperative palpation or transillumination via intraoperative enteroscopy of the bowel may be helpful.

Malignant Neoplasms

The most common malignant neoplasms are adenocarcinoma, carcinoid, sarcoma, and lymphoma. Patients usually complain of weight loss, diarrhea with mucus, or obstructive symptoms such as nausea, vomiting, or abdominal pain. Signs and symptoms of chronic blood loss (anemia and melena) may also occur. Treatment includes wide surgical resection with regional lymph node biopsy, palliative resection, or intestinal bypass to relieve symptoms or to prevent further complications. Radiation and chemotherapy have little role in adenocarcinoma but may improve survival rates in patients with lymphoma and

sarcoma. Prognosis is usually poor. For adenocarcinomas, the 5-year survival rate is less than 20%, and for leiomyosarcomas the 5-year survival rate is 30% to 40%.

Adenocarcinomas

Adenocarcinomas account for approximately one half of malignant small bowel tumors. There is a male-to-female ratio of 2:1, with a peak age of 50 years. These tumors are more common in the duodenum and jejunum. Approximately 50% of duodenal carcinomas involve the ampulla of Vater. Tumor location often will determine the symptoms. For example, if the tumor is periampullary, patients will have intermittent jaundice and heme-positive stools. If the tumor is jejunal, then patients will have symptoms of SBO. Survival rates are related to the stage of the disease at the time of diagnosis. Diagnosis is delayed secondary to vague symptoms or lack of symptoms, absence of physical findings, and the overall rarity of the disease.

Sarcoma

This mesenchymal neoplasm accounts for 2% of malignant small bowel tumors, with the most common type being leiomyosarcoma. These tumors have equal incidence in men and women, and diagnosis is usually made in the sixth decade. Small bowel sarcomas spread by several routes: direct invasion of adjacent tissues, hematogenous dissemination, and transperitoneal seeding leading to sarcomatosis. Other rare sarcomas include fibrosarcoma, Kaposi sarcoma, liposarcoma, and angiosarcoma. The most common indications for operative management include obstruction, bleeding, or perforation.

Lymphoma

Lymphomas account for 10% to 15% of small bowel malignant tumors. The ileum is the most common location, where the greatest concentration of gut-associated lymphoid tissue is also found. Lymphoma may be part of a generalized disease or an isolated primary bowel tumor. Criteria to help distinguish between primary and generalized disease include the absence of peripheral lymphadenopathy, lack of mediastinal lymphadenopathy on chest x-ray, normal white blood cell count and differential, a dominant small bowel mass as the principal tumor, and absence of metastatic disease to liver and spleen. More than 30% of patients with bowel lymphoma have generalized lymphoma.

Carcinoid

Small bowel carcinoid tumors account for somewhat less than one half of malignant small bowel neoplasms. Carcinoid tumors are derived from enterochromaffin (argentaffin) cells or Kulchitsky cells found in the crypts of Lieberkühn. About 90% of carcinoid tumors occur in the GI tract and have variable malignant potential. About 50% of carcinoid tumors occur in the appendix and 25% occur in the ileum. Carcinoid tumors of the ileum are much more frequently metastatic than appendiceal carcinoid. Small bowel carcinoid tumors are composed of multipotential cells, which have the ability to secrete substances such as serotonin and substance P. Approximately 5% of patients may present with episodes of cutaneous flushing, bronchospasm/asthma, diarrhea/malabsorption, vasomotor collapse, and right heart valvular disease, known together as malignant *carcinoid syndrome*. Malignant potential is related to size, location, depth, and growth pattern. Size, depth, and metastatic potential have a direct relationship. The histologic pattern is related to survival and has prognostic importance. Intraoperatively, the tumor appears slightly elevated, smooth, round, hard, and covered with normal mucosa. When transected, it has a characteristic yellow-gray appearance. The mesentery may be severely fibrotic secondary to an intense desmoplastic reaction caused by humoral agents (i.e., substance P) secreted by the tumor. Coexistence of another primary tumor of different histology has been found in one fourth of patients. About one third of patients may have multiple carcinoid neoplasms upon surgical exploration.

Diagnosis

The diagnosis is made by radiographic studies such as upper GI and SBFT, which show a filling defect that may result from tumor, kinking, or fibrotic bowel. Angiography of the mesenteric vessels may be used for tumor staging and to assess resectability. MRI may be used to evaluate for liver metastasis. Abnormal arrangements of the vessels, narrowing of the peripheral branches, and vascular insufficiency are often seen. About 30% to 70% of carcinoid tumors of the GI tract are found to be metastatic at the time of diagnosis.

Treatment

The surgical management is based on size and site of the neoplasm as well as the presence of metastatic disease (tumors up to 1 cm in greatest dimension require segmental resection; greater than 1 cm, multiple tumors, or regional lymph node metastases require wide excision; and duodenal lesions often require pancreaticoduodenectomy). If the tumor is localized, surgical resection is curative. If carcinoid has metastasized with malignant carcinoid syndrome, surgical resection may provide reasonable palliation. Chemotherapy (usually streptozotocin and 5-fluorouracil) may also be used for palliation. Long-term palliation is often possible as the tumors are slow growing and indolent. Appendiceal carcinoid usually occurs in individuals 20 to 40 years of age. If tumors are smaller than 1 cm and located at the tip, then a simple appendectomy is curative. However, if there is lymphovascular invasion present in the specimen, then a completion hemicolectomy is indicated even if the lesion is smaller than 1 cm. If the tumor is greater than 2 cm in dimension, then a right hemicolectomy is recommended because of increased metastatic potential.

Prognosis

The prognosis of small intestinal carcinoid tumors is related to the spread of the tumor. If tumor is localized, the survival rate is 75%. If the tumor is regional then survival is 60%; if the tumor is metastatic, survival approximates 20%. The type of growth pattern is an independent predictor of outcome.

Malignant Carcinoid Syndrome

The malignant carcinoid syndrome is found in only 6% to 9% of patients with metastatic carcinoid cancer. The primary tumor is usually in the small bowel and the syndrome is seen only in the context of functional liver metastases (the liver is unable to metabolize serotonin) or the primary tumor is either in the lung, ovary, or testicle (the serotonin enters the systemic venous system, therefore it bypasses the liver for metabolism). It is characterized by diarrhea, flushing, and hepatomegaly in approximately 80% of patients; right heart valvular disease in 50%; and bronchospasm/asthma in 25% of patients. The diarrhea is caused by elevated serum serotonin levels, and it is often postprandial and episodic in nature. It may be accompanied by severe abdominal pain secondary to intestinal ischemia caused by the mesenteric vessel fibrosis and by the vasoactive substances secreted by the tumor. Flushing and asthma may be caused by the secretion of serotonin, substance P, bradykinins, and prostaglandins E and F. Right heart valvular disease is the result of irreversible fibrosis of the endocardium, which is the same type of fibrosis found in the bowel wall and mesentery. Only the right-sided heart valves are affected (tricuspid and pulmonary valves), as the vasoactive agents are cleared efficiently by the lungs, therefore, sparing the mitral and the aortic valves. The most reliable test for diagnosis is made by repeated 5-hydroxyindoleacetic acid (5-HIAA; a metabolite of serotonin) secretion in the urine. Temporary treatment of the syndrome can include tumor resection and debulking of the liver (6 months of relief), hepatic dearterialization or embolization (5 months of relief) with chemotherapy (doxorubicin, cisplatin, 5-fluorouracil). Drug therapy (interferon, Sandostatin, somatostatin-14) may be used for prevention or relief of symptoms. Carcinoid crisis is a potentially catastrophic clinical state usually seen on induction of anesthesia for which immediate somatostatin analog treatment may be life-saving.

MISCELLANEOUS SMALL BOWEL DISEASES

Small Bowel Fistulae

The most common cause of small bowel fistula is surgery. Postoperative fistulae result principally from anastomotic leak or unrecognized injury to the bowel or its blood supply. Other causes include Crohn disease, inflammatory diseases, trauma, preoperative radiation, intestinal obstruction, vascular disease, and foreign bodies. Major complications from fistulae are sepsis, fluid and electrolyte derangements, necrosis of the soft tissue at the drainage site, and malnutrition. There is a 20% mortality despite TPN. Although the condition does not significantly reduce mortality, the best way to manage small bowel fistulae is to control sepsis and to prevent malnutrition.

Diagnosis

If the fistula is enterocutaneous in type, bowel contents are generally seen issuing from the site. Confirmation can be achieved using radiographic studies such as upper GI and SBFT, barium enemas, CT scans, contrast fistulograms, or oral ingestion of charcoal or nonabsorbable food coloring. It is important to identify if the fistula is proximal or distal and whether it is high or low output. These factors dictate the prognosis and the treatment plan. Proximal fistulae tend to have a greater impact on fluid and electrolyte balance as well as nutrition, since the bowel contents do not reach the distal bowel for absorption. High output fistulae, those secreting more than 500 mL per day, require even more diligent fluid and electrolyte replacement than do low output fistulae. Somatostatin analogs may decrease volume but do not affect duration of fistula closure. Five anatomic criteria have been described that lead to persistence of the fistula tract: distal bowel obstruction, intestinal discontinuity, the presence of an abscess, excessive inflammation or necrosis of the bowel, or other disease processes contributing to poor overall bowel condition.

Treatment

Control of sepsis is first and foremost the most important goal in the management of fistulae and may significantly affect eventual fistula closure. The decision to use appropriate antibiotics, drain the abscess, or débride devitalized tissue depends on the clinical situation. Volume and electrolyte repletion is critical and is obtained through bowel rest, judicious replacement of observed and insensible losses, and TPN. Skin protection to prevent further wound erosion is also needed. Conservative management should be maintained for up to 6 weeks with TPN if the patient is stable. TPN allows for healing, improves nutritional status, and permits optimization of the patient's status for future operative treatment. When the patient's condition is stabilized and the sepsis controlled, formal operative treatment of the chronic fistula is necessary in most cases. Surgical management can be accomplished by careful exploration to eliminate any factors contributing to fistula persistence (obstruction, foreign body, or intrinsic bowel pathology), to prevent further injury to the unaffected bowel, to identify and excise the fistula tract, and to resect the affected bowel. Proximal enterostomy may be required to protect tenuous anastomoses or if primary repair cannot be performed.

Blind Loop Syndrome

The blind loop syndrome is rare and clinically manifests as diarrhea/steatorrhea, abdominal pain, vitamin deficiency, neurologic symptoms, anemia, and weight loss. It is caused by bacterial overgrowth in a stagnant segment of small bowel. Stagnation of bowel may be caused by intrinsic stricture, adhesive obstruction, defunctionalized segments (as in jejuno-ileal bypass), or diverticula. Vitamin B_{12} deficiency is caused by increased bacterial consumption causing neurologic symptoms (demyelination of the posterior and lateral spinal columns) and megaloblastic anemia. Other nutrient malabsorption may be secondary to direct injury to the mucosa. Diagnosis is made by serum vitamin B_{12} levels or the Schilling test, in which labeled vitamin B_{12} is orally administered and then measured in the urine. Then the test is repeated with the addition of intrinsic factor. In true pernicious anemia, the urinary excretion is increased to normal levels. In blind loop syndrome, the urinary excretion is unchanged. The patient is then given a course of antibiotics such as tetracycline or doxycycline and the test is repeated. In blind loop syndrome, the urinary excretion should increase to normal. Medical management should be employed to optimize the patient for surgical treatment. Operative intervention is indicated and should include correction of the anatomic defects and resection of the diseased segment.

Radiation Enteritis

Adjuvant radiation therapy has been a common treatment for many abdominal and pelvic malignancies. Despite its beneficial effects, radiation-induced complications result in severe acute and chronic damage to the treated bowel. Damage is dependent on the dose of radiation (greater than 5,000 cGy), and other comorbidities (previous abdominal surgeries, diabetes, hypertension, vascular disease, and use of chemotherapeutic agents). Bowel epithelium is highly sensitive to irradiation but because of its high turnover rate the symptoms such as abdominal pain, diarrhea, and malabsorption are acute and self-limiting. Damage to the submucosa and its vessels produce the late symptoms of necrosis, perforation, fistula formation, stricture, and obstruction. Radiation injury to the submucosa progresses to submucosal fibrosis and obliterative arteritis, leading to bowel ischemia and necrosis. Radiation damage can be minimized or prevented by delivering the treatment in a limited treatment field, whether by adjusting the patient's position or adjusting the equipment. If preradiation laparotomy is performed, then the bowel can be protected by reperitonealization, omental transposition, or placement of mesh slings to exclude the bowel from the pelvis, if pelvic malignancies are targeted.

Treatment should be conservative and geared toward symptomatic relief. Operative management should be done with caution because the anatomy is distorted, and vascular injury is usually widespread making exploration and resection difficult. However, operation is required for symptomatic stricture, fistulae, and obstruction. Primary anastomosis of irradiated bowel has a higher anastomotic leak rate; therefore, adequate margin of resection must be balanced with prevention of short bowel syndrome. Grossly normal-appearing bowel may have sufficient microscopic damage to contribute to an anastomotic leak. If the affected bowel is fixed and rigid making resection technically difficult, intestinal bypass or proximal enterostomy may be indicated. Less than 25% of radiated patients die as a result of radiation enteritis and its complications. About one half of those patients undergoing their first operative procedure will likely need surgical intervention.

Short Bowel Syndrome

Short bowel syndrome is caused by massive surgical resection (emergent or staged) of the small bowel secondary to midgut volvulus, traumatic injury, vascular occlusion, or repeated resection. Clinical manifestations include diarrhea, malnutrition, and fluid and electrolyte abnormalities. Symptoms depend on the amount of small bowel resected, whether the ileocecal valve is intact, and whether the proximal or distal bowel is lost. Approximately 70% of the small bowel can be resected and be well tolerated if the ileocecal valve is intact. Resection of the proximal small bowel is better tolerated, as distal bowel can adapt to effectively increase absorptive abilities. Bowel adaptation is characterized by hyperplasia of the remaining enterocytes and lengthening of the villi, thereby creating a larger surface area, hypertrophy of the bowel wall, and increased caliber of the remaining bowel. The trigger for bowel adaptation may be from multiple factors that are currently being investigated. Enteral feeding and certain gut hormones (insulin-like growth factor 1, glucagon-like peptide 2, growth hormone, and neurotensin) have all been implicated.

Treatment

Conservative resections can prevent short bowel syndrome from occurring in most cases. If the syndrome is present, special enteral diets (elemental or polymeric) should be administered along with vitamins and GI prophylactic medications. Medium-chain fatty acids can also be added. Medications that slow bowel motility should be used sparingly. Surgical treatments are limited, and there are few clinical data to support the use of surgical procedures such as reversed intestinal segment, colonic interposition, or construction of an intestinal valve to slow intestinal transit time. In addition, long-term outcomes of small bowel transplantations have yet to be determined specifically for this disease process.

KEY POINTS

▲ *Small Bowel Crohn Disease:* Three fourths of patients with Crohn disease will eventually require surgical intervention. The indication for surgery parallels the incidence of local complications, with obstruction being the most common and fistula formation being second.

▲ *Small Bowel Obstruction:* One of the most important determinations the surgeon must make is whether small bowel obstruction is partial or complete. Management of complete small bowel obstruction is often surgical; management of partial bowel obstruction is initially nonoperative.

▲ *Small Bowel Fistulae:* The primary causes of death in patients with small bowel fistulae are malnutrition, electrolyte imbalance, and sepsis. Consequently, initial management priorities are provision of optimal nutrition, correction of the fluid and electrolyte imbalances, and control of sepsis with appropriate antibiotics and judicious surgical drainage.

▲ *Visceral Ischemia:* To favorably impact survival, the diagnosis of acute mesenteric ischemia must be made before bowel infarction develops. Selective mesenteric angiography is still considered the gold standard in diagnosis. In the presence of signs and symptoms of peritonitis, the high incidence of bowel infarction mandates laparotomy. Even in this setting, angiography may assist in the cause of bowel ischemia.

▲ *Small Bowel Neoplasms:* Nonneuroendocrine tumors of the small bowel are rare. Despite the fact that the small bowel comprises approximately four fifths of the inner surface area of the alimentary tract, tumors of the small bowel comprise only 5% to 7% of all gastrointestinal tumors. Malignant small bowel tumors are most commonly adenocarcinoma and carcinoid, in approximately equal proportions.

SUGGESTED READINGS

Behrns KE, Kircher AP, Galanko JA, et al. Prospective randomized trial of early initial and hospital discharge on a liquid diet following elective intestinal surgery. *Gastrointest Surg* 2000;4: 217–221.

Clavien PA, Richon J, Burgan S, et al. Gallstone ileus. *Br J Surg* 1990;77: 737–742.

Delaney CP, Fazin VW. Crohn's disease of the small bowel. *Surg Clin North Am* 2001;81(1):137–158.

Eriksen AS, Krasna MJ, Mast BA, et al. Use of gastrointestinal contrast studies in obstruction of the small and large bowel. *Dis Colon Rectum* 1990;33(1):56–64.

Evers BM, Townsend CM, Thompson JC. Small intestine. In: Schwartz SI, Shires GT, Spencer FC, eds. *Principles of surgery*, 7th ed. New York: McGraw-Hill, 1999.

Megibow AJ. Bowel obstruction: evaluation with CT. *Radiol Clin North Am* 1997;32(5):861–870.

Pickleman J, Lee RM. The management of patients with suspected early postoperative small bowel obstruction. *Ann Surg* 1989;210(2): 216–219.

Roggo A, Ottinger LW. Acute small bowel volvulus in adults: a sporadic form of strangulating intestinal obstruction. *Ann Surg* 1992; 216(2):135–141.

Song HK, Buzby GP. Nutritional support for Crohn's disease. *Surg Clin North Am* 2001;81(1):103–115.

The Colon, Rectum, and Anus

Leonard T. Su   *Robert Fry*

14

ANATOMY

Knowledge of the embryonic development of the colon, rectum and anus establishes a framework for understanding the important anatomical relationships of the large bowel, as well as its neurovascular supply. During development of the embryo, the midgut forms the proximal two thirds of the colon, while the hindgut develops into the rectum. During formation the gut actually herniates outside of the small embryonic abdominal cavity, and then returns to the developing abdomen with a counterclockwise rotation and subsequently becomes fixed in its final anatomical position. The colon itself is comprised of layers: mucosa, submucosa, an inner circular and outer longitudinal muscular layer, and serosa. The longitudinal muscular layer encircles the rectum, but it does not completely encircle the colon. Instead it consists of three distinct bands, the *teniae coli*. These longitudinal bands cause sacculations or *haustra*, which give the colon its typical radiographic appearance. The completely developed colon in an adult is a tube approximately 1.5 meters long, beginning as the cecum in the right lower quadrant of the abdomen. The cecum does not have its own mesentery, and thus can have a degree of mobility greater than that afforded to the other segments of the large bowel. The cecum is actually a spherical structure that connects to the tubular ascending colon and is the most capacious portion of the large bowel. The terminal ileum empties into this sac-like cecum at the ileocecal valve.

From the base of the cecum, within 2 to 3 cm of the ileocecal valve and at the convergence of the three tenia coli, arises the appendix, a blind-ended, 8 to 10 cm intraperitoneal tube that receives blood through its own mesentery, the "mesoappendix." The position of the tip of the appendix varies, most commonly (65%) lying posterior to the cecum (retrocecal), in the pelvis (31%) or many other positions including retrocolic or even in the left lower quadrant.

The ascending colon runs superiorly from the cecum to the hepatic flexure. Peritoneum covers its sides and anterior surface, but its posterior surface lies in a retroperitoneal position in close proximity to the right kidney and duodenum.

The transverse colon is an entirely intraperitoneal structure arising at the hepatic flexure on the right and ending at the splenic flexure on the left. This is a mobile loop of bowel that may descend between the two flexures as low as the pelvic brim. However, its mesentery has a broad base attached posteriorly at the inferior border of the pancreas, and this broad attachment prevents volvulus of this seemingly mobile organ. The transverse colon is also supported by the *gastrocolic ligament* arising from the greater curvature of the stomach. The gastrocolic ligament fuses with the peritoneal covering of the colon to form the *greater omentum*, a sheet of fat that appears to hang from the front of the transverse colon.

The descending colon courses inferiorly from the splenic flexure. Similar to the ascending colon, its posterior surface is retroperitoneal while its sides and anterior surface are covered with visceral peritoneum. The descending colon communicates with the entirely intraperitoneal sigmoid colon, which takes a sinuous course into the pelvis and joins the rectum. The sigmoid, supported by a mobile mesentery, is often redundant, even coursing to the right lower quadrant. Thus, sigmoid pathology may mimic acute appendicitis or pelvic inflammation. The sigmoid mesentery is closely associated with the left ureter, and care must be taken during mobilization of the sigmoid and its mesentery to avoid ureteral injury.

The longitudinal tenia coli converge to mark the rectosigmoid junction at approximately the level of the sacral promontory. The rectum is a partially intraperitoneal organ; as it descends into the pelvis, the posterior wall is in close proximity to the sacrum, and the peritoneum is reflected from its anterior surface to form the cul-de-sac and to invest the uterus in women and the bladder in men. Although the posterior rectum lies on the presacral fascia, the mesorectum is enveloped by a distinct mesothelial layer—the *fascia propria*. Dissection between fascia propria of the rectum and the sacrum preserves the integrity of the lymphatics contained in the mesorectum, an important principle of oncologic surgery. Mucosal infoldings project into the lumen as the *valves of Houston*. These structures are not true valves and provide excellent sites for mucosal biopsy with minimal risk of perforating the full thickness of the rectal wall. The rectum lies in the pelvis with a slight curve, and rectal mobilization may permit straightening of this curve which may provide as much as 5 cm of additional length above the anus, an important factor when fashioning an anastomosis deep within the pelvis.

The distensible rectum resides in the pelvic floor suspended by the *levator ani*, a funnel-shaped structure comprised of the *pubococcygeus, iliococcygeus,* and *puborectalis* muscles. The puborectalis acts as a sling around the terminal rectum to maintain a 90-degree bend, the anorectal angle. Relaxation of the puborectalis straightens this angle simultaneously with contraction of the sigmoid to permit defecation.

The anus (Fig. 14-1) runs approximately 4 cm from the anorectal junction to the skin of the anal verge. In the proximal anus the mucosa forms longitudinal folds called the *columns of Morgagni.* Anal glands lying in the plane between the internal sphincter and external sphincter (intersphincteric plane) connect with crypts lying between the columns of Morgagni. Infections in these glands can result in anorectal abscesses and fistulas.

The *dentate line* or pectinate line marks the transition from the columnar epithelium of the rectal mucosa to the squamous epithelium of the anoderm. The anorectum above the dentate line is supplied by visceral innervation, sensitive only to stretch. Somatic fibers via branches of the internal pudendal innervate below the dentate line, providing sensation of pain, touch and temperature. The *internal and external sphincters* surround the anus; the internal sphincter is involuntary smooth muscle continuous with the circular smooth muscle layer of the rectum. The external sphincter is composed of striated muscle fibers with voluntary control.

Blood Supply

The *superior mesenteric artery* (SMA) supplies midgut structures. It terminates in the *ileocolic artery* which supplies the terminal ileum, cecum and the appendix. The *right colic artery* originates from the SMA or occasionally from the ileocolic or middle colic arteries. It supplies the ascending colon and hepatic flexure. The *middle colic artery* branches into a right and left branch to supply the ascending colon and the proximal two thirds of the transverse colon. The *inferior mesenteric artery* (IMA) supplies the hindgut. Its first branch, the *left colic artery* runs superiorly to supply the distal transverse and descending colon. The sigmoidal branches originate from the IMA and anastomose with the left colic artery to supply the sigmoid colon. The IMA terminates in the *superior rectal artery,* which runs inferiorly in the mesorectum, supplying mainly the superior rectum along its course ending in the anal canal above the pectinate line. The *middle and inferior rectal arteries* are respectively branches of the internal iliac and internal pudendal arteries. They supply the middle and inferior rectum as well as the anus. The middle arteries anastomose with branches of the superior hemorrhoidal artery while inferior arteries do not. (Fig. 14-2.)

Arteries supplying the colon collateralize with each other creating considerable redundancy. The *marginal artery of Drummond* (Fig. 14-2) is a series of arterial arcades running along the mesenteric border of the entire colon. The *Arc of Riolan* connects the proximal SMA and the IMA. This important collateral maintains flow to the affected colon should one of these vessels become occluded or ligated. Increased size and tortuosity of this arc demonstrated on angiography suggest an obstruction in either the IMA or SMA. The supply of the splenic flexure is particularly at risk as it lies between IMA and SMA distributions and is mainly supplied by terminal branches of each. It thus is a watershed area and prone to vascular insult.

Venous drainage of the colon corresponds with arterial supply. The superior and inferior mesenteric veins (SMV, IMV) drain the distributions of the SMA and IMA respectively into the portal system. The IMV drains into the

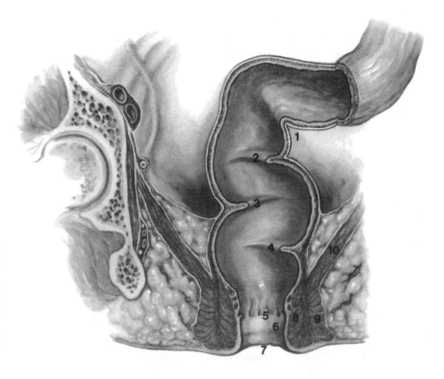

Figure 14-1 Coronal section of the rectum, anus, and perineum. 1, rectosigmoid junction; 2, superior valve of Houston; 3, middle valve of Houston; 4, inferior valve of Houston; 5, pectinate of dentate line; 6, pecten; 7, anal margin; 8, internal anal sphincter; 9, external anal sphincter; 10, levator ani muscle and puborectalis. (From Etala E, ed. *Atlas of gastrointestinal surgery.* Philadelphia: Williams & Wilkins, 1997:1737, with permission.)

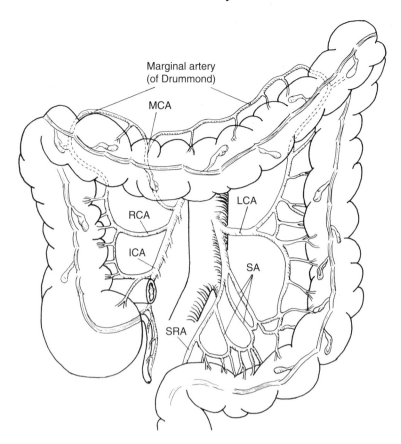

Figure 14-2 Arterial supply to the colon. ICA, ileo-colic artery; LCA, left colic artery; RCA, right colic artery; SA, sigmoid arteries; SRA, superior rectal artery. (From Monsen H. Anatomy of the colon. In: Nyhus LM, Baker RJ, eds. *Mastery of surgery.* Boston: Little, Brown and Company, 1992:1186, with permission.)

splenic vein, which subsequently joins the SMV to form the portal vein. Venous blood from the rectum can return via portal or systemic routes. The superior rectal vein communicates with the IMV, whereas the middle and inferior rectal veins drain into the vena cava via the internal iliac veins.

Lymphatics

Lymphatic drainage again mirrors the distribution of arterial supply. Lymphatic channels drain the submucosa, but not the mucosa, underscoring the importance of depth of invasion of colon cancers. Furthermore, lymphatics drain circumferentially and segmentally, limiting longitudinal lymphatic spread of cancers. Drainage proceeds to epiploic nodes within the wall of the colon. It continues into paracolic nodes of the marginal artery, then into intermediate nodes following main branches of arteries, then nodes of major arteries including superior and inferior mesenteric nodes. Lymphatics of the rectum, like venous routes, display bi-directional drainage both into inferior mesenteric nodes via drainage paralleling the superior rectal artery and into iliac nodes via middle and inferior rectal drainage.

Nerves

Innervation of the colon is by sympathetic and parasympathetic autonomic nerves. Sympathetic fibers from thoracic roots travel through the superior mesenteric plexus to innervate the ascending and transverse colon. Fibers from lumbar roots travel through the inferior mesenteric plexus to supply the descending colon and rectum. Parasympathetic fibers innervating the right and transverse colon originate from the vagus, while the left colon and rectum receive parasympathetic innervation from sacral roots (S2-4).

PHYSIOLOGY

The colon's functions include absorption, namely of water, secretion of electrolytes, and transit and storage of feces. One to 1.5 liters of water reach the colon daily with 90% being reabsorbed. Absorption occurs mainly passively down an osmotic gradient created by the active transport of sodium. This is maintained by a Na^+-K^+-ATPase pump at the basolateral membrane of the colonic epithelium. The colon can absorb up to 5 liters of water and 400 mEq of sodium daily. Concurrently, potassium is secreted into the lumen due to the gradient created by this active exchange. Chloride and bicarbonate are anions involved in exchange at the luminal border. Absorption takes place unevenly throughout the colon, with most occurring in the right colon. Short-chain fatty acids (SCFA) such as acetate, butyrate and propionate play an important role in colonic absorptive processes. These are mainly products of bacterial fermentation of nonabsorbed carbohydrates and fiber. These SCFA's, particularly *n*-butyrate, represent the main source of energy for the colon and its metabolic processes. They also play an important role in passive solute movement. Deficiency of SCFA's can result in abnormal absorption and diarrhea.

A dense population of colonic bacteria, the autochthonous flora, comprise up to 90% of the dry weight of feces.

Anaerobic species dominate, with *Bacteroides* species being most common. Colonic bacteria play important roles, including the metabolism of urea into ammonia, facilitating the enterohepatic circulation, and the production of vitamin K. Because of this large bacterial population, much attention has been paid to the need for preoperative bowel preparation for colonic procedures. Both mechanical cleansing and antibiotic regimens are employed. Although mechanical cleansing of stool from the colon greatly facilitates colonoscopy, experience with unprepared bowel in trauma surgery has indicated that mechanical preparation for segmental resections may not be necessary. Studies by European surgeons suggest that mechanical cleansing prior to colonic surgery provides no benefit in either intraabdominal or wound infection rates. Parenteral antibiotics administered immediately before colon surgery significantly reduce wound infection rates. Additional preparation with preoperative oral antibiotics likely does not add benefit.

Unlike small bowel, colonic motility is not characterized by peristalsis. Contractions called retrograde movements cause mixing and delay transit of colonic contents especially through the right colon, facilitating further absorption of water and sodium. Segmental contraction of the circular and longitudinal muscles propels contents forward through discrete segments of the colon, likely enhancing mixing. Finally, mass movements, consisting of strong contractions of long segments of colon with pressures rising as high as 200 mm Hg, aid propulsion into the distal colon and rectum. They occur approximately three times daily, typically in the morning and postprandially.

As fecal material reaches the rectum, receptive relaxation occurs in the rectal ampulla. This causes a relaxation of the internal anal sphincter allowing sensation at the transition zone, known as the sampling reflex. Continence is maintained by the external sphincter which contracts at default, a reflex mediated by neuronal control from sacral roots. Voluntary relaxation of the puborectalis and external sphincter allows expulsion of feces.

Overall control of colonic motility involves both neuronal and hormonal factors. Parasympathetic and sympathetic neurons supply extrinsic control, stimulating and inhibiting motility respectively. Intrinsic neurons within the wall of the colon form plexi including the myenteric (Auerbach) and submucosal (Meissner) plexi. Substance P, vasoactive intestinal peptide, and other substances have definite effects on colonic motility.

PATHOLOGIC PROCESSES OF THE COLON

Large Bowel Obstruction

Disorders of colonic motility are poorly understood and often multifactorial. Diet can play a role, as can electrolyte imbalances, especially potassium, calcium, and magnesium deficits. Systemic factors such as hypothyroidism, as well as diseases like scleroderma or amyloidosis, also affect motility. Colonic motility is often disturbed following surgery, a condition termed *postoperative ileus*. This decreased motility often resolves with the small bowel recovering first, followed by the stomach, and finally the colon. Ileus

most likely occurs due to a combination of factors such as direct bowel manipulation, anesthetic effects and the use of narcotics.

Constipation, usually defined as fewer than three bowel movements per week, can result from any of these reasons as well as a host of motility and pelvic floor disorders. New onset constipation or failure to respond to correction of these factors, however, requires further work up to rule out mechanical obstruction. Large bowel obstruction can present subacutely with a history of persistent or relapsing constipation. Often a more acute presentation includes nausea, pain, distention and obstipation (the complete lack of passing stool or flatus). The most common cause of large bowel obstruction is malignancy. Other causes include diverticulitis, volvulus, or inflammatory or ischemic processes. Prompt diagnosis and treatment may be required, given that the colon is a closed space in the presence of a competent ileocecal valve. Obstruction can lead to significant distension of the colon. The cecum, already the segment of largest diameter, is particularly susceptible to perforation. It experiences the highest wall tension as dictated by Laplace Law relating tension to the pressure and radius ($T = P \times R$). Increased pressure throughout the obstructed colon results in higher wall tension in the cecum. This can result in local ischemic necrosis and eventually perforation. Specific causes of large bowel obstruction are discussed here, as well as throughout the remainder of the chapter.

Volvulus

Colonic volvulus, which accounts for only 5% of large bowel obstruction in the U.S., results from bowel twisting upon its mesenteric axis, particularly long mesenteries with narrow bases. Torsion can cause partial to complete obstruction or a closed loop obstruction combined with varying degrees of vascular compromise. The sigmoid is most susceptible on its narrow mesenteric base, especially in the elderly where acquired redundancy of the sigmoid makes it freely mobile and prone to torsion. Diagnosis can be made radiographically with plain film (Fig. 14-3) showing the "bent inner tube" sign or with barium enema showing the classic "bird beak" or "ace of spades" sign. Sigmoidoscopy or colonoscopy can be both diagnostic and therapeutic; lower endoscopy is thus recommended initial therapy to reduce the volvulus and allow decompression. Endoscopic decompression has a high (50%) recurrence rate, owing to the fact that the underlying cause, a redundant sigmoid, remains. However, it does allow for resuscitation and bowel preparation prior to definitive surgical treatment. Operative therapy is urgently indicated should colonoscopic decompression fail, and elective definitive sigmoid resection is highly recommended following successful colonoscopic decompression in order to prevent recurrence in patients who can tolerate surgical intervention. Sigmoid resection should be performed as opposed to sigmoidopexy which has a high recurrence rate.

Cecal volvulus is far less common, and actually is not confined to the cecum but involves axial rotation of the cecum, ascending colon and terminal ileum. The cecum, which has no mesentery, can on rare occasion fold upon itself, a condition known as "cecal bascule." Presentation of cecal volvulus is similar to sigmoid volvulus, and diagnosis is usually made radiographically. However, colonoscopic decompression has a very low success rate; surgery is

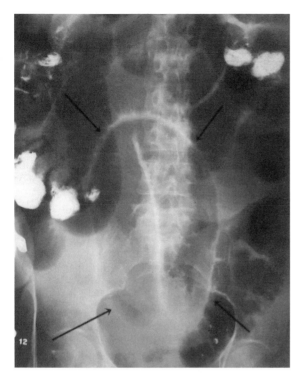

Figure 14-3 Plain supine abdominal film of a patient with sigmoid volvulus. The centrally located sigmoid loop is outlined by trapped air. (From Soybel DI. Ileus and bowel obstruction. In: Greenfield LJ, Mulholland MW, Oldham KT et al., eds. *Surgery: scientific principles and practice*, 3rd ed. Philadelphia: Lippincott Williams & Wilkins, 2001:803, with permission).

therefore the mainstay of therapy. Right hemicolectomy is preferred if tolerated by the patient, because simple reduction with or without cecopexy has high recurrence rates.

Colonic Pseudo-obstruction

Also known as *Ogilvie syndrome*, colonic pseudo-obstruction is a clinical entity involving signs and symptoms of colonic obstruction without mechanical cause. It should be a diagnosis of exclusion with mechanical causes as well as secondary causes of impaired motility aggressively ruled out. Treatment initially focuses on resuscitation and treating any underlying cause of decreased motility. Decompression via colonoscopy can resolve the condition. Intravenous administration of neostigmine, a parasympathomimetic agent, can abruptly enhance colonic motility and is fairly successful in treating pseudo-obstruction with low recurrence. However, mechanical obstruction must be ruled out to avoid excessively high intraluminal pressure after administration. Furthermore, cardiac monitoring is necessary because of the risk of bradycardia; atropine should be available. Surgery is reserved for refractory cases, or cases in which impending ischemia, necrosis, or perforation are suspected. Options include cecostomy for decompression, or segmental resection if bowel viability is compromised.

Lower Gastrointestinal Bleeding

Lower gastrointestinal (GI) bleeding, defined as bleeding originating distal to the ligament of Treitz, overwhelmingly originates in the colon rather than the small bowel, which accounts for only 1% of lower sources. Presentation may

involve melena or hematochezia. Blood loss can be significant; therefore, initial presentation requires prompt attention to large-bore intravenous access, fluid resuscitation, and early laboratory studies to rule out coagulopathy, to establish a baseline complete blood count, and to obtain cross-matched blood products.

Diagnosis focuses on localization of the source as this specifically directs treatment. Differentiation from an upper GI source is very important. Ruling out upper GI sources initially involves nasogastric tube lavage of non-bloody, bilious effluent. Ultimately, endoscopy may be necessary. While melena usually implies an upper source, lower GI bleeds that have slow transit through the colon, particularly from a right colon source, may present with melena. Localization of lower GI source requires proctoscopy to rule out anorectal sources such as hemorrhoids.

Further localization involves a combination of modalities based on the rate and amount of bleeding. Colonoscopy can identify and treat possible sources of colonic bleeding. However, significant active bleeding or inadequate bowel preparation may limit colonoscopy considerably. Nevertheless, colonoscopy gives the most precise localization of bleeding and can possibly provide treatment. In cases of active bleeding, *radionuclide scan* and *angiography* are important tools. Radionuclide scan involves two possible modalities: injection of labeled colloid or injection of autologous, Technetium-labeled "tagged" red blood cells. Labeled colloid scans can identify bleeding as low as 0.1 to 0.5 mL per min but require active bleeding at the time of injection. A tagged RBC scan requires bleeding at a rate of 1 mL per min but has the advantage of persistence of labeled RBC's for up to 24 hours. This allows for identification of intermittent bleeding. In either case, radionuclide scans are the least precise of modalities, giving regional localizing information only. Selective visceral angiography can give more specific information and offer therapeutic options. Accessing mesenteric vessels and their branches allows for identification of bleeding by visualizing extravasation of contrast. Angiography also requires active bleeding to detect the site, with rates at least 0.5 to 1 mL per minute. If no active bleeding is seen, angiography may still help identify lesions such as arteriovenous malformations, which might be likely sources of bleeding. Therapeutic options of angiography include catheter injection of vasopressin or catheter embolization. Risks of these therapies include colonic ischemia, myocardial ischemia, and general risks of angiography itself.

The etiology of lower GI bleeding includes diverticular disease, angiodysplasia, and less commonly, inflammatory bowel disease, neoplasms, and ischemic, infectious, or radiation induced colitis. Approximately half of *massive* lower GI bleeds result from diverticular disease. *Diverticula*, outpouchings of submucosa and mucosa through the bowel wall, occur at points where arterioles penetrate the colonic wall (Fig. 14-4). Therefore, the diverticulum is closely associated with the vessel and over time can erode into the vessel causing hemorrhage. Bleeding does not usually result from inflammation (diverticulitis). Most diverticular bleeds occur in the right colon. Only approximately 10% of patients with diverticulosis bleed, and 75% will stop spontaneously. Of those that stop, approximately 20% may rebleed, and among those who do, risk of subsequent recurrence is much higher.

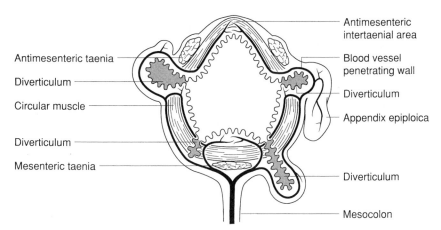

Figure 14-4 Colonic diverticula occur in the weak points in the colonic wall where mesenteric blood vessels penetrate the circular muscle layer. The close association of diverticula with these vessels can lead to significant hemorrhage. (From Telford GL, Otterson MF. Diverticular disease. In: Greenfield LJ, Mulholland MW, Oldham KT et al., eds. *Surgery: scientific principles and practice*, 2nd ed. Philadelphia: Lippincott-Raven, 1997:1152, with permission.)

Colonic angiodysplasia or AVM's are the second most common cause of lower GI bleeding (25%). These most likely occur with age and involve thin friable ectatic vessels, usually in the right colon. Most AVM's are asymptomatic, and bleeding from them usually is self-limited. However, once bleeding does occur, risk of recurrence usually increases with time.

Surgical intervention for massive lower GI bleed is reserved for patients whose bleeding persists despite exhaustive, nonoperative therapy. Overall, approximately 10% to 25% of patients with massive lower GI bleeding will ultimately require surgery. Ongoing transfusion requirements, typically greater than 6 units per 24 hours, usually indicate need for surgery. Prior to surgery the surgeon should endeavor to localize the source of bleeding in the patient to minimize the extent of surgery (i.e., segmental versus total colectomy), if possible, as well as to minimize the need for repeat surgery. Should such efforts fail, the patient may require subtotal colectomy, which can carry high morbidity and mortality in the emergent setting.

Infectious Colitis

Several infections of the colon have unique features. Amebic colitis results from the protozoan *Entamoeba histolytica*. The organism infects the colon primarily but may secondarily infect the liver. Presentation may vary from asymptomatic carriage to acute bloody diarrhea, similar to that in ulcerative colitis. *Metronidazole* is the treatment of choice. *Neutropenic enterocolitis* most commonly affects patients receiving chemotherapy. Tenderness, sepsis, and neutropenia are the most common presenting features, most often involving the cecum ("typhlitis"). Treatment is supportive, including broad-spectrum antibiotics; however, surgery may be indicated in cases of perforation. *Cytomegaloviral colitis* affects 10% of patients with acquired immunodeficiency syndrome (AIDS). Ganciclovir is the treatment of choice, and surgery is indicated in fulminant cases or in cases of perforation.

Pseudomembranous colitis is a syndrome with presentation varying from self-limited diarrhea to severe colitis, megacolon, and perforation. Mucosal inflammation leads to a characteristic exudative pseudomembrane seen on endoscopy. In most cases, previous or current antibiotic therapy alters the normal colonic flora, thereby allowing overgrowth of the bacterium *Clostridium difficile*. Use of antibiotic can cause such overgrowth, which can occur even up to 6 weeks after discontinuation. Clindamycin is the most common inciting antibiotic, whereas ampicillin and cephalosporins are also frequently to blame. *C. difficile* produces two exotoxins: a cytopathic toxin and an enteropathic toxin. A diagnostic assay that involves mixing a patient's stool sample with cultured fibroblasts is very sensitive and specific and can confirm the diagnosis (99% and 94% to 100%, respectively). However, a faster, commercially available immunoabsorbent assay exists with high specificity but lower sensitivity (70% to 90%); repeated samples may be required when clinical suspicion exists. Colonoscopic or sigmoidoscopic identification of pseudomembranes can also help confirm the diagnosis, but lower endoscopy is not absolutely necessary in cases of high clinical suspicion and confirmatory assays. Treatment begins with cessation of the inciting antibiotic. Metronidazole, either oral or intravenous, is first-line therapy for infections caused by *C. difficile*. Vancomycin given orally also eliminates the pathogen but is expensive. Cholestyramine, a resin that binds exotoxin, may also help, but it may bind therapeutic antibiotics as well. Antimotility agents are not indicated as they may lead to toxic dilation of the colon. Surgery is reserved for the rare cases of fulminant disease that fail to respond to antibiotics or cases involving perforation or sepsis.

Ischemic Colitis

The colon can undergo localized ischemia due to thrombosis, embolism, or ligation of a major vessel. However, in many instances no specific vascular abnormality is identified. Ischemic changes range from normal-appearing mucosa to edematous, hemorrhagic mucosa, or even to transmural ischemia with gangrene. A range of clinical presentation also exists. Pain is most common, often accompanied by passage of blood per rectum, mild fever, and leukocytosis. These patients may be treated with observation and hydration. More severe ischemia can lead to more marked pain and more pronounced leukocytosis. Such patients require close serial observation, bowel rest, and intravenous antibiotics. Transmural ischemia resulting in perforation will have signs of peritonitis, necessitating emergent surgery for resection, irrigation, and diversion. Occasionally patients with milder presentations may heal but later have ischemic stricture formation. Such strictures may present with obstructive symptoms and require resection.

Diverticular Disease

Diverticula of the colon are pouches protruding from the bowel wall (Fig. 14-4). They can be true diverticula consisting of all layers of the colon, or the far more common pseudodiverticula, in which only mucosa and submucosa protrude through the muscular layers. As stated in the preceding text, pseudodiverticula occur at the point in which colonic arterioles penetrate the muscular wall, particularly on the mesenteric side of each antimesenteric teniae. Pathogenesis involves increased intraluminal pressure causing herniation at these points. Risk factors for the development of colonic diverticula include a low-fiber diet, which is associated with generation of high intraluminal colonic pressure. The sigmoid, having the narrowest lumen of the colon, generates the highest pressure. Consequently, diverticula arise most commonly in the sigmoid colon (50% of patients) and second most commonly in the descending colon (40%), although the entire colon can harbor diverticula. Occurrence clearly increases with age; very few individuals are affected by age 30 but up to two thirds of the population has developed colonic diverticula by age 80.

Diverticulosis or diverticular disease implies the *presence of diverticula*, whereas the term *diverticulitis* denotes the pathologic inflammatory state that results from perforation of an obstructed diverticula. Diverticulosis is usually asymptomatic, although, as discussed previously, it is the most common cause of lower GI hemorrhage. Diverticulitis can occur in 20% of patients with diverticula. The perforation leads to localized inflammation and infection, which can result in a broad spectrum of sequelae ranging from localized abdominal pain associated with phlegmon or abscess formation, to free perforation with peritonitis, fistulization, or obstruction. Presentation usually includes pain, most often in the left lower quadrant. Significant inflammation can lead to fever, tachycardia, and leukocytosis. Further signs of systemic toxicity and sepsis may indicate free perforation. Obstruction may have an insidious or acute onset, further leading to a risk of perforation. Bleeding occurs rarely in diverticulitis but may frequently complicate diverticulosis.

Diagnosis of diverticulitis in the acute setting initially involves several modalities including clinical suspicion and corroborating laboratory evidence. Physical examination usually reveals left lower quadrant tenderness. Abdominal distention may indicate obstruction, and a mass noted on abdominal palpation or digital rectal examination may indicate an abscess. The differential diagnosis of diverticulitis includes but is not limited to acute colonic obstruction with or without perforation, inflammatory bowel disease, or ischemic colitis. Radiographic confirmation of the disease is best achieved by computerized tomographic (CT) scan, which can identify inflammation, abscess or phlegmon, obstruction, free intraperitoneal air, or other possible causes of abdominal pain. The instillation of barium or Gastrografin contrast per rectum (i.e., barium enema) carries the risk of causing free extravasation of dye and feces and has been mostly supplanted by the use of CT scan. Colonoscopy is an important diagnostic modality; however, it should not be employed during acute inflammation as high pressure from insufflation may lead to perforation. In some cases, limited sigmoidoscopy without insufflation

may help differentiate malignancy from diverticulitis in the case of rectal obstruction. In all cases, colonoscopy should be used to examine the extent of diverticular disease and to rule out malignancy after resolution of the inflammatory state, usually 6 weeks after the acute episode. This is especially important in the case of colonic obstruction presumed to be caused by diverticulitis.

In the uncomplicated setting (not involving free perforation, obstruction, or fistula), nonoperative management often suffices for acute diverticulitis. Mild cases may only require oral antibiotics in the outpatient setting. Signs of peritonitis, fever, or leukocytosis mandate hospitalization with intravenous antibiotics, fluids, and bowel rest. Most patients respond with this therapy alone, and risk of recurrence is only 25%. However, in patients in which the condition recurs, the recurrence risk increases to up to 50% and increases with further attacks. Thus, recurrent attacks of uncomplicated diverticulitis warrant elective sigmoid colectomy, usually 4 to 6 weeks after the acute inflammation subsides. Although the entire colon may contain diverticula, sigmoidectomy generally suffices to prevent recurrence. The extent of resection must include any thickened or grossly diseased segment of sigmoid, and the anastomosis should occur in distensible, pliable rectum. Failure to resect far enough distally into normal rectum is the cause for recurrent diverticulitis after sigmoid resection. Conversely, the proximal diverticula in a patient with pan diverticulosis do not require resection.

The presence of an abscess may not necessitate emergent surgery. In fact, laparotomy risks disturbing the abscess and exposing the entire abdominal cavity to purulent material. Abscesses larger than 2 cm should be drained percutaneously if possible. Following adequate drainage and administration of intravenous antibiotics, elective surgery can be performed several weeks after the acute episode to remove the diseased segment. The goal of this therapeutic strategy is to allow resolution of the acute inflammation and permit adequate bowel preparation such that resection with primary anastomosis may be performed and a temporary colostomy may be avoided.

Generalized peritonitis may occur with free perforation of a diverticulum or rupture of a previously localized, contained abscess. Diffuse abdominal tenderness with signs of infection and sepsis usually results, necessitating emergent surgery. After initial resuscitation, the goal of surgery is washout of infectious material and resection of the diseased segment of colon. In this setting, primary anastomosis is unsafe owing to the high risk of anastomotic breakdown in the face of infection. The procedure of choice is the *Hartmann procedure* of segmental resection, end-colostomy formation from the proximal segment, and closure of the distal stump. This removes the source of ongoing infection and soilage of the peritoneal cavity to allow for stabilization of the patient. Colostomy takedown and reanastomosis are subsequently performed in an elective setting approximately 6 to 8 weeks after the initial operation. Alternatively, in patients with diverticulitis associated with significant local peritonitis or infection, resection and primary anastomosis may be accompanied with a temporary proximal diverting loop colostomy or ileostomy.

The complication of fistula formation in the setting of diverticulitis can occur somewhat frequently. Most fistulas occur between the colon and the bladder, vagina, small bowel, or skin (especially after percutaneous abscess drainage). Enterovesical fistulas are most common, occurring more often in men (owing to the position of the uterus in females) and usually present with pneumaturia, fecaluria, and recurrent urinary tract infections. Other causes of enterovesical fistulas include Crohn disease and cancer, although diverticulitis is the most common cause. Diagnosis can be made by CT scan showing air in the bladder, whereas barium enema and cystoscopy are less reliable. Alternatively, hysteroscopy, fistulogram, or small bowel follow-through (SBFT) may help delineate fistula anatomy and distinguish communicating structures. In all cases of fistula, colonoscopy rules out other causes of fistulization, especially cancer. Fistulas are not indications for emergent surgery; they may serve to decompress an abscess and thus decrease a patient's symptoms. However, fistulas resulting from diverticulitis will generally not resolve with conservative, nonoperative management, because the diverticulum remains a source of infection. Therefore, treatment begins with broad spectrum intravenous antibiotics. After acute inflammation subsides, elective surgery entails resection of the diseased colon with primary anastomosis and fistula take-down. Surrounding structures involved in the fistula may be repaired if necessary, although these involved organs often heal once the inciting source of infection (the diseased colonic segment) is removed.

Obstruction is rare in the setting of diverticular disease and does not result from acute diverticulitis except in rare cases of small bowel obstruction due to inflammation. Rather, large bowel obstruction may result from stricture formation caused by previous inflammation and subsequent fibrosis. Presentation may range from subacute or partial obstruction to complete obstruction with colonic distention and bowel wall necrosis with perforation. The differential diagnosis for colonic obstruction must absolutely include carcinoma and, therefore, prompt further evaluation. Surgery is indicated to prevent progression to frank obstruction or to prevent complications of complete obstruction. Partial obstruction may allow for bowel preparation and preoperative colonoscopy or sigmoidoscopy to rule out malignancy. If possible, a one-stage resection and anastomosis is performed. However, complete obstruction prevents the possibility of preoperative bowel preparation and thus may necessitate a Hartmann procedure.

Inflammatory Bowel Disease of the Colon and Rectum

Inflammatory bowel disease (IBD) refers to ulcerative colitis and Crohn disease, two diseases of uncertain etiology that can affect the colon. Incidence is approximately 5 to 8 cases per 100,000 people per year. IBD occurs more often in whites, especially of Jewish descent, with roughly an equal male-to-female ratio. Age distribution shows peak occurrence at 15 to 40 years of age, with a smaller peak around 60 years.

No specific etiology has been proved, although several factors are implicated, and ultimately the cause is likely multifactorial. Immunologic mediation clearly plays a role, as best evidenced by the fact that immunosuppression modulates the disease. Several autoantibodies are often present [such as perinuclear antineutrophil cytoplasmic autoantibodies (pANCA) in patients with ulcerative

colitis]; however, there is no evidence of a direct autoimmune etiology. The inflammatory nature of the disease is apparent with alterations in cytokines levels including interferon-α (IFN-α), TNF-α, and a number of the interleukins. Genetic factors play a role as well, as 10% to 25% of patients have a first-degree relative with IBD, and twin–twin concordance is higher than that of nontwins. Several chromosomal linkages, for example, candidate genes on chromosome 16 in the case of Crohn disease, as well as many others have been studied. Infectious, dietary, and other environmental factors may also play a role.

Features of Ulcerative Colitis and Crohn colitis.

Although they have distinct pathologic and clinical features, ulcerative colitis and Crohn disease share many similarities, thus making a definitive diagnosis sometimes difficult. Distinguishing between these two diseases may indeed be challenging; however, the distinction is nonetheless important because surgical options will ultimately vary depending on the underlying pathophysiologic process.

On histopathologic examination, ulcerative colitis is characterized by friable, ulcerated, edematous mucosa. Edema causes formation of heaped-up inflammatory or "pseudo" polyps, whereas excessive inflammatory cells form crypt abscesses. The inflammation in ulcerative colitis is confined to the mucosa. Typically, the disease presents initially in the rectum with left-sided colonic predominance, but it can involve the entire colon. Diseased mucosa is continuous without "skip lesions" of intervening normal tissue. In contrast, the macroscopic characteristic feature of Crohn disease is deep linear ulcerations or fissures, whereas the microscopic feature is the granuloma. Although not always present in Crohn disease, granulomas rarely occur in ulcerative colitis. Furthermore, the presence of full-thickness, *transmural inflammation* distinguishes Crohn disease from ulcerative colitis, in which bowel wall inflammation is typically limited only to the mucosa. In addition, Crohn disease can affect any part of the alimentary track ("mouth to anus"), and skip lesions typically occur. Although 55% of cases of Crohn disease affect small and large bowel, 15% of cases involve only the colon. Of patients with Crohn colitis, only 50% to 75% have rectal involvement, whereas virtually 100% of UC cases will involve the rectum.

Presentation in ulcerative or Crohn colitis often correlates with the unique pathologic features of each. Generally, ulcerative colitis initially presents with bloody diarrhea. Mucosal ulceration combined with vascular engorgement results in characteristic bleeding. Affected epithelium loses absorptive capacity, leading to diarrhea. Pain is less common. Severity of presentation ranges from mild and relatively indolent flares to acute fulminant crises. Rarely, severe inflammation can lead to *toxic megacolon*, an acute surgical condition characterized by massive colonic distension, acute abdominal pain, and systemic signs of toxicity including fever, leukocytosis, and tachycardia. In contradistinction, Crohn symptoms correlate with the propensity for transmural inflammation. The most common initial symptom is abdominal pain. Acute inflammation may lead to edema and local obstruction. Further sequelae include stricture, perforation, abscess, and fistula. Obstruction from stricture can occur in ulcerative colitis owing to benign mucosal hypertrophy. However, any obstruction in this setting is more likely the result of malignancy and therefore necessitates a thorough evaluation. Furthermore, perforation in ulcerative colitis results specifically from toxic megacolon, and fistulae rarely occur. In both ulcerative colitis and Crohn disease, inflammation typically presents in a waxing and waning fashion, with intervening periods of remission.

Extraintestinal manifestations of inflammatory bowel disease are well known. Arthritides occur in the form of *ankylosing spondylitis* and *sacroiliitis*, occasionally associated with the human leukocyte antigen (HLA)-B27 haplotype. A peripheral nonrheumatoid arthritis may also appear. *Uveitis* and *episcleritis* are ocular manifestations of IBD, but not common. *Erythema nodosum* and *pyoderma gangrenosum* are skin lesions that may appear with both diseases. *Primary sclerosing cholangitis* is a serious extraintestinal disease seen far more often in ulcerative colitis than in Crohn disease.

The risk of malignancy (e.g., colon cancer) in patients with ulcerative colitis rises with duration of the disease. Relative risk of colon cancer in patients who have had ulcerative colitis for fewer than 10 years is low (0% to 3%), but risk subsequently rises to 2% per year after the tenth year of onset. The development of dysplasia can occur regardless of whether the disease takes a relatively active or asymptomatic course. Crohn colitis likely has a similar malignancy risk if the colon is involved primarily in the disease. Malignancy in colitis associated with IBD is often multicentric and can involve any portion of the colon.

Diagnosis

Diagnosis depends on history and physical examination findings first to establish a diagnosis of IBD and possibly to distinguish between ulcerative colitis and Crohn disease. Radiographic studies can help confirm the diagnosis. For example, barium enema may show a characteristic "stove pipe" appearance of the colon in ulcerative colitis owing to the loss of haustral markings. Obstruction series may reveal small bowel involvement, indicating Crohn disease as a likely diagnosis. Contrast studies with SBFT again may delineate small bowel pathology such as strictures or fistulae in Crohn disease. In both Crohn disease and ulcerative colitis, colonoscopy allows for tissue diagnosis and cancer surveillance. Although ulcerative colitis has a left-sided predominance, dysplasia can occur throughout the entire colon; colonoscopy is therefore preferred over sigmoidoscopy. Given the relatively low risk early in the disease course, recommendations for colonoscopic screening begin at 8 to 12 years after onset of ulcerative colitis. In addition to needing to differentiate ulcerative colitis from Crohn disease, other important differential diagnoses include infectious colitis (particularly pseudomembranous colitis), ischemic colitis, and radiation injury.

Medical Therapy

Treatment of inflammatory bowel disease initially involves medical therapy; surgery remains the definitive therapy, however, for ulcerative colitis. First-line medications include the aminosalicylates such as *sulfasalazine*. These act to modulate inflammation by decreasing mucosal prostaglandin synthesis, and they are effective in treating acute symptoms and maintaining remission. *Corticosteroids* remain important in treating IBD, as they can rapidly suppress active inflammation and provide significant relief of symptoms. However,

because of the adverse systemic effects of steroids, all efforts are made to taper them quickly, and they are not utilized as chronic maintenance therapy. For more severe cases or refractory cases, the immunosuppressive agents *6-mercaptopurine* and *azathioprine* are used. They help maintain remission in cases where aminosalicylates alone do not suffice, and they help spare steroid use. Other agents include the immunosuppressant *cyclosporine A* for refractory ulcerative colitis, and *infliximab*, a monoclonal anti-TNF-α antibody, useful in cases of severe Crohn disease.

Surgical Treatment, Ulcerative Colitis

Removal of the mucosa at risk (that of the colon and rectum) *cures* ulcerative colitis. Nevertheless, such a large operation involves significant morbidity and life alteration, and medical therapy remains first-line treatment. Indications for surgery include bleeding, toxic megacolon, intractable disease, obstruction, and suspicion, risk or evidence of malignancy. Ulcerative colitis rarely causes massive hemorrhage, and massive hemorrhage is the indication for only 5% of colectomies for ulcerative colitis. Patients with toxic megacolon may be acutely ill and require resuscitative and stabilizing efforts prior to surgery; evidence of perforation, however, may necessitate emergent operation. Intractable disease usually includes those patients who are poorly responsive to medical therapy, often involving a chronic debilitative course, or those for whom side effects of medical therapy are no longer tolerable. Occasionally, acute symptoms such as severe pain or diarrhea may not respond to even aggressive medical therapy for several days and thus warrant semi-elective surgery. Surgery for obstruction may be indicated either for obstructive symptoms or for the risk of malignancy. High-grade dysplasia or carcinoma are absolute indications for surgery, and surgery for low-grade dysplasia is now generally accepted.

In the emergent setting of intestinal perforation, patients benefit from the more conservative Hartmann procedure, with definitive surgery performed later under optimal circumstances. Nonemergent indications allow for surgery with curative intent—namely proctocolectomy with either continent ileostomy or permanent end-ileostomy, or proctocolectomy with sphincter-preserving ileal pouch–anal anastomosis (IPAA). Total colectomy with ileorectal anastomosis leaves a large portion of rectum, which remains at risk for ongoing inflammation, symptoms, and risk of malignancy. Therefore, this operation is rarely performed for ulcerative colitis and reserved for those who are of poor operative risk to undergo larger more definitive procedures. Proctocolectomy with continent (Kock) reservoir is rarely performed in light of the better results obtained with IPAA. Total proctocolectomy with permanent ileostomy still has a role for patients with poor sphincter function and for elderly patients. Disadvantages include permanent ostomy and the potential for perineal sinus.

Total proctocolectomy with IPAA is now the gold standard curative procedure for ulcerative colitis. The operation may be performed as a single operation or with temporary diverting loop ileostomy to allow full healing of the ileoanal anastomosis with decreased risk of leak and pelvic sepsis. Most surgeons prefer this two-staged approach, especially in the setting of ongoing inflammation or corticosteroid use. A minimal segment of rectal mucosa may be left in place to

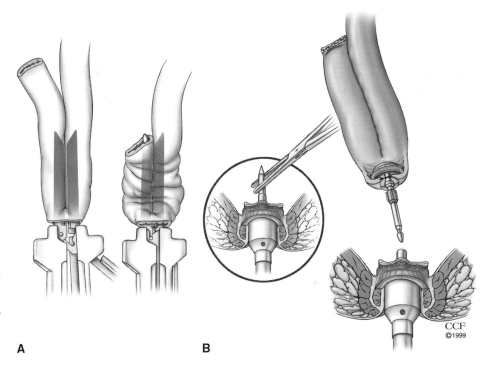

Figure 14-5 Formation of J-pouch **(A)**, and advancement of shaft/trocar and creation of double-stapled anastomosis **(B)**. (From Baker RJ, Fischer JE, eds. *Mastery of surgery*, 4th ed. Philadelphia: Lippincott Williams & Wilkins, 2001: 1511, with permission.)

A

B

allow a double-stapled anastomosis. Alternatively, rectal mucosectomy allows for removal of remaining rectal mucosa but requires a hand-sewn anastomosis. Mucosectomy removes all tissue at risk for inflammation, bleeding, or dysplasia. Disadvantages of mucosectomy, however, include incontinence, increased nocturnal staining, and the possibility of incomplete removal of rectal mucosa. Although there is still controversy over which method to use, any existing dysplasia or carcinoma in rectal mucosa is indication for mucosectomy. Creation of the ileal pouch requires adequate mobilization of small bowel, formation of a "J-," "S-," or "W-" pouch with stapling devices, and subsequent anastomosis to the anus. Because little functional difference exists among types of pouches, the J-pouch, which is technically easiest to create, is usually preferred. (Fig. 14-5.)

Complications of IPAA include those related to the anastomosis, postoperative bowel obstruction, anal stricture, and inflammation of the constructed pouch (*pouchitis*). Pouchitis likely results from bacterial overgrowth and stasis, although the exact etiology is unknown. Symptoms include increased frequency and urgency, pain, incontinence, and bleeding. It occurs in up to 30% of patients, usually within the first 2 years after surgery. A connection with the extraintestinal manifestations of the disease may exist, as those with prior manifestations are more likely to develop pouchitis, and symptoms may accompany pouchitis episodes. Treatment includes metronidazole with improvement usually within 24 to 48 hours. The use of probiotics, products containing living bacteria common to normal gut flora, has been effective in pouchitis, especially in refractory cases.

Surgical Treatment, Crohn Colitis

Unlike ulcerative colitis, surgery in Crohn colitis is only palliative. Owing to its highly recurrent nature and potential to affect the entire alimentary tract, curative resection is not possible. Surgery is reserved for intractable disease,

complications (abscess, obstruction, fistula, bleeding, and fulminant colitis), and to prevent malignancy. Because of the likelihood of future resections, the underlying goal of surgery in Crohn disease is *preservation of length of the gut*, resecting only grossly diseased bowel. Segmental colectomy may suffice if disease scope is limited. Disease in more than 50% of the colon often requires total colectomy with ileorectal anastomosis or total proctocolectomy if perianal disease exists.

Neoplastic Disease

Colorectal cancer is the fourth most common cause of cancer in the United States, with approximately 140,000 new cases per year, and it is the second most common cause of cancer death. Although sporadic development of colorectal cancer is the most common form of the disease, genetic factors clearly can play a role as colon cancer can present in hereditary or familial forms. Risk factors include high-fat diet, history of polyps, IBD, radiation, or previous colorectal carcinoma. Risk increases with age, especially age older than 50 years.

Genetics of Colorectal Cancer

A large body of evidence describes the genetic events that lead to colon cancer. Mutations within multiple genetic loci of colonic mucosal epithelium accumulate in a stepwise fashion. The *Fearon-Vogel model* describes the well-characterized progression from normal mucosa, to adenomatous polyp, to frank carcinoma. Understanding of this model and the well-characterized familial forms of colorectal cancer has elucidated these genetic steps (Fig. 14-6).

Several classes of genes have been identified as instrumental in colon carcinoma development: tumor suppressor genes, protooncogenes, and mismatch repair genes. *Tumor suppressor genes* control cell proliferation via inhibitory proteins. Loss of their function requires both alleles to be

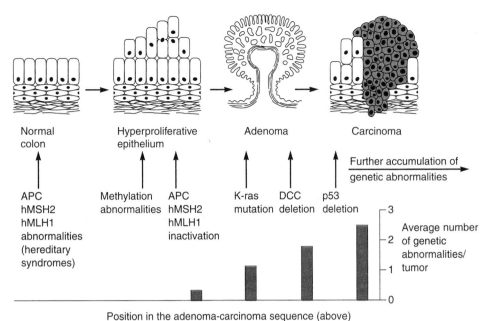

Figure 14-6 Molecular genetic events during the adenoma-to-carcinoma sequence. (From Bresalier RS, Toribara NW. In: Eastwood GL, ed. *Premalignant conditions of the gastrointestinal tract.* New York: Elsevier Science, 1991:238, with permission.)

deactivated, resulting in loss of this normal inhibition. Mutations of the adenomatous polyposis coli (APC) tumor suppressor gene on chromosome 5q21 occur in approximately 85% of sporadic cancers. APC mutations are likely the initiating step in adenoma formation. An inherited germline mutation in APC results in familial adenomatous polyposis (FAP), one of the polyposis syndromes. Other tumor suppressor genes include the "deleted in colon cancer" (DCC) gene and others on chromosome 18q, as well as the p53 gene on chromosome 17q. Mutation of p53 occurs in 75% of sporadic colon cancer and is a significant step in the progression from adenoma to carcinoma, resulting from a loss of the role of p53 in inducing normally programmed cell death, or apoptosis. *Protooncogenes* influence cell proliferation, and mutation in a single allele can lead to a "gain of function" resulting in abnormal cell proliferation. Mutation of the *ras* protooncogene on chromosome 12p occurs in up to 65% of sporadic colon cancer. These mutations likely result in the progression of adenomas, as large adenomas more frequently contain *ras* mutations than do small ones. Finally, mutation in *mismatch repair* (MMR) genes, which correct errors in genetic replication and thus maintain genomic integrity, can occur. Hereditary nonpolyposis colon cancer (HNPCC) results from mutation in the MMR genes, *hMLH1, hMSH2, hMSH3, hPMS1, hPMS2,* and *hMSH6.*

In summary, colon cancer results from mutations that can occur as sporadic events within mucosal cells incited by environmental insults on deoxyribonucleic acid (DNA). Alternatively, hereditary germline mutations lead to a genetic predisposition to polyps and colorectal cancer; further mutations within colonic DNA still must accumulate in the same progression.

Colonic Polyps

Colonic polyps are projections of cells beyond the normal mucosa into the lumen. They can be neoplastic, such as adenomas, or nonneoplastic including hyperplastic, juvenile, and inflammatory polyps. Hyperplastic polyps are heaped growths of normal mucosa that do not have cellular atypia or malignant potential. They are difficult to distinguish from adenomas and therefore must be biopsied. Juvenile polyps occur before 10 years of age. They are hamartomas and may occur as part of several polyposis syndromes. Although lacking malignant potential, they may present with bleeding or as a lead point for intussusception and therefore should be removed when encountered. Inflammatory polyps occur in the setting of IBD or some infections resulting in chronic inflammation.

Adenomas may be pedunculated (on a stalk) or sessile (flat). They are further classified according to their cellular architecture: *tubular* (65% to 80%), *villous,* containing frond-like networks of glands (5% to 10%), or *tubulovillous,* containing mixed features (10% to 15%). Sessile adenomas tend to have more villous elements than do pedunculated adenomas. Adenomas are precancerous lesions and, as described previously, progress through stepwise transformations: normal mucosa develops varying degrees of cellular atypia eventually leading to dysplasia, carcinoma *in situ,* and, finally, invasive carcinoma. The amount and severity of atypia is related directly to the amount of villous architecture present. Furthermore, the size of the adenoma determines the likelihood of invasive elements. Only 5% of tubular adenomas smaller than 1 cm are cancerous, whereas tubular adenomas larger than 2 cm have a 35% risk of cancer, and villous adenomas larger than 2 cm carry a 50% risk of cancer. Carcinoma limited to the mucosa is carcinoma *in situ,* whereas invasive carcinoma penetrates the muscularis mucosa of the polyp. Risk of metastasis depends on the level of extension through the head, the stalk (if present), and ultimately the submucosa of the bowel wall itself.

Polyps are usually asymptomatic, but can present with bleeding or, in rare instances of large villous adenomas, with hypokalemia. Colonoscopy remains the modality of choice for diagnosis and treatment. Colonoscopy allows for polypectomy and surveillance of the remainder of the colon for other lesions.

Because all adenomas are premalignant lesions, all warrant resection. Resected polyps containing carcinoma *in situ* are considered cured. Curative resection for those with invasive elements within the stalk require 2-mm margins and preferably favorable histology. Polyps with evidence of vascular or lymphatic invasion, positive margins, or poor histologic features require surgical treatment with segmental resection similar to that for frank carcinoma. Although pedunculated lesions usually can be endoscopically removed, removal of sessile lesions often poses risk of bowel wall perforation. Sessile adenomas, particularly those larger than 2 cm, therefore, may require surgical resection, especially given their higher malignant potential. Following any polypectomy, recurrence rates are high, with approximately 40% recurrence at 3 years. As a result of this high recurrence rate, it is recommended that patients with a history of colonic polyps undergo repeat colonoscopy within 3 years. Negative repeat studies dramatically decrease the risk of further recurrence.

Familial Syndromes

Familial adenomatous polyposis (FAP) results from an autosomal dominant mutation in the APC gene. Polyps can be extensive (up to 5,000 if untreated). They develop around puberty, and cancer develops in all patients if left untreated by the mean age of approximately 30 years. Differences in the location and type of mutation within the APC gene determine the severity and extent of disease, as well as the spectrum of variations of extraintestinal tumors. *Gardner syndrome* includes osteomas, sarcomas, and epidermoid inclusion cysts. *Turcot syndrome* involves brain tumors. Screening for all of the FAP variants in family members is recommended at around age 10, usually with sigmoidoscopy or proctoscopy, since most initial polyps present in the rectum. Treatment involves removing mucosa at risk, thus warranting total proctocolectomy with ileostomy [abdominoperineal resection (APR)]; however, IPAA with rectal mucosectomy has now gained favor. Alternatively, total colectomy with ileorectal anastomosis is technically more easily performed, but the remaining rectal mucosa remains at risk for neoplastic degeneration and therefore requires frequent surveillance. The cyclooxygenase 2 (COX-2) inhibitors such as Celebrex may cause some regression of rectal polyps through an unknown mechanism. Ultimately, the rectal tissue remains at risk for developing cancer. Occasionally in FAP, locally aggressive desmoid tumors can present intraabdominally. Furthermore, extracolonic polyps particularly in the duodenum are frequent, necessitating screening upper endoscopy and occasionally resection.

An important familial colorectal cancer syndrome without associated polyposis is *hereditary nonpolyposis colorectal cancer* (HNPCC), also known as *Lynch syndrome*. It occurs because of a mutation in the MMR genes as previously mentioned. Colon cancer arises at a mean age of 44 years, usually has poorly differentiated features, and often presents with metachronous or synchronous lesions. A detailed family history can often elicit the syndrome; the diagnosis is confirmed with genetic analysis. However, in up to 50% of clinically obvious cases, genetic analysis cannot detect any defect. Lynch class I involves early onset of colon cancer, whereas Lynch class II syndrome is also associated with endometrial, stomach, small bowel, biliary, urologic, or central nervous system (CNS) tumors. Presence of colon cancer warrants colectomy with ileorectal anastomosis; however, the role of prophylactic colectomy is not established.

Several polyposis syndromes involve hamartomas. *Peutz–Jeghers syndrome*, which also involves skin pigmentation lesions, presents with extensive polyps. These may present with obstruction or bleeding, but the malignant potential is low. Therefore, therapy is directed at symptoms rather than cancer prophylaxis and is preferably achieved endoscopically. *Juvenile polyposis* involves growths of lamina propria covered by normal epithelium. Colonoscopic surveillance is necessary because of the slightly increased risk of malignancy. *Cowden syndrome* involves hamartomas and facial lesions. *Cronkite–Canada syndrome*, although not familial but acquired, consists of polyps similar to those in juvenile polyposis, cutaneous lesions, and chronic diarrhea.

Clinical Features of Colorectal Cancer

Often asymptomatic and found upon screening, colorectal cancer may also present with vague abdominal symptoms such as pain, weight loss, or occult bleeding. Particular presentations vary with location: right-sided lesions may present with melena or anemia with fatigue, whereas left-sided lesions may constrict and cause change in stool character or obstruction. Patients with frank obstruction may present with acute colonic distention and even perforation. Advanced disease can involve extension into surrounding abdominal or pelvic structures. Distant metastasis occurs with the vast majority presenting in the liver secondary to the portal drainage of the colon. Metastasis can occur less commonly in the lung, especially from rectal cancers where portal and systemic venous drainage both exist. Magnetic resonance imaging (MRI) and CT scanning help identify lesions and can identify metastatic disease. Most importantly, colonoscopy establishes tissue diagnosis and also allows examination of the remainder of the colon. Carcinoembryonic antigen (CEA) level is an important marker for tumor recurrence and metastasis but is itself not specific enough to be used as an initial screening tool.

Colorectal cancer is an excellent disease for screening for several reasons: its high prevalence, the ability to identify premalignant lesions, and the ability to significantly alter the natural history of the disease with surgery. However, the ideal screening method has not been firmly established. Low-risk individuals currently should undergo yearly fecal occult blood testing (FOBT) and flexible sigmoidoscopy every 3 to 5 years after age 50. Moderate risk individuals (those with polyps before age 60 or with family members with colorectal cancer) should undergo routine screening starting at age 40. This combination is fairly inexpensive and can be done in the office setting, making it an attractive screening modality; however, it has been shown to miss 24% of proximal lesions. Alternatively, routine screening with colonoscopy for average or low risk patients may not be cost effective. Furthermore colonoscopy is more invasive and requires a separate visit to an endoscopy suite. Higher risk patients who have familial syndromes, particularly HNPCC, should undergo colonoscopy as early as age 20. Those with IBD should undergo screening colonoscopy after 8 to 15 years depending on severity.

Staging

Colorectal cancer spreads by direct, lymphatic, and hematogenous routes. Penetration of the bowel wall is not necessary for lymphatic spread to occur; staging must therefore reflect both depth of invasion and presence of nodes. This knowledge determined the Duke staging system and its modification based on the level of invasion through the muscularis propria (i.e., the modified Astler-Collier system). Similarly, the tumor, node, metastasis (TNM) system stages lesions based on these features (Table 14-1). Stage I tumors include T1 (mucosal) and T2 (into but not through the muscularis propria), and N0 tumors, and has a 5-year survival rate that approaches 90%. Stage II (similar to Duke B) also involves N0 tumors subdivided into IIa (T3, through the muscularis into serosa) and IIb (T4, through the visceral peritoneum or into adjacent structures). Stage II carries an overall 75% 5-year survival rate. Nodal involvement defines stage III disease (similar to Duke C) and carries a 20% to 50% survival with surgery alone. Subdivision is based on depth and number of nodes. Stage IV (Duke D) involves any distant metastasis and survival falls to less than 5% at 5 years (Table 14-1).

Treatment

Surgical resection is the mainstay of therapy. Traditionally, oncologic colorectal operations are performed through an abdominal incision, but this paradigm may be changing, as recent data from the Clinical Outcomes of Surgical Therapy Study Group show similar efficacy using laparoscopic-assisted surgery. Extent of resection is based on the natural course and spread of the disease, given that colonic lymphatics run circumferentially rather than longitudinally and subsequently follow arterial supply. Therefore, although a 5-cm longitudinal margin traditionally suffices for gross margins, the arterial supply of that region of colon (and thus its lymphatic drainage) determines the actual extent of colon resected (Fig. 14-7). Colonic segments supplied by

TABLE 14-1

AJCC STAGING FOR COLORECTAL CANCER

Stage	TNM	Duke (Modified Astler-Coller)
0	Tis, N0, M0	—
I	T1, N0, M0	A
	T2, N0, M0	B1
IIA	T3, N0, M0	B2
IIB	T4, N0, M0	B3
IIIA	T1, N1, M0	—
	T2, N1, M0	C1 (also T2, N2)
IIIB	T3, N1, M0	C2 (also T3, N2)
	T4, N1, M0	C3 (also T4, N2)
IIIC	ANY T, N2, M0	C(1-3)
IV	ANY T, ANY N, M1	D

TX, primary tumor cannot be assessed; T0, no evidence of primary tumor; Tis, carcinoma in situ—intraepithelial or invasion of the lamina propria; T1, tumor invades submucosa; T2, tumor invades muscularis propria; T3, tumor invades through the muscularis propria into the subserosa or into nonperitonealized pericolic or perirectal tissues; T4, tumor directly invades other organs or structures and/or perforates visceral peritoneum; N0, no regional lymph node metastasis; N1, metastasis in 1 to 3 regional lymph nodes; N2, metastasis in 4 or more regional lymph nodes; M0, no distant metastasis; M1, distant metastasis.

segmental arteries are resected as well as the mesentery and vessels themselves down to their origins. For example, tumors in the cecum and ascending colon require resection of the terminal ileum, and right and proximal transverse colon, such that the ileocolic, right colic, and right branch of the middle colic artery distributions are resected. Hepatic flexure and some transverse colon lesions require extended right hemicolectomy, including the transverse colon supplied by the middle colic artery. Resection of the left colon from splenic flexure to the rectosigmoid junction treats left colon tumors. Sigmoid colectomy suffices for sigmoid lesions. In most cases, continuity is reestablished with either hand-sewn or stapled anastomosis. Colon cancer that presents with obstruction may require emergent surgery if severe distention leads to necrosis or perforation. In such cases, resection of the tumor with a Hartmann procedure may be required.

Treatment of rectal cancer requires consideration of many factors. Specific management is determined by the depth of invasion and distance from the anal sphincters. Depth of invasion can best be determined by endoscopic ultrasonography (EUS) or MRI with endorectal coil. Rigid proctoscopy provides the most precise localization of tumor in relation to the internal and external anal sphincters.

Local transanal excision for T1 and occasionally T2 well-differentiated tumors within 4 cm from the anal verge and with no evidence of nodal metastasis may suffice but requires close follow-up to rule out recurrence. T2 lesions require adjuvant radiation with or without chemotherapy given the recurrence rate of up to 20%. In general, patients who do have recurrence and then undergo salvage resection of the rectum have poorer survival results than those who undergo resection of the rectum via an abdominal approach initially. However, local excision is an important option for patients who are at high risk for tolerating a more extensive operation.

Treatment of higher stage tumors or more proximal tumors requires resection of a part or all of the rectum. This can be achieved through low anterior resection (LAR) or APR. LAR involves resection of the sigmoid and proximal rectum with excision of the mesorectum to maintain the oncologic principle of removing the lymphatic basin for that cancer. Colorectal anastomosis restores intestinal continuity, usually with stapling devices. Alternatively, APR completely removes the rectum and anus with construction of a permanent ostomy. Traditionally, tumors lower than 5 cm from the anal verge required APR. Many surgeons now accept more aggressive criteria for LAR with newer stapling devices and the acceptance of 2- or 3-cm longitudinal margins. APR is now reserved for cases in which such a margin cannot be obtained or in which sphincter function is compromised. Disadvantages of LAR include possibility of anastomotic leak and significant changes in bowel habits, whereas APR involves a permanent ostomy and the possibility of poor perineal wound healing. Occasionally, sphincter-sparing coloanal anastomosis may be performed, especially in younger patients with favorable body habitus and good sphincter function.

Adjuvant Therapy

Colon cancer, although fairly chemoinsensitive, responds to the combination of 5-fluorouracil and leucovorin, and an established survival benefit exists for postoperative

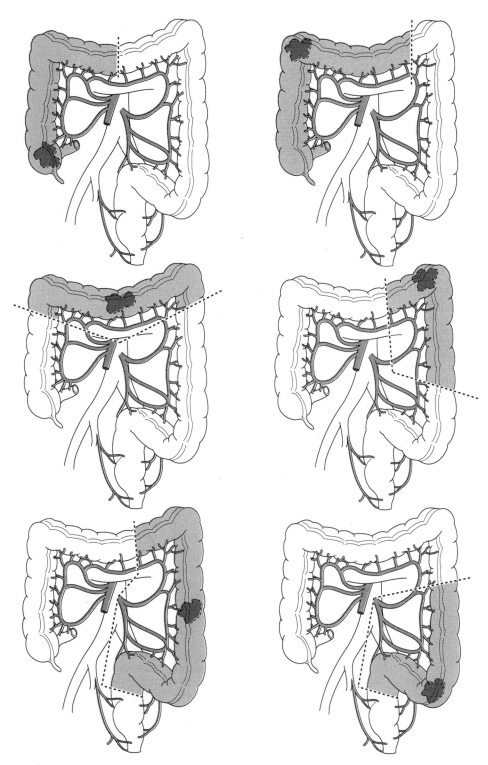

Figure 14-7 Segmental colonic resection including the vascular supply and lymphatics for various locations of colorectal cancer. (From Change AE. Colorectal cancer. In: Greenfield LJ, Mulholland MW, Oldham KT et al., eds. *Surgery: scientific principles and practice*, 2nd ed. Philadelphia: Lippincott-Raven, 1997:1139, with permission.)

chemotherapy in stage III tumors. Although adjuvant chemotherapy in stage II disease decreases recurrence, no survival benefit for stage II disease has been clearly demonstrated. Ongoing trials continue for this group of patients. Little benefit exists from radiation therapy except in certain cases of advanced or recurrent tumors.

Rectal cancer has a higher incidence of systemic and local recurrence than colon cancer in stage II disease; therefore, chemoadjuvant therapy is used for stage II or greater tumors. In addition, radiation therapy is employed for stage II patients pre- or postoperatively, especially given the propensity of rectal cancer for local recurrence. Both pre- and postoperative radiation decrease local recurrence, and there are advantages and disadvantages to each. However, only preoperative therapy has shown an improvement in overall survival in a limited number of studies, and the trend now clearly favors preoperative therapy.

Chemotherapeutic regimens include 5-fluorouracil with leucovorin in combination with irinotecan or oxaliplatin for metastatic disease (stage IV) and recurrent colon cancer. As stated previously, metastasis occurs mostly in the liver. Resection of hepatic metastases offers survival benefit in certain patients, and new regimens for intra-arterial hepatic delivery of chemotherapeutic agents show promise as well. The treatment of colorectal cancer metastatic to the liver is discussed in further detail in Chapter 15, "The Hepatobiliary System."

Follow-up

No firm data show benefit from any particular screening method for recurrence. As mentioned previously, CEA is a helpful marker for possible recurrence and metastatic disease, and colonoscopy can detect metachronous lesions. Approximately 80% of recurrences occur within 2 years, and 95% occur within 5 years. Surveillance through these methods and others such as liver chemistries or computerized tomography can be used. Recurrence may be locally resectable but most often presents as disseminated disease.

Other Tumors of the Colon and Rectum

Carcinoid tumors arise from neuroectoderm tissue. They can secrete a variety of hormones, but most are asymptomatic. The appendix is the most common site for carcinoid tumors, followed by small bowel and rectum. Metastasis may occur in the liver, but rarely from carcinoids smaller than 2 cm. Local resection usually suffices for these lesions, but those larger than 2 cm require larger resection such as segmental colectomy, and LAR or APR for carcinoid of the rectum.

Lymphoma occurs rarely in the colon. It is usually most responsive to systemic therapy, and surgery is reserved for local symptoms such as obstruction or bleeding. *Sarcomas* are rarer still, usually being leiomyosarcomas. Whenever possible, *en bloc* resection is indicated.

APPENDIX

The pathogenesis of *acute appendicitis* begins with luminal obstruction, usually from hypertrophied lymphoid tissue or other objects such as fecaliths, seeds, and rarely parasites or malignancy. Continued mucosal secretion within the obstructed appendix leads to increased pressure, which in turn can lead to lymphatic and venous congestion with subsequent edema and engorgement. Bacterial overgrowth within the appendix further distends the lumen. Early distention causes stimulation of visceral nerves of the abdomen with characteristic diffuse, vague abdominal pain often localized to the umbilicus. Further distention can trigger nausea and vomiting as pain increases. Because of continued obstruction, intraluminal pressure, and engorgement, the inflammation proceeds transmurally and eventually involves the surrounding parietal peritoneum. This produces the classic shift in presentation from the vague periumbilical visceral pain to sharp, right lower quadrant somatic pain. Ongoing obstruction eventually leads to necrosis and perforation.

Mild nausea and vomiting may also accompany symptoms. Anorexia is almost always present. Periappendicular inflammation of surrounding structures may result in diarrhea or urologic symptoms owing to irritation of the rectum and ureters, respectively. Presentation may mimic many other abdominal processes; therefore, the diagnosis of appendicitis must be entertained in the differential of many abdominal complaints. Conversely, the differential diagnosis for acute appendicitis is also very broad. Physical examination usually reveals tenderness over McBurney point (the point two thirds of the way laterally between the umbilicus and right anterior superior iliac spine), often with guarding and rebound. Rovsing sign (right lower quadrant pain with left lower quadrant palpation) may be present, as may the obturator sign (pain upon internal rotation of the hip, possibly indicating a pelvic appendix), and the psoas sign (pain upon extension of the thigh indicating a retrocecal appendix). A low or pelvic appendix may result in tenderness on rectal examination or cervical motion tenderness on pelvic bimanual examination.

Only approximately one half of patients present with classic signs of appendicitis, therefore necessitating further confirmatory studies. Fever and leukocytosis may accompany acute appendicitis; however, these are neither specific nor sensitive for the diagnosis. Plain films have a very limited role, as they may show nonspecific signs such as ileus and only rarely demonstrate an appendicolith, which itself may not be diagnostic for acute appendicitis. Ultrasonography can be very sensitive (approximately 90%) and also can identify other processes including gallbladder and ovarian pathology. However, it is operator dependent and occasionally limited by body habitus. Abdominal CT scan (Fig. 14-8) has excellent sensitivity and specificity (approaching 98%) for acute appendicitis and has become the diagnostic imaging modality of choice in recent years. CT scan may also help confirm other intra-abdominal pathology as suggested by the differential diagnosis. Despite the accuracy of these studies, the rate of negative appendectomy (normal appendix at time of resection) is still reported as high as 15%.

Treatment for appendicitis is surgery to remove the inflamed appendix. Options include laparoscopic or open appendectomy, which have been shown to have similar results. Open appendectomy is performed typically through an incision at McBurney point. Once in the abdomen, the cecum is partially delivered into the wound to allow visualization of the base of the appendix. The tip of the appendix is exteriorized. Ligation of the appendiceal artery in its mesoappendix and resection of the appendix then follows. The stump is usually cauterized to prevent mucus formation. Some surgeons bury the base of the appendix within the cecum; however, this step is likely unnecessary. The abdominal cavity, particularly the right lower quadrant and pelvis, is then irrigated, especially for cases of perforated appendicitis. A drain is unnecessary unless a cavity at risk for reaccumulation is present. The skin is closed, or may be left open in some cases of perforated appendicitis, where contamination may lead to wound infection.

Many surgeons advocate the use of laparoscopy, both for initial diagnosis and treatment. Laparoscopy allows visualization of other abdominal organs including those of the pelvis to rule out other processes. Results for simple appendicitis are similar to the open technique, although

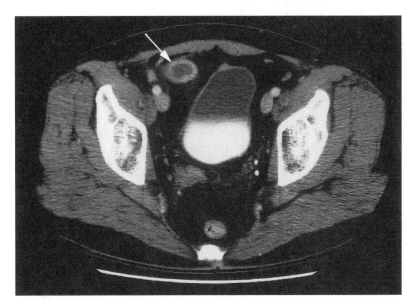

Figure 14-8 Acute appendicitis seen on abdominal computerized tomographic (CT) scan. Note the thick-walled, fluid-filled appendix with surrounding inflammation. (From Matthews JB and Hodin RA, Acute abdomen and appendix. In: Greenfield LJ, Mulholland MW, Oldham KT et al., eds. *Surgery: scientific principles and practice*, 3rd ed. Philadelphia: Lippincott Williams & Wilkins, 2001:1232, with permission.)

use of laparoscopy may be associated shorter hospital stays in advanced (e.g., perforated) cases. If a normal appendix is encountered, the cecum and small bowel should be inspected for other causes of right lower quadrant abdominal pain such as Meckel diverticulum or Crohn disease. If the base of the cecum appears normal, appendectomy should be performed to avoid diagnostic confusion in the future.

Special Considerations

Ruptured appendix may present as an appendiceal mass indicating phlegmon or abscess. Such walled-off structures usually present several days (5 or more) after initial presentation. These cases may be treated successfully with antibiotics, percutaneous drainage, and interval appendectomy several weeks later.

Appendicitis in the young often presents with diffuse peritonitis, as children often are not able to describe symptoms, leading to a delay in diagnosis. Furthermore, the inflammatory phlegmon that forms around the appendix and provides some protection against diffuse peritonitis is formed less efficiently in children. *Appendicitis in the elderly* similarly often has a delay in diagnosis owing to often vague symptoms, blunted tenderness, and diminished leukocytic responses. Thus, a higher index of suspicion is again required. The presence of a cecal malignancy must be seriously considered in the differential diagnosis of appendicitis in the elderly. Risk of perforation is greater, and because of advanced age, mortality and morbidity are elevated in the elderly. *Appendicitis in the pregnant patient* also presents important management considerations. Diagnosis is difficult as many of the symptoms mimic those associated with pregnancy. Furthermore, the position of the appendix shifts because of the growing uterus, gradually moving toward the right upper quadrant. Ultrasonography should be used as the first imaging modality as it can help rule out other common entities such as ovarian torsion or cholelithiasis. CT scan remains an important diagnostic modality, even in the pregnant patient owing to its high sensitivity and specificity. Although risk from ionizing radiation with single abdominal CT scan falls under levels that might cause harm to the fetus, CT should be reserved for cases in which

suspicion warrants confirmation prior to surgery. Because the risk of fetal mortality is 20% in perforated appendicitis compared to 5% fetal mortality with simple appendicitis, appendectomy is usually advocated. The operation carries an approximately 10% risk of miscarriage in the first trimester, which decreases during the second trimester. Appendectomy in the third trimester carries a 10% to 15% risk of premature labor.

Appendiceal Tumors

Occasionally appendiceal tumors are found incidentally by appendectomy or upon abdominal exploration for other reasons. Rarely, the mass may be the etiology of appendiceal obstruction. *Carcinoid* is most common, and 45% of all carcinoid tumors present in the appendix. Carcinoid tumors limited to the appendix rarely cause symptoms (e.g., carcinoid syndrome). Tumors smaller than 1.5 cm that do not involve the line of resection or have gross lymphadenopathy are treated with simple appendectomy. Those larger than 2 cm have higher malignant potential and should be treated with right hemicolectomy. *Adenocarcinoma* of the appendix behaves like that of the colon. Treatment usually involves right hemicolectomy, although simple appendectomy suffices for submucosal lesions with clear margins. *Mucoceles* may present as benign cystadenomas or malignant cystadenocarcinomas. *Cystadenomas*, which may rupture and produce mucinous ascites, are treated with simple appendectomy. Rupture of cystadenocarcinomas can lead to mucinous peritoneal implantation or *pseudomyxoma peritonei*. These tumors have an indolent course and may respond to appendectomy and tumor debulking. Occasionally mucinous ovarian tumors present synchronously, warranting oophorectomy.

ANORECTAL DISORDERS

A host of benign anorectal disorders exists usually resulting in a wide variety of symptoms such as pain, constipation, or bleeding. Despite being fairly common, a level of suspicion for other processes, particularly malignancy, must be maintained.

Hemorrhoids

The term hemorrhoids refers to well-vascularized subcutaneous tissues that cushion the anal lining during defecation. These are usually in the right anterior, right posterior, and left lateral ("2, 5, and 9 o'clock") positions. They may become engorged with blood following repetitive straining during defecation or with chronic increased abdominal pressure. Pathology develops from excessive engorgement of this naturally occurring tissue. *Internal hemorrhoids* lie above the dentate line deep to the rectal mucosa, whereas *external hemorrhoids* lie below the dentate line, deep to the anoderm (Fig. 14-9). This distinction affects the symptoms occurring from each.

Internal hemorrhoids present typically with bleeding or prolapse, but rarely pain. They are classified as follows: *first degree* present with bleeding only; *second degree* bleed and prolapse but spontaneously reduce; *third degree* require manual reduction; and *fourth degree* are not reducible. Symptoms may occur from prolapsed internal hemorrhoids, ranging from irritation and discomfort to severe pain from acute thrombosis of the hemorrhoid. Enlargement and thrombosis within the tissue can lead to severe pain. Workup for complaints of hemorrhoids, particularly bleeding or pain, requires distinction from other differential diagnoses, including anal fissures, fistulas, inflammatory bowel disease, and malignancy.

Treatment for bleeding first-degree hemorrhoids is primarily medical and includes stool softeners, dietary change, and counseling. Third-degree hemorrhoids and bleeding second-degree lesions may undergo elastic band ligation, an outpatient office procedure. Elastic ligations placed at the base of the hemorrhoidal tissue cause necrosis and tissue sloughing. Subsequent scarring prevents further bleeding and prolapsing of tissue. Care must be taken to avoid applying the band to skin below the dentate line, as this can cause significant pain in the richly innervated tissue. Furthermore, the bands may cause pain, spasm, or even urinary retention if placed on the internal sphincter. Complications of sepsis may happen

in immunocompromised patients or in patients in whom the full thickness of the wall is ligated. Rarely, bleeding requiring suture ligation may occur.

For external hemorrhoids that present with acute thrombosis, excision of the thrombosed tissue relieves pain. However, thrombosed external hemorrhoids will often resolve spontaneously over several weeks. Therefore, conservative therapy may suffice if tolerated by the patient.

Hemorrhoids not amenable to outpatient office therapy require operative excision. These include large third-degree and fourth-degree internal hemorrhoids or acutely thrombosed external hemorrhoids with severe pain. The procedure involves excising the hemorrhoidal tissue with an elliptical incision, carefully avoiding the underlying internal sphincter, followed by suture closure of the mucosa. The most common complication of this technique is urinary retention. Others include bleeding, infection, sphincter injury, and anal stenosis.

Rectal Prolapse

Rectal prolapse or *procidentia* is a protrusion of all layers of the rectum through the anus. It typically presents in patients with a long history of constipation and straining, rectal obstruction, or weakness of the pelvic floor. Women are more likely to have rectal prolapse, especially those older than 50 years. Anatomically, the defect likely occurs because of an unusually deep cul-de-sac, abnormal rectal fixation to the sacrum, diastasis of the levator ani, a redundant sigmoid, or a combination of these. The long-term result is an intussusception of the rectum. Symptoms usually involve a sensation of a mass, pain, bleeding, and discharge from the prolapsed mucosa, as well as incontinence. Furthermore, it may reduce spontaneously, may require manual reduction, or rarely may be irreducible. Physical examination often reveals the prolapsed segment protruding through the anus. A key finding is the appearance of *concentric* mucosal folds; this importantly distinguishes rectal prolapse from the prolapsing mucosa of internal hemorrhoids, where the mucosa

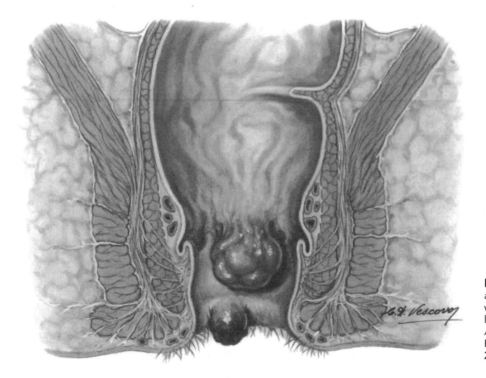

Figure 14-9   Internal hemorrhoids are located above the pectinate line whereas external hemorrhoids are located below. (From Etala E, ed. *Atlas of gastrointestinal surgery.* Philadelphia: Williams & Wilkins, 1997: 2309, with permission.)

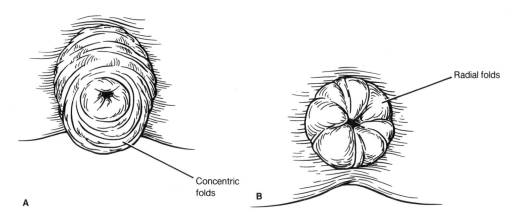

Figure 14-10   A: Full-thickness rectal prolapse involves more than just mucosa and is characterized by concentric mucosal folds. **B:** Rectal mucosal prolapse, however, is characterized by radial folds. (From Vernava AM III, Madoff RD. Anorectal disease. In: Bell RH, Rikkers LF, Mulholland MW, eds. *Digestive tract surgery: a text and atlas.* Philadelphia: Lippincott-Raven, 1996:1446, with permission.)

will have *longitudinal* folds (Fig. 14-10). Further workup should include studies to rule out a malignancy that may have acted as a lead point for intussusception.

In principle, the wide variety of surgical repairs reattach the rectum to the sacrum and resect redundant rectosigmoid. Use of mesh for rectopexy (e.g., Ripstein repair) is of historical interest, but is seldom done today because of the risk of increased constipation and erosion of the mesh into the bowel. The transabdominal approach entails resection of the sigmoid with suture of the rectal mesentery or lateral rectal stalks to the presacral fascia. It has low recurrence, avoids mesh, and may improve constipation and incontinence symptoms. Complications include obstruction or anastomotic leak. Transanal approach to rectosigmoid resection has gained favor, although higher recurrence rates are reported. This method is especially favorable in patients who may not tolerate transabdominal resection. For any type of prolapse repair, up to 50% of patients may have improved incontinence; however, no prolapse repair will reliably improve incontinence, especially in patients with long-standing symptoms.

Anal Fissure

A *fissure* is a painful linear tear in the anal canal. Most are associated with passage of hard stool causing local trauma. Whereas most tears heal spontaneously, continued nonhealing of a fissure can result, usually as a consequence of several factors. One such factor appears to be hypertrophy or hypertonicity of the internal sphincter, although manometric studies do not always demonstrate increased tone. Rather, a combination of fibrosis or spasm of the sphincter likely leads to local ischemia, resulting in poor healing. Fissures most commonly occur in the posterior midline (90%) where blood supply is most tenuous. Most other fissures occur in the anterior midline, and fissures in any other location should prompt a workup for other potential underlying disease processes, particularly Crohn disease. Pain is the most common presenting symptom of anal fissure and is occasionally accompanied by bleeding. Palpation on rectal examination or visualization with anoscopy usually establishes the diagnosis.

Initial therapy primarily is medical and is directed at treating pain and improving bowel habits by easing bowel movements with dietary changes and stool softeners. More directed therapy includes nitroglycerin ointment, which both relaxes the sphincter and improves blood supply, although this therapy may have untoward side effects related to systemic absorption of the nitroglycerin. Recently, injections of botulinum toxin into the sphincter have shown promise by relieving spasm. Overall, medical therapy succeeds in 90% of patients with initial anal fissures and 60% to 80% of patients who have recurrent episodes.

Operative treatment usually is reserved for chronic fissures that do not heal with medical therapy. The aim of relieving sphincter spasm/hypertrophy is achieved by lateral internal sphincterotomy. A lateral incision will heal better than a posterior midline incision for the same reason of decreased posterior blood supply. The procedure can be done under local anesthesia and be either closed or open. Closed sphincterotomy involves inserting a blade oriented parallel to the concentric sphincter, into the level of the dentate line (Fig. 14-11). The blade is then turned 90 degrees to divide the sphincter. The open technique involves visualization of the sphincter through a lateral incision. After splitting the sphincter, the wound is left open or closed. Both have excellent results with up to 95% initial success and only 10% recurrence.

Abscess and Fistula-in-ano

Anorectal abscesses most often result from inflammation and infection of the intersphincteric anal glands that drain into the anal crypts, resulting in an intersphincteric abscess. Infection then can spread most commonly inferiorly into the perianal space (*perianal abscess*). Other locations for spread include laterally through the external sphincter into the *ischiorectal space*, or superiorly above the levator ani into the *supralevator space*. (Fig. 14-12). Supralevator abscess may also form from upward extension of an ischiorectal abscess. Furthermore, ischiorectal abscesses may communicate posteriorly through the postanal space to the contralateral side to form a *horseshoe abscess*. Pain, at times severe, is almost universal, occasionally with fever, urinary retention, or sepsis. Examination may reveal a tender, possibly fluctuant mass, although an intersphincteric or ischiorectal abscess may be palpable only as a bulge on anorectal examination.

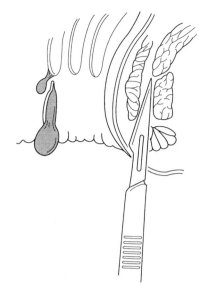

Figure 14-11 The closed technique of internal sphincterotomy involves selectively cutting the internal anal sphincter while the anal canal is stretched open. (From Nivatvongs S. Anorectal disorders. In: Greenfield LJ, Mulholland MW, Oldham KT et al., eds. *Surgery: scientific principles and practice,* 2nd ed. Philadelphia: Lippincott-Raven, 1997:1196, with permission.)

Treatment, as with any abscess, is drainage. Most commonly, incision of the skin overlying a perianal or ischiorectal abscess suffices. Horseshoe abscesses from communicating ischiorectal abscesses are drained through a posterior incision in the postanal space. Intersphincteric abscesses should be drained transanally with incision through the internal sphincter. Ischiorectal drainage treats supralevator abscesses of ischiorectal origin; however, in the extremely rare instance of supralevator abscess originating from the intersphincteric plane, transrectal drainage should be employed, because ischiorectal drainage can create a poorly healing fistula. Simple drainage under local or regional anesthesia often suffices, with antibiotic use reserved for patients with cellulitis, fever, or in patients with underlying immunocompromise.

Approximately one half of anal abscesses result in *fistula-in-ano*—the chronic result of inflammation and infection. The fistula drains internally in the cryptoglandular opening in the dentate line and externally through perianal skin. On the basis of the origin of the abscess, the fistula may be classified as an *intersphincteric, transsphincteric, suprasphincteric,* or *extrasphincteric* fistula. The relationship between the internal and external openings are described by *Goodsall rule* (Fig. 14-13). Fistulas anterior to a line bisecting the anus course directly to their internal openings, whereas posterior fistulas and those more than 3 cm from the anus curve to open internally in the posterior midline. This general rule aids the localization of the internal opening of the fistula.

Surgery is the mainstay of treatment, the underlying principles of which consist of providing adequate drainage and maintaining continence. In most cases, unroofing the fistulous tract over an inserted probe (*fistulotomy*) suffices. Resection of the fistulous tract (*fistulectomy*) is unnecessary and may result in excessive tissue loss and sphincter injury. Division of the internal sphincter usually is well tolerated, as is limited division of the external sphincter. Extensive division of the external sphincter, or division superior to

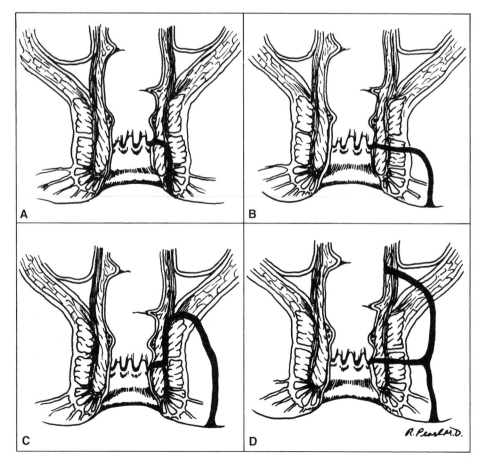

Figure 14-12 Classification of anal fistulae include **(A)** intersphincteric fistula, **(B)** *trans*sphincteric fistula, **(C)** suprasphincteric fistula, and **(D)** extrasphincteric fistula. (From Abcarian H. Surgical treatment of anal disorders. In: Nyhus LM, Baker RJ, eds. *Mastery of surgery,* 2nd ed. Boston: Little, Brown and Company, 1992:1359, with permission.)

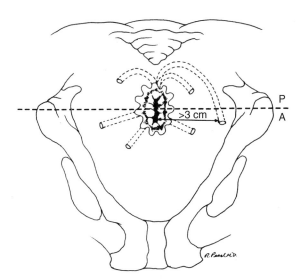

Figure 14-13 Goodsall rule describes the relationship between the internal and external openings of *fistula-in-ano*. (From Abcarian H. Surgical treatment of anal disorders. In: Nyhus LM, Baker RJ, eds. *Mastery of surgery*, 2nd ed. Boston: Little, Brown and Company, 1992:1358, with permission.)

the puborectalis muscle is better treated with placement of a *seton*, usually a vessel loop or suture placed through the tract and tied externally. Over several weeks, the seton is tightened progressively in the office, thereby cutting the encircled tissue slowly. The fistulous tract, therefore, progressively becomes more superficial as fibrosis and healing of the sphincters occurs behind the seton.

ANAL CANCER

Anal cancer is a rare form of cancer comprising only 1.5% of GI tumors. Generally it presents later in life, with a female-to-male ratio of 5:1. An association with human papillomavirus exists, particularly types 16 and 18. Anal cancer may affect the epithelium of the perianal skin and anal margin (generally defined as the perianal region extending from the anal verge laterally for 5 cm) or more commonly the anal canal (85%). Within the canal (generally defined from the anal verge to the anorectal ring), tumors arise in the nonkeratinized epithelium from the anal verge to the dentate line or the cuboidal cells that are continuous with rectal mucosa above the dentate line.

Anal Margin Tumors

In general, anal margin tumors are slow growing and may present late in their course. *Squamous cell* cancers of the anal margin act similarly to squamous carcinoma elsewhere in the body. Lesions often present with bleeding or itching. Treatment is similar to that for other squamous cell tumors, with wide local excision as the mainstay. *Basal cell* cancers also affect the anal margin and behave as basal cancers in other locations. Treatment again entails local resection; however, 30% of tumors recur which require reexcision. Larger or recurrent lesions may require APR. *Bowen disease* is a rare form of squamous cell carcinoma *in situ* in the elderly. The tumors are slow growing and local excision is treatment of choice. Perianal or extramammary *Paget disease* is a rare entity likely of apocrine origin which, if left untreated, can develop into an adenocarcinoma. Presentation often includes pruritus or burning, with a well-demarcated plaque. Treatment includes wide local excision and more aggressive excision including APR if malignancy is found.

Anal Canal Tumors

Tumors of the anal canal tend to be more aggressive. They often present with vague symptoms mimicking benign anorectal disorders. Metastasis occurs in 30% to 40% of patients. Lymphatic spread of tumors above the dentate line is primarily to the inferior mesenteric and to internal iliac nodes. Tumors below the dentate line may spread to inguinal or to internal iliac nodes. In general, a large variety of cancers including *squamous, basaloid, cloacogeneic,* or *transitional* are grouped as *epidermoid* cancers. These typically behave as nonkeratinizing squamous cancers. Workup of anal canal tumors includes physical examination, CT scan, and endorectal ultrasonography to assess depth of invasion. Historically APR was employed but had high recurrence rates. A protocol of chemoradiation with 5-fluorouracil, mitomycin C, and pelvic radiation, developed by Norman Nigro, is now the accepted first-line therapy. APR is reserved for salvage therapy.

Adenocarcinomas of the anal canal may occur rarely. They are usually associated with rectal cancers extending into the anus, with anal glandular epithelium, or with chronic fistulas. Treatment often is APR, although chemoradiation protocols may also be effective. *Melanoma* represents only 1% to 3% of anal cancers. Presentation often is late, with 40% having distant metastasis. Wide local excision and APR have been employed, although long-term outcomes are poor.

KEY POINTS

▲ The colon functions mainly as a site for absorption of water and sodium. Short chain fatty acids are a key source of energy for colonic epithelia; deficiency results in malabsorption and diarrhea. Colonic bacteria make up 90% of the dry weight of feces, but the role for mechanical bowel preparations prior to bowel surgery is not conclusive.

▲ Surgical treatment for ulcerative colitis includes total proctocolectomy; sphincter-sparing ileal pouch–anal anastomosis (IPAA) is used when feasible. Mucosectomy versus double-stapled rectal anastomosis remains controversial.

▲ The pathogenesis of colon cancer follows a stepwise progression from adenoma, through varying degrees of dysplasia, to frank carcinoma. Several specific genetic mutations are known to occur at these steps and may occur sporadically or in hereditary fashion. The complete stepwise progression must continue in both sporadic or hereditary forms of colon cancer.

▲ Anal canal tumors are treated initially with chemoradiation therapy. Abdominoperineal resection (APR) is second-line therapy given the high recurrence rates and morbidity.

SUGGESTED READINGS

Baker RJ, Fischer JE, eds. *Mastery of surgery*, 4th ed. Philadelphia: Lippincott Williams & Wilkins, 2001.

Beck DE, Wexner SD. *Fundamentals of anorectal surgery*, 2nd ed. London: Elsevier Science, 2002.

Cameron JL. *Current surgical therapy*, 7th ed. St. Louis: Mosby, 2001.

Clinical Outcomes of Surgical Therapy Study Group. A comparison of laparoscopically assisted and open colectomy for colon cancer. *N Engl J Med* 2004;350:2050–2059.

Greenfield LJ, Mulholland MW, Oldham KT et al., eds. *Surgery: scientific principles and practice*, 3rd ed. Philadelphia: Lippincott Williams & Wilkins, 2001.

Horton MD, Counter SF, Florence MG. A prospective trial of computed tomography and ultrasonography for diagnosing appendicitis in the atypical patient. *Am J Surg* 2000;179:379–381.

Martling A, Holm T, Johansson H, et al. The Stockholm II trial on preoperative radiotherapy in rectal carcinoma: long-term follow-up of a population-based study. *Cancer* 2001;92:896–902.

Schwarz SI, Spencer FC, Shires GT et al., eds. *Principles of surgery*, 7th ed. New York: McGraw-Hill, 1998.

Hepatobiliary System

15

Paige M. Porrett   Kim M. Olthoff

ANATOMY OF THE LIVER AND BILIARY SYSTEM

Located in the right upper quadrant, the *liver* is the predominant organ of the abdominal cavity. Constituting 2% of adult body weight and receiving 25% of cardiac output, this major organ plays a central role in digestion, detoxification, and metabolism as described in Chapter 16, "Nutrition, Digestion, and Absorption." The liver's physiologic importance is underscored by its anatomic complexity. The liver receives 70% of its blood supply from the *portal vein* (a confluence of the mesenteric and splenic veins) and the remaining 30% of its blood supply from the *hepatic artery*. This dual blood supply is drained by three large intraparenchymal hepatic veins that connect to the inferior vena cava. In addition to this intricate vascular lattice, a complicated network of bile canaliculi converge to form the extrahepatic bile ducts that drain bile via the *common bile duct* into the duodenum through the ampulla of Vater.

Two distinct classification schemes are commonly used to describe liver anatomy. The *morphologic* classification system divides the liver into four lobes. Upon inspection of the liver, these lobes are delineated by obvious fissures and/or ligaments (Fig. 15-1). The dominant right lobe is separated from the left lobe by the *falciform ligament*, whereas the smaller quadrate and caudate lobes are located on the inferior surface of the liver adjacent to the porta hepatis. Alternatively, the *functional* classification system as described by Couinaud (Fig. 15-2) divides the liver into eight segments that receive specific branches of the arterial and portal blood supply. This classification system is most frequently used by hepatobiliary surgeons. The liver segments are delineated internally by the vertically oriented *portal scissurae* containing the hepatic veins and the transversely oriented *portal pedicles* containing the portal vein branches. This classification scheme provides more relevant anatomic information to the surgeon, as the dissection planes involved in major liver resections follow this internal segmental anatomy. Segments 5, 6, 7, and 8 constitute the right hemiliver (resected in a formal right hepatectomy), whereas segments 2, 3, and 4 make up the left hemiliver (resected during a formal left hepatectomy). As it drains directly into the inferior vena cava, segment 1 (also known as the caudate lobe under the morphologic classification system) represents a functionally independent lobe and is not included as a component of either

hemiliver. The internal division of the liver into right and left hemilivers can be externally approximated by an imaginary line drawn anteriorly from the gallbladder bed posteriorly to the inferior vena cava . This is *Cantlie line*, and it represents the location of the *main portal scissura*, which envelops the middle hepatic vein.

Located on the inferior surface of the liver between segment 4 (the quadrate lobe) and the right hemiliver, the *gallbladder* stores bile produced by the liver. Following cholecystokinin stimulation, the gallbladder contracts and excretes bile into the *cystic duct*, which joins the *common hepatic duct* to form the *common bile duct* (CBD) (Fig. 15-3). A stone lodged in the infundibulum of the gallbladder or the proximal cystic duct will prevent egress of bile from the gallbladder, resulting in cholecystitis and necessitating cholecystectomy. The *cystic artery* that provides blood flow to the gallbladder must be ligated during this procedure. The

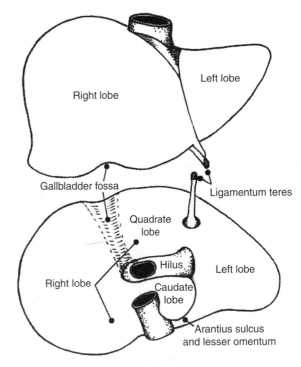

Figure 15-1 Lobar anatomy of the liver. (From Baker RJ, Fischer JE, eds. *Mastery of surgery*, 4th ed. Philadelphia: Lippincott Williams & Wilkins, 2001:1048, with permission.)

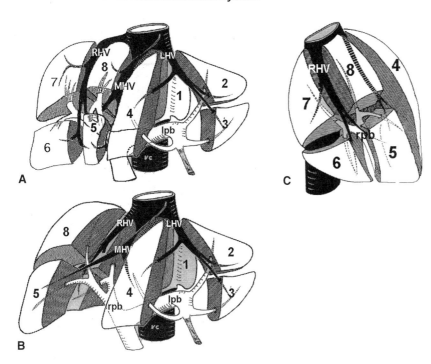

Figure 15-2 Couinaud segmental anatomy of the liver. **A:** Couinaud classic drawing of the liver in the autopsy or "bench" position. This depiction does not accurately portray the anterior–posterior dimension of the hepatic segments in relation to the inferior vena cava. **B:** A representation of the true anatomic position of the hepatic segments *in vivo*. Note the difference with **A**. **C:** Lateral schema of the *in vivo* lobar anatomy. Note the posterior position of segments 6 and 7. (From Baker RJ, Fischer JE, eds. *Mastery of surgery*, 4th ed. Philadelphia: Lippincott Williams & Wilkins, 2001:1049, with permission.)

cystic artery typically branches from the right hepatic artery and can be located upon dissection of the *triangle of Calot*, an anatomic construct composed of the inferior border of the liver, the common hepatic duct, and the cystic duct.

All surgeons must be familiar with the extraordinary degree of normal hepatobiliary anatomic variation present in humans. Approximately 50% of the population has the classic ductal and arterial anatomy commonly described in major surgical texts. Cadaveric dissections have revealed replaced or accessory right hepatic arteries in 20% of the population and similar anomalous left hepatic arteries in another 20% to 25% (Fig. 15-4). A replaced or accessory left hepatic artery can course from the left gastric artery through the hepatogastric ligament, and a replaced

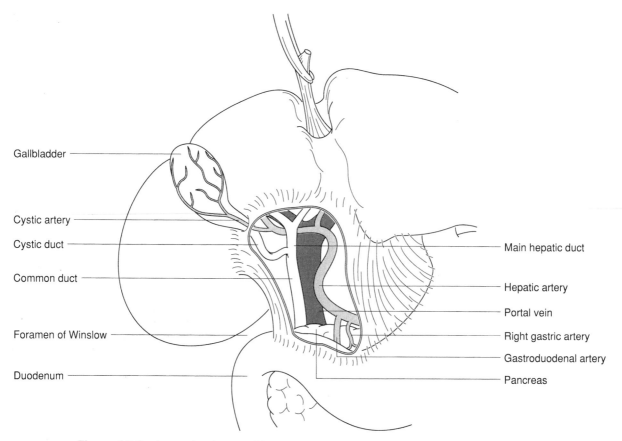

Figure 15-3 Anatomic relations of hepatic artery, portal vein, and common bile duct. (From Greenfield LJ, Mulholland MS, Oldham KT et al., eds. *Surgery: scientific principles and practice*, 2nd ed. Philadelphia: Lippincott-Raven, 1997:1025, with permission.)

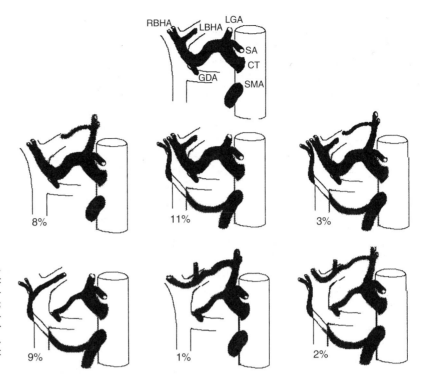

Figure 15-4 Variants of hepatic arterial anatomy. Percentages indicate the prevalence of anatomic variation. CT, celiac trunk; GDA, gastroduodenal artery; LBHA, left branch of middle hepatic artery; LGA, left gastric artery; RBHA, right branch of middle hepatic artery; SA, splenic artery; SMA, superior mesenteric artery. (From Baker RJ, Fischer JE, eds. *Mastery of surgery*, 4th ed. Philadelphia: Lippincott Williams & Wilkins, 2001:1051, with permission.)

or accessory right hepatic artery branching off the superior mesenteric artery can travel to the right of the CBD in the hepatoduodenal ligament. Because dissection of these ligaments is frequently performed in common biliary, pancreatic and gastric procedures, the surgeon may erroneously ligate these arteries if variants are not anticipated. Similarly, knowledge of the variable course of the cystic duct (Fig. 15-5) will also help the surgeon avoid injury to ductal structures such as the CBD that can be misinterpreted as the cystic duct during cholecystectomy.

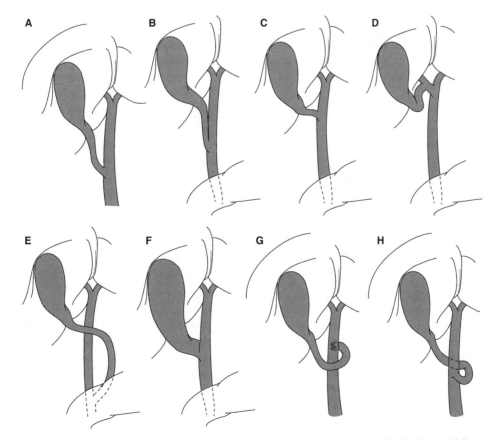

Figure 15-5 Anatomic variants of the cystic duct. (From Greenfield LJ, Mulholland MS, Oldham KT et al., eds. *Surgery: scientific principles and practice*, 3rd ed. Philadelphia: Lippincott Williams & Wilkins, 2001:1005, with permission.)

LABORATORY AND RADIOLOGIC EVALUATION OF THE HEPATOBILIARY SYSTEM

Hepatobiliary pathology may present in a multitude of ways, but common signs and symptoms include abdominal pain, mass, fever, nausea and vomiting, or jaundice. The patient's history and physical examination will provide important initial clues as to the underlying disease process and will guide appropriate laboratory and radiographic testing. Information gathered in the patient's history regarding the chronicity of illness, alcohol use, occupational exposures, and viral hepatitis infection will help differentiate the cause of symptoms. Physical examination findings such as the stigmata of portal hypertension (palmar erythema, *caput medusa*, etc.) or *Murphy sign* (right upper quadrant pain with palpation on inspiration) can further help narrow the differential diagnosis and indicate which tests the surgeon should perform. Finally, laboratory tests that represent liver synthetic function [such as serum albumin level and prothrombin time (PT)/partial thromboplastin time (PTT)] may yield important data regarding severity of hepatic disease in addition to providing diagnostic information.

Right upper quadrant (RUQ) abdominal pain due to hepatobiliary disease may result from (i) obstruction and distension of ductal structures or the gallbladder, (ii) stretching of the Glisson capsule that invests the liver, or (iii) inflammation of ductal structures or hepatocytes. Evaluation of pain should commence with a careful history, liver function tests (LFTs), and ultrasonography. Significant *transaminase elevation* [aspartate aminotransferase (AST) or alanine aminotransferase (ALT) of greater than 1,000 μg per L] frequently indicates hepatocyte inflammation and injury from drug toxicity (i.e., acetaminophen or alcohol) or viral infection (i.e., hepatitis B or C, cytomegalovirus) and is not usually associated with surgical disease. Cholangitis, a surgical disease discussed in subsequent text, can be associated with moderate transaminase elevation, although many patients with the disease do not have significant transaminase abnormalities. Of the serologic LFTs, *direct hyperbilirubinemia* is most likely to indicate surgical hepatobiliary disease. Although direct hyperbilirubinemia may have an intrahepatic, nonsurgical cause such as hepatitis or cirrhosis, posthepatic obstructive etiologies of direct hyperbilirubinemia such as choledocholithiasis, choledochal cysts, and pancreatic or biliary tumor may necessitate surgical intervention. Ultrasonography plays an important role in the evaluation of both RUQ pain and direct hyperbilirubinemia as it can demonstrate ductal dilation and confirm biliary obstruction.

Fever in the patient with RUQ pain suggests underlying hepatobiliary infection or tissue ischemia and necessitates urgent evaluation and treatment. *Acute cholecystitis* must be considered in the patient with fever and right upper quadrant pain.

Ultrasonographic findings of pericholecystic fluid, gallbladder wall thickening greater than 3 mm, and cholelithiasis will frequently confirm the diagnosis of acute cholecystitis in the appropriate clinical setting. However, although the sensitivity of ultrasonography is 96% to 98% for cholelithiasis, sensitivity for acute cholecystitis ranges from 50% to 80%, with the poorest sensitivity in cases of acalculous cholecystitis. Studies indicate that cholescintigraphy using technetium-99m *hepatobiliary iminodiacetic acid* (HIDA) *scan* remains the imaging modality of choice for the diagnosis of acute cholecystitis. Lack of visualization of nuclear tracer within the gallbladder during HIDA scan reflects obstruction of the cystic duct and yields greater than 90% sensitivity and specificity. HIDA scanning loses its reliability in the setting of hepatitis and cirrhosis, however, as hepatocyte dysfunction prevents proper uptake and excretion of the radiotracer in the bile.

Fever may also indicate the presence of *ascending cholangitis*, clinically suggested by Charcot triad of RUQ pain, jaundice, and fever. Cholangitis evolves in the setting of biliary obstruction, and urgent therapeutic decompression of obstructed bile is the treatment of choice to prevent progression to systemic sepsis. An *endoscopic retrograde cholangiopancreatogram* (ERCP) or antegrade evaluation of the biliary tree via *percutaneous transhepatic cholangiography* (PTC) will delineate the level of biliary obstruction and can also allow for therapeutic decompression of infected bile. Cross-sectional imaging such as *computerized tomographic* (CT) *scan* or *magnetic resonance imaging* (MRI) in this scenario can demonstrate pyogenic hepatic abscesses and help define extrinsic sources of biliary compression such as pancreatic tumor or lymphadenopathy.

A *hepatic mass* can be discovered either incidentally or during the evaluation of abdominal pain. Simple cysts are generally imaged easily by ultrasonography or CT scan. The morphology of more complex cystic lesions, such as cystadenomas and cystadenocarcinomas, are often better delineated on CT scan or MRI. Solid masses of the liver can represent benign or malignant pathology, and CT scan and MRI constitute the imaging modalities of choice for their evaluation. Table 15-1 characterizes the findings of solid hepatic masses using different imaging techniques. Modern cross-sectional imaging can frequently determine the etiology of the solid hepatic mass without the need for liver biopsy. Enhancement patterns on dynamic enhanced CT scan or MRI can distinguish malignant from benign lesions. Recently approved by the U.S. Food and Drug Administration (FDA), newer MRI contrast agents such as the superparamagnetic iron oxides (ferumoxides), which are taken up only by the reticuloendothelial cells of the liver, allow radiologists to differentiate metastatic nodules from liver parenchyma. By using a combination of imaging techniques, serum tumor markers, and clinical history to establish a preoperative diagnosis, there is an 85% to 95% accuracy rate when postoperative histology of resected tumors is compared to predicted pathology in both malignant and benign primary hepatic tumors. Given the complications of bleeding and needle tract seeding that have been well documented after percutaneous biopsy of both hepatocellular and metastatic cancers, the use of percutaneous fine needle or core biopsy is recommended only in cases of diagnostic uncertainty following employment of the less invasive methods described previously.

BENIGN TUMORS OF THE LIVER

Hemangiomas are the most common benign solid tumors of the liver. Only infrequently do hemangiomas necessitate surgical intervention as they rarely bleed. On occasion, however, these congenital vascular malformations may grow to a large size and become symptomatic. There

TABLE 15-1
RADIOGRAPHIC CHARACTERISTICS OF PRIMARY SOLID HEPATIC MASSES

Tumor	Ultrasound	CT	MRI
Hemangioma	Hyperechoic solid lesion	*Unenhanced:* Hypodense lesion *Enhanced:* Peripheral nodular enhancement with centripetal filling on delayed images	*T1 images:* Hypointense *T2 images:* Hyperintense *After gadolinium:* Similar to CT scan Diagnostic modality of choice
Focal nodular hyperplasia (FNH)	May or may not be visible. FNH has no specific characteristic features on ultrasonography	*Unenhanced:* Homogeneous & hypo/isodense to liver *Enhanced:* Characteristic pattern of early enhancement with washout on delayed images. Central scar noted in 50% of cases.	*T1 images:* Hypo/isointense *T2 images:* Iso/Hyperintense *After gadolinium:* Similar to CT scan
Hepatic adenoma	Nonspecific. Use of color Doppler technology may help distinguish from FNH	*Unenhanced:* Heterogeneous hypodense lesion *Enhanced:* Early variegated enhancement, well-defined border because of capsule	*T1 images:* Heterogeneous and hyperintense *T2 images:* Hyperintense *After gadolinium:* Similar to CT scan
Hepatocellular carcinoma	May be hypoechoic or hyperechoic Insensitive in screening studies in cirrhotic livers	*Unenhanced:* Hypodense lesion *Dual phase enhancement:* Enhancement in arterial phase 20 s after contrast administration Portal phase washout 60 s after administration Iodized oil more sensitive modality	*T1 images:* Hypo/hyperintense *T2 images:* Also variable *After gadolinium:* Similar to CT scan

CT, computerized tomographic; MRI, magnetic resonance imaging.

is no risk for rupture or malignant transformation. Retrospective studies indicate that patients usually present with abdominal pain or discomfort only after the hemangioma has grown to over 10 cm. Although surgery may be performed for symptomatic hemangiomas, it is rarely indicated. The outer rim of fibrous tissue associated with this tumor may permit enucleation of the mass with less operative blood loss and fewer intra-abdominal complications than anatomic resection. In addition to size or symptoms, the thrombocytopenia and consumptive coagulopathy that heralds *Kasabach–Merritt syndrome* is an indication for hemangioma resection. Although more common in children, this syndrome can occasionally plague adults and is associated with high mortality. Imaging with appropriate MRI techniques or a tagged red blood cell scan can verify the diagnosis.

Occurring in 7% of the population, simple *hepatic cysts* are commonly visualized during radiographic evaluation of the abdomen. They require no intervention but must be distinguished from *cystadenomas*, which can undergo malignant degeneration. Appreciation of internal septations within a cyst on ultrasound or CT scan suggests cystadenoma, and this lesion should be evaluated for resectability. If not resectable, open or laparoscopic biopsy of the cyst wall should be considered.

Discriminating *focal nodular hyperplasia* (FNH) from *hepatic adenoma* (HA) remains a surgical challenge despite advances in modern imaging techniques, as both of these tumors afflict young women of reproductive age and can appear very similar on CT scan. The distinction is nonetheless important as hepatic adenoma usually mandates surgical resection, whereas FNH requires no surgical intervention. MRI will most reliably distinguish between these lesions, although technetium-99m sulfur colloid scan may be used as a confirmatory study. The Kupffer cells of FNH will take up the radionuclide and become a "hot" nodule on scintigraphy. In contrast, HAs do not contain such reticuloendothelial cells and do not enhance. If a distinction cannot be made with imaging, resection or core biopsy is indicated.

As its name implies, FNH is a hyperplastic nodule formed by normal hepatocytes and Kupffer cells that congregate around a solid central artery without associated portal veins. The nodule forms in response to increased arterial flow, and nodules can change in size over time. These nodules do not hemorrhage, are not hormonally responsive, and are not associated with malignant change. Histopathologic examination of HA, however, demonstrates that 40% of these tumors do contain intraparenchymal hemorrhage. Rare cases of malignant degeneration of hepatic adenoma to hepatocellular carcinoma have also been reported in the literature. HA usually causes more symptoms than FNH does and is associated with hormonal influences such as pregnancy and the use of oral contraceptives (OCPs). Cessation of OCPs sometimes results in regression of HA tumor size and improvement of symptoms. It is important to note, however, that spontaneous intraabdominal hemorrhage of this tumor is not associated with size and is fatal in 5% to 10% of cases. Therefore, HA requires routine resection when discovered even incidentally. Arterial embolization of the tumor during an episode of spontaneous bleeding may arrest life-threatening hemorrhage until definitive surgical resection can be performed.

HEPATOBILIARY INFECTION

Although infrequently treated by surgeons during acute infection, the sequelae of chronic infection with *hepatitis B virus* (HBV) and *hepatitis C virus* (HCV) may necessitate surgical intervention. Clinical manifestations of disease result not from direct viral cytotoxicity but from immune response to these viruses, and such immune-mediated hepatic injury may result over time in the development of *hepatocellular carcinoma* (HCC) and/or end-stage liver disease.

Following acquisition of HBV through parenteral or sexual contact, carriers of this deoxyribonucleic acid (DNA) virus may be asymptomatic, or they may develop chronic active hepatitis with elevated transaminase levels and hepatic damage. Although most patients infected primarily with HBV eradicate the infection, 1% of patients will develop fulminant hepatic failure, and 5% of patients will become chronic carriers. Of note, 20% of chronic carriers will go on to develop cirrhosis over a period of years, and patients chronically infected with HBV have a 100-fold increased risk for developing HCC as compared to patients who have spontaneously cleared the virus. Chronic infection in HBV is associated with persistence of hepatitis B surface antigen and E antigen in the serum. Although interferon was previously the mainstay of therapy in the treatment of chronic HBV, newer nucleoside analogs such as lamivudine and adefovir developed initially to treat *human immunodeficiency virus* (HIV) infection have recently been approved by the FDA for the treatment of chronic hepatitis B. These efficacious agents demonstrate fewer side effects and have replaced interferon as first-line therapy by many practitioners.

Although the prevalence of hepatitis B is diminishing with time in the United States as a result of nationwide vaccination programs, infection with HCV has reached epidemic proportions. Approximately 2% of the general U.S. population and as many as one third of hemodialysis patients harbor this ribonucleic acid (RNA) virus, and 25% of these patients will develop end-stage liver disease over 10 to 30 years. Unlike HBV infection, chronic infection with HCV occurs in the majority of infected patients; some authorities estimate that as many as 70% to 80% of patients infected with HCV become chronic carriers. This devastating carriage rate explains why the majority of liver transplantations in the United States are performed for HCV cirrhosis. Combination therapy with pegylated interferon and ribavirin is the current standard of care for HCV infection. Reduction of circulating HCV RNA in the serum to undetectable levels constitutes a treatment response, but

prospective data correlating viral clearance from the serum with decreased rates of liver transplantation or overall patient survival are still lacking.

Although protracted viral infection of the liver can result in malignancy or cirrhosis, parenchymal hepatic infection with bacteria or parasites can generate *liver abscesses*. Patients with hepatic abscess frequently present with nonspecific laboratory tests and symptoms; most will present with fever, but only one half of patients will have abdominal pain, and jaundice is infrequent. CT scan is the most sensitive and specific test for diagnosis (Fig. 15-6). It is notable that neither the radiologic appearance of the abscess nor the patient's clinical symptoms will reliably distinguish the pyogenic bacterial abscess from a parasitic abscess. Nonetheless, this distinction must be made as treatment varies significantly with abscess etiology. Serologic testing employing indirect hemagglutination or enzyme-linked immunosorbent assay (ELISA) provides highly valuable information in this setting, as elevated antibody titers in cases of amebic abscess or hydatid cyst disease will differentiate these lesions from pyogenic abscesses.

Figure 15-7 illustrates the various causes of *pyogenic hepatic abscesses*. Historically, these abscesses most commonly formed via hematogenous portal venous seeding from intraabdominal infections such as diverticulitis and appendicitis. Within the last 50 years, however, cholangitis secondary to malignant obstruction has become the most common cause. Iatrogenic pyogenic liver abscesses can develop following therapeutic interventions such as radiofrequency ablation or hepatic artery chemoembolization, and can also complicate the postoperative course of liver transplantation should hepatic artery thrombosis occur. Abscesses are usually polymicrobial with *Klebsiella pneumoniae*, *Escherichia coli*, streptococci, and *Bacteroides fragilis* as the most likely causative organisms. Treatment consists of image-guided percutaneous drainage coupled with appropriate broad-spectrum antibiotic therapy. Open surgical

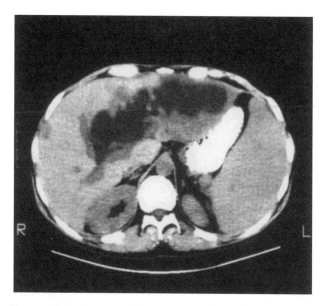

Figure 15-6 Computerized tomogram of the abdomen demonstrating a hepatic abscess. (From Greenfield LJ, Mulholland MS, Oldham KT et al., eds. *Surgery: scientific principles and practice*, 3rd ed. Philadelphia: Lippincott Williams & Wilkins, 2001:944, with permission.)

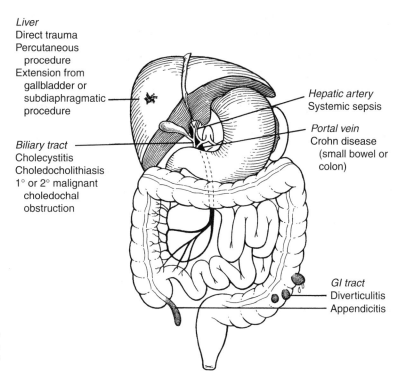

Figure 15-7 Etiology of pyogenic hepatic abscesses. (From Baker RJ, Fischer JE, eds. *Mastery of surgery*, 4th ed. Philadelphia: Lippincott Williams & Wilkins, 2001:1073, with permission.)

drainage of pyogenic abscess is reserved for septic patients whose conditions fail to respond to percutaneous drainage or for cases of free intraperitoneal rupture and contamination.

Entamoeba histolytica, an amoeba that infects 10% of the global population, may result in an *amebic liver abscess*. Most commonly infecting alcoholic patients or homosexuals in developed countries, trophozoites released by ingested cysts migrate from the intestine to reside in the liver. Medical instead of surgical management is the rule, and a 10 to 14 day course of metronidazole will usually provide adequate treatment. This contrasts with the therapy for *hydatid liver disease*, for which surgical resection of the hydatid cyst constitutes definitive therapy because only 50% of these cysts respond to antiparasitic albendazole treatment. A high index of suspicion is necessary to diagnose this lesion, and a recent or distant history of travel to endemic areas may be elicited during history taking. Although dogs are the definitive hosts for this tapeworm, humans become intermediate hosts after ingesting the eggs of *Echinococcus granulosum*. The eggs penetrate the small bowel wall and migrate via the portal bloodstream to the liver, where they hatch into larval scolices. The scolices are contained within the hydatid cyst until the cyst ruptures into the chest or abdomen. Because the fluid within the hydatid cyst is highly antigenic, cyst rupture may manifest as anaphylactic shock. Great care must therefore be taken intraoperatively to avoid inadvertent rupture of the cyst with spillage of antigenic fluid and infective scolices, which can adhere to other intraabdominal serosal surfaces. Controversy surrounds the surgical treatment of choice for hepatic hydatid cysts. Some clinicians advise decompression of the cyst followed by irrigation of the cyst cavity by a scolicidal agent such as silver nitrate and subsequent drainage of the pericystic cavity. Other experts recommend against puncture of the cyst and instead advocate total *cystopericystectomy*,

whereby the entire cyst is carefully dissected from the hepatic parenchyma and removed *in toto*. Alternatively, the intact, unmanipulated cyst may be removed by partial or complete hepatic lobectomy, depending on its anatomic intraparenchymal location.

BENIGN SURGICAL DISEASE OF THE GALLBLADDER AND BILIARY TREE

Although more commonly described in children, *choledochal cysts* may manifest in adulthood. Only a minority of patients afflicted with this rare disease will present with the classic triad of abdominal pain, jaundice, and a RUQ mass. More commonly, choledochal cysts are discovered in adults during the evaluation of complications such as cholangitis or pancreatitis known to occur with this disease. Choledochal cysts are classified according to their location along the biliary tree (Fig. 15-8). Although imaging modalities such as ultrasonography, CT scan, and ERCP may all diagnose choledochal cysts, magnetic resonance cholangiopancreatography (MRCP) has evolved into the imaging modality of choice. Given the high complication rate associated with this disease and the potential for malignant degeneration of the cysts, cyst excision with hepaticoenterostomy is the treatment of choice whenever possible. Type III and type V disease, however, deserve special therapeutic consideration. As the intrahepatic cysts of *Caroli disease* (type V) may not be amenable to resection, these patients may require partial hepatectomy or liver transplantation. Furthermore, in light of recent reports questioning the malignancy rate associated with type III cysts (choledochoceles), some authors advocate therapeutic transduodenal sphincteroplasty instead of cyst excision and biliary reconstruction. However, cholangiocarcinoma has been described in patients with choledochoceles in the

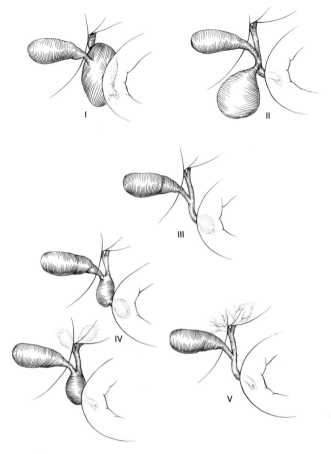

Figure 15-8 Choledochal cysts. (From Meyers WC, Jones RS. *Textbook of liver and biliary surgery*. Philadelphia: JB Lippincott, 1990:313, with permission.)

precipitate out of solution to form cholesterol stones, the most common stones afflicting patients (Fig. 15-9). The pathophysiology of pigment stone formation is similar; these stones are further subdivided into *black* or *brown pigment stones*. Patients with hemolytic blood dyscrasias may have increased concentrations of insoluble unconjugated bilirubin in the bile that predispose to black stone formation within the gallbladder. *Brown pigment stones* may form under infectious conditions when calcium concentrations within the bile increase and precipitate; these stones are therefore more frequently located in the bile duct.

Irrespective of their chemical etiology, gallstones become symptomatic when they obstruct or distend ductal structures. *Acute cholecystitis* can develop when a gallstone lodges in the cystic duct and obstructs bile flow from the gallbladder. Contraction of the gallbladder against this obstruction will create wall tension and lead to ischemia of the gallbladder wall with subsequent perforation. Occasionally the severe inflammation that accompanies cholecystitis will result in an *enterobiliary fistula*. In this situation, gallstones may erode directly from the gallbladder into the intestine; such gallstones may subsequently obstruct the bowel lumen (*gallstone ileus*). Plain radiographs in this condition will reveal small bowel obstruction associated with air in the biliary system. Gallstones also frequently cause complications when they migrate into the bile duct. *Choledocholithiasis* may cause ductal obstruction and ascending infection (*cholangitis*), and it may also result in pancreatic ductal obstruction with the development of *gallstone pancreatitis*. In suspected cases of choledocholithiasis, gallstones in the bile duct may be retrieved via urgent ERCP intervention. This is now the first intervention of choice if a skilled endoscopist trained in ERCP is available.

literature, so surveillance for the development of malignancy will remain critical in this population.

In stark contrast to the rarity of choledochal cyst disease in adults, the burden of disease associated with *cholelithiasis* in the United States is significant. Ten percent to 15% of the general population has gallstone disease, and 5% to 10% of these patients will become symptomatic at some point during their lifetime. Epidemiologic studies have defined subsets of the general population at highest risk for the development of cholelithiasis. Gallstones develop more frequently in women, the obese, and in patients who have had rapid weight loss or gain. The risk of developing cholelithiasis also increases with age, and prior reports described increased complication rates in the elderly as well as in traditionally high-risk populations such as diabetics and organ transplant recipients. In the past, cholecystectomy for asymptomatic diabetics and transplant recipients was recommended. However, recent data no longer support prophylactic cholecystectomy in these groups for asymptomatic disease. Intervention is instead reserved for all patients with symptoms of biliary colic or more serious complications such as acute cholecystitis, gallstone pancreatitis, or choledocholithiasis.

Gallstones are characterized by their composition into *cholesterol* or *pigment stones*. Under normal circumstances, cholesterol, bile salts, and lecithin remain in aqueous solution as bile-salt-lecithin micelles. However, when the concentration of bile salts or lecithin decreases, cholesterol may

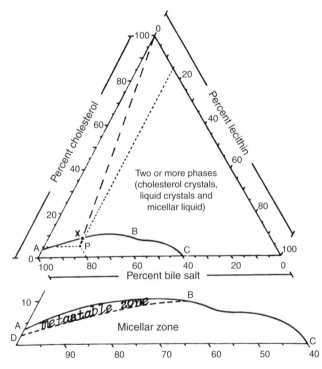

Figure 15-9 Cholesterol solubility decreases with decreasing bile-salt or lecithin concentration. (From Schoenfield LJ, Marks JW. Formation and treatment of gallstones. In: Schiff L, Schiff ER, eds. *Diseases of the liver*, 6th ed. Philadelphia: JB Lippincott, 1987:1268, with permission.)

Alternatively, the surgeon may explore the bile duct at the time of either laparoscopic or open cholecystectomy.

Laparoscopic cholecystectomy has revolutionized the treatment of gallbladder disease. Extensive study of this procedure during the 1990s has defined its safety profile and proved its superiority to open cholecystectomy, given the decreased length of hospital stay and shorter convalescence associated with the laparoscopic approach. Should the delineation of ductal anatomy prove difficult during laparoscopy, or in the event that significant bleeding develops, conversion to the traditional open cholecystectomy is recommended. In experienced hands, conversion rates from laparoscopy to laparotomy during elective cholecystectomy are usually less than 10%. However, conversion rates increase dramatically in the setting of *acute cholecystitis* as a result of the marked inflammation that can obscure anatomy in this condition; rates as high as 30% are commonly reported in the literature. Numerous studies indicate that early performance of laparoscopic cholecystectomy within 72 hours of symptoms of acute cholecystitis lowers conversion rates, decreases operative time, and results in a less costly procedure. This contrasts with the historical management of acute cholecystitis, whereby patients were "cooled off" for several days and then underwent interval cholecystectomy some 4 to 6 weeks later.

Although excellent outcomes generally prevail after laparoscopic cholecystectomy, complications of the procedure may significantly alter the patient's expected return to health. A *cystic duct stump leak* with resulting bile collection (*biloma*) can complicate 0.3% of laparoscopic cholecystectomies. Leaks usually occur when the clip on the cystic duct stump slips off, and patients with this problem present on average 3 days after the procedure with abdominal pain, fever, and/or vomiting. A HIDA scan or ERCP will confirm the diagnosis. Cystic duct stump leak is managed successfully with ERCP stenting of the CBD as well as percutaneous drainage of the resulting biloma to prevent abscess development. Recent analysis of this therapy indicates that more than 90% of cystic duct stump leaks seal with stenting and do not require additional operative intervention. A more serious complication than cystic duct leak, however, is iatrogenic injury to surrounding ductal structures. Published data suggest that *CBD injury* occurs more frequently during the laparoscopic than the open approach. Although ductal injury still remains rare (0.6% of cases), the injury rate during the laparoscopic approach is consistently higher than the injury rate historically reported for open cholecystectomy (0% to 0.5%). Ductal stenosis may result from electrocautery injuries that occur during ductal dissection, or the surgeon may inadvertently ligate the common bile or hepatic ducts when these structures are misidentified as the cystic duct. If the surgeon recognizes a ductal injury intraoperatively, most authorities advocate termination of the procedure and transfer of the patient to a tertiary care center for definitive management. If ductal injury occurs without knowledge of the surgeon at the time of laparoscopic cholecystectomy, ERCP can confirm the injury postoperatively when the patient develops symptoms (Fig. 15-10). In contrast to the conservative management of cystic duct stump leak, almost 90% of patients with bile duct injury require operative bile duct reconstruction. *Roux-en-y hepaticojejunostomy* remains the procedure of choice in experienced centers.

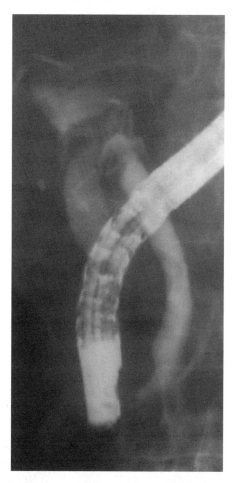

Figure 15-10   ERCP demonstrating extravasation of contrast from transected common bile duct after laparoscopic cholecystectomy. Note that the intrahepatic bile ducts cannot be visualized. (From Baker RJ, Fischer JE, eds. *Mastery of surgery*, 4th ed. Philadelphia: Lippincott Williams & Wilkins, 2001:1063, with permission.)

In addition to the aforementioned iatrogenic biliary strictures, surgeons may also employ biliary-enteric bypass for patients with distal biliary strictures resulting from chronic pancreatitis or as palliation for patients with pancreatic cancer obstructing the common bile duct. Much less frequently, biliary-enteric anastomosis is performed for *primary sclerosing cholangitis* (PSC). A disease of unknown etiology, PSC affects men more commonly than women and may progress to biliary cirrhosis and end-stage liver disease, thereby necessitating liver transplantation. This inflammatory condition of the bile ducts has an association with ulcerative colitis, although the majority of patients with PSC do not have ulcerative colitis. Currently, either ERCP or percutaneous biliary stenting may be utilized to treat dominant strictures. Avoidance of surgical intervention allows for less complicated liver transplantation should the patient develop end-stage biliary cirrhosis. ERCP has therefore become the treatment modality of choice in this disease. Ductal brushings obtained during ERCP can also provide cytology and permit surveillance for cholangiocarcinoma in this high-risk population. Patients with PSC should additionally be followed with serial serum CA 19-9 levels to attempt early detection of cholangiocarcinoma given their increased risk of development of this malignancy.

CIRRHOSIS AND PORTAL HYPERTENSION

Cirrhosis of the liver is a pathologic diagnosis whereby normal functioning hepatocytes are replaced by fibrous connective tissue and regenerative hepatic nodules. It represents the pathologic common end-point of severe hepatic injury. Common causes of cirrhosis include chronic HBV or HCV infection, exposure to hepatotoxins such as alcohol, and a variety of metabolic derangements including α_1-antitrypsin deficiency, hemochromatosis, and Wilson disease. As the pathologic representation of end-stage liver disease, cirrhosis has multiple clinical manifestations; patients may be relatively well compensated and asymptomatic, or they may have significant encephalopathy, jaundice, coagulopathy, and poor synthetic function associated with decompensated frank hepatic failure. The well-known complications of portal hypertension, such as gastroesophageal varices and ascites, may also afflict the cirrhotic patient. Although less frequently called upon to intervene for these complications since the advent of the *transjugular intrahepatic portosystemic shunt* (TIPS), surgeons still provide the only curative and definitive therapy for end-stage cirrhotic patients—liver transplantation.

The need to differentiate patients who would benefit from liver transplantation from such a diverse cirrhotic population has prompted the development of staging systems to estimate the severity of liver failure, predict mortality, and to determine the need for transplantation. Originally developed in the 1960s to estimate operative mortality in patients undergoing portosystemic shunt surgery, the classification system proposed by Child was the first of these staging schemas (Table 15-2). *Child class* is commonly employed today to estimate overall hepatic reserve. Clinicians have broadened its application to predict overall operative mortality in patients with cirrhosis following general surgical procedures as well as to identify patients who are at high risk for death following variceal hemorrhage or TIPS insertion. Furthermore, a modification of the Child classification system, the *Child-Turcotte-Pugh* (CTP) score, provided the foundation for the United Network of Organ Sharing (UNOS) donor liver allocation system for many years. However, given the subjective clinical criteria incorporated into CTP score

TABLE 15-2

CHILD CLASSIFICATION OF LIVER FAILURE ONE MODIFICATION

Criterion	Class A (good risk)	Class B (modest risk)	Class C (poor risk)
Serum bilirubin (mg/100 mL)	<2.0	2.0–3.0	>3.0
Serum albumin (g/100 mL)	>3.5	3.0–3.5	<3.0
Ascites	None	Easily controlled	Not easily controlled
Encephalopathy	None	Minimal	Advanced
Nutrition	Excellent	Good	Poor

From Meyers WC, Jones RS. *Textbook of liver and biliary surgery.* Philadelphia: JB Lippincott, 1990:213, with permission.

TABLE 15-3

MELD SCORE CALCULATION

MELD score = $0.957 \times \log_e[\text{creatinine (mg/dL)}]$
$+ 0.378 \times \log_e[\text{bilirubin (mg/dL)}]$
$+ 1.120 \times \log_e(\text{INR})$
$+ 0.643$

INR, international normalized ratio; MELD, model for end-stage liver disease.

(i.e., the assessment of encephalopathy and ascites), as well as its inability to discriminate severity of disease between thousands of patients, the CTP allocation system has been replaced by UNOS in favor of the *Model for End-Stage Liver Disease (MELD) system.* Calculated from a patient's creatinine, bilirubin, and international normalized ratio (INR) (Table 15-3), MELD score provides continuous numerical data that allow more objective ranking of patients by disease severity. First developed to assess risk and predict patient response to TIPS intervention, the MELD system has been validated in patients awaiting liver transplantation and was implemented by UNOS for liver allocation in 2002. A patient's risk of dying on the liver transplantation wait list is correlated closely with his or her MELD score, given that MELD score is predictive of 90-day mortality (Fig. 15-11). Current data indicate improvement in overall wait list survival to transplantation since the application of the MELD liver allocation system, as the MELD score more accurately estimates disease severity and allows for timely transplantation of the sickest patients.

Although most clinical manifestations of end-stage liver disease are neither incorporated directly into the MELD score nor influence an individual patient's rank on the transplant waiting list, a number of cirrhotic complications portend diminished survival. Univariate analyses of multiple retrospective studies indicate that the development of hepatic encephalopathy, the hepatorenal syndrome, or complications of portal hypertension all contribute to mortality in cirrhotic patients. *Hepatic encephalopathy* results from accumulation of cerebral toxins in the bloodstream, which are ordinarily removed by the functional liver. This occurs when venous collaterals shunt blood flow around the liver or when too few functioning hepatocytes remain to accomplish the detoxification process. The specific toxic agent responsible for this metabolic alteration in

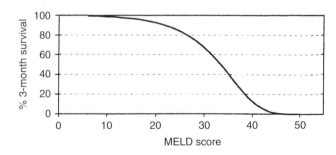

Figure 15-11 Estimated 3-month survival as a function of the Model for End-Stage Liver Disease (MELD) score. (From Wiesner R, Edwards E, Freeman R, et al. Model for End-Stage Liver Disease [MELD] and allocation of donor livers. *Gastroenterology* 2003;124:94, with permission.)

mental status remains unclear. Ammonia is frequently implicated in the pathogenesis of hepatic encephalopathy, but current data do not correlate ammonia levels with severity of symptoms. Encephalopathy can develop following shunting procedures such as TIPS or surgical portosystemic shunts and should be considered a contraindication for these procedures. The presentation of hepatic encephalopathy can range from mild confusion to severe coma. Treatment consists of a low protein diet and oral lactulose administration, which binds the alleged toxin intraluminally in the gut and allows its excretion in the feces.

The *hepatorenal syndrome* (HRS) may also complicate end-stage liver disease. HRS is a physiologic impairment in renal function associated with very high mortality in cirrhotic patients. The pathogenesis of HRS remains a mystery despite intense investigation. Some researchers currently theorize that the kidneys exist in a persistent prerenal state in the cirrhotic patient. The profound splanchnic vasodilation that develops in cirrhosis may result in sequestration of blood and contribute to a relative systemic hypovolemic state that subsequently affects renal function. Following liver transplantation, the patient with HRS will typically recover function of his or her native kidneys. Because serum creatinine level is the most heavily weighted objective data point that inputs into the MELD equation, HRS is accounted

for in the calculation of an individual patient's MELD score. The development of HRS will therefore increase the urgency of the patient's transplant listing status.

Portal hypertension is an increase in portal pressure that develops when fibrotic tissue within the cirrhotic liver impedes venous flow through the hepatic sinusoids. Pre- or postsinusoidal portal hypertension can also develop in noncirrhotic patients in the setting of portal venous or hepatic venous thrombosis (*Budd–Chiari syndrome*). Regardless of the etiology, the increased portal pressure can open venous collaterals that communicate with the systemic caval system, and *portosystemic varices* can therefore form at a number of locations throughout the body (Fig. 15-12). *Gastroesophageal variceal bleeding* is a major source of morbidity and mortality in the cirrhotic population. Studies have established that 25% to 35% of patients with cirrhosis will develop gastroesophageal variceal bleeding and that as many as 30% of initial bleeding episodes are fatal. Moreover, patients who survive the initial bleeding episode are at extremely high risk for bleeding recurrence. In light of these data, many authorities advocate endoscopic screening of all patients with cirrhosis to determine which patients are at highest risk for variceal bleeding episodes. Once these patients are identified, primary prophylaxis can be instituted. Randomized prospective trials have demonstrated that

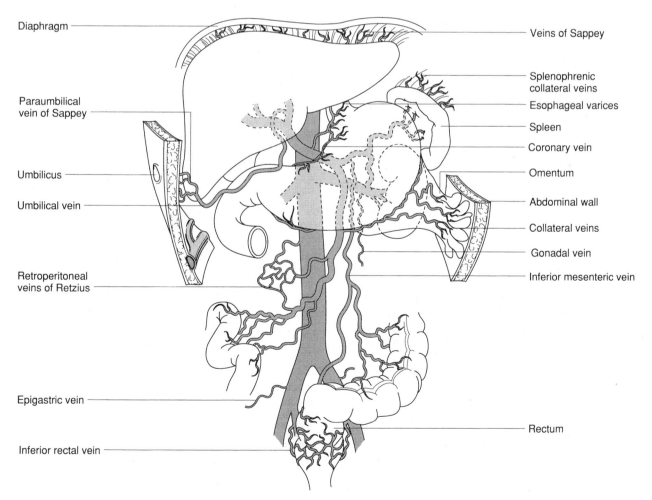

Figure 15-12 Sites of collateralization in portal hypertension. (From Greenfield LJ, Mulholland MS, Oldham KT et al., eds. *Surgery: scientific principles and practice*, 2nd ed. Philadelphia: Lippincott-Raven, 1997:888, with permission.)

nonselective β-blockade halves the risk of developing variceal bleeding. Endoscopic banding of esophageal varices may be employed as primary prophylaxis if the patient cannot tolerate β-blockade due to hypotension.

In the patient who develops an upper gastrointestinal bleed despite prophylaxis, emergent endoscopy is performed to establish the source and provide therapy. In patients suspected or known to have varices, clinicians should empirically administer octreotide intravenously, which will stop bleeding in up to 80% of patients. Placement of a Sengstaken-Blakemore tube emergently into the esophagus will tamponade life-threatening hemorrhage if necessary and can temporize the patient to definitive endoscopic therapy. At endoscopy, variceal band ligation has proven equivalent to endoscopic sclerotherapy in terms of efficacy, but it is associated with fewer complications. It has therefore become the therapeutic intervention of choice in the treatment of bleeding esophageal varices. Endoscopic band ligation (EBL) will terminate bleeding in 80% to 90% of patients, and serial endoscopy with banding should be performed until varices are eradicated.

Bleeding gastric varices provide a greater therapeutic challenge than esophageal varices because of their deeper submucosal position. It is important to note that this anatomic distinction frequently prevents effective endoscopic therapy. Gastric varices may result from portal hypertension in patients with cirrhosis, or they may occur from splenic vein thrombosis.

Knowledge of the specific etiology of gastric varices is extremely important in the development of an effective therapeutic intervention. Urgent *splenectomy* is required in patients with gastric variceal bleeding secondary to splenic vein thrombosis. In patients with gastric varices secondary to portal hypertension, however, insertion of a TIPS will more likely provide effective decompression and therapeutic intervention. TIPS is highly efficacious in decompressing the portal system and is indicated in virtually all cases of refractory gastroesophageal variceal bleeding secondary to portal hypertension. TIPS may also be used in the secondary prophylaxis of patients who cannot take β-blockers or undergo EBL. In addition, it has been employed in the treatment of refractory ascites. Complications of TIPS include the development of hepatic encephalopathy as well as shunt thrombosis. However, with routine surveillance of the shunt and angioplasty of the shunt when necessary, TIPS patency rates approach 80% to 90% over several years.

Given the overall efficacy of TIPS and EBL, *surgical portosystemic shunts* no longer play a prominent role in the treatment of gastroesophageal varices. However, surgical shunting may be required emergently in the extremely rare event that TIPS fails to stop bleeding or TIPS technology is not available. Although rarely indicated, surgical shunts may be performed for the prevention of recurrent variceal bleeding in patients with Child class A or B cirrhosis. *Nonselective portosystemic shunts*, such as the portocaval or mesocaval shunts, decompress the entire portal system (Fig. 15-13). Portocaval shunts not only shunt portal blood from the liver, but side-to-side portocaval shunts also result in retrograde decompression of the liver itself into the vena cava. Therefore, hepatic encephalopathy and even hepatic failure may develop after the placement of such a shunt. However, given the relative technical ease with which the portocaval shunt is performed, as well as its extreme effectiveness, the portocaval shunt is the surgical shunt of choice in the

emergent situation. *Selective* surgical shunts such as the distal splenorenal (Warren) shunt decompress the gastroesophageal bed only (Fig. 15-13). This shunt maintains portomesenteric flow through the liver and therefore results in less encephalopathy and a decreased risk of hepatic failure as compared to nonselective shunts. However, technical complexity may prevent the use of this shunt in the emergent situation. Furthermore, given that important peritoneal lymphatic channels may be ligated during mobilization of the left renal vein, the Warren shunt is contraindicated in patients with intractable ascites. Finally, it must be emphasized that any surgical shunt markedly increases the complexity and risk of future liver transplantation. Surgical portosystemic shunts should therefore be avoided in potential liver transplant recipients.

As modern surgeons rarely perform portosystemic shunts in the post-TIPS era, the general surgeon may lack the technical training to perform a surgical shunt when confronted with the emergent bleeding patient. Esophageal devascularization and transection procedures, such as the *Sugiura operation* and its modifications, provide the general surgeon with an alternative to shunt surgery in the case of uncontrolled gastroesophageal bleeding. Initially described in the 1970s, Sugiura detailed a two-stage operation performed through both thoracic and abdominal incisions whereby the distal 5 to 8 cm of the esophagus is devascularized and then subsequently transected and reanastomosed (Fig. 15-14). Of significance, the transection of the esophagus interrupts the submucosal venous collaterals that contribute to variceal bleeding, which are not treated by external devascularization of the esophagus alone. Although effective in arresting bleeding in the emergent situation, these transection procedures have been associated with significant morbidity and mortality as well as higher rebleeding rates (30% to 50%) than with portosystemic shunting. Therefore, the Sugiura procedure remains generally of historical interest only in the post-TIPS era and is performed in only very limited circumstances.

In addition to gastroesophageal variceal bleeding, portal hypertension contributes to the formation of *ascites*. Although ascites is usually treated medically by diuretics, large-volume paracentesis, or TIPS placement, surgeons may be involved in the treatment of ascites should the placement of a *LeVeen shunt* be required. This extra-anatomic peritoneovenous shunt drains ascitic fluid from the peritoneal cavity directly into the internal jugular vein (Fig. 15-15), and it is occasionally indicated for the treatment of ascites that is refractory to medical therapy. Complications include infection of the shunt or bleeding secondary to systemic fibrinolysis. Fibrinolysis can develop because the ascitic fluid contains high concentrations of tissue plasminogen activator (tPA), which is then infused directly into the bloodstream via the shunt and may result in a severe consumptive coagulopathy. Although an effective treatment for ascites, studies indicate that the LeVeen shunt does not confer survival benefit to cirrhotic patients with ascites, as many patients undergoing the procedure succumb to the aforementioned complications. In patients with refractory ascites who do not have hepatic encephalopathy, TIPS should be strongly considered.

Although surgical interventions for the complications of cirrhosis, as discussed in the preceding text, have become more and more infrequent with the success of less invasive techniques, the need for general surgical procedures

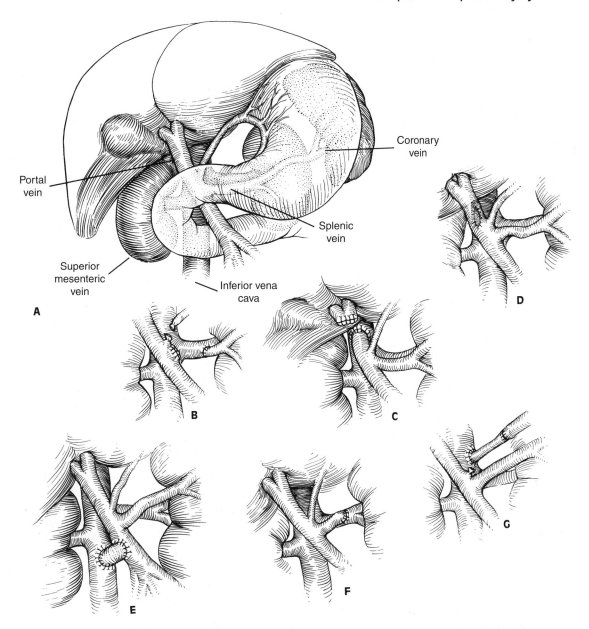

Figure 15-13 Portosystemic shunts. **A:** Intact portal venous anatomy. **B:** Distal splenorenal (Warren) shunt. **C:** End-to-side portacaval shunt. **D:** Side-to-side portacaval shunt. **E:** Mesocaval (H) shunt. **F:** Proximal splenorenal shunt. **G:** Coronary caval shunt. (From Meyers WC, Jones RS. *Textbook of liver and biliary surgery.* Philadelphia: JB Lippincott, 1990:184, with permission.)

in the patient with cirrhosis will persist well into the modern era. Certainly, these patients develop common surgical diseases such as cholecystitis, perforated viscus, or abdominal wall hernias. No specific technical modifications are required during such procedures in cirrhotic patients; however, a number of studies indicate that abdominal operations in patients with cirrhosis are associated with a much higher morbidity and mortality than in the general population. Published series describe increased mortality in patients who have ascites, elevated PTs, or encephalopathy. Overall, Child C classification and emergent operations are predictive of the worst survival—more than 80% of these patients will die perioperatively. Death results primarily from sepsis and rapid decompensation of hepatic function with the development of severe coagulopathy. Therefore, although patients with cirrhosis may indeed require surgical intervention, surgeons must recognize that

these patients have extremely limited physiologic reserve and generally do not tolerate any operation well. Recent data suggest that even under the best of circumstances, 10% of patients with class A cirrhosis will die following elective gastrointestinal procedures.

The decision to operate on any patient with cirrhosis, even those well-compensated patients with retained hepatic reserve who undergo uncomplicated elective procedures, must not therefore be entered into lightly. Such surgical intervention should be performed only in a center capable of supporting the patient through an anticipated difficult postoperative course. It is important that the anesthesia staff is knowledgeable in the management of patients with liver disease in order to minimize crystalloid use and administer required fresh–frozen plasma and platelets as necessary. In the postoperative period, careful attention must be paid to fluid and electrolyte balance,

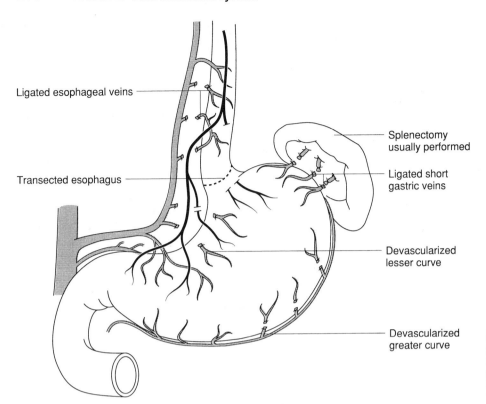

Ligated esophageal veins

Transected esophagus

Splenectomy
usually performed

Ligated short
gastric veins

Devascularized
lesser curve

Devascularized
greater curve

Figure 15-14 Sugiura procedure. (From Greenfield LJ, Mulholland MS, Oldham KT et al., eds. *Surgery: scientific principles and practice*, 2nd ed. Philadelphia: Lippincott-Raven, 1997: 1005, with permission.)

and the development and treatment of ascites, infection, and encephalopathy. If elective surgery must be performed, thought should be given to placement of preoperative TIPS as well as preoperative evaluation for liver transplantation.

HEPATOBILIARY MALIGNANCY

Cancer of the hepatobiliary system can be subdivided into primary or secondary malignancy, depending on the location and cell of origin. Metastatic tumors to the liver from the gastrointestinal tract, breast, or lung constitute the most common malignant hepatic neoplasms. Metastatic liver disease uniformly represents advanced cancer and usually precludes surgical intervention, as palliative resection of liver metastases is only rarely indicated. However, *liver metastases from colorectal cancer* defy this rule and are unique among solid organ malignancies. Data indicate that approximately 20% of patients with resectable lesions who undergo hepatic metastasectomy may be cured of their disease, and multiple studies have documented prolonged disease-free survival of 5 or even 10 years postoperatively. Such survival data have encouraged an aggressive surgical approach to the treatment of metastatic colorectal cancer over recent years, but many questions remain regarding selection of the population that would most benefit from hepatic resection, the specific procedure that provides the best disease-free survival, and the optimal timing of surgery for the 20% to 30% of patients with colorectal cancer who present with synchronous hepatic metastases.

Traditionally many patients with resectable synchronous lesions have undergone staged hepatic wedge resection. Proponents of this approach claim that a wedge resection with a 1 cm margin provides adequate oncologic therapy, and this procedure is performed 2 to 3 months after resection of the primary colon cancer so that patients with more indolent disease are selected from patients with aggressive disease to improve perioperative outcomes. However, more recent data from large cancer centers such as Memorial Sloan-Kettering have demonstrated a higher rate of positive surgical margins for nonanatomic wedge resections than anatomic segmentectomies or hepatic lobectomies. Moreover, these newer studies suggest that simultaneous hepatic and colonic resection does not result in higher surgical morbidity or mortality and actually results in fewer operative complications when compared to staged resection in experienced centers. These data have prompted some oncologic authorities to now advocate anatomic resection of hepatic colorectal metastases instead of wedge resection. Debate continues surrounding the timing of hepatic resection in patients with synchronous disease, although it is generally agreed that synchronous resection of colon and liver should not be performed if either procedure is complex or prolonged. In general, however, the paradigm may be shifting toward simultaneous resection of known coincident hepatic and colorectal malignancy in high-volume cancer centers experienced in surgical resection of metastatic colorectal cancer.

The development of new systemic and locoregional chemotherapeutic regimens will also continue to affect the timing of surgical resection for colorectal cancer metastatic to the liver. With the advent of more effective agents in recent years, the combination of systemic therapy followed by surgical resection has been advocated. Furthermore, at the time of resection, the surgeon may also implant an *hepatic arterial infusion pump* (HAIP) to deliver chemotherapy directly into the liver, as prospective randomized trials have demonstrated survival benefit of HAIP combined with systemic chemotherapy over systemic chemotherapy alone. However, HAIP does not improve survival in patients with number of new cases of HCC over the next decade, as many patients infected with HCV over the last 10 to 20 years will develop this complication of chronic hepatitis infection.

From an epidemiologic standpoint, cirrhosis of the liver of any etiology is the primary risk factor for the development of HCC. Eighty percent of patients in the United States with HCC have cirrhosis, and the risk for a patient with cirrhosis of developing HCC is 2% to 6% per year. Those at highest risk for developing HCC include men older than the age of 40 years with HCV cirrhosis. Despite the clear association of cirrhosis with the development of this cancer, researchers cannot yet fully explain how cirrhosis resulting from metabolic, viral, or toxic injury to the liver progresses to frank carcinoma. Although cirrhosis and HCC may be common endpoints of severe hepatic injury, the pathway of carcinogenesis likely varies with oncogenic agent. For example, the disruption of normal cellular function by the integration of HBV DNA into the host genome may play a role in carcinogenesis in patients with chronic HBV. However, this pathway cannot explain the oncogenic potential of HCV, as this RNA virus does not incorporate itself into the DNA of the hepatocyte. Whatever the pathway of oncogenesis, however, cirrhotic livers subjected to multiple carcinogenic agents have an even greater risk of developing cancer. Studies indicate that the risk of developing HCC is higher in patients who are coinfected with both HCV and HBV, as well as in patients infected with either virus who also consume alcohol.

The patient with hepatocellular carcinoma may present with a RUQ mass, or most commonly it is discovered incidentally on cross-sectional imaging performed for screening or the evaluation of some other complaint. The diagnosis of HCC can be made without biopsy if the patient has a liver mass and an elevated α-fetoprotein (AFP) level. As previously discussed, improvements in CT and MRI technology have increased the sensitivity and specificity of these modalities for the detection of HCC. Given the known association of HCC with cirrhosis of the liver, many physicians have maintained an interest in the development of screening programs targeting patients with cirrhosis. A number of prospective surveillance studies employing both ultrasonography and AFP levels at 6-month intervals have reported successful detection of HCC, but no randomized controlled trial of screening with these modalities has been performed that establishes a decrease in mortality from HCC following the institution of such a screening protocol. On the basis of the paucity of quality data regarding screening for HCC, the NCI does not recommend a standard screening protocol in any population for this disease. Debate continues regarding this issue, however, and most hepatologists as well as a number of consensus conferences have strongly recommended screening in high-risk cirrhotic populations, with AFP levels every 3 to 6 months and imaging with CT or MRI every 6 to 12 months.

Just as screening for HCC remains a debatable issue, uncertainty persists regarding the optimal surgical treatment of HCC as well. Because current chemotherapeutic regimens as primary treatment for HCC do not prolong survival in patients with this cancer, surgical resection of the disease has been the standard of care. However, the decision to either primarily resect the cancer or transplant the patient has remained controversial for many years and depends on a multitude of factors. In the 1980s, liver transplantation was generally reserved for those patients

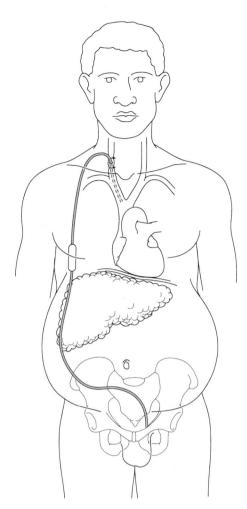

Figure 15-15   LeVeen peritoneovenous shunt. (From Greenfield LJ, Mulholland MS, Oldham KT et al., eds. *Surgery: scientific principles and practice*, 3rd ed. Philadelphia: Lippincott Williams & Wilkins, 2001:981, with permission.)

unresectable liver disease and is therefore not indicated for these patients. Patients who have unresectable colorectal cancer metastases to the liver instead can be palliated surgically with locally ablative modalities such as radiofrequency ablation or cryotherapy, as discussed further in the subsequent text for primary hepatocellular carcinoma.

Primary hepatobiliary cancers, such as hepatocellular carcinoma and cholangiocarcinoma, are the second most common malignancies involving the hepatobiliary tree. According to the National Cancer Institute (NCI), the incidence of primary *hepatocellular carcinoma* (HCC) of the liver in the United States in the year 2000 is 7 cases per 100,000 persons annually. Globally, HCC is a much more prevalent disease and is the fifth most common cancer in the world. In areas of sub-Saharan Africa and China, the incidence of HCC approaches that of breast or colon cancer in this country. Authorities correlate the burden of this disease worldwide with the high carriage rate of HBV infection in underdeveloped countries. In the United States, however, most cases of HCC are instead associated with chronic HCV infection and alcoholic cirrhosis. Despite the relatively low incidence of HCC in this country as compared to other malignancies, the incidence of HCC in the United States is indeed on the rise. The Centers for Disease Control and Prevention (CDC) projects a peak in the with unresectable cancers, but a high recurrence rate in the donor grafts made this strategy obsolete, and for some time surgeons abandoned liver transplantation for HCC in favor of primary resection. Unfortunately, many patients do not qualify for resection given the severity of their overall liver disease, and high recurrence rates of HCC in resected patients resulted in low survival rates of 30% to 50% at 5 years despite refinements in the technique of segmental liver resection. The overall poor performance of resected patients encouraged investigators to once again readdress the role of liver transplantation in the treatment of HCC. During the 1990s, a number of studies verified that revised patient selection criteria resulted in significantly improved outcomes of patients transplanted for HCC. Of note, these studies determined that patients who had solitary liver nodules less than 5 cm in diameter or who had fewer than three nodules all smaller than 3 cm (the *Milan criteria*) had impressive long-term survival that rivaled patients transplanted for nonmalignant disease. A published 5-year survival rate of 70% in patients with HCC far surpassed the results achieved with primary liver resection and reestablished liver transplantation as an acceptable treatment modality for HCC in patients who met these criteria. Furthermore, these criteria have been adopted by the UNOS in order to expedite the transplantation process. Patients who are listed for liver transplantation and meet the Milan criteria are afforded additional *MELD exception points* to help ensure timely transplantation before their disease progresses.

While these data suggest transplantation may be a superior therapy for HCC when compared to primary resection, limited organ availability and disease progression while awaiting transplantation do not necessarily make this treatment option viable for all patients. Furthermore, only a handful of studies have attempted to directly compare outcomes of transplantation versus resection, and these trials have been neither randomized nor controlled. Indeed, such trials may be difficult to design and implement, as most patients who undergo transplantation have more significant liver disease than those who are able to withstand resection, making comparison impossible. Nonetheless, available data indicate that the surgical treatment for HCC must be customized to the patient. In general, candidates for primary liver resection include noncirrhotic patients with anatomically favorable lesions, and Child A cirrhotic patients with preserved liver function and small peripheral solitary nodules. It must be remembered that HCC is often a multifocal disease and more than 50% of these resected patients will have recurrence by 2 years. Patients with Child B or C cirrhosis probably benefit most from liver transplantation provided they meet the Milan criteria. Living-donor liver transplantation has also become an option for treatment of HCC in patients with cirrhosis.

Despite the attention devoted to the controversy of resection versus transplantation, more than 80% of patients with HCC are neither transplant candidates nor do they have resectable disease, given the size or location of the primary tumor. For these unresectable patients, who constitute most patients afflicted with HCC, locally ablative therapies such as radiofrequency ablation (RFA) (Fig. 15-16), percutaneous ethanol injection (PEI), cryotherapy, transarterial chemoembolization (TACE), or combinations thereof constitute the main surgical treatment options. Although these ablative therapies hold promise for patients who have

unresectable HCC, a recent review of these procedures concluded that despite the abundance of case series in the literature that utilize these therapies, inadequate follow-up currently prevents physicians from drawing any definitive conclusions regarding an overall survival benefit provided by these procedures. Such techniques may also be employed as locoregional neoadjuvant therapy in patients awaiting either liver resection or transplantation, although preliminary data do not suggest improved survival in resectable patients when these strategies are implemented. Certainly, randomized controlled trials comparing these therapies are needed in order to define the standard of care in patients with HCC in the adjuvant setting.

Cholangiocarcinoma is an adenocarcinoma that arises from biliary ductal epithelium. With an incidence of 8 cases per 1,000,000 US citizens, this cancer is relatively rare in the United States, but its incidence is on the rise. Known risk factors for its development include congenital choledochal cysts, primary sclerosing cholangitis, and infection with the liver fluke *Clonorchis sinensis*. Cholangiocarcinoma can be subdivided into intrahepatic or extrahepatic disease; such anatomic distinction between these tumors influences presentation of disease, resectability, and overall survival.

Intrahepatic cholangiocarcinoma (ICC), also known as peripheral cholangiocarcinoma, constitutes 10% of primary hepatic malignancies. Of the primary hepatic malignancies, it is second only to HCC in prevalence and is frequently confused with HCC because of both its appearance as an intrahepatic mass on cross-sectional imaging and the lack of immunohistochemical markers that make it difficult to diagnose even after biopsy. By virtue of its location, ICC does not commonly result in obstructive jaundice, and patients therefore usually present late in the disease. Advanced disease at presentation results in poor outcome in these patients, with published 3-year survival rates of 15% to 40% postresection. Resection provides the only chance for long-term survival, but only approximately two thirds of patients are resectable at presentation, and most patients develop recurrent disease. Nonetheless, an

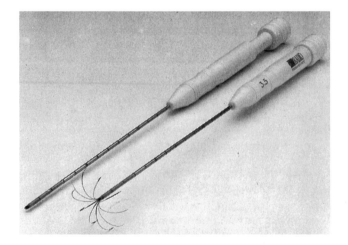

Figure 15-16 Radiofrequency ablation probe. The probe is inserted into the hepatic lesion to be ablated and the radial prongs are deployed. The surrounding tissue is superheated and necroses. (From Hurst RD, Fichera A, Michelassi F. Electrocautery, argon beam coagulation, cryotherapy, and other hemostatic and tissue ablative instruments. In: Baker RJ, Fischer JE, eds. *Mastery of Surgery*, 4th ed. Philadelphia: Lippincott Williams & Wilkins, 2001:247, with permission.)

aggressive surgical approach should be taken with any potentially resectable patient, as patients who have positive histologic margins postoperatively may still have improved survival when compared to unresectable patients.

Conversely, extrahepatic cholangiocarcinoma, also known as hilar cholangiocarcinoma or a *Klatskin tumor*, presents earlier with obstructive jaundice, given the location of this tumor at the confluence of the hepatic ducts. Despite earlier presentation, survival also remains poor with this cholangiocarcinoma as a result of its association with the major vascular structures of the liver at the hilum. Resection represents the only known curative modality, and patients fortunate enough to be diagnosed early with this disease have a definite chance of long-term cure provided they have resectable disease. Data published in small retrospective series confirm the importance of negative margins and suggest that increasing surgical radicality by extending the resection into the hepatic parenchyma instead of limiting it to the biliary ductal confluence improves median survival. Interestingly, studies also demonstrate that radical resection in these patients with the achievement of negative surgical margins influences overall survival more than the presence or absence of regional lymph node involvement.

Given the impact of resectability on survival and the importance of achievement of negative margins in patients with cholangiocarcinoma, orthotopic liver transplantation has been performed for certain patients with unresectable cholangiocarcinoma. Unfortunately, it has demonstrated poor outcome when compared to patients transplanted for HCC. However, there have been reported cases of long-term survival posttransplantation for patients with limited disease, and some centers are using a protocol of preoperative radiotherapy and exploratory staging laparotomy prior to transplantation for patients with small cholangiocarcinomas. Therefore, improved patient selection criteria and the development of more effective neoadjuvant therapies may improve outcomes following liver transplantation for cholangiocarcinoma in the future.

Angiosarcomas constitute a subset of primary hepatic sarcomas. Primary sarcomas involving the liver are exceedingly rare, and angiosarcomas have been associated with environmental exposure to vinyl chloride, Thorotrast contrast material, or arsenic. Cirrhosis is not a primary risk factor for this malignancy. Surgical resection remains the only curative treatment, but prognosis remains uniformly poor because of the late presentation of the majority of these tumors.

Finally, *hepatoblastomas* are the most common primary malignant liver tumors in children and have a peak incidence in children younger than 2 years of age. Most children present with some combination of abdominal pain, bloating, nausea, or vomiting, and jaundice is rare. Resection or transplantation remains the primary modality of therapy in these tumors, but neoadjuvant or adjuvant chemotherapy with cisplatin and doxorubicin regimens have resulted in cure rates of 60% to 70% and are considered the standard of care. Serum AFP level is usually elevated in children with this malignancy and measurement of this parameter is useful for both diagnosis and follow-up, since elevation of this tumor marker postresection is frequently the first indication of recurrent disease. Local recurrence in the liver and pulmonary metastases are the most common sites of disease recurrence.

KEY POINTS

▲ Hepatic arterial anatomic variation is prevalent and must be recognized—a recurrent or replaced hepatic artery may branch from the left gastric or superior mesenteric artery.

▲ Focal nodular hyperplasia (FNH) and hepatic adenoma (HA) affect the same population but have distinctly different treatments. FNH can be conservatively managed but HAs are resected primarily because of risk of rupture with consequent life-threatening bleeding.

▲ Liver abscesses and cysts are treated differently depending on the etiologic organism. Amebic abscesses are treated with metronidazole, whereas hydatid cyst disease will usually warrant liver resection, since it is refractory to medical therapy.

▲ Colorectal metastases to the liver are aggressively treated by surgery with anatomic resection.

▲ Noncirrhotic patients with preserved liver function and hepatocellular carcinoma (HCC) are treated with anatomic resection, but cirrhotic patients with HCC should be considered for liver transplantation given improved outcomes over recent years.

SUGGESTED READINGS

Baker RJ, Fischer JE, eds. *Mastery of surgery*, 4th ed. Philadelphia: Lippincott Williams & Wilkins, 2001.

Cameron JL, ed. *Current surgical therapy*, 7th ed. St. Louis: Mosby, 2001.

Ginès P, Cárdenas A, Arroyo V, et al. Management of cirrhosis and ascites. *N Engl J Med* 2004;350:1646–1654.

Greenfield LJ, Mulholland M, Oldham KT et al., eds. *Surgery: scientific principles and practice*, 2nd ed. Philadelphia: Lippincott-Raven Publishers, 1997.

Mansour A, Watson W, Shayani V, et al. Abdominal operations in patients with cirrhosis: still a major surgical challenge. *Surgery* 1997;122:730–735.

Martin R, Paty P, Fong Y, et al. Simultaneous liver and colorectal resections are safe for synchronous colorectal liver metastasis. *J Am Coll Surg* 2003;197:233–241.

Mazzaferro V, Regalia E, Doci R, et al. Liver transplantation for the treatment of small hepatocellular carcinomas in patients with cirrhosis. *N Engl J Med* 1996;334:693–700.

Seidenfeld J, Korn A, Aronson N. Radiofrequency ablation of unresectable primary liver cancer. *J Am Coll Surg* 2002;194:813–828.

U.S. Cancer Statistics Working Group. United States Cancer Statistics: 2000 Incidence Report. [updated 2003 Oct 29; cited 2004 May 8]. Available from: *http://www.cdc.gov/cancer/npcr/uscs/2000/index.htm.*

Wilmore DW, Cheung LY, Harken AH et al., eds. *ACS surgery: principles and practice.* New York: WebMD Corporation, 2002.

Nutrition, Digestion, and Absorption

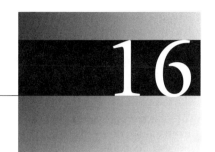

April Estelle Nedeau   Lisa D. Unger   John L. Rombeau

DIGESTION AND ABSORPTION

Introduction

The body has evolved the ability to break down and absorb food, while using the products as energy and building blocks for its own purpose. The gastrointestinal tract, along with several accessory organs, have been adapted for this use and also fulfill additional roles in fluid and electrolyte balance and immunity.

The anatomy and physiology of the gastrointestinal tract vary along its length in a coordinated serial fashion to optimize function. However, there are physical characteristics in common throughout. The intestinal wall is made up of several layers of specialized cells and tissues. The *mucosa* is the innermost epithelial layer and is often responsible for secretion and absorption. In general, it protrudes and invaginates to form villi and microvilli, thereby increasing its surface area. The *lamina propria* lies adjacent and external to the mucosa and is made up of loose connective tissue containing capillaries, enteric neurons, and immune cells, and it includes a ring of muscle called the *lamina muscularis*. The *submucosa* is the next layer and contains larger blood vessels and glands. It is surrounded by the *muscularis externa*, which consists of two or more layers of muscle arranged along a longitudinal or circular axis. Neurons of the *enteric nervous system* (ENS) lie between these two muscle layers. The *serosa* is the outermost layer and consists of connective tissue covered with squamous epithelium.

The Enteric Nervous System and the Gut–Brain Axis

The ENS is one of three divisions of the autonomic nervous system. It consists of two groups of neurons: the submucosal or Meissner plexus and the myenteric or Auerbach plexus. Meissner plexus lies within the submucosa of the small and large intestine only. Auerbach plexus exists between the two muscle layers of the muscularis externa from the proximal esophagus to the rectum. It is an independent and complete reflex circuit that includes afferent sensory neurons and efferent secretomotor neurons that stimulate smooth muscle, epithelial, and endocrine cells. Responses can be modified by brain and spinal cord input via autonomic ganglia, the main neurotransmitter of which is acetylcholine. Other important neurotransmitters include vasoactive intestinal peptide (VIP), enkephalins, somatostatin, substance P, serotonin, and nitrous oxide.

Extrinsic neuronal input originates from the other two branches of the autonomic nervous system. The vagus nerve innervates the gastrointestinal tract from the pharynx to the distal one third of the colon and it executes parasympathetic function. The sacral plexus innervates the remainder of the colon and rectum. Increased secretion and motility result from parasympathetic stimulation. The sympathetic branch initiates the *fight versus flight response*, thereby reducing blood flow and motility. This branch originates from centers in the medulla and cerebrum and contributes to the sensation of satiety.

Mouth and Pharynx

Digestion begins in the mouth through gross mechanical breakdown of food by the teeth and tongue. This provides an increase in the surface area for chemical digestion by salivary amylase. The salivary glands produce up to 1.0 to 1.5 L of saliva each day. The major glands include the parotid, submandibular, and sublingual glands. The minor glands are scattered throughout the submucosa of the mouth and pharynx. The functional unit of the salivary gland is a cluster of cells called acini, which empty into a collection of ducts. There are two populations of acinar cells. Serous cells produce a watery secretion containing α-amylase, a saccharidase secreted via exocytosis as zymogen granules. The second cell type produces mucin glycoproteins, which coat and lubricate the bolus in preparation for its entry into the esophagus. Other cell products include ribonuclease (RNase), deoxyribonuclease (DNase), lysozyme, peroxidase, and lingual lipase.

Saliva begins as an isotonic solution secreted by the acinar cells. It passes through the collection of ducts and is chemically altered along the course. The ductal cells absorb sodium and chloride, and to a lesser extent secrete potassium and bicarbonate. The degree of ion exchange is determined by the transit time of the saliva within the ducts. Slower rates increase exchange, producing hypotonicity and saliva rich in potassium and bicarbonate. Regulation of production and flow is controlled by the autonomic nervous system, with norepinephrine and acetylcholine as the two main agonists (Fig. 16-1).

The mouth and pharynx initiate the act of swallowing. The first of three phases is the oral or the *voluntary phase*, involving the propulsion of the bolus by the tongue toward the hypopharynx. Tactile receptors coordinate the transition to the *pharyngeal phase* as the bolus moves into the esophagus with reflex inhibition of respiration. The soft palate moves upward and the epiglottis covers the opening of the larynx to prevent aspiration into the nasopharynx and the trachea, respectively. Contraction of the superior pharyngeal muscles propels the bolus past the upper esophageal sphincter (UES) as it relaxes. This action is coordinated by the dorsal vagal nuclei and the nucleus ambiguus in the medulla and the lower pons. Failure of these muscles to relax properly may elevate intrapharyngeal pressure and lead to the formation of a Zenker diverticulum. The last of the three phases is the *esophageal phase*. The bolus passes beyond the UES into the esophagus and travels toward the stomach propelled by peristaltic waves (Fig. 16-2).

Esophagus

The esophagus is a passageway from the pharynx to the stomach. It is a hollow tube of muscle, approximately 25 to 30 cm long, beginning at the level of the cricoid cartilage and ending at the level of T11. Squamous epithelium lines the interior, except for the last few centimeters, which are covered by junctional columnar cells. The muscular layer is heterogeneous, with voluntary striated cells in the first one third and involuntary smooth muscle cells in the lower two thirds. Unique to , the esophagus is its lack of a serosa. The organ's primary function is to transport the food

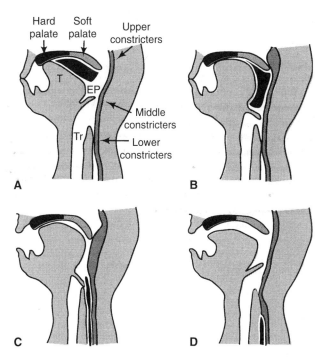

Figure 16-2 The oral and pharyngeal phases of swallowing involve the **(A)** separation of the bolus of food between the tongue and the soft and hard palate and **(B)** advancement of the bolus into the oropharynx. As respiration is inhibited, the bolus of food is propelled through the **(C)** pharynx by the sequential peristalsis of the superior, middle, and inferior constrictor muscles and advanced into the **(D)** upper esophagus, initiating the esophageal phase of swallowing. (From Johnson LR. Motility. In: Johnson LR, ed. *Essential medical physiology.* Philadelphia: Lippincott Williams & Wilkins, 1999:432, with permission.)

bolus, initiated by the act of swallowing. The UES relaxes, allowing passage of the bolus, and a primary peristaltic wave propels the bolus toward the stomach. If the bolus does not clear the esophagus, a second wave originating from the smooth, involuntary muscle, progresses. The muscle is stimulated by local distention and will continue to initiate waves until the bolus is delivered through the lower esophageal sphincter (LES) to the stomach. The LES is a high-pressure zone that serves as a functional sphincter and barrier against regurgitation of gastric contents. The high-pressure zone is established by its position between the positive pressure of the intraabdominal space and the negative pressure of the intrathoracic cavity. Tonic contraction is regulated by vagal cholinergic innervation. Chemicals shown to decrease local LES tone include atropine, caffeine, isoproterenol, secretin, calcium channel blockers, tobacco, ethanol, and prostaglandin E_2 (PGE_2). A decrease in tone may manifest in gastroesophageal reflux disease (GERD), whereas an increase in tone may play a role in the development of achalasia.

Stomach

The stomach is a reservoir in which mechanical digestion continues to completion in preparation for delivery to the small intestine. The organ can be divided into three main anatomic sections. The cardia is located just distal to the gastroesophageal junction and is devoid of the acid-secreting

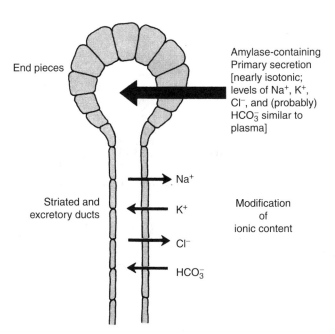

Figure 16-1 Salivary secretion. (From Berne RM, Levy MN, eds. *Physiology,* 2nd ed. St. Louis: Mosby, 1988, with permission.)

[Handwritten notes at top: Acid ⊕ → Parietal Cells → HCl; Gastrin ⊕ ↑⊕ ⊖ Somatostatin; Histamine]

parietal cells. The corpus, or body, is responsible for the storage of chyme and its proximal portion is called the fundus. The antrum is the distal portion, responsible for proper emptying of chyme into the intestine. The cardia and fundus are covered by columnar epithelium and gastric pits, which are lined by a variety of cell types. The mucous neck cells are located in the neck of the pit and produce a protective coat of mucus that shields the epithelium from the acidic environment. Parietal and chief cells are located deeper within the pit in varying proportions and they secrete acid and pepsinogen, respectively. In addition, the parietal cells secrete intrinsic factor, a significant protein in vitamin B_{12} absorption. The antral epithelium is dominated by mucus cells and gastrin secreting G cells (Fig. 16-3).

Gastric relaxation is a reflex triggered by the act of swallowing to receive the food bolus from the esophagus. It is regulated by the parasympathetic branch of the autonomic nervous system via the vagus nerve as a feedback loop called the vasovagal reflex. Relaxation of the proximal stomach and LES allow for an increase in volume without a proportional increase in pressure. The enteric nervous system contributes by stimulating active dilation of the fundus in response to gastric distention, termed gastric accommodation. Once the bolus is accepted into the stomach, it is churned vigorously into chyme. Ingested nutrients must be dissolved and solubilized in order to facilitate enzymatic digestion.

Although the majority of enzymatic digestion occurs in the small bowel, protein breakdown is initiated in the stomach by the chief cell product, pepsinogen. Pepsinogens are a group of aspartic proteinases secreted as zymogens that function as endopeptidases. There are eight different isoforms and they are secreted from the cell as inactive enzymes via compound exocytosis. Activation occurs by spontaneous cleavage of the N-terminus fragment within a specific pH range, optimal between 1.8 and 3.5. Secretion is stimulated through two second-messenger pathway systems. Secretin, β_2-adrenergic and PGE_2 receptors stimulate adenylate cyclase, whereas the M_3 muscarinic acetylcholine and gastrin/cholecystokinin (CCK) receptors stimulate calcium release from intracellular stores, utilizing the IP_3 pathway. The two most important agonists are acetylcholine, released as a vagal reflex in response to declining pH, and gastrin, secreted by antral G cells in response to the presence of amino acids. Secretin and CCK, produced by duodenal S cells and I cells, respectively, also stimulate pepsinogen release.

In addition to accommodating the food bolus, producing chyme, and initiating enzymatic digestion, the stomach provides a uniquely acidic environment. The acid serves as a barrier to pathogens and plays a regulatory role in digestion by activating enzymes and signaling the production of hormones. Acid is secreted by parietal cells via the hydrogen-potassium pump (H^+-K^+ pump), a member of the P-type adenosine triphosphatase (ATPase) gene family. The three acid secretogogues are acetylcholine, gastrin, and histamine, which bind to their respective receptors and function synergistically through a G-protein-coupled pathway. Acetylcholine and gastrin also act indirectly via histamine release from enterochromaffin-like (ECL) cells in the lamina propria. The four phases of acid secretion begin with the *basal phase*, occurring over the interdigestive periods. Acid secretion is maintained at a constant low level in the pH range between 3 and 7. The three remaining phases characterize acid secretion during a meal. The *cephalic phase* is initiated by stimulation of the senses, such as the smell and taste of food, as well as the act of swallowing. It is responsible for 30% of gastric acid production and is mediated by the vagus nerve and its neurotransmitter acetylcholine, which binds to the acetylcholine receptor causing acid production, histamine release and the production of GRP (gastrin-releasing protein) from local neurons. Finally, it inhibits the release of somatostatin, a gastrin inhibitor from antral D cells. The *gastric phase* is initiated by distention of the stomach and the presence of partially digested proteins, or peptones. It accounts for approximately 50% to 60% of the total gastric acid secretion and is mediated by a vasovagal reflex and local ENS pathways. Decreasing pH results in pepsinogen activation and production of peptones with subsequent gastrin release and acid secretion. The *intestinal phase* results in 5% to 10% of the gastric acid production. Gastrin is secreted by duodenal G cells in response to peptones and amino acids as they exit the stomach.

Inhibition of acid secretion is accomplished by a negative feedback loop. The delivery of acid, lipids, and hyperosmolar solution to the duodenum results in production of somatostatin by D cells. Somatostatin inhibits release of antral gastrin and downregulates parietal cell H^+-K^+ pump pump molecules. Duodenal enteroendocrine cells release CCK and gastrin-inhibitory protein (GIP), which both inhibit acid secretion directly. Aside from dampening excessive acid production, the stomach produces a layer of viscous mucus and a bicarbonate-rich microclimate that provide a diffusion barrier for the epithelium.

[Handwritten notes: Cells: Parietal Cell - HCl, IF; Chief Cells - pepsinogen; mucous neck cells - mucous; G-cells - gastrin]

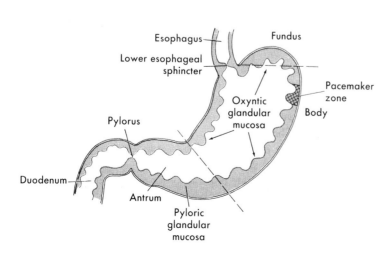

Figure 16-3 The stomach. (From Berne RM, Levy MN, eds. *Physiology*, 2nd ed. St. Louis: Mosby, 1988:633, with permission.)

Pancreas

The pancreas is a retroperitoneal endocrine gland embraced by a C-shaped loop of the duodenum. It weighs on average between 75 and 125 g and manufactures the vast majority of digestive enzymes, delivered to the duodenum through a branched ductal system. The ducts secrete a bicarbonate-rich solution that neutralizes the acidic chyme. The functional unit of the exocrine pancreas is the acinus, which is structurally defined by a collection of 15 to 100 acinar cells surrounding the proximal end of a small intercalated duct. These cells are highly polarized with a secretory apical end facing the duct lumen and a basolateral end adjacent to the blood supply. A lobule is formed by a group of acini that empties into an intralobular duct. These ducts coalesce to form larger interlobar ducts, which eventually form the main pancreatic duct (Wirsung) and the accessory duct (Santorini).

The pancreas generates more than 1.5 L of enzyme-rich fluid each day. The acinar cells produce an isotonic solution laden with approximately twenty different zymogens. These enzymes are classified by their substrates and include proteases, amylases, lipases, nucleases, and some less well-understood enzymes, such as glycoprotein 2, lithostathine, and pancreatic-associated protein. The proteases are categorized by the location of cleavage within the substrate molecule. Exopeptidases cleave protein molecules at the end of the amino acid chain and include carboxypeptidase A and B isoforms. Significant endopeptidases include trypsin, chymotrypsin, elastase, and kallikrein, which cleave between the inner amino acid molecules within the protein. These digestive enzymes form an efficient molecular tool for dissolution of ingested nutrients; however, protective mechanisms must be maintained, as they cannot discriminate between self and substrate. Initially, the enzymes are produced as inactive precursors and packaged within zymogen granules, isolated from the main cytoplasmic compartment. They are sequestered with inhibitory molecules in a low pH environment and dock on the apical membrane awaiting exocytosis. Within the small intestine, the duodenal mucosal enzyme enterokinase cleaves trypsinogen to produce its catalytic form. Trypsin subsequently activates the other zymogens, as well as additional trypsinogen molecules, by cleaving their inhibitory subunits. CCK is produced by neuroendocrine cells in the duodenal mucosa and it augments protein secretion from the acinar cells. It is released in the presence of peptones, amino acids, and especially lipids within the intestinal lumen. In addition to binding its own receptor on the acinar cell, it synergistically activates a parasympathetic cholinergic pathway. Binding to the CCK receptor and the muscarinic cholinergic receptor results in calcium-mediated upregulation of protein manufacture.

The centroacinar and intercalated duct cells contribute to the pancreatic secretory product by altering its composition as it travels through the ductal system. The final product is a clear, isotonic solution with an approximate pH of 8. Sodium and potassium are the major cations and their concentrations remain fairly constant. The concentrations of the major anions, chloride and bicarbonate, are dependent on the length of time they are exposed to the ductal epithelium (Fig. 16-4). As the fluid moves down the duct toward the duodenum, bicarbonate is exchanged for chloride via a protein pump on the apical membrane of the cells. As the rate of movement increases, less exchange occurs, resulting in a lower pH solution with a higher concentration of chloride (Fig. 16-5). Neurohumoral input also affects the fluid composition by stimulating the bicarbonate–chloride exchanger. The most potent pump stimulant is the hormone secretin, produced by S cells in the crypts of Lieberkühn. After secretin is released in response to bile or acid in the intestinal lumen, it circulates in the blood and binds to receptors on the ductal cell basolateral membrane. It modulates signal through a cyclic adenosine monophosphate (cAMP)-mediated second messenger mechanism. Parasympathetic innervation works synergistically via acetylcholine through a calcium second messenger system.

The three physiologic phases of pancreatic secretion are similar to the phases of acid secretion in the stomach. The *cephalic phase* causes a modest increase in fluid and electrolyte production but largely enhances enzyme secretion. Pancreatic stimulation in the *gastric phase* is modulated through several mechanisms including the release of hormones, neural mediation, altered pH, and the delivery of nutrients to the proximal intestine. Peptone-induced gastrin release and the vasovagal reflex are two prominent examples. The vasovagal reflex is initiated by gastric distention in this phase. The *intestinal phase* begins as chyme enters the duodenum, with secretin and CCK-mediated hormonal stimulation and a vasovagal enteropancreatic reflex. The pattern and strength of the pancreatic response is influenced by the specific contents of the chyme. A liquid meal is evacuated from the stomach rapidly and therefore elicits about 60% of the maximum secretory potential (Fig. 16-6).

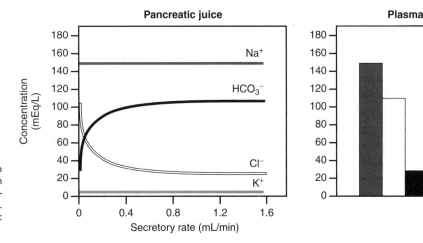

Figure 16-4 Ionic composition of pancreatic secretion. (From Greenfield L, ed. *Surgery: scientific principles and practice*, 1st ed. Philadelphia: JB Lippincott, 1993: 784, with permission.)

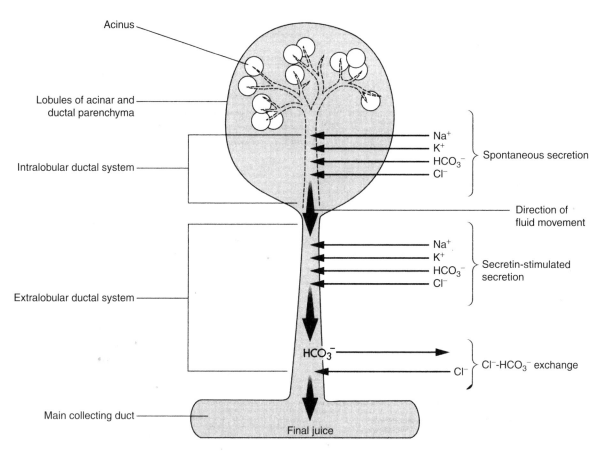

Figure 16-5   Pancreatic secretion. (From Savage E, Fishman S, Miller L. *Essentials of basic science in surgery*. Philadelphia: JB Lippincott, 1993:189, with permission.)

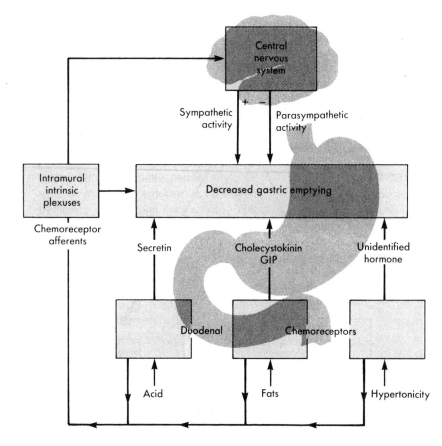

Figure 16-6   Regulation of gastric emptying. (From Berne RM, Levy MN, eds. *Physiology*, 2nd ed. St. Louis: Mosby, 1988:639, with permission.)

Evacuation of a solid meal is slower and results in a prolonged pancreatic response. Carbohydrates elicit little effect, whereas energy rich foods, such as long chain fatty acids, are the most potent.

Biliary System

Enzymatic digestion and intestinal absorption are both dependent on solubilization and dissolution of ingested nutrients into a hydrophilic solution. Bile is a mixture of phospholipids, salts, cholesterol, and pigments synthesized by hepatocytes and stored in the gallbladder. Bile functions to dissolve fat through organization into micelles, making them vulnerable to lipases. As bile passes through the canaliculi and bile ducts, it is altered by the addition of bicarbonate, a process augmented by exposure to secretin. After entering the gallbladder, it is refined further into an isoosmotic concentration of 10- to 20-fold. This process affects the solubility of calcium and cholesterol, inclining precipitation and stone formation. The main functions of the gallbladder are to concentrate and store bile during fasting and to deliver bile to the duodenum during meals. Its epithelium secretes mucus glycoproteins that form a protective barrier against detergent effects of the bile salt. Hydrogen ions are also secreted to acidify the solution and increase calcium solubility. During fasting, the gallbladder is filled by tonic contraction of the ampullary sphincter with periods of relaxation and partial emptying. During digestion, CCK is released from the duodenal mucosa and stimulates the gallbladder to contract while relaxing the sphincter of Oddi. Fifty percent to 70% of the bile is introduced to the duodenum within 30 to 40 minutes (Fig. 16-7). When its contribution to digestion is complete, 95% is actively absorbed by the terminal ileum, and the bile is carried through the portal blood by albumin and lipoprotein to the liver where it is extracted and reused. Bile that enters the colon is deconjugated by local bacteria via 7α-dehydroxylation to form the secondary bile acids, deoxycholate and lithocholate. A portion is absorbed and reprocessed while the remainder is defecated (Fig. 16-8).

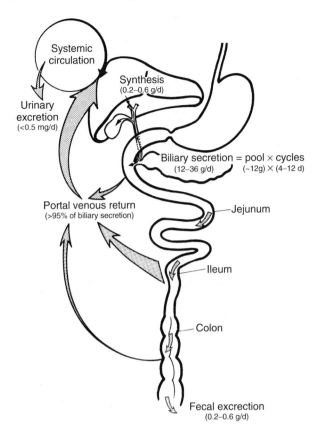

Figure 16-8 Enterohepatic circulation of bile acids. (From Carey MC, Cahalane MJ. In: Arias IM, Jakoby WB, Popper H et al., eds. *The liver: biology and pathobiology*, 2nd ed. New York: Raven Press, 1988, with permission.)

Small Bowel

The small bowel is a hollow muscular organ in which most enzymatic digestion and nutrient absorption occurs. Its large surface area is accomplished by two anatomic features: the plicae circulares or concentric circular folds and finger-like epithelial projections called villi. The duodenum begins at the pylorus and is approximately 20 cm in length. Its junction with the jejunum is supported by a strand of peritoneum called the ligament of Treitz. The jejunum is about 150 cm length and is followed by the ileum, making up the remaining three fifths of the small intestine. The epithelium forms microvilli and blankets a landscape of villi and crypts, increasing the enteric surface area and absorptive power. Enterocytes are one of the four main cell types populating the mucosa. They are the most numerous type and are responsible for nutrient absorption. Goblet cells secrete mucus. Paneth cells secrete lysozyme, tumor necrosis factor (TNF), and cryptidins, which are homologs of leukocyte defensins. The remaining cells are enteroendocrine in origin and include a constellation of ten different populations that produce distinct gastrointestinal hormones.

The semipermeable membrane of the small intestine is ideal for both secretion and absorption of simple molecules such as water, carbohydrates, lipids, proteins, minerals, and vitamins. Approximately 9 L of fluid pass through the small intestine each day, with only 500 to 1,000 mL reaching the cecum. Seven of the 9 L are endogenous, originating from intestinal tract secretions (i.e., salivary, gastric, hepatic, and pancreatic secretions) (Fig. 16-9). The

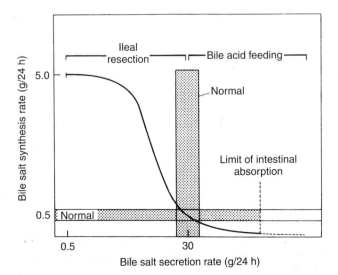

Figure 16-7 Regulation of bile acid secretion and synthesis. (From Carey MC, Cahalane MJ. In: Arias IM, Jakoby WB, Popper H et al., eds. *The liver: biology and pathobiology*, 2nd ed. New York: Raven Press, 1988, with permission.)

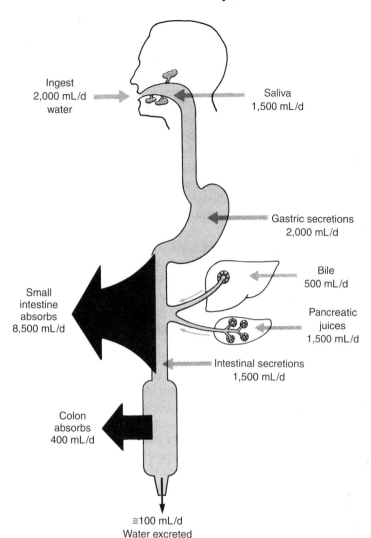

Ingest
2,000 mL/d
water

Saliva
1,500 mL/d

Gastric secretions
2,000 mL/d

Bile
500 mL/d

Small
intestine
absorbs
8,500 mL/d

Pancreatic
juices
1,500 mL/d

Intestinal secretions
1,500 mL/d

Colon
absorbs
400 mL/d

≅100 mL/d
Water excreted

Figure 16-9   Fluid balance in the gastrointestinal tract. (From Berne RM, Levy MN, eds. *Physiology*, 2nd ed. St. Louis: Mosby, 1988:697, with permission.)

jejunum is the most active site of water absorption and is coupled to the movement of solutes and nutrients across the membrane. Passive diffusion, solvent drag, and active transport are the three mechanisms of electrolyte absorption. Passive diffusion is the energy-free movement of electrolytes down an electrochemical gradient through a protein channel or between cells, and occurs mostly in the jejunum. Solvent drag is the coupling of solute absorption with the movement of water across the membrane. Active transport is an energy-dependent mechanism that moves simple molecules against the electrochemical gradient and is usually accomplished by an ATPase protein pump.

Carbohydrates

Carbohydrate ingestion in North America averages between 350 and 400 g/person/day and exists in the form of starch and monosaccharides. Amylose and amylopectin are the two major dietary starch varieties, making up 20% and 80%, respectively. Amylose is a long chain of glucose molecules connected by α-1, 4 carbon bonds, where it is broken down by salivary and pancreatic amylase to form maltotriose and maltose. Amylopectin is similar to amylose in structure with the exception of an α-1, 6 carbon bond every 2.5 molecules. Oligosaccharides are reduced to monosaccharides by the brush-border enzymes of the small intestine mucosa.

Galactose and glucose are absorbed by a carrier-mediated active transport mechanism dependent on sodium movement into the cell. Fructose molecules are passively absorbed via a carrier-mediated facilitated diffusion (Fig. 16-10). Carbohydrate deficiencies are uncommon, but intolerance can occur from an enzyme deficiency. Lactose intolerance occurs with the absence of lactase on the intestinal brush border and results in malabsorptive diarrhea upon ingestion of milk-based products. It appears to have a genetic component and often affects those of Asian and African-American descent.

Protein

Protein digestion begins with denaturation in the acidic environment of the stomach and exposure to the chief cell product pepsin. Endopeptidases continue the process of protein breakdown within the duodenum, forming peptones. Exopeptidases serially remove single amino acids from the peptones yielding about 70% short chain peptides and 30% amino acids. Oligopeptidases on the intestinal brush border complete digestion. These enzymes are efficient, and 50% of the protein is absorbed after the chyme passes through the duodenum. Absorption of amino acids, and di- and tripeptides occur by carrier-mediated active transport. This process prefers dipeptides and is

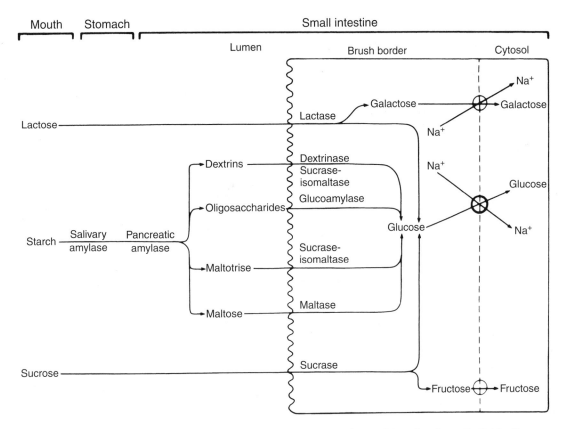

Figure 16-10   Carbohydrate digestion in the gastrointestinal tract. (From Rombeau JL, Caldwell MD, eds. *Clinical nutrition: enteral and tube feeding*, 2nd ed. Philadelphia: WB Saunders, 1990:25, with permission.)

variable depending on the amino acid. Eighty percent of ingested protein is absorbed after passing through the jejunum. Protein malabsorption is rare, even with extensive resection of the intestine, because absorption occurs throughout.

Lipids

Fat ingestion averaging between 60 and 100 g/person/day is typical for the Western diet. Gastric churning emulsifies the lipid, and pancreatic lipase removes fatty acids from the glycerol backbone in the duodenum. The water solubility of free fatty acids and monoglycerides is poor, preventing their access to transport molecules in the intestinal mucosa. This problem is overcome by the formation of micelles, facilitated by their combination with bile salt, and may include cholesterol, fat-soluble vitamins, and phospholipids. Lecithin is an important phospholipid that greatly enhances micelle formation. Micelles are highly organized, providing a hydrophobic core with a water-soluble hydrophilic exterior, allowing lipid movement within the aqueous environment (Fig. 16-11). Fatty acids and monoglycerides are carried by micelles to the mucosa and transported passively across the membrane leaving the micelle behind. Within the cell, long chain fatty acids are resynthesized into triglycerides and processed into chylomicrons, which are absorbed into the lymphatic system via intestinal lacteals. Eventually, they return to the central circulation through the thoracic duct for metabolism or storage in the periphery. Short and medium chain fatty acids are absorbed directly into the capillary system.

Vitamins, Minerals, and Trace Elements

The mechanism of vitamin absorption within the small intestine depends on their solubility in fat versus water. The fat-soluble vitamins are carried within micelles, absorbed like lipid, processed into chylomicrons, and travel through the thoracic duct to the central circulation. They include vitamins A, D, E, and K. The water-soluble vitamins have a more complex absorptive process and include vitamins C, B_6, thiamine, riboflavin, B_{12}, and others. Vitamin B_{12} is synthesized by microorganisms and also ingested in the diet from primary sources such as meat, fish, shellfish, and eggs. It is not present in vegetable matter and therefore strict vegetarians are more susceptible to deficiencies. In human physiology, there are two vitamin B_{12}–dependent enzymatic reactions. Methionine synthase converts homocysteine to methionine, an amino acid required for the synthesis of S-adenosylmethionine. This molecule plays an important role in several methylation reactions, including DNA and RNA synthesis, and therefore affects rapidly dividing cells. Folate is an intermediate in the pathway and its deficiency has the same result. The second dependent enzyme is l-methylmalonyl-CoA mutase, which catalyzes the conversion of l-methylmalonyl-CoA to succinyl CoA, an important intermediate in fat and protein metabolism, as well as the in production of hemoglobin. Vitamin B_{12} and folate deficiencies affect the bone marrow early, resulting in the immature, hemoglobin-poor red blood cells of megaloblastic anemia. Neurologic manifestations, such as extremity numbness and tingling, memory loss, disorientation, and dementia occur only with vitamin B_{12} deficiency.

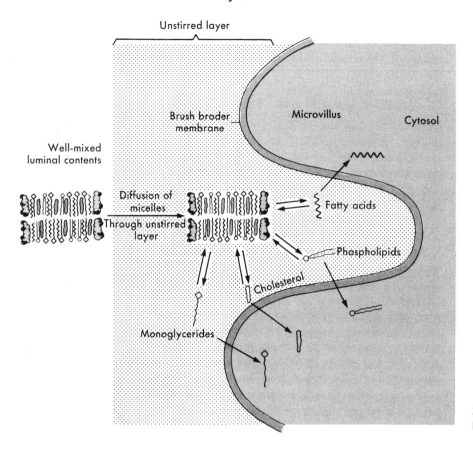

Figure 16-11 Lipid absorption. (From Berne RM, Levy MN, eds. Physiology, 2nd ed. St. Louis: Mosby, 1988:712, with permission.)

The mechanism is poorly understood but damage to neuronal myelin sheaths is suspected.

Vitamin B_{12} reaches the stomach bound to ingested protein. It is released when the protein is denatured in the acid environment and binds to the salivary gland product, haptocorrin (R protein). Haptocorrin protects vitamin B_{12} until it is degraded by pancreatic proteases and releases cobalamin. Finally, Vitamin B_{12} binds to intrinsic factor and is absorbed by the terminal ileum as a complex.

With the aid of Vitamin D, calcium is absorbed across the brush border of the duodenum and jejunum. Once it enters the cytosol, calcium binds to CaBP (calcium-binding protein), which transports it to the basolateral membrane. The calcium ATPase and the Na^+–Ca^{2+} exchanger move calcium ions into the circulatory system. Vitamin D enhances absorption through several mechanisms. It increases absorption across the brush border of the small intestine, and acting as a hormone, it upregulates the calcium exchangers in the basolateral membrane. Vitamin D is a molecule derived from cholesterol and is obtained by either dietary sources or from the skin after activation by sunlight. Initially, it is biologically inactive and must be activated by two separate hydroxylation reactions. The first enzymatic reaction occurs in the liver and the second in the kidneys, resulting in the molecule 1, 25-(OH)2-vitamin D3. Parathyroid hormone (PTH) stimulates the renal enzymes in response to decreasing serum calcium levels.

The average daily diet includes about 20 mg of iron per day, but only 1.0 to 1.5 mg is absorbed. The majority is absorbed in the duodenum and the mechanism is not completely understood. Iron exists in the form of ferric iron (Fe^{3+}) when ingested as food and it is insoluble in water when the pH is greater than 3. In the stomach, acid reduces ferric iron to ferrous iron (Fe^{2+}), making it soluble and therefore easier to absorb. Iron binds to transferrin in the lumen of the small intestine and is absorbed as a complex by endocytosis. After it enters the cytosol, it is released from transferrin and travels to the basolateral membrane where it is transported across into the circulation. It is carried in the serum via the plasma form of transferrin. Iron binds ferritin within the brush border cells in times of excess and once bound it cannot be relinquished. It is lost when the cells are desquamated.

Other important dietary elements include magnesium, zinc, copper, and selenium, but their absorption is not well understood. Zinc and copper are absorbed actively and copper absorption occurs mainly in the proximal intestine. Magnesium is absorbed along the entire length of the intestine, but the mechanism is unclear.

Colon

The colon is approximately 1.5 m in length and it follows the small intestine in sequence. It is responsible for water and electrolyte absorption, as well as the storage and elimination of nonabsorbable fecal material. Although one liter of chyme reaches the cecum each day, the body defecates only about 100 to 200 mL. Similar to the small intestine, the sodium–potassium ATPase pump plays a critical role in water and electrolyte absorption. It exchanges sodium and potassium across the basolateral membrane. This creates an electrochemical gradient that enables sodium and chloride ion movement from the lumen into the cell cytosol, in exchange for potassium and bicarbonate ions, respectively. Water is coupled to electrolyte absorption through the process of solvent drag.

Immunology

Beneath the mucosal surfaces of the gastrointestinal and respiratory tracts lies 50% to 60% of the body's total immunity. Within the lamina propria, 70% to 80% of antibody is produced, mostly in the form of immunoglobulin (Ig)A. Immunoglobulin is transported by the overlying epithelial cells onto the mucosal surface. It binds to bacteria, preventing local attachment and infection. The surface area of the gastrointestinal tract is approximately 300 m^2 and protective barriers have evolved to prevent infection. The mucous coat, glycocalyx, resident microflora, peristalsis, proteolytic gastrointestinal secretions, and IgA prevent invasion and allow a symbiotic relationship between host and bacteria. Peyer patches are lymphocytic collections located in the distal small bowel and are the principal site for sensitization. The *common mucosal barrier immune hypothesis* is a theory that explains the interaction between separate mucosal departments in the attempt to share immunity between them. It utilizes the circulatory system to provide generalized mucosal protection, initiated by local immunization. Antigen is transported to underlying dendritic and macrophage populations in the Peyer patches, which are subsequently presented to CD4$^+$ T cells and naïve B cells. When mature, these cells proliferate in the mesenteric lymph nodes and migrate through the thoracic duct to the circulation, homing to distant mucosal lamina propria sites.

Both the route and type of nutrition affect the histology, cytokines, IgA levels, and the effectiveness of the gastrointestinal and respiratory tract mucosal immunity. Studies have demonstrated a reduction in gastric mucosa–associated lymphoid tissue (GALT) lymphocyte number within the lamina propria of long-term total parenteral nutrition (TPN)–fed rats. Burke et al. (1989) showed that glutamine supplementation of parenteral nutrition elevated IgA and decreased bacterial translocation. A 2% glutamine-supplemented parenteral solution was shown to maintain relatively normal numbers of T and B cells within the Peyer patches. However, IgA levels in both respiratory and gastrointestinal tract mucosa were lower as compared to those in chow-fed animals. Lastly, Li et al. (1997) suggested that it is not enteral nutrients that determine immunologic integrity. ENS release of neuropeptides in response to gut feeding may play a more significant role then exposure to nutrients alone. Kudsk et al. used bombesin, a GRP analog, as a supplement in parenteral nutrition and demonstrated normalized GALT cell population in Peyer patches and the lamina propria, consistent with chow-fed levels. IgA levels also remained normal.

NUTRITION AND METABOLISM

Assessment

In the 1930s, the relationship between disease-related malnutrition and postoperative morbidity and mortality was recognized. Postoperative complications may include impaired respiratory muscle function resulting in reintubation, reduced cardiac contractility, impaired renal function, nonhealing wounds, apathy, and impairment of functional recovery. A number of assessment methods have been designed to identify and aid those patients at risk. No single current method is ideal, but in combination they derive useful information for the practitioner.

A comprehensive assessment should begin with a thorough history and physical examination. The history and review of systems should expose impediments to appropriate oral intake or efficient intestinal absorption. These obstacles may include the inability to chew or swallow, severe alcoholism, and disorders of malabsorption, such as Crohn disease. Recent history of surgery or trauma and chronic medical issues are also significant. During the examination, peripheral edema, ascites, and signs of vitamin and mineral deficiency should be noted. Severe caloric deficiency, or *marasmus*, may be manifested as decreased subcutaneous fat and a cachectic appearance with muscle wasting. Weight measurements alone are not recommended to assess nutritional status. They do not encompass critical factors such as age, height, and gender, which help reflect the lean body mass more accurately. They also compare individual patients to a chart of "normal" values derived from one specific and limited population. However, inquiry into recent weight loss is critical and predicts higher risk when in excess of 15%. Body mass index (BMI; kg per m^2) is a more optimal nutritional indicator, but shares similar limitations, particularly in the obese population. *Kwashiorkor*, an isolated protein deficiency, common in the obese and postsurgical populations can be difficult to detect. Notably, a low BMI, especially if less then 18 kg per m^2, has been associated with significant postoperative morbidity and mortality.

The inaccuracy of using weight alone to assess nutritional status has led to the development and implementation of other techniques. Anthropometry is the measurement of mid-arm circumference and triceps skin-fold thickness. It can provide valuable data regarding muscle mass and body fat index respectively, but it cannot account for age-related changes in lean body mass, observer variance, edema, and arm/hand dominance. Serum transport proteins such as albumin, prealbumin, and transferrin are a useful measure of visceral protein mass. Albumin has a half-life in the serum of 18.2 days and therefore is limited in its ability to indicate acute changes in the critically ill patient. Because of their shorter half-lives, prealbumin (1.3 days) and transferrin (8.5 days) have increased sensitivity in the detection of acute protein loss.

The use of a combination of measures to assess nutritional status is currently the most accurate and reliable method in identifying malnourished patients. The subjective global assessment (SGA) incorporates elements of the history, physical examination, and subjective analysis. It separates patients into well-nourished, moderately nourished, and malnourished categories and includes factors such as weight loss, calorie counts, gastrointestinal symptoms that impair oral intake or absorption, functional capacity, and subcutaneous fat and muscle loss. The SGA in combination with obtainable objective data, such as BMI and albumin level, is used at many institutions as a ruler of nutritional health.

Metabolism

Caloric Requirements

In order to assure adequate caloric and nutritional intake, it is necessary to obtain or estimate energy and protein requirements. A practical and accurate approximation of caloric needs can be assessed via indirect calorimetry. After the patient breathes into a spirometer or metabolic cart, energy expenditure is calculated by measuring oxygen consumption and carbon dioxide production. These values are inserted into an equation to yield the metabolic rate.

$$\text{Metabolic rate (kcal/m}^2/\text{h}) = [3.9 \times \text{VO}_2 \text{ (L/min)}]$$
$$+ 1.1 \times \text{VCO}_2 \text{ (L/min)}$$
$$\times 60 \text{ (min/h)/body surface}$$
$$\text{area (m}^2)$$

These values can also be used to derive the *respiratory quotient* (RQ), which is the ratio between expired carbon dioxide and consumed oxygen. The RQ supplies information on substrate utilization; for example, an RQ of 1.0 is indicative of glucose oxidation, 0.8 for protein oxidation, and 0.7 for fat. Of note, this measurement is made at only one time-point on a continuum. Frequent reassessment is required, especially in the acutely ill patient with rapidly changing metabolism.

Unfortunately, indirect calorimetry using the metabolic cart is not available at many institutions because it is labor-intensive and expensive. Although less accurate, a variety of other calculations based on weight, age, and gender may be employed. The **Harris-Benedict equation** estimates basal energy expenditure (BEE) and can be adjusted to estimate total energy expenditure (TEE) with a multiplication factor that reflects an individual's activity level.

$$\text{BEE (women)} = 655 + (9.6W) + (1.8H) - (4.7A)$$
$$\text{BEE (men)} = 66 + (13.7W) + (5H) - (6.8A)$$

where W is weight in kilograms, H is height in centimeters, and A is age in years. The Harris-Benedict equation was derived for basal energy levels using healthy people. The TEE can be estimated by multiplying an activity factor of 1.3 for hospitalized patients and 1.5 for outpatients.

Protein

Protein is responsible for the enzymatic function and the structural integrity of the entire human form. It is not stored, only utilized or wasted. Proteins are made of functional units called amino acids, of which 20 varieties exist, which can be separated into two categories. *Essential amino acids* must be obtained exogenously from the diet because the body cannot synthesize them. Synthesis of nonessential amino acids occurs regularly. Amino acids can be utilized in one of three ways: protein synthesis; catabolic reactions that lead to energy production; or synthesis of *nonessential amino acids*, purines or pyrimidines. The liver regulates the distribution of absorbed amino acids, with only 25% reaching the general circulation. Sixty percent is converted to urea, 6% is used for plasma protein synthesis, and 14% becomes liver protein. Plasma amino acids are exchanged among muscle, gut, and viscera, especially in times of need when serum glucose is low and glycogen stores are deficient. In muscle, branched chain amino acids are transaminated to alanine and glutamine with pyruvate or α-ketoglutamate as the usual amine receptor. Alanine is deaminated by the liver to form pyruvate which then undergoes gluconeogenesis. The amino group generated from the deamination is eliminated via the urea cycle. The gut metabolizes glutamine into alanine for final hepatic conversion to glucose. The kidney uses glutamine to form ammonia for its regulation of acid–base balance in the argininosuccinate cycle. It is important to note that the degradation of protein yields

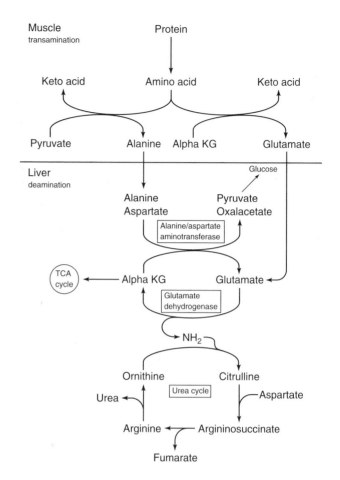

Figure 16-12 Protein metabolism.

only 25% of the energy used to synthesize it and therefore is a poor energy source (Fig. 16-12).

The **protein requirement** for an average healthy adult is approximately 0.8 g/kg/d, with approximately 20% of consumed protein as essential amino acids. Each gram of protein yields 4 kcal. In the acutely ill patient, the requirement may be substantially higher owing to protein wasting. The increased requirement is usually estimated, but it can be assessed and followed more accurately by measuring nitrogen balance. Nitrogen output, or the sum of all nitrogen found in excretions and secretions, including urine, feces, or fistula drainage is subtracted from nitrogen intake, or the sum of all nitrogen consumed via enteral or parenteral means. Nitrogen balance can be estimated on the basis of the urine urea nitrogen excreted in a 24-hour period of urine collection and also on a correction factor (4 g per 24 hours), to approximate insensible nonurea urinary nitrogen and fecal losses. Additional correction factors can be used to estimate nitrogen output from other sources such as fistulas. One gram of nitrogen composes 6.25 g of protein.

$$\text{Nitrogen balance} = \text{(protein intake in grams/6.25)}$$
$$- \text{(urinary urea nitrogen} + 4 \text{ g)}$$

In general, a positive nitrogen balance suggests an anabolic state, whereas a negative balance suggests catabolism, or protein wasting. Most healthy individuals will present with a nitrogen balance in equilibrium.

Carbohydrates

Glucose is the monosaccharide molecule chiefly responsible for the production of energy fueling the vast majority of metabolic processes. The oxidation of glucose yields approximately 3.4 kcal per g. After absorption by the intestine, glucose is converted into fat, stored as glycogen in muscle and liver cells, or immediately oxidized for energy in the form of adenosine triphosphate (ATP). Once glucose enters the cell, it is phosphorylated to glucose-6-phosphate (G6P) and thereby confined to the cytosol. In conditions of excess, G6P is polymerized into glycogen via glycogen synthetase in muscle and liver cells. However, only liver glycogen stores can be systemically used because these cells alone are able to dephosphorylate G6P to form glucose, which can readily leave the cell. Once glycogen stores are repleted, excess glucose is converted into fat. ATP is the currency of energy and it is required for many enzymatic reactions. Along with water and carbon dioxide (CO_2), it is the final product of the oxidation of glucose. Through glycolysis, a series of chemical reactions, G6P is processed into pyruvate. It is subsequently converted into acetyl-CoA and enters the tricarboxylic acid cycle (TCA) to yield CO_2, hydrogen, water, and electrons. These molecules enter the electron transport chain (ETC) to yield the final product. The TCA and ETC are aerobic reactions that together are the final common pathway for the oxidation of amino acids, fatty acids, and glucose.

Systemic glycogen reserve can sustain appropriate levels of serum glucose for about 24 hours in times of starvation. Approximately 100 g is stored in the liver and 200 to 250 g in skeletal muscle. After these stores are depleted, the body must rely on lipolysis and proteolysis for energy supply and the maintenance of serum glucose levels via gluconeogenesis (Fig. 16-13). Red and white blood cells require glucose because of their limited cellular machinery and the brain prefers glucose but can adapt to other fuel sources over time. The primary source of substrate for gluconeogenesis is amino acid molecules from proteolysis. Fat molecules can contribute only glycerol backbones because acetyl-CoA molecules from fatty acid oxidation must react with oxaloacetate for progression to the TCA cycle, and its supply is limited. Therefore, protein breakdown is required to sustain gluconeogenesis in times of starvation.

Lipids

Lipids are essential nutrients that provide the most efficient energy reserve; their oxidation yields 9 kcal per g. They are also processed into important biochemical molecules or structures, such as myelin sheaths around axons. Lipids are stored in adipose cells as triglyceride molecules, the structure of which is composed of a glycerol backbone with three covalently bound fatty acids. The heart, liver, and skeletal muscle use fatty acids as a major fuel source.

The storage of energy as fat begins with fatty acid synthesis in the cell cytosol. Acetyl-CoA is converted into malonyl-CoA, which is subsequently and repetitively elongated by the addition of a two-carbon unit also derived from acetyl-CoA. When glycogen stores are depleted, triglycerides are mobilized via lipolysis and fatty acid molecules are oxidized for energy. After absorption into the cell, fatty acids are combined with coenzyme A (CoA) and ATP to yield fatty acyl-CoA. This molecule enters the mitochondria and undergoes a process called β-oxidation involving a cycle of reactions. With each cycle, a two-carbon acetyl-CoA molecule is cleaved from the end of the fatty acyl-CoA and enters the TCA. It leaves behind the fatty acyl-CoA, two carbon atoms shorter, to reenter the cycle. The glycerol molecule can be converted into pyruvate for gluconeogenesis (Fig. 16-14).

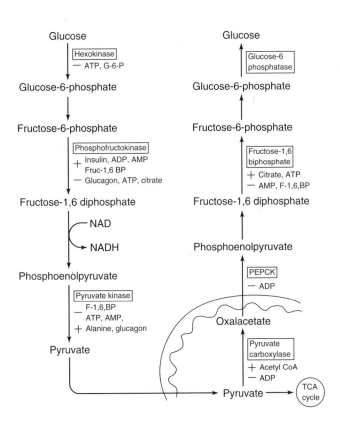

Figure 16-13 Glycolysis, gluconeogenesis.

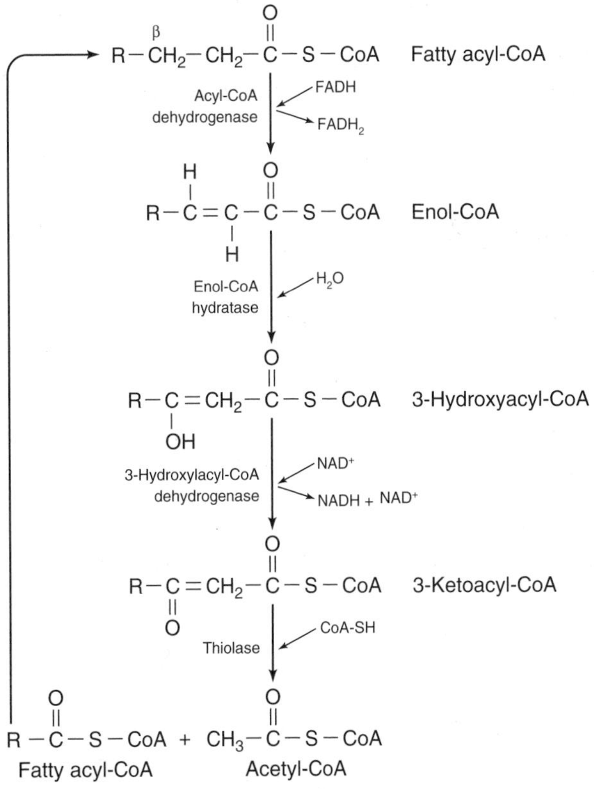

Figure 16-14 Fatty acid β-oxidation.

Certain tissues, such as heart, brain, and skeletal muscle are also able to use ketone bodies as energy in times of starvation. Acetoacetate and β-hydroxybutyrate are synthesized by the liver when oxaloacetate levels are low. Acetyl-CoA is shunted from the TCA and toward the formation of ketones.

Vitamins

Vitamins serve as crucial cofactors for many biochemical pathways and are necessary for growth, maintenance, and reproduction. There are four fat-soluble and nine water-soluble vitamins. Their functions and deficiency states are listed in Table 16-1. The fat-soluble vitamins include A, D, E, and K. Vitamin A limits the keratinization of the epithelium in the eye and is therefore important in maintaining sight by preserving these membranes. It also promotes wound healing. Vitamin D is essential in the intestinal absorption of calcium and phosphorus. Vitamin E is a family of tocopherols with seven members that serve in many biochemical functions. Finally, vitamin K is a critical cofactor in the synthesis of several clotting factors produced by the liver, specifically factors II, VII, IX, and X. These factors participate in the clotting cascade measured via the prothrombin time. Fat-soluble vitamins in particular are dependent on the presence of bile for absorption, and vitamin K is sensitive to intestinal overgrowth of bacteria because the colon produces and absorbs a considerable amount.

The water-soluble vitamins include the B complex vitamins, and ascorbic acid (vitamin C). Vitamin B_{12} is vital for DNA synthesis. It is the only water-soluble vitamin that can be stored in the liver and recycled for a substantial length of time. Therefore, it is a rare deficiency except in patients with certain disease states, such as pernicious anemia or after intestinal bypass surgery, without supplemented injections. Vitamin B_{12} may manifest as macrocytic anemia and neuropathy. Folate is the most common water-soluble vitamin deficiency and it is also needed for DNA synthesis. Folate deficiency may manifest as leukopenia, megaloblastic anemia, steatorrhea, sprue, and glossitis.

Trace Elements

The trace elements include iron, iodine, cobalt, zinc, copper, selenium, manganese, and chromium. They comprise less than 0.1% of the diet but facilitate metabolism, immune function, and wound healing. Zinc is vital for wound healing and 60% of its stores are found in muscle. During proteolysis zinc is mobilized and wasted in the urine. Patients who are acutely ill are susceptible to zinc deficiency presenting as diarrhea, CNS disturbances, eczematoid dermatitis, and alopecia. Chromium is a cofactor for insulin and its deficiency causes glucose intolerance and peripheral sensory neuropathy. Selenium is a component of the red blood cell enzyme glutathione peroxidase, which plays an important role in protecting the red blood cells from peroxidation of polyunsaturated fats. Chromium deficiency is rare, but skeletal and cardiomyopathies have been reported (Table 16-2).

Fluid and Electrolytes

The human body comprises approximately 60% water in men and 50% in women. Forty percent is intracellular and 20% is contained either within the vasculature as plasma (4.5%) or within the interstitium as lymphatic fluid (15.7%). Sodium and chloride account for the majority of serum osmoles in the plasma. Serum osmolality can be calculated using serum glucose, sodium, and urea values.

$$Serum\ osmolality = [2Na^+ + urea/2.8] + [glucose/18]$$

Sodium

Hyponatremia is defined as a serum sodium level of less than 130 mEq per L. Declining levels should be monitored cautiously if severe fluid shifts are expected, such as with shock, high-output enteric fistulas, or aggressive diuresis. When serum values fall to less than 120 mEq per L, patients are at high risk of neuropsychiatric symptoms, including lethargy, anorexia, vomiting, and decreased consciousness. When values decline below 110 mEq per L,

TABLE 16-1

VITAMINS

Vitamin	Function	Deficiency State
Fat Soluble		
A (retinol)	Rhodopsin synthesis	Xerophthalmia, keratomalacia
D (cholecalciferol)	Intestinal calcium absorption, bone remodeling	Rickets (children), osteomalacia (adults)
E (α-tocopherol)	Antioxidant	Hemolytic anemia, neurologic damage
K (naphthoquinone)	τ-Carboxylation of glutamate in clotting factors	Coagulopathy (deficiency in factors II, VII, IX, and X)
Water Soluble		
B_1 (thiamide)	Decarboxylation and aldehyde transfer reactions	Beriberi, neuropathy, fatigue, heart failure
B_2 (riboflavin)	Oxidation-reduction reactions	Dermatitis, glossitis
B_5 (niacin)	Oxidation-reduction reactions	Pellagra (dermatitis, diarrhea, dementia, death)
B_6 (pyridoxal phosphate)	Transamination and decarboxylation reactions	Neuropathy, glossitis, anemia
B_7 (biotin)	Carboxylation reactions	Dermatitis, alopecia
B_9 (folate)	DNA synthesis	Megaloblastic anemia, glossitis
B_{12} (cyanocobalamin)	DNA synthesis, myelination	Megaloblastic anemia, neuropathy
C (ascorbic acid)	Hydroxylation of hormones, hydroxylation of proline in collagen synthesis, antioxidant	Scurvy

TABLE 16-2
TRACE ELEMENTS

Trace Element	Function	Deficiency
Chromium	Promotes normal glucose utilization in combination with insulin	Glucose intolerance, peripheral neuropathy
Copper	Component of enzymes	Hypochromic microcytic anemia, neutropenia, bone demineralization, diarrhea
Fluorine	Essential for normal structure of bones and teeth	Caries
Iodine	Thyroid hormone production	Endemic goiter, hypothyroidism, myxedema, cretinism
Iron	Hemoglobin synthesis	Hypochromic microcytic anemia, glossitis, stomatitis
Manganese	Component of enzymes, essential for normal bone structure	Dermatitis, weight loss, nausea, vomiting, coagulopathy
Molybdenum	Component of enzymes	Neurologic abnormalities, night blindness
Selenium	Component of enzymes, antioxidant	Cardiomyopathy
Zinc	Component of enzymes involved in metabolism of lipids, proteins, carbohydrates, nucleic acids	Alopecia, hypogonadism, olfactory and gustatory dysfunction, impaired wound healing, acrodermatitis enteropathica, growth arrest

life-threatening seizures may ensue. A serum sodium level less than 130 mEq per L necessitates assessment and correction. The most common cause of hyponatremia is volume overload, although it can occur in a volume deficit or a euvolemic state as well. Hypotonic hyponatremia is associated with low plasma osmolality and can occur postoperatively or postinjury from excessive antidiuretic hormone (ADH) release. It is worsened by infusions of hyposmolar fluids. Hypertonic hyponatremia is caused by an abundance of solutes within the intravascular space resulting in large fluid shifts. This may occur with mannitol infusions or hyperglycemia. Isotonic hyponatremia is most commonly seen with the use of isotonic sodium-free solutions such as the irrigant used during a transurethral prostatectomy (TURP). *Pseudohyponatremia* is a falsely low serum sodium laboratory value caused by hyperglycemia or hyperlipidemia.

Serum and urine sodium levels are valuable in the assessment of hyponatremia. If the circulating volume is low and the urine sodium level is greater than 20 mEq per L, hyponatremia is typically caused by renal wasting caused by diuretic use or renal dysfunction. A urine sodium concentration less than 20 mEq per L suggests an extrarenal source of sodium loss, such as diarrhea, nasogastric suction, or enteric fistula. Hyponatremia and euvolemia are associated most commonly with syndrome of inappropriate antidiuretic hormone secretion (SIADH). Hypovolemic patients should be resuscitated with isotonic saline or lactated ringers, whereas those with hypervolemia or SIADH should be treated with fluid restriction. Rapid correction of hyponatremia may result in central pontine myelinolysis.

Hypernatremia occurs when a net negative water balance is sustained and the total body water content contracts, with a serum sodium concentration greater than 145 mEq per L. Symptoms include lethargy, weakness, and irritability. Major gastrointestinal losses or massive burns are frequent causes of hypovolemic hypernatremia. Sodium bicarbonate infusion or excessive exogenous sodium administration is the usual cause of hypervolemic hypernatremia. Finally, isovolemic hypernatremia may occur when hypotonic losses are replaced with isotonic solutions such as in TPN administration. It may also occur

with fever or head injury causing diabetes insipidus. Free water deficit can be calculated with the following equation.

Total Body Water (TBW) deficit
$$= 0.6W - [0.6W \times (140/P_{Na})]$$

W is weight in kilograms, 0.6 or 60% is the percentage of water in men, and 0.5 should be used for women. P_{Na} is the current serum sodium concentration and TBW is measured in liters. Aggressive correction of hypernatremia may result in cerebral edema, and, therefore, correction should be made slowly over 48 to 72 hours. The treatment for diabetes insipidus is the administration of intranasal or parenteral desmopressin (DDAVP).

Potassium

Potassium is the dominant intracellular cation and only 2% of total body potassium resides in the extracellular space. The Na^+–K^+ pump ensures the intracellular sequestration of potassium while extruding sodium into the extracellular compartment. It contributes significantly to maintaining homeostasis across cell membranes. The movement of potassium across cell membranes contributes to a vast number of physiologic reactions, such as axon depolarization. Although potassium balance is under renal regulation, small amounts are also excreted by the gastrointestinal tract. Increased excretion is stimulated by high plasma concentrations, alkalosis, ADH, aldosterone, and elevated sodium delivery to the distal renal tubules. Serum concentrations may vary with potassium flux across membranes as can occur with increasing insulin levels that drive glucose intracellularly. Alkalosis also drives potassium into the cell in exchange for proton ions.

Hypokalemia is defined as a serum potassium concentration of less than 3.3 mEq per L. It is frequently caused by excessive renal loss from aggressive diuretic administration. Extrarenal loss via the gastrointestinal tract, decreased oral intake, and certain medications may also lead to low serum concentrations. Mild hypokalemia is generally asymptomatic, but when the concentration falls below 3.0 mEq per L, muscle weakness, ileus, and alterations in cardiac conduction may result. Possible electrocardiographic (ECG) changes include T-wave depression, prominent U waves and prolongation of the QT interval. Oral formulations can be used to correct mild hypokalemia, unless oral repletion is contraindicated. Parenteral formulations can be administered safely at a rate of 10 to 20 mEq/L/h and should be used if severe or symptomatic hypokalemia is present. Hypomagnesemia antagonizes the correction of hypokalemia, which is remedied by magnesium repletion.

A potassium serum concentration in excess of 5.5 mEq per L defines hyperkalemia. Renal dysfunction is the most common etiology, but other common causes include crush injuries, cell lysis such as in rhabdomyolysis, reperfusion injury, adrenal insufficiency, and certain drugs including succinylcholine, β-receptor agonists, and digitalis. The most feared complication of hyperkalemia is cardiac arrhythmia, which occurs with severe hyperkalemia, especially when levels reach higher than 6.5 mEq per L. One of the early ECG changes is peaking of the T wave, which may forebode a life-threatening arrhythmia. Other possible ECG changes include prolongation of the QRS interval and deepening of the S wave into a sinusoidal pattern. Mild hyperkalemia can be treated with the combination of oral intake restriction and loop diuretics, such as furosemide. Severe hyperkalemia, especially in the presence of ECG changes, must be addressed urgently. Calcium gluconate infusion is frequently administered to stabilize the myocardial membrane. There are two methods of driving potassium intracellularly for an immediate, albeit temporary, solution. Sodium bicarbonate injection causes serum alkalization requiring cells to exchange intracellular proton ions for serum potassium. Intravenous insulin and glucose injection will also produce an intracellular shift. These methods do not permanently eliminate potassium, and therefore the administration of oral or rectal potassium binding resins is necessary to achieve excretion. The most rapid and definitive treatment is hemodialysis and may be initiated if hyperkalemia is life-threatening or in those patients with renal failure.

Calcium

Calcium is a divalent cation with significant roles in muscle contraction, coagulation, cell division, and renal tubular and neuron function. It is especially critical to cell-signaling mechanisms and often serves as a second messenger. It conveys and amplifies outside communication to the cell machinery and its nucleus. Approximately 99% of calcium resides within bone and its balance among bone exchange, intestinal absorption, and renal excretion is controlled by PTH and calcitonin. Forty-five percent of serum calcium exists in its biologically active, ionized form. Otherwise, it is bound to albumin and other plasma proteins. When assessing laboratory values of serum calcium it is important to note that most laboratories sum the ionized and plasma-bound fractions. Because a large fraction of serum calcium is bound to albumin, the assay is sensitive to albumin depletion. The ionized fraction is physiologically significant and is unchanged by fluctuations in the albumin concentration.

PTH is the main modulator of calcium homeostasis and is released from the parathyroid gland when serum concentrations of calcium decline. PTH increases serum calcium by three separate mechanisms involving bone resorption, renal reabsorption, and intestinal absorption. Bone resorption is accomplished by the PTH stimulation of osteoclast cells within bone. They dissolve bone and release calcium into the serum. In the kidney, PTH alters renal tubular function to increase reabsorption of filtered calcium. However, there is a reciprocal increase in renal phosphate excretion. Finally, PTH promotes conversion of vitamin D to its active form. 7-Dehydrocholesterol (provitamin D_3) obtained in the diet is converted to previtamin D_3 by ultraviolet (UV) light and into vitamin D_3 by a spontaneous reaction. Conversion into 1–25, dihydroxycholecalciferol occurs via several hydroxylation reactions within the liver and kidneys. Vitamin D contributes to osteoclast activation and renal calcium reabsorption, but it is the chief stimulus of enteric calcium absorption (Fig. 16-15).

Parathyroidectomy or thyroid surgery is the primary cause of hypocalcemia in the postsurgical population. This may occur because of bruising, unintentional excision of the parathyroid glands, or compromise of its blood supply during thyroidectomy, or because of atrophy in the remaining glands following resection of a parathyroid adenoma. The result is a precipitous drop in PTH level. Hypocalcemia can also occur after vitamin D deficiency secondary to malnutrition or malabsorption. Other causes of hypocalcemia include hypomagnesemia, which impairs PTH release and function, chronic renal failure, which can lead to a derangement of vitamin D metabolism, and pancreatitis caused by sequestration. Hypocalcemia manifests as hyperactivity of muscle contraction and reflexes, with muscle cramps and perioral tingling as early warning signs. If severe, tetany and/or ventricular arrhythmias may ensue. The Chvostek sign is a facial muscle spasm upon tapping of the facial nerve and Trousseau sign is carpal-pedal spasm after application of a blood pressure cuff on the limb. ECG changes demonstrate a prolonged QT interval and ST segment. If hypocalcemia is severe, immediate treatment with intravenous calcium gluconate is appropriate. In some circumstances long-term oral calcium/vitamin D supplementation is recommended.

Although the most common etiology of hypercalcemia is primary hyperparathyroidism, it is one of many causes. Another frequent etiology, especially in the hospital setting, is malignancy with associated metastatic disease or parathormone activity. Cancers associated with parathormone secretion are tumors of the lung, breast, thyroid, kidney, and parathyroid. Other causes include thiazide diuretics, multiple myeloma, Paget disease, hyperthyroidism, sudden immobilization, and sarcoidosis. Severe hypercalcemia occurs when serum levels rise greater than 12 mg per dL. Severe hypercalcemia can be associated with renal stones; polyuria; gastrointestinal symptoms that include nausea, vomiting, ileus, and pancreatitis; cardiovascular manifestations, such as hypotension, and shortened QT intervals on electrocardiography; and neurologic symptoms that include confusion and coma. If severe, hypercalcemia deserves immediate attention and treatment should aim to maximize renal excretion via normal saline infusion and loop diuretics. Calcitonin, a hormone involved in the inhibition of calcium resorption, has been used effectively in malignancy-induced hypercalcemia. Mithramycin may also be used on a long-term basis to treat those with malignancy to inhibit bone resorption.

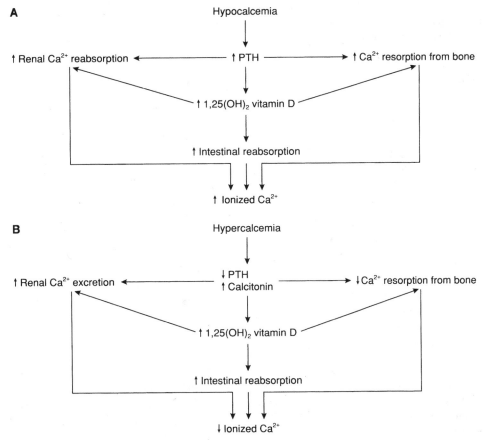

Figure 16-15 Physiologic compensatory effects of **(A)** hypocalcemia and **(B)** hypercalcemia. (From Wait RB, Kahng KU, Mustafa IA. Fluids, electrolytes and acid-base balance. In: Greenfield LJ, Mulholand MW, Oldham KT et al., eds. *Surgery: scientific principles and practice*, 3rd ed. Philadelphia: Lippincott Williams & Wilkins, 2001: 260, with permission.)

The treatment of hyperparathyroid-induced hypercalcemia is resection of the adenoma or tumor. Calcium regulation is discussed further in the endocrine section of the textbook (see Chapter 30).

Magnesium

Magnesium is second only to potassium as the most abundant intracellular cation. It often serves as a cofactor in enzymatic reactions and plays an important role in the activity of electrically excitable cells. In addition, magnesium facilitates the movement of calcium into muscle and thereby is pivotal to muscle contraction. Magnesium is absorbed in the small intestine and 50% is stored in bone reserves. It is renally excreted and is not under any known hormonal control.

Hypomagnesemia is caused by excessive renal loss, due to diuretic therapy, primary hyperaldosteronism, or renal dysfunction; gastrointestinal loss as seen in malabsorptive states; and nutrition deficiency, such as chronic alcoholism. The presentation of hypomagnesemia is similar to hypocalcemia in its manifestation of muscle weakness, spasm, and hyperreflexia. Widening of the QRS and prolongation of the QT interval may be evident on ECG findings. Mild deficiencies can be treated with oral supplementation but levels below 1 mEq per L should be repleted with intravenous magnesium sulfate at a rate no greater than 1 to 2 g per hour.

The primary cause of hypermagnesemia is renal failure and is otherwise extremely rare. Other causes of hypermagnesemia include severe crush injury, rhabdomyolysis, and severe dehydration and metabolic acidosis. Depression of deep tendon reflexes and neuromuscular activity may occur with severe hypermagnesemia, and may progress to paralysis, coma, and cardiac arrhythmia. Sinus bradycardia and prolongation of the PR, QRS, and QT intervals may be seen. Treatment includes the infusion of normal saline in combination with a loop diuretic. The infusion of calcium gluconate may play a role in antagonizing arrhythmic side-effects. However, hemodialysis may be necessary to rapidly lower the serum concentration.

Phosphorus

The organic form of phosphorus contributes significantly to many important metabolic intermediates, such as the energy molecule ATP. Its inorganic form, representing 85% of its stores, resides in the bone, contributing strength and structure. Hypophosphatemia can be the result of gastrointestinal loss, excessive renal excretion, or intracellular electrolyte shifts. It is usually clinically silent but could potentially cause skeletal and cardiac muscle weakness resulting in weak respiratory effort and decreased cardiac output. If the deficiency is mild, oral replacement is sufficient. Intravenous replacement is reserved for severe deficiencies, especially with the previously noted symptoms, or if oral replacement is contraindicated. Hyperphosphatemia is exceedingly rare outside of renal failure but may be caused by severe cell lysis from tumor or rhabdomyolysis. If mild, sucralfate or aluminum-containing antacids can be used as binders. If severe, or in the case of renal failure, hemodialysis is necessary.

Metabolism in Starvation

The physiology of starvation is an evolutionary defense strategy developed for the purpose of survival in times of famine. Unfortunately, this condition is a frequent necessity while treating patients in the surgical population, both pre- and postoperatively. It may be necessary to withhold oral intake in preparation for an operation or a diagnostic study or patients may have nutritional deficits secondary to poor oral intake because of illness or therapy. Nutritional support in this subset of patients has increasingly become a priority.

It is vital that adequate serum glucose concentration be maintained, as various tissues such as brain and red blood cells depend on glucose. After approximately 24 hours of starvation, liver glycogen stores are depleted and gluconeogenesis occurs. As glucose levels begin to fall, insulin follows suit and thereby withdraws the stimulus for protein and lipid synthesis. This fall in serum insulin coupled with a rise in the glucagon level results in triglyceride breakdown. The glycerol backbone and the amino acid products of proteolysis become the substrates for hepatic gluconeogenesis. The fatty acid molecules cannot be used as substrate, but their energy rich stores provide fuel for the process.

Proteolysis is dominant in early starvation, with urinary nitrogen losses between 8 and 12 g per day. The urinary losses are equivalent to 340 g of tissue per day. The body must quickly adapt to retard proteolysis and conserve protein, or patient survival would not last beyond a month. When this goal of adaptation is achieved, an unstressed chronically starved patient may survive several additional months. This adaptation involves the increased utilization of fatty acid molecules as a fuel source by peripheral tissues.

In addition, the brain is able to alter its preference for glucose to that of ketone bodies. Therefore, the need for gluconeogenesis and its required proteolytic substrates is reduced and a more efficient use of fat-derived energy is achieved.

Metabolism in Stress/Injury/Sepsis

The physiologic response to starvation in times of stress or injury is maladaptive. The ability of the body to adapt and temporarily overcome the obstacles of simple starvation is overwhelmed by the neuroendocrine-mediated inflammatory response.

The altered metabolism of starvation under stress is a two-phase process. During the initial hours immediately following injury, energy expenditure is either normal or decreased and hyperglycemia is prominent as the restoration of tissue perfusion ensues. These events characterize the *ebb phase*. The next phase can last from days to weeks and is characterized by hypermetabolism, negative nitrogen balance, glucose intolerance, and lipolysis. It is called the *flow phase* and was later separated into subdivisions comprising a prolonged catabolic phase, despite correction of the underlying injury, and an anabolic phase with eventual restoration of normal physiology (Fig. 16-16).

Unlike starvation without stress, starvation after injury results in dramatic increases of the basal metabolic rate in an attempt to mount an inflammatory/stress response and heal wounds. The most exaggerated response is seen after thermal burn injuries. This hypermetabolic response is catecholamine induced and mediated by sympathetic nerve discharge.

The maladaptive stress response is largely mediated by neuroendocrine mechanisms. Rising levels of adrenocorticotropic hormone, cortisol, catecholamines, glucagon, and growth hormone all contribute to a state of hyperglycemia with peripheral glucose intolerance, despite elevated serum insulin. Glucagon is chiefly responsible for driving ongoing hepatic gluconeogenesis, while peripheral intolerance is strongly enhanced by cortisol and catecholamines. The brain and peripheral tissues fail to "ketoadapt" and continue their preference for glucose. Therefore, demand for

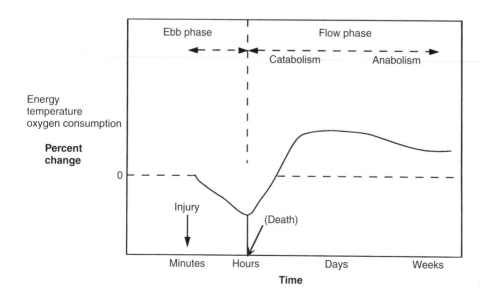

Figure 16-16 Metabolism following injury. (From Schwartz SI, Shires GT, Spencer FC, eds. *Principles of surgery*, 7th ed. New York: McGraw Hill, 1994:27, with permission.)

glucose remains high and the only supply is through breakdown of valuable and functional protein molecules.

The derangement in glucose metabolism is not the only force behind increasing proteolysis and its corresponding nitrogen loss. Amino acids are required by the liver for synthesis of inflammatory molecules and acute phase reactants involved in the clotting cascade, coagulation, and opsonization. The bone marrow also demands substrate for production of hematopoietic cells needed for mounting immunity and healing wounds. In addition, the protein-sparing effect of glucose administration is lost. Because of the inefficient utilization of structural and visceral protein for energy substrates and protein synthesis, exogenous protein requirements may increase by up to threefold.

Fat metabolism is accelerated by the sympathetic nervous system in times of stress or injury. Although lipolysis increases substantially, free plasma levels remain normal demonstrating their massive consumption by the tissues. Unlike simple starvation, ketone production decreases. This is probably because of the elevation of molecules inhibitory to ketogenesis, including insulin, glucagons, glucose, alanine, and lactate.

Burns

The state of hypermetabolism is both pronounced and prolonged after severe thermal injury. The oxygen consumption and metabolic rate increase in proportion to the surface area of the burn, and can rise as high as 100% to 200% greater than normal. As discussed previously, neuroendocrine influences drive the antagonistic metabolism that results in carbohydrate intolerance, protein wasting, and the inflammatory response. This process proceeds until complete closure of the wounds has been accomplished. Without proper nutritional support, organ function and wound healing are impaired. The optimal formulation contains 1 to 2 g/kg/d of protein to augment protein-sparing and provide synthetic precursors.

A common method of calculating the elevated energy requirement has been to use the Harris-Benedict equation and multiply it by 2.0 for burns covering 40% of the total body surface area. Studies measuring BEE by using indirect calorimetry suggest that this calculation is an overestimate. By multiplying the BEE by 1.4 instead of 2.0, a more accurate estimate may be obtained.

Cancer

Patients with neoplastic disease experience weight loss and cachexia for many reasons. The interference of cerebral satiety centers by tumor products, mechanical obstruction of the gastrointestinal tract, and chemotherapy-induced nausea are several examples. Nutritional support research in cancer patients during the last 20 years suggests that supplemental nutrition may be detrimental in some groups of patients. Laboratory evidence implies a relationship between the provision of supplemental protein and calories with accelerated tumor growth. Biologic variability in the cancer patient population is diverse and comparative studies are difficult to interpret. However, benefit has been demonstrated in at least one subset of patients receiving

preoperative support. Randomized prospective trials have shown a survival advantage, as well as a diminished complication rate, in severely malnourished patients with upper gastrointestinal tumors who are undergoing operative therapy. Finally, recent trials present evidence in support of using enteral nutrition with immunologically active solutions (e.g., arginine and omega-3) postoperatively, in patients undergoing large gastrointestinal operations.

NUTRITIONAL SUPPORT

Routes of Administration

Nutritional support is administered either enterally, parenterally or in combination. Total enteral nutrition (TEN) is delivered into the stomach or the jejunum. This method does not bypass the liver and allows hepatic processing of nutrients before entrance into the systemic circulation. In several recent prospective, randomized studies TEN has been associated with decreased mortality and septic complications as compared to TPN. Although the mechanism is unclear, nutritional support via enteral access when compared to parenteral feedings appears to result in better outcomes, especially in posttraumatic patients. One hypothesis supported by animal studies is that TEN may improve the integrity of the gut mucosal barrier and therefore decrease the rate of bacterial translocation. For these reasons, enteral access is the preferred route of nutritional support.

Long-term enteral access can be achieved via a gastrostomy tube or a jejunostomy tube. The gastrostomy tube is generally placed percutaneously into the stomach by interventional radiology or by using endoscopic guidance, but it can also be placed in an open fashion. It should be reserved for patients with a low aspiration risk and a competent lower esophageal sphincter. In patients who are more susceptible to aspiration, enteral access should be obtained distal to the ligament of Treitz. The jejunostomy tube is sewn into the jejunum about 20 to 30 cm distal to the ligament of Treitz with the Witzel technique. Although the position of the tube may help to prevent aspiration, potential complications may still develop including bowel obstruction, volvulus, perforation, and ischemia.

Parenteral Nutrition

Parenteral nutrition is recommended when the gut cannot be used safely. Although less physiologic than oral or enteral feeding, nutrition can be delivered parenterally and provide optimal support. TPN is also used to supplement enteral nutrition when TEN is poorly tolerated. When compared to enteral feeding, TPN is associated with a higher rate of morbidity and mortality, probably because of potential sepsis-related complications, and is much more expensive then TEN.

With central TPN, venous access can be obtained by using a percutaneous or an open technique through the axilla. The tip usually terminates in the superior vena cava. The catheters may be temporary or long-term indwelling lines, such as the Broviac or Hickman catheters. Two possible life-threatening complications include line-related sepsis and pneumothorax.

KEY POINTS

▲ *Starvation During Injury:* The response to starvation in times of stress or injury is maladaptive. It is characterized by hypermetabolism, negative nitrogen balance, glucose intolerance, and lipolysis, fueled by adrenocorticoids, catecholamines, and glucagon. The protein-sparing effect of glucose administration is lost and tissues fail to ketoadapt, resulting in ongoing proteolysis. A prolonged catabolic phase occurs, despite correction of the underlying injury, and an anabolic phase follows with eventual restoration.

▲ *Gastric Acid Secretion:* Acid is secreted by parietal cells via the hydrogen–potassium pump (H^+–K^+ pump). The three acid secretogogues are acetylcholine, gastrin, and histamine, which bind to their respective receptors and function synergistically through a G-protein coupled pathway. Acetylcholine and gastrin also act indirectly via histamine release from enterochromaffin-like (ECL) cells in the lamina propria.

▲ The Harris-Benedict equation estimates basal energy expenditure (BEE).

BEE (women) = $655 + (9.6W) + (1.8H) - (4.7A)$
BEE (men) = $66 + (13.7W) + (5H) - (6.8A)$

▲ The TEE (total energy expenditure) can be calculated by multiplying an activity factor of 1.3 for hospitalized patients and 1.5 for outpatients.

▲ *Nutrient Oxidation Energy:* The protein requirement for the average healthy adult is approximately 0.8 g/kg/d with 19% to 20% of consumed protein as essential amino acids. Each gram yields 4 kcal. The oxidation of glucose yields approximately 3.4 kcal per g. Lipids are essential nutrients that provide the most efficient energy reserve, and their oxidation yields 9 kcal.

▲ *Vitamin B_{12} Metabolism:* Vitamin B_{12} reaches the stomach bound to ingested protein. It is released when the protein is denatured in the acidic environment and binds to the salivary gland product, haptocorrin (R protein.) Haptocorrin protects vitamin B_{12} until it is degraded by pancreatic proteases and releases cobalamin. Finally, Vitamin B_{12} binds to intrinsic factor and is absorbed by the terminal ileum as a complex.

▲ *Pancreatic Protein Digestion:* The duodenal mucosal enzyme enterokinase cleaves trypsinogen to produce its catalytic form trypsin, which activates the other zymogens. Cholecystokinin (CCK) is produced by neuroendocrine cells in the duodenum in response to lipids, peptones, and amino acids and augments protein secretion from the acinar cells. CCK receptor and the muscarinic cholinergic receptor activation result in calcium-mediated upregulation of protein manufacture.

SUGGESTED READINGS

Boron WF, Boulpaep EL, eds. *Medical physiology: a cellular and molecular approach,* 1st ed. Philadelphia: WB Saunders, 2003.

Burke DJ, Alverdy JC, Aoys E, et al. Glutamine-supplemented total parenteral nutrition improves gut function. *Arch Surg* 1989;124: 1396–1399.

Carney DE, Meguild MM. Current concepts in nutritional assessment. *Arch Surg* 2002;137:42–45.

DeWitt RC, Wu Y, Renegar KB, et al. Bombesin recovers gut-associated lymphoid tissue (GALT) and preserves immunity to bacterial pneumonia in TPN-fed mice. *Ann Surg* 2000;231:1–8.

Li J, Kudsk KA, Janu P, et al. Effect of glutamine-enriched TPN on small intestine gut-associated lymphoid tissue (GALT) and upper respiratory tract immunity. *Surgery* 1997;121:542–549.

Townsend CM, Beauchamp DR, Evers MB et al., eds. *Sabiston textbook of surgery: the biological basis of modern surgical practice,* 16th ed. Philadelphia: WB Saunders, 2001.

Trauma Evaluation and Resuscitation, Shock, and Acid–Base Disturbances

17

Benjamin M. Jackson   Stephen C. Gale   C. William Schwab

EVALUATION AND RESUSCITATION OF THE TRAUMA PATIENT

Background

Injuries comprise the leading cause of death in persons ages 1 to 34 years. As a consequence, trauma constitutes the leading cause of loss of potential, unrealized life. Following traumatic injury there is a trimodal distribution in fatalities. Fifty percent of all deaths due to trauma occur in minutes; 30% occur in hours; and 20% occur in days to weeks later. In general, little can be done to treat those who die within minutes of injury: these patients die from aortic rupture or devastating central nervous system (CNS) injury resulting in cardiovascular and respiratory collapse. It was the aim of the Advanced Trauma Life Support (ATLS) program, at the outset, to reduce the mortality of those patients who would die in hours to days.

Salvage of the critically injured is optimized by a coordinated team effort in an organized trauma system. Management of life-threatening injuries must be initiated according to physiologic necessity for survival; that is, active efforts to support airway, breathing, and circulation (the ABCs) are usually initiated before a specific diagnosis is established.

Organizational Aspects

Evaluation and resuscitation of trauma patients begin at the scene of the injury. However, the goal in trauma is to get the right patient to the right hospital at the right time. When possible, critically injured patients should be taken directly to a designated level I facility (Regional Resource Trauma Center) or to a level II facility (a Regional Trauma Center).

The trauma team is composed of a variety of members with a range of backgrounds. The surgical staff, including the attending trauma surgeon, is responsible for the evaluation and resuscitation of, and any operations performed on trauma patients. The emergency department staff, including the attending emergency physician, performs an important role in supporting the trauma patient and in assisting the surgical staff. In many trauma centers the emergency staff is responsible for initial airway management until the need for a surgical airway is established. In addition, radiologists, neurosurgeons, orthopedists, and anesthesiologists are important adjuncts to the primary trauma team.

The ubiquitous use of universal or standard precautions must be stressed. All personnel in the trauma bay should use goggles, gloves, fluid-impervious gowns, shoe covers and impervious leggings, masks, and head coverings. In addition, all members of the trauma team should be immunized against hepatitis B.

Primary Survey and Initial Resuscitation

Upon the trauma patient's arrival to the emergency department, the protocols set forth in the ATLS program are initiated. The goal of evaluation and therapy is to establish adequate oxygen delivery to vital organs. To this end, adherence to the "ABCDE" acronym (airway, breathing, circulation, disability, exposure) is suggested. During procession through this algorithm, *life-threatening problems are treated as they are discovered*. For example, recognition of a tension pneumothorax during the evaluation of *Breathing* requires immediate tube or needle thoracostomy.

Airway control is essential to oxygenation of blood and therefore to the maintenance of adequate oxygen supply to tissues. Primary respiratory failure is most often caused by airway obstruction in the injured patient. Assessment of the airway in a responsive patient can often be accomplished by asking a simple question, such as, "How are you?" or, "What happened?" A garbled, hoarse, or inaudible response suggests airway compromise. In blunt trauma, efforts to gain control of the airway should proceed under the assumption that cervical spine fracture exists; movement of the neck should therefore be avoided. The upper airway is cleared of debris and suctioned. Supplemental oxygen is applied. In the patient with decreased alertness, pharyngeal obstruction by the tongue can be alleviated by elevating the angle of the mandible or by use of an oropharyngeal or nasopharyngeal airway. Bag-mask ventilation can be a useful means of temporarily ventilating and oxygenating the patient, but may result in air insufflation into the stomach, may be resisted by the awake patient, and is ineffective in the patient with significant maxillofacial injuries. In the patient with evidence of airway compromise or with diminished alertness, the decision should be made quickly to obtain a definitive airway (an endotracheal tube with its cuff inflated): orotracheal intubation (preferred), nasotracheal intubation (occasionally), cricothyroidotomy (uncommonly) (Fig. 17-1), or tracheostomy (rarely) are the usual procedures of choice. This decision is based on clinical evaluation of the patient; there is not usually time to obtain an arterial blood gas. Patients with expanding neck hematomas, deteriorating vital signs, evidence of severe head trauma, or a Glasgow coma score of less than 8 should generally be managed with a definitive airway. Rapid sequence orotracheal intubation with in-line immobilization of the cervical spine is the standard approach.

Breathing is assessed after the airway is secured; airway patency does not ensure adequate oxygenation and ventilation. Observation, percussion, palpation, and auscultation are the requirements of the chest physical examination. Poor air exchange at the mouth and nose, decreased breath sounds, and diminished chest wall excursion are signs of hypoventilation; head injury, cervical spinal cord transection, pneumothorax, flail chest, and profound shock are the most likely etiologies. In the unstable patient, the response to any

physical findings suggestive of hemothorax or pneumothorax, including absent breath sounds unilaterally, should be immediate placement of a large-bore chest tube.

Tension pneumothorax, simple and open (or "sucking chest wound") pneumothorax, flail chest, and hemothorax are all entities that can result in dramatic compromise to breathing in the trauma patient necessitating emergent intervention. The pathophysiology and management of these conditions are discussed in greater detail in the section on thoracic trauma in Chapter 18, "Traumatic Injuries."

Circulation should be evaluated next. Heart rate; blood pressure; and the presence of femoral, carotid, and brachial or radial pulses should all be interrogated. Generally, the carotid pulse is palpable at a systolic blood pressure of 60 mm Hg, the femoral pulse is palpable at 70 mm Hg, and the radial pulse is palpable at 80 mm Hg. Any immediately life-threatening problems must be identified and treated. The primary objective of the treatment of shock in the trauma patient should be identifying and controlling hemorrhage, followed by restoration of blood volume with fluid and blood resuscitation. Time to control of bleeding has been identified as the most important prognostic indicator in the patient with hemorrhagic shock.

Exsanguination can occur into the thoracic cavity, the peritoneum, the retroperitoneum (abdominal great vessels or massive pelvic fracture), a groin or thigh, or from open wounds. Other conditions can also cause hemodynamic collapse, including tension pneumothorax and pericardial tamponade, as discussed in the preceding text. Cardiac tamponade occurs as a result of cardiac rupture from blunt injury or penetrating injury traversing the pericardium; the condition classically presents as unexplained shock and occasionally results in Beck triad: hypotension, distended neck veins, and distant heart sounds.

Hypotension is most likely caused by hemorrhage in the injured patient; therefore, large-bore intravenous catheters should be placed in the bilateral antecubital fossae, and crystalloid infusion initiated. Alternative means of intravenous access include saphenous vein cutdown at the medial ankle anterior to the medial malleolus, femoral or subclavian vein cannulation via the Seldinger technique, or intraosseous access to the medullary cavity of the tibia in children age 6 years and younger. All intravenous catheters should be short and large bore (the internal diameter determines flow). With initial venous access, blood samples for blood typing, screening, and cross-matching, coagulation profile, hematocrit, white blood cell count, amylase, electrolytes, and toxicology should be obtained. The choice of fluid for resuscitation is discussed in the subsequent text, as is the classification and grading of hemorrhagic shock.

All sources of external bleeding must be controlled. Bleeding arteries should be treated with direct digital pressure. If this measure fails to control the hemorrhage, manual pressure at the nearest proximal location of normally palpable pulses should be attempted. In the rare occasion that these two maneuvers fail to control bleeding from an extremity, a tourniquet may be applied to the proximal edge of the wound; the time of application must be recorded. Control of bleeding in deep wounds by means of surgical clamps should be avoided in order to avoid damage to vessels and nerves. Bleeding from the scalp can be profuse and is often initially unrecognized. It is best initially treated with direct suturing of the bleeding site,

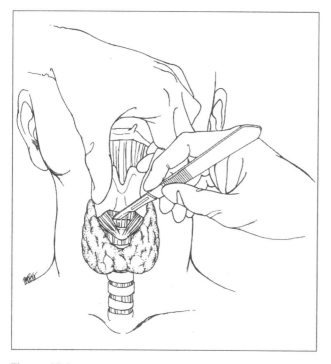

Figure 17-1 Technique of cricothyroidotomy. (From ACS Surgery section 5 chapter 1.)

skin staples applied to the laceration, or with neurosurgical (Rainey) scalp clips.

In the case of life-threatening hypotension from pericardial tamponade in the patient with either blunt or penetrating chest trauma, consideration should be given to left anterior thoracotomy to enable direct drainage of the pericardial sac, inspection, and repair of any cardiac wound. Left thoracotomy has the added advantage of allowing access to the descending thoracic aorta for temporary aortic tamponade and control of exsanguinating intraabdominal bleeding. Suspected pericardial tamponade can usually be diagnosed by ultrasonography (FAST, focused abdominal ultrasonography for trauma, discussed in subsequent text) or occasionally by needle pericardiocentesis via the subxiphoid approach.

Myocardial contusion should be suspected in any victim of blunt trauma with unexplained hemodynamic instability or arrhythmia. Definitive diagnosis is difficult, given the nonspecificity of electrocardiographic (ECG) findings. In all patients with suspected myocardial contusion, acidosis should be corrected, hypoxia treated, electrolyte abnormalities addressed, and arrhythmias treated pharmacologically.

If major pelvic fracture is suspected as a cause of hypotension—that is, in patients who have sustained injury in auto-pedestrian, motor vehicle, or motorcycle crashes; or falls from heights—mechanical stability of the pelvic ring should be tested by downward anterior and bilateral inward compression, and an anteroposterior pelvic radiograph should be obtained. If pelvic instability is confirmed, measures to splint the unstable pelvic fracture and close the internal pelvic volume should be undertaken. Application of a sheet wrapped around the pelvis, use of a pneumatic anti-shock garment, or placement of a temporary external compression device (TPOD) are all effective and accepted strategies. If the patient's hemodynamic status does not stabilize with such measures and with resuscitation, and if no other sources of hemorrhage (in the setting of negative chest radiograph and negative diagnostic peritoneal lavage or FAST) are identified on primary and secondary surveys, the patient should undergo angiography and embolization to diagnose and treat ongoing bleeding from the pelvic arterial plexus.

Intravenous fluid therapy should be initiated immediately upon presentation of the trauma patient. The crystalloid solution of choice is warmed Ringer lactate (Table 17-1). Continued administration of electrolyte compositions alone in the patient with massive bleeding may result in increased blood loss from dilution of coagulation proteins and platelets. After crystalloid infusion of 2 to 3 L for the adult male, blood products should be administered if blood pressure and pulse do not trend toward normal. In most cases, type-specific blood can be available within 20 to 30 minutes after the patient's arrival; if blood is needed more urgently, type O-negative packed red blood cells should be administered. Acidosis associated with hypovolemic shock should be treated with volume resuscitation and blood products: administration of steroids, vasopressors, or sodium bicarbonate is usually not indicated in hypovolemic shock. Patients who require early administration of blood usually need immediate operative or angiographic control of hemorrhage.

Disability or neurologic evaluation should proceed expeditiously with the aim of establishing the patient's level of consciousness. This assessment provides the opportunity to revisit the potential need for intubation: an altered level of consciousness can alert the examiner to defects in oxygenation, ventilation, or cerebral perfusion. If hypoxia and hypotension are excluded, altered mental status should be attributed to CNS injury until proven otherwise. The Glasgow coma scale (Table 17-1) is a simple neurologic assessment that is predictive of the need for certain therapies (e.g., GCS ≤8 and intubation) and predictive of patient outcome. Patients should also be asked to move the lower extremities, especially to dorsiflex and plantarflex the foot to rule out spinal cord injury.

Exposure and *environmental control* are accomplished by cutting away all of the patient's clothing, examining the patient's back by means of log roll with cervical spine immobilization, and covering the patient with warm blankets or a warming device to prevent hypothermia. In addition, all intravenous fluids should also be warmed to between 37°C and 40°C prior to infusion. Exposure is necessary to accomplish the full head-to-toe physical examination comprising the secondary survey. However, all means to warm the hypothermic patient are necessary to prevent acidosis, arrhythmias, and coagulopathy.

Adjuncts to Primary Survey

Continuous ECG monitoring, is useful in the trauma bay, as it provides a continuous readout of heart rate and rhythm. Automated plesthmography allows intermittent blood pressure measurement. Pulse oximetry is a valuable adjunct to vital sign measurement. Temperature is a key physiologic determinant and any hypothermia calls for rapid treatment. Arterial blood gas measurement may provide useful information early in the process of resuscitation.

Placement of a urinary catheter should be considered upon completion of the primary survey because urinary output is a sensitive indicator of renal perfusion or genitourinary injury. Examination of the rectum and genitalia should be undertaken prior to transurethral catheterization, which is contraindicated in patients with urethral injury. Urethral injury is suspected on the basis of (i) blood at the urethral meatus, (ii) perineal ecchymosis, (iii) blood in the scrotum, (iv) a high-riding or nonpalpable prostate, or (v) a pelvic fracture. If urethral injury is suspected, retrograde urethrogram should be performed prior to catheterization; alternatively, suprapubic bladder catheterization may be performed.

Gastric catheterization should be considered following the primary survey: decompression of the stomach reduces the risk of aspiration. However, if fracture of the anterior

TABLE 17-1

RINGER LACTATE SOLUTION COMPOSITION

	(1 L)
Sodium	130 mEq
Chloride	109 mEq
Calcium	3 mEq
Potassium	4 mEq
Lactate	28 mEq

skull, skull base, or midface is suspected, any gastric tube must be inserted orally to prevent passage of the catheter intracranially. In addition, insertion of a nasogastric tube may induce emesis, causing the very problem its placement is intended to prevent.

The chest x-ray [anteroposterior (AP), supine] is of considerable utility early in the evaluation of the trauma patient. This film may reveal life-threatening injuries requiring immediate therapy or further diagnostic study, such as pneumothorax, hemothorax, or a widened mediastinum suggestive of aortic rupture.

Cervical spine assessment is integral to developing an airway management plan and in evaluating for potential spinal cord injury. (The majority of significant spinal cord injuries in adults arriving to the emergency department are at the C5 to C7 levels; in children the most frequent location of spinal cord injury is in the region between the occiput and C3.) A good-quality cross-table lateral cervical spine film will reveal only approximately 80% of unstable fractures in the adult; three-view plain films (cross-table lateral, AP, and open mouth odontoid) will reveal approximately about 90%. Fine-cut computerized tomographic (CT) scan of the entire cervical spine has become the standard because of its accuracy.

An AP pelvic film may assist in evaluating the trauma patient by identifying a pelvic fracture causing pelvic hemorrhage, identifying or confirming a hip dislocation, or visualizing a retained foreign body (bullet). In general, stable awake patients without pelvic or hip injury symptoms do not need a pelvic x-ray if they are going to have an abdominal-pelvic CT scan.

Two studies directed at identifying intraperitoneal hemorrhage are considered at this stage in evaluation of the patient. Diagnostic peritoneal lavage (DPL) can be performed in either a percutaneous or open fashion. Aspiration of gross blood on placement of the catheter constitutes a positive result and mandates surgical exploration. Second, 10 mL per kg of body weight warmed crystalloid is instilled into the peritoneum and allowed to remain for 5 to 10 minutes. It is then drained by gravity: either a red blood cell concentration greater than 10^5 per mm^3 or a white blood cell count greater than 500 per mm^3 indicates the need for exploration. Alternatively, abdominal ultrasonography or FAST can be performed to assess for intraperitoneal hemorrhage; FAST also can be used to identify pericardial tamponade. Four anatomic windows are generally examined: the pericardium (subxiphoid), the hepatorenal fossa, the splenorenal fossa, and the pelvis. A positive FAST in the unstable patient mandates operative exploration; in the stable patient, contrast-enhanced abdominal and pelvic CT scan is obtained following a positive FAST.

Patient Transfer

At the completion of the primary survey, the attending physician often has sufficient information to indicate the need for transfer to another facility. This situation is typified by circumstances requiring definitive care from a speciality center (pediatric burn, spinal cord, or a level I trauma center). In particular, injuries should not be managed expectantly, thus patients may require definitive care in a different setting; for example, solid visceral injury from blunt abdominal trauma should not be managed conservatively at a hospital without 24-hour operating room capabilities. Once the need for transfer is identified, transfer should not be delayed for any further diagnositic study that will not change the immediate plan of care. All records and x-rays should be sent with the patient to the receiving facility.

Secondary Survey

The secondary survey should be a complete head-to-toe physical examination including reevaluation of the ABC and D's evaluated in the primary survey. It should also include an in-depth medical history and details of the mechanism of injury. The mnemonic AMPLE—for allergies, medications, past illnesses and surgeries, last meal, and events related to the injury—provides an algorithm for acquisition of the early key elements of a history. Key elements and possible pitfalls of the physical examination are discussed herein; an expanded discussion of the diagnosis and management of particular injuries is presented in Chapter 18.

Description of the mechanism of injury (MOI) may lead the trauma surgeon to suspect particular patterns of injury. For example, a pedestrian hit by an automobile will frequently sustain injuries to the lower extremeties and torso. An unrestrained driver in a front-impact collision should be suspected of having blunt cardiac injury. High-speed deceleration injuries, either in automobiles or falls, predispose the patient to aortic injury. Patients undergoing a fall from height, ejection from a vehicle, crush injury, or cervical spine fracture should be suspected of having thoracic or lumbar spine injuries and should be evaluated comprehensively for such.

The *head* is examined first. The eyes are examined for direct trauma, foreign bodies, visual acuity, and pupillary size and reactions. Bruising behind the ears (Battle sign) or around the eyes (raccoon eyes), hemotympanum, and drainage of cerebrospinal fluid (CSF) from the nose or ears are all suggestive of basilar skull fracture.

The *neck* is examined after removal of the cervical collar, with in-line stabilization. The cervical spine can be cleared clinically only in those patients who are awake and alert and without eveidence of intoxication or distracting injuries. In a patient who does not meet these criteria, or who has any cervical spine tenderness, muscle spasm, or radicular signs or symptoms, three-view radiographs of the cervical spine should be obtained. Pitfalls here include failure to image completely from C1 to T1 on the lateral film and failure to obtain an open-mouth odontoid view. Neck wounds are difficult to assess and manage because of the vital repiratory, vascular, and digestive structures in this region. Wounds to zone II of the neck, from the cricoid cartilage inferiorly to the angle of the mandible superiorly (Fig. 17-2), may be managed by operative exploration or assessed with a combination of angiography, esophagoscopy, and bronchoscopy. Wounds to zones I (from the suprasternal notch to the cricoid cartilage) and zone III (from the angle of the mandible to the base of the skull) are best managed initially by endoscopy and angiography (with possible embolization), not operative exploration, given the possiblity of damage to intrathoracic and mediastinal structures in the former case, and the difficulty of operative access and exploration in the latter (see Chapter 18).

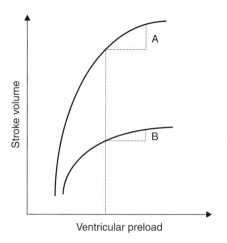

Figure 17-2 Frank-Starling relationship, in a normal heart **(A)** and in a failing heart **(B)**. Note that in heart failure, there is limited capacity for recruitment of cardiac function by increasing preload. (From The Critical Care Forum, *www.ccforum.com*.)

The *chest* examination is repeated, and if not yet performed, a portable AP chest radiograph should be obtained. Patients who sustain blunt trauma, especially if subjected to high-speed deceleration injury, and found to have a widened mediastinum, pleural cap, leftward tracheal deviation, elevation of the left mainstem bronchus, or left-sided hemothorax should be evaluated for aortic transection. In addition, 7% of patients with aortic injury have a normal chest radiograph; therefore, if the history and mechanism of injury are suggestive of possible aortic injury, diagnostic steps should be undertaken. Contrast chest CT scan is the study most often used to evaluate the widened mediastinum; in the unstable patient, the patient already in the operating room, or the patient with elevated serum creatinine, transesophageal echocardiogram (TEE) is an excellent alternate to screen for aortic injury. Contrast aortography is the gold-standard for detection of thoracic aortic injury and should be performed in the case that a CT or TEE is equivocable.

The *abdomen* and *back* are examined, with special attention to penetrating wounds. In the unstable patient with a penetrating abdominal wound, emergent exploratory laparotomy is indicated. In the stable patient with a stab wound to the anterior abdominal wall, local wound exploration is performed; if the anterior fascia is violated, exploration in the operating room is mandated. In the case of a stab wound to the back or flank, contrast-enhanced CT scan is used to identify retroperitoneal and intraperitoneal injuries. In any patient with localized tenderness over the thoracic or lumbar spines, AP and lateral radiographs of the thoracic and lumbar spine should be obtained.

The *pelvis* and *perineum* are evaluated next. The stability of the pelvic ring is assessed by medial and anteroposterior compression, or—if questionable—by AP pelvic radiograph. Rectal tone is assessed to evaluate for spinal cord injury and the position of the prostate in males. In females, the vagina and genitalia are examined.

All four *extremities* should be examined for deformity, bruising, lacerations, penetrating injuries, soft tissue injury, peripheral pulses, and neurologic function. External bleeding must be addressed if not adequately treated during the primary survey and resuscitation. Femur fractures—in particular—can be characterized by significant internal bleeding; application of traction or immobilization splints should be undertaken expediently. Compartment syndrome must be recognized early. Etiologic factors include soft tissue injury, hematomas, fractures, arterial injuries, and massive fluid resuscitation. Consequences of compartment syndrome include muscle necrosis, myoglobinuria, renal failure, and limb loss. Signs and symptoms of increased interstitial tissue pressure and decreased tissue perfusion include pain (especially with passive motion), paresthesias, palpably swollen tense extremity, paresis or paralysis, and, very late, diminution of peripheral pulses. Compartment pressures can be measured using a needle inserted into the compartment of concern; a pressure greater than 25 mm Hg associated with clinical suspicion of decreased tissue perfusion should prompt emergent fasciotomy. Clear cases of vascular injury—with pulsatile bleeding, expanding hematoma, regional ischemia, or absent pulses—should undergo operative exploration and repair, without delay for further diagnostic studies; intraoperative angiography may be performed prior to or following repair in any case. In less obvious circumstances, angiography or duplex ultrasonography should be used to detect any arterial injury.

A complete *neurologic* examination should be completed in all cases. All 12 cranial nerves should be evaluated. Spinal cord and peripheral nerve function are determined with both proximal and distal sensory and motor examinations of all extremities. Patients with spinal cord injury detected within 8 hours are treated with methylprednisolone: 30 mg per kg bolus followed by 5.4 mg/kg/h continuous infusion for 23 hours is required if started within 3 hours of injury. Longer duration is recommended if begun more than 3 hours after injury. All traumatic CNS injuries should be evaluated by the neurosurgical team. These injuries and their treatment have been discussed in Chapter 1, "Neurosurgery."

Emergency Department Thoracotomy

Resuscitative thoracotomy or emergency department (ED) thoracotomy is a technique of emergency department or trauma bay management, which is extreme in its invasiveness and appropriate in a narrow set of circumstances. Indications for its utility and technical considerations of its performance are discussed in more depth in Chapter 18.

Resuscitation

Initial intravenous fluid administration is accomplished with isotonic electrolyte solutions. Lactated Ringer solution is the initial solution of choice. Normal saline has the potential to cause hyperchloremic acidosis, especially in patients with imparied renal function. Solutions containing glucose should not be used in initial resuscitative efforts: most patients are hyperglycemic as a result of high serum concentrations of epinephrine and cortisol, and excessive serum glucose levels can induce an osmotic diuresis. During the initial evaluation and resuscitation of the trauma patient, intravenous fluids are administered as rapidly as possible. This requires immediate and repetitive assessment of the hemodynamic status in response to serial volume resuscitation.

TABLE 17-2

HYPOVOLEMIC SHOCK CLASSES; ESTIMATED FLUID AND BLOOD LOSSES—BASED ON THE PATIENT'S INITIAL PRESENTATION

	Class I	Class II	Class III	Class IV
Blood loss (mL)	≤750	750–1500	1,500–2,000	>2000
Blood loss (% blood volume)	≤15%	15%–30%	30%–40%	>40%
Heart rate	<100	>100	>120	>140
Blood pressure	Normal	Normal	Decreased	Decreased
Pulse pressure	Normal	Decreased	Decreased	Decreased
Respiratory rate	14–20	20–30	30–40	>35
Urine output (mL/h)	>30	20–30	5–15	Negligible
Mental status	Slightly anxious	Mildly anxious	Anxious, confused	Confused, lethargic
Replacement fluid	Crystalloid	Crystalloid	Crystalloid and blood	Crystalloid and blood

From Committee on Trauma of the American College of Surgeons. *ATLS for Doctors—Student Course Manual.* Chicago: American College of Surgeons, 1997, with permission.

In the patient with shock, the dose of the initial fluid bolus is 1 to 2 L in the adult patient and 20 mL per kg in the pediatric patient. Although the total amount of fluid required to reestablish a patient's intravascular volume is difficult to predict, guidelines can be inferred from Table 17-2. Note that crystalloid administration should be guided by the "3:1 rule," such that each milliliter of suspected blood loss must be replaced initially by 3 mL of crystalloid solution. This rule is consistent with the fact that the intravascular volume of sodium (and associated water) represents approximately one third of total body extracellular sodium (and water).

Regardless of the initial assessment of the patient's intravascular volume deficit, the most important measure in resuscitation is early and repeated assessment of the patient's response to fluid administration. The surgeon must evaluate the patient's end-organ perfusion and oxygenation, taking measure of level of consciousness, blood pressure, peripheral pulses and tissue capillary refill, urinary output, and acid–base status (as determined by repeated blood gases).

According to the guidelines of the Committee on Trauma of the American College of Surgeons, the initial response to fluid resuscitation can be classified in one of three categories: rapid response, transient response, and minimal or no response.

Patients with *rapid response* to initial fluid bolus quickly normalize their blood pressure and heart rate. These patients have usually lost less than 20% of their total blood volume and have minimal ongoing losses. That said, they must continue to be observed for signs of further bleeding or occult shock, and typed and cross-matched packed red blood cells should be kept available.

Patients who initially or *transiently respond* to bolus administration of intravenous fluids but who demonstrate subsequent deterioration in indices of perfusion and hemodynamic stability most likely have ongoing blood loss or have been inadequately resuscitated. These patients have likely lost 20% to 40% of their intravascular volume. Continued rapid fluid administration, the initiation of transfusion, and continued aggressive search for sources of hemorrhage should be undertaken.

A third group of patients will *fail to respond* to crystalloid fluid bolus. These patients should be considered to have greater than 40% intravascular volume loss and ongoing hemorrhage. They should be transfused early. Very aggressive and focused search for ongoing massive bleeding is key. Appropriate surgical therapy must be undertaken for any identified sources of bleeding. Simultaneously, the diagnosis of nonhemorrhagic shock should be entertained (e.g., tension pneumothorax, pericardial tamponade, myocardial contusion, and spinal cord injury). FAST examination or diagnostic peritoneal lavage is helpful.

In general, most institutions today administer only separate blood components rather than whole blood. In the trauma patient, restoration of volume by crystalloid administration and restitution of oxygen-carrying capacity by transfusion of packed red blood cells are the current standards of hypovolemic resuscitative therapy. Ideally cross-matched blood is available; however, the cross-matching process generally requires approximately 1 hour. Type-specific blood is appropriate for most patients classified as *transient responders* to initial crystalloid resuscitation. In the nonresponder or hemodynamically unstable patient with suspected or identified exsanguinating blood loss, type O packed red blood cells should be administered and, as it becomes available (20 to 30 minutes), type specific red blood cells subsequently given. In females of childbearing age, Rh-negative type O blood should be administered.

All fluids and blood products should be warmed prior to or during administration, in concordance with efforts to warm the trauma bay and thereby further prevent heat loss from the patient. Crystalloid solutions should be kept in a warmer (40°C to 45°C) or heated in a microwave oven prior to administration. Blood products can neither be stored at body temperature nor heated in a microwave oven, but can be warmed via passage through a rapid-infuser fluid warmer during transfusion.

In the patient who has hemorrhagic shock with hemothorax, the drained blood can be given by autotransfusion via thoracostomy tube and reservoir collection devices capable of collecting blood in a sterile manner.

Coagulopathy

It is uncommon for the trauma patient to demonstrate significant coagulopathy on arrival. More commonly, early coagulopathy is caused by a patient's medications, which alter coagulation or platelet function, such as warfarin and aspirin. Following exsanguination, class IV shock and its resuscitation, multiple factors contribute to the consumption and dilutional coagulopathy frequently seen in a delayed fashion. Hypothermia contributes to platelet dysfunction and disordered coagulation cascade enzymatic activity. Dilution of platelets and clotting factors in the process of massive resuscitation also contributes to bleeding. Transfusion of platelets, fresh frozen plasma, and cryoprecipitate should be guided by measurements of serum fibrinogen, partial thromboplastin time, prothrombin time, and platelet count in the patient with coagulopathy. Of note, patients who have sustained severe injury to the CNS are especially prone to coagulopathy because of the release of endogenous anticoagulants such as tissue thromboplastin from the damaged neural tissues.

SHOCK

Definition and Classification of Shock

Shock is the clinical syndrome that arises from the inadequate perfusion of tissues and cells. When tissue perfusion diminishes to the point that oxygen delivery is inadequate to meet the demands of cellular metabolism, shock ensues. Alterations in cellular metabolism lead to cellular dysfunction, expression of inflammatory mediators, and cellular injury. In general, when the oxygen demands of the cell are not met, there is an uncoupling of oxidative phosphorylation and the cell begins to metabolize glucose anaerobically, which leads to a buildup of lactic acid. Cellular efficiency is impaired and the cell membrane loses the ability to maintain its sodium gradient via the active ionic pump, thereby leading to cellular swelling. If perfusion is quickly restored, cellular injury is limited and the progression of shock can be halted. However, if oxygen delivery remains inadequate, irreversible cellular injury occurs and end-organ damage can result. The recognition that both trauma resuscitation and postoperative patient care are primarily the responsibility of the surgeon demands that the training resident becomes familiar with the treatment of shock.

The signs and symptoms of shock include skin changes (pale, cool, and mottled), mental status change, hypotension, tacchycardia or bradycardia, tachypnea, or hypoxemia (measured via arterial blood gas). In addition, oliguria or other end-organ dysfunction can be observed.

Recognizing that shock may present with varying degrees of severity is paramount to initiating treatment. Timely restoration of perfusion is the core concept when treating shock regardless of the etiology. Even when the cause of shock is not immediately apparent, treatment—to include volume resuscitation—is initiated immediately to halt the progression of the shock syndrome and prevent the onset of multisystem organ failure (MSOF).

Essential in the initial response to the shock patient is identifying and treating the conditions precipitating a shock state. In this regard, MOI and a brief history of how the patient was injured and a physical examination are invaluable. These alone usually identify the loss of airway, inadequate ventilation or oxygenation, pericardial tamponade, tension pneumothorax, or site of hemorrhage. More complete history taking may reveal more uncommon causes of shock such as pelvic fracture, spinal cord injury, anaphylaxis, severe electrolyte abnormalities, or hypoglycemia. Next, transfer of the patient in a shock state to the OR for definitive control of bleeding or occasionally for angioembolization is common. Less common, transfer to an intensive care unit, with invasive monitoring, and appropriate life support measures is warranted for further diagnostic steps intended to elucidate the etiology of shock (e.g., blunt myocardial injury).

Shock can be usefully classified according to its etiology. Discussion follows of hypovolemic, cardiogenic, neurogenic, and septic or vasogenic shock states and their respective treatments. Subsequent to this is a discussion of diagnostic measures intended to differentiate between the types of shock and therefore to guide therapy. Physiologic features of each class of type of shock are presented and contrasted in Table 17-3.

Hypovolemic shock is the most common type of shock following injury and results from bleeding. Fundamentally, hypovolemic shock results in the inability of the heart to generate sufficient cardiac output ($CO = HR \times SV$) as a result of impaired diastolic ventricular filling, where CO is cardiac output, HR is heart rate, and SV is stroke volume. This failure of the cardiac pump mechanism is predicted by the Frank-Starling mechanism, as represented in Figure 17-2. The most frequent cause of hypovolemic shock is hemorrhage. Other forms of hypovolemic shock ensue from excessive third-space plasma losses, as might occur from severe burns or excessive gastrointestinal or other insensible losses. The clinical signs and symptoms of hypovolemic shock depend on the severity of the intravascular volume deficit (how much blood is lost) and the rate of bleeding. The treatment of hypovolemic shock is predicated on the

TABLE 17-3
PHYSIOLOGIC CHARACTERISTICS OF THE VARIOUS FORMS OF SHOCK

Type of Shock	CVP & PCWP	Cardiac Output	Systemic Vascular Resistance	Mixed Venous O$_2$ Saturation
Hypovolemic	↓	↓	↑	↓
Cardiogenic	↑	↓	↑	↓
Septic	↓ or ↑	↓ or ↑	↓	↑
Neurogenic	↓	↓	↓	↓

CVP, central venous pressure; PCWP, pulmonary capillary wedge pressure.

reestablishment of adequate circulating blood volume and oxygen carrying capacity.

In the trauma patient, hemorrhagic shock is treated in the emergent manner as discussed in the preceding text. Often, in the exsanguinating (the loss of blood volume in minutes) patient, identification of the class of hemorrhagic shock is less vitally important than the expedient identification of bleeding site and resuscitation. That said, in the metastable patient (transient responder), signs and symptoms can reliably predict the amount of blood loss in most bleeding patients, including those patients with gastrointestinal bleeding, postsurgical bleeding, retroperitoneal bleeding, or other hemorrhagic conditions. The classification of hemorrhagic or hypovolemic shock is presented in the preceding text in the section of this chapter on resuscitation in trauma.

Cardiogenic shock is the result of pump failure. Both extrinsic and intrinsic mechanisms of diminished cardiac output are incorporated into this classification of shock. Extrinsic cardiogenic shock is sometimes referred to as *compressive* (or obstructive) cardiogenic shock and occurs due to increased extracardiac forces, which limit blood return to the heart. Tension pneumothorax, pericardial tamponade, and extreme levels of positive end-expiratory pressure (PEEP) are examples of forces that may limit blood return to the heart and result in shock. These syndromes and their treatment have already been addressed.

Intrinsic cardiogenic shock may result from primary myocardial dysfunction such as ischemic or other cardiomyopathy, myocardial ischemia or infarction, cardiac arrhythmia, valvular insufficiency or stenosis, papillary muscle rupture, myocarditis, or myocardial contusion. Right-sided heart failure may ensue after a large pulmonary embolus that causes an acute increase in right ventricular pressure.

The treatment of cardiogenic shock depends on the exact etiology of the cardiac failure. In the common case of myocardial ischemia, oral aspirin, intravenous heparin, supplemental inhaled oxygen, intravenous β-blockers, and either intravenous or oral morphine and nitroglycerin should be administered. In many cases of cardiogenic shock, diuresis may be effective in alleviating symptoms of pulmonary compromise from left-sided heart failure and pulmonary edema. Dopamine, dobutamine, or milrinone are frequently utilized to temporarily augment cardiac output but may be relatively contraindicated in the case of ongoing myocardial ischemia if myocardial oxygen demand is increased by their administration. Efforts should be made to transfuse those patients with myocardial ischemia to a hemoglobin concentration of at least 10 g per dL. Finally, for those patients with myocardial ischemia or infarction, coronary angiogram and endovascular intervention are appropriate and necessary. Following coronary catheterization, coronary artery bypass grafting or valvular replacement or repair may be indicated. Cardiogenic shock from severe blunt myocardial injury is treated in a similar fashion to cardiogenic shock after a myocardial infarction. Anticoagulation is probably best avoided after acute injury, especially in the setting of multiple traumatic injuries.

Finally, mechanical support of cardiac function should be considered in the patient in profound or recalcitrant cardiogenic shock: Intraaortic balloon counterpulsation

can be life-saving in these patients, especiallly in cases of clear coronary insufficiency, mitral insufficiency (frequently caused by myocardial ischemia), and a competent aortic valve. Ventricular assist devices can also be considered by the cardiac surgery team; they provide temporary "bridges" to either cardiac transplantation or to cardiac recovery, especially in the case of infectious myocarditis.

Sympathetic denervation from spinal cord injury, spinal anesthesia, or severe head injury produces generalized arteriolar vasodilation and venodilation resulting in *neurogenic shock*. Traumatic spinal cord injuries generally must occur above the level of T6 to cause disruption of the sympathetic outflow tract, resulting in this shock syndrome. Relative hypovolemia results when the normal blood volume is suddenly insufficient to fill the acutely increased intravascular space. These patients present with the characteristic findings of warm extremities and normal to decreased heart rate despite hypotension. The initial therapy is directed at restoring sympathetic tone by using volume repletion and vasopressors. Dopamine, at various doses, is the usual agent selected, especially in the cases with bradycardia. Norepinephrine or neosynephrine can also be used.

Vasogenic or *septic shock* is similar to neurogenic shock in that it results from a sudden decrease in vascular tone, thereby resulting in relative hypovolemia; however, the mechanisms are quite different. Vasoactive mediators are responsible for this type of shock, and causative mechanisms include systemic inflammatory response syndrome (SIRS), infection or sepsis, anaphylaxis, acute hypoadrenal states, traumatic injury, or ischemia–reperfusion injury. In addition to the loss of vascular tone, the patient in septic shock suffers a generalized injury to the endothelium resulting in leakage of plasma into the interstitium, compounding the effective hypovolemia. Septic shock is easily distinguished from neurogenic shock in that sympathetic outflow is intact, and these patients are tachycardic and often refractory to volume resuscitation.

The initial therapy of septic shock is the administration of intravenous fluid to reestablish adequate intravascular volume. Vasoactive drugs or pressors may be necessary to maintain an adequate blood pressure and tissue perfusion pressure. However, the physician must be cautious to reserve the use of pressors until adequate intravascular volume is reestablished; if not, a cardiogenic shock state may ensue from the confounding of preload deficits with afterload increases. Finally, the cause of the septicemia must be addressed: Débridement of necrotic or gangrenous tissue, drainage of purulent collections, and administration of broad spectrum antibiotics are all necessary.

Shock due to *adrenocortical insufficiency* is a rare form of vasogenic shock. This entity should be considered in any patient who has a history of glucocorticoid use and in severely ill patients, especially the elderly, who are refractory to volume resuscitation and pressors. The patient may be hypoglycemic, hyponatremic, and hyperkalemic. Eosinophilia has also been reported in association with adrenal insufficiency in the intensive care unit setting. This form of shock responds rapidly to the intravenous administration of corticosteroids. It is usually a diagnosis of exclusion and occasionally requires corticosteroid treatment prophylactically.

Response to the Shock State

Every organ system when faced with decreased supply and tissue hypoxemia undergoes compensatory physiologic changes and sustains damage if the shock state is not treated expediently. Especially important to the maintenance of life and severely affected by the shock state are the circulatory, pulmonary, and renal systems. When the shock state results in end-organ damage in multiple (three or more) physiologic systems, survival is dismally poor. These patients are said to have MSOF or multiorgan dysfunction syndrome (MODS).

The circulatory system has compensatory mechanisms that initially maintain blood pressure, cardiac output, and redirect flow to the vital organs. The venous system contains two thirds of the total circulating blood volume, including 20% to 30% within the splanchnic venous system. Most of this blood volume resides within the small venous capacitance vessels, which tend to collapse or empty with hypotension, passively shunting blood toward the heart. Selective arteriole vasoconstriction also occurs via α-adrenergic stimulation in response to shock. Blood flow to the skin is sacrificed early, followed by muscle beds, the splanchnic viscera, and kidneys in an attempt to maintain perfusion to the brain, heart, and lungs. The resultant increase in systemic vascular resistance helps to transiently maintain the arterial pressure despite decreasing cardiac output. As long as the systolic arterial pressure remains greater than 70 mm Hg, autoregulatory mechanisms maintain blood flow to the cerebral and coronary vessels.

Acutely, pulmonary compensation is manifest in tachypnea, occurring largely in response to the increased sympathetic tone as well as any metabolic acidosis. Subsequently, especially in prolonged shock or septic shock, damage to lung parenchyma may result in acute respiratory distress syndrome (ARDS), a continuum of progressive intrinsic lung injury. The hallmark of ARDS is the occurrence of pulmonary edema, despite normal or even decreased left heart pressures. Intrapulmonary shunting results in hypoxemia as underventilated or collapsed lung segments are perfused. Decreased levels of surfactant and pulmonary edema lead to a decrease in lung compliance. Chest x-ray findings may lag behind the clinical picture by as much as 24 hours and are of little value early in the course of ARDS. In established ARDS, chest radiography will demonstrate alveolar-interstitial infiltrates in the central lung fields early and then diffusely later in the clinical course.

When subjected to shock, the kidney will preserve salt and water. A drop in blood flow to the kidney causes a reflex constriction of the renal afferent arteriole, which results in a drop in the glomerular filtration rate (GFR). As GFR decreases, circulating antidiuretic hormone (ADH) and aldosterone levels rise, producing oliguria. Back-diffusion of filtered urea causes a rise in the serum urea nitrogen level out of proportion to the creatinine level, which is known as *prerenal azotemia*. At this point, the process is reversible if adequate volume resuscitation is initiated. Prolonged decreases in renal blood flow may result in ischemia and acute tubular necrosis (ATN). Restoration of renal blood flow at this point results in a reperfusion injury. This may present as a loss of renal concentrating ability such that urine output is no longer an accurate measure of adequate perfusion (high-output ATN). Conversely, if the ischemic injury was profound, the renal tubules may be clogged with cellular debris so that urine output remains low despite adequate resuscitation (oliguric or anuric ATN). Most renal failure from ATN resolves over time but permanent renal insufficiency or failure can occur, especially in the elderly or those with antecedent renal disease.

Approach to the Diagnosis and Treatment of Shock

The goal in the management of shock is to restore perfusion and coincident oxygen delivery to tissues. The determination of the type of shock afflicting a particular patient is tantamount to diagnosing their disease state and essential to determining the appropriate therapy. After the initiation of resuscitation, transfer to an intensive care unit, and placement of telemetry and intermittent or continuous (arterial line) blood pressure monitoring, consideration must be given to investigation of the physiologic status of the patient and the causation of shock.

Initial consideration should be given to placement of a central venous catheter. This will allow administration of pressors and inotropes centrally, eliminating the risk of extravasation and skin necrosis or compartment syndrome inherent in peripheral administration of intravenous vasoactive medications. A central line will also permit the measurement of the central venous pressure (CVP), allowing the clinician to differentiate between cardiogenic shock and other shock states.

However, distinguishing among the various shock states characterized by low CVP, and assessing other standard and fundamental measures of cardiovascular and metabolic physiology, will require either pulmonary artery catheterization or echocardiogram. Pulmonary artery catheterization provides—in general—more information and allows serial evaluation of the patients physiologic status as treatments are implemented and the patient's condition improves or deteriorates. However, the pulmonary artery catheter is an invasive monitor and its insertion a procedure not without risk. Therefore, consideration should always be given to the use of either transthoracic or transesophageal echocardiogram to obtain an assessment of the immediate physiologic and cardiovascular state of the patient.

The pulmonary artery, or Swan-Ganz, catheter provides a number of measures of physiologic status that are invaluable to the critical care physician. First, it provides an estimate of left ventricular end-diastolic volume (LVEDV), or preload. Because the shock state is manifested by decreased cardiac output and decreased blood pressure, and because one principal determinant of left ventricular function is preload (according to the Frank-Starling mechanism), knowledge of the LVEDV is invaluable in assessing the patient's condition. Second, the pulmonary artery catheter provides a measure of cardiac output or cardiac index (cardiac output divided by total body surface area) by means of thermodilution. Finally, blood can be aspirated from a port in the right ventricle or pulmonary artery, providing a measure of the oxygen saturation of mixed venous blood ($S\bar{v}O_2$) and thus an index of physiologic and cardiovascular status and reserve. Modern Swan-Ganz catheters have incorporated a laser oximeter in the distal end of the catheter to permit continuous and almost instantaneous measurement of $S\bar{v}O_2$.

It deserves mention that use of the pulmonary artery catheter and knowledge of the parameters elucidated in the preceding text, allow *complete* specification of the cardio-vascular state.

$$CO = HR \times SV$$

of the patient, as follows. HR is measured by telemetry or arterial line and CO is measured by Fick thermodilution. Therefore, SV can be calculated:

Likewise, given SV, preload (from LVEDV), and after-load (from an arterial line), cardiac contractility can be de-termined:

$$SV = f(preload, afterload, contractility)$$

Finally, sytemic vascular resistance (SVR) reflecting va-somotor tone of the systemic circulation can be assessed:

$$SVR = \frac{MAP - CVP}{CO}$$

Evidently, with reference to Table 17-3, these measures of physiologic parameters can be utilized to define the par-ticular etiology of shock in any particular patient.

Again it is important to note that an echocardiogram provides much the same information as the Swan-Ganz catheter, including a more direct measure of left ventricular preload, a measure of SV and thereby CO, and a *direct* as-sessment of cardiac contractility. But it does not allow serial assessment of these same parameters nor the interval evalu-ation of physiologic state with therapeutic interventions.

ACID–BASE PHYSIOLOGY AND INTERPRETATION OF BLOOD GASES

Normal Acid–Base Physiology

The maintenance of the concentration of hydrogen ions within a narrow range is vitally important to physiologic homeostatis and cellular viability. An acid is a chemical that donates hydrogen ion (H^+) and a base is a chemical that accepts H^+. The pH is defined as the negative loga-rithm of the concentration of hydrogen ions:

$$pH = -\log[H^+]$$

The normal extracellular fluid pH is between 7.35 and 7.45; note that a pH of 7.4 corresponds to a hydrogen ion concentration of 40 nEq per L. Normal respiratory metab-olism of glucose and fatty acids produces approximately 20×10^3 mmol of carbon dioxide per day; in aqueous so-lution the carbon dioxide forms carbonic acid, H_2CO_3. This acid load must be buffered in order to maintain acid–base homeostasis.

Intracellularly, organic phosphates, bicarbonate, and proteins—especially histidine moieties—serve as buffers. Two extracellular buffering systems normally function to maintain normal $[H^+]$: the bicarbonate system and bone. The bone buffering reservoir has the capacity to exchange hydrogen ions for sodium and potassium ions, and can re-lease alkali salts to further decrease body pH, but bone plays little role in acute acid—base physiology or derange-ments. Meanwhile, the bicarbonate buffering system is the

principal extracellur buffering system. The bicarbonate ion, HCO_3^- acts to buffer H^+ according to the equilibrium:

$$CO_2 (gas) \leftrightarrow CO_2 (aqueous) + H_2O$$
$$\leftrightarrow H_2CO_3 \leftrightarrow H^+ + HCO_3^-$$

The Henderson-Hasselbach equation is simply a state-ment of the equilibrium existing between carbon dioxide at one extreme of this chemical equation and hydrogen and bicarbonate ions at the other extreme:

$$\left[H^+ = \frac{24 \times P_{CO_2}}{[HCO_3^-]} \right]$$

This relationship illustrates that any alteration in car-bon dioxide partial pressure, for instance, must result in a compensatory change in bicarbonate concentration or the body fluid pH will become abnormal. In practical clinical circumstances, the Henderson–Hasselbach equation serves to calculate the serum bicarbonate concentration from the measured P_{CO_2} and pH.

It is immediately evident that the bicarbonate buffer sys-tem also drives the mechanism of acid excretion via carbon dioxide elimination by the lungs. Total body bicarbonate supply and hydrogen ion concentration is simultaneously regulated by the kidneys. The nephron reclaims approxi-mately 4,500 mEq of bicarbonate filtered by the glomerulus daily. This reabsorption occurs primarily in the proximal tubule, and is accomplished with luminal membrane car-bonic anhydrase. Meanwhile, H^+ is secreted in the distal tubule, largely in exchange for sodium ions absorbed under the influence of aldosterone. Hydrogen ion secretion in the distal tubule serves to eliminate nonvolatile acids. Phos-phates and ammonia filtered in the glomerulus are poorly reabsorbed and so "trap" H^+ in the urine.

Interpretation of Arterial Blood Gases

The evaluations of a patient's condition with regard to acid–base physiology begins with an arterial blood gas (ABG) and serum electrolyte concentrations. The ABG provides measurement of pH, P_{O_2}, and P_{CO_2} (normal 38 to 42 mm Hg). The bicarbonate concentration (normal range, 22 to 28 mmol per L) is then calculated by using the Henderson-Hasselbach equation. In addition, total serum carbon dioxide—including serum bicarbonate—is meas-ured as part of the electrolyte panel; however, gaseous car-bon dioxide has a very low solubility in water, such that total serum carbon dioxide represents serum bicarbonate with considerable accuracy (such that the ABG calculated value of $[HCO_3^-]$ should differ by no more than 2 mEq per L).

Initially, the clinician must ascertain whether the pa-tient is acidemic or alkalemic by consideration of the pH alone. In general, the variety of primary (as opposed to compensatory) disorders can be recognized by the devia-tion in pH: Any physiologic compensation will return the pH toward normal, but not completely correct (or over-compenste for) the underlying acidosis or alkalosis. Note that a patient *may* have an acid–base disorder even with a *normal* pH (in this case both serum bicarbonate and P_{CO_2} will be abnormal), but this would be indicative of a *mixed* disorder because—again—compensation for primary dis-orders will not in general fully correct the pH.

Next, the physician assesses whether the primary disturbance is respiratory or metabolic, and thereby obtain a "minimum" diagnosis. In acidosis, the bicarbonate concentration will be decreased in a metabolic disorder, whereas the P_{CO_2} will be increased in a respiratory disorder. Meanwhile, in alkalosis, the bicarbonate will be increased in a metabolic disorder, whereas the P_{CO_2} will be decreased in a respiratory disorder. At this stage in the evaluation of the patient, recourse should be made to the history and physical examination: Clues to the nature and mechanism of the acid–base disturbance can greatly aid in the interpretation of the patient's condition and direct the clinician to identify, for instance, a mixed disorder.

Detection of any second primary disorder—that is, a mixed disorder—next proceeds by determination of the appropriateness of compensation of the primary disorder. In the case of primary respiratory disorders, great distinction must be made between acute and chronic disorders, because of the time course of renal metabolic compensation. In acute respiratory acidosis, one can expect 1 mEq per L increase in $[HCO_3^-]$ per 10 mm Hg increase in P_{CO_2}; in chronic respiratory acidosis, on the other hand, there will be a full 3.5 mEq per L increase in $[HCO_3^-]$ per 10 mm Hg increase in P_{CO_2}. Meanwhile, in acute respiratory alkalosis, there will be a 2 mEq per L decrease in $[HCO_3^-]$ per 10 mm Hg decrease in P_{CO_2}; in chronic respiratory alkalosis, one can expect a full 5 mEq per L decrease in $[HCO_3^-]$ per 10 mm Hg decrease in P_{CO_2}.

The respiratory response—and resulting partial pressure of carbon dioxide—to metabolic acidosis is predicted by Winter fomula:

$$P_{CO_2} = 1.5 \times [HCO_3^-] + 8 \pm 2.$$

Meanwhile, the expected respiratory compensation for a metabolic alkalosis is usually expressed as a change in P_{CO_2} from normal:

$$\Delta P_{CO_2} = 0.6\Delta[HCO_3^-].$$

In the case of a metabolic acidosis, one must determine the anion gap. When an organic acid, for instance, lactic acid, is added to the extracellular fluid, the acid is buffered and the bicarbonate concentration falls, without concomitant alterations in the concentration of the primary serum elemental ions, Na^+ and Cl^-. The anion gap

$$Ag = [Na^+] - ([HCO_3^-] + [Cl^-])$$

is normally 8 to 12; a larger anion gap in metabolic acidosis is indicative of ketoacidosis, lactic acidosis, toxin ingestion (most commonly methanol, ethylene glycol, or salicylates), or renal failure. In contrast, nongap acidosis is characteristic of renal tubular acidosis, diarrhea, and sometimes chronic renal failure.

Finally, and only in the setting of a gap acidosis, the anion gap can be compared to the decrement in bicarbonate concentration to assess whether a concomitant metabolic alkalosis exists. Explicitly, one can calculate the "delta ratio" as the increase in anion gap (from its normal value of 10), divided by the decrease in $[HCO_3^-]$ (from its normal value of 24). A delta ratio greater than 2.0 indicates an abnormally elevated "initial" bicarbonate concentration, resulting in a smaller than expected "decrease" in $[HCO_3^-]$,

being diagnostic of a metabolic alkalosis. (Alternatively, a concommitant compensated chronic respiratory acidosis could also result in the same elevated delta ratio.)

It is important to recognize that, as discussed thus far, knowledge of serum electrolyte concentrations is integral to interpretation of the ABG. First, the bicarbonate concentration is confirmed by measurement of total serum carbon dioxide. Second, the anion gap cannot be calculated without knowledge of the serum concentrations of sodium and chloride ions.

Frequently the base deficit (or excess) will be reported by the laboratory with the ABG results. This is a calculated quantity that does not provide any information above and beyond the three primary determinants of the Henderson-Hasselbach relationship. It represents the number of mEq per liter of base (or acid) that would be required to titrate serum pH back to normal if the patient's respiratory compensation were ignored, that is, if the P_{CO_2} were 40 mm Hg. This measure, therefore, purely reflects the patient's *metabolic* acid–base state, and as such is considered useful by many clinicians. Base deficit can be especially revealing as a marker of hypovolemic shock and poor cellular perfusion (anaerobic metabolism) leading to an occult lactic acidosis.

Finally, note that the ABG provides the serum partial pressure of oxygen, P_{O_2}. This is useful as a measure of oxygenation, for calculation of alveolar–arterial gradient, and as a measure of transpulmonary shunting, but does not play a direct role in interpretation of acid–base status.

Specific Acid–Base Disorders

Metabolic acidosis is diagnosed by a decrease in serum bicarbonate concentration. This results either from excretion of bicarbonate-rich fluids (e.g., diarrhea or ileostomy output), or by buffering of abnormal acids. In the setting of renal failure, metabolic acidosis frequently results as a consequence of the kidneys' inability to reabsorb bicarbonate. The classification of metabolic acidoses into "gap" and "nongap" has been briefly addressed in the preceding text, as have the conditions typically responsible for each classification.

The treatment of metabolic acidosis depends on the underlying disease and on the severity of the acidosis. Except in the setting of an ACLS-protocol resuscitation from cardiac arrest, bicarbonate administration is generally reserved for any patient who is hemodynamically unstable and has a pH less than 7.1. In diabetic ketoacidosis, fluid resuscitation and insulin administration are the hallmarks of therapy. The treatment of lactic acidosis consists of improving tissue perfusion and thereby ameliorating the shock state. Methanol and ethylene glycol poisoning are treated with ethanol (which competitively inhibits alcohol dehydrogenase conversion of the ingestants into their toxic metabolites), fomepizole (an intravenous inhibitor of alcohol dehydrogenase), and hemodialysis.

Metabolic alkalosis results from excess serum bicarbonate. Normally, excess $[HCO_3^-]$ is corrected by renal excretion of the anion. The maintenance of metabolic alkalosis, therefore, requires a defect in renal excretion. The most common cause is vomiting or gastric tube drainage: The alkalosis is initiated by the gastrointestinal loss of hydogen ions but maintained because the accompanying hypovolemia results in secretion of aldosterone and increased renal tubule sodium reabsorption, in turn causing distal tubule H^+ secretion. Similarly, other etiologies of hypovolemia, including underresuscitation in the postoperative patient and diuretic administration, can result in decreased renal bicarbonate excretion and metabolic alkalosis. Loop and thiazide diuretics are most commonly implicated in this "contraction alkalosis." Note that hypokalemia coexists with any hypovolemic alkalosis and exacerbates the tendency towards renal H^+ excretion. All of the aforementioned causes of metabolic alkalosis are classified as chloride-sensitive because the mainstays of therapy are volume expansion with sodium chloride and repletion with potassium chloride.

The chloride-resistant metabolic alkaloses result from primary or apparent mineralocorticoid excess, Bartter syndrome, and excessive alkali administration or ingestion in the setting of impaired renal function. Apparent mineralocorticoid excess is characteristic both of the rare inherited disorder Liddle syndrome and of excessive licorice ingestion. Excessive alkali ingestion occurs classically in milk-alkali syndrome, initially recognized in the 1920s as a consequence of the Sippy regimen, consisting of milk and bicarbonate administration, for the treatment of peptic ulcer disease.

Respiratory acidosis results from impaired alveolar ventilation. The most common etiologies of acute respiratory acidosis include narcotic overdose, respiratory muscle paralysis (e.g., muscle relaxants in anesthesia), airway obstruction, or inappropriate ventilator settings in the intubated and sedated or paralyzed patient. Acute increases in P_{CO_2} can result in somnolence, confusion, and eventually unresponsiveness. Chronic respiratory acidosis is most commonly caused by chronic pulmonary disease, such as emphysema, kyphoscoliosis, or severe obesity (Pickwickian syndrome). The approach to management of acute respiratory acidosis consists of establishment and maintenance of a patent airway, mechanical support of ventilation if necessary, and treatment of the underlying disorder. In patients with chronic respiratory acidosis who develop a new increase in P_{CO_2}, efforts should be made to identify aggravating conditions such as a new pneumonia or bronchitis.

Respiratory alkalosis is caused by hyperventilation. Common etiologies include pain, anxiety, hypoxia, inappropriate ventilator settings in the intubated patient, salicylate poisoning, and fever. In addition, various cardiopulmonary processes, including pneumonia, pulmonary embolus, and congestive heart failure, can result in hyperventilation and respiratory alkalosis.

CONCLUSION

The evaluation and resuscitation of the trauma patient occur simultaneously and follow the principles of the ATLS put forth by the American College of Surgeons. The ABCDE scheme is important and—in severe injury—allows rapid determination and treatment of those injuries that are most deadly.

This chapter has also addressed two topics of importance to those surgeons caring for patients in the intensive care unit: shock and acid–base physiology. Shock is a common consequence of severe illnesses, and its evaluation and treatment are essential elements in the care of critically ill patients. Likewise, an understanding of acid–base physiology and an ability to interpret arterial blood gas values are crucial for the physician and surgeon.

KEY POINTS

▲ Injuries comprise the leading cause of death in persons ages 1 to 34 years. As a consequence, trauma constitutes the leading cause of loss of potential, unrealized life.

▲ The Advanced Trauma Life Support (ATLS) system proposes the "ABCDE" (airway, breathing, circulation, disability, and exposure) protocol for the "primary survey" in the evaluation, resuscitation, and treatment of the injured patient. During procession through this algorithm, life-threatening problems are treated as they are discovered.

▲ Initial intravenous fluid administration is accomplished with isotonic electrolyte solutions; lactated Ringer solution is the initial solution of choice. The most important measure in resuscitation is early and repeated assessment of the patient's response to fluid administration. In patients who either respond transiently or who do not respond to fluid resuscitation, both transfusion and continued aggressive search for sources of ongoing bleeding should be undertaken.

▲ Shock is the clinical syndrome that arises from the inadequate perfusion of tissues and cells; it can be classified as hypovolemic, cardiogenic, neurogenic, or vasogenic. Differentiation between the various etiologies of shock—and assessment of response to therapy—frequently requires Swan-Ganz catheter monitoring.

▲ An understanding of acid–base physiology is crucial for physicians and surgeons. The evaluation of a patient's condition with regard to acid–base physiology begins with measurement of the arterial blood gas (ABG) and serum electrolyte concentrations.

SUGGESTED READINGS

Committee on Trauma of the American College of Surgeons. *ATLS for doctors—student course manual.* Chicago: American College of Surgeons, 1997.

Peitzman AB, Rhodes M, Schwab CW, et al. *The trauma manual,* 2nd ed. Philadelphia: Lippincott Williams & Wilkins, 2002.

Specter SA, Rabinovici R. Initial evaluation and resuscitation of the trauma patient. In: Cameron JL, ed. *Current surgical therapy.* St. Louis: Mosby, 2001.

Traumatic Injuries

18

Stephen C. Gale   Patrick K. Kim   Vicente H. Gracias   C. William Schwab

SPECIFIC INJURIES BY ANATOMIC REGION AND SPINAL CONDITIONS

Traumatic Brain Injury

Traumatic brain injury (TBI) is very common in patients who sustain blunt trauma and is the most common cause of death from injury. TBI is classified both by the specific parenchymal lesion and the patient's clinical neurologic function. Although the latter is more predictive of neurologic outcome, effective treatment is based on both components. Therefore, irrespective of clinical findings at presentation, patients suspected of sustaining a TBI should undergo head computerized tomographic (CT) scan as soon as possible after arrival to the trauma center.

The clinical classification of TBI is based on the Glasgow coma scale (GCS): mild (13–15), moderate (9–12), and severe (8 or less) (see Table 1-1). The motor component of the GCS is the most important predictor of neurologic severity and recovery. For patients with mild TBI who have had a brief loss of consciousness but no focal neurologic deficit, prognosis is excellent and mortality is rare. Patients with moderate TBI often have confusion, amnesia of the event, and occasionally focal neurologic findings. However, they are usually able to follow simple commands and have an overall good prognosis. Patients with coma (GCS ≤8) have usually sustained severe TBI. Mortality approaches 40% and many survivors have a significant persistent neurologic deficit. Admission to the intensive care unit (ICU), intracranial pressure monitoring, and craniotomy are often required in these patients. Parenchymal lesions are diagnosed anatomically on the basis of CT scan findings. Concussion is the *absence* of parenchymal damage in a patient with a documented loss of consciousness. This is a clinical diagnosis with variable neurologic symptoms. Postconcussive symptoms are common and include headache, inattention, short-term memory loss, and mood swings. Although these symptoms rarely persist for more than a few months, patients and their families must be advised of these potential sequelae before discharge.

A cerebral contusion is essentially a "brain bruise" with localized intracerebral hemorrhage and edema adjacent to an area of impact. Depending on the degree of trauma sustained, these lesions can enlarge with time and may coalesce into an intracerebral hematoma and occasionally result in a mass effect. Similarly, subarachnoid hemorrhage (SAH) is often localized anatomically but more often represents a shearing mechanism with local vascular disruption. SAH lesions typically do not cause mass effect.

Space-occupying intracranial hematomas are usually characterized by their relationship to the dural lining as epidural (superficial to the dura) or subdural (deep to the dura). Epidural hematomas are most often seen after a direct lateral impact to the temporal region with skull fracture and laceration to the middle meningeal artery. Blood accumulates between the skull and the dura. There may be little direct trauma to the brain parenchyma. Classically patients experience a brief loss of consciousness and a subsequent lucid interval in which they may appear normal, sleepy, or even intoxicated. After a short time they lose consciousness again as the lesion expands and produces cerebral compression. Ipsilateral pupillary dilation indicates impending uncal herniation secondary to elevated intracranial pressure and occurs as a result of direct compression of the third cranial nerve. Immediate evacuation is indicated in any patient with altered mental status, a lesion greater than 1 cm in diameter, or with evidence of midline shift on CT scan. With early evacuation, prognosis is excellent and depends mostly on the degree of underlying cerebral trauma and the time delay to hematoma evacuation.

Subdural hematomas accumulate between the dura and the brain itself. The shearing or tearing of dural bridging veins is the most common underlying cause and generally suggests a significant force of impact. In addition to the parenchymal compression of the hematoma, significant direct brain injury and axonal shearing are present. Therefore, patients with subdural hematomas have worse prognosis and greater residual functional deficits. Occasionally patients will present in coma (GCS ≤8) but there are minimal findings on initial CT scan. These patients may have sustained a diffuse axonal injury (DAI), which is an axonal shearing due to rapid deceleration. There may be little or no evidence of trauma on CT scan. Some patients with DAI will have scattered punctuate hemorrhages, loss of gray–white matter differentiation, diffuse edema with brainstem compression, and loss of basolateral cisterns or compression of cerebral gyri/sulci. The prognosis for DAI is poor, with a high incidence of residual neurologic deficit and high mortality.

Traumatic Brain Injury Management

These various lesions describe the primary brain injury sustained during the traumatic event. That event cannot be altered. The basic management of TBI strives to prevent *secondary* injury that might further compromise neural tissue and further limit neurologic recovery. This secondary neurologic injury is the result of brain tissue ischemia from either hypoxia or impaired perfusion pressure. Treatment strategies emphasize prevention of hypoxia at the cellular level and center on the concept that the cranium is a closed space with a fixed volume. Typically, intravascular blood, brain tissue, and cerebrospinal fluid (CSF) are the only intracranial contents. Brain swelling or mass lesions, such as hematomas, occupy space and raise intracranial pressure. Once a critical volume has been reached, autoregulation mechanisms fail and intracranial pressure (ICP) increases markedly. Cerebral perfusion pressure (CPP) is the differential between mean arterial pressure (MAP) and ICP (CPP = MAP − ICP). As ICP increases for a given MAP, CPP falls. Below a CPP of 60 mm Hg, tissue hypoxia occurs and causes secondary brain injury. Furthermore, conditions that lead to increased cellular metabolism may lead to a relative hypoxia as oxygen demand surpasses supply. These metabolic alterations must be controlled. Table 18-1 summarizes the various causes of primary and secondary brain injury after trauma.

After the initial resuscitation, the initial management of elevated ICP involves evacuating clinically significant hematomas, reducing intracranial swelling, and optimizing cerebral perfusion (Fig. 18-1). Euvolemia is an important goal and 0.9% (normal) saline is the maintenance fluid of choice; hypotonic solutions are contraindicated in TBI resuscitation as they may worsen cerebral edema. The head of the patient's bed should be elevated 30 degrees

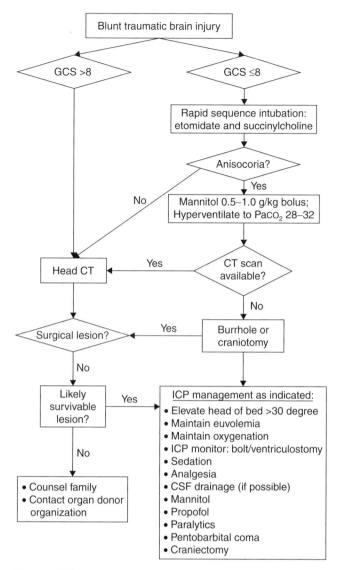

Figure 18-1 Initial management of blunt traumatic brain injury. GCS, Glasgow coma scale; ICP, intracranial pressure; CSF, cerebrospinal fluid.

and adequate pain control and sedation given. Chronic prolonged hyperventilation should not be utilized to control ICP; a Paco$_2$ of 35 to 40 mm Hg should be maintained. Of note, hyperventilation does play a role in the acute setting of elevated ICP with clinical deterioration. In the ICU or operating room, if the clinical examination cannot be followed, ICP must be monitored and is accomplished with either an intraventricular (ventriculostomy) or extradural (bolt) monitor. The ventriculostomy has the advantage of allowing not only ICP monitoring but also ICP treatment by CSF drainage. An ICP of greater than 20 mm Hg typically requires treatment.

Pharmacologic reduction of intracranial swelling is achieved transiently with mannitol or hypertonic saline. Mannitol is administered as a large bolus (1 g per kg) in the acute setting and is supplemented with smaller boluses (0.25 g per kg) every few hours as needed. Serum osmolarity must be monitored closely and maintained below 320 mOsm. In some centers, hypertonic saline is used. Hypertonic saline is administered as either 30-mL boluses of 7.5% solution or a continuous infusion of 3% solution with a goal of maintaining serum sodium levels

---

TABLE 18-1

PRIMARY AND SECONDARY CAUSES OF TRAUMATIC BRAIN INJURY

Primary brain injury

- Diffuse
  - Diffuse axonal injury (DAI)
- Focal
  - Vascular injury
    - Intracerebral hemorrhage
    - Subdural hemorrhage
    - Epidural hemorrhage
    - Subarachnoid hemorrhage
  - Parenchymal
    - Contusion
    - Laceration

Secondary brain injury

- Intracranial causes (compression)
  - Hemorrhage (mass effect)
  - Swelling
    - Venous congestion
    - Edema
  - Infection
  - Extracranial causes
  - Hypoxia
  - Hypotension
  - Hyponatremia
  - Hyperthermia
  - Hypoglycemia

at approximately 155 to 160 mEq per L. Hypertonic saline has the advantage of maintaining intravascular volume, whereas mannitol can lead to hypovolemia due to osmotic diuresis thereby compromising cerebral perfusion.

In the most severe cases of intractably elevated ICP, adjunctive measures such vasopressor agents to increase MAP, as well as neuromuscular blockade and barbiturate coma to reduce cerebral metabolism, are also used. Decompressive craniectomy may have a role in the treatment of select patients with severe intracranial hypertension but has not yet been rigorously studied. Anticonvulsants such as phenytoin are often administered during the first week after TBI treatment. Corticosteroids have no role in TBI management.

Because of the variability in injury patterns, the optimal management of penetrating gun shot wound (GSW) injuries to the brain is less well established. Shock waves created by the passing missile cause significant cavitation and severe parenchyma disruption both in and away from the missile tract. Subsequent hemorrhage and edema are often the cause of fatal intracranial hypertension with herniation. Transcranial tracts that damage both hemispheres cause devastating injury with early herniation and carry an extremely high mortality rate.

In penetrating brain injury, surgical intervention is indicated to evacuate hematomas caused by the laceration of cerebral vessels, to débride devitalized tissues, and to remove bone fragments from the wound. Extensive débridement or tract exploration is discouraged, however, as it may cause further neurologic damage. In general, bullets are not retrieved unless they are infected or are very easily accessible.

Spinal Cord Injury

The initial management of patients with spinal cord injury (SCI) is identical to that of most other trauma patients. Crystalloid resuscitation is initiated with the goal of euvolemia. If evidence of neurogenic shock exists, dopamine is used to further support the patient's physiology. Phenylephrine should be avoided because of the risk of reflex bradycardia in an already sympatholytic patient. Absolute spinal precautions must be maintained and the entire spine (thoracic, lumbar, and sacral) must be imaged owing to the high (10% to 15%) incidence of synchronous fractures present elsewhere in patients with a known spinal fracture.

Although controversial, the use of high-dose corticosteroids in spinal cord injury is still common practice. The rationale behind this practice is the potential further loss of function related to inflammation and edema that occurs postinjury. Patients with neurologic deficit who present less than 8 hours from the time of injury are candidates for treatment. Exclusions include pregnancy, penetrating injury, children, and isolated peripheral nerve deficits/cauda equina symptoms. The initial bolus of methylprednisolone is 30 mg per kg intravenous given over 15 minutes. If presentation is 3 hours or less from the time of injury, patients are subsequently given 5.4 mg/kg/h for the next 23 hours. If presentation is between 3 and 8 hours, therapy should continue for a total of 48 hours. Neurologic deficits suggesting SCI also require early neurosurgical consultation to expedite possible operative decompression.

Neck Injury

The high density of vital structures in the neck makes injury to this region highly morbid and often fatal. The trachea, esophagus, carotid and vertebral arteries, cervical spine and spinal cord, phrenic nerve, and brachial plexus are all vulnerable to injury with neck trauma. Each of these is a vital structure, and delays in diagnosis and treatment of injuries can be devastating. Penetrating neck injuries are generally from stab or GSWs. In contrast, blunt injury results from either direct impact to the neck or torsion from stretch of vital structures after decelerating impact to the head or chest. Because of the different injury constellations associated with a penetrating versus blunt mechanism, pattern recognition is used to initiate the appropriate diagnostic and therapeutic algorithms. The anatomic complexity of this region makes surgical intervention hazardous and requires a highly organized approach based on the surgeon's experience and the patient's clinical condition.

Penetrating Neck Injury

Anatomic considerations are very important in evaluating penetrating neck injuries. Trajectory of the knife or bullet determines anatomic injury. The platysma serves as an important superficial landmark, as patients without violation of this layer are unlikely to have significant injury to deeper structures. If the platysma has been violated or if violation cannot be excluded, further workup is needed and is generally guided with neck exploration; however, diagnosis and therapy is directed by the anatomic "zone of injury" (Fig. 18-2). The importance of zone differentiation relates primarily to the surgical accessibility for control of vascular injuries. Zone I extends from the clavicles to the cricoid cartilage and includes the thoracic outlet and subclavian vessels. Zone II includes all structures between the cricoid and the angle of mandible, including the carotid and vertebral arteries and the jugular veins. Zone III is the area between the angle of the mandible and the skull base and contains the distal internal carotid artery. Not surprisingly, zones I and III require advanced operative techniques to

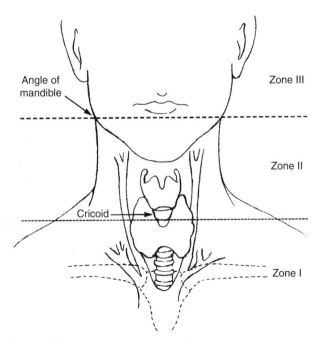

Figure 18-2 Anatomic neck zones for penetrating injury. (From Maxwell RA. Penetrating neck injury. In: Peitzman AB, Rhodes M, Schwab CW et al., eds. *The trauma manual*, 2nd ed. Philadelphia: Lippincott Williams & Wilkins, 2002:192, with permission.)

TABLE 18-2

INDICATIONS FOR IMMEDIATE SURGERY AFTTER PENETRATING NECK TRAUMA

- Airway compromise
- Extensive subcutaneous emphysema
- Pulsatile hematoma
- Active bleeding
- Shock

obtain vascular control in the chest (sternotomy) or skull base (mandibular dislocation), respectively. The aerodigestive structures obviously traverse all three zones.

As with any injury, clinical presentation guides workup and therapy. Irrespective of the location of injury, immediate surgical exploration is required in patients who present with hard signs of vascular injury, pulsatile hematoma, active bleeding or shock (Table 18-2). Airway control is always the primary concern and is usually accomplished with use of oral endotracheal intubation. Surgical airway control below the level of injury with emergent cricothyroidotomy or tracheostomy is sometimes required. Bleeding is initially controlled with direct manual pressure; wounds should not be blindly probed nor should any attempt be made to blindly clamp bleeding vessels. With profuse bleeding, the compressing hand should be "prepped" into the operative field and removed only when formal surgical exploration begins.

In contrast, patients without an indication for immediate surgery are candidates for selective management. Careful consideration must be given to identify and exclude injury to the aerodigestive structures or to the vascular system. The traditional approach to diagnostic testing is based primarily on the anatomic zone of injury. This management strategy is summarized in Figure 18-3. Patients with Zone I penetrations should undergo aortic arch and great vessel angiography, tracheobronchoscopy, and either barium swallow or esophagoscopy for diagnosis. Positive findings are followed by appropriate surgical management. The evaluation of Zone II injuries has traditionally been operative, requiring complete surgical exploration to exclude vascular, esophageal, or tracheobronchial injury. More recently, an increasingly selective approach is used for zone II penetrations as well with angiography, esophagoscopy/barium swallow, and bronchoscopy replacing neck exploration in stable patients. Similarly, zone III injuries require angiography, bronchoscopy, and rigid esophagoscopy/barium swallow for injury identification and exclusion. Some centers have begun using imaging triage with CT angiography to identify missile trajectory and to guide further workup. This technique is attractive, accurate, and efficient and can be used for the evaluation of stable patients with penetrating neck injury.

Blunt Cervical Injury

Blunt traumatic injury results from either direct impact, crush injury, or torsion and stretch of vital structures caused by a decelerating impact to the head or chest. A

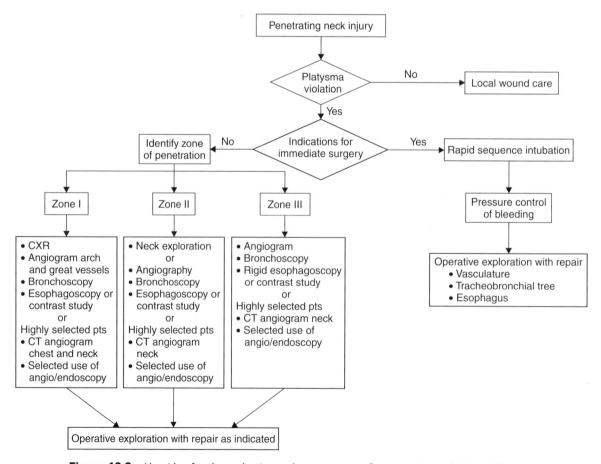

Figure 18-3 Algorithm for the evaluation and management of penetrating neck injury. CT, computerized tomographic; CXR, chest x-ray.

high index of suspicion is needed to avoid missing injuries in this region. Important injuries sometimes delayed in diagnosis include spinal cord injury due to traumatic instability of the cervical spine, crushing tracheal injury and fracture, and blunt cerebrovascular injury.

Until systematic evaluation is complete, cervical spine immobilization should be maintained in all blunt trauma victims. The burden is on the trauma surgeon to prove that no injury exists before removing the cervical collar. Some patients who meet all of the appropriate clinical criteria may have their cervical spine "cleared" without radiographic evaluation. These criteria include: no midline tenderness, normal mental status, no painful distracting injury, no clinical intoxication, and no neurologic deficits (transient or permanent) (Table 18-3). All other patients require complete cervical spine radiography from C1 to T1. Current guidelines recommend a combination of plain films and CT scans as needed. Traditional three-view cervical radiographs include an open-mouth odontoid view, an anteroposterior view, and a lateral view. Inadequate visualization of the cervical spine must be supplemented by either swimmer's view or, preferably, CT scan of the appropriate levels. Suspected areas of fracture should prompt imaging with CT scan. Because of the ease and efficiency of modern CT technology, some centers have abandoned the use of plain cervical radiographs in favor of complete cervical CT scan.

The examining physician should review cervical radiographs personally and make sure to inspect the films for adequacy (C1 to T1), alignment, vertebral height and cortical integrity, and soft tissue characteristics. Clinicians should err on the side of caution, and questionable areas should be evaluated further with use of CT scan or magnetic resonance imaging (MRI) as needed. Patients who continue to have midline tenderness or pain with movement despite normal radiographs should undergo flexion-extension radiographs or MRI to help exclude soft tissue injury and instability. Patients with neurologic deficits or documented fracture on plain films should undergo CT scanning of the entire cervical spine. MRI is then used to evaluate spinal cord injury or soft tissue injury such as ligamentous injury.

Blunt Cerebrovascular Injury

Cerebrovascular injury (carotid and vertebral artery) due to blunt trauma is increasingly being recognized. This diagnosis should be entertained in the presence of neurologic deficits that cannot be explained by the head CT findings, thus leading to cerebral angiography. However, these lesions can usually be occult with no neurologic deficits. Recent guidelines for diagnosis and treatment of occult cerebrovascular injuries have emerged. Because of the devastating potential of a missed injury and subsequent stroke, patients with injuries that suggest either direct trauma to the cerebrovascular structures or evidence of severe hyperextension, rotation, or flexion should undergo a four-vessel screening procedure. Such injuries include neck bruising (seat belt mark) or swelling from direct trauma, upper cervical spine (C1 to C3) fractures or cervical spine fractures with extension into the transverse foramina, basilar skull fractures through the petrous portion of the temporal bone, severe facial or mandibular trauma, or hanging/near hanging. Screening should also occur in patients who have neurologic deficits not explained by head CT scan or SCI. Although angiogram is the gold standard for diagnosing vascular abnormalities, magnetic resonance angiography (MRA) has emerged as an acceptable noninvasive screening modality. CT angiography is also being used in some centers. In most cases, treatment consists of heparin anticoagulation with transition to Coumadin when safe. Surgery or stenting are rarely indicated. Patients who have contraindications to systemic anticoagulation may be treated with antiplatelet therapy as an alternative.

Tracheal Injury

Tracheal crush injury is usually not subtle in presentation. Airway compromise is detected in the primary survey. Emergent airway control is usually indicated and may require a surgical approach. Operative repair of tracheal injuries requires débridement and end-to-end anastomosis with 4-0 absorbable suture. Well-vascularized tissue such as omohyoid muscle should be used to cover the anastomosis to help prevent breakdown or fistulization.

Thoracic Injury

Thoracic injury is extremely common after both blunt and penetrating trauma. Thoracic injuries are responsible for 25% of all trauma deaths and occur in a trimodal distribution. Immediate deaths usually involve cardiac or great vessel trauma. Deaths within the first few hours after injury are often caused by airway compromise, tension pneumothorax, or cardiac tamponade. Complications such as pulmonary sepsis account for most late deaths and are often related to chest wall trauma, with pulmonary contusion and poor pulmonary toilet, and subsequent pneumonia. Despite the potential for significant injury with thoracic trauma, greater than 85% of all chest injuries can be managed nonoperatively with appropriate analgesia, aggressive pulmonary toilet, tube thoracostomy, and selective endotracheal intubation. All patients require complete evaluation of their chest with physical examination and chest x-ray. Some require ABG determination, CT scan, or angiography.

Indications for urgent thoracotomy include both emergent and nonemergent conditions defined most consistently by the patient's clinical presentation. Immediate surgery is indicated for massive hemothorax (greater than 1,500 mL blood upon chest tube insertion), cardiac tamponade, acute deterioration after penetrating chest injury, major tracheobronchial injury, and chest wall disruption. Emergency department thoracotomy (EDT) is a distinct entity reserved for the patient *in extremis* and is discussed in greater detail in subsequent text. Urgent surgery is required in the stable patient with ongoing thoracic bleeding (greater than 200 mL per hour for 4 hours), massive persistent air leak, evidence of tracheal or esophageal injury after transmediastinal chest wound, evidence of great vessel injury, and impalement

---

TABLE 18-3

CRITERIA FOR CLINICAL CERVICAL SPINE "CLEARANCE"

- Absence of midline tenderness
- Normal mental status
- Absence of intoxication
- Absence of significant distracting injury
- Absence of neurologic deficit

wounds to the chest. Nonacute indications for thoracotomy after trauma include evacuation of retained hemothorax, decortication and drainage of empyema, repair of chronic diaphragmatic hernia, and repair of fistulous communications between aerodigestive and vascular structures after initial repair or missed injury. Video-assisted thoracoscopic surgery (VATS) is often utilized as an effective less-invasive alternative in the non-acute setting for conditions like retained hemothorax. A summary of the indications for thoracotomy after trauma is given in Table 18-4.

The initial evaluation of chest trauma, either blunt or penetrating, proceeds according to Advanced Trauma Life Support (ATLS) guidelines with attention directed at identifying and treating the imminently lethal chest injuries such as tension pneumothorax, pericardial tamponade, open pneumothorax, massive hemothorax, and flail chest. Subsequent evaluation must identify or exclude other "hidden" causes of death in thoracic trauma: aortic disruption, tracheobronchial disruption, blunt cardiac injury, diaphragmatic tear, esophageal perforation, and pulmonary contusion. The index of suspicion for these injuries is formulated from pattern recognition based on the mechanism of injury and the patient's clinical presentation.

Specific Conditions in Thoracic Trauma

Tension Pneumothorax

Tension pneumothorax can occur after both blunt and penetrating trauma and is caused by progressive air entry into the pleural space without a route of escape from either lung parenchymal or chest wall injury. Pressure develops as the air volume builds and with subsequent compression of the lung and mediastinum. Mediastinal shift causes a kinking of the superior and inferior vena cavae with impaired venous return and progressively diminished cardiac output. If unrelieved, cardiac arrest eventually occurs. There are varying presentations but all patients will have severe

respiratory distress, hypotension, and unilaterally diminished breath sounds. Although not present in all cases, there may also be unilateral hyper-resonance to percussion over the affected hemithorax, neck vein distention, and tracheal deviation away from the injured side.

Treatment requires immediate decompression, which is accomplished by inserting a 12- or 14-gauge intravenous catheter into the second intercostal space in the midclavicular line; this converts the tension pneumothorax into a simple pneumothorax. Decompression must then be followed immediately by tube thoracostomy.

Massive Hemothorax

Massive hemothorax is uncommon and occurs more often with penetrating trauma rather than blunt trauma. Etiologies include intercostal or internal mammary arterial bleeding, hilar vessel injury, great vessel injury, and cardiac injury. The presentation includes hemorrhagic shock and unilateral absence of breath sounds. Neck veins may be flat secondary to hypovolemia or distended because of the mechanical effects of intrathoracic blood compressing the mediastinum. A chest radiograph will demonstrate a completely opacified hemithorax and mediastinal shift in the most severe cases. Airway control and large-bore intravenous access and volume infusion should be begun before decompression. A large chest tube (36 or 40 French) is needed and should be attached to a collecting system with an autotransfusion setup. Thoracotomy is indicated for hemodynamic instability due to chest bleeding, greater than 1,500 mL initial blood loss, ongoing bleeding of greater than 200 mL per hour for more than 4 hours, or failure of a hemothorax to drain despite at least two functioning and well-positioned chest tubes.

Pericardial Tamponade

Pericardial tamponade occurs most commonly after penetrating trauma to the heart, but it can also be seen in blunt chest trauma. Because the pericardial sac does not acutely distend, as little as 75 to 100 mL of blood may produce tamponade in the adult. Classic signs such as distended neck veins, hypotension, and muffled heart tones (*Beck triad*) are present in only a few patients with confirmed tamponade. *Pulsus paradoxus*, a decrease in systolic pressure of more than 10 mm Hg during inspiration and *Kussmaul sign*, a rise in venous pressure with inspiration, are rarely seen. More commonly, patients are extremely anxious with a sense of "impending doom," and may appear "death-like." The presence of persistent hypotension and acidosis despite adequate blood and fluid resuscitation require consideration of the diagnosis of tamponade. Shock plus the presence of an elevated CVP is highly suggestive. If available, an ultrasonographic examination focussed abdominal ultrasound for trauma (FAST) or (ECHO) should be performed to detect pericardial fluid. A *positive* pericardial view in the setting of hemodynamic instability is an indication for immediate operative decompression with thoracotomy or median sternotomy. An equivocal pericardial view with FAST in an unstable patient or a positive examination in a stable patient necessitates an operative pericardial window. Although a negative FAST in the unstable patient is usually satisfactory to exclude tamponade, *in the presence of hemothorax*, tamponade cannot be excluded as pericardial fluid can decompress into the pleural space.

Treatment consists of immediate decompression and repair of the underlying injury. Pericardiocentesis may be

---

TABLE 18-4

INDICATIONS FOR THORACOTOMY AFTER TRAUMA

- Emergency department thoracotomy
  - Cardiac arrest after blunt trauma with signs of life in the trauma bay
  - Cardiac arrest after penetrating trauma with signs of life in the field or in the trauma bay
- Emergent
  - Massive hemothorax >1,500 mL
  - Pericardial effusion after penetrating chest injury
  - Acute deterioration after penetrating chest injury
  - Major tracheobronchial injury
  - Chest wall disruption
- Urgent
  - Ongoing thoracic bleeding >200 mL/h × 4 h
  - Ongoing massive parenchymal air leak
  - Radiographic evidence of vascular, tracheal, or esophageal injury after mediastinal traverse
  - Impalement
- Nonacute
  - Evacuation of retained hemothorax
  - Decortication/drainage of empyema
  - Repair chronic diaphragmatic hernia
  - Repair fistulous aerodigestive tract connection

used as a temporizing maneuver to relieve tamponade until definitive repair is possible. If the patient is *in extremis*, an emergent left anterolateral thoracotomy can also be performed to relieve the tamponade as described in the following text. In the unstable patient, urgent sternotomy should be performed in the operating room (OR). Stable patients with pericardial fluid evident on FAST should undergo a diagnostic pericardial window in the OR to confirm the diagnosis. A positive finding during pericardial window mandates extension to median sternotomy for evaluation and repair of cardiac injury.

Open Pneumothorax

An open pneumothorax or "sucking chest wound" is most often caused by an impalement injury or destructive penetrating wound (shotgun). A large open defect in the chest wall (greater than 3 cm diameter) allows equilibration between intrathoracic and atmospheric pressure. When the defect is greater than two thirds the tracheal diameter, air flows preferentially through the chest wall with each inspiration leading to profound hypoventilation and hypoxia.

Any patient with respiratory distress or hemodynamic instability should undergo immediate endotracheal intubation. The chest wall defect should be temporarily occluded with the gloved hand and then closed with an occlusive dressing taped on three sides to act as a flutter valve. This maneuver allows the spontaneously breathing patient to preferentially breathe though the trachea but prevents development of this into a tension pneumothorax. After temporary occlusion, a tube thoracostomy should be placed and the wound completely occluded with a sterile dressing. The chest tube placement should be through clean tissue and away from the traumatic wound. Thereafter, patients with large chest wounds should undergo formal operative thoracotomy to evacuate blood clot, debride devitalized tissue, and close the chest wall defect. Very large defects may require flap closure.

Chest Wall Injury

Direct injuries to the chest wall are very common in trauma victims. Specific manifestations of chest wall trauma are pain, tenderness, pain with inspiration, and chest wall instability. Rib fractures and chest wall contusion are painful injuries and carry significant morbidity. Poor pulmonary performance caused by "splinting" from pain, coupled with the presence of underlying pulmonary contusion, often leads to the development of pneumonia—especially in the elderly population. Adequate analgesia is the hallmark of successful treatment and allows aggressive pulmonary toilet and early mobilization. Pain control is the key to preventing complications and is achieved with *scheduled* nonsteroidal anti-inflammatory drugs (NSAIDs) and oral narcotics with liberal use of parenteral or epidural analgesia as required.

Bleeding from direct chest trauma is associated with rib fractures and lacerated intercostal vessels and musculature. This is a common cause of traumatic hemothorax; extrapleural hematomas due to rib fractures are less common. Typically, bleeding is self-limited and tube thoracostomy alone is adequate treatment. Occasionally patients require thoracotomy with direct ligation of bleeding chest wall vessels or lung.

The presence of chest wall instability or "flail chest" implies a large energy force imparted to the patient. A flail segment exists when two or more ribs are fractured in two or more locations. Although paradoxical motion occurs and contributes to the respiratory compromise of flail chest, the underlying *pulmonary contusion* is the most important clinical factor causing morbidity and mortality. Splinting due to pain further exacerbates the condition, and patients with flail chest often require epidural analgesia. Initial care should occur in the ICU with monitoring to detect clinical deterioration, progressive hypoxia, or hypercapnia. Many patients require endotracheal intubation and positive pressure ventilation. There is currently no role for mechanical stabilization of the flail segment.

Blunt Cardiac Injury

Blunt cardiac injury describes a spectrum of injury that includes myocardial muscle contusion to blunt rupture of the heart. Most blunt cardiac injury that is clinically significant presents with arrhythmias or acute heart failure. Although blunt cardiac injury causing hemodynamic instability is rare, new-onset arrhythmia or cardiac failure in a patient after significant blunt trauma raises the suspicion of blunt myocardial injury. Sinus tachycardia is the most common arrhythmia seen with myocardial contusion followed by premature atrial contractions, atrial fibrillation, right bundle branch block, ST-segment elevation, and premature ventricular contractions.

Diagnosis requires a high index of suspicion based on mechanism of injury. Twelve-lead electrocardiogram is obtained first; completely normal electrocardiographic (ECG) findings exclude clinically significant blunt cardiac injury. An echocardiogram is usually performed to detect myocardial dyskinesia or akinesia and most commonly follows the and electrocardiogram as the second confirmatory test. Findings of new-onset murmur or with hemodynamic instability require expedited ECHO evaluation. Transthoracic echocardiogram (TTE) is convenient and noninvasive and is adequate in most cases. Transesophageal echocardiography (TEE) can be used when the TTE is technically inadequate. Cardiac enzyme [creatine kinase (CK) and troponin-I] levels do *not* to correlate with the severity of blunt myocardial injury nor do they predict complications and, in general, should not be checked. Myocardial enzyme levels continue to be useful in diagnosing cardiac *ischemia* in trauma patients. Therefore, if a patient is suspected of a myocardial infarction before or after injury, they are necessary.

Patients with *any* new abnormal findings on electrocardiogram require admission with 24 hours of telemetric monitoring. Echocardiographic-proven contusion (hypokinesis or abnormal wall movement) mandates admission to the ICU. Invasive monitoring with a pulmonary artery catheter may be indicated to help guide therapy in patients who develop signs and symptoms of acute heart failure. Dobutamine may be useful in overcoming the impaired contractility experienced after blunt cardiac injury. Follow-up of an ECHO-proven myocardial injury is normally with a cardiologist.

Traumatic Aortic Injury

Traumatic rupture of the aorta (TRA) occurs after rapid deceleration injury, such as a fall from significant height or high-speed motor vehicle crash. The majority of individuals with this injury die at the scene. In survivors, there is typically a tear in the wall of the aorta that is contained by the adventitia and the parietal pleura. These patients are at risk for delayed free rupture into the mediastinum or pleural space with near-instant death. Because free rupture of the transected aorta is rapidly fatal, persistent or recurring nonlethal hypotension must be assumed to be from a different cause than the aortic injury.

In 85% of patients, aortic laceration is located just distal to the ligamentum arteriosum, past the left subclavian artery. Less often, this injury occurs in the ascending aorta, at the diaphragm, or in the mid-descending thoracic aorta. Physical findings that increase suspicion of TRA include asymmetry of upper extremity blood pressures, chest wall contusion, intrascapular pain, and intrascapular murmur. Importantly, half of all patients with TRA have no external signs of blunt chest injury. Radiographic signs on chest x-ray (Table 18-5) include *widened mediastinum* (greater than 8 cm), obliteration of aortic knob, deviation of trachea to right, presence of an apical pleural cap, depression of the left mainstem bronchus, obliteration of the aortopulmonary window, and deviation of esophagus (nasogastric tube) to the right. No single sign on chest radiograph reliably confirms or excludes aortic injury, although mediastinal widening is the most consistent finding. Further, radiographic evidence of fractures of the first rib, sternum, and scapula are not specific for TRA but do imply a large force applied to the thorax. A high index of suspicion based on mechanism of injury and the presence of any of the previously noted findings should prompt further evaluation.

Aortography is the gold standard for diagnosis of TRA. Although invasive with well-described complications, aortography clearly demonstrates disruptions and their anatomic characteristics. More recently, technologic advances have allowed contrasted chest CT scan to become a valuable diagnostic tool. Currently in many centers, high-speed multidetector helical CT scan provides definitive diagnosis of aortic injury allowing thoracic surgeons to proceed to repair without angiographic confirmation. Mediastinal screening with chest CT scan should be used liberally in patients whose clinical or radiographic findings are suspicious for aortic injury.

Once the diagnosis of TRA has been made, blood pressure must be lowered and tightly controlled to prevent any hypertension that may lead to rupture. Typically this is accomplished with a β-blockade (esmolol) infusion. Interestingly, with the multiply injured patient, management may be complicated by competing interests such as maintaining cerebral perfusion while hoping to stave off aortic rupture. Once the diagnosis of TRA has been made, a thoracic surgeon should be consulted and, if no competing priorities exist, immediate repair should be accomplished.

TABLE 18-5

CHEST RADIOGRAPHIC FINDINGS SUGGESTIVE OF TRAUMATIC RUPTURE OF THE AORTA

- Widened mediastinum (>8 cm)
- Obliteration of aortic knob
- Obliteration of aortopulmonary window
- Deviation of trachea to right
- Presence of pleural cap
- Depression of the left mainstem bronchus (>4 cm)
- Deviation of esophagus (nasogastric tube) to right

Transmediastinal Penetrating Injury

Missile injuries that traverse the mediastinum require special mention because of the complexity of their evaluation and the potential for devastating complications with any delay in diagnosis. One must remember that the heart, great vessels, tracheobronchial tree, and esophagus are all at risk with mediastinal traverse and an evaluation of *each* of these structures must be performed in *all* patients. The evaluation proceeds according to the patient's clinical condition summarized in Figure 18-4. Patients in *extremis* will undergo immediate median sternotomy or left anterolateral thoracotomy to control hemorrhage or relieve cardiac tamponade; if successful, further evaluation of the tracheobronchial structures and esophagus will continue in the OR. In the *unstable patient* with hypotension, a chest x-ray should be obtained and chest tubes should be placed on one or both sides as needed for pneumothorax or hemothorax. A rapid *FAST examination* is performed to exclude pericardial effusion. OR thoracotomy is performed as indicated on the basis of FAST examination findings, the volume of chest tube return, and the patient's hemodynamic status. In the OR, after control of major hemorrhage, flexible esophagoscopy and bronchoscopy are performed to diagnose aerodigestive tract injuries. If hemodynamic stability was achieved in the trauma bay but great vessel injury is suspected, formal *angiography* embolization and possibly endovascular stent placement can be performed followed by panendoscopy in the OR or ICU.

In the *stable patient*, evaluation must proceed in an organized and deliberate fashion to exclude injury to the heart, great vessels, esophagus, and tracheobronchial tree. Workup begins with a chest x-ray and FAST examination or ultrasonographic examination. If ultrasonography is not available and there is concern for cardiac injury, one must proceed to the OR for pericardial window. Angiography is then performed to rule out vascular injury. If injuries are found requiring operation, esophagoscopy and bronchoscopy can be performed in the OR or they can be completed in the ICU. Esophagography can be used as a complement to esophagoscopy. Combined, these two tests are used to exclude esophageal injury. When used together overall sensitivity increases to 90%.

More recently, an alternative algorithm has arisen for the evaluation of mediastinal traversing injuries in highly selected *stable* patients, which includes computed tomography (CT) angiography as an imaging triage tool. If CT angiography is rapidly available, this modality can be used to determine missile trajectory and guide further workup. Angiography, bronchoscopy, and/or esophagoscopy are then performed selectively as needed based on proximity of missile tract to individual structures. Computerized tomography is best used to exclude injury based on trajectory and proximity rather than identify individual injuries.

Emergency Department Thoracotomy and Cardiac Penetration

Emergency Department Thoracotomy (EDT) can be lifesaving in properly selected trauma patients; therefore, the trauma center and its staff must be prepared to perform this procedure. EDT must be considered heroic and has only few indications. EDT may waste valuable resources and risks injuring the staff and exposing them to various blood-borne infectious diseases; therefore, decision to perform EDT is made carefully.

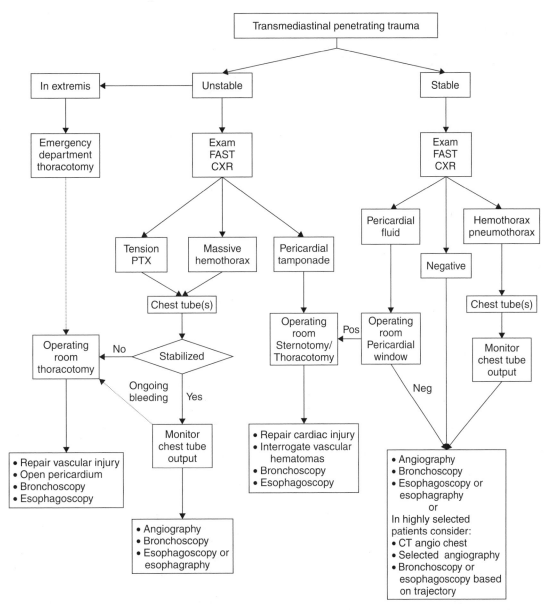

Figure 18-4 Evaluation and management of transmediastinal penetrating trauma. CT, computerized tomographic; CXR, chest x-ray; FAST, focused abdominal sonography for trauma, PTX, pneumothorax.

The goals of EDT are to relieve pericardial tamponade and/or to stop bleeding to allow definitive operative repair to take place and to temporarily occlude the descending aorta in cases of severe hypovolemic shock. The presence and timing of witnessed signs of life, as reported by prehospital personnel, determines the usefulness of EDT after trauma. Accepted signs of life are palpable pulse, spontaneous movement, pupillary response, spontaneous respirations, and ECG-determined narrow complex electrical rhythm of greater than 40 beats per minute (Table 18-6). The witnessed absence of signs of life by medical personnel precludes EDT regardless of mechanism.

After blunt trauma, patients with cardiac arrest in the field or *en route* to the hospital are usually *not* candidates for EDT and should be declared dead on arrival. With blunt mechanism, thoracotomy should be performed *only* after acute deterioration of signs of life *in the* ED; EDT should not be performed with acute deterioration due to massive head trauma. The indications for EDT after penetrating trauma are slightly more liberal and reflect a greater potential for recovery. EDT should be *considered* after loss of signs of life in the field witnessed by prehospital personnel. The evaluating surgeon must determine the amount of time elapsed since loss of signs of life before arriving to the ED and the presence of lethal injuries such as massive head injury or occasionally the presence of other patients requiring care before proceeding with EDT.

The technique for EDT (Table 18-7) involves a left anterolateral thoracotomy below the nipple at the fourth

TABLE 18-6

SIGNS OF LIFE

- Palpable pulse
- Spontaneous movement
- Pupillary response
- Spontaneous respirations
- Narrow complex electrical rhythm >40 bpm

TABLE 18-7

STEPS IN EMERGENCY DEPARTMENT THORACOTOMY TECHNIQUE

1. Incise skin/subcutaneous tissue in fourth intercostal space/ inframammary crease from midline to posterior axillary line
2. Divide intercostal muscles and pleura with heavy scissors
3. Insert rib spreader (handle toward axilla)
4. Extend to right side if needed
5. Perform pericardiotomy with scissors
   - Incise anterior and parallel to phrenic nerve
   - Evacuate clots
6. Repair/control any cardiac injuries present
   - Digital pressure
   - Pledgeted mattress suture
7. Cardiac life support
   - Ventricular fibrillation: internal cardioversion
   - Asystole: epinephrine 1 mg and internal bimanual massage
8. If #7 is unsuccessful:
   - Release left inferior pulmonary ligament
   - Gain digital control of aorta anterior to spine
   - Clamp with large vascular instrument to increase coronary perfusion
   - Repeat #7
9. Pulmonary hilar occlusion as needed for bleeding
   - Release affected inferior pulmonary ligament
   - Clamp hilum or perform 180-degree hilar twist
10. Cross-clamp aorta for intraabdominal exsanguinations
    - Release left inferior pulmonary ligament
    - Gain digital control of aorta anterior to spine
    - Clamp with large vascular instrument
11. Proceed to operating room for definitive repairs/control
    - Ligate internal mammary arteries as needed

---

intercostal space or in the inframammary crease in females. A generous incision should be made from the posterior axillary line to just across the midline to the right side of the sternum. The initial incision should be through all subcutaneous tissues and onto the chest wall. The intercostal muscles are incised with scissors and a large rib spreader is inserted with the crossbar downward toward the stretcher. The pericardium is then incised longitudinally, anterior and parallel to the phrenic nerve. The heart is delivered from the pericardial sac, which relieves any tamponade and allows for more effective internal compressions. If the heart is not beating, internal massage is performed while resuscitation with fluids proceeds. If the heart is fibrillating, internal cardioversion is performed at 20 J initially, followed by 30 J. If these maneuvers fail, temporary occlusion of the ascending aorta with gentle cardiac compression may augment perfusion of the coronary arteries and should be followed with another attempt at cardioversion.

If the heart is lacerated, gentle wound compression with a finger usually controls bleeding. If possible, definitive repair should occur in the OR with the surgeon's finger prepped into the wound. If not feasible, immediate closure is performed with a 2-0 pledgeted, monofilament, nonabsorbable suture. Balloon catheters should *not* be inserted into cardiac holes nor should attempts should be made at clamping ventricular wounds. These maneuvers will often fail to control bleeding while only enlarging the hole in the myocardium. Atrial wounds may be controlled by vascular clamp occlusion followed by suture repair.

Access to the thoracic aorta requires incising the inferior pulmonary ligament to retract the lung anteriorly and superiorly. Partial injury to the descending aorta may be controlled with manual compression or with a side-biting vascular clamp. Effective occlusive clamping is difficult, risking injury to the esophagus, and should be performed by blunt dissection around the aorta and then clamp placement. On occasion, with arrest after penetrating injury to the abdomen, temporary occlusion of the descending aorta will slow abdominal bleeding to allow transport to the OR for laparotomy. Survival after EDT for penetrating *abdominal* injury is very rare. Massive bleeding from the pulmonary parenchyma or hilum is controlled with a large hilar clamp or by finger occlusion. The surgeon must be mindful that in the absence of tamponade or easily controllable thoracic bleeding, survival after EDT for cardiac arrest is very poor.

Abdominal Trauma

Blunt Abdominal Trauma: General Considerations

The elements of the abdominal examination are detailed elsewhere and guide the subsequent evaluation and management. Physicians evaluating trauma victims must recall that the physical examination for abdominal trauma is unreliable. Blunt trauma patients who remain hemodynamically stable and in whom abdominal injury is suspected should have contrast enhanced abdominal and pelvic CT scanning. This is sensitive and specific for detecting solid organ injury after blunt trauma. CT is less sensitive for hollow viscus injuries, but, in general, a *completely normal* abdominopelvic CT scan reliably excludes solid organ and hollow viscus injuries. If CT scanning is unavailable or the patient cannot undergo the procedure, and the patient is alert and hemodynamically stable they can undergo a 24-hour period of observation and serial examinations. Serial FAST examinations by an experienced ultrasonographer can also be used to exclude injury in select patients. Deterioration of vital signs or the development of new signs (fever, tachycardia, or abdominal pain or tenderness) or leukocytosis should prompt repeat CT scanning or exploratory laparotomy.

Victims of blunt trauma who are hemodynamically unstable or who have considerable ongoing fluid requirements should be considered to have an uncontrolled source of hemorrhage. Management of such patients requires rapid decision-making. These patients are not candidates for CT scanning and should undergo cavitary triage with chest x-ray and either diagnostic peritoneal lavage (DPL) or FAST. DPL is very sensitive for intraabdominal hemorrhage but has a poor specificity (i.e., a positive DPL merely confirms intraperitoneal blood without yielding further information about its source). The technique involves open or percutaneous catheter placement into the pelvis with the instillation of 1 L of crystalloid with subsequent retrieval of the effluent and microscopic examination. Before proceeding with DPL, the stomach and urinary bladder must be decompressed with appropriate catherization. In blunt trauma, a positive test is the presence of greater than 100,000 RBCs per mL; greater than 500 WBCs per mL; amylase greater than or equal to 20 IU; or the presence of bile, bacteria or vegetable matter. In penetrating trauma, the positive indicators are the same but the bleeding threshold is much lower at greater than or equal to 10,000 RBCs per mL. Given the appropriate clinical setting, these findings should prompt operative intervention. A supra-umbilical approach should be used for patients with known or suspected pelvic fractures or suspected pregnancy.

Relative contraindications to DPL include pregnancy, prior abdominal operations, and pelvic fractures. The only absolute contraindication to DPL is the need for laparotomy. FAST is well-accepted in the initial evaluation of trauma patients and has great utility in unstable patients. FAST has excellent specificity for hemoperitoneum, but does not have either specificity or sensitivity for hollow viscus injury. By demonstrating the presence or absence of fluid (blood) in either the pericardium or abdominal cavity, FAST facilitates surgical decision-making. In the unstable patient, a FAST examination showing fluid in any of the three abdominal views and absence of pericardial fluid should prompt urgent abdominal exploration.

Penetrating Abdominal Trauma: General Considerations

In general, the safest course of action in penetrating injury to the anterior abdomen is laparotomy. Only in select cases where violation of the anterior abdominal fascia is excluded can laparotomy be safely avoided. A safe alternative to wound exploration in stable patients is exploratory laparoscopy simply to diagnose abdominal penetration. Once peritoneal violation is seen on laparoscopy, open exploratory laparotomy is indicated. Hemodynamically normal patients with penetration to the back or flanks, who have no abdominal tenderness, may undergo CT to identify trajectory, abdominal penetration, and visceral injury. Laparotomy can be avoided in some patients who have trajectory that is clearly away from all abdominal or retroperitoneal organs. In this setting, CT is not used to identify specific injuries but only to safely exclude them. Proximity to vital structures or questionable findings on CT scanning should prompt operative exploration and evaluation.

Trauma Laparotomy

Patients who require urgent laparotomy for trauma should have tetanus status updated and receive preoperative broad-spectrum antibiotics such as ampicillin/sulbactam that cover skin flora, enteric organisms, and anaerobes. In addition, a nasogastric tube, Foley catheter, and calf compression boots should be placed before commencing surgery. Skin preparation and towel draping should routinely be from the chin to the knees and to both sides of the operating table irrespective of the area of injury. A consistently wide operative field allows the trauma surgeon to be prepared for any contingency and to explore any cavity, or harvest a leg vein without repreping or draping.

In general a midline incision from xiphoid to pubis is used and affords the greatest exposure and flexibility. Consideration to possible stoma placement should be given when incising around the umbilicus. In those patients with previous laparotomy and presumed midline adhesions, when immediate access to control hemorrhage is needed, a bilateral subcostal incision can be used and gives adequate exposure, except for the pelvic structures.

Hepatic Trauma

The liver is the most commonly injured organ in blunt injury. Hepatic lacerations, hematomas, or active bleeding may be demonstrated by abdominopelvic CT scanning with intravenous contrast. Most hepatic hemorrhage is venous in nature and is self-limited. Therefore, assuming no concomitant abdominal injuries requiring operation, hemodynamically stable patients with liver laceration or hematoma, regardless of grade, may be considered candidates for nonoperative management. The decision to pursue nonoperative management after blunt hepatic injury requires the patient be hemodynamically monitored, serially examined, and to undergo frequent hemoglobin determination. The presence of hepatic contrast extravasation ("blush") on initial CT scan suggests active hemorrhage and an increased risk of failing nonoperative management. These patients should be considered for evaluation by an interventional radiologist for angioembolization. Among patients who are managed nonoperatively, a falling hemoglobin concentration should prompt repeat abdominal CT scan to exclude ongoing hepatic hemorrhage with consideration of angiographic intervention. In addition, if signs of peritoneal irritation develop, laparotomy is required to explore for hollow visceral injury.

Laparotomy or angioembolization must be considered in any blunt trauma patient who becomes unstable, develops peritonitis, or has ongoing transfusion requirements. At laparotomy, most liver injuries are controlled by suture ligation, cautery, or topical hemostatic agents. Finger fracture may be used to expose specific vessels in deeper injuries. Selective ligation of injured vessels and bile ducts is preferable to mass ligation of liver tissue, which increases hepatic necrosis. In hepatic trauma, nonanatomic débridement and resection is preferable to formal anatomic resection. With massive hemoperitoneum from hepatic hemorrhage, opening the peritoneum may release tamponade and precipitate profound hemodynamic instability. In this situation, the liver should be compressed manually until the anesthesia team can "catch up." In severe liver trauma, the Pringle maneuver, occlusion of the portal triad at the hepatoduodenal ligament manually or with a vascular clamp, will occlude hepatic arterial and portal venous flow and significantly reduce bleeding. Ongoing hemorrhage after a Pringle maneuver suggests retrohepatic vena caval injury or hepatic venous avulsion. These complex injuries carry a very high mortality and may necessitate total hepatic vascular isolation with control of both the suprahepatic and infrahepatic vena cavae in addition to the hepatic artery and portal vein. Sternotomy or thoracotomy may be necessary to gain access to the suprahepatic vena cava. Atriocaval (Schrock) shunting has been described, but despite its theoretical appeal, is rarely successful. Venovenous bypass has also been described, but few hospitals have round-the-clock capability. Massive hepatic trauma quickly leads to physiologic derangements as described above. The development of coagulopathy, hypothermia, or metabolic acidosis should prompt the application of damage control principles of abbreviated laparotomy and subsequent abdominal angiography and selective embolization of intrahepatic bleeding vessels to avoid irreversible physiologic debt.

After repair of hepatic injuries, closed suction drainage is generally used to control biliary leakage. Postoperative complications after hepatic surgery or embolization include recurrent bleeding, intrahepatic or perihepatic abscess formation, biloma, and hemobilia. Recurrent bleeding or hemobilia may require reoperation or angioembolization. Abscess and biloma are diagnosed by CT scan and are generally treated by percutaneous drainage. Biliary leak may also require endoscopic retrograde cholangiogram with sphincterotomy and/or stent placement or even transhepatic biliary drainage.

Splenic Trauma

Many of the concepts of the management of blunt hepatic injury also apply to blunt splenic injury. Nonoperative management of blunt splenic injury is well-validated, and the same limitations apply. The patient must be hemodynamically stable and must not have another indication for laparotomy. Success of nonoperative management depends on the severity of splenic injury and the patient's clinical status. Nonoperative management requires a commitment to serial examination, close monitoring of vital signs, and serial hemoglobin evaluation. Most importantly the surgeon must be able to objectively evaluate changes in the patient's condition and undertake an operative course if there is clinical deterioration. Advanced age, severe traumatic brain injury, unreliable physical examination, multiple injuries, and likely noncompliance with postdischarge activity restrictions are all relative contraindications to nonoperative management of splenic injury. If nonoperative management is pursued, after a period of inpatient observation dictated by the degree of injury, the patient may be discharged with limited physical activity (especially contact sports) for several weeks. Splenic injuries are not typically followed by serial imaging.

If the decision has been made to operate for splenic injury, either blunt or penetrating, the safest management is splenectomy via midline laparotomy. If a minor or non-bleeding splenic injury is discovered, splenic salvage may be considered. Splenic salvage techniques include splenorrhaphy and partial splenectomy. Splenorrhaphy may be performed using mesh to wrap the spleen. Partial splenic resection is performed with pledgeted mattress sutures. If there is significant splenic trauma or if there hemodynamic compromise, splenectomy is the safest option. The time required for splenic salvage is prohibitive in this setting, and there is also risk of further bleeding in an already compromised patient. Patients who undergo splenectomy should receive vaccinations to pneumococci, meningococci, and *Haemophilus influenzae* postoperatively. The optimal time for immunization is 2 weeks after splenectomy but in general vaccinations are given just prior to discharge. This practice limits but does not completely prevent overwhelming postsplenectomy sepsis (OPSS), which is a rare but grave complication of total splenectomy. The patient should also be given written confirmation of splenectomy, vaccination, and date.

Pancreatic Injury

Pancreatic injury is rare but it is more common after penetrating abdominal trauma. Furthermore, this organ is rarely injured in isolation and hemorrhage from injury to the surrounding vascular structures usually takes precedence during the laparotomy. Therefore, a high index of suspicion is needed when evaluating the pancreas after trauma to avoid missed injuries. During the trauma laparotomy, if injury to the pancreas is suspected based on missile trajectory or the presence of central hematoma, the entire length of the pancreas must be inspected and palpated utilizing wide mobilization techniques.

Once an injury to the pancreas is identified, the critical issue is to determine if the major pancreatic duct has been disrupted. This can usually be accomplished by inspection and palpation; intraoperative ductal imaging is rarely indicated or necessary. Operative management is then based on the status of the duct itself. The operative principles of managing pancreatic injuries are hemorrhage control, débridement of devitalized tissue, wide closed-suction drainage, and feeding jejunostomy with severe injuries. In addition, injuries involving the pancreatic duct typically require distal pancreatectomy at the point of ductal injury. Severe injuries to the pancreatic head and duodenum that involve the ampulla call for a pancreaticoduodenectomy, which should be performed in a staged fashion according to the operative complexity. Pancreatic fistulae are common after pancreatic trauma and are usually managed successfully with nonoperative management.

Genitourinary Tract

Hematuria, either gross or microscopic, is the most common presenting sign of the patient with genitourinary tract trauma. Although present in most cases, the *absence* of hematuria does not necessarily exclude genitourinary tract trauma. Therefore, renal injury should be considered in any blunt trauma victim with impact to the back and flanks, or complaint of costovertebral angle (CVA) or flank pain, especially in the presence of posterior rib fractures. Renal injuries after blunt trauma are most commonly diagnosed by CT scan, which may demonstrate renal laceration, contusion, perinephric hematoma, collecting system disruption, or segmental or complete devascularization. In the absence of active hemorrhage, nearly all renal injuries, even those with urinary extravasation, heal without intervention. Gross hematuria typically resolves rapidly. Arteriography and selective embolization should be considered for those patients with persistent gross hematuria. Renovascular injury may result in thrombosis and segmental or complete infarction. Traditionally, nephrectomy has been advocated for hemodynamically unstable patients with severe grade V renal injury ("shattered kidney") or renal infarction. However, expectant management of renal infarction is well tolerated and has not revealed significant rates of hemorrhage, abscess, or hypertension. Therefore, immediate nephrectomy is not mandatory in stable patients. Injury to the collecting system may result in urinoma, which is usually treated effectively by percutaneous drainage.

Physical findings of lower genitourinary tract trauma to the urethra or bladder include blood at the penile meatus, scrotal hematoma, and/or abnormal position of the prostate on rectal examination. Although these signs are often present, injury to theses organs should be considered in all patients with severe pelvic trauma or straddle type injuries. If any of these signs are present, retrograde urethrogram should be performed prior to placement of a Foley catheter. If no urethral injury is identified, bladder catheterization is safe to perform. Return of gross hematuria should prompt cystogram to rule out bladder injury. Classically, a plain film cystogram is utilized with two views of the contrast-filled bladder (AP and oblique) followed by a postvoid film. Recently CT cystogram has emerged as an option. Extraperitoneal bladder injury is typically managed by Foley catheter drainage alone, whereas intraperitoneal bladder injury requires formal operative repair followed by Foley catheter drainage. Bladder injuries are repaired in layers (two or three) with absorbable suture to create a watertight seal. A suprapubic catheter is occasionally needed to supplement Foley catheter urethral drainage after bladder repair, especially if there is bladder contusion and continuous hematuria.

At trauma laparotomy for either blunt or penetrating injury, if renal injury is suspected, the lateral retroperitoneum (zone 2) should be examined for hematoma. An expanding hematoma irrespective of mechanism indicates major vascular injury and mandates exploration. The presence of a functioning contralateral kidney should be confirmed by palpitation. The decision of whether or not to gain proximal vascular control prior to opening Gerota fascia is highly controversial. Proximal and distal aortic and inferior vena cava (IVC) control should be done quickly if the hematoma obscures the hilum of the injured kidney. A finding of significant hilar injury on exploration should prompt nephrectomy, as should significant renal injury in the face of hemodynamic instability. Although renal revascularization has a theoretical appeal, it is rare to achieve diagnosis and revascularization before the onset of irreversible nephron loss because of warm ischemia. Destructive lesions of the renal parenchyma, where the hilum is intact, may require partial nephrectomy and renorrhaphy with use of pledgeted horizontal mattress suture. Injury to the collecting system should be repaired with absorbable suture (permanent suture is a nidus for stone formation) and drained by ureteral stent (double J) or nephrostomy tube.

There is general consensus that in blunt trauma patients, nonexpanding hematomas of the lateral retroperitoneum should not be routinely explored. For victims of penetrating trauma, this remains controversial. Because injury to the collecting system cannot be excluded, the safest approach in penetrating trauma is to evaluate the kidney directly by exploring the organ.

Ureteral injury is rare in blunt injury but should be suspected in patients with microscopic hematuria and no other genitourinary tract injury. It is more common in penetrating injury and requires evaluation and even exploration if the bullet passes near its course. Ureteral transection is more common after penetrating injury. Ureteral injury should be repaired primarily with absorbable suture over a double J stent after débriding and spatulating the cut ends to avoid stricture. If primary ureteroureterostomy is not feasible because of tension, kidney and bladder mobilization, a psoas bladder hitch, a Boari flap (bladder tube neoureter), or transureteroureterostomy are options for tension-free repair.

Hollow Viscus Injury

Hollow viscus injury due to blunt trauma is difficult to diagnose in the acute setting. Physical examination may be unreliable because of altered mental status, head injury or distracting injuries, and trauma evaluation many times occurs before the development of peritoneal irritation. The presence of an abdominopelvic "seat belt sign" should alert the physician to possible intestinal and mesenteric injury caused by deceleration with the creation of shearing forces. Injuries to duodenum and proximal jejunum (and pancreas) should be suspected in the presence of lumbar spine anterior compression fracture due to hyperflexion (Chance fracture). This is especially true in children. CT signs suggestive of hollow viscus injury include bowel wall thickening, free intraabdominal fluid (in the absence of solid organ injury), mesenteric stranding, and extraluminal air. In sudden deceleration injuries, the intraabdominal viscera can be avulsed from the mesentery, especially near the relatively fixed ileocecal valve. CT scan is evolving to evaluate hollow viscous injury but with certain key caveats; a *completely* normal abdominopelvic CT is sufficiently accurate to rule out hollow viscus injury with a negative predictive value of 99.6%. CT findings consistent with bowel injury warrant surgical exploration. Stable patients with any equivocal CT signs of bowel injury should be admitted for 24-hour observation including serial physical examination and serial amylase and white blood cell determination. Patients with fever, changes in vital signs or physical examination findings, or leukocytosis should undergo urgent exploration.

All victims of penetrating injury to the anterior abdomen should be considered to have bowel injury. Although various treatment algorithms have been proposed in recent literature, exploratory laparotomy should be the default management of penetrating abdominal trauma. CT scan is not indicated in this setting and FAST and DPL may be falsely negative in the immediate postinjury patient.

At laparotomy the bowel should be examined in its entirety including both sides of the stomach, the entire small intestine, the colon, the visible rectum, and, if indicated by missile trajectory or by adjacent hematoma, the entire duodenum. Contamination by enteric contents should be rapidly controlled with figure-of-eight sutures or Babcock clamps until all injuries are identified. Definitive repair begins with débridement of nonviable edges. Primary repair may be considered if the resulting defect is less than 50% of the circumference of the bowel. Defects should be closed transversely to avoid luminal compromise. More extensive injury or concern on the part of the surgeon should prompt segmental resection with anastomosis. Either stapled or hand-sewn anastomoses are appropriate and can be performed in a one- or two-layer closure at the surgeon's discretion. Serosal tears and bowel wall hematomas are imbricated with Lembert silk suture.

Colon injuries are common after penetrating injuries but can also occur after blunt trauma. During exploration, the entire colon is inspected and small injuries with minimal contamination can be débrided and repaired as with small bowel. More significant injuries require segmental or anatomic resection and primary anastomosis. In the presence of shock, heavy contamination, or destructive injury, resection and colostomy may be indicated. Traditionally, the threshold for performing colostomy for left colon injuries is lower than for right colon injuries, although there is no difference in anastomotic breakdown after trauma. If there is doubt about primary repair or diverting colostomy, the surgeon is best advised to perform colostomy after resection. Colostomy is best done out of the zone of injury.

Intraperitoneal rectal injuries are managed identical to colonic injuries. Minor injuries can be débrided and repaired primarily. Significant injuries require resection and performance of a Hartmann procedure, creating an end colostomy. More distal extraperitoneal rectal injuries require the "three Ds" of rectal injury management: diversion, distal washout, and presacral drainage. In addition, if the rectal injury can be visualized through the anoscope or proctoscope it should be closed. Diversion can be either loop or end colostomy. Presacral drainage and distal rectal washout are recommended by some but have recently been called into question as to their efficacy in preventing pelvic sepsis.

Extremity Trauma

The extremities are commonly injured by both blunt and penetrating mechanisms. Blunt mechanisms are very common and when high-energy transfer occurs (e.g., "bumper

TABLE 18-8

HARD/SOFT SIGNS OF VASCULAR SURGERY

- Hard Signs
  - Pulsatile bleeding
  - Expanding or pulsatile hematoma
  - Absent distal pulse
  - Palpable thrill or audible bruit
  - Signs of distal ischemia (six Ps)
    - Pain
    - Pallor
    - Pulselessness
    - Paresthesias
    - Poikilothermia (temperature change)
    - Paralysis
- Soft signs
  - Proximity to known vessel
  - History of pulsatile bleeding
  - Neurologic deficit
  - Small, nonpulsatile hematoma

injury"), often lead to severe complex injuries known as the "mangled extremity." Extremity gunshot woundings and stabbings are extremely common. From the perspective of the trauma surgeon, irrespective of mechanism, vascular integrity and neurologic function must be rapidly assessed. In penetrating extremity trauma, a high index of suspicion is required to avoid the morbidity of missed neurovascular injuries. Fortunately, with simple physical examination techniques, most vascular injuries are easily diagnosed. Trauma surgeons must be attentive to the presence of "hard" and "soft" signs of vascular injury (Table 18-8). Hard signs mandate immediate diagnosis and intervention and include absent or diminished pulses, pulsatile bleeding, expanding or pulsatile hematoma, palpable thrill or bruit, and signs of distal ischemia (six Ps). Soft signs include wound proximity to a named artery, small nonpulsatile hematoma, neurologic deficit, and prehospital history of "pulsatile bleeding." Although these signs do not require immediate intervention in the absence of a deficit, they should increase the surgeon's awareness of possible vascular injury and lead to further evaluation or serial examination.

Diagnostic maneuvers include comparing blood pressures between extremities (ankle-brachial index or ABI), formal angiography, and operative angiography. ABI compares the systolic pressure of the affected extremity to that of an uninjured extremity. This should be performed by a trauma physician using a hand-held Doppler and manual blood pressure cuff. A normal ABI is 1.0 or greater and usually requires no further workup. An ABI less than 0.9 indicates a high probability of a vascular injury requiring operative intervention. In patients who have hard signs of injury and obvious operative indications, angiographic confirmation of injury prior to operation is often not necessary. However when needed before vascular exploration, angiography can be performed in the OR by the operative surgeon. This allows the surgeon to plan the incision and repair. Interventional angiography is reserved for those patients with ABIs of 0.9 to 1.0 who may have soft signs of injury, multilevel injury (gun shot), or in the rare case where clinical suspicion is high. Vascular injury after blunt trauma is most often caused by long bone fracture or joint dislocation (e.g., knee) with arterial compromise from compression between bony fragments. Occasionally, fracture or dislocation relocation restores an absent pulse and requires prompt evaluation. ABI should be performed after reduction with subsequent workup as needed. The surgeon must be mindful that intimal injuries may be present and serial vascular examination must be performed with liberal use of angiography in suspicious cases.

Penetrating extremity injuries require rapid determination of trajectory by examination of wound locations and radiographic localization of any foreign bodies. Physical examination including ABI measurement guides the workup. Hard signs of vascular injury lead the surgeon directly to the operating room. Direct pressure is used to control external hemorrhage until operative proximal control can be obtained. Tourniquets and blind clamping should be avoided.

When needed diagnostic operative "on-table" angiogram is performed from the proximal artery and, if available, digital subtraction angiography is recommended. A direct approach to the injured vessel with an incision directly over the area of injury is used for vascular exploration. After identifying the injury, proximal and distal vascular control allows bidirectional embolectomy, local heparinization, and subsequent repair. Proximal, large vessel injuries can be repaired with interpositions of either artificial material such as polytetrafluoroethylene (PTFE) or autogenous reversed saphenous vein with relatively equal outcomes. Distal vascular repairs and "bypasses" should use autogenous saphenous vein. A completion angiogram must be performed after every repair with the surgeon prepared to redo any unsatisfactory anastomosis. If necessary, wide debridement of damaged tissue is then carried out. Figure 18-5 summarizes the evaluation and management of both blunt and penetrating extremity trauma.

Mangled Extremity/Crush Syndrome

The mangled extremity deserves special mention owing to the tremendous complexity of care and the great potential for associated complications. These devastating injuries are those with concomitant soft tissue, bony, vascular, and often nervous injury. They are seen with farm machinery and industrial mishaps, high-speed motorcycle crashes, and in explosive combat injuries and mostly involve the lower leg and foot.

Although most severely injured extremities can be salvaged with an aggressive multidisciplinary approach, the trauma surgeon, as the team leader, must keep the patient's overall condition as the central focus. Factors predictive of a poor outcome include prolonged ischemia (longer than 6 hours), age older than 50 years, crush injury, significant comorbidities (diabetes, smoking, and heart disease), and major neurologic injury to the extremity. Prolonged ischemia is the only absolute contraindication to limb salvage. In the presence of these factors, limb salvage may be more detrimental than early amputation. Further, the development of the crush syndrome may make limb salvage impossible (see subsequent text).

If the decision is made to proceed with limb salvage, early restoration of blood flow must be a priority and preoperative discussions between the orthopedic, vascular, and trauma specialists are needed to plan the best approach. Depending on the clinical scenario, surgeons must decide between immediate revascularization versus temporary shunting and internal versus external fixation. The patient's clinical condition and the amount of contamination present

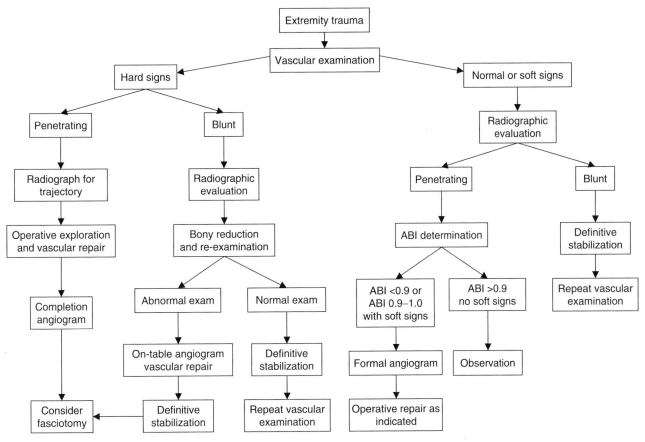

Figure 18-5 Evaluation and management of extremity trauma. ABI, ankle-brachial index.

guide these decisions. Typically these injuries will require multiple surgeries and washout procedures with eventual muscle flap and skin-graft closure of remaining wounds. In general, named nerve disruption with an insensate foot, ischemia, and large soft tissue and bone defects predict very poor long-term outcome and the need for amputation.

The crush syndrome refers to metabolic derangements that occur after restoration of blood flow after vascular injury or prolonged extremity ischemia from a crushing mechanism. It is caused by rhabdomyolysis with systemic manifestations of ischemia–reperfusion including shock, acidosis, hyperkalemia, myoglobinuria, and, at times, acute renal failure from the liberation of intracellular toxins as muscle cells die. In severe cases, multiorgan failure occurs with cardiac dysfunction, respiratory failure, and dialysis dependence.

The diagnosis is made by having a high index of suspicion, noting discolored urine, and testing the urine for myoglobin. Following serial labs (CK and electrolyte levels, and the patient's acid–base status) is necessary. Worrisome trends should prompt preemptive intervention with aggressive crystalloid resuscitation, mannitol diuresis, urine alkalinization with bicarbonate, and early dialysis as indicated. Muscle beds should be examined for devitalized tissue requiring debridement and, in some cases, amputation will be life saving.

Compartment Syndrome and Fasciotomy

The compartment syndrome occurs when pressures within fascia-restricted compartments exceed the perfusion pressure therein causing tissue ischemia. In extremity trauma, swelling and bleeding are the most common factors causing

elevated pressures; vascular injury, crush injury, and fractures are the usual underlying etiologies. Muscle and nerve cell death occur and result in a devastating loss of function with significant morbidity. The true tragedy with compartment syndrome is that in most cases, this complication of extremity trauma is preventable with early recognition and treatment.

The keys to preventing compartment syndrome after extremity trauma are a high index of suspicion, pattern recognition, and liberal use of fasciotomy in the appropriate clinical setting. In reality the morbidity of fasciotomy is low compared to that of the compartment syndrome and certain injury constellations should lead the surgeon to perform prophylactic fasciotomy at the time of the initial surgery. These include patients with crush injuries, prolonged ischemia time (longer than 4 hours) prior to reestablishing perfusion, and combined arterial and venous injuries.

In patients with extremity trauma who have not undergone fasciotomy, recognition of compartment syndrome can be difficult. Typical symptoms and signs occur late after tissue death has occurred and are related to the classic six Ps of distal ischemia. Symptoms are pain (out of proportion to examination) and paresthesias. Signs include a cool and tense swollen extremity, pain on passive stretch, sensory nerve deficits, and progressive motor weakness. In the lower extremity, the first sign may be numbness in the first digital web space due to compression of the deep peroneal nerve in the anterior compartment.

Of importance is pulselessness, which is a very late sign and indicates extremely high compartment pressure. Because tissue perfusion pressure is only 25 mm Hg, compartment pressures of only 30 mm Hg cause muscle ischemia while allowing a normal blood pressure to be transmitted to the distal extremity. Therefore, a palpable pulse does not exclude the compartment syndrome. If clinical suspicion suggests elevated compartment pressures, they should be quantified with a special monitoring device (Stryker) or with a modified arterial-line transducer setup. If compartment pressures exceed 25 to 30 mm Hg or if clinical suspicion is high fasciotomies should be performed.

When performing fasciotomies, surgeons should release all compartments of the affected extremity with generous full-length fascial incisions. Compartment syndrome can occur in any part of any extremity but the lower leg is by far the most common site. It has four compartments that are generally accessed by a two-incision fasciotomy. The anterior and lateral compartments are accessible through a lateral incision, whereas the superficial and deep posterior compartments can be released through a medial incision. Incisions should be generous to decompress the entire compartment as inadequate fasciotomies may not prevent compartment syndrome. The muscle should be assessed at the time of fasciotomy but only grossly necrotic tissue should be debrided. All other tissues can be reinspected at a later time to assess recovery and viability utilizing conservative debridement. Postoperatively, leg elevation and nonrestrictive circumferential bandaging is done.

Fasciotomy incisions can often be closed within 5 to 10 days. The goal is to provide skin coverage of the muscle; fascial closure is not necessary. Techniques include primary skin closure or split-thickness skin grafting. Often only one side can be closed primarily owing to excessive tension. In this setting, the lateral incision should be closed primarily for cosmetic purposes and to allow comfort when crossing one's legs. The medial side can then undergo skin grafting.

DAMAGE CONTROL

Damage control is recognized as one of the major advances in surgical care in recent history. This concept evolved from the realization that, in exsanguinating hemorrhage, patients die from a triad of coagulopathy, hypothermia, and metabolic acidosis. Once this metabolic failure has developed it is often intractable and terminal. From this knowledge arose the theory that early operative termination, with retreat to the ICU for physiologic and metabolic recovery, would allow patients to recover metabolic stability and survive to complete a staged operative repair of their injuries.

Because it challenged the fundamental surgical tenet that definitive operation is best for the patient, the principle of damage control was slow to be accepted. However, it is now well known that victims of multiple trauma and other acute surgical emergencies are more likely to die from metabolic failure than from a failure to achieve a technically complete operation. Trauma surgeons have led the way to a paradigm shift that places metabolic recovery and overall patient survival above the gratification of individual surgical achievement.

The trauma surgeon must rely on pattern recognition to help him or her identify, as rapidly as possible, those patients who require an abbreviated procedure to prevent metabolic failure. Pattern recognition incorporates certain "conditions, complexes, and critical factors" (Table 18-9) that serve to alert the surgeon that prolonged operative

TABLE 18-9
FACTORS FOR PATTERN RECOGNITION LEADING TO DAMAGE CONTROL APPLICATION

- Conditions
  - High energy blunt torso trauma
  - Multiple torso penetrations
  - Hemodynamic instability
  - Coagulopathy or hypothermia at presentation
- Complexes
  - Combined major abdominal vascular injury and major visceral injury
  - Multifocal or multicavitary bleeding with concomitant visceral injury
  - Multiregional injury with competing priorities
- Critical Factors
  - Severe metabolic acidosis (pH <7.30)
  - Hypothermia (Temp <35°C)
  - Resuscitation and operative time >90 min
  - Coagulopathy (nonmechanical bleeding)

efforts to achieve technical completion of all repairs may be detrimental. Patients with high energy mechanism or abnormal physiologic status on presentation, severe combined vascular and visceral injuries, multicavitary bleeding, or prolonged operative times should all be considered for staged procedures. These hemodynamic parameters, injury patterns, and intraoperative physiologic factors must be integrated by the trauma surgeon with rapid decision-making to perform damage control.

The damage control approach to the severely injured patient is a three-stage procedure (Table 18-10). In the first stage of damage control the priorities are *rapid and simple* control of hemorrhage and contamination. Once the decision is made to abbreviate the initial procedure, all efforts must concentrate on this goal. Simple techniques, such as "stapling off" injured bowel segments rather than restoring bowel continuity and ligating or shunting bleeding vessels rather than repairing them, help to keep operative times short. Liberal packing of nonarterial bleeding and rapid temporary abdominal closure complete the initial procedure.

The second stage of damage control is a retreat to the ICU for aggressive rewarming, resuscitation, and restoration of

TABLE 18-10
PHASES OF DAMAGE CONTROL FROM ABDOMINAL TRAUMA

1. Operative control of hemorrhage and contamination
   a. Control of active hemorrhage
   b. Pack solid organ injuries
   c. Resect injured bowel without anastomosis
   d. Rapid temporary abdominal closure
2. Retreat to surgical intensive care unit (SICU)
   a. Aggressive resuscitation with blood products
   b. Active rewarming
   c. Correction of coagulopathy
3. Reoperation
   a. Complete reexploration
   b. Remove packing
   c. Complete vascular repairs
   d. Restore gastrointestinal continuity
   e. Fascial closure (if possible)

normal physiology. Correction of metabolic acidosis and coagulopathy with biologically active colloid blood products is performed with frequent laboratory monitoring to assess progress. Failure of metabolic parameters to normalize may indicate ongoing surgical bleeding from inadequate hemorrhage control and should lead the surgeon back to the OR.

After correction of the metabolic derangement, which typically takes 24 to 48 hours, patients are ready to be returned to the OR. This third stage of damage control requires careful and complete abdominal reexploration with removal of packing, definitive repair of injuries, restoration of intestinal continuity, and abdominal wall closure provided that the patient's physiologic status remains normal. If there is evidence of recurrent metabolic failure, the surgeon must have the confidence to terminate the procedure and again retreat to the ICU. In most cases, successful abdominal closure is accomplished in this setting. Occasionally, patients require prolonged "open" abdominal management and eventually require absorbable mesh closure with split-thickness skin grafting. Abdominal wall reconstruction can be contemplated in the *years* after recovery.

Lastly, it is important to note than although most commonly applied to abdominal trauma, the concept of damage control can be applied to any traumatic or emergent surgical situation were metabolic failure occurs. The same tenets of pattern recognition and early decision-making can be used to achieve survival when persistence would lead to death. Septic abdominal catastrophe from perforated viscus and ruptured aortic aneurysm are common examples; interestingly, damage control techniques have been described in orthopedic and neurologic surgery as well.

THE PREGNANT TRAUMA VICTIM

Trauma complicates an estimated 1 in 10 pregnancies and is the leading nonobstetric cause of maternal death. Although the initial evaluation and treatment priorities of the pregnant trauma patient do not differ from trauma management in general, there are a few important maternal–fetal issues of which the trauma surgeon should be aware. Further, patients may present to the trauma center unaware of their pregnancy or unable to convey their condition to the trauma team. Therefore, pregnancy should be considered possible in all women of child-bearing age (10 to 50 years) with liberal use of pregnancy testing.

In evaluating and treating the injured pregnant patient, the surgeon must recognize that to "save the fetus, one must save the mother." Although unnecessary interventions should be avoided in all patients, essential diagnostic or therapeutic procedures must not be withheld from the pregnant patient solely for fear of harming the fetus. The best possible outcome for both the patient and fetus is early, rapid and efficient diagnosis and treatment of sustained injuries. Delays in diagnosis or missed injuries lead to significantly increased maternal–fetal morbidity and mortality. In general, the indications for operative intervention in pregnant patients are not different from those in other trauma patients.

Anatomic and Physiologic Changes in Pregnancy

During pregnancy, physiologic changes occur that alter the physical findings and response to injury after trauma.

Cardiovascular changes stem from the altered hormonal milieu, which leads to total body fluid retention with a 6 to 8 L increase in total body water. This results in a 30% to 40% increase in plasma volume and is accompanied by a 15% increase in red blood cell mass. The result is a dilutional "physiologic anemia" of pregnancy in which hemoglobin may be as low as 11 g per dL. In addition, a 10 to 15 bpm increase in pulse rate is present throughout the pregnancy. Hormone-mediated vasodilation results in relative hypotension (systolic blood pressure of approximately 105 mm Hg). This increased preload and decreased afterload creates a 25% increase in cardiac output. Importantly, late in pregnancy, the weight of the gravid uterus in the supine position may occlude the vena cava, thereby reducing venous return and dramatically limiting cardiac output. An additional important change includes decreased pulmonary functional residual capacity (FRC) as the uterus displaces the diaphragm and lungs. In addition, estrogen and progesterone significantly impair gastrointestinal motility leading to increased gastric distention and risk of aspiration with emergent intubation.

Assessment and Management

The initial evaluation and management of the pregnant patient are identical to that for other trauma victims. Airway, breathing, and circulation are assessed and interventions are initiated to quickly gain cardiopulmonary stability. Early relief of inferior vena cava compression by the gravid uterus by adjusting the patient to the left lateral decubitus position, when possible, augments circulatory stability. One must remember that with the expanded intravascular volume of the pregnant patient, significant blood loss may occur before signs of shock are present. Furthermore, during early shock, the maternal circulation will shunt blood away from the uterus depriving the fetal perfusion as a compensatory mechanism. The fetus may be in distress while the mother is relatively asymptomatic.

A thorough prenatal history, obstetric examination, and fetal evaluation including monitoring are a part of the secondary survey in the pregnant patient. A comprehensive prenatal history should identify pregnancy-induced hypertension, gestational diabetes, or other complicating factors as well as any prenatal care received and the name of the patient's obstetrician. The last menstrual period, the expected delivery date, and the date of perception of fetal movement should also be recorded. The measurement of uterine fundal height serves as a surrogate to estimate fetal age: at 20 weeks the uterus is at the level of the umbilicus and grows roughly 1 cm per week thereafter. Examination of the mother and fetus must also detect or exclude the following: vaginal bleeding, premature rupture of membranes, perineal bulging, uterine contractions, or an abnormal fetal heart rate or rhythm. The abnormal presence of amniotic fluid or blood on vaginal examination and the degree of cervical effacement or dilation must be noted.

Secondary testing is an important adjunct in the evaluation of the gravid trauma patient. Ultrasonography is performed early to confirm or modify fetal age estimations, to assess the fetal position, and to examine the placenta for evidence of abruption. In addition, beyond 20 to 24 weeks of gestation, cardiotocographic (CTM) monitoring is indicated to correlate any maternal contractions with changes in fetal heart rate. Bradycardia (less than 120 bpm) is indicative of fetal distress. Patients with frequent contractions (more than 6 per hour), abdominal pain, vaginal bleeding, hypotension, or an altered cervical examination should have a minimum 24 hours of CTM. Although radiation exposure is an important concern in the first 8 weeks of gestation (the period of organogenesis), it is much less important as the fetus enters the second and third trimesters. The accepted limit for direct fetal radiation exposure is less than 10 rads (0.10 Gy) and the risk to the fetus with direct exposure of less than 5 rads (0.05 Gy) is extremely small. Furthermore, with proper shielding of the abdomen and pelvis, actual direct fetal exposure with nonregional radiography is quite limited. Therefore, it must be stressed again that despite any concerns on the part of the mother or trauma team members about fetal radiation exposure, essential radiographic studies should not be withheld during the trauma evaluation. This includes abdominopelvic CT scans in patients in whom there is concern for intraabdominal injury; the direct fetal radiation exposure is estimated at only 0.5 rads (0.005 Gy).

The Kleihauer-Betke (K-B) test is used to detect the presence of fetal blood in the maternal circulation after injury and should be performed in all Rh-negative gravidas. Fetal hemoglobin F (HbF) can be detected in a maternal sample by using commercial kits that rely on differential staining between HbF and adult hemoglobin A (HbA). The test is quantitative and is used to estimate the volume of fetomaternal transfusion. A positive test indicates the possibility of maternal sensitization to fetal blood in the Rh-negative mother and should prompt the administration of Rh-immune globulin (RhoGAM) 300 μg per 30 mL of estimated fetomaternal transfusion.

Because the likelihood of fetal viability is high after a gestational age greater than 20 to 24 weeks, early obstetric consultation is indicated in such patients. Furthermore, most patients in this group, irrespective of injury or mechanism, will be monitored for cardiotocographic changes for 24 hours on an obstetric ward and are typically released at the discretion of the evaluating obstetrician. Evidence of placental abruption in a gestationally viable pregnancy will typically prompt immediate operative delivery.

KEY POINTS

▲ In patients with traumatic brain injury, the primary injury cannot be undone; the goal of therapy is to prevent secondary brain injury by maintaining tissue oxygenation to uninjured but at-risk brain parenchyma.

▲ Stable patients with penetrating neck injuries require both vasculature and aerodigestive tract evaluation. Classically zones I and III are managed by angiography and endoscopy, whereas zone II is managed operatively. Unstable patients require exploration irrespective of the zone of injury.

▲ All blunt trauma patients require cervical spine evaluation either by physical examination or with radiography.

▲ Many life-threatening chest injuries, either blunt or penetrating, have subtle presentations—physical examination and/or chest x-ray can reliably identify or exclude most injuries.

▲ Essentially all patients with penetrating trauma to the anterior abdomen must undergo exploratory laparotomy. Rare exceptions require advanced decision-making and extensive clinical experience.

▲ All patients with blunt abdominal trauma must have objective evaluation to exclude intraabdominal injury. Serial examinations, serial ultrasounds, diagnostic peritoneal lavage (DPL), and computerized tomographic

(CT) scan are accepted options.

▲ DPL is an invasive objective test for excluding intraabdominal injury. It is very sensitive but not specific and currently has a limited role. Focused abdominal sonography for trauma (FAST) is more commonly used and identifies free fluid in the dependent portions of the abdomen; it also lacks specificity.

▲ All patients with extremity trauma require special attention to the vascular examination. Signs of vascular injury require angiogram or operative exploration.

▲ Surgeons must learn to recognize "conditions, complexes, and critical factors" that place patients at risk for hypothermia, coagulopathy, and acidosis. Early termination of procedures after control of life-threatening hemorrhage "damage control" will prevent death in severely injured patients.

▲ Pregnant trauma patients are evaluated initially in the same manner as nonpregnant patients. Early obstetric consultation in pregnancies greater than 20 weeks of gestation is encouraged. Secondary testing should be utilized as needed as maternal missed injuries are more detrimental to the fetus than the theoretical risk of moderate radiation exposure.

SUGGESTED READINGS

Ivatury RR, Cayten CG, eds. *The textbook of penetrating trauma*, Baltimore: Williams & Wilkins, 1996.

Moore EE, Mattox ML, Feliciano DV, eds. *Trauma*, 5th ed. New York: McGraw-Hill, 2004.

Peitzman AB, Rhodes M, Schwab CW, et al., eds. *The trauma manual*, 2nd ed. Philadelphia: Lippincott Williams & Wilkins, 2002.

Rotondo MF, Schwab CW, McGonigal MD, et al. Damage control and approach for improved survival in exsanguinating penetrating abdominal trauma. *J Trauma* 1993;49:969–978.

Trauma and Emergency Care. In: Cameron J, ed. *Current surgical therapy*, 8th ed. Philadelphia: Elsevier-Mosby, 2004:897–1041.

Burn Management

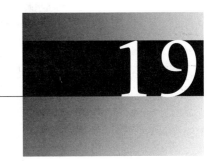

19

Mark F. Berry   James H. Holmes IV
C. William Schwab

INTRODUCTION

Approximately 1.25 million burn injuries occur each year in the United States. The majority of burns are thermal injuries, although electricity, chemical contact, and frostbite can also cause injury. Most burns are of limited extent and managed on an outpatient basis. However, burns result in approximately 45,000 hospital admissions and 4,000 deaths each year, mostly involving young children and the elderly, who have the greatest difficulty escaping from a fire. Approximately 25% of serious burns are work related. More than 90% of burns are considered preventable, and about one half involve substance abuse, including alcohol and smoking.

Burn treatment advances have improved patient survival and quality of life considerably over the last few decades. Advances in understanding the need for appropriate fluid resuscitation and early burn wound excision and grafting have significantly improved mortality rates. The median lethal dose (LD_{50}) for burns was 80% total body surface area (TBSA) in the year 2000, compared to 30% TBSA in 1970. The most recent advances in burn care over the last decade have focused on improving the long-term functional and cosmetic outcomes of burn wound treatment.

THERMAL BURNS

Incidence and Etiology

Most thermal burns are caused by scalds from hot substances. These burns generally have a low mortality but can have a high morbidity. Approximately one third of burns are caused by fire and flame sources. Unattended and/or improperly positioned cooking and heating devices are the leading causes of residential fires. Careless smoking is the most common cause of residential fire deaths (25%), followed by arson and defective or inappropriately used heating devices. Playing with matches or lighters is the cause of approximately 10% of residential fire deaths. Most burn deaths occur in residential fires during cold winter months when heating and lighting devices are most commonly used, especially in low income areas and multifamily dwellings.

Pathophysiology

Local Burn Wound Injury

Adult skin has a surface area of 1.5 to 2.0 m^2 with a depth of 1 to 2 mm. Skin has an outer layer of epidermis and an inner layer of dermis (Fig. 19-1). The epidermis consists of a keratinized squamous epithelium that extends into underlying dermal appendages. The dermis lies underneath the basal layer of the epidermis to provide flexibility, support, and strength through its attachment to subcutaneous tissues. Skin functions as a protective barrier and contributes to protein, fluid, and electrolyte balance. Skin also has thermoregulatory, neurosensory, immunologic, and metabolic functions, and plays a key role in social interactions.

Burns damage skin in several ways. The initial heat energy causes cell damage, denaturing of proteins, and surface vessel thrombosis. The depth of thermal injury depends on contact time with and the temperature of the source. Wet heat travels more rapidly into tissue than dry heat. Burns caused by grease or asphalt have prolonged contact times that contribute to deeper injury. An inflammatory process follows the initial heat-mediated injury and can cause further local tissue destruction as well as systemic changes, as described in the subsequent text.

A burn wound has three histologic zones of injury. The zone of coagulation is the central, most severely damaged area of tissue where cells are necrotic and unsalvageable. The zone of stasis is deep and peripheral to the zone of coagulation, where cells are viable but vulnerable to further injury. Local perfusion defects caused by systemic hypovolemia, edema, vasoconstriction, and vascular thrombosis from both the burn and the subsequent inflammatory process can cause ischemia in the zone of stasis and extend the amount of tissue injured. The zone of hyperemia is an area deep and peripheral to the zone of stasis with vasodilation and minimal cell injury.

Burn wounds are classified according to the depth of injury into skin and subcutaneous tissues as *superficial*, *partial-thickness*, or *full-thickness* burns. A *superficial* burn, formerly classified as first-degree, involves only superficial

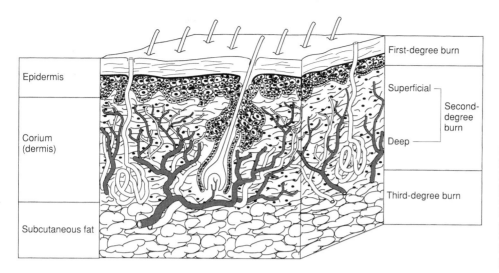

Figure 19-1 Depiction of skin. Degree of burn injury is classified based on depth of penetration. (From Sheridan RL, Tompkins RG. Burns. In: Greenfield LJ, Mulholand MW, Oldham KT et al., eds. *Surgery: scientific principles and practice*, 2nd ed. Philadelphia: Lippincott-Raven Publishers, 1997:423, with permission.)

epidermal damage in which the epidermis remains intact and is equivalent to "sunburn." The area is erythematous and painful, but does not contain any blisters. *Partial-thickness* burns, formerly called second-degree, involve both the epidermis and dermis and are categorized as either superficial or deep. A superficial partial-thickness burn appears moist and pink, is extremely painful, and blanches with pressure. Blisters are usually present as fluid accumulates at the epidermal-dermal junction. Nerve endings and dermal appendages remain intact. Deep partial-thickness burns also blister, but have a wound surface that appears red with patchy white areas or as a dry white area. Some sensation and pain is preserved, but these wounds are not exquisitely tender. *Full-thickness burns*, formerly classified as third-degree, involve loss of the entire dermis and epidermis. The area is firm and depressed compared to adjacent normal skin, is insensate owing to complete destruction of nerve endings, and appears whitish-gray with a leathery appearance. Wounds are classified as greater than full-thickness if the underlying subcutaneous fat, muscle, connective tissue, or bone is also damaged.

Burn wounds heal by a combination of wound contraction and reepithelialization from epidermal cells lining both the periphery of the wound as well as dermal appendages. Superficial burns generally heal within 5 days without scarring. Superficial partial-thickness burns usually heal spontaneously within 3 weeks without excessive scarring. Deeper wounds require more than 3 weeks for spontaneous healing because of a significant loss of skin appendages. Primary healing of deep burns is universally associated with scarring and frequently complicated by hypertrophic scarring and contractures that have undesirable functional/cosmetic outcomes. Only very small areas, generally less than 2 cm in diameter, can heal by contraction within acceptable time frames and with reasonable cosmetic outcomes.

Burn wounds are initially sterile but quickly become colonized by endogenous bacteria within 72 hours of injury. At first, gram-positive bacteria predominate, but by the fifth postburn day, gram-negative organisms colonize the burn. Bacteria proliferate and penetrate the avascular zone of coagulation until reaching the nonviable/viable tissue interface. Systemic invasion can occur if host defense is compromised, resulting in burn wound sepsis.

Burn Shock and Cardiovascular Effects

Burns greater than 35% to 40% TBSA usually result in severe cardiovascular derangements known as burn shock. Burn shock is hemodynamically characterized by low cardiac output, a reduced effective arterial blood volume, decreased urine output, and increased systemic vascular resistance (SVR), which collectively lead to microvascular hypoperfusion. Cardiac output decreases within minutes after injury in proportion to burn size, although the heart is typically hyperdynamic during this period. The reduction in cardiac output after burn injury is a result of cellular shock, hypovolemic shock, and increased SVR due to sympathetic stimulation from the release of multiple mediators. The cardiac myocyte shock state is a result of impaired calcium homeostasis and subsequent intracellular signaling dysregulation. This is likely caused by the burn trauma itself as well as induction of tumor necrosis factor, which leads to a significant increase in myocyte cytosolic free calcium ion concentrations. Following successful resuscitation, cardiac output normalizes within 24 to 72 hours and then increases to supranormal levels during the wound-healing phase.

Thermal injury causes hypovolemia due to a massive fluid shift from the intravascular to the interstitial space. Capillary endothelial injury and precipitation of protein leads to edema in the burned tissue within 15 to 30 minutes. Thermal injury also causes the release of inflammatory mediators from injured mast cells in the skin and activated neutrophils and macrophages. These mediators cause edema in nonburned tissue both directly by altering vascular permeability and indirectly by causing vasodilation that increases microvascular hydrostatic pressure. This systemic capillary leak increases sharply over the first 6 hours and more slowly over the next 18 hours until equilibrium is reached and edema formation stops approximately 24 hours after injury.

Many inflammatory mediators are implicated in the pathogenesis of burn shock. Histamine is thought to be the mediator responsible for the increased capillary permeability seen early after a burn, by disrupting venular endothelial tight junctions. Other mediators that play a role include arachidonic acid metabolites, bradykinin, serotonin, catecholamines, and multiple cytokines.

Pulmonary Effects

Burns have multiple effects on the pulmonary system. In the absence of chest wall or inhalation injury, burns generally cause predictable changes in a patient's pulmonary status. The initial hypovolemic state usually results in tachypneic, shallow breathing. A few days after a burn, adequately resuscitated patients are hypermetabolic and typically have a hyperventilation breathing pattern with a respiratory alkalosis. Resuscitated patients can also have mild hypoxemia secondary to pulmonary edema from significant fluid resuscitation.

Chest wall and inhalation injury cause further pulmonary dysfunction. Circumferential burns of the thorax lead to loss of tissue elasticity that can restrict chest wall excursion and impair ventilation, particularly as edema develops with resuscitation. Inhalation injury occurs in almost 20% of patients with a 50% TBSA burn and significantly increases mortality above that which would be expected based on TBSA alone for any given burn severity. Inhalation injury is generally divided into upper airway and lower airway patterns. Upper airway injury results in acute mortality, whereas lower airway injury generally results in delayed mortality.

Direct thermal injury to structures above and including the vocal cords leads to rapid upper airway edema that can cause obstruction. This edema typically increases progressively over the first 24 to 36 hours, after which it subsides. Because of efficient upper airway heat dissipation, lower airway inhalation injury is not caused by direct thermal damage, but rather by toxic products of incomplete thermal combustion. Type I pneumocyte damage causes gas exchange difficulties, whereas type II pneumocyte damage leads to inefficient surfactant secretion and small airway collapse. The cumulative result is airway obstruction, intrapulmonary shunting, compromised endobronchial debris clearance, and progressive hypoxia with respiratory failure. Clinically, the patient may show signs of respiratory distress at any time up to approximately 48 hours after the time of injury. Approximately 40% of those with an inhalation injury will develop pneumonia.

Neurologic Effects

Exposure to combustion products such as carbon monoxide (CO) can lead to tissue anoxia and death, which is initially manifested by neurological changes. CO, an odorless product of hypoxic combustion, has an affinity for hemoglobin 200 times that of oxygen and leads to tissue hypoxia by displacing oxygen from its binding site on the hemoglobin molecule. The CO half-life of 4 hours breathing room air is decreased to 40 to 60 minutes by the administration of 100% oxygen. Hyperbaric oxygen therapy at 2 to 3 atm of pressure reduces the half-life further to approximately 30 minutes. Normal blood CO levels range from 3% to 5% in nonsmokers and 7% to 10% in smokers. Symptoms of CO poisoning can occur when levels are 10% to 20%, with mortality occurring at levels greater than 50% to 60%. Symptoms range from headache and nausea and vomiting at lower levels to syncope, confusion, coma, and cardiorespiratory collapse at higher levels. Postexposure neurologic sequelae include parkinsonism, cortical blindness, deafness, memory deficits, and frank psychosis that can persist in up to 10% of individuals who have CO poisoning. However, very few patients develop permanent impairment, as most either die or fully recover from their symptoms.

Hydrogen cyanide (CN) is a combustion product of nitrogen-containing polymers often present in closed-space industrial fires. CN combines with the cytochrome complex to inhibit oxidative phosphorylation and halt mitochondrial aerobic activity. Lactic acidosis and tissue anoxia are seen despite normal blood oxygen content. Symptoms include lethargy, weakness, headache, nausea, and an altered level of consciousness. CN poisoning rarely occurs without CO poisoning.

Metabolic Effects

The metabolic response to thermal injury is biphasic. The immediate, or ebb phase, is a 12 to 24 hour period of hypometabolism. After resuscitation, the patient enters the flow phase, where cardiac output and metabolic rate can be double that of resting values. Elevated oxygen consumption and increased body temperature to as high as 38.5°C is often seen. This process, driven mainly by catecholamines, cortisol, and glucagon stimulated by the needs of the burn wound, results in protein catabolism with muscle wasting, lipolysis with futile fatty acid cycling and hepatic steatosis, and profound weight loss if the patient does not receive adequate nutritional support.

Gastrointestinal Effects

The initial decrease in cardiac output leads to decreased splanchnic blood flow, which weakens gastrointestinal mucosal defenses and can result in ulceration (Curling ulcer). Even when fluid resuscitation restores normal blood flow, focal gastric and duodenal mucosal ischemia can be observed as early as 3 to 5 hours postburn. Small bowel and colonic hypoperfusion can also result in mucosal alteration and increased permeability. Although perforation is rare, bacterial translocation is frequent in the burn patient. An ileus persisting for 3 to 5 days postburn may occur in patients with larger burns unless early, aggressive enteral nutrition is provided.

Renal Effects

Changes in renal function after burns are typically a result of the initial hypovolemic state and the subsequent fluid resuscitation. However, patients with high-voltage electrical injury or those with burns involving extensive muscle destruction can have significant myoglobinemia, which can lead to renal dysfunction if a brisk diuresis is not achieved.

Immunologic and Hematologic Effects

The integument is the largest immunologic organ in the body. As such, major burn injury causes immunosuppression to a degree directly proportional to burn size. Alterations in cellular and humoral immunity are seen with T-cell and neutrophil dysfunction, and a depletion of complement and immunoglobulins. This immunosuppression combined with protective skin loss significantly increases susceptibility to infections, ranging from suppurative thrombophlebitis at intravenous line sites to invasive burn wound sepsis. The most common organism isolated from the blood of the burned patient is *Staphylococcus aureus*. Burn wound sepsis caused by *Pseudomonas aeruginosa*, formerly very common, is now rare because of aggressive wound management involving early excision and grafting. Pneumonia is the most common infectious complication in the burn patient, and accounts for approximately 50% of burn fatalities. Pneumonia in the burn patient is most commonly caused by *S. aureus* or gram-negative opportunistic bacteria that colonize the burn patient. Immune function generally returns to normal 2 to 3 weeks after a burn in uncomplicated courses.

Burns result in biphasic changes to the clotting factors. At first, the microthrombi that form both locally and systemically as a result of the burn cause a consumptive coagulopathy characterized by a relative thrombocytopenia, a drop in fibrinogen level, and an increase in fibrin split products. Following resuscitation, there is a prompt return to normal and even supranormal levels of platelets, fibrinogen, and other coagulation proteins. Despite this apparent pro-thrombotic state, clinically significant thromboembolic phenomena are surprisingly infrequent in the burn population.

Treatment of the Burn Patient

Management of the burn patient can be divided into stages of initial assessment, initiation of resuscitation, secondary survey, burn wound assessment, wound care, and wound coverage.

Initial Assessment

The first treatment step is removing the patient from the source of injury and stopping the burning process. If the burned tissue has not cooled spontaneously, cool tap water or saline is poured directly on the burned area to cool the area and potentially reduce the depth of the burn and pain, although cooling measures must never cause hypothermia. Ice can potentiate injury via local vasoconstriction and should not be used. After cooling, burned areas are covered with a clean dressing or sheet to control pain and heat loss. Initial management of a burned patient is then the same as for any trauma patient, starting with a primary survey to rapidly identify any life-threatening conditions, followed by a thorough head-to-toe secondary survey.

Initial care of a burned victim starts with the ABCs – airway, breathing, circulation. Focusing on the surface manifestation of the burn, no matter how horrific, can cause the care provider to overlook other life-threatening injuries. An adequate airway and ventilation must be ensured, which can be problematic in patients with inhalation injury or cervicofacial injuries. The presence of singed eyebrows or facial hair, evidence of burns in and around the mouth and nose, hoarseness or any other change in voice quality, and carbonaceous sputum are signs of possible inhalation injury. History of confinement in a closed space should also raise the physician's suspicion for inhalation injury. Any patient who has respiratory distress, stridor, progressive hoarseness, or significant burns of the face or neck should be endotracheally intubated for airway protection as early as possible. All patients, even those without respiratory distress, are given 100% humidified oxygen during transport and during initial treatment in the emergency department. Individuals with minor upper airway injuries can be managed expectantly without intubation, but respiratory status in all patients must be continually monitored and assessed. Progressive airway edema can rapidly develop after fluid resuscitation is started and requires delayed intubation or an emergent surgical airway.

Every patient's chest must be exposed and assessed for adequate chest wall excursion with respiration, as the eschar of circumferential full-thickness burns can restrict chest movement. Escharotomy is needed if ventilation is impaired or if airway pressures are significantly elevated. This procedure can be performed painlessly at the bedside with minimal blood loss. The eschar is incised in the bilateral anterior axillary lines, extending from the clavicle to below the costal margin (Fig. 19-2). Electrocautery is preferred but a scalpel can be used. The anterior axillary escharotomies can

be connected by a subcostal incision if chest wall motion is still inadequate.

Intravenous access for pain control and fluid resuscitation should be established in all patients with burns greater than 10% to 20% TBSA, inhalation injury, or concomitant nonthermal trauma. Peripheral large-bore catheters are preferred and should be placed through normal skin if possible, although placement through the burn wound is acceptable if the only option. Central access is obtained if no peripheral site is available or invasive hemodynamic monitoring is needed.

Resuscitation

Appropriate fluid resuscitation of the hypovolemic state that results from fluid sequestration due to the initial burn is critical to the survival and overall outcome of the burn patient.

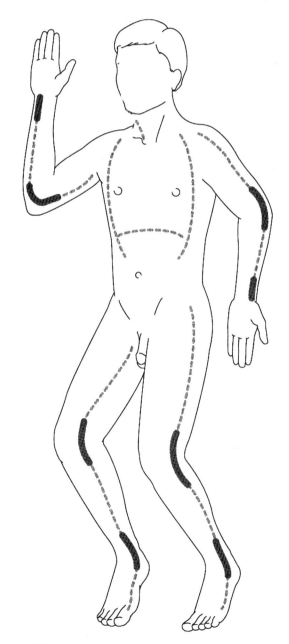

Figure 19-2   Preferred sites for escharotomy incisions. (From Moylan JA, Wellford WJ, Pruitt BA. Circulatory changes following circumferential extremity burns evaluated by the ultrasonic flowmeter: an analysis of 60 thermally injured limbs. *J Trauma* 1971;11:767, with permission.)

Formal fluid resuscitation is needed for adults with a greater than 20% TBSA burn or children with a greater than 10% TBSA burn. Patients with smaller burns generally can be "orally resuscitated." After the primary and secondary surveys exclude the presence of immediate life-threatening conditions, a more careful evaluation of the burn wounds with an accurate determination of severity is performed.

The extent of a burn can be estimated by using various techniques, including the Rule of 9s. The body is divided into 11 parts, each making up 9% of the TBSA (head, left arm, right arm, anterior chest, posterior chest, anterior abdomen, lower back, left upper leg, left lower leg, right upper leg, and right lower leg) with the perineum making up 1% of TBSA. However, the Rule of 9s is notoriously inaccurate in young children, as their head and thighs represent a much greater percentage of the TBSA relative to adults. Formal burn diagrams, available in any emergency department, are more accurate and can help avoid serious miscalculations (Fig. 19-3).

Various types of fluid and several formulas for estimating needs have been used for burn patient resuscitation. The most commonly used formula is the Parkland formula, which calculates the total fluid requirement as follows:

Parkland formula: (4 mL lactated Ringer solution)
$\times$ (body weight in kg) $\times$ (% TBSA burned)

Only partial-thickness, indeterminate, and full-thickness burns are used in calculating fluid requirements. One half of the calculated fluid requirement is given in the first 8 hours from the time of injury, and the remainder is given over the following 16 hours. Additional, appropriately calculated, dextrose-based maintenance fluid should be added for children weighing less than 20 kg, as their glycogen stores are insufficient to maintain euglycemia during formal resuscitation.

Any resuscitation formula should function only as a guide. The patient's physiologic response to fluid administration should ultimately direct therapy to avoid both over and under resuscitation. Of note, patients with inhalation injury typically require resuscitation volumes in excess of those calculated. The goal of resuscitation is normalization of hemodynamics and adequate end-organ perfusion. Resuscitation beyond this point will only lead to additional edema which may compromise care. The best monitor of the adequacy of resuscitation is following the hourly urine output. A Foley catheter is required and should be placed early. The goal is a urine output of 0.5 to 1.0 mL/kg/h in adults and 1.0 to 1.5 mL/kg/h in children averaged over 2 to 3 hours. Inadequate urine output is responded to by increasing the intravenous fluid rate, not by administering fluid boluses. Invasive hemodynamic monitoring with a pulmonary artery catheter is generally not indicated, although it may be useful in patients with preexisting cardiopulmonary disease or other complicating factors.

Diuretics are not indicated to improve urine output in burn patients. Patients with myoglobinuria secondary to electrical injury or crush injury are the only possible exceptions, but fluid should first be administered above resuscitation protocols in such patients to achieve a urine output of 75 to 100 mL per hour. Failure to achieve adequate output despite additional fluid administration is an indication for a diuretic during the resuscitation phase. The patient is preferably given mannitol until the desired urine output is achieved, and pigment clears from the urine. Because myoglobin is more soluble in an alkaline solution, some clinicians advocate alkalinizing the urine to enhance renal clearance by the addition of sodium bicarbonate to the resuscitation fluid. Once a diuretic is administered, urine output is no longer a safe indicator of intravascular volume status and central monitoring should be used to guide resuscitation.

Colloid should generally not be administered in the first 24 hours, as the capillary leak that initially occurs after thermal injury makes it no better than crystalloid. After the first 24 hours, patients who have a low serum oncotic pressure due to intravascular protein depletion can have protein repletion with albumin. Recommendations for albumin administration vary over the second 24 hours. Patients should also begin to receive dextrose-based maintenance fluids following their resuscitation, with electrolytes being monitored and corrected as necessary.

Secondary Survey

The secondary survey involves a thorough history, including the mechanism and time of injury, a description of the surrounding environment, whether the burn occurred in an enclosed space, the possibility of smoke inhalation, the presence of any chemicals, and any related nonthermal trauma. Loss of consciousness or an explosion could signal closed head or other bodily injuries. Comorbid medical conditions, current medications, allergies, and tetanus status must be determined. A complete head-to-toe examination is performed.

CO exposure should always be suspected, particularly for burns that occurred within an enclosed space or in any patient with neurologic signs or symptoms. Normal transcutaneous oxygen saturation does not preclude CO poisoning, and the level of carboxyhemoglobin (COHgb) must be measured. CO treatment should be empiric in the field, and administration of 100% oxygen by face mask or endotracheal tube usually reduces CO levels significantly by the time the patient arrives in the emergency department. Hyperbaric oxygen therapy should be considered in patients with neurologic signs or symptoms or COHgb levels greater than 25% without major concomitant burns. The cumbersome resuscitation of the burned patient in an enclosed hyperbaric chamber, however, precludes its general use. Treatment for CN poisoning should also be based on clinical suspicion (injury history and profound lactic acidosis),

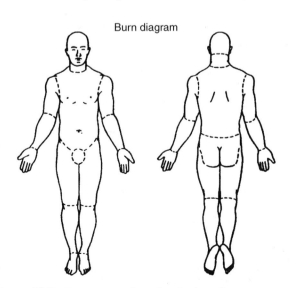

Burn diagram

Figure 19-3 Burn estimate based on body surface area.

as standard CN level testing can take hours to perform, and the symptoms of CN poisoning are indistinguishable from that of CO poisoning. The patient should be given 100% oxygen along with intravenous sodium thiosulfate (125 to 250 mg per kg) and hydroxocobalamin (4 g).

The patient's respiratory status should be continually monitored and reassessed, particularly since patients with a lower airway inhalation injury may not manifest signs and symptoms until a few days after the initial injury. The workup of the patient with suspicion for inhalation injury begins with a thorough oronasopharyngeal inspection. The supraglottic passages are examined for signs of upper airway injury, which include edema, erythema, or a carbonaceous coating. Bronchoscopy may aid diagnosis in selected patients with equivocal physical examination findings. Bronchoscopic evidence of mucosal inflammation, ulceration, deposition of carbon particles, or loss of definition of the septa dividing the bronchial orifices is indicative of lower airway injury. A false-negative bronchoscopy can result from insufficient resuscitation and failure of inflammatory changes to develop in the underperfused mucosa. Bronchoscopy can be risky in an irritated airway, and intubation should be performed before bronchoscopy if there are any concerns regarding the patient's airway status.

The treatment of inhalation injury is supportive. Patients with progressive hypoxia or respiratory distress may require mechanical ventilation, with attention paid to avoiding barotrauma and further injury. The use of appropriate levels of positive end-expiratory pressure can reduce the fraction of inspired oxygen required, and high frequency oscillating/jet ventilation may decrease the incidence of barotrauma and facilitate the clearance of secretions. Patients who do not require mechanical ventilation should be given supplemental oxygen with therapeutic coughing, chest physiotherapy, early ambulation, and tracheobronchial suctioning performed to assist airway clearance of debris and reduce the chance of developing pneumonia. Rarely therapeutic bronchoscopy may be required to clear airway secretions if these less invasive measures fail.

Assessment of peripheral extremity perfusion with a thorough pulse examination must be performed both initially and during the first few days after the burn. Edema of constricting circumferential eschar can compromise blood flow to the arms and legs. Escharotomy may be required if pulses are diminished or absent by Doppler examination or if the patient has any signs or symptoms of compartment syndrome. The five Ps of a compartment syndrome (pain, paresthesia, pallor, pulselessness, and poikilothermia) can be difficult to assess in a charred extremity, and clinical suspicion is sufficient reason for an escharotomy. Escharotomy is typically performed at the bedside, but can be done in the operating room depending on institutional protocols. Incisions through the eschar are made along planes designed to avoid major vessels and nerves, preferably with electrocautery (Fig. 19-2). Care must be taken not to incise viable subcutaneous tissue, as this may precipitate extensive hemorrhaging. Fasciotomy is rarely needed and performed only when escharotomies do not decompress the limb in patients with deep thermal or electrical burns.

The burned patient must be carefully monitored for any sign of infection. Because patients with inhalation injury are particularly susceptible to pneumonia, sputum cultures and gram stains should be obtained at the first sign of clinical deterioration to guide antimicrobial therapy. Atelectasis frequently precedes pneumonia and can be seen gradually developing on chest x-ray as an ill-defined pneumonic process. In contrast, the sudden appearance of a solitary, round infiltrate on a routine chest x-ray can be the first indication of a hematogenous pneumonia, and the patient should be examined closely for an infected wound (see subsequent text) or a vein harboring an area of septic thrombophlebitis, which must be completely drained.

Successful support of severely burned patients through the early hypodynamic phase must be followed with adequate nutritional support through the subsequent hyperdynamic phase, when the patient's resting energy expenditure is 1.5 to 2.5 times the normal basal level. Although patients with large burns may develop an ileus, this can be thwarted by starting appropriate high-protein enteral nutrition as soon as possible following injury. Glutamine (Gln) supplementation, in particular, appears to be important following major thermal injury. Gln is the preferred metabolic substrate of both small intestinal enterocytes and lymphocytes. Exogenous Gln supplementation at approximately 30 g per day has been shown to reduce infectious morbidity and overall mortality after major burns. Early enteral nutrition not only helps support the increased metabolic needs of the burn patient, but also preserves gastrointestinal integrity, decreases bacterial translocation and wasting of visceral protein, and limits acalculous cholecystitis. Total parenteral nutrition is rarely indicated in burn patients and is associated with increased mortality. Sudden onset of ileus or hyperglycemia in a patient previously tolerating enteral feeds is an early sign of systemic infection, and requires cessation of feedings and aggressive investigation to identify a septic focus.

All burn patients must be followed for any signs of gastrointestinal ulceration. Patients with large burns likely require initial stress ulcer prophylaxis with sucralfate, H_2-blockers, proton-pump inhibitors, or antacids. Early institution of total enteral nutrition and/or gastric acid control has virtually eliminated the incidence of perforation of and bleeding from Curling ulcers, which had been the most life-threatening gastrointestinal complications seen after burn. Although burn patients have a lower than expected incidence of deep venous thrombi after injury, patients with a prolonged hospital course need some form of prophylaxis, either with compression devices or heparin.

Indications for inpatient care depend on both the size of the burn as well as the circumstances surrounding the injury. Patients with partial- and full-thickness burns involving more than 10% to 20% TBSA should be admitted for fluid resuscitation, pain control, and management of the wound. Lesser burns with associated inhalation injury, concurrent trauma, or preexisting medical conditions are also better managed in a hospital setting. Electrical injury, including lightning injury, carries the added risk of dysrhythmias. In addition, any patient for whom outpatient therapy fails should be admitted. Table 19-1 lists the criteria for transfer to a burn center.

Cases of suspected child abuse and neglect should be admitted no matter what the extent of the actual burn. Caregivers are obligated to report their suspicions to the appropriate local agency for proper investigation. A high level of awareness is required to identify child or elder abuse. The physician's suspicions should be aroused whenever an odd mechanism, inconsistent history, sharply defined borders, or circumferential injury is involved in the burn of a dependent child or elderly person. Accidental

TABLE 19-1

AMERICAN BURN ASSOCIATION CRITERIA FOR TRANSFER TO A BURN CENTER

Burn involving TBSA >20% in patients ages 10–50 years

Burn involving TBSA >10% in patients younger than 10 or older than 50 years

Full-thickness burns >5% in patients of any age

Burns that involve the face, hands, feet, eyes, ears, or perineum

High voltage electrical injury

Significant chemical burns

Multiple trauma patients in whom the burn is thought to pose the greatest risk of morbidity and mortality

Inhalation injury

Patients with significant comorbidities that can potentially complicate treatment

Patients with burns who are expected to require extensive social or rehabilitative support (e.g., substance abuse, child abuse)

TBSA, total body surface area.

burns should always manifest an unequal pattern of injury as the child or elder moves away from the heat. Any burn that conforms exactly to the shape of an object or is uniform in all directions because of prolonged contact may have been intentional.

Burn Wound Assessment

Initial care and assessment of the burn wound should include gentle cleaning with soap and water and removal of loose nonviable skin. In contrast to the assessment of the burn size, initial evaluation of burn depth is notoriously inaccurate. Determining the depth of burns that fall between very shallow and very deep burns is difficult, particularly during the early period of resuscitation. The clinical assessment of burn depth will change frequently during the first postinjury week as a result of an inaccurate initial observation or because of progressive injury in the zone of stasis, either inevitable or due to inadequate resuscitation. Fortunately, accurate burn depth estimation is not necessary for resuscitation because partial- and full-thickness burns are treated the same. However, accurate evaluation of burn wound depth becomes very important in the first few days following successful resuscitation, as burn wound depth guides burn wound care, as described in subsequent text. Although numerous technical aids such as laser Doppler flowmeter, vital dyes, and staining have been devised to aid in this determination, clinical observation remains the standard for the assessment of burn wound depth.

All burn wounds are tetanus-prone. If the patient is within 10 years of his or her last tetanus immunization, 0.5 mL of tetanus toxoid should be administered. If the patient is improperly immunized, tetanus toxin antibody should be given concurrently in the contralateral arm. Any patient whose immunization status is unknown or whose last booster was more than 10 years ago should also receive 250 U of tetanus immunoglobulin.

Burn Wound Care

Expectant Management

The primary objective of burn wound care is to have all wounds healed within 1 month. Modern treatment involves excision of wounds not expected to heal spontaneously within 3 weeks. As described previously, shallow burns will generally heal within 3 weeks and therefore are managed nonoperatively. Superficial burns with an intact epidermis require neither topical agents nor dressings. Superficial partial-thickness burns are managed with daily wound care consisting of loose skin débridement, cleansing with soap and water, topical antimicrobials, and sterile dressing application. Although recommendations vary, a reasonable policy for managing blisters is to leave intact blisters alone unless they limit extremity range of motion, as unroofing blisters exposes a painful underlying wound that is potentially more susceptible to infection.

Systemically administrated antibiotics generally do not achieve therapeutic levels at the burn wound surface and prophylactic administration has no role in burn wound treatment. Topically applied agents, in contrast, provide high drug concentrations at the wound surface to control the bacterial population, although the burn wound is not sterilized. Three topical antimicrobial agents are currently used in routine burn wound care: silver sulfadiazine (Silvadene), mafenide acetate (Sulfamylon), and silver nitrate. Silvadene is most commonly used. Each agent is bacteriostatic and has specific advantages and side effects as described in Table 19-2. Both Sulfamylon and Silvadene contain a sulfa moiety as an active ingredient and should be used with caution on patients with a documented sulfa allergy or glucose-6-phosphate dehydrogenase deficiency. In addition, topical bacitracin is often used, particularly on facial burns as Silvadene treatment may result in pigmentation changes or corneal irritation.

Burns involving "critical" areas such as the face, eyes, ears, hands, feet, and perineum are ultimately managed as any other thermal injury of similar severity. However, the complexity and protracted nature of their successful management warrants referral to a dedicated burn center.

An occlusive burn dressing, generally consisting of cotton gauze, protects underlying tissue, reduces evaporative heat loss, and improves comfort by limiting air currents from the very sensitive wound surface. Dressings should generally be changed at least daily for inspection and cleansing of the wound, and to allow early identification of infection and prevention of systemic complications. Conversion of a partial-thickness to a full-thickness burn, early eschar separation, and dark-brown or black discoloration of the burn wound are all signs of invasive wound infection. Histologic examination of a burn wound biopsy is the most accurate way to confirm the diagnosis of invasive infections. A tissue sample of the eschar and underlying unburned tissue is obtained using a scalpel. A portion of the sample is sent to the microbiology laboratory for identification of the organisms and a portion is sent to pathology for frozen section analysis. Quantitative counts of greater than 10^5 organisms per gram of tissue indicate the presence of invasive infection, particularly if microorganisms are seen extending into viable uninjured tissue. Vascular or lymphatic invasion may also indicate systemic infection. Therapy should be switched to mafenide acetate for increased eschar penetration if a nonpenetrating antimicrobial agent is being used. Systemic antibiotics are promptly administered based on microbial sensitivity, and the patient is scheduled for immediate wound excision.

An alternative to classic wound care for the treatment of superficial partial-thickness burns is thorough cleansing

TABLE 19-2

TOPICAL ANTIBIOTICS USED IN BURN WOUND CARE

Agent	Advantages	Disadvantages
Silver sulfadiazine (Silvadene) 1% cream	Well tolerated Painless application	Poor eschar penetration Transient leukopenia in 5% to 15% of cases Rash in 5% of cases Limited activity against *Pseudomonas* and *Enterobacter cloacae*
Mafenide acetate (Sulfamylon) 11% cream and 5% solution	Eschar penetration Broad spectrum of activity	Painful application (especially with cream) Carbonic anhydrase inhibition can cause hyperchloremic metabolic acidosis Rash in 5% of cases No fungal coverage
Silver nitrate 0.5% suspension	Painless application Broad spectrum of activity, including fungi	Difficult to apply, stains everything black Bulky dressings limit joint motion Poor eschar penetration Can cause electrolyte disturbances by leaching sodium, potassium, chloride, and calcium from wound

followed by the immediate application of a biologic dressing that is left in place until healing is complete. Examples of biologic dressings are Trans-cyte, BGC-matrix, Biobrane, porcine xenograft, and cadaveric allograft. Biobrane is a bilaminate composed of an inner layer of knitted nylon threads coated with porcine collagen and an outer layer of silicone pervious to gases but not liquids. Biobrane, which can be applied to fresh moist wounds free of necrotic debris and left in place until reepithelialization, may result in less pain and shorter healing times. Another alternative dressing is Acticoat, which is a nonadherent, silver impregnated antimicrobial barrier that can be left in place up to 3 to 7 days. These dressings are fairly expensive but, if successful, eliminate the need for frequent dressing changes. However, these dressings must be used with care as underlying infection can be masked, and a learning curve is associated with the use of each dressing.

Patients treated on an outpatient basis should be seen frequently in follow-up. If the area remains free of infection, the patient is monitored as an outpatient until the wound heals. Any sign of wound infection mandates immediate hospitalization and the initiation of systemic antibiotics.

Operative Management

Elucidation of the deleterious systemic effects of burn eschar due to mediator release and recognition that delayed wound healing results in hypertrophic scarring with adverse functional and cosmetic outcomes has led to a policy of early excision and coverage for those wounds not expected to heal spontaneously within 3 weeks. The advantages of early excision include increased survival, reduced pain, a shortened duration of hypermetabolism, earlier reversal of immunosuppression, decreased incidence of burn wound sepsis, and less hypertrophic scarring—all leading to shorter hospitalization and an earlier return to school or work. Wounds that benefit from early excision and grafting include virtually all full-thickness, most deep partial-thickness, and occasional superficial partial-thickness burns.

Tangential excision is the most commonly used technique for burn wound excision. The goal is to remove all nonviable tissue down to a healthy bed, which is characterized by brisk bleeding from patent vessels. Various dermatomes are used to sequentially remove thin layers until all nonviable tissue is excised. Fascial excision, employing electrocautery, involves removal of all tissue down to muscular fascia and is reserved for full-thickness burns involving substantial subcutaneous tissue death. Fascial excision is associated with less blood loss than tangential excision, but the cosmetic results are inferior. Excision is performed within 7 days of injury. Waiting longer diminishes the benefits of early excision and allows for the progression of burn wound colonization to infection, although delay is often necessary in patients with concomitant nonthermal trauma, multiorgan dysfunction, or inhalation injury. A limitation of tangential excision is the potentially excessive blood loss. Use of tourniquets and/or topical hemostatic agents such as thrombin or epinephrine decreases bleeding. Prolonged operating time and extensive excision can lead to massive blood loss and systemic hypothermia, so operations using tangential excision are generally limited to a few hours and excision of 10% to 20% TBSA. Patients are brought back to the operating room every few days until all nonviable tissue is removed.

Burn Wound Coverage

The benefits of early excision of the burn injury are realized only if the wound is properly covered. Both biologic and synthetic dressings have been developed for this purpose and can be grouped as either permanent or temporary coverage.

Autologous skin grafting is the best choice for wound coverage and is classically the first choice for immediate surgical reconstruction. Although full-thickness skin grafts significantly reduce wound contraction and therefore yield the best cosmetic results, split-thickness grafts consisting of epidermis and a variable proportion of dermis are usually necessary to attain coverage in extensive burns. Split-thickness autografts of 0.010 to 0.016 in. thick can be harvested from almost any site of unburned skin. Sites preferred for harvest include the thigh, upper arm, and flat portions of the torso. Because the harvest of a split-thickness skin graft leaves intact dermal elements, donor sites do not require surgical closure, and reepithelialization of the donor site is typically complete within 14 to 21 days. The same site can be used for multiple harvests, but grafts become thinner and poorer in quality with each successive harvest.

Skin grafts initially adhere weakly to subgraft tissue and receive nutrients by a process of imbibition. Revascularization is achieved by the growth of capillary buds from the recipient area to the undersurface of the graft, initially by inosculation and subsequently by neovascularization. Revascularization is well advanced by day 3 and fibroblasts invade the fibrin clot to form the definitive connection within 1 week. Care must be taken to avoid shear forces to the graft or the formation of subgraft seromas or hematomas, all of which can compromise graft survival. Graft failure can also result from heavy bacterial colonization and subsequent infection. The graft is usually meshed, in a ratio ranging from 1:1 up to 9:1, to expand the surface area covered and also reduce the chance of subgraft seroma or hematoma formation. Reepithelialization occurs from the small bridges of skin centrally to cover the entire wound. Because the meshed pattern never fully disappears, areas of cosmetic concern such as the face and dorsum of the hand should be covered with unmeshed graft.

Patients with burns sufficiently extensive that the immediate use of autologous skin is not feasible require alternative methods of wound coverage. Decades of research have finally produced viable, albeit imperfect, skin substitutes. Three such skin substitutes are currently available in the United States: Integra, Alloderm, and Dermagraft. These products are fundamentally similar in that they allow for the creation of a "neodermis" populated by the patient's own mesenchymal cells upon which an ultra-thin graft is placed. The use of an ultra-thin graft (0.006 to 0.008 in) allows for earlier recropping of donor sites, quicker closure of the complete burn, and less donor site scarring. Successful use of any one of the available skin substitutes is technique-dependent and associated with a learning curve. Integra is a bilaminate membrane composed of a bovine collagen matrix impregnated with chondroitin 6-sulfate covered by a thin silicone epidermal analog. Integra is applied to the excised wound same as an autograft. When neovascularization is completed by approximately 14 days, the silicone layer is removed, and the neodermis is covered with an ultra-thin graft. Alloderm is a cryopreserved allogeneic dermis from which the epithelial elements have been removed with hypertonic saline prior to freeze-drying. This results in a theoretically antigen-free, complete dermal scaffolding with intact epidermal basement membrane proteins. Immediately following excision to viable tissue, Alloderm is rehydrated and applied to the wound bed. It is designed to be immediately autografted with an ultra-thin graft. Dermagraft consists of human neonatal fibroblasts cultured on Biobrane. Following excision, Dermagraft is applied to the wound. Approximately 2 weeks after application, the membrane is removed and the neodermis is grafted.

Cultured epithelial autograft (CEAs), which are commercially grown sheets of autologous keratinocytes cultured from skin biopsies of the burned patient, have also been used to close extensive burns. CEAs lack a supporting dermis and epithelial appendages. The staggering cost to cover a large body surface, low resistance to mechanical trauma, late wound contracture, and overall fragility limit clinical usefulness. In addition, approximately 2 weeks are required to grow CEA, during which time patients require temporary wound coverage.

Temporary coverage of an excised wound often must be provided while waiting for permanent coverage in the form of regenerating autograft sites or CEA. This can be achieved by using one of the skin substitutes as previously mentioned, allograft, or xenograft. Cutaneous allograft (homograft) harvested from appropriate cadavers is placed over the wound in a manner similar to that of an autologous split-thickness graft. Recognition and rejection of the foreign graft by the host's immune system occur within several weeks as the graft sloughs. The allograft provides durable biologic cover by preventing wound desiccation, limits bacterial proliferation, and conditions the wound bed by promoting granulation tissue until the graft is rejected by the host or removed for autografting. Cutaneous allograft limitations include a finite shelf life and potential disease transmission. Cutaneous porcine xenograft has an advantage over human allograft in that there is no shortage of supply. Xenografts do not vascularize but adhere to a clean wound and provide excellent pain control while preventing desiccation. Amniotic tissue can also be used to cover the burn wound, but carries the same disease transmission risk as allograft and requires frequent replacement due to desiccation.

ELECTRICAL BURNS

Electrical injury is responsible for approximately 1,000 deaths and 5% of burn center admissions annually. Injury results from the conversion of electrical energy to heat with the passage of current through tissue, a function of the tissue resistance, as well as from electrical arc flash burns. Less than 1,000 volts is defined as low-voltage. Alternating current as low as 120 volts can cause tonic muscle contractions that do not allow victims to release the energy source. Paraspinal muscle tetany can cause spinal compression fractures, and a complete spine series is indicated for any electrical injury greater than 380 volts. Alternating current at frequencies of 50 to 60 cycles per second and lightning injury often result in ventricular fibrillation or asystole. All electrical injuries can produce dysrhythmias, and a 12-lead electrocardiogram should be obtained with immediate continuous cardiac monitoring. Patients with documented asystole, dysrhythmias, or an abnormal electrocardiographic (ECG) findings should have prolonged cardiac monitoring, generally for at least 24 hours.

The pattern of injury seen with low-voltage electricity is similar to that of a thermal burn. High voltage injury can have a large amount of muscle and soft tissue destruction underlying a small cutaneous injury, with myoglobinuria and hyperkalemia often seen as a result. Myoglobinuria can cause acute renal failure, and mannitol may be required if aggressive fluid infusion does not maintain an adequate urinary output. Surgical treatment of the wound is staged. The first stage involves prompt wound exploration and decompression with fasciotomies in any patient who develops signs or symptoms of compartment syndrome. The second stage involves excision of nonviable tissue and definitive wound closure, usually within a week of injury.

Deep burns of the oral cavity and lips are the most common electrical burn in young children, often the result of chewing on an electrical cord. Significant bleeding can occur from the labial artery 10 to 14 days after injury, and families need to be carefully instructed to apply pressure to the bleeding point and return to the hospital immediately if bleeding occurs. Even extensive injuries can heal with good cosmetic results, although elective reconstruction is sometimes needed.

Neurologic changes can occur after an electrical injury. Immediate neuropathy results from electrical injury directly and usually resolves with time. Late manifestations, including localized deficits, ascending paralysis, or even quadriplegia, are more permanent and result from the thrombosis of nutrient vessels to the spinal cord or large nerve trunks. The delayed formation of cataracts can result from any electrical injury, particularly high-voltage injuries.

CHEMICAL BURNS

Strong acid or base destroys tissue by protein denaturation and thermal energy liberation. Injury occurs for as long as the offending agent maintains skin contact. The mainstay of initial treatment is the prompt removal of all contaminated clothing and continuous, copious irrigation with water for at least 30 minutes after acid exposure, and even longer with alkali exposure due to deeper tissue penetration, with care taken to avoid hypothermia. Neutralization of the acid or base is avoided because the resulting exothermic reaction can cause further thermal damage. The chemical burn is then treated like any other burn wound.

Hydrofluoric acid is a very strong acid commonly used in industry that directly destroys tissue via pH changes, and also penetrates deeply into tissue to precipitate with calcium and magnesium. Severe pain accompanies tissue injury. Topical application, subcutaneous injection, or intraarterial infusion of calcium gluconate limits damage and relieves pain. The patient must be monitored for development of systemic hypocalcemia, which is treated by intravenous repletion.

FROSTBITE

Treatment of cold injury differs significantly from that of a burn. Cutaneous microvasculature has alternating periods of vasoconstriction and vasodilation when tissue temperatures drop below 10°C to protect extremities from cooling, a response known as the "hunting reaction." However, systemic hypothermia abolishes this mechanism and tissue freezes when tissue temperature falls to approximately −2°C or −3°C. Intracellular ice crystal formation and distortion of cellular architecture causes cellular damage and death. Unlike a burn, damage is unevenly distributed owing to variable tissue tolerance to cold. Skin is relatively resistant to freezing, but other tissue such as nerves and blood vessels are quite sensitive. Vascular endothelial damage leads to platelet aggregates that occlude the microvasculature. This obstruction opens arteriovenous shunts that increase flow to the frozen extremity upon rewarming but decrease flow to the damaged tissue.

Frostbite is treated with rewarming by placing the injured area into a circulating water bath at 40°C within 30 minutes of injury. Tissue edema is often evident upon thawing but rarely sufficiently extensive to require fluid resuscitation. The depth of frostbite is classified, similar to a burn, into three levels. Unlike a burn, mummified tissue over a frostbite injury does not result in physiologic alterations and serves as a protective covering for underlying tissue. Demarcation can take several weeks to months and premature debridement can lead to the loss of potentially viable tissue. Local care focuses on preventing infection via cleansing and topical antimicrobials while the tissue demarcates, with avoidance of early eschar excision.

KEY POINTS

▲ No matter how bad a burn, initial assessment of all burn victims must focus on airway, breathing, and circulation (the ABCs) to identify and treat any immediate life-threatening injuries.

▲ Burn shock is a result of hypovolemia due to fluid shifts, and most adults with burns greater than 15% to 20% of their total body surface area (TBSA) require fluid resuscitation. The amount of fluid infused is initially calculated from the Parkland formula (4 mL Lactated Ringer solution/kg/%TBSA), but should be adjusted based on the patient's hemodynamic status and urine output.

▲ Inhalation injury should be suspected in all burn patients and can greatly increase fluid resuscitation needs. Upper airway injuries can be immediately life-threatening, and caregivers must have a low threshold to intubate burn victims early for airway protection. Lower airway injuries are generally responsible for delayed mortality.

▲ Early excision and grafting of any wound that will not heal within 3 weeks (deep partial- and full-thickness burns) decrease mortality and improve functional and cosmetic outcomes. Autologous skin is the first choice for wound coverage.

▲ Burn victims require adequate nutrition to fuel the metabolic response to the burn. Enteral nutrition should be provided as soon as possible. High protein and high calorie enteral nutrition improves wound healing and anabolism, although it has had no proven direct effect on mortality.

SUGGESTED READINGS

Carrougher GJ, ed. *Burn care and therapy*. St. Louis: Mosby, 1998.
Farrell K, Haith LR. Burns/inhalation. In: Peitzman AB, Rhodes M, Schwab CW et al., eds. *The trauma manual*, 2nd ed. Philadelphia: Lippincott Williams & Wilkins, 2002.
Herndon D, ed. *Total burn care*, 2nd ed. London: WB Saunders, 2002.
Holmes JH, Heimbach DM. Burns. In: *Schwartz's principles of surgery*, 8th ed. New York: McGraw-Hill, 2004.
American Burn Association. *http://www.ameriburn.org*. Accessed June 2004.

Hemostasis and Coagulation

20

Lee J. Goldstein   Jeffrey P. Carpenter

The human vascular system maintains tight control over the volume of blood that travels through it. Hemostasis refers to the interruption of blood loss, whereas thrombosis refers specifically to the formation of clot within the cardiovascular system. Coagulation, or clotting, describes the transition of fluid blood from a liquid to a thick gel. An exquisite mechanism of hemostasis exists where blood remains fluid throughout the vasculature and clots once it exits a vessel. A constant balance between procoagulants, anticoagulants, and the various cellular components present in the blood ensure the integrity of this system, and act to prevent thrombosis when functioning properly.

An understanding of the mechanisms responsible for hemostasis and coagulation is essential to the practicing surgeon, as disruptions in these systems are regularly seen both in the operating room and perioperatively.

THE ENDOTHELIUM

A layer of endothelial cells collectively referred to as *the endothelium* lines the cardiovascular system. This lining maintains fluid blood within the vessels and creates a barrier between the blood cells and the subendothelial surfaces and interstitium. Endothelial cells were once thought only to locally replicate when covering defects in the lining of the vascular system or developing new vessels. It is now accepted that endothelial cells, both at sites of wound healing and in the neovasculature of malignancy, are partly derived from a population of bone marrow stem cells known as *endothelial progenitor cells* (EPCs). The endothelium possesses the unique attribute of being a completely nonthrombogenic surface. Endothelial cells accomplish this by several mechanisms: a continuous smooth surface that prevents contact activation, a mucopolysaccharide glycocalyx lining that prevents coagulation, and a continual production of both pro- and anticoagulants. (Table 20-1) These properties allow the endothelium to modulate the coagulation system and its proteins (called factors), and the cells responsible for hemostasis.

Procoagulant activity by endothelial cells is stimulated by thrombin (the primary naturally occurring procoagulant), cytokines (IL-1), endotoxin, and other mediators resulting from infection, surgery, or trauma. These agonists cause expression of tissue factor (TF, also factor III) and synthesis of plasminogen activator inhibitors (PAIs), which regulate tissue plasminogen activator (tPA). These agonists also stimulate expression of various integrin-adhesive receptors for fibronectin, collagen, laminin, and vitronectin. Endothelial cells produce the powerful vasoconstrictor endothelin-1, and express E and P selectin, which bind leukocytes.

TABLE 20-1

PROCOAGULANTS AND ANTICOAGULANTS PRODUCED BY ENDOTHELIAL CELLS

Procoagulant	Anticoagulant
Produces types IV, V, and VIII collagen	Produces PGI₂
Produces laminin, thrombospondin, fibronectin	Produces nitric oxide
Produces von Willebrand factor	Produces heparan sulfate, dermatan sulfate
Produces plasminogen activator inhibitor-1 (PAI-1)	Produces protein S
Produces platelet-activating factor (PAF)	Inactivates platelet secreted ADP, ATP
Produces endothelin-1, renin, and angiotensin-converting enzyme	Produces thrombomodulin
Activates platelets	Produces tissue factor pathway inhibitor
Expresses tissue factor (TF)	Produces tissue plasminogen activator (tPA)
Binds vWF, factor IXa, factor Xa, HMWK, and vitronectin	Produces protease nexin-1
Inactivates bradykinin	

ADP, adenosine diphosphate; ATP, adenosine triphosphate; HMWK, high-molecular-weight kininogen; PGI₂, prostacyclin.

Anticoagulant activities of endothelial cells include production of antithrombin (AT), heparan sulfate and dermatan sulfate, thrombomodulin, proteins C and S, TF protein inhibitor, tPA, and protease nexin-1. Endothelial cells inactivate platelet-secreted adenosine triphosphate (ATP) and adenosine diphosphate (ADP) and produce adenosine.

Liver and endothelium produce AT, the primary naturally occurring anticoagulant, which functions to inactivate thrombin (factor IIa). Heparan sulfate produced on the endothelial surface acts as a cofactor for AT. *Thrombomodulin* is an endothelial membrane-bound receptor for thrombin. Thrombomodulin binds thrombin, removing it from the circulation, and the receptor–ligand complex greatly accelerates the activation of protein C. Activated protein C acts as an anticoagulant by inactivating factor Va and VIIIa. Protein S acts as a cofactor for protein C, thereby enhancing its action. *Prostacyclin* (PGI$_2$) is a product of cyclooxygenase and arachidonic acid metabolism, primarily produced by endothelium in response to thrombin, ADP, ATP, histamine, and kallikrein. PGI$_2$ causes vasodilation and inhibits platelet activation and adhesion by increasing intracellular platelet cAMP. PGI$_2$ is synthesized and secreted at the borders of hemostatic plugs, preventing intravascular platelet aggregation. *Nitric oxide* (NO), produced by endothelial cells via l-arginine metabolism, functions as a potent local vasodilator and platelet inhibitor. The NO molecule inhibits platelet function by raising cyclic guanosine monophosphate (cGMP) levels. NO has a half-life of less than 1 second.

Endothelial cells and platelets are negatively charged and therefore resist adhesion, whereas the subendothelium contains adhesive proteins that make up the basement membrane and the extracellular matrix, including collagen, TF, fibronectin, and von Willebrand factor (vWF). These adhesive proteins form a nidus for the formation of a platelet plug when the endothelium is disrupted.

HEMOSTASIS

Once the integrity of the vascular system has been violated, the mechanism that has evolved to establish hemostasis involves several key steps: (i) vascular spasm (vasoconstriction), (ii) formation of the platelet plug, (iii) formation of clot by coagulation, and (iv) permanent closure of the opening by fibrous tissue.

Vasoconstriction

Once a blood vessel has sustained an injury and blood loss ensues, immediate vasoconstriction takes place via myogenic, humoral, and neurogenic mechanisms. Vasoconstriction is produced by vascular smooth muscle cell (SMC) contraction at the level of the arterioles and arteries. Once platelets present in the serum attach to the area of injury, they release substances including ADP, thromboxane A$_2$ (a potent vasoconstrictor), and serotonin, all of which further potentiate SMC contraction. This contraction is the first step the body takes to stem the loss of blood from a site of injury. Vasoconstriction is proportional to the amount of vessel injury; a crushed vessel will constrict more, whereas a sharply cut vessel will bleed more. Local

vascular spasm can last minutes or even hours, allowing the platelet plug to form and coagulation to occur.

The Platelet Plug

Platelets play a central role in hemostasis (Fig 20-1). Produced in the bone marrow by fragmentation from megakaryocytes, platelets are cells that are 3 to 4 μm in diameter and have lifespans of 9 to 12 days. Blood normally contains approximately 150,000 to 400,000 platelets per mL, with approximately one third sequestered within the spleen. Platelets do not contain nuclei and cannot reproduce. A system of canaliculi, which functions much like the sarcoplasmic reticulum in muscle cells, regulates rapid influx of calcium into the cytoplasm and provides for rapid secretory product egress. Platelet cytoplasm contains contractile proteins including actin, myosin, and thrombosthenin to control shape and granule movement when activated.

When a platelet encounters a damaged endothelial cell or damaged vascular surface, such as a collagen fibril, a cascade begins leading to platelet activation. The platelet will change in shape (expressing many pseudopods), release secretory granules, and become "sticky" by the secretion of active factors and expression of receptors. The major agonists for activation of platelets are *ADP, thromboxane A$_2$, collagen, thrombin, epinephrine, and platelet-activating factor.* ADP may be released from damaged red cells, endothelial cells, or activated platelets. Platelets have specific receptors for activating agonists, which activate platelets by lowering cyclic adenosine monophosphate (cAMP) or cGMP. Three classes of phosphodiesterases that either inhibit or stimulate metabolism of the cyclic nucleotides regulate cAMP and cGMP concentrations in the platelet.

Upon activation, platelets express various glycoprotein (GP) receptors on the membrane surface and interact with other platelets and subendothelial structures to produce aggregation and adhesion. These GP receptors include GPIb, GPIIb, GPIIIa, GPIV, and GPV, which interact with substances such as vWF, fibrinogen, fibronectin, vitronectin, and collagen. GPIb is the primary receptor for vWF, which allows binding to subendothelial surfaces, and GPIIb/IIIa bind vitronectin, fibronectin, vWF, and, fibrinogen, thereby allowing platelets to bind other platelets. Platelets also express receptors for procoagulant proteins such as thrombin, and facilitate formation of both the tenase (VIIIa, IXa, Ca) and prothrombinase (Va, Xa, Ca) complexes to produce yet more thrombin. All of these reactions focus aggregation and adhesion of platelets and production of fibrin at the site of vascular injury to quickly stem the exit of blood into the extravascular space.

The Coagulation System

The blood contains a number of proteins involved in the clotting mechanism collectively called "coagulation factors." These proteins circulate as inactive zymogens that become serine proteases or cofactors when activated. Most of these proteins are glycoproteins, and are generally indicated by Roman numerals, with a lowercase *a* appended to indicate an active form. The liver synthesizes all coagulation factors except factor VIII and vWF, which are produced by endothelial cells. The liver produces factors II, VII, IX, and X

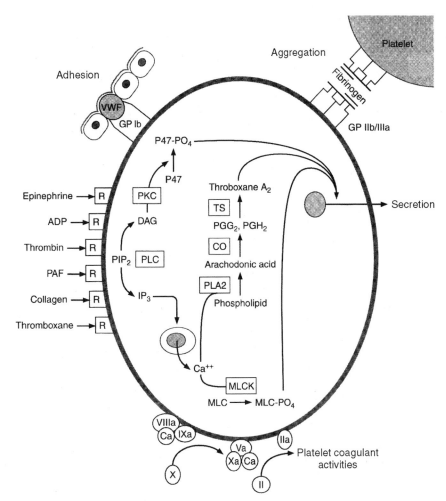

Figure 20-1 Overview of platelet function (see text for details). (From Coleman RW, Hirsh J, Marder VJ, et al. *Hemostasis and thrombosis: basic principles and clinical practice.* Philadelphia: J.B. Lippincott Co, 1994, with permission.)

through a vitamin K–dependent reaction. Carboxylation of precursors (blocked by warfarin) forms γ-carboxylated glutamic acid residues that, via a calcium cofactor, bind to phospholipid membranes.

More than one pathway exists by which blood can coagulate, but all pathways ultimately result in cross-linked fibrin. (Fig. 20-2) Regardless of the pathway taken to produce a clot, there are a series of consistent steps: (i) a cascade of reactions between coagulation factors resulting in activation of factor X, (ii) factor Xa–mediated conversion of prothrombin to thrombin, and (iii) thrombin-mediated conversion of fibrinogen to fibrin, which polymerizes to stabilize clot. The contact activation system, the intrinsic coagulation pathway, and the extrinsic coagulation pathway converge after the activation of factor X to Xa (step 1). Steps 2 and 3 after this point are referred to as the *common pathway.*

The Contact Activation System

The coagulation system has four zymogens called the contact proteins: factor XII (Hageman factor), prekallikrein (Fletcher factor), high-molecular-weight kininogen (HMWK), and factor XI. When blood contacts a nonendothelial cell surface, plasma proteins are adsorbed onto that surface. On the surface, these adsorbed proteins (such as factor XII) undergo conformational changes to expose reactive sites.

Upon contact with an activating surface, factor XII is converted into XIIa and XIIf in the presence of cofactors HMWK and prekallikrein (Fig. 20-2). Factor XIIa then cleaves prekallikrein to kallikrein, an important agonist for activating neutrophils. Factor XIIa also cleaves HMWK to produce bradykinin, a vasodilator and inflammatory mediator. Importantly, factor XIIa catalyzes cleavage of factor XI to XIa to initiate the *intrinsic coagulation pathway.* Congenital absence of factor XII, prekallikrein, or HMWK does not produce symptoms. Absence of factor XI causes a mild bleeding disorder.

The Intrinsic Coagulation Pathway

Factor XIa activates factor IX to factor IXa. Factor IXa in combination with factor VIIIa, Ca^{2+}, and a phospholipid surface forms the tenase complex, which cleaves factor X to factor Xa. Factor VIII is activated by thrombin, as are factors V and VII. Phospholipid surfaces greatly accelerate reactions between coagulation proteins and are provided primarily by platelets, monocytes, and endothelial cells.

The Extrinsic Coagulation Pathway

A specialized contact pathway exists if the nonendothelial surface blood is exposed to is a wound. Most of the cells in the wound express tissue factor (TF, also factor III),

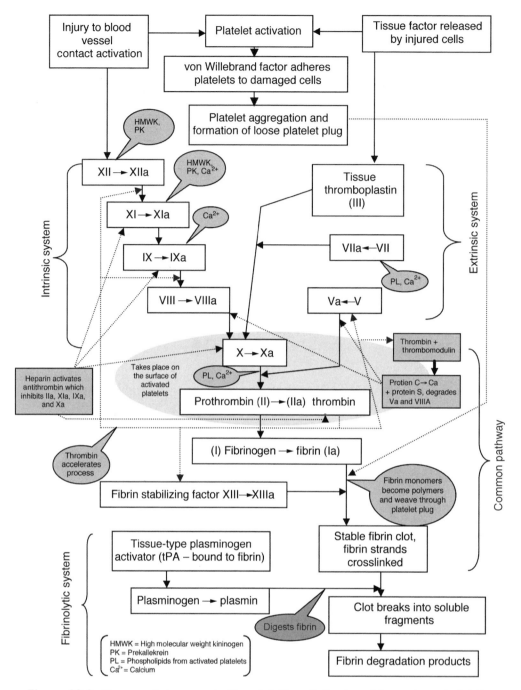

Figure 20-2   The coagulation cascade [From Lab Tests Online (*www.labtestsonline.org*), © 2004 American Association for Clinical Chemistry, with permission.]

which initiates the extrinsic coagulation cascade. TF, a membrane-bound protein that is constitutively expressed in an active form on cells of most tissues (muscle, fat, adventitia, epicardium, among others), initiates the extrinsic coagulation pathway. TF in the presence of factor VIIa, Ca^{2+}, and a phospholipid surface directly cleaves factor X to factor Xa. Thrombin increases TF expression in both monocytes and endothelial cells, whereas interleukin-1 (IL-1) and tumor necrosis factor (TNF) stimulate its expression in many others. The combination of TF, factor VIIa, Ca^{2+}, and a phospholipid surface also activates factor IX, thereby leading to the formation of the tenase complex, cleaving factor X to factor Xa, and demonstrating more overlap between the intrinsic and extrinsic

pathways. Both the intrinsic and extrinsic coagulation pathways converge and produce factor Xa, but the extrinsic pathway is the most relevant with regard to surgical procedures and trauma victims.

The Common Pathway

Once factor Xa has been activated, the coagulation pathways converge. On a phospholipid surface, factor Xa with cofactors Va and Ca^{2+} (the prothrombinase complex) cleaves prothrombin (factor II) to thrombin (factor IIa). Prothrombin fragment F1.2 is formed in the process, and can be a useful marker of thrombin generation. Thrombin is a powerful procoagulant, directly activating platelets and factors V, VII, and VIII. In addition, thrombin can act directly on prothrombin to generate yet more thrombin—a cycle that results in expansion of the clot. Thrombin ultimately cleaves fibrinopeptides A and B from fibrinogen to form polymerized fibrin. Thrombin also activates factor XIII, which cross-links adjacent fibrin molecules. Cross-linked fibrin molecules woven through platelet plugs constitute a stable clot.

Fibrinolysis

As thrombin is generated and clot expansion begins there are several checks in place that are meant to limit the amount of expansion, thereby preventing excessive spread. Up to 90% of the thrombin formed will be adsorbed to the polymerizing fibrin strands, whereas the remaining amount will combine with the alpha globulin *antithrombin III* (ATIII). ATIII will prevent thrombin from propagating clot and eventually inactivate the thrombin.

When a clot develops, many plasma proteins are incorporated into the rapidly forming polymer. Included in these proteins is *plasminogen*—an inactive precursor to *plasmin*, the enzyme responsible for dissolution of clot. Bound plasminogen is activated to plasmin via tissue tPA, which endothelial cells and injured tissues slowly release in response to thrombin. tPA is regulated by PAI-1. Once formed, plasmin digests fibrin, fibrinogen, factor V, factor VIII, factor XII, and prothrombin.

Small amounts of circulating plasmin are continually produced and would be a severe impediment to the appropriate functioning of the coagulation cascade if not for α_2-antiplasmin. This circulating enzyme inhibits plasmin in the vasculature, keeping it in check until a critical threshold is reached where plasmin will become effective. Plasmin is also inhibited by the much slower α_2-macroglobulin.

DISORDERS OF COAGULATION

Many disorders exist in which the body cannot accomplish effective hemostasis. These can be genetic (congenital) disorders, or acquired disorders, and can affect the proteins of the coagulation cascade, or the cells responsible for hemostasis.

Hemophilia

Two major types of hemophilia exist. *Hemophilia A* (classic hemophilia) is a sex-linked recessive disease with approximately 1 per 10,000 to 1 per 25,000 males in the United States affected. Hemophilia A is characterized by a deficiency in factor VIII. These patients tend to have spontaneous bleeding, including hemarthroses, and excessive bleeding following relatively minor trauma. Most concerning in these patients is the risk of a devastating central nervous system (CNS) hemorrhage. Treatment involves administration of cryoprecipitate or purified factor VIII. *Hemophilia B* (Christmas Disease), also sex-linked recessive, is a milder form of the disease caused by a deficiency of factor IX. This variant is treated with fresh-frozen plasma or purified factor IX concentrate. Laboratory abnormalities in hemophilia include elevated activated partial thromboplastin time (aPTT) and reduced factor VIII or IX levels. Other tests

of coagulation are usually normal. Treatment for surgery or life-threatening hemorrhage should include transfusion to 80% to 100% of normal concentrations of these factors.

von Willebrand Disease

A carrier protein for factor VIII, vWF participates in platelet adhesion to collagen. *von Willebrand disease* has many variations, and can be transmitted as autosomal recessive (homozygous) or autosomal dominant (heterozygous). Clinical manifestations include petechiae, epistaxis, and menorrhagia; however, hemarthroses occur less frequently compared to their occurrence in hemophilia. Laboratory findings include prolonged aPTT, prolonged bleeding time, decreased factor VIII activity, decreased vWF level, and abnormal platelet aggregation as measured by ristocetin assay. Treatment involves transfusion with cryoprecipitate or factor VIII concentrates, which contain vWF, or administration of D-deoxy desmopressin arginine vasopressin (DDAVP).

Factor V Leiden

Factor V Leiden is a mutation in the gene for factor V that results in an increased risk of venous thrombosis. It is the most common hereditary coagulation disorder, present in 5% of white Americans and 1.2% of African Americans. Patients usually discover the mutation after onset of a clot; however, many live their entire life without a thrombotic event. Treatment is short-term anticoagulation to resolve clots, and long-term anticoagulation for severe or refractory cases. The severity of this disorder increases substantially in homozygotes, and those with superimposed risk factors (e.g., smoking, oral contraceptives, or prothrombin 20210 mutation).

Protein C Deficiency

Protein C (responsible for neutralizing factors V and VIII) and protein S (a cofactor that helps stabilize protein C on a phospholipid membrane) are both dependent on vitamin K for their synthesis. Congenital protein C deficiency is autosomal dominant, and venous thrombosis is the most common complication. Arterial thromboses, including myocardial infarction, have also been reported. Homozygous mutation is lethal, heterozygous mutation manifests between 15 and 30 years of age.

Protein C has a short half-life. As such, administration of a vitamin K–inhibiting anticoagulant such as warfarin can result in a precipitous drop in protein C levels. This deficiency can result in microvascular thrombi, usually to the skin. For this reason, systemic heparinization is recommended prior to warfarin initiation.

Antithrombin-III Deficiency

Deficiency in ATIII usually manifests itself early in adult life with widespread venous and/or arterial thromboses. These patients are resistant to heparin anticoagulation, as ATIII is the enzyme upon which heparin acts. Treatment involves replacement of ATIII with fresh-frozen plasma to allow heparinization, and then long-term warfarin anticoagulation.

Heparin-induced Thrombocytopenia

Heparin-induced thrombocytopenia (HIT) is a potentially catastrophic complication affecting 1% to 3% of patients receiving heparin. HIT is characterized by the formation of platelet-activating antibodies after heparin administration, and significantly lowered platelet levels (as low as 10,000 per mm^3). Heparin interacts with *platelet factor 4* (PF4), a positively charged protein tetramer released from platelet storage granules during activation, forming an immunogenic complex. These complexes, composed of antibodies, heparin, and PF4, activate platelets through the FcγIIa receptor. PF4 is present on endothelium as well, causing antibody activation and thrombin generation at the endothelium as well as at the platelet. Platelet activation and thrombin generation puts these patients at significant risk of venous thrombosis and potentially life-threatening thromboembolic events. Recognition of thrombocytopenia during heparin therapy mandates immediate intervention to prevent devastating injury.

Once the clinician suspects HIT, several laboratory tests exist to help confirm the diagnosis. These tests fall into two major groups: functional assays and antigen assays. Functional assays include the C-14 serotonin release assay (SRA), and the heparin-induced platelet aggregation assay (HIPA). Both functional tests have a sensitivity of less than 90%, but approach nearly 100% specificity. The SRA involves mixing C-14 radiolabeled donor platelets with patient serum in the presence of heparin. Radiolabeled serotonin release is measured, indicating activation of platelets. Unfortunately, this test is technically demanding, time-consuming, and uses radioactivity. The HIPA study mixes donor platelets with patient serum and heparin, and measures platelet aggregation. The HIPA is fast and inexpensive, but operator dependent, and has a low sensitivity. The antigen assay is an enzyme-linked immunosorbent assay (ELISA) to detect patient antibodies to the heparin-PF4 complex. This assay has the highest sensitivity, but produces false-positive results, with up to 50% of postcardiac surgery patients having ELISA detectable HIT antibodies. For the most accurate diagnosis of HIT, the clinician must combine clinical suspicion, ELISA results, and the results of one of the functional assays.

Treatment for HIT requires immediate cessation of heparin therapy. In addition, any and all potential exposure to heparin must be stopped, including prophylactic injections, flushes, and coated catheters. Alternative methods for anticoagulation with direct thrombin inhibitors should be investigated based on the patient's clinical condition.

Disseminated Intravascular Coagulation

Disseminated intravascular coagulation (DIC) describes the clinical scenario of uncontrolled, widespread activation of coagulation with intravascular generation of thrombin and fibrin. As a result of the consumption of platelets and coagulation factors, severe bleeding can ensue. This devastating situation can be initiated by a variety of stimuli, including sepsis, massive trauma and/or head injury, certain uncontrolled cancers, severe immunologic disorders, and reactions to snake venom and other toxins. The diffuse activation of the coagulation system is coupled with a simultaneous suppression of natural anticoagulants

including AT III and the protein C pathway. The clinical diagnosis is made using the following criteria: the presence of an initiating condition, a platelet count of less than 100,000 per μL, prolonged prothrombin time (PT) and aPTT, and the presence of fibrin-degradation products (such as fibrinopeptide A). A lowered level of AT III strengthens the diagnosis. Treatment is geared toward addressing the inciting pathology and replacing consumed platelets and coagulation factors through transfusion. Heparin can be used to inhibit thrombin activity, but is often contraindicated in patients with DIC (e.g., postoperative patients). Patients with sepsis often have associated organ dysfunction secondary to DIC and the microvascular thrombi that ensue. Administration of human recombinant activated protein C (*Xigris*) to restore microvascular anticoagulant pathways and reduce systemic inflammation has been shown to help improve outcomes in these patients.

Iatrogenic Coagulopathy

Patients subjected to massive blood loss and transfusion often exhibit drastic disorganization of the coagulation system. The most common complication is hypothermic coagulopathy, which can be treated by warming both the patient and the blood products being infused. Care must be taken to replace coagulation factors and platelets in addition to red cell requirements.

Cardiopulmonary bypass (CPB) requires the use of an anticoagulant. Thrombin is formed continuously both in the wound and perfusion circuit, despite high doses of anticoagulant. CPB causes platelet activation, as well as qualitative platelet dysfunction. Soluble coagulation factors are diluted during CPB, but concentrations remain sufficient to maintain clot formation.

COAGULATION PHARMACOLOGY AND TRANSFUSION THERAPY

Our understanding of the intricacies of the coagulation system has allowed the development of numerous interventions to treat disorders of coagulation. Advances in transfusion medicine and hematologic pharmacology permit routine manipulation of the blood components and their interactions.

Drugs Affecting Platelet Function

Aspirin acts by irreversibly binding cyclooxygenase (CO) in platelets (see CO in Fig. 20–1). This prevents formation of the products of this pathway, notably thromboxane A_2, and ultimately results in severely decreased platelet aggregation and prolonged template bleeding times. The inhibition does not prevent platelet activation. Platelet turnover returns function within 7 to 10 days. Aspirin also inhibits formation of prostacyclin by blocking cyclooxygenase in endothelial cells. Endothelial cells can overcome this effect by producing new cyclooxygenase. Low-dose aspirin (81 mg per day) is an effective long-term dose for permanently blocking platelet arachidonic acid metabolism and minimizing side effects. Nonsteroidal anti-inflammatory drugs (NSAIDs) reversibly inhibit cyclooxygenase with platelets recovering full function in 2 to 3 days after cessation of NSAID therapy.

Dipyridamole (Persantine) inhibits platelet uptake of adenosine, which increases intraplatelet cAMP, thereby inhibiting platelet aggregation. Aggrenox is a commercially available oral formulation combining aspirin with extended release dipyridamole.

Glycoprotein IIb/IIIa receptor blockers are a class of drugs that block the final step of platelet aggregation by interfering with the ability of platelets to aggregate around fibrinogen. These drugs are used primarily in patients with acute coronary syndromes, or those undergoing percutaneous coronary interventions. *Abciximab* (ReoPro) is a chimeric monoclonal antibody Fab fragment against the platelet IIb/IIIa receptor, with rapid onset and effects lasting more than 12 hours. *Tirofiban* (Aggrastat) is a nonpeptide molecule with a plasma half-life of approximately 1.6 hours. It reversibly inhibits the IIb/IIIa receptor. *Eptifibatide* (Integrilin) is a small molecule that also reversibly inhibits the IIb/IIIa receptor, with platelet aggregation returning to normal function approximately 4 to 8 hours after cessation of the infusion.

Thienopyridines, such as *ticlopidine* (Ticlid), and *clopidogrel* (Plavix), block ADP-mediated platelet activation, preventing platelet aggregation. Ticlopidine has been associated with neutropenia.

Drugs Affecting the Coagulation Cascade

Heparin is a negatively charged conjugated polysaccharide produced by many different cell types. Pericapillary basophilic mast cells and plasma basophils produce the highest amounts, but the naturally occurring blood level is still extremely low. Heparin combines with AT III increasing its activity up to a thousandfold. The heparin–ATIII complex inactivates thrombin, factor XIIa, XIa, IXa, and Xa. Exogenous administration of a heparin infusion allows for near instantaneous removal of plasma thrombin, and effective anticoagulation of the patient. Heparin can be administered intravenously or subcutaneously. Commercial unfractionated heparin is obtained from pork or beef lung and intestine. Heparin infusion requires laboratory monitoring via aPTT, and its effects can be reversed with protamine, which binds the heparin molecules.

Low-Molecular-Weight Heparin (LMWH) (e.g., Lovenox) contains smaller molecules isolated from unfractionated heparin, and is also administered intravenously or subcutaneously. The effectiveness of LMWH is in its ability to inhibit factor Xa. Because of their pharmacology, LMWHs produce more predictable anticoagulation and do not require laboratory monitoring. Antifactor Xa levels can be measured if there is a question of effective dosing. LMWH has a much lower incidence of HIT.

Oral anticoagulants such as *warfarin* act by competing with vitamin K, a cofactor needed for carboxylation of factors II, VII, IX, and X in the liver. Warfarin levels can be adjusted on the basis of PT. Warfarin can be reversed in about 24 hours with intramuscular or intravenous vitamin K injections. Patients should be advised to stop taking oral anticoagulation at least 4 days before invasive surgery, with the possibility of needing inpatient anticoagulation via an agent with a shorter half-life, if warranted by the clinical situation. Warfarin is teratogenic and should not be used in pregnancy.

Alternative anticoagulants include *lepirudin* (Refludan) and *argatroban* (Argatroban). Lepirudin is a recombinant form of medicinal leech hirudin. Care should be taken in patients with renal dysfunction, as it can prolong the effects of lepirudin. Argatroban, a synthetic peptide, has the advantages of nonrenal (hepatic) clearance, and short half-life, but the disadvantage of prolonging the PT, making transition to warfarin anticoagulation more difficult. Both of these drugs are approved for the treatment of HIT, are administered as a continuous infusion, and act by direct inhibition of thrombin.

A new oral direct thrombin inhibitor, ximelagatran (Exanta), has been submitted to the U.S. Food and Drug Administration (FDA) for the indications of stroke prevention in atrial fibrillation, and venous thromboembolism prevention, and has already been approved in Europe. This drug has several advantages over warfarin including fewer drug interactions, fixed dosing without need for monitoring and adjustment, and fewer incidences of bleeding in clinical trials. As the first fixed-dose anticoagulant to be marketed since the introduction of warfarin, expect this class of drugs to expand and play a prominent role in future outpatient anticoagulation.

Procoagulants

Antifibrinolytic medications aim to block the action of plasmin and slow bleeding. *Aprotinin* (Trasylol) is a naturally occurring inhibitor of plasmin and kallikrein harvested from bovine lung. Aprotinin preserves the GP receptors on platelets and slows the turnover of coagulation factors that is seen during fibrinolysis. Test doses must be given prior to administering aprotinin as anaphylaxis has been reported, especially in those previously sensitized. *ε-Aminocaproic acid* (Amicar), another inhibitor of fibrinolysis, acts by inhibiting plasminogen activators and also by direct antiplasmin activity.

D-deoxy desmopressin arginine vasopressin (desmopressin acetate, DDAVP) is a polypeptide with structural homology to vasopressin (antidiuretic hormone, ADH). DDAVP is used to treat hemophilia A, von Willebrand disease, and uremic coagulopathy by causing vWF release from endothelium.

NovoSeven (recombinant factor VIIa, rFVIIa) is used to treat bleeding episodes in hemophiliac patients with inhibitors present to factors VII and IX. NovoSeven exerts its effect by activating the extrinsic coagulation cascade. As a recombinant therapeutic it poses no infectious risk. rFVIIa is increasingly employed off-label in blood loss unresponsive to conventional transfusion therapy, or surgical situations associated with excessive bleeding.

Therapeutic Fibrinolytics

Knowledge of the fibrinolysis system has allowed the development of drugs to exploit this system. Fibrinolytics can be administered intravascularly (either systemically or locally) in order to combat detrimental thromboses such as during cerebrovascular accidents, myocardial infarctions, major pulmonary embolisms, proximal deep venous thromboses, or acute arterial thromboses. First-generation fibrinolytics include streptokinase and urokinase. Recombinant streptokinase, a glycoprotein from the *Streptococci* bacterium, is a plasminogen activator able to lyse both bound plasminogen as well as circulating plasminogen. As a bacterial protein, streptokinase is antigenic, and febrile reactions have been reported. Urokinase, a serine-protease plasminogen activator found in the urine, is commercially available from cultured neonatal human kidney cells and indicated for treatment of significant pulmonary embolism (although often employed in other clinical scenarios). The major morbidity associated with these drugs is bleeding, most significantly intracerebral hemorrhage.

In an attempt to generate more specific thrombolytics and reduce the incidence of extraneous bleeding, second-generation drugs were developed. Recombinant tissue plasminogen activator (rtPA) is commercially available and acts to dissolve fibrin clots as tPA does physiologically in humans. After much review, there has not been overwhelming evidence that second-generation thrombolytics are superior to earlier compounds. In fact, there is some evidence that fewer episodes of bleeding are seen with urokinase. Expect further refinement of these therapeutics as recombinant techniques improve. These compounds are contraindicated in recent trauma or surgery (14 days or less), severe hypertension, known active bleeding, pregnancy, severe liver or kidney disease, or intracranial pathology. They can be reversed with fresh-frozen plasma and ε-aminocaproic acid.

Topical Hemostatic Agents

There are many topical hemostatic agents available for use during surgical procedures, provided as woven fabrics, gels, and liquids. One of the most commonly employed agents, oxidized regenerated cellulose (*Surgicel, Surgicel fibrillar*), derived from plant material, acts by providing a scaffold for coagulation. Gelatin sponges (*Surgifoam, Gelfoam)*, contain collagen, and can be used with or without prior saturation with a thrombin solution. Several newer biologic glues have been introduced that contain synthetic hemostatic agents, as well as animal products including thrombin, fibrinogen, and serum.

Transfusion Medicine

In many cases the best way to treat blood loss or coagulopathy is by transfusion. Various blood products are available including whole blood, packed red blood cells (with a hematocrit of approximately 70%), fresh-frozen plasma (providing coagulation factors), cryoprecipitate (the best source of factor VIII and fibrinogen), platelets, and specific factor concentrates. Whole blood, although infrequently used, has the advantages of retaining factors V and VII, having less free potassium, and having a lower acidity. Although the risk of transfusion-related infectious disease is extremely low, it is not zero. The United States increased its stringency by testing its blood supply for human immunodeficiency virus (HIV) and hepatitis C virus (HCV) in 1999 by nucleic acid tests, in place of antibody tests.

Over time, banked blood will deteriorate. Stored blood is kept anticoagulated with citrate, a calcium binder. In addition, the pH of stored blood will decrease, owing in part to the presence of citrate. By about one month, the pH is approximately 6.5, the potassium level has risen to almost 8, 2,3 diphosphoglycerate (2,3 DPG) levels decrease, approximately 1% of erythrocytes have lysed, and most of the labile blood factors have diminished.

The most common complication of transfusion is a febrile reaction, which occurs in about 1 per 100. Other complications include fatal hemolytic reactions (1 per 250,000 to 600,000) and nonfatal hemolytic reactions (1 per 6,000 to 33,000). TRALI (transfusion-related acute lung injury) affects 1 per 2,000 to 5,000 patients causing pulmonary edema and inflammation, with a reported mortality as high as 10%. One per 500 U of platelets is found to have positive bacterial cultures.

TESTING AND PREOPERATIVE ASSESSMENT

Tests of Coagulation

Whole blood clot retraction testing can be done to check for coagulopathy caused by thrombocytopenia or platelet dysfunction. Modern platelet-specific laboratory tests make this a rarely used test.

Bleeding time is checked by making a standard small superficial incision on the forearm, inflating a blood pressure cuff to 40 mm Hg (Ivy Method), and recording the time required for bleeding to stop. Blood is wiped clean from the incision every 30 seconds, and less than 10 minutes is considered a normal bleeding time. Prolonged bleeding times usually indicate a problem with platelet number or function, but can be related to syndromes of increased capillary fragility.

PT is used to measure the function of the extrinsic and common pathways of the coagulation system. PT measures the clotting ability of factors I, II, V, VII, and X. It is commonly employed to measure hepatic dysfunction or the effect of oral anticoagulation with warfarin (which affects factor VII function most owing to its short half-life). The absolute value reported will vary by laboratory because of differences in thromboplastin reagents and measuring devices. As such, the *international normalized ratio* (INR) has been developed to allow standardized measurements comparable across institutions, independent of reagents or methods. Normal INR is 1.0.

aPTT is used to assess the intrinsic and common coagulation pathway, evaluating factors I, II, V, VIII, IX, X, XI, and XII. The original PTT test has had activating reagents added to shorten the clotting time, and narrow the normal window; therefore, the test is now referred to as aPTT. As heparin inactivates factor IIa (via ATIII), it prolongs the aPTT, making aPTT the test for monitoring heparin levels.

Activated clotting time (ACT) measures whole blood clotting time in the presence of an activator. ACT is used as a real-time measure of the ability of blood to clot, especially during and after cardiopulmonary bypass or vascular surgery.

Preoperative Screening

Any preoperative workup should start with careful history taking and physical examination. The preoperative history should include a family history of bleeding problems, prior episodes of excessive bleeding or bruising, and medications. Anticoagulant medications, especially those taken sporadically such as aspirin or NSAIDs should be reviewed. Patients should be specifically asked about herbal supplement use. Some herbal medicines and supplements that can affect coagulation include: danshen, dong quai, fever-few, garlic, ginkgo, and ginseng. Be sure to include any adverse reactions patients may have had with previous anticoagulation, which would prompt an investigation into the presence of antiheparin antibodies. Physical examination should look for excessive bruising, petechiae, hepatosplenomegaly, or occult gastrointestinal blood loss.

For minor surgery with a noncontributory history and physical, no further workup is needed. For more invasive procedures, especially those involving invasive monitoring, routine coagulation studies including a platelet count, PT, and aPTT are indicated. Abnormal findings mandate a workup for disorders of coagulation, potentially with the involvement of a hematologist.

KEY POINTS

▲ Heparin acts via antithrombin-III (ATIII) and inactivates thrombin, factor XIIa, XIa, IXa, and Xa.

▲ Warfarin acts by competing with vitamin K, a cofactor needed for carboxylation of factors II, VII, IX, and X in the liver.

▲ Warfarin-induced skin necrosis occurs by rapid depletion of protein C after warfarin administration and a transient hypercoagulable state.

▲ Banked blood exhibits lowered calcium, lowered pH, lowered 2,3 diphosphoglycerate (DPG), increased potassium, and about 1% red blood cell lysis at 1 month.

SUGGESTED READINGS

Calaitges JG, Silver D. Principles of hemostasis. In: Rutherford RB, Cronenwett JL, Gloviczki P et al., eds. *Vascular surgery,* Philadelphia: WB Saunders, 2000.

Hoffman R, Blanz EJ Jr, Shattil SJ, eds. *Hematology: basic principles and practice,* 3rd ed. New York: Churchill Livingstone, 2000.

Levi M. Current understanding of disseminated intravascular coagulation. *Br J Haematol* 2004;124(5):567–576.

Pagana KD, Pagana TJ. *Mosby's diagnostic and laboratory test reference,* 6th ed. St. Louis: Mosby, 2003.

Roberts HR, Monroe DM, Escobar MA. Current concepts of hemostasis: implications for therapy. *Anesthesiology* 2004;100(3): 722–730.

Coagulation-Factors. *http://www.coagulation-factors.com.* Accessed May 2005.

DocMD. *http://www.bleedingweb.com.* Accessed May 2005.

The Cardiovascular System

21

Pavan Atluri   *Y. Joseph Woo*

The heart is the center of the cardiovascular system. The primary function of the cardiovascular system includes the supply of oxygen and metabolites at the cellular and organ level as well as the removal of toxic waste products (including carbon dioxide). There exists a complex interaction between the various components of the cardiovascular system to maintain homeostasis. A thorough understanding of this system includes a detailed understanding of the development and anatomy as well as organ and cellular physiology.

EMBRYOLOGY

The cardiovascular system appears in the third week of development when the developing embryo outgrows the ability to maintain homeostasis by diffusion alone and requires an active system for delivery of nutrients and removal of toxic metabolites. Angioblastic tissue (primitive cardiac tissue) arises from splanchnic mesoderm. Initially, islands of angiogenic tissue form clusters known as angiocysts. These angiocysts are located both on the lateral sides and in the midline of the developing embryo. The lateral angiocysts spread in the cephalic and medial directions and with time form a uniting horseshoe-shaped plexus forming peripheral vascular tissue. The midline angiocysts form the dorsal aorta and paired endocardial heart tubes.

These two heart tubes fuse in the midline cardiogenic area to form the primitive heart tube. The heart begins to bulge at its central aspect with simultaneous expansion of the mesoderm to form the myocardium. Eventually, the heart wall is composed of three layers: (i) an inner endothelial cell lined endothelium, (ii) a middle myocardial layer, and (iii) a mesothelial cell–derived epicardium, which is also known as the visceral pericardium.

The heart tube continues to elongate with the cephalic (ventricular) portion bending in a ventral and caudal direction. The caudal (atrial) portion moves in a dorsocranial direction to the left creating a cardiac loop. As seen in Figure 21-1, the 4-week heart consists of a common atria (which becomes incorporated into the pericardium), a narrow atrioventricular junction (atrioventricular canal), the narrow proximal *bulbus cordis* (primitive trabeculated right ventricle), the middle *conus cordis* (outflow for both ventricles), and the distal *truncus arteriosus* (roots, proximal aorta, and pulmonary artery).

At this stage the *sinus venosus*, origin to the primitive common atrium, receives blood from three paired veins: (i) vitelline (omphalomesenteric vein), (ii) umbilical vein, and (iii) common cardinal vein. By 5 weeks the umbilical vein and left vitelline vein are obliterated. At 10 weeks the left common cardinal vein is obliterated. Eventually, the remaining sinus venosus forms the smooth wall of the right atrium, valve of the inferior vena cava, and valve of the coronary sinus. Between 27 and 37 days the major cardiac septa are formed (Fig. 21-2). At this stage, endocardial cushions develop and actively grow in the atrioventricular and conotruncal regions, thereby assisting in the formation of the atrial and ventricular (membranous septa), aortic and pulmonary channels, and atrioventricular canals.

During the end of the fourth week the *septum primum* grows from the roof of the common atrium toward the atrioventricular endocardial cushion (Fig. 21-2). The opening between the endocardial cushion and septum primum is the *ostium primum*. Before the atrioventricular endocardial cushion and septum primum are able to meet and obliterate the ostium primum, cell death forms perforations in the septum primum, thereby forming the *ostium secundum*. The ostium secundum allows for requisite right-to-left flow of blood across the atria. A second growth cushion arises from the roof of the primitive right atria, *septum secundum*, which allows closure of the *foramen ovale*. In approximately 20% of neonates the septum primum and septum secundum fail to fuse, leaving a narrow opening between the atria, a patent foramen ovale.

At the end of the fourth week septum formation in the common atrioventricular canal begins partitioning into left and right circulations. This is accomplished with the fusion of four endocardial cushions—superior, inferior, and two lateral endocardial cushions. Mesenchymal cells invade the endocardial cushions as they approach each other to divide the atrioventricular canal into right and left by the end of the fifth week. Malformation at this stage will

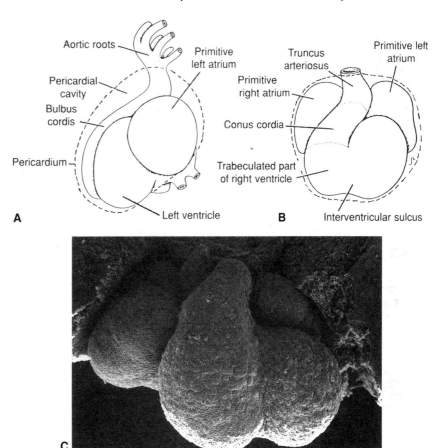

Figure 21-1 The heart of a 5-mm embryo (28 days). **A:** Viewed from the left. **B:** Frontal view. Note that the bulbus cordis is divided into the truncus arteriosus, conus cordis, and trabeculated part of the right ventricle. **C:** Scanning electron microscope of a 28-day mouse embryo heart. *Broken line*, pericardium. (From Sadler TW. *Langman's Medical Embryology*, 7th ed. J.B. Lippincott, 1995:190, with permission.)

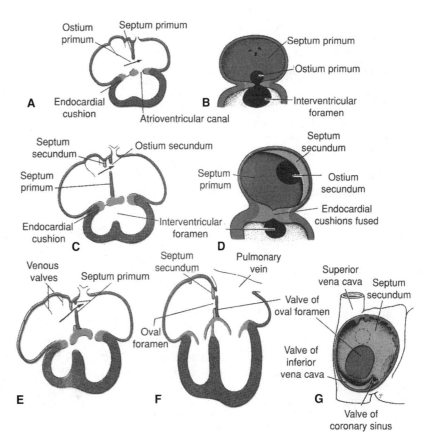

Figure 21-2 Schematic representation of the atrial septa at various stages of development. **A:** 30 days (6 mm). **B:** Same stage as in **A** but viewed from the right. **C:** 33 days (9 mm). **D:** Same stage as in **C** but viewed from the right. **E:** 37 days (14 mm). **F:** Newborn. **G:** View of the atrial septum from the right; same stage as in **F**. (From Sadler TW. *Langman's medical embryology*, 7th ed. JB Lippincott, 1995:195, with permission.)

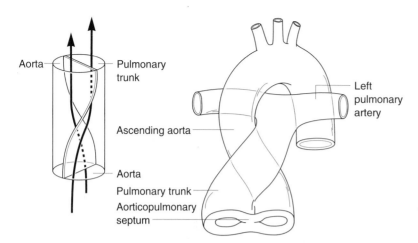

Figure 21-3 Partitioning of the truncus arteriosus by the aortopulmonary septum separates the aorta from the pulmonary trunk. (From The cardiovascular system. In: Moore KL, Persaud TVN. *The developing human*, 6th ed. Philadelphia: WB Saunders, 1998:373, with permission.)

result in abnormal atrioventricular valvular anatomy. After the atrioventricular endocardial cushions fuse, the atrioventricular valvular orifices are surrounded by localized mesenchymal proliferations. These mesenchymal cushions will eventually remodel forming the atrioventricular, tricuspid, and mitral valves, and associated chordae tendineae attached to papillary muscles.

By the end of the fourth week the two ventricles begin to expand. The medial walls of the ventricles appose forming the muscular interventricular septum. The ventricles are not isolated until the end of the seventh week. There is a crescent shaped *interventricular foramen* between the free edge of the interventricular septum and fused endocardial cushions. During the seventh week, the right and left bulbar edges and endocardial cushions fuse closing the interventricular foramen and separating the ventricles.

Formation of the aorta and pulmonary artery involves mesenchymal cell proliferation in the bulbus cordis as well as truncus swellings. Truncus swellings appear opposite each other (right superior and left inferior truncus swellings) in the truncus arteriosus. The right superior grows distally to the left and the left inferior grows proximally to the right. The swellings twist around each other forming the spiraling aorticopulmonary septum between the pulmonary trunk and aorta (Fig. 21-3). Once the truncus arteriosus is nearly divided, tubercles are formed in the aortic and pulmonary channels that will form the aortic and pulmonary valves respectively.

FETAL CIRCULATION

Oxygenated blood from the placenta is brought to the fetus via the umbilical vein. Roughly half of the blood from the placenta passes through hepatic sinusoids, whereas the remainder bypasses hepatic circulation flowing directly into the inferior vena cava via the *ductus venosus*. In the inferior vena cava, oxygenated placental blood mixes with deoxygenated venous blood returning from the lower extremities before entering the right atrium. Once in the right atrium, the majority of blood passes directly to the left atrium via the foramen ovale, bypassing the pulmonary circulation (Fig. 21-4). Left atrial blood mixes with the small amount of deoxygenated blood in

the fetal pulmonary circulation before entering the left ventricle and ultimately the ascending aorta.

A small portion of right atrial blood mixes with superior vena caval blood from the head and upper extremities as well as coronary sinus blood and passes into the right ventricle, which accounts for 5% to 10% of total cardiac output. Because there is very high pulmonary vascular resistance in the fetus, the majority of right ventricular blood enters the pulmonary artery and is shunted to the descending aorta via a patent ductus arteriosus. Roughly half of the descending aortic blood passes into paired umbilical arteries and is returned to the placenta (oxygen saturation of roughly 58%) for reoxygenation. It is these two fetal shunts, patent foramen ovale and patent ductus arteriosus, which allow many neonates born with cyanotic congenital heart disease to survive. Figure 21-5 illustrates the fetal circulation.

At birth, because the placental circulation is no longer present and the neonatal lungs are expanded, the pulmonary vascular resistance is greatly reduced, a state that allows increased pulmonary blood flow. With increased

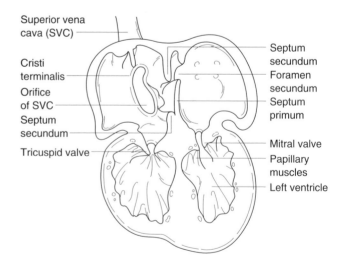

Figure 21-4 After about 8 weeks, the heart is partitioned into four chambers. Well-oxygenated blood bypasses the pulmonary circulation through the foramen secundum. (From The cardiovascular system. In: Moore KL, Persaud TVN. *The developing human*, 6th ed. Philadelphia: WB Saunders, 1998:362, with permission.)

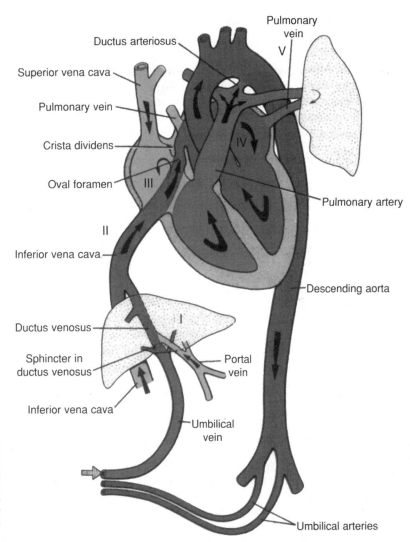

Figure 21-5 Diagram of the human circulation before birth. Arrows indicate the direction of blood flow. Note where oxygenated blood mixed with deoxygenated blood: in the liver (*I*), in the inferior vena cava (*II*), in the right atrium (*III*), in the left atrium (*IV*), and at the entrance of the ductus arteriosus into the descending aorta (*V*). (From Sadler TW. *Langman's medical embryology*, 7th ed. JB Lippincott, 1995:225, with permission.)

pulmonary blood flow, left atrial pressure is greater than right atrial pressure. This difference in pressure allows closure of the foramen ovale by pressing the septum primum against the septum secundum. During the first days of life this closure is reversible. When an infant cries, an increase in pulmonary pressure with a right-to-left shunt through the foramen ovale may be present. This is manifested as cyanosis in newborns.

Closure of the ductus arteriosus is a result of bradykinin release from the lung. Bradykinin mediates contraction of the muscular ductus wall. Functional closure of the ductus typically occurs within the first 15 hours after birth and anatomic closure occurs by day 12 of parturition. Prior to birth, locally produced prostaglandins maintain patency of the ductus. The fibrotic, atrophied remnant of the ductus arteriosus is referred to as the ligamentum arteriosum.

In premature and cyanotic infants the ductus arteriosus frequently remains patent. In most instances cyclooxygenase inhibitors such as indomethacin can be used to reduce production of the prostaglandins that maintain ductus patency. The decreased concentration of local prostaglandins allows closure of the ductus arteriosus. If this medical treatment modality is unsuccessful, surgical intervention may be indicated. Surgical ligation of the patent ductus arteriosus can be

performed via minimally invasive video-assisted thoracoscopic means through the left chest.

ANATOMY

The human cardiovascular system is composed of the systemic circulatory system, the pulmonary circulation, and a four-chamber heart pump at the center of the circulatory system. The heart is situated obliquely within the pericardial sac, with one third of the heart situated to the right of the median plane and two thirds to the left. The right ventricle abuts the sternocostal surface and forms the anterior surface of the heart. The right side of the heart receives deoxygenated systemic blood via the superior and inferior vena cava as well as deoxygenated blood from the coronary circulation via the coronary sinus. The right heart then pumps this blood through the low pressure, high flow pulmonary arteries. Once the blood has circulated through the pulmonary circulation it is returned to the left heart via four posteriorly situated pulmonary veins (two superior and two inferior pulmonary veins). Blood from the left heart is ejected from the left ventricle into the systemic circulation via the aorta.

Valvular Anatomy

The mammalian heart is composed of four one-way valves. Two atrioventricular valves (mitral and tricuspid) provide unidirectional diastolic flow from the atria to the ventricles and allow a systolic pressure gradient between the atria and ventricles. The semilunar valves (aortic and pulmonary) allow systolic flow and maintain a diastolic pressure gradient between the ventricles and outflow circulations.

The tricuspid and mitral valves are fibrous endocardium-lined valves. The tricuspid valve separates the right atria from the right ventricle and consists of a large anterior leaflet attached to the anterior wall of the heart, a posterior leaflet at the right margin, and a septal leaflet attached to the septum. Three chordae tendineae are attached to the free surface of the leaflets and to the papillary muscles at the right ventricular base. This apparatus prevents prolapse of the tricuspid valve leaflets into the right atrium during systole. The mitral valve, located at the orifice of the left ventricle, consists of a large anterior leaflet in continuity with the posterior wall of the aorta and a smaller posterior leaflet. The anterior leaflet of the mitral valve is anatomically in proximity to the aortic valve. Chordae tendineae (Fig. 21-6) secure the leaflets to the anterior and posterior papillary muscles and ensure coaptation of the valve leaflets during systole.

Infarction of the papillary muscles as can occur following a myocardial infarction results in mitral insufficiency. When assessing the ejection fraction of a patient with mitral regurgitation, one must keep in mind the bidirectional flow of left ventricular flow in this pathologic condition. An average ejection fraction in a patient with mitral regurgitation actually represents a low forward flow of blood into the systemic circulation.

The aortic and pulmonic valves are situated at the outflow of the left and right ventricles, respectively. The aortic valve is a tri-leaflet valve. These leaflets are named according to the origin of the coronary arteries, namely, the right coronary, left coronary, and noncoronary leaflets (Fig. 21-7). Similarly, the pulmonic valve is a tri-leaflet valve with a right, left, and noncoronary leaflet.

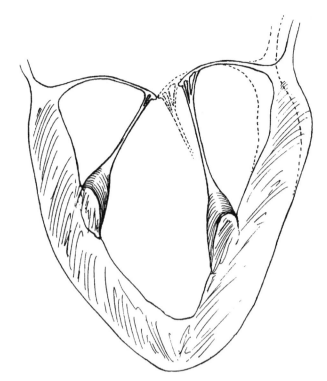

Figure 21-6 Chordae tendineae tether the leaflets of the mitral and tricuspid valves, allowing precise coaptation during systole. (From Chitwood WR Jr. Mitral valve repair: ischemic. In: Kaiser LR, Kron IL, Spray TL, eds. *Mastery of cardiothoracic surgery.* Philadelphia: Lippincott Williams & Wilkins, 1998:312, with permission.)

Coronary Anatomy

The coronary circulation (Fig. 21-8) supplies the myocardium and epicardium. The endocardium is in continuous contact with intracardiac blood and does not require additional blood flow. The right and left coronary arteries of the heart arise just superior to the aortic valve and are the first branches of the aorta.

The *right coronary artery* arises from the anterior (right) *sinus of Valsalva* in the aorta and runs along the atrioven-

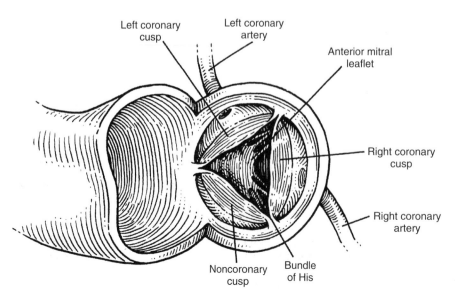

Figure 21-7 Normal aortic valve from a surgeon's point of view. (From Damiano RJ. Aortic valve replacement: prosthesis. In: Kaiser LR, Kron IL, Spray TL, eds. *Mastery of cardiothoracic surgery.* Philadelphia: Lippincott Williams & Wilkins, 1998:362, with permission.)

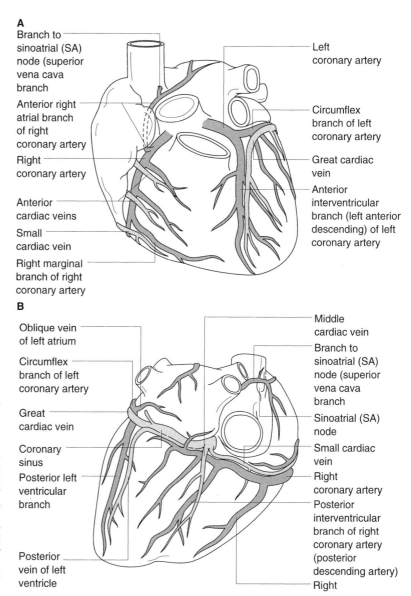

A
Branch to sinoatrial (SA) node (superior vena cava branch

Anterior right atrial branch of right coronary artery

Right coronary artery

Anterior cardiac veins

Small cardiac vein

Right marginal branch of right coronary artery

Left coronary artery

Circumflex branch of left coronary artery

Great cardiac vein

Anterior interventricular branch (left anterior descending) of left coronary artery

B
Oblique vein of left atrium

Circumflex branch of left coronary artery

Great cardiac vein

Coronary sinus

Posterior left ventricular branch

Posterior vein of left ventricle

Middle cardiac vein

Branch to sinoatrial (SA) node (superior vena cava branch

Sinoatrial (SA) node

Small cardiac vein

Right coronary artery

Posterior interventricular branch of right coronary artery (posterior descending artery)

Right

Figure 21-8 Anatomy of the coronary arteries and cardiac veins. **(A)** Anterior view. The origin of the left main coronary artery is left lateral and somewhat posterior with respect to the aorta; it courses behind the pulmonary artery and then divides into the left anterior descending and circumflex coronary arteries. The origin of the right coronary artery is almost directly anterior, and it runs in the atrioventricular groove. **(B)** Posterior view. The great, middle, and small cardiac veins come together at the level of the coronary sinus, which lies in the left inferior atrioventricular groove and empties into the right atrium. (From Greenfield LJ, Mulholland MW, Oldham KT et al., eds. *Surgery: scientific principles and practice*, 3rd ed. Philadelphia: Lippincott Williams & Wilkins, 2001:1487, with permission.)

tricular (coronary) groove. Roughly 60% of the time the right coronary artery gives off a sinoatrial branch near its origin to supply the sinoatrial (SA) node. It traverses posteriorly toward the apex of the heart, and gives off a *right marginal artery*, which supplies the right ventricle. After giving off this branch it continues in the posterior interventricular groove. In roughly 85% of patients the *posterior descending artery* arises from the right coronary artery and defines a *right-side dominant circulation*. In approximately 5% of patients, a balanced pattern exists in which the right coronary and circumflex coronary arteries supply the posterior descending artery, branches to the septum, and atrioventricular node (Fig. 21-9).

The *left coronary artery* arises from the left *sinus of Valsalva* and passes between the left auricle (atrial appendage) and pulmonary trunk toward the anterior atrioventricular groove. In 40% of the patients, the sinoatrial branch arises from the left coronary artery. The left coronary artery divides at the atrioventricular groove to give off the *left anterior descending artery* (LAD) and the *circumflex coronary artery* (Fig. 21-9). The LAD passes anteriorly along the interventricular groove to the apex and provides: (i) septal branches that supply the

anterior two thirds of the interventricular septum and (ii) diagonals that supply the anterolateral wall of the left ventricle. The circumflex coronary artery follows the atrioventricular groove around the left border of the heart to the posterior surface of the heart and provides marginal branches (i.e., obtuse marginal) that supply the posterior left ventricle. In 10% of patients the circumflex coronary artery ends in the posterior descending artery, providing blood flow to the posterior one third of the interventricular septum and atrioventricular node, defining a left-side dominant circulation.

Malperfusion of the conduction system following a myocardial infarction can result in the development of atrial or ventricular conduction abnormalities and dysrhythmias. The presence of conduction abnormalities and/or arrhythmias should prompt evaluation for myocardial ischemia or infarction.

The venous drainage of the heart occurs by means of veins that drain into the coronary sinus as well as smaller venae cordis minimae and anterior cardiac veins that drain into the right atrium. The coronary sinus is a large vein that receives coronary venous blood from the left (great cardiac, left marginal, and left posterior ventricular veins) and right

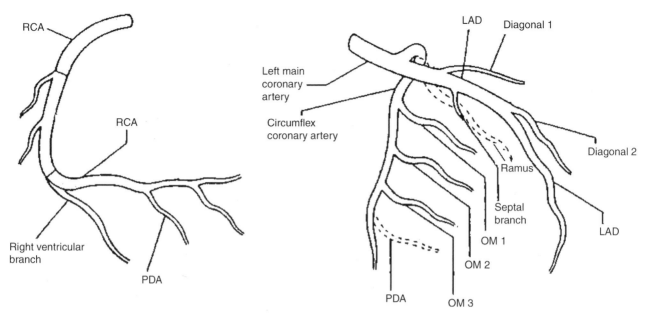

Figure 21-9 Coronary anatomy. RCA, right coronary artery; PDA, posterior descending artery; LAD, left anterior descending artery; OM, obtuse marginal artery.

(middle and small cardiac veins) side veins. It runs in the posterior atrioventricular groove.

The coronary sinus is often used to provide optimal myocardial protection during prolonged periods of cardiopulmonary bypass. A retrograde cardioplegia catheter is inserted into the coronary sinus. The myocardial protective cardioplegia solution then flows retrograde into the coronary circulation, thereby providing enhanced protection that cannot be provided by traditional antegrade cardioplegia via the coronary ostia.

ELECTROPHYSIOLOGY

As with any striated muscle, cardiac muscle contraction is initiated by action potentials. Action potentials mediate rapid voltage changes of the cell membrane. Certain cells within the cardiac muscle are capable of acting as the pacemaker and spontaneously initiate action potentials. The action potentials of cardiac muscle are special in that they can self-generate, conduct from cell to cell via gap junctions, and are of long duration.

Action potentials of the myocardium can be classified as either fast action potentials or slow action potentials. *Fast action potentials* occur in normal myocardium of atria, ventricles, bundle of His, and Purkinje fibers. *Slow action potentials* are seen in the pacemaker cells of the sinoatrial (SA) and atrioventricular (AV) nodes. As seen in Figure 21-10 (solid line), fast action potentials are characterized by a rapid depolarization (phase 0, –transient increase in Na^+ conductance), partial repolarization (phase 1, –outward movement of K^+), a plateau (phase 2, –inward movement of Ca^{2+}), membrane repolarization (phase 3, –decreased Ca^{2+} conductance and increased K^+ conductance), and a resting membrane potential (phase 4, –equal inward and outward currents). In contrast, slow action potentials demonstrate a slower depolarization phase (phase 0), and shorter plateau and repolarization (phase 3) to an unstable slow depolarization resting phase (phase 4). The alterations in the membrane potential are a factor of the

permeability of a cell membrane to particular ions (Na^+, K^+, and Ca^{2+}) and the resulting gradients that exists.

During an action potential, cardiac myocytes are in an effective refractory period (ERP) and cannot be stimulated by another action potential. This occurs during phases 1, 2, and the beginning of phase 3. Shortly after this period is a relative refractory period (RRP, late phase 3), during which a supranormal action potential is needed for excitation. Immediately after the action potential, before return to a normal resting state (phase 4), is the supranormal period (SNP) during which the cells are hyperexcitable and require a lower than normal action potential for stimulation.

Once an action potential arises it is conducted across the cell membrane to adjacent cells via gap junctions. The speed of transmission of the action potential is determined by a combination of cell size and rate of depolarization. The smaller cells of the pacemaker cells demonstrate a slower conduction velocity than the larger Purkinje cells. Similarly, the slow response of the pacemaker cells mediates a slower conduction velocity when compared to the fast response of ventricular myocardial cells.

SA nodal cells demonstrate the most rapid spontaneous depolarization and hence act as the pacemaker under routine conditions. This tissue lies within the wall of the right atrium at the junction of the right atrium and superior vena cava. Once the action potential is initiated in the SA node it is propagated via the atria to the AV node. The AV node is located in the interatrial septum above the tricuspid valve near the coronary sinus. In pathologic conditions with SA nodal discontinuity the AV node can act as a pacemaker. The AV node protects the ventricle from excess stimulation in the case of increased atrial rates, allowing the ventricle adequate diastolic filling. From the AV node the action potential is sent to the ventricle via the bundle of His. The bundle of His splits into right and left bundle branches and ultimately into Purkinje fibers, which conduct to the subendocardial surfaces (Fig. 21-11).

The autonomic nervous system (sympathetic and parasympathetic nervous systems) both innervates the SA

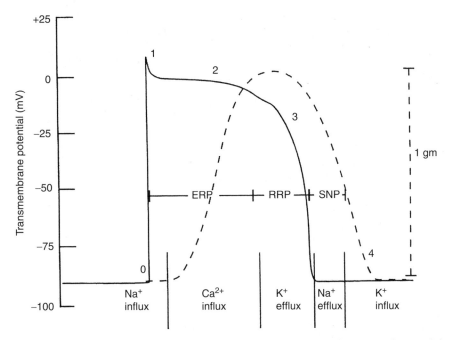

Figure 21-10 Schematic fast action potential of human ventricular myocardium (*solid line*) with electrolyte movements, refractory periods (see text), and force generated (*dashed line*). The five phases of fast cardiac action potential are indicated as numbers. *Phase 4*: the resting membrane potential. Potassium conductance is high and sodium conductance is low. *Phase 0*: Upstroke of the action potential due to membrane depolarization. An increase in sodium conductance due to the opening of voltage dependent fast sodium channels causes depolarization. There is a simultaneous decrease in potassium conductance. *Phase 1*: Period of partial repolarization due to a dramatic decrease in sodium conductance and a brief increase in chloride conductance. *Phase 2*: Plateau phase during which changes in potassium efflux (conductance decrease and then plateaus) are matched by calcium influx (conductance increases and then plateaus). *Phase 3*: Membrane repolarization phase due to an increase in potassium efflux (increase potassium conductance) and a decrease in calcium influx (decreased calcium conductance).

node and controls heart rate by modifying SA nodal activity. The sympathetic nervous system increases heart rate by increasing the rate of depolarization. In contrast, the parasympathetic nervous system increases potassium conductance, increases the magnitude of hyperpolarization, slows the rate of spontaneous depolarization, decreases the rate of closure of potassium channels, and

slows the heart rate. In addition, to increasing heart rate (positive chronotropic effect) the sympathetic nervous system increases the rate of conduction of action potentials through the conduction system. The parasympathetic nervous system slows conduction.

The electrical activity of the heart can be interpreted by utilizing an *electrocardiogram* (ECG). The normal electrocar-

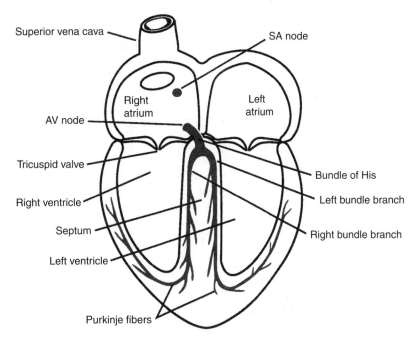

Figure 21-11 Structure of conduction system of the heart. (From Johnson LR. *Essential medical physiology*, 2nd ed. Philadelphia: Lippincott Williams & Wilkins, 1998:166, with permission.)

diogram demonstrates *P* and *QRS* complexes, which represent atrial and ventricular depolarization, respectively. Ventricular repolarization is demonstrated by the *T* wave.

CARDIAC PACEMAKERS

Pacemakers are devices that provide electrical stimuli to cause cardiac contraction during periods of slow or absent intrinsic cardiac electrical activity. The pacing system consists of a pulse generator and pacing leads. Pulse generators contain a sensor, timer, output circuit, and battery. For permanent pacemakers, the generator is placed subcutaneously, usually in the region of the deltopectoral groove. In the case of traditional permanent pacemakers, the pacing leads are directed via the venous circulation to the right ventricle and/or atrium. Alternatively, epicardial pacing leads can be placed directly on the heart surface surgically. Newer pacing schemes utilize an additional left atrial pacing lead (biatrial pacing) to minimize atrial fibrillation. An additional ventricular lead can be placed on the left ventricle (biventricular pacing) to maximize efficiency of cardiac activity in a failing or cardiomyopathic heart. Most pacemakers use lithium-iodide batteries that have a lifespan of 5 to 8 years depending on the energy output.

Temporary pacing can use epicardial pacing leads (placed surgically, usually following cardiac surgery), transcutaneous pacing pads that can be connected to most defibrillators (utilized in emergency bradycardic circumstances), or emergent transvenous pacing wires placed through the central venous circulation into the right ventricle.

Pulse generators can be set to a fixed firing rate (asynchronous) or can work with the intrinsic cardiac electrical activity and fire only when needed (synchronous). Asynchronous activity carries a risk of firing during ventricular repolarization, "r on t", thereby producing malignant arrhythmias. The chamber to pace and sense and the response to the sensed impulse can all be regulated. These various coding options are illustrated in Table 21-1. For example, in the VVI mode, the ventricle is paced and sensed, and a pacemaker stimulus is inhibited when a ventricular response is sensed. In the DDD mode, both atria and ventricle are paced and sensed, and stimuli to both chambers are inhibited in the presence of a detected stimulus. Other settings on the pacemaker include the minimum threshold at which an impulse is detected and the pulse amplitude (mA) generated by the pacemaker.

CARDIOVASCULAR PHYSIOLOGY

The cardiovascular system is in a continuous state of flux to maintain normal homeostasis. There are complex intrinsic and extrinsic regulatory mechanisms that work in concert to ensure that adequate perfusion is maintained to end organs. A thorough understanding of cardiovascular physiology begins at the cellular level.

Cardiac Muscle Physiology

Cardiac myocytes (groups of cardiac muscle cells) are the building blocks of cardiac muscle. There are three essential muscle bundles within the myocardium: (i) the conducting Purkinje fibers of the heart; (ii) sinoatrial and atrioventricular

TABLE 21-1
PACEMAKER CODING SYSTEM

Paced Chamber (First Letter)	Sensed Chamber (Second Letter)	Response to Sensed Impulse (Third Letter)
V	V	I
A	A	I
D	D	D
O	O	O

V, ventricle; A, atrium; D, both chambers/dual; O, none; I, inhibited.

nodal tissue, which are specialized to initiate and propagate the heart beat; and (iii) the contractile atrial and ventricular muscle masses.

The highly specialized contractile ventricular muscle cells are branching, nucleated cells 10 to 15 μm in greatest dimension (compared to 100 μm for skeletal muscle). They adjoin each other via intercalated discs. The majority of the cell is composed of myofilaments and mitochondria. Mitochondria comprise 30% to 40% of cellular volume, reflecting the highly aerobic nature of cardiac tissue. The small cell size allows for rapid diffusion of substances from the extracellular space into the cardiac cellular compartment. Within the intercalated discs are large surface area interdigitating connections between adjacent cells that allow for conduction of electrical impulses (**gap junctions**) as well as tight mechanical connections that allow for transmission of mechanical impulses (**desmosomes**). This allows both electrical and mechanical synchrony during myocardial contraction.

Regulation of contractility of the cardiac muscle is a calcium-mediated process. Increased cellular/stored calcium results in increased *inotropic* activity. Inotropy is the intrinsic ability of cardiac muscle to develop force at a given muscle length. Cellular calcium is stored in both the *sarcoplasmic reticulum* as well as in the *sarcolemma* (cell membrane and associated connective tissue structures). Once the action potential arrives at the cell surface it is conducted intracellularly to the sarcoplasmic reticulum via the *transverse tubules (t-tubules)* resulting in intracellular calcium release. At the same time cell membrane depolarization mediates release of calcium from the sarcolemma to the intracellular compartment. Extracellular calcium entry further augments intracellular calcium levels and plays a role in *calcium-induced calcium release* from intracellular stores. In this phenomenon, extracellular calcium induces calcium release from the sarcoplasmic reticulum. Extracellular calcium does not play a role in current muscle contraction, but it does increase the cellular calcium available for storage in the sarcoplasmic reticulum for subsequent muscle contractions.

Cardiac muscle is a specialized form of skeletal muscle with contractility dependent on actin–myosin binding. During contraction intracellular calcium binds to troponin-C on thin filaments, removing the inhibitory action of tropomysin. This allows for the cross-bridging of actin (on thin filaments) and myosin (on thick filaments) and the subsequent adenosine triphosphate (ATP)–mediated contraction that results from the sliding of the actin and myosin filaments past each other. The magnitude of tension generated is proportional to the intracellular calcium concentration. In addition to sodium–calcium exchange on the sarcolemma that extrudes calcium extracellularly; active calcium-ATPase pumps on the sarcoplasmic reticulum and sarcolemma mediate reaccumulation of the intracellular calcium and subsequent cardiac muscle relaxation.

Circulatory Physiology

As previously stated the cardiovascular system is composed of: (i) the pulmonary circulation to provide perfusion to the lung parenchyma and (ii) systemic circulation to provide systemic perfusion (and a very small degree of pulmonary circulation via the bronchial vessels). The pulmonary circuit is a low pressure (mean pulmonary artery [PA] pressure of 15 mm Hg), high flow system. As compared to the systemic circulation the pulmonary vessels contain very little smooth muscle and are much shorter. This results in highly compliant [compliance (mL/mm Hg) = volume (mL)/pressure (mm Hg); inversely proportional to elastance], low resistance vessels. It should be remembered that the pulmonary circulation must be capable of handling the same volume as the systemic circulation. Right heart output is equal to left heart output.

The pulmonary circulation is capable of handling increased cardiac output as seen with exercise by both recruiting additional pulmonary capillaries that are not normally utilized as well as distending the pulmonary vessels. Pulmonary vascular resistance decreases with increasing cardiac output by these two mechanisms. This drop in resistance maintains low pulmonary artery pressures. Low pulmonary artery pressures decrease right heart cardiac work, thereby preventing pulmonary edema. Other regulators of pulmonary blood flow are lung volume, hypoxia (which causes pulmonary vasoconstriction), and hypercapnia (which results in pulmonary vasodilation).

In contrast to the pulmonary circuit, the systemic circulation operates at a high pressure, with high resistance to blood flow. The flow of blood is from the left heart (left ventricle) to the aorta. From the aorta blood flows down a pressure gradient through various branches to arterioles and capillary beds. The large and small arteries are thick-walled vessels with extensive elastic tissue and smooth muscle. They are under high pressure but offer little resistance to blood flow. Resistance can be calculated by using the following equation derived from the work of Jean Leonard Marie Poiseuille on flow mechanics:

$$\text{Resistance} = \frac{8 \, (\text{viscosity of blood})(\text{length of vessel})}{\text{II} \, (\text{radius of blood vessel})^4}$$

Aortic and arterial elasticity maintains perfusion during the diastolic–filling phase of left ventricular cycling. *Arterioles*, the short, terminal branches of the arteries, are the principal resistance vessels of the systemic circulation. They contain a large amount of vascular smooth muscle innervated by the autonomic nervous system within the vessel wall that can impede the flow of blood. Arterioles provide the largest pressure drop in the circulation. Arteriolar resistance is regulated by the autonomic nervous system.

As arterial structures progressively branch from the aorta ultimately to the capillary bed, cross-sectional area of the vascular bed continues to increase. On the outflow side of the capillary bed the cross-sectional area decreases as capillaries drain into venules, which merge into small veins, large veins, and ultimately the vena cava. The velocity of blood flow is directly proportional to blood flow and inversely proportional to cross-sectional area.

Velocity of blood flow (cm/s) =

$$\text{flow (cm}^3\text{/s)/cross-sectional area (cm}^2)$$

As illustrated in Figure 21-12, there is a decrease in the velocity of blood flow as the cross-sectional area of the vascular bed increases. This is ideal at the capillary level (high surface area, low velocity), in which a high contact surface and low velocity provide for optimal exchange of metabolic products at a cellular level.

Cardiac Mechanics

The heart is a biomechanical pump. The mechanical force generated by the heart is utilized to eject blood from the

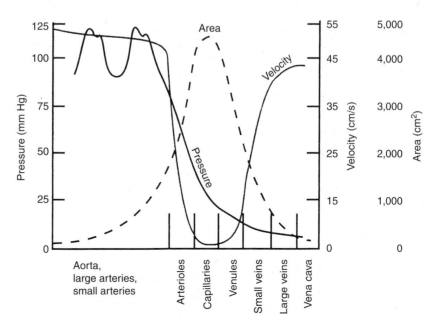

Figure 21-12 Pressure, area, and velocity relationship across the systemic circulation.

heart to either the pulmonary or systemic circulations, thereby providing perfusion to end organs. There must be synchrony of the cardiac myocytes, valves, and four chambers of the heart for maximum efficiency. The heart is in a constant state of flux to ensure that adequate end-organ perfusion is achieved. The primary variables that alter cardiac function are preload, afterload, and autonomic nervous system stimulation. A proper understanding of these forces is a prerequisite to an adequate understanding of cardiac mechanics. Figure 21-13 demonstrates the flow of blood during the various stages of the cardiac cycle.

The left and right ventricles function in a cyclical manner. Contraction and ejection of blood occurs during *systole*. Myocardial perfusion as well as filling of the ventricles occurs during the relaxation phase known as *diastole*. To simplify the explanation all discussions will focus on left ventricular mechanics.

The left ventricular intracavitary volume and pressure at end-diastole (immediately prior to contraction) determines the *preload* of the heart. There are several factors that affect preload. Increasing venous return increases preload. Fibrotic, hypertrophied, and aging hearts become increasingly stiff and limit left ventricular filling and preload. As described earlier, relaxation is an energy-dependent process (calcium-ATPase), which is augmented by adrenergic stimulation, but is impaired in ischemia, hypothyroidism, and congestive heart failure—all conditions that limit preload.

The afterload of a muscle is the pressure against which it must contract. For the left ventricle, this is equivalent to the aortic pressure against which it must eject blood during systole. Afterload for the right ventricle is equal to the pulmonary artery pressure. The greater the afterload, the greater the potential energy the heart must generate to provide adequate ejection into the aorta, and subsequently the greater the cardiac work (described in subsequent text). Maximal velocity of contraction is achieved when afterload is minimal.

Within normal physiologic ranges the heart is able to accommodate a broad range of end-diastolic volume by altering contractility. This dynamic activity is described by the *Frank-Starling* relationship, which describes the interplay between ventricular filling and contractility. With increased ventricular filling the sarcomeres are stretched to an optimal length, thereby facilitating increased contractility. Adrenergic stimulation can further increase contractility (inotropy) of the heart, thereby increasing the

stroke volume (volume of blood ejected from the heart with each beat). Parasympathetic innervation decreases inotropy. In addition, right atrial stretch leads to an increase in heart rate with subsequent increase in cardiac output.

$$\text{Cardiac output (L/min)} = \text{stroke volume (L/beat)} \\ \times \text{heart rate (beats/min)}$$

The cardiac cycle, as well as the interplay between preload and afterload on stroke volume, can best be described by using pressure-volume loops (Fig. 21-14). These pressure-volume loops are constructed by combining systolic and diastolic pressure curves. The diastolic component (dotted line) is determined by diastolic filling (preload). The shape of the loop is determined by both contractility and the afterload against which the ventricle must contract. The cardiac cycle begins at end-diastole when the left ventricle is filled with left atrial blood and the cardiac muscle is relaxed. Upon excitation the muscle begins to contract and generate force against closed valves (isovolumetric contraction). Once the pressure in the left ventricle exceeds aortic pressure the blood is ejected into circulation during systole. This volume ejected is the stroke volume (depicted by the width of the pressure-volume loop). The remaining volume at the end of contraction is the end-systolic volume. At the end of contraction the ventricle begins to relax (isovolumetric relaxation) and the aortic valve closes as the pressure in the aorta exceeds that of the left ventricle. With a drop in left ventricular pressure the mitral valve opens and left atrial blood begins to fill the left ventricle during diastole. It should be noted that in the ideal system following passive flow of atrial blood, atrial contraction near the end of diastole optimizes filling of the left ventricle (*atrial kick*), thereby optimizing the Frank-Starling relationship. Loss of this end-diastolic atrial contraction as in atrial fibrillation in a heart with diminished function can have adverse systemic hemodynamic consequences.

There are several factors that affect the pressure-volume loops. Increasing preload increases end-diastolic volume and stroke volume. Increased afterload increases pressure needed to be generated during isovolumetric contraction to eject blood and decreases the stroke volume. Increased contractility, as with adrenergic stimulation, increases stroke volume and decreases end-systolic volume. The ability of a hypertrophic heart to increase stroke volume is severely limited by its decreased diastolic compliance.

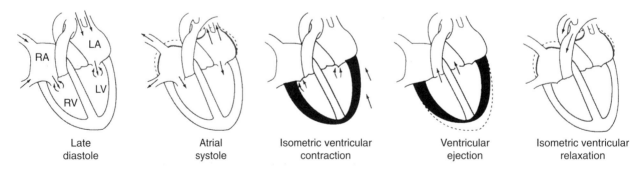

| Late diastole | Atrial systole | Isometric ventricular contraction | Ventricular ejection | Isometric ventricular relaxation |

Figure 21-13 Blood flow in the heart, great veins, aorta, and pulmonary arteries during a single cardiac cycle. Atrial and ventricular contractions are symbolized by *shading* of the wall. Right and left atria are designated *RA* and *LA* and right and left ventricles *RV* and *LV*. (From Johnson LR. *Essential medical physiology*, 2nd ed. Philadelphia: Lippincott Williams & Wilkins, 1998:189, with permission.)

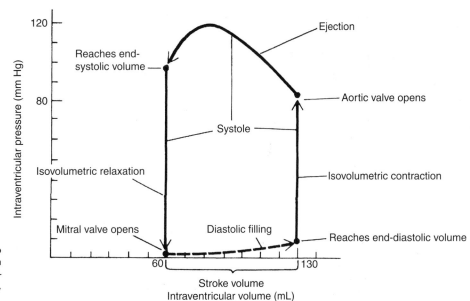

Figure 21-14 Pressure-volume loop of one cardiac cycle. (From Mohrman DE, Heller LJ. *Cardiovascular physiology*, 3rd ed. New York: McGraw Hill, 1991:54, with permission.)

Oxygen utilization by the heart is twofold. A small amount of oxygen is used for cellular homeostasis and a large amount during contraction. Changes in myocardial oxygen consumption are directly related to the work of the heart and changes in contractility. Cardiac work can be quantified as *stroke work,* or work which the heart performs with each beat (stroke work = aortic pressure × stroke volume). The *minute work* of the heart is equal to the product of heart rate times the stroke volume multiplied by the aortic pressure (or cardiac output × aortic pressure), so an increase in any of these three variables will increase cardiac work and ultimately increase myocardial oxygen consumption and demand.

The major determinant of oxygen demand is *myocardial wall tension.* Tension in the wall of the ventricle is determined by both the pressure in the ventricle and the geometry of the ventricle. The normal left ventricle is a pressurized irregularly shaped chamber. If we were to consider the ventricle as a cylinder then the *law of Laplace* states that wall tension is proportional to internal pressure times the radius. Increasing the wall thickness decreases the wall tension by distributing the internal pressure over a greater number of muscle fibers. In other words, wall tension equals pressure times radius divided by wall thickness. Altering the geometric configuration of the ventricle (as with cardiomyopathy) increases the radius, decreases the wall thickness and increases ventricular pressure all increasing wall tension and myocardial oxygen demand. Changing the geometry of the ventricle requires extra energy consumption to realign the myocytes prior to each systolic contraction.

As stated previously, cardiac output is equal to the product of stroke volume multiplied by the heart rate. A clinically feasible means of calculating cardiac output is to use the Fick equation:

$$Cardiac\ output = \frac{total\ body\ oxygen\ consumption}{[O_2]\ arterial\ blood - [O_2]\ venous\ blood}$$

Dye dilution and thermal dilution of heat are other clinically used methods of calculating cardiac output (described later in this chapter). Given the varied sizes of patients (varying body surface area) simply calculating a cardiac output may not provide enough information regarding cardiac function and adequate systemic perfusion. The calculated parameter of *cardiac index* factors in patient size and expresses cardiac output per square meter of surface area, thereby eliminating the variable of patient size (cardiac index = cardiac output/body surface area). A cardiac index greater than 2 L/min/m² is accepted as adequate. Figure 21-15 demonstrates the mechanical and electrical events during the various phases of the cardiac cycle.

Coronary Physiology

Coronary blood flow follows the major vessels into smaller penetrating arteries that provide the majority of the resistance to blood flow. There is a dense capillary network by which the extensive metabolic demands of the heart can be provided. At rest coronary blood flow is approximately 1 mL per gram of myocardium, but with demand this flow is capable of increasing nearly fourfold. The increase in blood flow is accomplished with a combination of local vasodilatation of the penetrating arteries as well as recruitment of vessels that are collapsed at rest. Because nearly 70% of the oxygen is derived from delivered coronary blood, there exists a very tight regulatory system to ensure adequate perfusion of the myocardium. The myocardial tissue functions most optimally under aerobic conditions and is capable of sustaining only a few minutes of anaerobic activity.

Coronary perfusion is accomplished during the relaxing diastolic phase. During systole the compressive forces within the myocardial wall are powerful enough to collapse the penetrating vessels and prevent myocardial perfusion. Therefore, increasing heart rate will not only increase myocardial oxygen demand but will also decrease myocardial perfusion. Regulation of coronary blood flow is accomplished by a combination of the (i) autonomic nervous system, (ii) metabolic vascular mediators, and (iii) vascular endothelium–mediated vasodilatation. There are a combination of α and β receptors on the conductance vessels that regulate nervous system–mediated vasoconstriction and vasodilatation, respectively. *Adenosine* is produced by

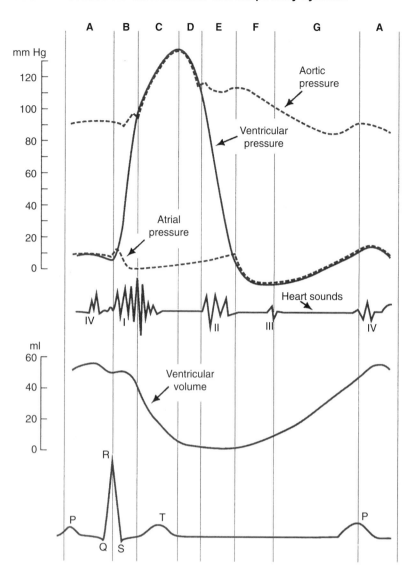

Figure 21-15 Mechanical and electrical events during a single cardiac cycle. The seven phases are denoted by letters as follows: **(A)** atrial systole, **(B)** isovolumetric ventricular contraction, **(C)** rapid ventricular ejection, **(D)** reduced ventricular ejection, **(E)** isovolumetric ventricular relaxation, **(F)** rapid ventricular filling, and **(G)** reduced ventricular filling. (From Johnson LR. *Essential medical physiology*, 2nd ed. Philadelphia: Lippincott Williams & Wilkins, 1998:190, with permission.)

cardiac myocytes in response to ischemia. It acts locally on vascular smooth muscle to cause vasodilatation. Adenosine is the primary metabolic vascular mediator. The endothelium is capable of releasing both vasodilatory and vasoconstricting mediators.

PULMONARY ARTERY CATHETERS

Assessment of hemodynamic parameters can be vital in managing the critically ill patient. Pulmonary artery catheters (Swan-Ganz catheters) can provide quantitative data of vital hemodynamic variables. The pulmonary artery catheter is a flow-directed catheter that is inserted via a central vein through the vena cava, right atrium, and right ventricle into the pulmonary arterial circulation. The right internal jugular and left subclavian veins are the preferred entry points into the central venous circulation. These two vessels provide the smoothest angles for the PA catheter to follow. There is a balloon on the end of the PA catheter that allows it to follow the flow of blood passively until it lodges within the pulmonary arterial circulation. PA catheters provide many valuable hemodynamic parameters that help manage both cardiac and noncardiac surgical patients.

The Swan-Ganz catheter provides measures of central venous pressure (CVP), right ventricular pressure, pulmonary artery pressure, pulmonary capillary wedge pressure (PCWP), and cardiac output (CO). Normal cardiac pressure ranges are illustrated in Table 21-2. The PCWP is measured when the balloon on the end of the PA catheter is inflated, thus occluding pulmonary circulation. This results

TABLE 21-2	
NORMAL HEMODYNAMIC PARAMETERS	
Cardiac output	4.0–8.0 L/min
Cardiac index	2.5–4.5 L/min/m^2
Stroke volume	60–130 mL
Systemic blood pressure	100–130/60–90 mm Hg
Mean arterial pressure (MAP)	70–105 mm Hg
Right atria/central venous pressure	2–10 mm Hg
Right ventricular pressure	15–30/0–18 mm Hg
Pulmonary artery pressure	15–30/6–12 mm Hg
Pulmonary capillary wedge pressure	5–12 mm Hg
Systemic vascular resistance (SVR)	700–1600 dynes/s/cm^2
Pulmonary vascular resistance	20–130 dynes/s/cm^2

in the ability to measure the pressure in the pulmonary capillary bed. At the end of diastole the pulmonary capillary circulation, left atria, and left ventricle can all be thought of as a single column filled with fluid. Hence, PCWP is a measure of left ventricular end-diastolic pressure, or in other words a measure of left ventricular preload.

Cardiac output can be measured by either the Fick formula or the dilution method. The Fick method requires one to measure the arterial-venous oxygen difference as well as oxygen consumption. It requires the measurement of a peripheral arterial blood gas, pulmonary artery venous blood gas, and oxygen consumption derived from inspired and expired oxygen concentrations.

The dilution method mathematically calculates cardiac output based on how fast the flowing blood can dilute a marker substance. Early dilution methods used dyes. More modern techniques utilize a thermodilution technique. In standard PA catheters cold or room temperature saline is infused via an infusion port, and the temperature downstream at a thermistor is measured. Continuous cardiac output catheters (CCO) incorporate a pulse-heating current filament on the PA catheter that cycles over a specified period. The heat is generated proximally and the diluted, cooled blood is measured distally allowing for a thermodilution measure of cardiac output. Because each person has a different body mass, we can standardize the cardiac output to body mass to derive cardiac index (cardiac output/body surface area = cardiac index).

Modern PA catheters often incorporate a fiberoptic pulse oximeter at the end of the catheter that measures mixed venous oxygen saturation ($S\bar{v}O_2$), which is an indirect measure of cardiac output. With diminished cardiac output peripheral tissues will extract more oxygen from circulating blood. Ultimately, this results in a diminished mixed $S\bar{v}O_2$. Hence, in situations of severely decreased cardiac output the $S\bar{v}O_2$ will be significantly lowered. $S\bar{v}O_2$ is a more accurate measure of cardiac output than is thermodilution in patients with tricuspid regurgitation. Other factors that lower $S\bar{v}O_2$ include lowered oxygen carrying capacity (decreased hemoglobin level), compromised oxygen saturation (hypoxemia), and increased tissue oxygen consumption (i.e., awakening after anesthesia).

VASOACTIVE MEDICATIONS

There are a wide variety of vasoactive medications that are available to both aide the failing heart and help maintain perfusion pressure. Vasoactive medications can be classified into two subsets: (i) medications that augment perfusion and (ii) medications that treat hypertension (reduce afterload). Medications that augment perfusion can either act centrally on the heart and/or peripherally on the systemic circulation. The majority of centrally acting agents exert their effects by interacting with the β_1-adrenergic receptors (epinephrine, norepinephrine, dopamine, dobutamine, isoproterenol). This interaction with the β_1 receptor elevates intracellular cyclic adenosine monophosphate (cAMP) levels. The second class of centrally acting agents is the phosphodiesterase inhibitors (amrinone and milrinone). Phosphodiesterase inhibitors elevate cAMP levels by inhibiting cAMP degradation. cAMP augments influx of calcium into cardiac cells and enhances contractility.

A brief description of each of these agents will be presented. Epinephrine acts primarily on β_1 receptors, but it also binds β_2 receptors to a lesser degree. It is a potent inotrope that increases cardiac output by increasing cardiac output and heart rate. Norepinephrine has predominantly α-adrenergic activity and mild β-adrenergic activity. The strong α activity makes norepinephrine a better peripherally acting agent by which to increase systemic vascular resistance and blood pressure. The hemodynamic effects of dopamine are dose-dependent: at low doses (2 to 3 μg/kg/min), it dilates renal arteries and increases urine output; at medium doses (3 to 8 μg/kg/min), β-adrenergic activity predominates; and at high doses (greater than 8 μg/kg/min), α-adrenergic activity predominates. Dobutamine exerts its effects via β_1 and β_2 receptors. Therefore, it increases heart rate and contractility while reducing SVR and afterload. Isoproterenol has strong β_1 effects that produce an increase in contractility and a marked increase in heart rate. It also exhibits β_2 activity that lowers pulmonary vascular resistance, thereby reducing right heart afterload. Milrinone and the older amrinone are phosphodiesterase inhibitors with very long half-lives of 2.3 and 3.6 hours, respectively. They exhibit inotropic activity in addition to pulmonary and systemic vasodilation. This vasodilation may result in hypotension, thereby limiting utilization of these agents.

Peripherally acting agents include phenylephrine and vasopressin, in addition to norepinephrine, dopamine, and dobutamine. Phenylephrine is a pure α-agonist that increases blood pressure by increasing SVR; a reflex decrease in heart rate may result. Vasopressin is a potent vasoconstrictor that interacts with vasopressin-1a receptors on vascular smooth muscle. Decreased vasopressin levels have been shown in conditions of sepsis and systemic illness. Recent literature supports the use of "physiologic dose" infusions of vasopressin in these situations.

The subject of selection of vasodilators and antihypertensive medications is extensive and beyond the scope of this chapter.

CARDIOPULMONARY BYPASS

The cardiopulmonary bypass (CPB) circuit is used to isolate the cardiopulmonary system and thereby provide optimal, blood-free, operative exposure for cardiovascular surgery. The CPB circuit must perform the functions of the cardiovascular system. It must oxygenate blood, remove carbon dioxide, and provide adequate perfusion to end organs. The cardiovascular surgeon can use either total or partial cardiopulmonary bypass. During total CPB, the venous return of the heart is circulated through the CPB circuit in its entirety, whereas during partial CPB, a fraction of the blood is allowed to circulate to the right ventricle and pulmonary circulation.

The basic components of the CPB circuit include the venous reservoir, oxygenator, heat exchanger, and pump. The venous reservoir stores systemic venous return. The oxygenator both adds oxygen and removes carbon dioxide from the blood. Thermoregulation of blood is controlled by the heat exchanger. Blood is returned to the systemic circulation via the ascending aorta or femoral artery by the pump. The pump can either be a kinetic centrifugal pump or the more common electric motor driven, load-independent roller pump.

During cardiopulmonary bypass blood flow generated by either centrifugal or roller pumps is nonpulsatile. At the same time, the pulmonary artery and central venous pressure are nearly zero, since the inflow to these systems is diverted via venous cannulas to the venous reservoir of the cardiopulmonary bypass system. There is much controversy over the necessity for pulsatile flow and hence cyclically elevated systolic pressures as opposed to a steady mean arterial pressure.

INTRAAORTIC BALLOON PUMPS

A failing heart often requires both decreased myocardial work, thereby decreasing myocardial oxygen demand, as well as increased perfusion. An intraaortic balloon pump (IABP) can help satisfy these needs. The IABP is positioned in the descending thoracic aorta just distal the left subclavian artery take-off. The IABP is timed to inflate during diastole. This allows for increased retrograde flow of aortic blood through the coronary ostia enhancing coronary perfusion. During systole the IABP deflates, allowing increased empty space and consequent decrease in afterload and thereby a decrease in myocardial work. This results in a diminished myocardial oxygen demand and consumption. IABP can provide considerable myocardial support when utilized properly (see Table 21-3). Unfortunately, IABP utilization can carry significant risk; namely, exacerbation of aortic insufficiency, lower extremity malperfusion, aortic dissection, or embolic disease. IABP is good treatment for left heart dysfunction, but unfortunately it affords little benefit in treating isolated right ventricular failure.

TABLE 21-3

INDICATIONS AND CONTRAINDICATIONS FOR PLACEMENT OF INTRAAORTIC BALLOON PUMP

Indications	Contraindications
Refractory unstable angina	Aortic insufficiency
Complications of myocardial infarction	Acute aortic dissection
Mitral regurgitation	Peripheral vascular disease (relative)
Ventriculoseptal defect	
Refractory arrhythmias	Abdominal aortic aneurysm (relative); thoracic aortic aneurysm
Ventricular aneurysm	
Cardiogenic shock	
Severe left main coronary disease prior to revascularization	
Pump failure after cardiac surgery	
Septic shock (rare cases)	

KEY POINTS

▲ Upon taking initial breaths the neonatal pulmonary vascular resistance drops, pressure in the left atria exceeds that in the right atria, and spontaneous closure of the foramen ovale occurs.

▲ The anterior leaflet of the mitral valve is in proximity to the aortic valve.

▲ The coronary arteries are the first branches of the aorta.

▲ Cardiac cells can maintain prolonged action potentials, conduct from cell to cell via gap junctions, and self-generate.

▲ Coronary perfusion occurs during diastole.

▲ The major resistance to blood flow occurs at the level of penetrating arteries.

▲ Myocardial oxygen demand is dependent on myocardial oxygen tension.

SUGGESTED READINGS

Berne RM, Levy MN. *Cardiovascular Physiology*, 8th ed. St.Louis, Mosby, 2001.

Cohn LH, Edmonds LH. *Cardiac surgery in the adult*, 2nd ed. New York McGraw-Hill, 2003.

Constanzo LS. *Physiology*, 2nd ed. PhiladelphiaWB Saunders, 2002.

Kaiser LR, Kron IL, Spray TL. *Mastery of cardiothoracic surgery*. Philadelphia: Lippincott-Raven, 1997.

Mohrman DE, Heller LJ. *Cardiovascular physiology*, 4th ed. New York: McGraw-Hill, 1996.

Moore KL. *Essential clinical anatomy*, 2nd ed. Philadelphia: Lippincott Williams & Wilkins, 2002.

Rhoades RA. *Medical physiology*, 2nd ed. Philadelphia: Lippincott Williams & Wilkins, 2003.

Sadler TW, Langman J. *Langman's medical embryology*, 8th ed. Philadelphia: Lippincott Williams & Wilkins, 2000.

Cardiovascular Pathophysiology and Treatment

Vasant Jayasankar   Michael A. Acker

Cardiovascular diseases are the predominant cause of disability and death in industrialized nations. In the United States, cardiovascular diseases account for approximately 40% of all deaths, almost twice the number of deaths caused by all forms of cancer combined. Diseases of the cardiovascular system encompass a diverse array of pathologic processes, including congenital malformations, acquired lesions of the coronary circulation and aorta, valvular diseases, and inflammatory and autoimmune processes. Because of the importance of the cardiovascular system for perfusion of all tissues of the body, clinical presentation of many of these disorders can be precipitous and severe. This chapter reviews the major cardiovascular disorders and their surgical management.

CONGENITAL HEART DISEASE

Congenital heart defects occur in 4 to 9 per 1,000 live-births. A useful classification system organizes the congenital heart defects into three general physiologic disturbances: left-to-right shunt, right-to-left shunt, and ventricular outflow obstruction. In addition, there are several complex congenital defects that can be classified as bidirectional shunts.

Left-to-right Shunts

This condition is characterized by the absence of cyanosis and increased pulmonary blood flow. Communication between pulmonary and systemic circulations may occur at the level of the atria, ventricles, or great vessels. Lesions leading to this condition are common and represent 40% of anomalies diagnosed in the first year of life.

Atrial Septal Defect

Atrial septal defect (ASD) is one of the most common congenital heart anomalies. It accounts for 10% to 15% of patients with congenital heart disease and is the most common congenital heart lesion in adults. ASDs are commonly observed with other heart anomalies and are associated with genetically determined syndromes such as Down, Turner, Marfan, and Ehlers-Danlos. Maternal rubella exposure or ingestion of thalidomide is also associated with development of ASDs. The male-to-female ratio is approximately 1:2.

Approximately 20% of healthy individuals have a patent foramen ovale. This usually is of no consequence because the flap mechanism formed by the septum primum prevents interatrial shunting unless there are high right atrial pressures. Defects or deficiencies in the septum primum lead to ostium secundum–type ASDs (Fig. 22-1).

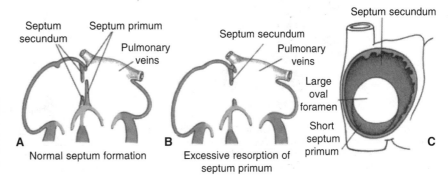

Figure 22-1 Normal atrial septum formation **(A)** and ostium secundum type atrial septal defect caused by excessive resorption of the septum primum **(B,C)**. (From Sadler TW. *Langman's medical embryology,* 5th ed. Baltimore: Williams & Wilkins, 1985, with permission.)

Spontaneous closure of ASDs is rare after 2 years of age. Operative closure of ASDs by primary repair or with a pericardial or prosthetic patch is indicated in patients with Q_p:Q_s ratio of greater than 1.5. More commonly these repairs are being undertaken using percutaneous techniques with catheter-based devices.

Ventricular Septal Defect

Ventricular septal defect (VSD) is one of the most common congenital heart lesions and accounts for approximately one fourth of all congenital heart defects. It is present as an isolated anomaly approximately once per every 1,000 live-births. In addition, approximately one half of patients with a VSD have associated anomalies.

VSDs are categorized according to their anatomic location in the ventricular septum (Fig. 22-2). A VSD is considered large when its diameter is equal to or greater than the diameter of the aortic valve ring. In the setting of low pulmonary vascular resistance after the first few months of life, a large defect may lead to high pulmonary blood flow (Q_p:Q_s ratio of greater than 2), left ventricular (LV) diastolic overload, and congestive heart failure (CHF). Ultimately, high pulmonary blood flow results in medial thickening of the pulmonary vasculature, pulmonary hypertension, and right heart failure.

Early surgical repair is indicated for infants with large defects (Q_p:Q_s ratio of greater than 2) who have severe symptoms. Otherwise, repair of large defects is usually deferred until between 1 and 2 years of age. Repair of moderate-sized defects (Q_p:Q_s ratio of 1.5 to 2) is generally done in childhood because of the likelihood of spontaneous size reduction or closure.

Patent Ductus Arteriosus

Patent ductus arteriosus (PDA) is a common congenital heart lesion, particularly in premature infants, in whom the incidence may exceed 15%. For this reason, PDA is not considered to be abnormal until after 3 months of age. Maternal exposure to rubella, high-altitude living, polygenic inheritance, prematurity, neonatal hypoxia, and respiratory distress of the newborn have all been found to be associated with this lesion. The male-to-female ratio is approximately 1:2. Failure of this closure is thought to be caused by immaturity of the thick medial layer of smooth muscle of the ductus arteriosus and biochemical unresponsiveness to stimuli. The decrease in pulmonary vascular resistance combined with the increase in systemic vascular resistance that occurs shortly after birth leads to reversal of blood flow through a PDA and left-to-right shunting.

Closure of a PDA in newborns can be attempted medically with prostaglandin synthase inhibition using acetylsalicylic acid or indomethacin. If this fails, operative division via a posterolateral thoracotomy is indicated in all patients whether they are symptomatic or not because of the long-term risk for development of medial hypertrophy of the pulmonary vasculature and subsequent pulmonary hypertension. Catheter-based percutaneous techniques are also being employed to treat these lesions.

Right-to-left Shunts

This condition results from obstruction of pulmonary blood flow in combination with an intracardiac defect that leads to right-to-left shunting and systemic hypoxia.

Tetralogy of Fallot

Tetralogy of Fallot is the most common of the cyanotic congenital heart lesions, accounting for up to 50% of such lesions. In most cases, the cause of the condition is not known. However, it has been associated with maternal exposure to rubella and thalidomide and diabetic embryopathy. Tetralogy also occurs in association with Down, XXX, Turner, Klippel-Feil, and Noonan syndromes. There is a slight preponderance of men affected by this lesion.

Tetralogy of Fallot consists of VSD, right ventricular outflow tract obstruction, an overriding aorta, and right ventricular hypertrophy (Fig. 22-3). The additional presence of an ASD is referred to as "pentalogy" of Fallot. Right-sided aortic arch is present in 25% of patients and abnormalities of the coronary circulation, such as origin of the left anterior

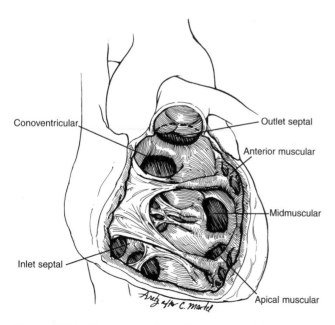

Figure 22-2   Major types of ventricular septal defects categorized by anatomic location. (From Kaiser LR, Kron IL, Spray TL, eds. *Mastery of cardiothoracic surgery.* Philadelphia: Lippincott Williams & Wilkins, 1998, with permission.)

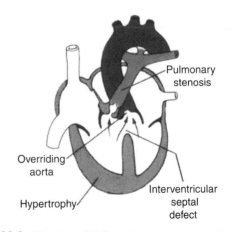

Figure 22-3   Tetralogy of Fallot: schematic drawing. (From Sadler TW. *Langman's medical embryology*, 5th ed. Baltimore: Williams & Wilkins, 1985, with permission.)

descending coronary artery from the right coronary artery, are present in 5%.

With severe right ventricular (RV) outflow obstruction, there is considerable early right-to-left shunting with greatly reduced pulmonary blood flow that is dependent on a patent ductus arteriosus. With mild obstruction, there may be mixed intracardiac shunting initially with left-to-right predominance, resulting in increased pulmonary blood flow and only mild oxygen desaturation. This has been referred to as the "pink" tetralogy. In severe cases, most patients present with cyanosis within the first 6 months. Older children with tetralogy may squat for relief of symptoms or develop "blue spells," which are thought to result from spasm of the right ventricular outflow tract. Physical examination reveals a systolic murmur over the left sternal border and an accentuated aortic second heart sound. A common finding on electrocardiogram is right axis deviation and right ventricular hypertrophy. Cardiac catheterization is still considered necessary for preoperative evaluation.

Surgical treatment of tetralogy of Fallot is indicated because of the long-term risk for CHF, cerebrovascular accidents secondary to polycythemia, and bacterial endocarditis.

Tricuspid Atresia

Tricuspid atresia is characterized by lack of communication between the right atrium and right ventricle. Associated anomalies include interatrial communication, enlargement of the mitral valve and left ventricle, and right ventricular hypoplasia. Tricuspid atresia is the third most common cyanotic heart lesion, following tetralogy of Fallot and transposition of the great arteries. Surgical therapy is indicated because of the poor prognosis, even for patients with near-normal pulmonary blood flow. The Fontan procedure achieves separation of the pulmonary and systemic circulations by diverting systemic venous return directly to the lungs, relying on the right atrium to provide pulmonary perfusion pressure. This results in increased systemic arterial saturation and decreased LV work.

Eisenmenger Syndrome

Longstanding left-to-right shunting of blood flow, as occurs with VSD, can lead to medial hypertrophy of the pulmonary vasculature and a progressive increase in pulmonary vascular resistance. Subsequent reversal of blood flow through the shunt causes cyanosis and decreased pulmonary blood flow. Repair of the underlying defect at this stage is usually contraindicated because of the likelihood of right heart failure.

Ventricular Outflow Obstruction

This group consists of congenital heart anomalies that cause obstruction to right and/or left ventricular outflow.

Aortic Stenosis

Congenital aortic stenosis collectively describes all lesions that cause LV outflow obstruction and includes supravalvar stenosis, valvar stenosis, subaortic stenosis, and LV outflow obstruction. All of these forms of aortic stenosis occur predominantly in men, with a male-to-female ratio of approximately 4:1. Idiopathic hypertrophic subaortic stenosis and to a lesser extent supravalvar aortic stenosis

have been recognized to occur in families and are, in some cases, thought to have a genetic component.

Severe LV outflow obstruction caused by aortic stenosis leads to pulmonary congestion, pulmonary venous hypertension, systemic hypoperfusion, and metabolic acidosis. Patients presenting in childhood may have infective endocarditis, LV failure, and sudden death. On physical examination, aortic stenosis is characterized by a systolic murmur over the aortic area. Chest x-ray findings include LV and aortic enlargement and pulmonary venous congestion. Cardiac catheterization provides pressure gradient measurements, allows calculation of valve areas, and reliably distinguishes between the different anatomic types of aortic stenosis.

Aortic valvotomy is indicated for young children with severe aortic stenosis (gradient greater than 75 mm Hg) whether or not they are symptomatic. This procedure may also be indicated for older children with moderate aortic stenosis (gradient between 50 and 75 mm Hg) who have angina, syncope, exercise intolerance, or evidence of LV hypertrophy with strain on electrocardiogram.

Coarctation of the Aorta

Coarctation of the aorta is characterized by a discrete narrowing or hypoplasia of the proximal descending thoracic aorta at the site of entrance of the ductus arteriosus. It is a relatively common lesion and accounts for 5% to 8% of all congenital heart anomalies. It may be associated with VSD, congenital aortic stenosis, hypoplastic left ventricle, or congenital mitral valve stenosis. In addition, bicuspid aortic valve is reported to be present in about one third of patients with coarctation.

Coarctation has historically been categorized into two groups: infantile and adult. In infantile coarctation, the aortic obstruction is most often preductal and leads to separation of LV flow (which is directed to the head and arms) from pulmonary artery flow (which is directed to the lower body). This type of coarctation results in early LV failure and death if not surgically corrected. The more common adult type of coarctation is postductal and leads to proximal hypertension and eventual CHF over time, although patients may remain asymptomatic and appear healthy into adulthood.

Approximately 15% of patients with coarctation present with severe CHF requiring early surgical intervention within the first few months of life. In the remainder, coarctation is most frequently detected during workup for a heart murmur or for hypertension noted during routine physical examinations. Patients who are symptomatic at the time of presentation may complain of dyspnea, headache, and nosebleeds. Physical examination findings include upper extremity systolic hypertension, absent or decreased lower extremity pulses, prominent pulsations at the sternal notch, and a systolic heart murmur over the left sternal border that may be transmitted to the back. Chest x-rays may reveal rib notching by the age of 10 years secondary to enlarged intercostal artery collaterals. Other x-ray findings include an indentation over the left border of the heart at the site of coarctation, which gives the "3" sign.

Patients presenting early with severe CHF are treated with prostaglandin E_1 to maintain ductal patency, which improves blood flow to the descending aorta until surgical repair can be attempted. In older children, end-to-end anastomosis is appropriate. Repair in adults may be hazardous because of the presence of large, friable intercostal artery collaterals. Bypass using a prosthetic tube graft may be performed in this setting and also in the case of recurrent coarctation.

Bidirectional Shunts

These complex congenital defects have also been termed *admixing lesions* because they result in both left-to-right and right-to-left shunts. Patients with these lesions commonly present with CHF because of increased pulmonary blood flow and volume overload.

Transposition of the Great Arteries

Transposition of the great arteries is the most frequent congenital heart lesion causing cyanosis in the newborn period and accounts for 8% to 10% of all congenital heart defects. There is a distinct male preponderance in patients presenting with this condition. In complete transposition, the aorta arises anteriorly from the right ventricle and the pulmonary artery arises posteriorly from the left ventricle (Fig. 22-4). Patent ductus arteriosus, VSD, and patent foramen ovale are usually associated with transposition.

The physiologic effect of complete transposition is separation of the pulmonary and systemic circulations so that they exist in parallel rather than in series. Absence of intracirculatory shunts that allow admixture of oxygenated pulmonary circulation blood with deoxygenated systemic circulation blood is incompatible with life. The most common clinical features of complete transposition are cyanosis, which is usually present at birth, and CHF, which develops in the neonatal period as the pulmonary vascular resistance decreases. Physical examination reveals a systolic murmur and loud single second heart sound. Classic chest roentgenogram findings are an oval or egg-shaped heart, a narrow superior mediastinum, and increased pulmonary vascular markings.

Successful physiologic correction of complete transposition by use of an intraatrial baffle was first reported in 1964 by Mustard. This procedure uses the right ventricle as the source of systemic flow but at late follow-up has been associated with progressive right ventricular failure. The modern standard of care is the arterial switch procedure, which involves switching the great vessels to their appropriate ventricles and reimplanting the coronary arteries into the neoaorta. The 5-year actuarial survival following this procedure approaches 90%.

Total Anomalous Pulmonary Venous Connection

Total anomalous pulmonary venous connection (TAPVC) describes a condition in which the pulmonary veins do not communicate with the left atrium but rather with the right atrium, coronary sinus, or a major systemic vein. The left atrium receives blood via a patent foramen ovale or ASD in those patients who survive beyond birth. A PDA is also present in 25% to 50% of cases. The male-to-female ratio among patients with this lesion is nearly 2:1. TAPVC and other severe congenital heart defects may be associated with the asplenia syndrome. In approximately 50% of cases of TAPVC, the site of pulmonary venous connection is supracardiac, most commonly a left anomalous vertical vein draining to the innominate vein. In approximately 25% of cases, the connection is intracardiac, with the coronary sinus being the most common site of connection in this group. More than 80% of infants born with TAPVC die before the age of 1 year. Early surgical intervention is therefore indicated, even in those patients with unobstructed connections and only mild cyanosis. Surgical repair involves redirecting flow from the pulmonary venous chamber to the left atrium and, if successful, is associated with only rare long-term complications.

Hypoplastic Left Heart Syndrome

Hypoplastic left heart syndrome is a complex anomaly characterized by marked hypoplasia or atresia of the left ventricle, hypoplasia of the ascending aorta, intact ventricular septum, and mitral valve atresia or hypoplasia. The cause of hypoplastic left heart syndrome in most cases is felt to be severe underdevelopment of LV outflow secondary to isolated aortic valve atresia or double outlet right ventricle with aortic valve atresia. Hypoplastic left heart syndrome is relatively common, making up 7% of congenital heart malformations presenting in the first year of life.

In this condition, the left ventricle is nonfunctional and the systemic circulation is dependent on a patent ductus arteriosus. Newborns typically present within the first 24 to 48 hours of life with cyanosis and tachypnea. As the ductus closes, systemic perfusion decreases and metabolic acidosis develops. Definitive diagnosis of this lesion is made by echocardiography. Cardiac catheterization is generally not indicated for diagnostic or therapeutic purposes.

Initial management consists of prostaglandin E_1 infusion to maintain patency of the ductus arteriosus and allow systemic perfusion through this structure. Early surgical intervention is required because this lesion is uniformly fatal without reconstructive surgery or heart transplantation. The Norwood procedure involves application of a Fontan-like reconstruction to this malformation in two stages. Because of the high mortality associated with this procedure, particularly the first stage, cardiac transplantation has been advanced as a potential alternative for the management of this syndrome. This strategy is limited by the inadequate supply of donor hearts, the need for chronic immunosuppression, and unknown long-term outlook. Using modern techniques the results of the Norwood procedure have been improving.

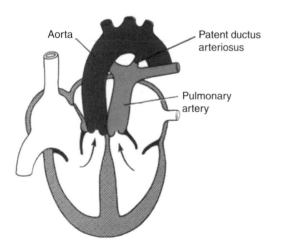

Figure 22-4   Transposition of the great vessels: schematic drawing. (From Sadler TW. *Langman's medical embryology*, 5th ed. Baltimore: Williams & Wilkins, 1985, with permission.)

ACQUIRED HEART DISEASE

Functional classification has been useful in stratifying patients with acquired heart disease for prognostic and therapeutic purposes. The two most commonly used classification systems are the New York Heart Association (NYHA) heart failure functional classification, which is a general subjective classification of symptoms (Table 22-1), and the Canadian Cardiovascular Society functional classification, which classifies angina symptoms related to coronary artery disease (Table 22-2).

Coronary Artery Disease

Coronary artery disease is the leading cause of death in the United States. It is caused by atherosclerotic narrowing of the arteries. Risk factors include inappropriate diet, hypertension, diabetes, smoking, sedentary lifestyle, and family history. Men are at higher risk for developing premature coronary artery disease than women, for whom the risk after menopause increases to that of men. Anatomically, the most severe atherosclerotic changes occur in the proximal third of the coronary arteries, making therapeutic bypass of such lesions feasible. Diffuse atherosclerotic disease of the coronary arteries does occur occasionally, however, and may be associated with diabetes mellitus and hyperlipidemia disorders.

Patients with coronary artery disease may present with angina pectoris, myocardial infarction (MI), or sudden death secondary to ventricular arrhythmias. Severe manifestations of this disease are not necessarily preceded by angina. Indeed, one half of all fatal heart attacks occur in previously asymptomatic individuals. Individuals at risk for cardiac events can be identified by use of stress electrocardiogram and thallium tests, stress echocardiography, or intravenous dipyridamole thallium-201 scintigraphy (DTS). The ability to identify patients at high risk for cardiac events is of particular interest to surgeons, as the leading cause of death after major surgery is cardiac. It has been estimated that more than 10% of patients undergoing surgical procedures in this country are at risk for coronary disease,

---

TABLE 22-1

NEW YORK HEART ASSOCIATION HEART FAILURE FUNCTIONAL CLASSIFICATION

Class I	Patients with cardiac disease but without resulting limitation of physical activity.
Class II	Patients with cardiac disease resulting in slight limitation of physical activity. Ordinary physical activity causes fatigue, palpitations, dyspnea, or angina. No symptoms at rest.
Class III	Patients with cardiac disease resulting in marked limitation of physical activity. Less than ordinary physical activity results in fatigue, palpitations, dyspnea, or angina. No symptoms at rest.
Class IV	Patients with cardiac disease who are unable to carry on any physical activity without discomfort. Symptoms of cardiac insufficiency or angina may be present even at rest. Any physical activity increases discomfort.

From Braunwald E. The history. In: Braunwald E, ed. *Heart Disease: a textbook of cardiovascular medicine*, 5th ed. Philadelphia: WB Saunders, 1997:1–14, with permission.

TABLE 22-2

CANADIAN CARDIOVASCULAR SOCIETY FUNCTIONAL CLASSIFICATION

Class I	Ordinary physical activity does not cause angina. Angina may occur with strenuous or prolonged exertion.
Class II	Slight limitation of ordinary activity. Angina may occur with walking or climbing stairs rapidly, walking uphill, walking or stair climbing after meals or in the cold, in the wind, or under emotional stress, or walking more than two blocks on the level or climbing more than one flight of stairs under normal conditions at a normal pace.
Class III	Marked limitation of ordinary physical activity. Angina may occur after walking one or two blocks on level ground or climbing one flight of stairs under normal conditions at a normal place.
Class IV	Inability to carry out any physical activity without anginal discomfort; angina may be present at rest.

From Braunwald E. The history. In: Braunwald E, ed. *Heart disease: a textbook of cardiovascular medicine*, 5th ed. Philadelphia: WB Saunders, 1997:1–14, with permission.

---

and of these patients at risk up to 15% subsequently suffer significant cardiac complications. The group at highest risk for cardiac morbidity are patients undergoing surgery for peripheral vascular disease. This group has been found to have associated severe coronary artery disease in up to one third of patients.

Intravenous DTS is now thought to be the best preoperative noninvasive screening test for patients at risk for cardiac events. It is particularly useful for patients who are unable to undergo exercise stress testing because of peripheral vascular, orthopedic, neurologic, or other debilitating conditions. The finding of positive DTS results (an initial myocardial perfusion defect followed by delayed reperfusion of this region) is associated with increased risk for cardiac events and should be followed by coronary angiography and appropriate therapy. Conversely, negative DTS results are associated with a low incidence of perioperative cardiac events. The average sensitivity of DTS is approximately 90%, whereas the specificity is approximately 75%.

Clinical risk factors associated with increased risk for significant coronary artery disease include history of angina, Q waves on electrocardiogram, age older than 70 years, ventricular ectopy requiring medical therapy, diabetes mellitus, and clinical evidence of LV failure. Patients with none of these risk factors have been found to have a 3% incidence of perioperative cardiac events versus a 50% incidence for patients with three or more clinical risk factors. DTS has been found to be most useful as a screening tool for patients with one or two clinical risk factors who are at intermediate risk. In this group, patients with negative DTS results had a 3% incidence of cardiac events versus 30% for patients with positive DTS results.

Indications for Intervention

General indications for revascularization of the coronary circulation include increasing symptoms, and revascularization is undertaken to prevent myocardial damage in high-risk patients and to prolong life. Because the long-term benefits of coronary artery bypass grafting (CABG) decrease with time, surgery is usually not recommended for patients presenting with mild-to-moderate symptoms who do not have evidence of life-threatening coronary artery disease and do not have LV dysfunction. These patients can be treated medically until symptoms become unmanageable.

Patients with progressive or unstable angina despite maximal medical therapy frequently have considerable amounts of myocardium at risk and are candidates for urgent revascularization. For one- or two-vessel disease, percutaneous transluminal coronary angioplasty (PTCA) is frequently attempted, with surgery reserved for patients with early failure. In most centers where angioplasty is a common procedure, the incidence of patients requiring emergency surgery after early PTCA failure is less than 3%. In addition to early failure, an additional 20% to 30% of patients with initially successful angioplasties develop restenosis within 6 to 12 months, requiring further intervention. The randomized trials of PTCA versus CABG have demonstrated that percutaneous interventions are a reasonable approach, and may be preferred as the initial therapeutic modality in most patients. There is a higher incidence of recurrent angina and restenosis in PTCA versus CABG; however, PTCA does not appear to increase the rate of MI or death. In addition, the advent of drug-eluting stents may significantly improve long-term patency of this approach, although long-term follow-up is still needed in these studies.

Indications for elective CABG have been developed on the basis of results of large randomized trials of CABG versus medical therapy (Table 22-3). Improved survival with surgery has led to the following clear indications for CABG: NYHA class III or greater with angina unresponsive to medical therapy, unstable angina, left main coronary artery disease, three-vessel disease or two-vessel disease where the left anterior descending has a severe obstruction proximal to the first septal perforator, and failed PTCA. Possible indications for CABG are postmyocardial infarction patients with positive stress test results at low workload and patients in cardiogenic shock with viable myocardium to salvage. No survival benefit has been demonstrated for single vessel disease.

The decrease in long-term benefits of CABG over time is related primarily to the development of vein graft disease. After 10 years, only 50% to 60% of saphenous vein grafts remain patent. In contrast, the internal mammary artery appears to be relatively resistant to late atherosclerosis and

---

TABLE 22-3

INDICATIONS FOR CORONARY ARTERY BYPASS GRAFTING

New York Heart Association class III angina unresponsive to
   medical therapy
Unstable angina
Left main coronary artery disease
Symptomatic patient with three-vessel coronary artery disease
Failed percutaneous transluminal coronary angioplasty
Postmyocardial infarction patient with positive stress test results at
   low workload
Acute myocardial infarction with cardiogenic shock

From Franco KL, Hammond GL. Surgical indications for coronary revascularization. In: Baue AE, Geha AS, Hammond GL et al., eds. *Glenn's thoracic and cardiovascular surgery*, 6th ed. Stamford: Appleton & Lange, 1996:2073–2079, with permission.

---

graft disease, leading to a greater than 95% patency rate even after 20 years. Significant improvement in survival and freedom from cardiac events has been demonstrated in patients receiving internal mammary artery bypass grafts to the LAD. Long-term benefits of CABG are also limited by progression of atherosclerotic changes in the native vessels. Postoperative care therefore includes patient education, diet control, cessation of smoking, control of hypertension, and use of cholesterol-lowering agents if indicated.

Alternatives to Traditional Coronary Artery Bypass Grafting

There have been a number of technologic advancements in cardiothoracic surgery that offer alternatives to the traditional on-pump CABG via median sternotomy. These include minimally invasive direct coronary artery bypass grafting (MIDCAB), off-pump CABG (OPCAB), and robotics.

MIDCAB stemmed from the trends toward noninvasive and less-invasive techniques in other areas of surgical intervention (such as laparoscopy and video-assisted thoracic surgery). Coronary grafting without the benefit of bypass dates back to the 1960s; however, the inherent technical difficulties of operating on the beating heart made it unpopular for many years. MIDCAB has been used for single-, double- and triple-vessel disease, and for both primary and reoperations. However, it is most suited for primary grafting of isolated left anterior descending lesions. Relative contraindications include severe pulmonary disease, circumflex disease, poor LV function, and arrhythmias. The approach is via a left anterior minithoracotomy, and the left internal mammary artery is dissected and skeletonized under direct visualization. Stabilization devices can be employed to assist. Although the MIDCAB offers the distinct advantage of avoiding cardiopulmonary bypass, its value for treating primarily single-vessel disease, the advancement of coronary stenting, and the questionable benefit of thoracotomy versus sternotomy has limited its widespread use in favor of OPCAB.

OPCAB was developed with the recognition that cardiac arrest with cold cardioplegia and cardiopulmonary-bypass were associated with significant potential morbidity. The recognition of improved outcomes in some patients that underwent CABG without cardiopulmonary bypass lent further impetus to refine the techniques of off-pump coronary grafting. Currently, up to 25% of bypass operations in the United States are performed off-pump. Contraindications to this approach include hemodynamic or electrical instability. Multivessel disease is amenable to OPCAB, and it is particularly well-suited to patients with low ejection fractions where weaning from bypass may be difficult. A median sternotomy is performed, and specialized stabilization and retraction devices are utilized to facilitate positioning of the heart. A misted carbon dioxide blower is generally employed to maintain a bloodless field. The sequence of graft construction is extremely important, and collateralized vessels should be grafted before the feeding collateralizing arteries. Proximal control is obtained with soft silastic tape, whereas distal control is obtained only if needed. Intracoronary shunts may be used to preserve flow during the anastamoses. In randomized trials OPCAB has been shown to significantly decrease transfusion requirement and systemic inflammatory response compared to on-pump CABG. Further studies are needed to assess the potential benefits on mortality, stroke rates, MI, hospital stay and total costs. Although off-pump coronary surgery is technically challenging, it is likely that its use will further increase in the near future.

Robotic cardiac surgery is currently in its infancy. It has been used to harvest the internal mammary artery, to perform coronary anastamoses, and for complex valvular operations. This evolving technology provides a high degree of control and stereoscopic vision to allow complex and delicate manipulations, including suturing. Further development of feedback mechanisms to help guide the surgeon will add to its usefullness. This cutting-edge technology offers the benefits of reduced incision size and the potential to avoid a median sternotomy, and significant advances are likely in the near future.

Myocardial Infarction

Current management of acute MI includes early reperfusion within the first 3 to 6 hours after onset. Angioplasty of the infarcted vessel has may be successful in approximately 95% of cases, and is the current preferred approach over thrombolytic therapy. Trials have demonstrated superior success and patency rates of angioplasty versus lysis.

Although CABG has not been shown to prolong survival for patients who are asymptomatic after recovery from MI, studies have identified subgroups of patients who are at high risk for death in the postinfarction period and who may benefit from bypass surgery. For postinfarction patients who have positive stress test results or angina at a low workload, have mechanical complications, or those with cardiogenic shock, CABG may prolong survival and in some instances be lifesaving. An important factor in the immediate and long-term prognosis of such patients for whom surgery is considered is the amount of residual functioning myocardium that remains after the patient has sustained an infarction. Early results in patients with LV ejection fractions of less than 25% have been discouraging.

Surgical Complications of Myocardial Infarction

MI may lead to a number of sequelae that require surgical intervention in the early or late postinfarction period. These include VSD, free wall rupture, LV aneurysm, and ischemic mitral regurgitation. Overall mechanical complications are responsible for 15% to 20% of the deaths following MI.

Ventricular Septal Defect

Rupture of the interventricular septum is a rare complication following MI, with an incidence of approximately 1% on autopsy. The clinical presentation can vary from an asymptomatic murmur to full blown cardiogenic shock. The average time from infarction to rupture is approximately 2 to 4 days, but it may present as far out as 2 weeks. VSD occurs more commonly in men than in women, with a ratio of 3:2. Postinfarction VSD is associated with a significant area of necrosis, and usually occurs following a first-time MI with poorly developed collaterals. The VSD may be a simple rupture with communication between the ventricles, or may involve the development of a serpiginous dissection tract. The most important determinant for early outcome is the development of heart failure, which portends a poor prognosis. The natural history, if left untreated, is death in 25% of patients within 24 hours, 50%

within 1 week, and 80% within 4 weeks. Only 7% of patients survive longer than one year if untreated.

The diagnosis can be made with the presence of a harsh pansystolic murmur, and is confirmed with transthoracic and/or transesophageal echocardiography. The necessity of preoperative cardiac catheterization is not clear, but may provide important information about concomitant coronary artery disease that can benefit from revascularization. The definitive management is surgical correction of the VSD. Those in cardiogenic shock require emergent repair, whereas those requiring minimal or no support may defer repair to an elective basis. Preoperative management centers on reducing systemic vascular resistance while maintaining cardiac output and mean arterial pressure, which in some patients may require placement of an intraaortic balloon pump. Deaths in most patients occur from multisystem organ failure. Operative repair depends upon the location of the defect, but in general involves endocardial patch repair with possible exclusion of the infarct. Operative mortality averages 15% to 30% for anterior lesions and 30% to 50% for inferior VSDs. The increased mortality for inferior defects is secondary to right ventricular dysfunction and increased rates of mitral insufficiency caused by right coronary disease.

Ventricular Free Wall Rupture

Ventricular free wall rupture following an MI occurs in approximately 11% of patients overall, but may be as high as 30% in patients with large anterior infarctions. LV rupture and cardiogenic shock are the leading causes of death following acute MI. Rupture occurs more commonly in elderly women, and usually occurs within 5 days of the first transmural infarction. Older studies have documented a preponderance of anterior wall rupture, whereas more recent studies suggest that lateral and posterior wall ruptures occur more commonly. LV ruptures are divided into three categories of chronicity: acute, subacute, and chronic. Acute ruptures usually lead to profound shock, pulseless electrical activity, and death within minutes. A subacute rupture is the result of a smaller defect, and may be sealed temporarily by clot or fibrin, allowing time for workup and treatment. These usually present with signs and symptoms of cardiac tamponade, and may allow survival for hours or days before intervention. A chronic rupture usually presents as a false aneurysm of the LV, where adhesions form that contain the rupture. These patients usually present with CHF. The diagnosis of rupture is best made with echocardiography. Patients with tamponade should undergo pericardiocentesis, and aspiration of uncoagulated blood is diagnostic of subacute rupture. The natural history of the disease is invariably fatal if left untreated. Operative closure of the rupture involves mattress closure buttressed with Teflon felt, or use of a Dacron patch.

Left Ventricular Aneurysm

The incidence of LV aneurysm following MI is between 10% and 35%. Asymptomatic patients generally have an excellent prognosis, with 90% survival at 10 years versus 46% in symptomatic patients. Development of an aneurysm within 48 hours of infarction leads to diminished survival and a poorer prognosis. In the absence of known thrombus, the risk of thromboembolic complications is generally low, approximately 0.35% per patient-year, and anticoagulation is not recommended for the long-term. In 50% of patients, however, considerable LV mural thrombus or diminished function is seen on echocardiography, and in these patients careful follow-up and long-term anticoagulation is indicated. The presenting symptom of LV aneurysm is most frequently angina, which is unsurprising in that 60% of these patients will present with three-vessel coronary artery disease. Atrial and/or ventricular arrhythmias may be present in up to 33% of patients. Aneurysms are thought to form from infarct scar expansion following an MI, and are differentiated from false aneurysms by the lack of communication with the pericardial space (Fig. 22-5). The diagnosis can be made on the basis of electrocardiographic findings, which demonstrates anterior lead Q waves with persistent ST elevation. Chest radiograph may demonstrate LV enlargement or obvious bulge (Fig. 22-6). Paradoxical bulge of the aneurysm during systole can be seen on echocardiography. The gold standard for diagnosis is left ventriculography, which demonstrates a large area of dyskinesia or hypokinesia usually in the anteroseptal-apical walls.

There are no absolute indications for operative treatment of asymptomatic LV aneurysms given the overall good prognosis. For symptomatic patients with angina, CHF, or arrhythmias, operative intervention offers a better long-term outcome than medical management. Operative techniques include simple plication of the aneurysm, which is usually reserved for very small aneurysms that do not contain mural thrombus. Linear closure of the LV may be performed after resection of the aneurysm and removal of any thrombus, which is best performed on the anterior

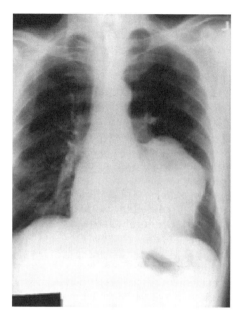

Figure 22-6 Chest radiograph demonstrating large ventricular aneurysm. (From Kaiser LR, Kron IL, Spray TL, eds. *Mastery of cardiothoracic surgery.* Philadelphia: Lippincott Williams & Wilkins, 1998, with permission.)

wall. Inferior or posterior aneurysms require circular Dacron patch closure, and this technique can be applied to anterior aneurysms as well. In-hospital mortality for repair is 7% to 9%, with LV failure being the most common cause

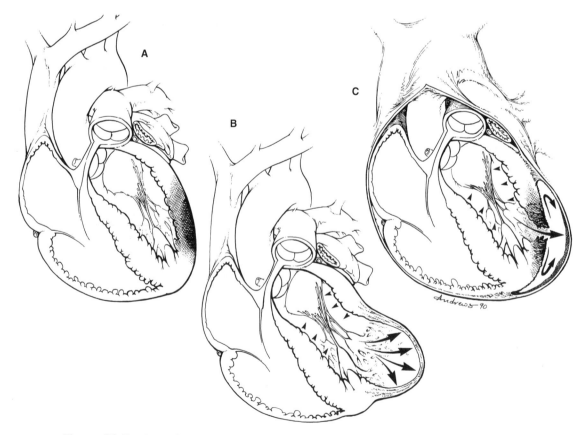

Figure 22-5 The pathophysiology of LV aneurysm formation. **A:** Area of infarction. **B:** True aneurysm. **C:** False aneurysm. (From Kaiser LR, Kron IL, Spray TL, eds. *Mastery of cardiothoracic surgery.* Philadelphia: Lippinccott Williams & Wilkins, 1998, with permission.)

of death overall. Overall 5-year survival is 58% to 80%, whereas 10-year survival is only 34%. Studies have consistently shown an improvement in patient symptoms following aneurysm repair relative to preoperative symptoms.

Ischemic Mitral Regurgitation

Chronic ischemic mitral regurgitation (MR) is always preceded by MI or significant myocardial ischemia, and, by definition, the valvular leaflets and subvalvular apparatus are normal. It is primarily a disease of the myocardium that in turn perturbs normal valvular function (as opposed to primary valvular disease that in turn leads to dysfunctional myocardium). The incidence of ischemic MR following MI is between 17% and 55%, with up to 18% of patients having evidence of MR within 6 hours of the onset of MI symptoms. In many patients, however, the MR is mild and may be transient with improvement over time. Infarct location predisposes to ischemic MR, with posteroinferior MIs having the highest likelihood secondary to papillary muscle dysfunction. Ruptured papillary muscles can lead to life-threatening acute MR, with the posterior papillary muscle involved 3 to 6 times more commonly than the anterior. Complete rupture usually occurs within the first 7 days after MI, but may be delayed by up to 3 months. The presence of MR after MI has not been shown to independently increase early mortality. However, it does significantly increase the 30-day and 3-year mortality to 15% and 20% respectively, which is approximately double that for patients without MR. The natural history of untreated papillary muscle rupture is death within 3 to 4 days, although with partial rupture patients may survive for weeks. Acute severe MR following MI causes LV volume overload, and CO is maintained by significant increases in stroke volume. Patients usually present with acute chest pain and shortness of breath, and typically have a loud apical holosystolic murmur that radiates to the left axilla. Transesophageal echocardiography (TEE) is the diagnostic tool of choice and can document the degree of MR, wall motion abnormalities, and papillary muscle function.

Surgical therapy should not be unnecessarily delayed with acute ischemic MR in the face of cardiogenic shock, with prompt surgery conferring the best chance for survival. Operative therapy consists of mitral valve repair or replacement, with or without revascularization of the coronary circulation. Concomitant coronary bypass surgery may confer improved mitral valve function by limiting infarct extension and improving papillary function. With acute, severe MR, replacement of the valve is the most reliable option. Intraoperative TEE is helpful to assess myocardial function and valvular competence when weaning from bypass. Intraaortic balloon pump placement may be necessary in these patients, and hospital mortality varies from 30% to 70%. For patients with chronic ischemic MR, indications for surgery include symptomatic coronary disease, severe MR (3+ or 4+), or significant LV dysfunction secondary to MR. Valve replacement is usually indicated in older patients with severe LV dysfunction who cannot tolerate a long bypass run. In select patients mitral valve repair has a 97% efficacy in preventing MR, and ring annuloplasty is usually employed (and may be the sole intervention in up to 80% of patients) (Fig. 22-7). In select patients reimplantation of the papillary muscles may improve leaflet function (Fig. 22-8).

Acquired Valve Disease

Aortic Stenosis

Obstruction of the LV outflow tract may occur at the subvalvular, valvular, and supravalvular levels. In the adult population, most patients present with obstruction at the valvular level, which results from congenital or degenerative abnormalities of the aortic valve. A bicuspid configuration is generally responsible for the congenital type and has an incidence of 0.9% to 2.0% in the general population and approximately 50% in patients with aortic stenosis. Both congenital and degenerative aortic stenosis are associated with progressive calcification and loss of cusp mobility.

The common hemodynamic effect of these lesions is decreased valvular area, which necessitates a large transvalvular gradient to maintain LV outflow. Most patients become symptomatic at valve areas of less than 1.0 cm^2, and areas of less than 0.7 cm^2 represent critical stenosis (normal aortic valve area equals 2.5 to 3.5 cm^2). The adaptive response of the left ventricle to outflow obstruction is progressive hypertrophy, which is accompanied by decreased diastolic compliance. Because of the capacity of the left ventricle to adapt to the outflow obstruction, gradients as high as 90 to 120 mm Hg may be present in severe aortic stenosis. Eventually, the ventricle is unable to compensate and dilates, which results in decreased cardiac output, increased pulmonary artery pressures, and CHF. LV changes associated with aortic stenosis also may lead to myocardial ischemia, even in the presence of normal coronary arteries. Myocardial oxygen demand is increased with increased ventricular mass and high systolic pressure, whereas oxygen delivery is decreased by high end-diastolic pressures. This mismatch in myocardial oxygen supply and demand may lead to effort-related angina or an anginal equivalent, such as dyspnea.

Because of the capacity of the left ventricle to adapt for long periods to the demands of outflow obstruction, patients may remain asymptomatic for many years. As the valve area progressively decreases, however, they typically experience CHF, angina, or syncope. After the appearance of symptoms, the clinical course of aortic stenosis may become progressively severe. Aortic stenosis is the most frequently fatal valvular lesion, and sudden death may occur in up to 20% of patients. Physical examination reveals a loud, harsh systolic aortic murmur, which may be transmitted to the neck. The second heart sound is usually split. An S_4 is commonly heard with decreased LV compliance and adaptive left atrial hypertrophy. The electrocardiogram demonstrates LV hypertrophy and left atrial enlargement. Echocardiography is useful in demonstrating the configuration of the aortic valve and motion of the leaflets; however, cardiac catheterization is necessary to directly measure pressure and flow across the valve. Coronary arteriography is also recommended, even in patients without ischemic symptoms, to assess the need for combined valve replacement and coronary bypass. Indications for aortic valve replacement are patients with aortic stenosis who have symptoms of angina, CHF, or syncope, and asymptomatic patients with severe aortic stenosis demonstrated by an aortic valve area of less than 0.7 cm^2.

Aortic Regurgitation

Aortic regurgitation (AR) has historically resulted most commonly from rheumatic fever; however, with modern

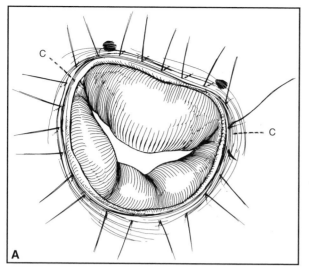

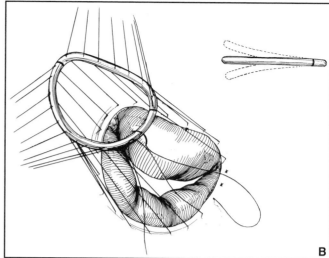

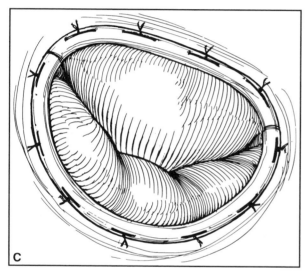

Figure 22-7 Technique of mitral ring annuloplasty. **A:** Placement of annular sutures. **B:** Placement of sutures on the annular ring prosthesis. **C:** completed ring annuloplasty. (From Kaiser LR, Kron IL, Spray TL, eds. *Mastery of cardiothoracic surgery.* Philadelphia: Lippincott Williams & Wilkins, 1998, with permission.)

antibiotic therapy the most common etiologies are now bicuspid aortic valve, dilation of the aortic root, or aortic dissection. Other more rare causes of AR include infective endocarditis, cuspal avulsion, or laceration following blunt chest trauma, myxomatous degeneration, rheumatoid arthritis, and systemic lupus erythematosus. AR from dilation of the aortic root in the presence of a histologically normal aortic valve occurs with tertiary syphilis and Marfan syndrome, which is an autosomal dominant (rarely autosomal recessive) disorder characterized by a basic defect in the formation of elastic fibers. Acute aortic dissection may cause detachment of the valve cusps, thereby leading to AR.

The size of regurgitant orifices leading to significant AR range from 0.5 to 1.0 cm^2. Up to 60% to 70% of stroke volume in such cases may regurgitate into the left ventricle during diastole. To maintain normal forward flow, the left ventricle increases stroke volume and work. Chronic changes include hypertrophy, which is followed by the gradual onset of ventricular dilation. Patients with moderate or severe AR may remain asymptomatic for many years because of LV adaptation. Eventually, however, ejection

fraction and cardiac output decrease and patients experience symptoms of CHF. In contrast to that of aortic stenosis, the course of AR after the onset of symptoms is prolonged, and 50% of patients may survive 10 years. Physical examination reveals a widened pulse pressure and a blowing diastolic murmur along the left sternal border. An S$_3$ may be present in patients with deteriorating ventricular function. Electrocardiograms and chest x-rays demonstrate LV hypertrophy and left atrial enlargement in some cases. Echocardiography is useful in documenting the degree of dilation and hypertrophy of the left ventricle but does not accurately quantitate the degree of regurgitation. The best method for demonstrating the dynamics and severity of AR is echocardiography. Coronary angiography should be performed when aortic valve replacement is considered.

Aortic valve replacement is indicated for symptomatic patients with AR. Asymptomatic patients should be treated medically until they experience symptoms or noninvasive studies demonstrate significant LV dilation or deteriorating function. Patients with severe acute AR and CHF should be operated on as soon as possible.

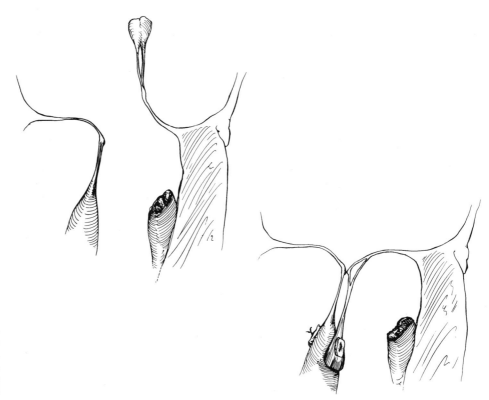

Figure 22-8 Technique of papillary muscle reimplantation. (From Kaiser LR, Kron IL, Spray TL, eds. *Mastery of cardiothoracic surgery.* Philadelphia: Lippincott Williams & Wilkins, 1998, with permission.)

Idiopathic Hypertrophic Subaortic Stenosis

Idiopathic hypertrophic subaortic stenosis (IHSS) is an asymmetrical obstructive hypertrophic cardiomyopathy in which anatomic and physiologic obstruction of the LV outflow tract results in presentation similar to that of aortic stenosis. The male-to-female ratio is approximately 2:1. In some cases, IHSS has been demonstrated to be inherited in an autosomal dominant pattern. Anatomically, IHSS results in marked thickening of the middle and upper ventricular septum. Histologic examination reveals a bizarre, whorled configuration of myocytes and connective tissue elements described as myocardial disarray.

LV outflow obstruction is dynamic, increasing with factors that decrease ventricular volume, such as inotropes, or that decrease afterload or venous return. In patients who are symptomatic, dyspnea and angina are common. IHSS may also present as sudden death, which accounts for more than 50% of deaths in patients with this condition. On physical examination, a systolic murmur usually is heard over the left sternal border. Electrocardiograms and chest roentgenograms show LV hypertrophy. Echocardiograms display various patterns of hypertrophy and mitral valve function. Cardiac catheterizations provide pullback gradient measurements across the outflow tract as well as coronary arteriograms.

Symptomatic patients usually can be treated medically with β blockers and calcium channel blockers. Surgery is reserved for patients with severe symptoms and resting or provocative gradients, despite maximal medical therapy and patients who have survived sudden death episodes and have significant resting or provocative gradients. Surgical treatment of IHSS may involve LV myotomy and myomectomy by Morrow technique, or, in certain cases, elimination of systolic anterior motion of the mitral valve by mitral valve replacement. Modern innovations also include alcohol ablation of the hypertrophic septum by injection into the first septal perforator using percutaneous techniques, and synchronized atrioventricular (AV) pacing to reduce dynamic outflow obstruction.

Mitral Stenosis

Despite its dramatic decrease in incidence in most industrialized nations, chronic rheumatic disease remains the most common cause of mitral stenosis. Approximately 55% of patients have a documented history of group A streptococcal pharyngitis. Although the pathogenesis of rheumatic heart disease remains unclear, patients typically have high antistreptolysin O (ASO) titers, and valvular lesions are believed to result from autoimmune damage. Rare causes of mitral stenosis include degenerative calcification in the elderly, myxoma, malignant carcinoid, systemic lupus erythematosus, and rheumatoid arthritis.

Anatomically, rheumatic mitral valve stenosis is caused by fibrous fusion of the valve commissures. In advanced cases, fibrosis progresses to involve the leaflets and chordae, giving the valve a funnel-like appearance. The hemodynamic effect of mitral stenosis is chronic pulmonary venous obstruction. Left atrial pressures are elevated, and, in severe cases, reactive pulmonary hypertension, right ventricular enlargement, and CHF may develop. If there is a documented history of acute rheumatic fever, symptoms typically develop after a long asymptomatic latent period. The most common presenting symptom is dyspnea, which initially occurs with exertion but then progresses to occur at rest. Classic physical examination findings are an opening snap, a loud first heart sound, and a diastolic rumble. Signs of right heart failure may be present. Electrocardiograms frequently show atrial fibrillation and chest x-rays show left atrial enlargement. Echocardiography is useful in delineating anatomy and flow dynamics across the mitral valve. Cardiac catheterization is reserved for patients for whom noninvasive studies are inadequate or coronary angiography is indicated.

The normal mitral valve area is 4 to 6 cm^2. Patients typically develop symptoms secondary to mitral stenosis when valve areas reach 1.5 to 2 cm^2. Valve areas of less than 1.0 cm^2 are usually associated with severe symptoms. Surgery is indicated for patients with hemodynamically significant valve obstruction and NYHA class III to IV symptoms, onset of atrial fibrillation regardless of symptoms, increasing pulmonary hypertension, episodes of systemic embolization, or infective endocarditis. Choice of procedure is highly dependent on individual valvular anatomy and includes open commissurotomy, more complex valve repair techniques, and mitral valve replacement.

Mitral Regurgitation

Mitral valve competence depends on the coordinated function of the annulus, leaflets, chordae tendineae, papillary muscles, and ventricular wall. Disease processes affecting any of these elements may lead to valvular incompetence. Common etiologies include degenerative (myxomatous), ischemic, and ventricular remodeling with annular dilation. Blunt chest trauma may also led to chordal rupture and mitral regurgitation. Rheumatic heart disease is no longer a common cause of MR.

As in mitral stenosis, left atrial pressures are elevated and lead to chronic pulmonary venous obstruction. Reactive pulmonary hypertension may ensue, and, in severe cases, there may be right heart failure and functional tricuspid incompetence. In contrast to mitral stenosis, the left ventricle is subject to chronic volume overload, which may cause left ventricle dilation, diminished ejection fraction, and left heart failure. Symptoms, which typically include dyspnea, occur when the regurgitant volume approaches 50% of stroke volume. Physical examination reveals an apical pansystolic murmur, which is accompanied in severe cases by an S$_3$ gallop. Chest x-rays show enlargement of cardiac chambers, and electrocardiograms frequently indicate atrial fibrillation. As in mitral stenosis, echocardiography provides useful information on valvular anatomy, flow dynamics across the mitral valve, and ventricular function.

Surgical intervention is indicated for patients with hemodynamically significant lesions who have symptoms that compromise their lifestyle (usually NYHA class III or IV). For asymptomatic patients, surgery is recommended for progression of pulmonary hypertension, onset of atrial fibrillation, or LV dilation. Acute mitral regurgitation resulting from infective endocarditis or myocardial ischemia leads to rapid clinical deterioration, and urgent operation is indicated. Prosthetic ring annuloplasty, complex mitral valve repair, or mitral valve replacement may be performed depending on the patient's valve anatomy and clinical setting.

Tricuspid and Pulmonary Valves

Acquired tricuspid valve disease most commonly occurs in the setting of annular dilation leading to tricuspid incompetence. More rarely, rheumatic involvement leads to tricuspid stenosis, which may be associated with regurgitation as in rheumatic disease of the mitral valve. Acquired pulmonary valve disease is rare, although rheumatic involvement can occur. Valve fibrosis secondary to carcinoid syndrome most commonly affects right-sided valves.

Infective Endocarditis

Invasion of the endocardium of the heart by microorganisms most commonly occurs on the valves. The infectious agent can be bacterial, fungal, or viral. Predisposing factors for development of infective endocarditis include previous congenital or acquired heart lesions, immunocompromised status, intravenous catheters, and intravenous drug abuse. The male-to-female ratio is 2:1. Gram-positive organisms remain the most common cause of bacterial endocarditis, specifically *Staphylococcus aureus*, *Staphylococcus epidermidis*, and the viridans group of streptococci. With the increasing use of broad-spectrum antibiotics in the treatment of critically ill patients, gram-negative bacterial endocarditis has increased in frequency in recent years. Broad-spectrum antibiotics, prosthetic valve endocarditis, nosocomial infection, and intravenous hyperalimentation are all factors in the increasing frequency of fungal endocarditis as well.

Fever, weakness, night sweats, and anorexia are common presenting complaints. Physical examination commonly reveals a cardiac murmur; splinter hemorrhages, Osler nodes, Janeway lesions, and Roth spots are classic findings. Blood cultures are positive in 85% to 95% of patients owing to persistent bacteremia from seeding of the bloodstream from vegetations, which can be visualized by echocardiography in many cases. Cardiac catheterization is useful for demonstration of hemodynamic and anatomic abnormalities caused by infective endocarditis; however, catheterization is generally not necessary for patients with acute hemodynamic instability and may cause embolization in patients with aortic valve endocarditis. Medical management with appropriate intravenous antibiotics is the treatment of choice for most patients with infective endocarditis. Valve replacement is reserved for prosthetic valve endocarditis, failure of medical management, life-threatening emboli, severe valvular insufficiency or obstruction, and CHF.

Valve Prostheses

The three general types of prosthetic valves used for valve replacement are (i) mechanical valves, which include caged ball, tilting disk, and bileaflet designs; (ii) tissue heterograft valves, which include glutaraldehyde-preserved native porcine valves and fabricated bovine pericardial prostheses; and (iii) aortic valve homografts, which are cryopreserved after being harvested from human cadaveric hearts. In general, the advantages of mechanical valves reside in their durability, and in the case of tilting disk and bileaflet designs, the low profile of the prosthesis. Disadvantages of mechanical valves include a higher incidence of thromboembolic events, anticoagulation-related complications, hemolysis, and perivalvular leaks. In contrast, tissue valves do not require permanent anticoagulation and have fewer thromboembolic and perivalvular leak complications but degenerate over time and have a tendency to calcify. Many tissue heterograft valves will require replacement after 10 to 14 years. Calcific degeneration is accelerated in younger patients, and the use of tissue valves is generally contraindicated in pediatric and adolescent patients for this reason.

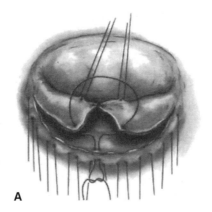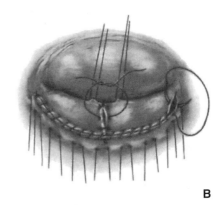

Figure 22-9 Quadrangular resection of the posterior mitral valve leaflet and mitral valve annuloplasty for mitral valve prolapse. The free edges of the resected margin are reapproximated in the midline and the posterior valve is sutured to the annulus. (From Kaiser LR, Kron IL, Spray TL, eds. *Mastery of cardiothoracic surgery.* Philadelphia: Lippincott Williams & Wilkins, 1998, with permission.)

A   **B**

Current recommendations are that tissue valves be reserved for patients with a limited life expectancy (those older than 60 to 65 years of age for the aortic position, and 65 to 70 years for the mitral position) or for those who have contraindications to permanent anticoagulation. The St. Jude mechanical valve (bileaflet design) is recommended for pediatric and young adult patients because of durability and superior hemodynamics. Homograft valves are commonly used for the repair of complex congenital malformations or in patients with native or prosthetic valve endocarditis. Long-term follow-up of patients with cryopreserved homograft valves is limited; however, durability of these grafts up to 15 years has been reported.

Valve Repair

The significant consequences of valve replacement with prostheses—including thromboembolism, valve dysfunction, infection, anticoagulation, and bleeding—have led to efforts to develop techniques for valve repair. Currently, tricuspid and mitral valvuloplasty are considered preferable to valve replacement when technically feasible because of lower morbidity and mortality. Conversely, operative repair and balloon valvuloplasty of the aortic valve have had disappointing results.

Prosthetic ring annuloplasty is a central technique for valve repair and is required in most cases of mitral insufficiency. The basic principle is to reduce the size and restore the shape of the dilated annulus. More complex repairs involving chordal transposition, cuneiform resection of elongated papillary muscles, resection of secondary or marginal chordae, and chordal replacement with Gore-Tex suture are tailored to the individual lesion. Figure 22-9 illustrates a quadrangular resection of the posterior leaflet of the mitral valve and annuloplasty to correct mitral valve prolapse. Competency of repaired valves is tested by saline injection and intraoperative TEE, thereby allowing immediate evaluation and revision of repairs at the same operation.

A number of factors are thought to contribute to the lower morbidity and mortality associated with valve repair. The ability to perform valve repair, as opposed to valve replacement, has prompted earlier referrals, which allows better long-term results. LV function is improved with valve repair, possibly because the continuity between the mitral valve and the ventricular wall is maintained via the chordae and papillary muscles, which are thought to play an important role during isometric contraction and results in increased stroke volume. Endocarditis and

thromboembolism are rare following valve repair, and anticoagulation is not required. Long-term follow-up has demonstrated that mitral valve repair is durable, particularly for patients with myxomatous or degenerative disease, as compared to patients with rheumatic valve disease who tend to have more subvalvular scarring and patients with ischemic mitral regurgitation in whom papillary muscle or regional ventricular wall dysfunction may be seen.

Arrhythmia Surgery and Pacemakers

Endocardial catheter and surgical procedures have been developed for the treatment of medically refractory supraventricular and ventricular tachyarrhythmia. Although diagnosis of these arrhythmias can frequently be made by routine electrocardiography, further electrophysiologic evaluation is generally necessary before intervention.

Insertion of a permanent pacemaker is frequently necessary for the treatment of patients with bradyarrhythmia. Generally accepted indications for permanent pacing are given in Table 22-4. The most commonly used pacing systems are ventricular demand (VVI) and dual chamber sensing and pacing (DDD) systems. VVI systems sense and pace only the ventricle and therefore lack atrioventricular (A-V) synchrony, which may not be important in patients with slow atrial fibrillation and who are not able to respond to increased physiologic stress by increasing heart rate. DDD systems maintain A-V synchrony, which has been associated with a 20% to 25% increase in cardiac output, and

---

TABLE 22-4

INDICATIONS FOR PERMANENT PACEMAKER INSERTION

Sick sinus syndrome
Symptomatic type II arteriovenous block
Complete arteriovenous block
Bilateral bundle branch block following acute myocardial infarction
Bifascicular or trifascicular block with symptomatic bradycardia or with intermittent type II arteriovenous block
Carotid sinus syncope
Intractable low cardiac output syndrome benefited by temporary pacing

From Lowe JE, Wharton JM. Cardiac pacemakers and implantable cardioverter-defibrillators. In: Sabiston DC Jr, Spencer FC, eds. *Surgery of the chest*, 6th ed. Philadelphia: WB Saunders, 1995:1763–1813, with permission.

which can increase heart rate with increasing physiologic demand.

Atrial fibrillation is present in 1% of the general population, and 6% of those older than the age of 65. The loss of synchronous A-V contraction diminishes cardiac output, since the atrial "kick" is lost, whereas left atrial stasis leads to increased risk of thromboembolism. Optimal medical management of chronic fibrillation includes adequate rate control to slow ventricular response, since antiarrhythmics often fail to provide long-term conversion to sinus rhythm. In addition, patients must be maintained on long-term anticoagulation, which is particularly dangerous for older patients. The electrophysiologic basis of atrial fibrillation includes macro-reentrant circuits, passive atrial conduction, and atrioventricular conduction. These three phenomena result in a spectrum of dysrhythmia from atrial flutter to complex atrial fibrillation. The major indication for surgical intervention is intolerance of the arrhythmia including symptoms of dyspnea on exertion, lethargy, and malaise during bouts of fibrillation, or distal thromboembolic events. The current standard operative approach is the Maze-III procedure, wherein electrical conductivity of the atrium is interrupted by a series of surgically constructed impediments. This was originally accomplished by performing atrial incisions that, after closure, lead to electrically nonconducting scars (Fig. 22-10). More recent approaches involve cryosurgical and radiofrequency ablation techniques to avoid the added time and morbidity of opening both atria. The Maze procedure is amenable to minimally invasive and off-pump surgical approaches, and is often combined with valvular or coronary procedures. Long-term results are extremely good, with 98% of patients free from fibrillation by 3 months. The long-term stroke rate is 0.1% per year. Overall 15% of patients require pacemakers postoperatively, usually due to preexisting sick

sinus syndrome or abnormal sinoatrial nodes masked by atrial fibrillation.

Heart Failure

Heart failure (HF) is responsible for more than 700,000 US deaths annually, and affects more than 5 million people in the United States. Approximately one third of these patients have severe symptomatic failure, NYHA class III or IV. Although systolic dysfunction is a central finding in heart failure, it is now thought that chamber dilation and ventricular remodeling are central to the development of contractile dysfunction, which is an effect rather than a cause in this model. Medical treatment with angiotensin-converting enzyme (ACE) inhibitors and β-blockers can improve survival and inhibit the remodeling process. Despite these advances in our understanding of heart failure, the mortality and hospitalization rates remain high. Surgical treatment of heart failure with transplantation, reversal of remodeling, mechanical assistance, and resynchronization hold promise for improved survival and decreased morbidity.

Heart Transplantation

Cardiac transplantation is the gold standard of surgical therapy for advanced and end-stage heart failure. The absolute contraindications include age older than 70, fixed pulmonary hypertension, neoplasm other than skin cancer, human immunodeficiency virus (HIV) and acquired immunodeficiency syndrome (AIDS), and irreversible hepatic or renal dysfunction. More recent expansion of eligibility criteria has led to an escalating donor shortage. In general, the recipient prognosis for 1-year survival without transplantation should be less than 50%. Organ allocation is determined by priority status (IA, IB, or II), duration on the

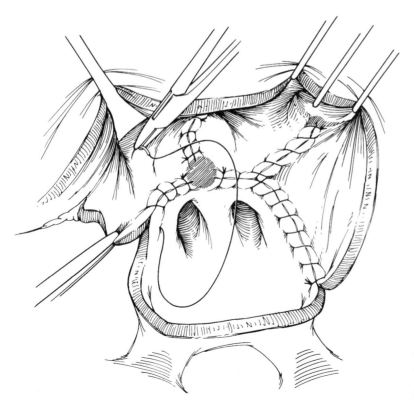

Figure 22-10 Closure of atrial incisions around the right-sided pulmonary veins in the Maze-III procedure. (From Kaiser LR, Kron IL, Spray TL, eds. *Mastery of cardiothoracic surgery.* Philadelphia: Lippincott Williams & Wilkins, 1998, with permission.)

waiting list, and geographic distance between donor and potential recipient. Using current techniques, cardiac allografts may be safely preserved for 4 to 6 hours of cold ischemia. ABO compatibility barriers should not be crossed, as this frequently results in fatal hyperacute rejection.

Orthotopic heart transplantation is the procedure of choice, and involves replacement of the recipient's heart with a healthy donor allograft (Fig. 22-11). Immunosuppressive regimens in most centers include cyclosporine or tacrolimus, steroids, and mycophenolate mofetil. Acute rejection generally occurs within the first 3 months after transplantation, and corticosteroids are the cornerstone of management. The 30-day mortality following transplantation is 5% to 10%, with primary graft failure being the most frequent cause of early death. Overall 1-year survival is approximately 80%, and 10-year survival is approximately 50%. Infection and rejection are the most common causes of death within the first 6 months, whereas accelerated coronary artery disease claims most lives thereafter. Advancements in organ preservation, immunosuppressive regimens, and mechanical assist devices hold promise for future improvements.

Reversal of Remodeling

The concept of surgical restoration of ventricular geometry for patients with severe HF was first introduced by Batista

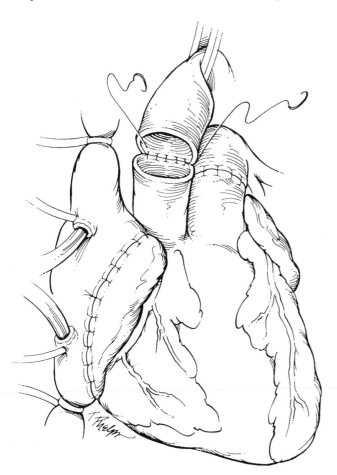

Figure 22-11 Orthotopic implantation of a cardiac allograft. The aortic anastomosis is being completed. (From Kaiser LR, Kron IL, Spray TL, eds. *Mastery of cardiothoracic surgery*. Philadelphia: Lippincott Williams & Wilkins, 1998, with permission.)

et al. in 1996. This procedure involved resection of normal muscle between the anterior and posterior papillary muscles, with concomitant mitral valve repair or replacement. The goal of this procedure is to restore the ventricle to a more normal volume/mass/diameter relationship. Despite initially high success rates, many patients reverted to significant recurrent ventricular dilation, whereas the perioperative mortality was greater than 20% in many studies. This concept has evolved over the intervening years to a modification of the Dor procedure for LV aneurysm repair, termed endoventricular circular patch plasty or surgical ventricular restoration (SVR). This procedure is amenable to patients who have sustained a large anterior wall MI, with a significant area of akinesia or dyskinesia. An endoventricular Dacron patch is used to exclude the nonfunctional portions of the anterior LV wall and septum so as to restore a more normal elliptical rather than spherical ventricular geometry (Fig. 22-12). Recent studies have reported objective improvement of systolic volume index and LV ejection fraction following this procedure.

An alternative or complementary approach uses girdling devices to limit or reverse ventricular remodeling following an ischemic insult. There have been a number of promising studies in animal models, suggesting that this approach results in reduced ventricular dilation and improved myocardial performance and energetics following implantation. The Acorn Cardiac Support Device (ACSD) is a polyester mesh fabric and can reduce ventricular wall stress by providing external support to the heart. The ACSD is sized and placed around the ventricle, with suture fixation to the base of the heart. A snug fit is obtained by accumulating excess fabric anteriorly and placating it in place. Early clinical data suggest that LV chamber dimensions are reduced and ejection fraction is improved after implantation.

Mechanical Assistance

Mechanical assistance of ventricular function is an established therapy that serves as a bridge to transplantation. More than 70% of patients placed on LV mechanical assistance subsequently undergo successful transplantation. These devices allow patients in cardiogenic shock not only to live but to be mobile and rehabilitated prior to transplantation. The expert use of a variety of ventricular assist devices for left, right, and biventricular support is mandatory for any cardiac transplantation center today. More recently devices have been used as a bridge to recovery and even as destination therapy for permanent long-term heart support or replacement. Several investigators have reported prolonged (weeks to months) use of LV-assist devices as a bridge to recovery. Although some feel that this approach in patients with chronic heart failure is unpredictable and rarely successful, in patients presenting with fulminant acute myocarditis such support has been particularly successful, resulting in full cardiac recovery in many cases.

Most assist systems are prone to forming clots in the pumping devices, thereby increasing the risk of stroke and necessitating anticoagulation. The rate of mechanical failure is less than 10% with devices employed for greater than 1 year. Infectious complications including driveline exit site, pump pocket, or true endocarditis occur with a 30% to 50% incidence and are the cause of most severe adverse events. Until these complications are drastically

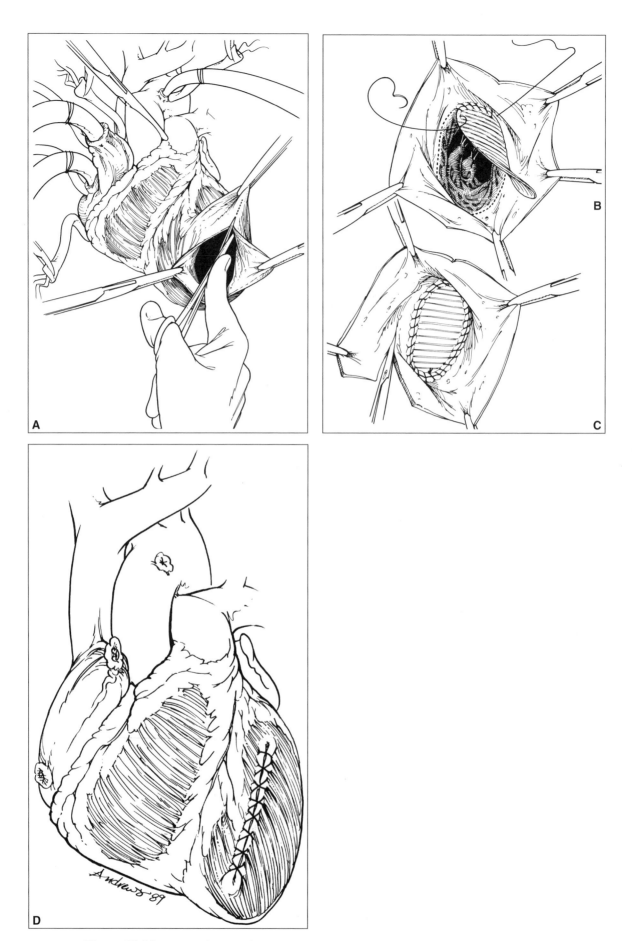

Figure 22-12 Repair of ventricular aneurysm using endoventricular circular patch plasty. (From Kaiser LR, Kron IL, Spray TL, eds. *Mastery of cardiothoracic surgery*. Philadelphia: Lippincott Williams & Wilkins, 1998, with permission.)

reduced, these devices cannot be considered for permanent placement.

The HeartMate LV assist device (LVAD) is an implantable pulsatile device, originally pneumatic in design, which now offers a vented electric model that allows greater patient mobility with a portable battery. Patients take an aspirin daily, primarily as an antiinflammatory rather than anticoagulant, since the blood-contacting surface of this device forms a biologic pseudoneointima that is not thrombotic. This device has the lowest incidence of stroke, approximately 7.4%. In the REMATCH trial of 129 patients in 20 centers comparing medical management to HeartMate placement, there was a reduction of 48% in the risk of death in the LVAD treatment group. In addition, there were significant improvements in quality of life in the LVAD group, although the rates of adverse events and hospital days were increased.

A new generation of assist devices will soon be entering initial phase I and II studies. Axial flow pumps have been developed that are tiny relative to present general pulsatile pumps, yet still capable of up to 10 L of flow. The LionHeart (Arrow International), currently undergoing phase I U.S. Food and Drug Administration (FDA) evaluation, is a destination device that is a totally intracorporeal LVAD, powered by transcutaneous energy transmission with no driveline crossing the skin. Total artificial hearts (Abiocor—Abiomed) will very soon enter clinical trials. Further technologic and surgical enhancements will likely lead to greater use of mechanical support as both temporary and permanent treatment for heart failure.

Cardiac Resynchronization Therapy

Cardiac resynchronization therapy (CRT) has been recently used as a treatment for heart failure patients with significant ventricular conduction delay. Approximately 30% of these patients exhibit ventricular dyssynchrony, manifested by widened QRS complexes on electrocardiographic findings. This further impairs ventricular function, and may worsen mitral regurgitation and increase the risk of death. Prospective randomized trials have demonstrated improvements in LV function, clinical symptoms, exercise tolerance, and quality of life with CRT. The success of this therapy relies upon proper LV lead placement, with the posterobasal wall providing the most effective hemodynamic augmentation compared to either anterior or lateral positioned leads. The benefit of CRT appears to lie in normalizing septal wall movement and advancing lateral wall activation in relation to the septum. Approximately 10% to 15% of attempted LV lead placements fail in the cardiac catheterization laboratory, necessitating open placement using traditional open or minimally invasive surgical techniques.

Cardiac Neoplasms

Primary cardiac neoplasms are rare, with an incidence of less than 0.25% in autopsy series. Nevertheless, because they represent one of the potentially curable forms of cardiac disease, their early diagnosis and management has assumed increasing emphasis.

Approximately 70% to 80% of primary cardiac neoplasms are benign, with myxoma being by far the most common lesion in this group, except in children. Myxomas account for approximately 75% of benign cardiac neoplasms and 50% of all primary cardiac tumors. They are derived from multipotential mesenchymal cells and grossly present as polypoid masses projecting into the cardiac chamber from the endocardium. Approximately 75% of myxomas occur in the left atrium, typically arising from the limbus of the fossa ovalis. Twenty percent of myxomas occur in the right atrium, and 5% in more than one chamber. Myxomas arising from the ventricles are extremely rare. These tumors have been reported in all age groups; however, they are most frequently seen in women in the fourth, fifth, and sixth decades of life. Rarely, familial forms may be inherited in an autosomal-dominant fashion. These lesions are most commonly asymptomatic and are incidentally discovered. When symptomatic, myxomas most frequently present with generalized weakness and malaise, but can result in mitral valve obstruction and embolism. Surgical resection is indicated after diagnosis is confirmed, usually by echocardiography. Preoperative coronary angiography should be considered in patients older than 40 years if the clinical setting allows. Rhabdomyomas account for approximately 20% of benign cardiac neoplasms and are the most common tumor in pediatric populations. These lesions are typically of ventricular origin, poorly encapsulated, multicentric, and may not be resectable.

Almost all malignant primary cardiac neoplasms are sarcomas. The most common types are angiosarcoma, rhabdomyosarcoma, and fibrosarcoma. These tumors tend to grow rapidly, with invasion and displacement of cardiac and mediastinal structures leading to progressive CHF. Metastases are present at the time of diagnosis in up to 80% of cases. The prognosis for this disease is poor, with the median survival in surgically treated patients being less than 1 year. Metastatic tumors to the heart are the most common cardiac neoplasms. The major types secondarily invading the heart are bronchogenic carcinoma, melanoma, leukemia, lymphoma, and carcinoma of the breast.

Aortic Dissection

Aortic dissection refers to development of a hematoma within the middle to outer third of the media of the aorta. In approximately 95% of cases, this hematoma originates from a tear in the aortic intima and media and can extend around the circumference of the aorta as well as proximally and distally from the site of the tear. Aortic dissection commonly is associated with cystic medial necrosis, a tissue factor defect associated with Marfan syndrome that may also occur sporadically. Dissection of the aorta is also associated with aortic stenosis, particularly the bicuspid type, and a history of hypertension. The most common symptom of dissection is severe back pain. Occlusion of arteries by extension of the hematoma can lead to loss of pulses, stroke, and limb or end-organ ischemia.

Aortic dissections are classified by duration and anatomy. Acute dissections are defined as being less than 2 weeks old, whereas chronic dissections have occurred 2 weeks or more earlier. The most useful anatomic classification system is the Stanford system because initial surgical versus medical management generally follows this system. In the Stanford classification, type A dissections involve the ascending aorta and type B dissections do not (Fig. 22-13). Emergent

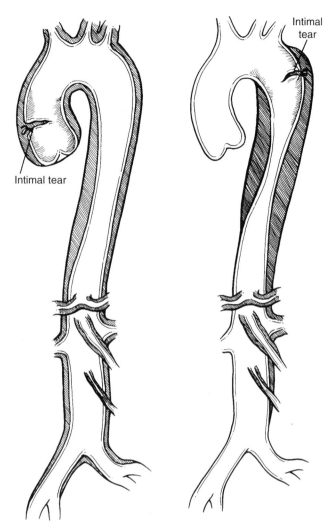

Figure 22-13   The Stanford classification of aortic dissections. (From Kaiser LR, Kron IL, Spray TL, eds. *Mastery of cardiothoracic surgery.* Philadelphia: Lippincott Williams & Wilkins, 1998, with permission.)

surgical repair of acute type A dissections is indicated because of the high mortality associated with this lesion (Fig. 22-14). Approximately 80% of these patients die within the first week because of free rupture, pericardial tamponade, MI secondary to extension to the coronary ostia, or massive aortic insufficiency and CHF. Acute type B dissections are initially treated medically with control of hypertension unless there is evidence of aortic rupture into the left chest or severe major organ or limb ischemia from aortic branch obstruction.

The indications for surgical repair of chronic dissections differ. Type A dissections, which are not diagnosed acutely, are repaired for late development of aortic insufficiency and CHF or aneurysmal dilation of the ascending aorta exceeding 5 cm. Chronic type B dissections are repaired for aneurysmal dilation of the descending aorta greater than 6 cm or end-organ malperfusion.

A goal of surgical repair is to replace the segment of aorta containing the intimal tear with a prosthetic graft whenever possible. For acute type A dissections, aortic replacement is limited to the ascending aorta and proximal aortic arch, even when the dissection extends distally. This procedure effectively eliminates the causes of death related to type A dissection without exposing the patient to the hazards of replacement of the entire aorta. Lifetime follow-up with serial magnetic resonance imaging (MRI) or computerized tomographic (CT) scans is necessary to identify the significant portion of patients who develop aneurysmal dilation of the aorta at other points of reentry distal to the original intimal tear.

Aneurysms of the Thoracic Aorta

Aortic aneurysms are the 13th leading cause of mortality in the United States. Risk factors include smoking, hypertension, atherosclerosis, cystic medial degeneration, and the inherited Marfan and Ehlers–Danlos syndromes. Syphilis, once a common cause, is a decidedly rare etiology in the modern era. The proximal aorta is rich in elastin, which allows the ascending aorta to expand during systole to store energy, with recoil during diastole to drive forward flow of blood. With any weakening of the aortic wall and/or loss of elasticity progressive dilation then ensues. The law of Laplace dictates that wall tension increases with increasing radius and decreasing aortic wall thickness.

Ascending Aortic Aneurysms

Many ascending aortic aneurysms are asymptomatic, but they may present with anterior chest pain. Asymptomatic aneurysms may be detected on routine chest radiographs. Ascending aneurysms are the most frequent cause of isolated aortic insufficiency, and therefore may be detected with TEE. Aortography allows accurate assessment of the aneurysm with respect to the great vessels, and can assist in detecting aotic insufficiency. Computerized tomography provides rapid and accurate evaluation of the ascending aorta, and can identify concomitant dissections and mural thrombus, making it the initial imaging test of choice for most patients. Magnetic resonance imaging may also be employed for patients in whom intranveous contrast may be contraindicated. The indications for emergent operative intervention in ascending aneurysms is acute rupture or dissection. Symptomatic aortic insufficiency and stenosis are indications for operative repair as well, whereas an aneurysm size of 4 to 5 cm for the aortic root is the cutoff for replacement. In the absence of valvular dysfunction, an absolute size of 5 cm or growth of greater than 1 cm per year are indications for intervention. There are a variety of surgical procedures than can be performed, depending on the extent of the aneurysm, condition of the aortic valve, underlying pathology, life expectancy, and potential contraindications to anticoagulation. These range from simple tube-graft replacement to composite valve-graft conduit, with more recent advances including valve-sparing procedures. In the absence of involvement of the arch, these procedures are undertaken with cardiopulmonary bypass.

Aortic Arch Aneurysms

The risk factors for arch aneurysms are the same as those for ascending aortic aneurysms. Evaluation of the arch aneurysm is usually performed with contrast enhanced CT scanning, although MRI can also be used. Elective repair is

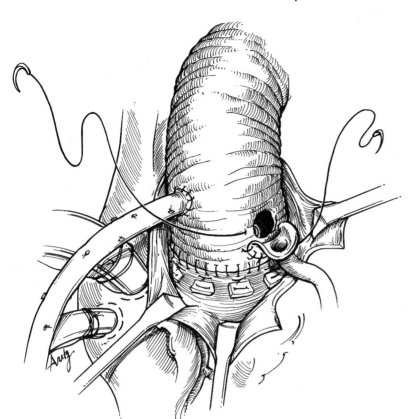

Figure 22-14 Repair of acute type A aortic dissection with root reconstruction and composite valve graft. (From Kaiser LR, Kron IL, Spray TL, eds. *Mastery of cardiothoracic surgery.* Philadelphia: Lippincott Williams & Wilkins, 1998, with permission.)

indicated for a diameter exceeding 6 to 7 cm, although surgical intervention may be undertaken earlier based on unfavorable geometry (such a saccular aneurysms or severe asymmetry). Unlike other aortic aneurysm repairs, these procedures necessitate a period of deep hypothermic circulatory arrest (DHCA), wherein the core body temperature is lowered to 10°C to 15°C core temperature by using cardiopulmonary bypass. Cerebral protection can be enhanced by either antegrade or retrograde cold blood perfusion to reduce the incidence of neurologic complications. The aneurysmal portion of the aorta is resected, leaving an island containing the origins of the arch branches. These are anastamosed to a tube graft, which is sewn to the proximal and distal aortic cuffs (Fig. 22-15). Long-term results are acceptable, with approximately 84% survival at 1 year, and 75% survival at 5 years.

Descending Thoracic and Thoracoabdominal Aneurysms

Descending thoracic and thoracoabdominal aneurysms result from atherosclerosis or degenerative disease in most cases. Other etiologies include chronic dissections, contained traumatic transections, cystic medial necrosis, and aortitis. Patients may present with upper back pain, or more rarely with hoarseness when the aneurysm compresses the recurrent laryngeal nerve. Approximately 50% of patients are symptomatic at the time of diagnosis. Aortogram is the gold standard to evaluate the anatomic extent of the lesion; however, with modern advances in imaging technology CT scan and MRI are more commonly used for preoperative evaluation. Thoracoabdominal aneurysms can be classified by the extent of their involvement, most

commonly using the Crawford system (Fig. 22-16). Type I aneurysms are confined to the thoracic aorta, whereas types II, III, and IV involve the visceral portion of the aorta as well.

The size indications for surgical repair are controversial; however, repair is usually recommended for asymptomatic patients with aneurysms greater than 6 to 8 cm in diameter. This is because of the poor prognosis of patients after diagnosis of descending thoracic aneurysm. Up to 60% to

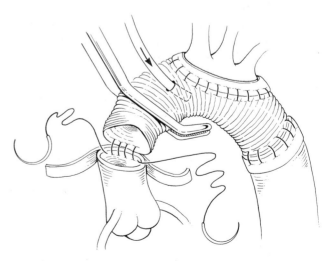

Figure 22-15 Completion of the proximal aortic anastomosis in an aortic arch aneurysm repair. (From Kaiser LR, Kron IL, Spray TL, eds. *Mastery of cardiothoracic surgery.* Philadelphia: Lippincott Williams & Wilkins, 1998, with permission.)

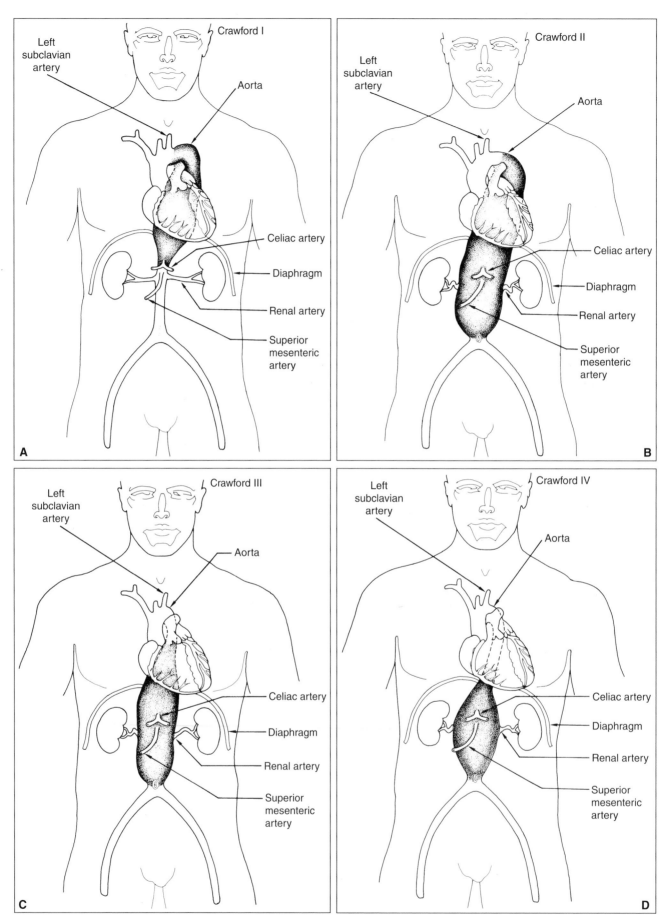

Figure 22-16 Crawford classification of thoracoabdominal aneurysms. (From Kaiser LR, Kron IL, Spray TL, eds. *Mastery of cardiothoracic surgery.* Philadelphia: Lippincott Williams & Wilkins, 1998, with permission.)

70% of patients with aneurysms larger than 6 cm die within 2 years of diagnosis and at least one half of these deaths result from rupture. Symptomatic aneurysms should be repaired irrespective of size.

Circulatory management during repair typically involves some method of distal perfusion. This may be accomplished with the use of left atrial to femoral artery bypass or a heparin-bonded shunt to the distal aorta or femoral artery. A major source of morbidity is spinal cord ischemia leading to paraplegia. The arteria magna provides most of the blood supply to the region of the spinal cord at risk and arises variably between the T8 and L4 vertebral bodies. Because of this, every attempt is made to preserve all large intercostals not involved in the aneurysm. Use of the clamp-and-sew technique has been associated with a higher incidence of spinal cord ischemia, particularly when clamp times exceed 30 minutes. Intraoperative spinal cord monitoring by measurement of somatosensory or motor evoked potentials has been used in an attempt to limit this complication. Postoperative management to reduce ischemia includes mantaining high mean arterial blood pressure and reducing cord pressure with lumbar drain placement to enhance perfusion pressure. Thoracoabdominal aortic aneurysms involving the abdominal aorta are repaired by using a branch inclusion technique with direct anastomosis of branch vessels to the graft. Aneurysms involving the visceral vessels may be best repaired with selective perfusion intraoperatively by using balloon cannulas.

Endovascular Repair of Thoracic Aortic Aneurysms

The first clinical use of stent grafts for endovascular thoracic aortic repair was reported in 1994. This technology has also been used for repair of traumatic, mycotic and ruptured aneurysms of the descending thoracic aorta. Anatomic criteria for stent graft repair includes a normal 2-cm proximal arterial segment distal to the left common carotid artery, a normal 2-cm segment proximal to the celiac artery, and iliac arteries greater than 8 mm in diameter. A minimally invasive approach to thoracic aortic disease is very desirable given the significant comorbities of these often elderly patients. Long-term clinical data have not yet been fully established, and there are several ongoing trials for a number of devices. FDA approval for one or more of these devices is expected in the very near future. One recent review out of Stanford University of 103 patients treated between 1992 and 1997 demonstrated actuarial survival of 49% at 5 years in the stent graft group versus 78% in the open repair cohort. However, in this trial, stent grafts were reserved primarily for high-risk surgical candidates with significant comorbidities, and therefore results were likely skewed toward poorer outcomes. As endovascular technology and techniques improve, there will likely be an expanding role for stent graft repair of thoracic aortic disease. As it stands now, stent graft repair is not appropriate for younger patients without significant comorbidities. The long-term durability has yet to be established.

KEY POINTS

▲ Ventricular septal defect (VSD) is the most common congenital heart defect.

▲ Tetralogy of Fallot is the most common cause of cyanosis in an infant; transposition of the great arteries is the most common cause of cyanosis in a newborn.

▲ The treatment of an acute myocardial infarction (MI) consists of aspirin, heparin, and possible angioplasty within the first 4 to 6 hours.

▲ A post-MI patient with decreased blood pressure and a holosystolic murmur most likely has acute mitral regurgitation due to papillary muscle dysfunction/rupture.

SUGGESTED READINGS

Alexander RW, Schlant RC, Fuster V, eds. *Hurst's the heart, arteries and veins*, 9th ed. New York: McGraw-Hill, 1998.

Baue AE, Geha AS, Hammond GL et al., eds. *Glenn's thoracic and cardiovascular surgery*, 6th ed. Stamford: Appleton & Lange, 1996.

Braunwald E, ed. *Heart disease: a textbook of cardiovascular medicine*, 5th ed. Philadelphia: WB Saunders, 1997.

Cohn LH, Edmunds LH Jr, eds. *Cardiac surgery in the adult*, 2nd ed. New York: McGraw-Hill, 2003.

Kaiser LR, Kron IL, Spray TL, eds. *Mastery of cardiothoracic surgery*. Philadelphia: Lippincott Williams & Wilkins, 1998.

Sabiston DC Jr, Spencer FC, eds. *Surgery of the chest*, 6th ed. Philadelphia: WB Saunders, 1995.

Vascular Disease and Vascular Surgery

23

Mireille Astrid Moise   *Ronald M. Fairman*

Vascular diseases are responsible for more morbidity and mortality than any other category of human disease. Atherosclerosis, which affects large and medium-sized vessels, is characterized by endothelial cell dysfunction leading to vascular inflammation and damage. Atherosclerotic vessels contain atheromatous plaques within the tunica intima layer. These plaques contain a necrotic lipid core framed by lipid-laden macrophages, topped with a fibrous cap. These lesions can cause vascular disease by either encroaching upon the lumen of the vessels causing narrowing or stenosis, or by plaque rupture leading to thrombosis and occlusion of the vessel. Moreover, these plaques can also lead to weakening of the vessel wall and aneurysmal degeneration.

VASCULAR ANATOMY

The normal blood vessel wall contains three layers: the tunica intima, tunica media, and tunica adventitia. Veins and arteries differ in that arteries have a thicker wall and a greater wall thickness-to-lumen diameter ratio. Two thirds of systemic blood is contained in the venous circulation at any one time, making the venous system a large capacity system. Larger veins will often contain muscular valves that aid in the movement of blood back to the heart by propelling blood against gravity.

The tunica intima is composed of a thin layer of endothelial cells overlying a thin subendothelial surface of connective tissue. The endothelial cell, which forms the inner lining of the blood vessel, has a number of important functions and is crucial to maintaining vascular homeostasis. Endothelial cells modulate vascular tone, caliber, and blood flow with the secretion of the vasoactive mediator nitric oxide (NO), which is a vasodilator, anti-inflammatory mediator, and antithrombotic agent. NO also inhibits vascular smooth muscle cell proliferation responsible for dysfunctional neointima formation seen with recurrent stenosis. NO release is stimulated via acetylcholine receptor stimulation, and it is generated by nitric oxide synthase using L-arginine as the substrate. An isoform of nitric oxide NOSIII (eNOS) is constitutively expressed. NO-induced vasodilation is mediated by increased production of cyclic

guanosine monophosphate (cGMP) through activation of guanylate cyclase. The end result is a reduction in intracellular calcium. Other key functions of NO include an antiinflammatory and antithrombotic effect by preventing leukocyte adhesion, vascular smooth muscle cell proliferation, and platelet aggregation.

The tunica media layer is the muscular layer of the vessel wall comprising smooth muscle cells. It is separated from the tunica intima by the internal elastic lamina composed of the protein elastin. It is well-developed in arteries in order to withstand the pulsatile flow and higher blood pressure of arterial blood. It is demarcated from the adventitial layer by the external elastic lamina. The tunica adventitia is a collection of adipose and other supportive connective tissue. The vaso vasorum, a collection of feeding vessels, if present, is contained within this layer and supplies a tunic media with more than 28 elastic layers (Fig. 23-1).

There are three different types of arteries. The largest arteries are the elastic arteries, which consist of the aorta and its major branches such as the subclavian, brachiocephalic, and common carotid arteries. Distributing arteries are the second largest and consist of the coronary and the renal arteries. Finally, the smallest arteries are contained within the substance of organs and tissues.

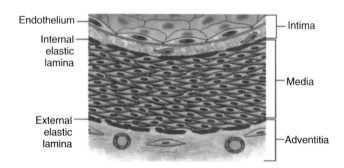

Figure 23-1 Structure of the vascular wall. (From Robbins SL. *Pathologic basis of disease*, 6th ed. Philadelphia: WB Saunders, 1999:494, with permission.)

Arterioles are the smallest arteries and can dramatically affect the distribution of blood flow and systemic arterial pressure simply by dilating or constricting. Richly supplied with nerve fibers, the tunica media layer is exquisitely responsive to hormonal and chemical mediators that affect vascular tone. Because resistance to blood flow is inversely related to the fourth power of the radius, relatively small changes in diameter can have dramatic effects on distribution of blood flow. Arterioles tend to be most vulnerable to hypertensive damage as they bear the brunt of stresses associated with elevated blood pressure. Conversely, large elastic and muscular arteries tend to feel the effects of atherosclerotic changes that will be discussed in subsequent text. With aging, the elastic arteries lose their elasticity, and, hence, vessels tend to become progressively tortuous and dilated in older individuals. In particular, the external elastic lamina, which is already thinner than the internal elastic lamina, begins to diminish with age.

Briefly, capillaries are small diameter vessels, usually the size of a single red blood cell, which are responsible for diffusion of nutrients and wastes within tissue beds. Capillaries arise at the end of arterioles and eventually coalesce into postcapillary venules and progressively larger veins as the blood makes its way back to the heart.

Lymphatic vessels found within interstitial tissues are thin-walled endothelium-lined structures. These conduits aid in mobilizing extracellular fluid back to the vasculature and eventually to the heart. As with veins, the larger vessels are outfitted with valves to prevent retrograde flow of fluid.

PATHOGENESIS OF ATHEROGENESIS

Although numerous theories have been proposed to explain the development of atherosclerosis, compelling evidence has propelled one theory to predominance. Atherosclerosis can essentially be defined as an inflammatory disease.

Endothelial injury causes the expression of surface-selective adhesion molecules such as vascular cell adhesion molecule 1 VCAM-1 that allow binding of leukocytes. One pathway that appears to mediate expression of many genes during endothelial activation is the transcription factor *nuclear factor* kappa B (NFκB)—a common intermediate in a number of inflammatory pathways. The presence of leukocytes infiltrating the tunica intima leads to the expression of proinflammatory cytokines, which signal the migration of monocytes into the tunica intima which then go on to differentiate into macrophages. Monocyte chemoattract protein (MCP) and monocyte colony-stimulating factor (MCSF) are known monocyte chemokines expressed in these lesions. MCP is produced by endothelial cells in a paracrine manner and macrophages in an autocrine manner. These macrophages begin to engulf lipids resulting in lipid-laden cells called foam cells. B and T cells also promote the migration and proliferation of smooth muscle cells. The result is an atheromatous plaque. The key components of these plaques are a lipid-rich necrotic core containing foam cells as well as extracellular lipid covered by a fibrous cap made up of smooth muscle cells, lymphocytes, and connective tissue (Fig. 23-2). The plaque lies within the intima with the potential to enlarge and intrude upon the lumen occluding the vessel lumen. Other complications of atheromatous plaques that could occur in addition to stenosis include calcification, plaque rupture with subsequent hemorrhage, ulceration, or superimposed thrombosis. Calcification of atheromas can produce vessels with eggshell brittleness and is felt as a nodularity in the vessel wall. Plaque rupture can occur when activated macrophages, and smooth muscle cells produce collagenases that degrade the elastin and collagen of the fibrous cap. An unstable plaque can then develop, which is subsequently prone to rupture and subsequent hemorrhage or ulceration. Rupture can also result in the release of tissue factor—a prothrombotic substance, initiating thrombosis and an acute event (Fig. 23-3).

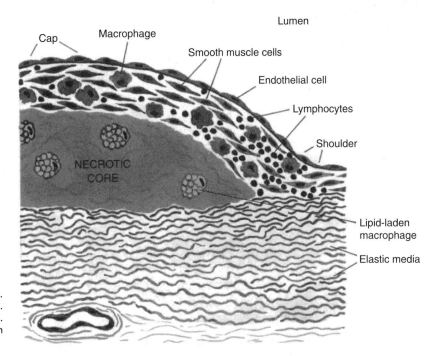

Figure 23-2 Plaque in atherosclerosis. (From Benditt EP, Schwartz SM. Blood vessels. In: Rubin E, Farber JL, eds. *Pathology*, 2nd ed. Philadelphia: JB Lippincott, 1994:472, with permission.)

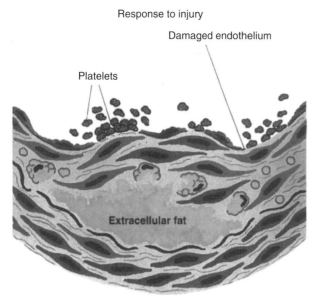

Figure 23-3 Reaction to injury. (From Benditt EP, Schwartz SM. Blood vessels. In: Rubin E, Farber JL, eds. *Pathology*, 2nd ed. Philadelphia: JB Lippincott, 1994:469, with permission.)

The earliest lesions present even in childhood are that of a fatty streak. Fatty streaks are flat lesions composed of T lymphocytes, lipid-filled macrophages or foam cells, and extracellular lipid. Fatty streaks seen in childhood often lie in the abdominal aorta. It is important to note that although fatty steaks may be precursors to atherosclerotic plaques, they do not all progress down that pathway. The mechanism behind progression of the disease is under intense study.

Branch points in arteries are sites in the arterial tree that tend to develop atheromas. At these branch points, absence of normal laminar shear stress leads to the breakdown of normal endothelial cell defenses (Fig. 23-4).

Risk Factors

Risk factors can be divided into two main groups: non-modifiable and modifiable. Age, sex, family history, and genetic abnormalities are the nonmodifiable risk factors. With advancing age, the risk of developing atherosclerosis rises. Men are more prone than women to develop atherosclerosis. Some evidence suggests that estrogen has a protective effect, as these differences in vascular and especially cardiovascular disease incidence seem to decline postmenopause. A family history also seems to predispose patients to the development of plaques and their subsequent complications. Family clustering of such modifiable factors as hypertension, diabetes, and hyperlipidemia may be the reason. Finally, genetic factors such as disordered lipid metabolism can lead to accelerated atherosclerosis.

The modifiable risk factors are described below:

Hyperlipidemia—The total cholesterol level is the determining factor with regard to pathogenesis of atherosclerosis, particularly the low-density cholesterol level, low-density lipoprotein (LDL). Numerous studies have demonstrated a causal relationship between high cholesterol diets and the development of atheromatous plaques. The oxidation hypothesis of atherosclerosis states that LDLs undergo oxidative modification and localize in the lipid atheroma.

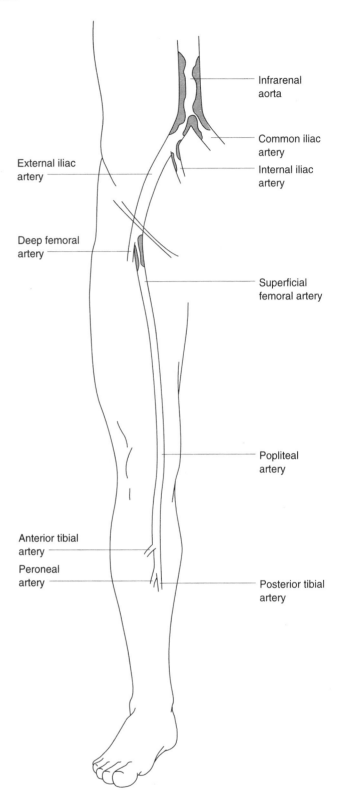

Figure 23-4 Atherosclerotic sites in aortoiliac region. (From Brewster DC. Aortoiliac disease. In: Greenfield LJ, Mulholland MW, Oldham KT et al., eds. *Surgery: scientific principles and practice*, 1st ed. Philadelphia: JB Lippincott, 1993:1645, with permission.)

The oxidized endproducts, of which oxLDL is the most important, function as inflammatory mediators. oxLDL can induce adhesion molecule expression from endothelial cells. oxLDL is also a potent macrophage chemokine and promotes its migration into the tunica intima. High-density cholesterol, or high-density lipoprotein (HDL), another component of the total cholesterol level, also plays a key role. HDL exerts a protective effect against atherosclerosis. HDL is involved in transporting cholesterol back from the periphery to the liver. Exercise and moderate consumption of alcohol raise the HDL level, whereas obesity and smoking lower it. The level of total cholesterol should be in the range of 140 to 200 mg per dL. LDL level ideally should be maintained below 130 mg per dL and HDL level should be above 40 mg per dL.

Hypertension—After the age of 45, hypertension plays more of a role than hypercholesterolemia in the death rates attributed to stroke and ischemic heart disease. Both elevated systolic and diastolic pressure increase risk. A link between hypertension and inflammation most likely lies with angiotensin II (AII), a potent vasoconstrictor. AII is a pro-oxidant in that it promotes the production of superoxide anion from arterial endothelial cells and smooth muscle cells. AII also acts on smooth muscle cells to secrete proinflammatory cytokines such as interleukin 6 (IL-6), MCP-1, and VCAM-1.

Diabetes Mellitus—Accumulating evidence points to endothelial dysfunction as the mechanism behind the vasculopathy that develops in diabetics. Diabetic patients have impaired endothelium-dependent vasodilation, impaired function of endothelial NOS, and increased production of endothelin-1, a potent vasoconstrictor. Platelet dysfunction has also been described in diabetic patients. Platelets are larger, with an increased number of glycoprotein (GP) IIb-IIIa receptors in the membrane, and are hyperreactive.

Hyperglycemia not only induces the formation of reactive oxygen species, but also contributes to the formation of proinflammatory mediators. Hyperglycemia leads to the addition of advanced glycation endproducts (AGEs) to macromolecules. AGE-modified proteins bind to RAGE (receptor for AGE) surface molecules that then lead to the inflammatory pathways.

Obesity is linked to several of the other risk factors. Obesity increases the risk of developing hypertension and insulin resistance. In addition, obesity is associated with elevated levels of circulating LDLs.

Smoking is a major modifiable risk factor associated with atherosclerosis. A pack or more of cigarettes per day increases the death rate from ischemic heart disease by up to 200%. Cessation of smoking approximately halves this increased risk.

Finally, although not proved to be a definitive risk factor, an association between infectious agents and atherosclerosis has been identified. The presence of *Chlamydia pneumoniae* has been demonstrated in a number of atherosclerotic lesions; however, no studies have been able to prove that infection with this agent is a causative factor for these lesions. Nonetheless, the presence of an infectious agent in the blood vessel wall can serve as an inflammatory stimuli.

THEORIES OF ANGIOGENESIS

Research in angiogenesis is being conducted with much fervor among cancer researchers who are searching for ways to circumvent angiogenesis in tumors, whereas cardiac and vascular researchers are striving to promote it. For this reason, we will discuss briefly several angiogenesis mediators.

Vasculogenesis, in early development, occurs when endothelial cells proliferate *in situ* and then come together to form tubular structures or nascent blood vessels. Angiogenic remodeling is the process of branching of vessels and involves both pruning and vessel enlargement. Finally, angiogenic sprouting refers to new vessel formation in adults as well as revascularization of tissue in the developing embryo.

Vascular endothelial growth factor (VEGF), the first characterized vascular-specific growth factor, is instrumental in both vasculogenesis and angiogeneic sprouting. Two other factors AngI and ephrin-B2 help to mature this nascent vasculature. Ephrin-B2 serves to distinguish developing arterial from venous vessels. Ang1 continues to play a role by stabilizing the mature vasculature. Ang2, a natural antagonist of Ang1, counteracts these effects by destabilizing the vasculature initiating new vessel growth as occurs in tumors.

The VEGF family consists of three types of tyrosine-kinase receptors. VEGFR-2 appears to be the major mediator of endothelial cell growth and the arrangement of this growth into tubular structures. Mutations in VEGFR-1 result in endothelial cell proliferation but in a disorganized assembly into primitive vessels. VEGFR-3 appears to play a role in the development of lymphatic vessels. Finally, the ligand VEGF-B appears to be central in coronary vessel development, whereas VEGF-C, which binds to VEGFR-3, may be important for lymphatic vessel formation.

VEGF works in conjunction with angiopoeitins. The angiopoeitin family interacts with the Tie-2 receptor family. Angiopoeitins aid in the maturation of early blood vessels by allowing proper signaling and interactions between endothelial cells and their supporting cells. Although transgenic expression of VEGF led to the development of immature, leaky, and hemorrhagic vessels, transgenic expression of Ang1 led to the development of leak-resistant vessels.

Neointimal Formation

Graft failure can occur for many reasons. If it occurs between 6 months and 2 years, it is due to restenosis via neointimal formation. After 2 years, graft failure is attributed to progressive atherosclerosis. Before 6 months, graft failure is generally the result of a technical failure in the operating room or a hypercoaguable state. Restenosis can occur after angioplasties, vein bypass grafting, and endarterectomies. Neointima formation is the term used to describe the process by which a once patent vessel becomes occluded. This little-understood complex process is initiated after endothelial cell injury. Thrombus formation and infiltration of neutrophils and monocytes release cytokines and other factors, which then stimulate migration of medial smooth muscle cells into the intima. Smooth muscle cell migration persists despite the presence of an intact endothelium. A thickened wall is the end-result with subsequent luminal narrowing.

PERIPHERAL ARTERIAL OCCLUSIVE DISEASE

Introduction and Epidemiology

Peripheral arterial occlusive disease (PAD) or chronic lower extremity ischemia affects roughly 5% of men and women 55 to 74 years of age. The prevalence of the disease increases with age. PAD can be attributed to progressive atherosclerotic disease. Most patients are asymptomatic despite having objective evidence of atherosclerotic disease. The more common symptoms that result from chronic ischemia to the lower extremities include intermittent claudication, rest pain, and ischemic ulcers. In general, claudication alone, as will be discussed in subsequent text, is rarely limb-threatening. In contrast, rest pain and tissue loss will likely progress to limb loss if untreated.

Diagnosis

The symptoms of chronic lower extremity ischemia, when they occur, are fairly classic. Claudication, usually the first manifestation of PAD, is described by patients as pain or cramping in the buttock, thigh, or calf muscles after walking a predictable distance. This pain is relieved upon rest, but reliably recurs once activity is reinitiated.

Pain of this nature and pattern that occurs in the hip, buttock, or thigh is usually reflective of aortoiliac disease. Men may complain of difficulty achieving or maintaining an erection or both as a result of decreased perfusion through the internal pudendal arteries, which originate from the internal iliac arteries. On physical examination, these patients may have evidence of leg muscle atrophy and diminished or absent femoral pulses. This syndrome described by *Leriche* now bears his name. In general, patients complaining of claudication due to isolated aortoiliac disease tend to be younger than those whose claudication caused by disease of the femoropopliteal system. In addition, lesions of the aortoiliac system, regardless of lumen diameter, are at risk for distal embolization. This complication has been described as the "blue toe syndrome." It is for these reasons, as well as the excellent long-term results obtained with this patient population (primary unassisted patency approaching 95% at 4 years), that a more aggressive approach to claudication due to aortoiliac disease is taken.

Pain in the calf usually represents superficial femoral artery disease. For the most part, multiple lesions at various levels are required to progress to limb-threatening ischemia. As discussed earlier, most patients complaining of intermittent calf claudication can be safely observed until symptoms of critical ischemia provide an absolute indication for revascularization.

Diminished peripheral pulses will make the diagnosis of vascular disease more likely; however, nonvascular causes of claudication need to be considered. The most common conflicting diagnosis is that of neurogenic leg pain. Because spinal stenosis and nerve compression can occur concomitantly with vascular occlusion, the absence of distal pulses does not rule out a spinal problem. Symptoms that begin with a change in position and are relieved only by assuming the recumbent position must be suspected to be of neurogenic origin. In addition, a normal systolic pressure response to exercise, despite the occurrence of symptoms with exercise, effectively excludes claudication on a vascular basis. Further studies to evaluate patients with atypical symptoms thought likely to be neurogenic in origin include lumbosacral spine films, electromyography, lumbosacral spinal magnetic resonance imaging (MRI) or computerized tomographic (CT) scanning, and myelography. In addition, patients in whom symptoms do not resolve following revascularization should be evaluated for a neurogenic process.

Critical limb ischemia occurs when the arterial blood supply is insufficient to meet the metabolic demands of resting muscle or tissue. This is the most common indication for lower extremity arterial reconstruction. Chronic ischemia is manifested as imminent or actual tissue loss in the form of rest pain, ischemic ulcers, or gangrene. In contradistinction to the often benign natural history of mild and moderate claudication, the natural history of limb-threatening ischemia is progression to amputation unless intervention occurs with improvement of arterial perfusion.

Ischemic rest pain or diffuse pedal ischemia can be described as severe pain not readily controlled by analgesics, which is usually localized in the forefoot and toes of the chronically ischemic extremity. If the pain is also felt more proximally, it usually does not spare the distal sites. This pain is brought on or made worse by elevation of the extremity and is relieved or improved by dependency. Therefore, it is often experienced only at night or while the patient is reclining. Diffuse pedal ischemia is commonly associated with ankle pressures less than 40 mm Hg and toe pressures less than 30 mm Hg.

Ischemic ulcers are often the result of minor traumatic wounds failing to heal because of reduced blood supply that is insufficient to meet the increased demands of healing tissue. The ulcers are often painful and associated with other manifestations of chronic ischemia including rest pain, pallor, hair loss, skin atrophy, and nail hypertrophy. These ulcers often form at sites of increased focal pressure such as the lateral malleolus, tips of toes, metatarsal heads, and bunion area. Ischemic ulcers are usually dry and punctate and need to be distinguished from ulceration as a result of venous insufficiency. Venous ulcers are more commonly located superior to the medial ankle and are often moist, superficial, and diffuse. They are often associated with hemosiderin pigmentation and other evidence of venous insufficiency such as varicosities and worsening symptoms with dependency. Patients may have combined arterial and venous disease and manifest signs of both arterial and venous insufficiency.

Gangrene is characterized by cyanotic anesthetic tissue associated with necrosis owing to reduction of arterial blood supply below the level necessary to meet minimal metabolic requirements. Gangrene can be described as either dry or wet. Dry gangrene is more common in patients with atherosclerotic disease that frequently results from embolization to the toe or forefoot. Wet gangrene is a true emergency, often occurring in diabetic patients who sustain an unrecognized trauma to the toe or foot. If sufficient viable tissue is present to maintain a functional foot, emergent debridement of all affected tissue usually results in a healed foot. If the wet gangrene involves an extensive portion of the foot, emergent guillotine amputation may be warranted, with revision to below-the-knee or above-the-knee amputation 72 hours later.

Acute ischemia can be manifest in the form of distal embolization of proximal atheromatous material to the toes, resulting in the blue toe syndrome, or result from a large embolus or sudden occlusion of a previously stenotic area, causing diffuse acute ischemia.

Blue toe syndrome consists of the sudden appearance of a cool painful cyanotic toe or forefoot in the often perplexing presence of strong pedal pulses and a warm foot. This clinical situation results most often from embolic occlusion of digital arteries with atherothrombotic material from proximal arterial sources. These episodes portend both similar and more severe episodes in the future. Therefore, location and eradication of the embolic source is usually indicated.

Diffuse acute ischemia is characterized by the sudden onset of pain progressing to numbness and finally paralysis of the extremity accompanied by pallor, coolness, and absence of palpable pulses. Acute ischemia is usually caused by embolic or thrombotic occlusions of native arteries, sometimes in conjunction with previous vascular occlusions. Factors that predict a favorable prognosis include a preexisting history of claudication or other factors suggesting the formation of collaterals before the acute event, audible arterial flow at the time of presentation, and the absence of neurologic changes at the time of presentation. Absence of the previously noted factors suggests a poorer prognosis. It is important that limb-revascularization procedures in the form of thrombolysis, embolectomy, or bypass be performed early and expeditiously in the face of deteriorating clinical findings and is withheld in the face of irreversible ischemic changes with extensive gangrene.

Patient evaluation begins with a detailed history and careful physical examination. Rare is the patient complaining of limb-threatening ischemia that does not have some evidence of underlying medical disease including heart disease, diabetes, kidney disease, hypertension, chronic pulmonary disease, or extracranial cerebral vascular disease. Maximal therapy of these conditions must be provided preoperatively, intraoperatively, and postoperatively to ensure the best possible outcome. The physical examination must be complete, including a careful search for bruits, aneurysms, and malignancies. Additional time must be dedicated to the examination of the extremities for a careful evaluation of pulses, tissue changes, and evidence of prior vascular intervention.

Because physical examination findings are neither specific nor sensitive enough to design operative therapy, patients with evidence of peripheral ischemia should undergo objective testing. Two simple tests include the measurement of segmental systolic pressures and the ankle–brachial index (ABI). Normally, Doppler segmental pressures increase 20 mm Hg from the brachial artery to the proximal femoral artery. Any change less than a 20-mm Hg increase indicates significant aortoiliac disease. A pressure drop of greater than 30 mm Hg between any two successive cuffs normally placed at the arm, proximal thigh, distal thigh, proximal calf, and distal calf signifies a significant arterial obstruction. The ABI is also a helpful test that can be performed at the bedside. The ABI is the ratio of the ankle blood pressure to the brachial blood pressure. An ABI of greater than 1.0 is considered normal. An ABI of 0.5 to 0.84 suggests that the degree of arterial obstruction is associated with claudication, and an ABI of less than 0.50 suggests severe arterial obstruction often associated with critical ischemia. A more rigid objective determination of claudication severity uses exercise testing. The standard exercise test is a treadmill test for 5 minutes at 2 mph on a 12% incline. Severe claudication can be defined as an inability to complete the treadmill exercise due to leg symptoms, and ankle pressures of less than 50 mm Hg following exercise. Exercise testing is often required for patients with a convincing history but with normal examination results and resting ankle

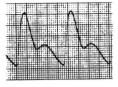 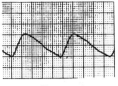

Normal   Abnormal

Figure 23-5 Normal and abnormal pulse volume recordings at ankle level. (From Rutherford RB. *Vascular surgery*, 4th ed. Philadelphia: WB Saunders, 1995:86, with permission.)

pressures. In these patients, segmental Doppler pressures and ABIs performed both before and after exercise may unmask the severity and location of the obstruction.

Pulse volume recordings (PVRs) involve placement of cuffs at the levels of the proximal and distal thigh, calf, and ankle, to help localize the site of obstructive lesions. The PVR is a calibrated air plethysmographic waveform recording system that can also be performed at the metatarsal and toe levels, which is particularly helpful in diabetic patients with relatively incompressible proximal vessels (Fig. 23-5)

Duplex imaging is a useful tool that in experienced hands can provide accurate localization and quantification of lesions, as well as help differentiate stenoses from occlusions, which is an advantage over segmental Doppler pressures or PVRs. However, the time, equipment, and expertise required to perform a complete screening examination of the lower extremity vessels with duplex imaging makes it an impractical replacement for segmental pressures and PVRs. Its ability to answer precise questions about specific arterial segments and measure flow velocities in bypass grafts makes Duplex imaging a useful tool in following known lesions for evidence of progression.

Magnetic resonance angiography (MRA) is becoming increasingly popular in the evaluation of lower extremity ischemia, particularly for patients who have a contraindication to standard angiography. Its use as a replacement for angiography requires careful evaluation and significant experience with MRA.

Currently, contrast angiography remains the gold standard in the evaluation of lower extremity ischemia. A complete study of the aorta, iliac, femoral, popliteal, and runoff vessels is usually performed on both the affected and contralateral sides, as atherosclerotic disease is most commonly bilateral and occurs at multiple levels. However, angiography should be reserved for patients who are expected to undergo revascularization and who do not have contraindications for this imaging modality, such as renal failure.

Natural History

The risk of limb loss is approximately 1% to 2% for patients with claudication within 5 years of diagnosis. For those who smoke, the risk can be as high as 11%. With respect to diabetics approximately 21% will require amputations, compared to 3% of nondiabetics. It is important to note that although the risk of limb loss is fairly low, the risk of a cardiovascular event or death is elevated. Approximately one half of patients will die from coronary artery disease and 10% of patients with claudication will die of stroke in 5 years. Less than 10% will succumb to a vascular event such as a ruptured abdominal aortic aneurysm. Finally, 25% will die of a nonvascular related cause.

Patients with critical limb ischemia rarely improve without intervention. The mortality rate is 25% within one year of the onset of critical limb ischemia. Fifty percent will go on to undergo amputation of the affected limb.

Management

Because the risk of limb loss is low in patients with claudication, initial conservative management is appropriate for these patients. Modification of risk factors is essential and includes weight loss and discontinuation of smoking. In addition, claudication, even asymptomatic, is a marker for cardiovascular disease, and interventions with regard to risk reduction of myocardial infarctions should be considered. Unfortunately, even strict control of diabetes cannot prevent the development or progression of peripheral vascular disease. In addition, patients should be placed on an exercise regimen. Patients should be encouraged to walk to the point of pain, rest, and then continue walking again. This should be continued for 30 minutes daily. With conservative management, 75% of patients will improve or stabilize. Only 5% will need further invasive treatment. Because the risk of limb loss is low, invasive treatment is reserved for patients who face a drastic reduction in their quality of life or performance of their occupation. Critical limb ischemia is an ominous symptom and patients require consideration for revascularization.

Endovascular therapies play a role in the treatment of chronic lower extremity ischemia despite potential inferior long-term patency rates relative to that of open surgical procedures. Endovascular therapies are less invasive, which benefits patients who are of high operative risk, and, most importantly, endovascular failures are rarely accompanied by clinical or angiographic failures that render the procedures repeatable. A meta-analysis of more than 2,000 patients who underwent percutaneous transluminal angioplasty (PTA) and stent placement for aortoiliac lesions found a 30-day mortality rate of less than 1% and a 3-year patency rate of 86%. The patency rate was higher for treated aortoiliac stenoses rather than occlusions. Three-year patency rates for infrainguinal disease were less than 60%. Although surgical revascularization provides more durable results than endovascular therapy, for appropriate lesions, a risk-benefit analysis might suggest endovascular therapy over surgery.

Aortoiliac Occlusive Disease

For patients with aortoiliac occlusive disease, an aortofemoral bypass with prosthetic graft has been the operation of choice. The TransAtlantic Inter-Society Consensus (TASC) devised a classification scheme of certain atherosclerotic lesions and their treatment. TASC A lesions are those for which endovascular therapy is appropriate. TASC A lesions include a single stenosis of the common iliac artery (CIA) or external iliac artery (EIA) of less than 3 cm in length. TASC B lesions are those with no clear superior treatment strategy, but one in which endovascular therapies are more commonly performed. Examples of those lesions include single stenosis of the CIA between 3 and 10 cm in length, two isolated stenosis of less than 5 cm in the CIA and/or EIA, and a single CIA occlusion. Angioplasty alone often produces successful

sustainable results. Pressure gradients with a catheter should be checked before and after therapy to document the severity of a lesion and to ensure that no residual stenosis exists after PTA. Stenting is performed in cases of residual stenoses, dissection, and in lesions that might embolize. Four-year patency of angioplasty alone for claudication due to stenosis is 65% compared to 77% for stenting. For claudication due to occlusive lesions, angioplasty has a success rate of 54% compared to 65% with the addition of stenting. Finally, for critical limb ischemia, patency rates for angioplasty are 53% compared to 67% with the addition of stenting.

For TASC-C and TASC-D lesions, which are characterized by multiple, long segments of stenoses or occlusions, surgery is the treatment of choice. Aortobifemoral bypasses enjoy a higher success rate than other surgical bypass procedures, but the procedure isassociated with a high degree of morbidity and mortality. Overall 5-year cumulative patency rates approach 88%, with 10-year rates approaching 75%. When further categorized by the severity of disease, cumulative patency rates of aortofemoral bypass grafts in patients with rest pain or gangrenous tissue loss are 60% to 70% at 5 years and 50% to 60% at 10 years.

For isolated iliac disease, a femorofemoral bypass can be performed. Some surgeons will attempt an endovascular repair of these lesions as they do not interfere with eventual surgery if one is needed. EIA disease is associated with recurrent stenosis and the need for repeated interventions. Disease extending into the common femoral artery (CFA) can be treated with endarterectomy of the CFA followed by PTA and stent of the proximal iliac disease. For high-risk patients, an axillobifemoral bypass can be performed; however, it is associated with a higher failure rate than aortobifemoral bypass.

Femoropopliteal Disease

For patients with infrainguinal disease, autologous vein grafts are preferable, as their patency rates remain superior to prosthetic material. Prosthetic material is still considered an acceptable bypass conduit as long as it is performed above the knee. Endovascular therapies are best performed in no more than two focal stenotic lesions less than 3 cm. Endovascular therapies are generally less successful with longer lesions, occlusions versus stenosis, and in patients with diseased run-off. The role for infrainguinal primary stenting is unclear. Three-year patency rates for angioplasty and stenting are 51% and 58%, respectively. Five-year patency rates in claudicants for a femopopliteal bypass with vein is 80%, for polytetrafluoroethylene (PTFE) above the knee is 75% and below the knee 65%.

Tibial Disease

The role of percutaneous angioplasty and stenting for tibial disease remains controversial and is reserved for high-risk patients and those for whom revascularization is otherwise not possible. The optimal choice for treatment of tibial disease is a femoral-distal bypass. The 4-year patency rates for infrapopliteal bypass are approximately 50% with autogenous vein grafts and only 12% with prosthetic grafts. Hence, prosthetic material has less of a role for this type of arterial reconstruction.

The generally accepted order of preference for the infrapopliteal anastomosis is the posterior tibial artery, the anterior tibial artery, and lastly the peroneal artery, based on the fact that the peroneal artery is not directly continuous with the pedal arteries, and, therefore, may produce an inferior result. However, more importantly, the choice of outflow vessel should be based on the overall quality of the vessel and its runoff. If two vessels of excellent quality are available, the preference should go to the vessel with the greatest degree of direct continuity with the foot.

Fortunately, most patients presenting with even critical ischemia can be offered a reasonable attempt at limb salvage. However, there are situations in which the best option remains primary amputation. In cases in which gangrene extends into the deeper tissues of the tarsal region of the foot, primary amputation at the below-the-knee level is indicated. If the patient was previously reasonably healthy, a well-fitting prosthesis will provide excellent functionality. The functional outcome following below-the-knee amputation is far better than that following amputation at the ankle despite the higher level. In cases in which the patient has severe depression of mental status such that he or she is unable to ambulate, stand and pivot, communicate, or provide self care, an above-the-knee primary amputation should be considered. Severe, long-standing contractures can occur with below-the-knee amputations in this patient group, and often the below-the-knee amputation wound may break down because of contact with the mattress.

Postoperative Graft Surveillance

There are three major causes of graft failure. Failure in the immediate postoperative period (less than 30 days) is most often the result of technical or judgmental errors. Other causes include inadequate outflow, infection, or an unrecognized hypercoagulable state. Failure between 30 days and 2 years is most often caused by myointimal hyperplasia within the vein graft or at anastomotic sites. Late graft failure is usually caused by the natural progression of atherosclerotic disease. It is estimated that strictures develop in 20% to 30% of infrainguinal vein bypasses during the first year. Careful surveillance is justified because intervention based on a duplex ultrasound surveillance protocol can result in 5-year assisted patency rates of 82% to 93% for all infrainguinal grafts studied, significantly higher than the 30% to 50% secondary patency rates of thrombosed vein grafts. A typical surveillance protocol would include duplex ultrasonography to measure flow velocity and the velocity ratio across a stenosis. Further workup would be indicated in vein grafts with less than 45 cm per second flow velocity and a velocity ratio of more than 3.5 across a stenosis. In addition, ABIs can be easily measured, with a decrease of more than 0.15 between examinations considered significant. Examinations should be performed perioperatively, at 6 weeks, and then at 3-month intervals for 2 years and every 6 months thereafter.

Considerable progress has been made over the last 10 years in the treatment of limb-threatening ischemia, particularly with the success of distal bypass grafts. Patients with limb-threatening ischemia are most likely to do well if they receive an aggressive approach with revascularization if indicated.

ACUTE LOWER EXTREMITY ISCHEMIA

Etiology

The etiology of acute lower extremity ischemia is either an embolus (clot from a distant source) or thrombus (*in situ* clot formation). A recent large-center trial, TOPAS, established that thrombus was the etiology in 85%, whereas an embolus was causative in 15%. In the native artery, acute occlusion is usually caused by thrombosis secondary to atherosclerotic disease. Occlusions of prosthetic material from bypass grafts generally start with a stenotic lesion, a reduced inflow, or an obstructed outflow. In addition, in patients with valvular disease, an embolus of cardiac origin can often precipitate acute lower extremity ischemia. Delineating between two etiologies, however, is not always possible. Acute lower extremity ischemia can occur in the absence of atherosclerotic disease and include such etiologies as arterial trauma, dissection, embolus from a popliteal artery aneurysm, and spontaneous thrombosis associated with a hypercoagulable state.

Diagnosis: Acute lower extremity ischemia often creates a painful, pale, cool extremity with absent or weak distal pulses. The six Ps of pallor, pain, pulselessness, poikilothermia, paresthesias, and paralysis are present in some variation in these patients. Patients with a history of atherosclerotic disease may not have such a dramatic presentation. Because their peripheral vascular disease progressed through the years, development of collateral circulation to overcome the reduced blood flow can mitigate some of the symptoms from an acute thrombus. Often it is the patient who sustains an embolus to a normal or near-normal circulation who will have the most striking presentation and potentially worse outcome.

Natural History

Outcome is related to the proportion of ischemia. Left untreated, patients will progress to limb loss and potentially death. Tissue ischemia can lead to acidosis, rhabdomyolysis with subsequent renal failure, sepsis, and death. Prompt treatment while the limb is salvageable can stave off these complications. However, revascularization comes with its own set of potential complications including reperfusion syndrome.

A 30-day mortality is approximately 15%, with amputation rates ranging from between 10% to 15%. In one study, the amputation rate was found to be proportional to the interval between onset of acute limb ischemia and exploration: 6% if within 12 hours, 12% within 13 to 24 hours, and 20% after 24 hours.

Management

Immediate systemic anticoagulation with therapeutic levels of heparin is imperative as it prevents clotting of distal blood and reduces morbidity and mortality. Catheter-direct thrombolysis has emerged as a successful alternative to surgical therapies. In addition to being less invasive, gradual reperfusion with thrombolysis potentially reduces the risk of reperfusion syndrome and compartment syndrome. Indications and contraindications for thrombolysis are listed in Table 23-1. Situations in which thrombolysis

TABLE 23-1

INDICATIONS AND CONTRAINDICATIONS FOR THROMBOLYSIS

Indications for Thrombolysis	Contraindications for Thrombolysis
Acute (<14 d duration) thrombosis of previously patent graft or native artery	*Absolute*
	Bleeding diathesis
	Gastrointestinal bleeding within the last 10 d
Arterial embolus lesion not accessible to embolectomy	Neurosurgery within the last 3 mo
	Intracranial tumor within last 3 mo
	History of stroke within the last 2 mo
Acute thrombosis of popliteal artery aneurysm and distal run-off	
	Relative
Risk of high surgical mortality	Recent major nonvascular surgery or trauma within last 10 d
	Cardiopulmonary resuscitation within the last 10 d
	Uncontrolled hypertension, systolic >185 mm Hg or diastolic >110 mm Hg
	Recent eye surgery
	Known aneurysm, especially intracerebral aneurysm
	Mitral valve disease
	Intracranial neoplasm
	Puncture of uncompressible vessel

is unlikely to be effective include cases of irreversible ischemia, early postoperative bypass graft thrombus, large-vessel thrombus easily accessible to surgery, and mild-to-moderate ischemia with claudication.

The thrombolysis catheter is introduced through the femoral artery in the groin. For patients with iliofemoral occlusion, the contralateral artery is accessed. For more distal vessels such as the superficial femoral, popliteal, or tibial arteries, the ipsilateral femoral artery is accessed. The choice of lytic agent includes streptokinase, urokinase, and tissue plasminogen activator. Recombinant proteins have recently been developed. Urokinase is used preferentially over streptokinase, as it has a higher clinical success rate with a lower incidence of bleeding complications. New agents are under developments that are more fibrin-specific, in an attempt to reduce the complication rate of bleeding.

Outcome is related to whether a prosthetic graft is being lysed and whether an arterial or venous lesion is being treated. The order of successful outcome is as follows: prosthetic grafts (78%), native arterial occlusions (72%), and vein graft thromboses (53%). Patients who do not have diabetes tend to do better than those with diabetes (80% and 52%, respectively.) Long-term management following successful thrombolysis involves full systemic anticoagulation with heparin and then Coumadin.

Some minor complications include pericatheter thrombosis, either from reduced flow or an occlusive catheter. Pericatheter thrombosis is combated by anticoagulation initiated prior and during thrombolysis. Three percent to 17% of adequately anticoagulated patients have this complication. Pseudoaneurysm formation can occur from catheter-related trauma in approximately 1% to 2% of patients. The major complication of thrombolysis is bleeding.

The incidence of hemorrhagic stroke is 1%, whereas that of another major bleed resulting in hypotension and requiring transfusion is 5%. Minor bleeding complications such as oozing from puncture sites or groin hematomas occur in approximately 10% to 15% of patients. Other complications include distal embolization of fragments in about 5% of patients. Treatment is continued thrombolysis with eventual resolution.

Compartment syndrome arises in approximately 2% of patients and is caused by reperfusion injury. Patients will complain first of pain with passive stretch, and on examination the anterior component of the calf will be tense. Four-compartment fasciotomy is indicated in these cases.

Rare complications (less than 0.5%) that have been reported to occur include the development of acute renal failure, serious allergic reactions, and death. Not surprisingly, the risk of major complications increases with the duration of thrombolysis therapy, approximately 4% for 8 hours, increasing to 35% for 40 hours.

The surgical options include revascularization in the profoundly ischemic limb, embolectomy in the case of severe acute ischemia, and, finally, amputation if ischemia is irreversible. Irreversible ischemia is manifested by cyanotic discoloration, firm calf muscles, anesthesia, and paralysis of the extremity. Severe ischemia is indicated by loss of sensitivity, decreased skin temperature, skin discoloration, and moderate muscle rigor. As with thrombolysis therapy, heparin is administered immediately with the goal of achieving full anticoagulation as soon as possible. Embolectomy is performed via a small incision in the groin and introduction of a Fogarty balloon catheter with several passes to remove clot. A completion angiography must be performed to look for evidence of any residual thrombus. In the case of thrombus, arterial reconstruction is necessary. In the case of a thrombosed popliteal aneurysm, the aneurysm must be excluded and bypassed.

Three major trials were performed comparing the outcome of patients who underwent thrombolysis or primary surgical therapy for acute limb ischemia. Both the National Institutes of Health (NIH)–sponsored University of Rochester (Rochester) trial and Surgery or Thrombolysis for the Ischemic Lower Extremity (STILE) trial found equivalent outcomes in terms of the rate of limb salvage between the two groups. In terms of major morbidity and death, the Rochester trial found a higher death rate in the surgery group, which they attributed to postoperative deaths. In contrast, although mortality among the two groups was not significantly different, patients in the thrombolysis group had a higher rate of major morbidity. The Thrombolysis and Peripheral Arterial Surgery (TOPAS) trial provided the most conflicting results. The issue was raised of whether initial surgery instead of thrombolysis might be more cost-effective. Roughly two thirds of patients who presented with acute ischemia and who were treated with thrombolysis eventually underwent surgery within 6 months. As with most therapies, proper patient selection is needed to ensure that patients will have the best outcome.

ANEURYSMAL VASCULAR DISEASE

Aneurysmal dilatation is defined as dilation of the vessel wall diameter to 1.5 times its normal diameter. Although associated with atherosclerotic disease, the exact cause of arterial degeneration is unknown. Other etiologies of aneurysms include syphilis, cystic medial necrosis, and dissection.

Pseudoaneurysms, also known as a false aneurysm, occur from rupture of blood through all three layers of the blood vessel wall. There is a persistent communication between the originating artery and the blood-filled cavity. A fibrous wall develops over top this cavity. Some pseudoaneurysms resolve spontaneously, whereas others require repair to prevent rupture and hemorrhage. Pseudoaneurysms most commonly occur after an arterial puncture and are most commonly seen in the common femoral artery after an endovascular procedure. The incidence ranges from 0.5% to 2% after such procedures. Diagnosis is made by the physical examination finding of a pulsatile hematoma. Duplex sonography can make a definitive diagnosis. A pseudoaneurysm appears as a cystic structure in gray-scale image. Color Doppler will demonstrate flow from the artery into the cavity. Treatment consists of either duplex compression or ultrasound-guided thrombin injection. Surgery is necessary for pseudoaneurysms associated with bypass grafts, as they are often associated with a defect in the graft.

Inflammatory aneurysms are another distinct entity comprising 3% to 10% of all abdominal aortic aneurysms. Excessive thickening of the aneurysmal wall accompanied by a dense inflammatory fibrotic reaction in the retroperitoneum is a feature of this type of aneurysm. The retroperitoneum becomes progressively encased, with compression of visceral organs. Hydronephrosis and duodenal obstruction have been known to occur. Symptoms include back pain and weight loss. The erythrocyte sedimentation rate (ESR) will often be elevated. CT findings include a thickened, calcified aortic wall and a mass of periaortic inflammatory tissue. Treatment is surgical repair of the aneurysm, but is often made difficult by dense adhesions and fibrotic tissue.

Abdominal Aortic Aneurysms

Epidemiology and Natural History

Abdominal aortic aneurysms (AAAs) are the 13th leading cause of death, causing approximately 15,000 deaths per year in the United States secondary to rupture. AAAs are estimated to be present in 9% of patients older than the age of 65 years. There is a male-to-female preponderance of 6:1. White men are 3.5 times more likely than black men to have aneurysms. AAAs most often occur in the setting of atherosclerosis, but mounting evidence suggests that this may only be part of the picture. For example, the various rates at which aneurysms expand are not fully explained by this disease process. AAAs are known to grow at an average rate of 0.5 cm per year. There is clearly loss of elastin and support proteins in the walls of AAAs, presumably by the action of proteases. Recent research has been focused on the role of matrix metalloproteinase in aneurysmal degeneration.

The risk factors for aneurysmal disease are family history, previous aneurysm repair such as a popliteal artery aneurysm, coronary artery disease, smoking, and hypertension. A family history of aneurysmal disease is seen in 25% of patients who present with an AAA. Patients with popliteal artery aneurysms have a high incidence of coexistent AAAs (25% to 50%).

The natural history of AAAs is to cause death by rupture. A 5-cm abdominal aortic aneurysm has a 10% risk of rupture per year. Other independent risk factors for rupture aside from size include family history, chronic obstructive pulmonary disease, smoking, higher mean arterial pressure, and gender. Women have a higher risk of rupture than men for smaller aneurysm diameters. In other words, a woman with a 5.5-cm aneurysm has an equivalent rupture risk of a man with a 6-cm aneurysm. Finally, increased wall stress and a very eccentric aneurysm are also associated with a higher rupture risk.

Pathology

The aortic wall has the same basic structure as any other blood vessel. The tunica media is the largest layer in terms of diameter and contains elastin lamellae units in addition to smooth muscle cells. Within the adventitia is a network of collagen fibers that is responsible for the tensile strength of the aortic wall, once the level of mechanical strain exceeds the capacity of medial elastic fibers. With the development of aneurysmal dilation, the collagen fibers become maximally linear aligned reaching the limits of their tensile strength.

Ninety-five percent of AAAs are infrarenal. Five percent are located above the level of the renal arteries. Juxtarenal describes those aneurysms with no normal segment of infrarenal aorta. Finally, those that involve the renal artery origins but not the superior mesenteric artery are termed "pararenal." Iliac artery involvement is seen in up to one half of AAAs. A thoracic aortic aneurysm is seen in association with an AAA in 12% of patients.

Diagnosis

Physical examination to detect AAAs is unreliable as it is very insensitive. The typical finding is that of a pulsatile abdominal mass. Rare symptoms arise from obstruction or compression of the aneurysm on adjacent structures. Examples include hydronephrosis, duodenal compression, and venous thrombosis. Other manifestations of aneurysmal disease include:

- Peripheral emboli—Distal embolus originating from small AAAs can produce livedo reticularis of the feet or the blue toe syndrome.
- Acute aortic occlusion—Claudication symptoms can arise from thrombosis of small AAAs.
- Aortocaval fistulae—Rupture into the vena cavae results in a large arteriovenous fistula. High-output cardiac failure develops with tachycardia and lower extremity edema.
- Aortoduodenal fistulae—Finally, AAA may rupture into the fourth portion of the duodenum. These patients may present with a herald upper gastrointestinal bleed followed by an exsanguinating hemorrhage.

AAAs are rarely symptomatic unless rupturing. The sudden onset of back pain is generally the presenting symptom. Physical signs include hypotension; cold, clammy extremities; and other signs of shock. Diagnosis must be made quickly in these situations as the mortality of this condition can reach up to 90%. The mortality rate for ruptured AAA has not changed significantly over the last 30 years.

In the majority of cases, the discovery of an AAA is an act of serendipity, found on an abdominal ultrasonography or abdominal CT scan ordered for an unrelated reason. Ultrasonography, CT scan of the abdomen and pelvis, and MRA are all 100% sensitive in the detection of AAA. Because of its low cost, ultrasonography is often used for surveillance purposes.

Ultrasonography is useful for its wide availability, inexpensiveness, and portability. It is 100% sensitive in detecting the presence of an aneurysm and provides a fair estimate on size. Hence, its role is mainly in establishing the presence of an AAA in the acute setting and in observing an increase in size of a known aneurysm over time. For the purposes of planning operative repair, ultrasonography has a number of limitations. The relation of the AAA and the renal arteries cannot be reliably determined. In addition, the images produced by ultrasonography are adversely affected by patient factors such as obesity and the presence of gas or barium in the bowel.

A CT angiogram is the diagnostic procedure of choice. (Fig. 23-6) It is very useful in planning operative repair as information regarding size, extent, and relation to the renal arteries is easily obtained. Multiplanar analysis and reconstruction of CT images can also be made and provide an additional level of detail that is used for endovascular stent graft repair planning. In the subacute setting, CT scan can detect the presence of small leaks and contained ruptures. However, in the acute setting, a CT scan may not be readily available.

Finally, MRI can produce highly accurate images in longitudinal, transverse, and coronal planes without the use of ionizing radiation. However, the technology is expensive and not widely available. In addition, this technology can not be applied universally to all patients, as patients with intracorporeal metal implants and a history of claustrophobia must be excluded. The major limitation of MRI is that it does not reveal extent of calcification, which is somewhat crucial in planning for endograft repair.

Invasive angiography is no longer widely used. Because of the mural thrombus present in almost all AAAs, the size of the aneurysm can not be accurately assessed by angiography. The use of angiography is reserved, for the most part, when there is suspected concomitant aneurysmal

lesions elsewhere in the body, an anatomic renal abnormality such as horseshoe kidney or pelvic kidney, or question of renal or visceral involvement.

Management

Large randomized prospective trials in both the United Kingdom and the United States indicate that patients with aneurysms as large as 4.5 cm can be attended to by careful surveillance. There was no long-term survival advantage to operating early. Currently, there is no consensus for routine screening of patients via ultrasonography, and current practice is to survey patients with known disease. Once the aneurysm has reached a size of 4.5 to 5.5 cm, operative repair is considered. The decision to operate involves many variables including not only aneurysm size and recent expansion, but operative risk, medical comorbidities, life expectancy, gender, and family history of rupture. Preoperative testing includes standard laboratory blood tests as well as a cardiac stress test with or without an echocardiogram and pulmonary function tests to assess risk. More than 45,000 operations are performed for this indication each year in the United States alone. In the case of a suspected ruptured aneurysm, time is of the essence. In patient with a known history of an aneurysm, signs and symptoms of shock should prompt a quick trip to the operating room in the absence of time-consuming diagnostic tests. For those patients with a high clinical suspicion for a ruptured aneurysm but no clear history, ultrasonography can quickly document the presence of an aneurysm.

Definitive Treatment

Conventional AAA repair consists of "open" repair by either a retroperitoneal approach through the left flank or a transabdominal approach via a midline incision. Juxtarenal and suprarenal aneurysms are best approached through the left retroperitoneal space. Upon clamping of the aorta proximally, the aneurysm sac is entered. A prosthetic graft, the length of the aneurysm, is sewn proximally and distally to normal aorta. The aneurysm sac is closed over the graft in an attempt to prevent aortoenteric fistulas from erosion of the duodenal wall by friction from the prosthetic graft. Special operative considerations include establishing proximal control. The left renal vein must be identified. With regard to pelvic outflow, if the inferior mesenteric artery (IMA) is to be sacrificed, then at least one hypogastric (internal iliac) artery must have good flow to prevent colon ischemia. If both hypogastric arteries are sacrificed secondary to aneurysmal disease, the IMA must be reimplanted into the aorta. Finally, in the case of an inflammatory aneurysm with dense adhesive disease, supraceliac arterial control must be obtained. This can be established via first dividing the ligaments attached to the left lateral segment of the liver. Once this segment of the liver is retracted, the crura of the diaphragm are separated.

With the introduction of endovascular therapies for repair of AAAs by Parodi in 1991 and the subsequent U.S. Food and Drug Administration (FDA) approval of two stent-graft devices in 2000, this technology has spread widely. (Fig. 23-7) Evidence supports that endovascular repair of AAA can be accomplished with decreased length of stay and decreased morbidity compared to open repairs. Mortality rates between the two types of repairs remain similar. Initially, endovascular repair was believed to be able to

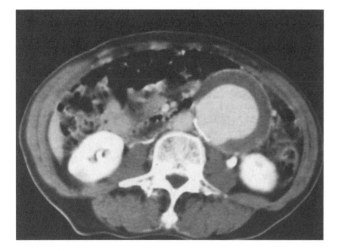

Figure 23-6 Abdominal computerized tomographic scan demonstrating abdominal aortic aneurysm with mural thrombus. (From Goldstone J. Abdominal aortic aneurysms. In: Greenfield LJ, Mulholland MW, Oldham KT et al., eds. *Surgery: scientific principles and practice*, 1st ed. Philadelphia: JB Lippincott, 1993:1715, with permission.)

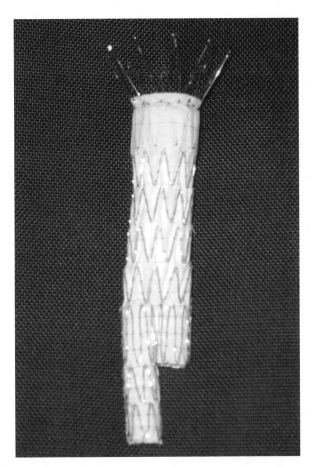

Figure 23-7 Zenith stent graft for treatment of endovascular repair of abdominal aortic aneurysms (AAAs). Note the barbs for suprarenal aorta fixation.

benefit most patients with prohibitive operative risk for open repair, however, now the technology is being offered to all patients. Not all patients who desire endovascular repair, however, are candidates. The aneurysm neck (or distance between the lowest renal artery and the beginning of aneurysmal dilation), and the size and tortuosity of access vessels, namely, the femoral and iliac vessels, are the main anatomic factors. An adequate neck length is necessary to ensure proper fixation of the device without compromising flow to the renal arteries. Hypogastric artery (internal iliac) outflow is also important as loss of blood flow can lead to impotence in men and sigmoid colon ischemia in all.

Endovascular repair is not without its own set of unique risks and complications. Difficulties with the stent graft device itself can occur, such as migration of the stent graft, kinking, occlusion, and modular junctional separations. Most worrisome is the development of an endoleak, which signals incomplete exclusion of the aneurysm. Persistent endoleaks can lead to continued AAA enlargement, continued AAA rupture risk, and, of course, eventual rupture. With regards to endovascular repair, up to 10% of patients will require a second intervention. A persistent endoleak may require coil embolization or placement of a second graft to "seal" the leak. Introduction of a second extension graft may also be necessary in the case of a migrated stent graft. Fortunately, a large number of these interventions are catheter-based and do not require an open repair. This need for another procedure after endovascular repair, is in

striking contrast to conventional repair with a secondary intervention rate of less than 2% in the first 5 years. Finally, after endovascular repair, patients still have a 1% chance of rupture per year.

Postoperative Care and Complications

Complication rates for open repair in the literature range from 1% to 8% of all patients. In patients with select risk factors such as elevated serum creatinine of greater than 1.8 mg per dL, advanced age, ischemic heart disease, congestive heart failure (CHF), or COPD, the 30-day mortality rate can reach upward of 50%. Women have a higher mortality rate than men, with an odds ratio of 1.5 greater risk. High volume centers (11 aneurysm repair per year) have a lower mortality rate than low volume centers. Finally, anatomic characteristics of aneurysms will also affect outcomes. Inflammatory aneurysms, which can adhere to adjacent structures, will often have a worse outcome. In addition, juxtarenal aneurysms requiring suprarenal clamping are also associated with increased morbidity and mortality. Surgery for a ruptured aneurysm is associated with an increased rate of complications across the board. Hence, elective repair should be performed when possible.

The most common complication following AAA repair is coronary ischemia or arrhythmia. Cardiac events are seen in 3% to 16% of postoperative patients. Myocardial infarction is the most common cause of postoperative death. Renal dysfunction is the second most common complication and occurs in up to 5% of patients.

Renal failure can result from intraoperative hypotension, suprarenal aortic clamping, atheromatous embolization, and, finally, preoperative aortography. Twenty percent of patients who undergo emergent repair for a ruptured aneurysm will develop some degree of renal failure. Pneumonia is seen in approximately 5% of patients and is the third most common complication.

Ischemic colitis can occur in 1% of patients and presents as bloody diarrhea, abdominal pain, and abdominal distention. This is an ominous sign, as mortality reaches up to 50%. Full-thickness gangrene and peritonitis is uniformly fatal. Spinal cord ischemia is a rare complication. It is seen more commonly in repairs of thoracoabdominal aneurysms and ruptured AAAs. Fortunately, full recovery of neurologic function is seen in one half of patients with this complication.

Paralytic ileus is common and lasts approximately 2 to 3 days. Occasionally, a small bowel obstruction may occur, which usually resolves with conservative treatment.

Impotence is also fairly common and results from hypogastric artery malperfusion or nerve injury.

Late complications can occur in the months to years following aneurysm repair and include graft infection, graft thrombosis, and pseudoaneurysm formation from dehisced suture lines. Incisional hernias are also fairly common especially in sick, debilitated patients.

Other Aneurysms

Popliteal artery aneurysms are the most common peripheral arterial aneurysms accounting for only about 80%. They are most prevalent in elderly white men. Eighty percent are bilateral and 50% are associated with an abdominal aortic aneurysm. Fifty percent are asymptomatic and present with rather acute symptoms. Symptomatic aneurysms are associated with a 20% amputation rate. Popliteal artery aneurysms can cause acute limb ischemia secondary to propagation of distal emboli or acute thrombosis. These aneurysms can also rupture. Chronic symptoms can be attributed to compression of adjacent structures such as veins or nerves. When diagnosed, the aneurysm should be treated. The operation of choice is ligation with revascularization via a femoropopliteal bypass.

Femoral artery aneurysms are the second most common peripheral arterial aneurysm. Pseudoaneurysms are more common than true aneurysms. These lesions are typically found in elderly male smokers. Femoral artery aneurysms are often bilateral and their discovery should prompt an investigation for other aneurysms such as those of the abdominal aorta or popliteal artery. The complications of femoral artery aneurysms include thrombosis, embolization, and rupture. Distal embolization occurs in 0% to 26% of patients, thrombosis in approximately 15%, and rupture in between 10% and 15%. Surgical options include excision and interposition grafting.

Renal artery aneurysms, in contrast to femoral artery aneurysm and renal artery occlusive disease are seen in younger patients without any significant atherosclerotic disease. The only risk factor of atherosclerosis associated with these aneurysms is hypertension; however, the renal artery aneurysm may be causal. The main complication of renal artery aneurysm is rupture, which is increased in peripartum females. Operative therapy is primarily *in situ* aneurysmectomy or exclusion and bypass, usually with autologous conduit. Saccular renal artery aneurysms are increasingly treated by endovascular coil embolization.

Asymptomatic splenic artery aneurysms are rare but have been increasing in frequency. Often detected incidentally, they can present with life-threatening hemorrhage. Management is controversial. Resection can be performed; however, splenic function is compromised. Acceptable treatment modalities include aneurysmectomy, exclusion, and bypass; however, endovascular approaches are increasingly gaining acceptance.

CAROTID STENOSIS

Epidemiology

Stroke is the third leading cause of death among Americans behind heart disease and cancer. Numerous studies have incontrovertibly proved an increased risk of stroke in patients with carotid artery disease, specifically carotid artery stenosis. The risk of stroke is increased in symptomatic patients and in patients with increasing degrees of stenosis. For asymptomatic patients with a degree of stenosis of less than 75%, the annual rate of stroke is 1.3%. In patients with a degree of stenosis is 75% or less, the annual risk of stroke triples to 3.3%. In patients who were symptom-free, the annual rate of ipsilateral stroke for degree of stenosis greater than 75% is slightly lower at 2.5%.

Pathophysiology

The pathogenesis of carotid artery disease is similar to the progression of atherosclerotic disease elsewhere in the body as described earlier in this chapter.

Atherosclerosis and stenosis are typically seen at the carotid bifurcation, where presumably turbulent flow contributes to endothelial injury and plaque formation. The cumulative effect is decreased vessel lumen diameter and in some cases total occlusion.

Risk Factors

With regard to risk factors, the previously described risk factors for atherosclerotic disease such as hyperlipidemia, smoking, and types 1 and 2 diabetes mellitus play a role in carotid stenosis as well. Isolated systolic hypertension is associated with the degree and progression of carotid artery stenosis. In addition, *C. pneumoniae* strain TWAR had a significant cross-sectional association with asymptomatic carotid artery atherosclerosis. Finally, smoking also significantly increases the prevalence of internal carotid artery stenosis greater than 50% from 4.4% in those who had never smoked to 7.3% in former smokers and 9.5% in current smokers.

Diagnosis

Carotid artery disease is insidious in its development and is often not accompanied with symptoms. The only objective clinical finding is that of a carotid bruit—a thrill heard with a stethoscope upon auscultation of the carotid artery. The presence of a carotid bruit in patients enrolled in the North American Symptomatic Carotid Endarterectomy Trial (NASCET) only had a sensitivity of 63% and specificity of 61% for high grade stenosis. In patient with symptoms, 75% were found to have moderate-to-severe stenosis upon further evaluation.

Clinical symptoms range from a transient ischemic attack (TIA) (stroke symptoms that generally last for less than 24 hours), reversible ischemic deficits (which last from 1 day to 3 weeks), stroke, and amaurosis fugax. None of these are specific for carotid artery disease.

Carotid artery duplex ultrasonography (CDUS) is the most widely used noninvasive test for carotid artery stenosis. The two components of CDUS include B-mode ultrasonographic scanning, which provides a longitudinal section of the carotid artery from the proximal common carotid artery to beyond the bifurcation. Duplex ultrasonography estimates the degree of stenosis based on flow velocity. Although incredibly useful, CDUS does have its limitations. It is not as precise with stenoses of greater than 50%. On the other extreme, CDUS can not reliably distinguish high-grade stenotic lesions with occluded vessels. In addition, CDUS is limited to evaluation of the extracranial portion of the carotid artery system. Finally, it is highly operator dependent.

MRA is gaining a larger role in diagnosing carotid artery disease. Its advantages include visualization of the entire carotid circulation. However, MRA is not permissible for use in patients with metallic implants and not practical in patients who are critically ill or claustrophobic.

Conventional contrast angiography remains the gold standard. It allows for visualization of the entire carotid artery circulation as well as the vertebrobasilar circulations. In addition, information about plaque structure, ulceration, and dissection is also provided. This test, however, is limited by its 4% risk of all neurologic complications and its 1% risk of major stroke or death. In addition, the use of

TABLE 23-2

COMPARISON OF CAROTID ANGIOGRAPHY, CAROTID DUPLEX ULTRASONOGRAPHY, AND MAGNETIC RESONANCE ANGIOGRAPHY

	Carotid Duplex Ultrasonography	MRA	Carotid Angiography
Sensitivity	86%	94%	Gold standard
Specificity	90%	86%	Gold standard
Cost	Low	High	High
Advantages	Low cost, portable	Visualization of entire carotid circulation	Gold standard
Disadvantages	Operator-dependent, not helpful in estimating degree of stenosis in patients with stenosis <50%	Expensive	Higher complication rate
Contraindications	None	Metal implants, claustrophobia	Renal insufficiency, vascular access
Stroke risk	0%	0%	1%

contrast dye limits its use in patients with renal insufficiency. Comparisons of the three studies are included in Table 23-2.

The recommended protocol to evaluate patients for carotid artery stenosis is CDUS plus MRA, if those modalities are available. Angiography should be reserved in cases of disparate or equivocal findings.

Treatment

Medical Therapy

Aspirin is the most widely studied and, until recently, the only drug used broadly for this purpose. Clinical trial results now indicate that ticlopidine, clopidogrel, and dipyridamole are also effective in preventing stroke and other vascular events in patients who have cerebrovascular disease.

Based on 2 meta-analysis, aspirin reduced the risk of stroke by 25% in patients with a known history of atherosclerosis and by 16% in patients with a past history of TIAs or stroke. However, it has been proved that surgical treatment is superior to medical treatment. Hence, medical treatment is reserved for those patients who are believed to be at high risk for complications if undergoing the surgical procedure.

Surgical Therapy: Carotid Endarterectomy

A number of large prospective studies have demonstrated a significant risk reduction in incidence of stroke in patients with symptomatic carotid artery stenosis and select patients with asymptomatic carotid artery stenosis. A summary of those studies is included in Tables 23-3 and 23-4. It is important to note that women and minorities were not routinely included in these studies and hence were not fairly represented.

These results have led the American Heart Association (AHA) to put forth recommendations on symptomatic patients with carotid stenosis who might benefit from carotid endarterectomy (CEA). Patients with carotid stenosis greater than 70% and a history of mild stroke or transient TIA within the past 6 months have proven benefit from CEA. In symptomatic patients with 50% to 70% carotid stenosis, performing a CEA is acceptable but of no proven benefit as is performing simultaneous CEA and coronary artery bypass grafting (CABG). For asymptomatic patients, the AHA has put forth these recommendations. With a surgical complication risk of less than 3%, patients with greater than 60% carotid artery stenosis should undergo CEA to effect a risk reduction in their incidence of stroke. There is no proven benefit, but it is acceptable to perform a unilateral CEA with simultaneous CABG for carotid artery stenosis of greater than 60%. In patients with surgical risk of between 3% and 5%, there is no proven benefit to performing CEAs on any patient population; however, it is acceptable to perform CEAs in patients with greater than 75% stenosis.

Endovascular Therapies

Endovascular techniques have been proposed as an alternative therapy to treat carotid stenosis, particularly in those patients with severe cardiopulmonary risk factors or a

TABLE 23-3

MAJOR TRIALS OF CAROTID ENDARTERECTOMY (CEA) IN PATIENTS WITH SYMPTOMS

Trial/Patients (n)	Degree of Ipsilateral Carotid Artery Stenosis	Risk of Stroke After CEA	Risk of Stroke After Medical Treatment	Length of Follow-up (yr)
NASCET (659)	70%–90%	9%	26%	2
ESCT (2518)	All degrees	2.8%[a]	16.8%[a]	3
VA cooperative trial (193)	50%	7.7%	19.4%	11.9 mo

[a] In patients who have 70% to 90% carotid artery stenosis.

TABLE 23-4

MAJOR TRIALS OF CARTOID ENDARTERECTOMY IN PATIENTS WITHOUT SYMPTOMS

Trial/patients (n)	Carotid Artery Stenosis (%)	Risk of Stroke After CEA	Risk of Stroke After Medical Treatment	Length of Follow-up (yr)
CASANOVA (410)	50%–90%	10.7%	11.3%	3
VAAST (444)	>50%	8.0%	20.6%	3
ACAS (1662)	>60%	5.1%	11%	5

Note: In CASANOVA, more than one half of those in the medical treatment group underwent CEA during 3-year follow-up, thereby limiting that statistical validity of the results. This flawed design is the likely explanation for the lack of difference in the rates of death and stroke seen between the medical and surgical groups.

hostile neck secondary to previous surgery or radiation. Experience with percutaneous angioplasty has not been sufficiently consistent to predict any success. In the North American Cerebral Percutaneous Thrombosis Angioplasty Registry, difficulties with vessel wall recoil, angiographically documented intimal dissection, and plaque dislodgement with subsequent embolization were seen. In addition, the incidence of death and stroke were high.

Stent-assisted balloon angioplasty has emerged to combat the problems seen with PTA alone. Intimal dissection, elastic recoil, and restenosis can all potentially be reduced. Small, nonrandomized cohort studies in high surgical risk patients have been promising, and large, multicenter randomized trials are currently underway.

Data from the Schneider WALLSTENT trial were recently released. Of 223 patients enrolled in the study, 108 were treated with stents and 115 were treated with CEA. Complications such as ipsilateral stroke and death were significantly higher in the stent group, 6.5% vs. 0.9% at 2 days, and at 1 year, 12% vs. 3.5%. The trial was prematurely stopped by the company. The steep learning curve to master the technique of carotid artery stenting was felt to negatively impact the results of the study. A number of recently performed industry sponsored FDA-approved clinical trials have demonstrated highly favorable results with carotid PTA/stenting, and this procedure is likely to gain increasing acceptance.

THORACIC OUTLET SYNDROME

Thoracic outlet syndrome (TOS) is a clinical entity described by a constellation of vascular and/or neurologic symptoms, often without any objective evidence. The condition is caused by compression of the subclavian artery, vein, or branches of the brachial plexus. Symptoms described by patients are vague and numerous: weakness, numbness, paresthesias, pain, atrophy of intrinsic hand muscles, as well as swelling of face and arms. Symptoms caused by compression of the brachial plexus outweigh symptoms caused by compression of the subclavian artery or vein. TOS is a controversial subject in that symptoms are not always accompanied by objective tests and treatment is not always met with symptomatic improvement.

Anatomy

Although the thoracic inlet is defined as the region between the scalene muscles and the first rib, TOS can occur in three distinct regions. The first, the scalene triangle, has as its three boundaries: the middle scalene muscle, the anterior scalene, and the first rib. Both the brachial plexus and the subclavian artery pass over the first rib between the anterior and middle scalene muscles. The subclavian vein also passes over the first rib but is external to the scalene triangle. The costoclavicular space, which contains all three structures, is bordered by the clavicle and the first rib. The costoclavicular ligament is anterior to this space, whereas the edge of the middle scalene lies posterior. Finally, the subcoracoid space, which is traversed by the brachial plexus, lies beneath the pectoralis muscle, the coracoid process, and the ribs posteriorly. The most commonly identified sites of compression in patients with TOS are the scalene triangle and the subcoracoid space.

The presence of a cervical rib can compress the lower trunk of the brachial plexus as well as cause arterial compression. Anomalous cervical ribs are seen in 0.17% to 0.74% in the general population; with a higher percentage seen in women. Rudimentary first ribs are seen in 0.29% to 0.76% of the general population. Only 10% of patients with cervical ribs will experience TOS symptoms, and symptoms usually arise after trauma of the cervical spine. Other anatomic anomalies such as congenital bands and ligaments in the "thoracic outlet" area can also cause compression of neurovascular structures. These bands, which lie either within or on the anterior surface of the middle scalene, extend from the transverse process of C7 or tip of the cervical rib and attach to the first rib.

Neurologic Symptoms

Most of the complaints related to TOS are of neurogenic origin. Patients with TOS will describe symptoms ranging from pain and paresthesias, to weakness with activity, and rarely frank atrophy of hand muscles. Pain is generally described in the subscapular, scapular, and cervical regions, often in association with occipital headaches. Patients will also describe a tired, heavy aching sensation in their arms. Paresthesias and numbness occur in the hands and medial forearms most commonly. Elevation of the arm will often exacerbate symptoms.

There are no objective tests to diagnose the neurogenic aspects of this syndrome, hence it is purely a clinical diagnosis based on history, physical examination, and exclusion of other causative conditions. Sensorimotor testing can often point to the site of compression. For example, isolated compression of the lower trunk of the brachial plexus will produce sensory symptoms in the ulnar nerve distributions. Similarly, sensory complaints in the thumb, index finger, and middle finger are likely caused by compression of the upper trunk.

The mainstay of treatment is conservative with exercise and physical and occupational therapy effecting symptomatic relief. Surgical treatment of TOS, which should be reserved for cases refractory to conservative management, include the following options: The transaxillary approach for first rib resection or a supraclavicular approach for anterior and middle scalenectomies with or without first rib resections. Major neurovascular complications are a risk with both procedures. Nonetheless success rates defined as symptomatic relief of 90% to 95% have been reported within 1 year. However, the success rate trails off to 70% by 5 years.

Vascular Symptoms

Both arterial and venous compression is often seen in patients with a history of vigorous arm activity. Subclavian vein thrombosis is often described as Paget-Schroetter syndrome. Common in younger men with a history of strenuous upper extremity activity, it presents as painful swelling of the dominant arm. The risk of gangrene and pulmonary emboli is low. In younger patients, anomalous ribs and ligamentous bands should be suspected for arterial compression. Finally, patients with previous fractures may subsequently develop this condition. Complications of vascular compression include stenosis, aneurysm formation, ulceration, and, finally, limb-threatening ischemia. Arterial collateralization will often compensate for ischemia producing only mild symptoms. Patients tend to present with late manifestations of ischemia from embolization or proximal arterial thrombosis such as gangrene or Raynaud phenomenon.

The diagnosis of venous compression is made through venous duplex studies or venography. Measurement of blood pressure in both arms and auscultation of bruits with the arm in both the elevated and dependent positions can be helpful. Obliteration of the radial pulse in the arm-elevated position is not a very sensitive test as this can be present in many asymptomatic patients. Arteriogram is also helpful in diagnosis if results of noninvasive tests such as segmental pressures or duplex are equivocal.

Subclavian vein thrombosis is treated with thrombolysis with urokinase followed by first rib resection. Medical treatment with anticoagulation often left patients with functional impairment of the affected arm and is not recommended. The need for and timing of surgical decompression via thrombectomy remains controversial with no clear consensus. Arterial compression leading to compromise requires urgent intervention. Thromboembolic events require decompression of the artery and restoration of distal perfusion. This is accomplished by release of the scalene muscles and resection of any bony abnormalities. Embolizing lesions and or aneurysms require repair. Acute ischemia is best treated with prompt anticoagulation followed by thrombectomy. Chronic occlusions require distal bypass.

VENOUS DISEASE

Superficial venous thrombosis is termed thrombophlebitis. Thrombophlebitis can occur in association with trauma, usually from the site of intravenous infusion. It is characterized by a tender cord along the course of the vein. Ecchymosis may be present. Migratory thrombophlebitis is characterized by repeated bouts of thrombosis in superficial veins, usually in the lower extremity. Migratory thrombophlebitis is seen in patients with malignancy and various vasculitides. Thrombophlebitis of the superficial veins of the breast and the anterior chest wall is termed Mondor disease. Septic phlebitis can occur in association with the long-term use of an intravenous cannula. Suppurative thrombophlebitis is characterized by purulence within the vein. Diagnosis is predominantly clinical. The intravenous catheter, if present, should be removed. Treatment consists of elevation of the extremity and application of hot, wet compresses. Antibiotics and potential excision of the inflammatory process is reserved for cases of suppurative thrombophlebitis.

Thrombosis of the deep venous system can be asymptomatic, but when symptomatic is clinically manifest as pain in the calf or thigh. In the case of an upper extremity deep venous thrombosis (DVT), the pain is felt in the upper or lower arm. The hand and feet are generally spared. In some patients, swelling may be the only complaint. Unilateral swelling in a limb is one of the best clinical indicators of DVT. Calf pain upon sudden dorsiflexion of the foot, or Homan sign, is insensitive and nonspecific. The differential diagnosis of a DVT includes musculoskeletal disorders such as muscle or tendon tears, edema due to inactivity, a lymphatic disorder, venous reflux, or a Baker cyst.

Phlegmasia alba dolens is characterized by diffuse swelling of the entire extremity, pallor, and moderate pain. In association with tenderness over the common femoral vein, these findings are almost diagnostic of iliofemoral venous thrombosis. Phlegmasia cerulean dolens refers to a deeply cyanotic, severely painful, swollen limb. Virtually the entire superficial and deep venous systems are thrombosed. Pedal pulses may be reduced or absent. In severe cases, the distal tissues become ischemic and gangrene can develop.

Of the three elements of Virchow triad: endothelial damage, stasis, and hypercoagulability, stasis is the most likely causative factor of DVT. A major risk factor for venous thrombosis includes scenarios in which prolonged immobility occur such as with recovery after major operations and long automobile or airplane rides. Venodilation from the induction of anesthesia is another cause of stasis that leads to the development of DVT. Other conditions that predispose to venous thrombosis include malignancy, obesity, heart failure, a history of venous thrombosis, and the postpartum state. Patients with antithrombin III, protein C, and protein S deficiencies can also develop DVT.

Confirmation of the diagnosis of DVT is made radiographically. B-mode ultrasonography and Doppler ultrasonography are the mainstay of objective diagnosis. Although venography remains the gold standard for diagnosis, it is rarely used as the initial test given its invasive nature and the need for exposure to contrast dye. B-mode imaging selects and identifies veins for study as well as detects intraluminal echoes signaling clot. Real-time color flow assesses blood flow and aids in the recognition of partially occluding versus occlusive clots. In a symptomatic patient, an inability to fully compress a vein and thereby obliterate its lumen is a clear sign (greater than 95% sensitivity and specificity) of proximal DVT. This test is less sensitive for the detection of calf vein thrombosis. In addition, the distinction between chronic versus acute clot is not always readily made by this modality. With regards to laboratory analysis, a negative D-dimer test can be useful in excluding a diagnosis of DVT. Elevated D-dimer levels are found in nearly all patients with venous thromboembolic disease, as well as in patients with active cardiopulmonary disease or malignancy. In patients who are clinically suspected of having DVT, a D-dimer level of less than 500 ng per mL on enzyme-linked immunosorbent assay (ELISA) has a negative predictive value of 95%.

The acute complication of DVT is pulmonary embolism. Seventy percent of pulmonary emboli arise from embolus from the pelvic and deep veins of the lower extremity. Chronic venous insufficiency is a late complication of venous thromboembolism and is also termed postthrombotic syndrome. The venous hypertension of postthrombotic syndrome is caused by residual venous obstruction and valvular incompetence.

Treatment of acute DVT is anticoagulation. Intravenous therapy with heparin is instituted first. Heparin is a large polysaccharide molecule that binds to antithrombin III, resulting in the inactivation of factor Xa and IIa (thrombin). Therapeutic levels of anticoagulation via heparin are assessed via the partial thromboplastin time (PTT). The goal PTT is 1.5 to 2.5 times the control value. Failure to achieve that PTT is associated with a high risk of recurrent venous thromboembolism.

Low-molecular-weight heparin (LMWH) has a similar mechanism of action to that of unfractionated heparin. The difference is that LMWH has a longer plasma half-life owing to its lesser degree of nonspecific binding to proteins. Laboratory monitoring is usually not necessary but can be performed with an anti-Xa assay. LMWH can be given on an outpatient basis as it is administered subcutaneously every 12 hours. Studies have demonstrated similar efficacies between unfractionated and fractionated heparin in the treatment of DVT and pulmonary embolus (PE). Although not a contraindication, care must be taken in administering this agent to patients with renal insufficiency because of its renal clearance.

Oral anticoagulation with warfarin can be initiated at time of heparin therapy. Warfarin inhibits γ-carboxylation of vitamin K–dependent coagulation factors II, VII, IX, and X. A full anticoagulant effect from warfarin is usually seen in 72 hours, the half-life of factor II. Because warfarin also inhibits carboxylation of natural anticoagulant proteins C and S, patients with deficient levels of protein C and S can exhibit hypercoagulability in the first days of treatment with warfarin. For this reason, concomitant treatment of heparin and warfarin is recommended. The optimal duration of intravenous anticoagulation is not fully resolved; however, oral anticoagulation should be maintained from between 3 and 6 months. A therapeutic level of warfarin therapy is assessed via the INR (international normalized ratio). The INR was developed in response to the significant variability in thromboplastin reagents used in determining the prothrombin time. The goal INR in the treatment of DVT and PE is between 2.0 and 3.0.

The role of thrombolytic therapy remains controversial. Thrombolysis is usually reserved in cases of iliofemoral DVT, in which phlegmasia cerulean dolens is present. Thrombolysis is achieved via a plasminogen activator: streptokinase, urokinase, or tissue plasminogen activator.

For those patients who (i) have a contraindication to anticoagulation, i.e., fall risk or previous gastrointestinal bleed; (ii) recurrent DVT on therapeutic levels of anticoagulation; or (iii) pulmonary embolism despite therapeutic levels of anticoagulation, venal caval interruption procedures should be considered. The most common method of venal caval interruption is via an inferior vena cava (IVC) filter. A number of devices have been FDA approved for the prevention of pulmonary embolus. The filter acts as a "basket" that collects emboli emanating from the lower extremity and prevents them from traveling to the lung. The filter is inserted via approaching the common femoral vein or the internal jugular vein. The filter is seated in the IVC, generally underneath the renal veins. Complications are not uncommon. Thrombosis of the vena cava is reported in up to 10% to 20% of cases; recurrent pulmonary emboli despite filters occurs in 5% to 10% of cases. Tilting of the filter, malposition, or migration can also occur. Breakage and caval perforation of struts are reported in up to 5% to 9% of cases.

LYMPHATIC DISEASES

Lymphedema is caused by an obstruction or interruption of lymphatic vessels and lymph nodes, leading to the accumulation of lymph fluid in subcutaneous tissue resulting in edema of the affected limb. Primary and secondary lymphatic vessels parallel the superficial veins and drain into a third layer of lymphatic vessels contained in the subcutaneous fat. This deeper layer of lymphatic vessels parallels the deep venous system. Lymph fluid from the lower extremity drains into lumbar trunks into the cisterna chyli, travels up the thoracic duct, and then empties into the left subclavian vein. Lymphatic channels from the upper extremity drain into subclavian trunks and eventually enter the venous system via the subclavian vein.

Primary lymphedema is a rare inherited condition characterized by a congenital absence or malformation of lymphatic vessels. The most common form of lymphedema, however, is secondary lymphedema, which is caused by an interruption of normal flow of lymph fluid through lymphatic vessels. Secondary lymphedema can be caused by obstruction of lymphatic flow from tumor infiltration and compression, scarring from radiation therapy or infection and via interruption of lymphatic flow secondary to surgical removal of the lymph nodes. The most common cause worldwide of lymphedema is filariasis, a parasitic infection caused by *Wucheria bancrofti*. In North America and Europe, the most common cause of lymphedema is malignancy. Not all patients who undergo nodal dissection or radiation go on to develop lymphedema. In addition, those who do develop lymphedema may not do so until many years after surgery or radiation. Avoidance of venipuncture in the operated limb as well as heavy lifting may preserve lymphatic vessel function and stave off the development of this complication.

Complications of lymphedema include recurrent cellulitis, fibrosis, and neoplasia. Lymphedematous limbs are susceptible to infection from even minor trauma. In addition, the high protein content of lymph fluid leads to the release of a host of inflammatory mediators that cause fibrous proliferation and scarring. Finally, the development of lymphangiosarcoma is a well-known sequela of peripheral lymphedema.

Chronic lymphedema is a progressive, usually painless, swelling of the extremity. Patients will describe the affected limb as heavy and may describe difficulties with performing activities of daily living or ambulating. Two thirds of the cases will be unilateral. Diagnosis can be confirmed by history and physical examination accompanied by a number of radiographic modalities. A complete history and physical examination to determine if there is a history of malignancy, previous node dissection, or trauma to the affected limb is necessary. The differential diagnosis of an edematous extremity includes acute or chronic deep venous thrombosis, volume overload secondary to heart or renal failure, and lipedema (lipomatosis of the legs). Initially, pitting edema is present but with chronic lymphedema, progressive fibrosis sets in and the edema is nonpitting.

Lymphoscintigraphy is the gold standard for diagnosis of lymphedema. A technetium Tc-99m-labeled colloid allows measurement of lymphatic function, movement, drainage, and response to treatment. Computerized tomography and Doppler ultrasonography are useful diagnostic adjuncts that differentiate between a venous etiology for lower limb swelling versus a lymphatic one. In addition, CT scan is helpful in detecting the presence of lymphatic obstruction via tumor. MRI is also helpful with the differential diagnosis. MRI can distinguish among lipedema, lymphedema, and phlebedema. Findings of lymphedema on MRI include circumferential edema, increased volume of subcutaneous tissue, and a honeycomb pattern above the fascia between the muscle and subcutis with marked thickening of the dermis. Differentiating between primary and secondary lymphedema is generally unreliable using MRI. Lymphangiogram has largely been abandoned as a diagnostic modality given its invasive nature and potential for infection.

Early treatment is conservative consisting of manual lymphatic drainage, compression bandaging, exercise therapy, and meticulous skin care. Benzopyrone has emerged as a pharmacologic option. Benzopyrones function by increasing the number of macrophages, thereby enhancing proteolysis and resulting in removal of protein and edema. Use of benzopyrones results in reduction of the number of secondary infections seen. Surgical options exist but are reserved for refractory cases. Debulking procedures involve radical excision of subcutaneous tissue together with primary or staged skin grafting. This involves removal of the skin, subcutaneous tissue, and deep fascia *en bloc*. Good functional results have been reported with reduced incidence of secondary infection. Bypass procedures involving anastomosis of the lymphatic and venous systems have been reported but only work well in patients with no coexisting venous disease.

ACCESS

The vascular surgeon is often called upon to create two-way circulatory access for the implementation of continuous arteriovenous hemofiltration indicated for dialysis or plasmapheresis. Access can be maintained via a percutaneous cannulation, arteriovenous (AV) fistula or an AV graft.

Percutaneous central venous cannulation is reserved for patients for acute poisonings, anticipated short-term need for hemodialysis, or for those in whom long-term dialysis is expected but alternative methods of access have been exhausted. For long-term access, in-dwelling catheters are tunneled subcutaneously with a Dacron cuff. In-dwelling catheters function on average 3 months but can last as long as 28 months. Access via the subclavian is associated with subclavian vein stenosis with reported rates as high as 50%. Access via the internal jugular veins is the preferred cannulation site and is associated with a lower incidence of associated stenosis but can be uncomfortable for the patient. The catheter is positioned in the superior vena cava (SVC), ideally at the second intercostal space, the largest portion of the SVC, The proximal arterial port is best positioned in the center of the SVC, minimizing obstruction against the caval wall during dialysis.

Fifteen percent of catheters will require eventual removal secondary to infection or thrombosis. Thrombosis is the most common complication and can be treated with streptokinase or urokinase infusion. Catheter-related bacteremia is treated with parenteral antibiotics. In 25% of the cases, the line can be sterilized with antibiotics, but catheter removal is needed in most cases. Other complications related to placement include pneumothorax, hemothorax, hemomediastinum, subclavian vein or SVC perforation, right atrial thrombus, air embolism, and exit-site hematoma. Collectively, these complications account for 3% of cases.

An autogenous AV fistula remains the best form of hemodialysis access. The Brescia-Cimino fistula, a direct anastomosis between the radial artery and usually the cephalic vein, was described in 1966. Before undertaking fistula formation, the Allen test is performed to determine the adequacy of ulnar blood supply to the hand, which will be the sole supplier of blood flow to the hand postprocedure. Patency of the cephalic vein is determined by gentle percussion of the vein at the wrist and looking for transmitted pressure at the antecubital fossa. Duplex scanning, angiography, and or sequential pressures are useful adjuncts to the physical examination. The subclavian vein should also be studied for patency. An occult subclavian stenosis can manifest itself with venous hypertension during dialysis. In patients with a history of a previous dialysis catheter in the subclavian vein, a duplex should be performed. Side to side anastomosis is the easiest to construct and has the highest flow, although a higher risk of venous hypertension. A thrill should be heard, a transmitted pulse in the fistula indicates outflow obstruction or clotted fistula.

At least 3 weeks should be allowed before accessing the fistula to allow for resolution of edema, wound healing, dilation of the vein, and development of a hypertrophied muscular vein wall. If early venipuncture is performed, bleeding, hematoma, and false aneurysms are more likely to occur.

AV grafts are constructed in the case of either a failed Brescia-Cimino fistula or if the distal circulation is inadequate to perform a fistula. PTFE has emerged as the widely accepted conduit of choice given its availability, ease of handling, and comparatively low failure and complication rate. As described previously for fistula construction, preoperative imaging to determine patency of distal veins as well as the central venous system is recommended to ensure success. Distal radial artery to the cephalic or brachial vein is the ideal first choice. As peripheral sites are spent in the case of graft failure, more proximal configurations using the brachial artery can be employed.

Thrombosis is the most common complication of AV fistulas and grafts. Early thrombosis (less than 3 months) is greater in the Brescia-Cimino fistula compared to PTFE grafts; however, long-term patency is higher with the fistula. Early thrombosis is usually caused by technical errors. Late thrombosis of PTFE grafts is most often caused by stenosis of the venous anastomosis, whereas fistula thrombosis results from fibrosis and stenosis caused by repeated needle punctures. Diagnosis of a thrombosed graft is made by palpation of a strong pulse at the arterial limb. Doppler ultrasonography or angiography can confirm the diagnosis. Thrombectomy can be performed in cases of early thrombosis, but late thrombosis often requires revision of the graft. Thrombolysis and PTA are alternative approaches. Recanalization after thrombolysis can be followed by dilation of hemodynamically significant stenoses by PTA.

Infection is the second most common complication and occurs in approximately 10% of PTFE grafts. The most common pathogen is *Staphylococcus aureus*. Infections range from a localized cellulitis to abscess formation and bacteremia. Antibiotic therapy with gram-positive coverage should be instituted promptly. If the entire graft is involved or systemic infection sets in, the entire graft should be excised. A full course of antibiotic therapy must be completed prior to constructing a new graft.

Venous hypertension can arise from retrograde venous flow from venous arterialization. Edema of the arm causing pain and discoloration are often the presenting symptoms. Venography can detect potential venous stenoses requiring repair. If no stenoses are present, ligation of the arterialized venous tributary distal to the graft anastomosis can often relieve the venous hypertension.

Finally, arterial insufficiency or steal can result from excessive shunting of arterial blood through the low-pressure fistula, reversal of flow in the artery distal to the anastomosis, or inadequate arterial collateral flow. Patients often complain of pain, coldness, numbness, and occasionally decreased motor function of the fingers and hand. Digital and forearm blood pressures with plethysmography or Doppler can confirm the diagnosis. In many cases, removal of the fistula is the only solution. Ligation of the fistula can sometimes exacerbate ischemia. In cases of reversal of flow, revision of the fistula to create an end-to-side anastomosis by ligation of the radial artery distal to the fistula eliminates ischemia and preserves the fistula.

ACKNOWLEDGMENTS

Special thanks to previous edition chapter authors, David G. Neschis, MD and Michael A. Golden, MD.

KEY POINTS

▲ Endothelial cells modulate vascular tone, caliber, and blood flow with the secretion of the vasoactive mediator nitric oxide (NO). NO is generated by nitric oxide synthase (NOS) using L-arginine as the substrate.

▲ An ankle–brachial index (ABI) of greater than 1.0 is normal. Claudication is usually present with an ABI of between 0.5 and 0.84, whereas rest pain and/or tissue loss are usually present in the setting of an ABI of less than 0.5

▲ The mainstay of treatment for claudication is conservative therapy with elimination of risk factors and exercise. Critical limb ischemia with rest pain and/or tissue loss mandates intervention.

▲ Endovascular intervention, or percutaneous transluminal angioplasty (PTA), for claudication and critical limb ischemia is best reserved for focal stenotic lesions (less than 3 cm) in the aortoiliac system and femoral popliteal system. Although stenting, in addition to PTA, is approved for use in the iliac system, there is no clear benefit to stenting of infrainguinal lesions.

▲ Acute limb ischemia with a viable limb is treated via thrombolysis.

▲ Autologous vein graft has a higher patency by far for femoral-distal bypass than polytetrafluoroethylene (PTFE). PTFE should be avoided in femoral-distal bypasses.

▲ Major limitation to abdominal aortic aneurysm (AAA) stent graft repair is neck anatomy, with necks less than 15 mm and greater than 26 mm in diameter being prohibitive.

▲ For asymptomatic patients with an operative risk of less than 3%, carotid endarterectomy is indicated for lesions greater than 60%. For symptomatic patients [previous ipsilateral stroke or transient ischemic attack (TIA)], carotid endarterectomy is indicated for lesions greater than 70%.

▲ Treatment of a subclavian vein thrombosis is **thrombolysis** followed by first rib resection.

▲ The most common cause of lymphedema worldwide is filiaris. The most common cause of lymphedema in North America and Europe is malignancy.

▲ The Brescia-Cimino fistula, a direct anastomosis between the radial artery and usually the cephalic vein remains the best option for hemodialysis access.

SUGGESTED READINGS

Ernst CB, Stanley JC. *Current therapy in vascular surgery,* 4th ed. St. Louis: Mosby, 2001.

Geroulakos G, Van Urk H, Hobson RW, et al. *Vascular surgery: cases, questions, and commentaries.* New York: Springer-Verlag, 2003.

Moore WS. *Vascular surgery: a comprehensive review,* 6th ed. Philadelphia: WB Saunders, 2001.

Ouriel K, Rutherford RB. *Atlas of vascular surgery: operative procedures,* 1st ed. Philadelphia: WB Saunders, 1998.

Rutherford RB, ed. *Vascular surgery,* 5th ed. Philadelphia: WB Saunders, 2000.

Pulmonary Physiology

24

Bradley G. Leshnower   Joseph B. Shrager

Respiration is a process that is essential to human life. In humans, the main organ of the respiratory system is the lung, which serves as a gas exchange system that allows the transfer of atmospheric oxygen to the red blood cells and concomitantly disposes of carbon dioxide, the byproduct of aerobic metabolism. This highly efficient system has three components: ventilation, perfusion, and the blood–gas interface. Atmospheric oxygen reaches the alveoli by a process referred to as *ventilation; gas exchange* occurs at the alveolar–pulmonary capillary membrane, known as the *blood–gas interface; perfusion* describes the process whereby blood reaches the blood–gas interface. A defect in any of these three components will affect the system as a whole and may result in respiratory failure. Therefore, it is essential that the surgeon understands the physiology behind each component in order to effectively treat pathophysiology of the respiratory system. This chapter discusses the physiology of air movement, pulmonary blood flow, and the blood–gas interface, as well as describes derangements in respiratory physiology that result in hypoxemia and/or hypoventilation. In addition, the treatment of respiratory failure with mechanical support will be reviewed.

AIR MOVEMENT

Airways

Air enters the upper airways (pharynx and larynx) through the mouth and nose and then enters the tracheobronchial tree. The tracheobronchial tree is formed from successive divisions of hollow tubes, which progressively decrease in diameter with each division. Despite this progressive narrowing, the number and total cross-sectional area of the airways increase at each division. This design, which is also mimicked by the pulmonary vascular tree, creates a vast surface area for gas exchange. The trachea extends from C6 or C7 to T4 or T5 and connects the larynx to the right and left main *bronchi*. The right main bronchus gives rise to the upper lobar bronchus and the bronchus intermedius, which subsequently splits into the middle and lower lobar bronchi. On the left, the main bronchus bifurcates directly to give rise to the upper and lower bronchi. Segmental bronchi continue to divide until they reach the most distal airways, which are called the *terminal bronchioles*. These first 16 divisions of the airway tree, also known as the *conducting*

zone of the lung, are responsible only for gas transport. These airways, along with the pharynx, larynx, and trachea, constitute the *anatomic dead space* because gas exchange does not occur within them. Anatomic dead space volume in a normal upright human is approximately 150 mL. The *acinus* is the respiratory unit of the lung and consists of approximately the last seven divisions of the airway. The 17th to 19th generations consist of the respiratory bronchioles, from which the first alveoli emerge. This region is termed the *transitional zone* of the lung. Subsequent generations are lined with alveolar ducts and sacs and are known collectively as the *respiratory zone* whose primary function is gas exchange (Fig. 24-1).

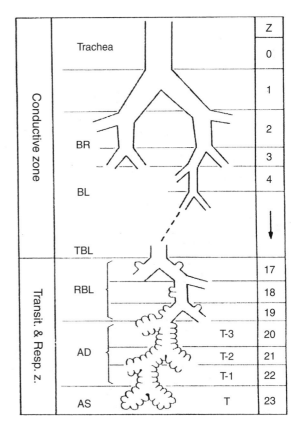

Figure 24-1 Lung zones. BR, bronchi; BL, bronchioles; TBL, terminal bronchioles; RBL, respiratory bronchioles; AD, alveolar ducts; AS, alveolar sacs. (From Weibel ER. *Morphometry of the human lung.* Berlin: Springer-Verlag, 1963:111, with permission.)

The conducting airways distal to the pharynx to the level of the terminal bronchioles are lined with ciliated epithelium interspersed with mucus-secreting goblet cells (Fig. 24-2). The cilia and mucus are involved in the clearance of inhaled or aspirated particles. The mucociliary escalator carries particles in the tracheobronchial tree to the pharynx, where they are either swallowed or expectorated. Smokers demonstrate abnormalities in both mucous production and ciliary motility that contribute to their difficulties with secretion clearance. In addition, some smokers will develop frank metaplasia of the tracheobronchial epithelium to nonciliated squamous epithelium, further compromising secretion clearance mechanisms. Following pulmonary surgery, there is transient dysfunction of the mucociliary escalator, which predisposes this population of patients to postoperative atelectasis and/or pneumonia.

The structure and function of the bronchi and bronchioles are closely related and differ at various levels of the tracheobronchial tree. The trachea and first three generations of the conducting zone contain cartilage as part of their structure. The anatomy of the trachea, with its C-shaped cartilaginous rings anterolaterally, prevents airway collapse when significant intrathoracic pressure is generated such as during forced expiration. The amount of cartilage in the airways decreases as the conducting zone transitions into the respiratory zone, where the presence of cartilage would hinder gas exchange. Cartilaginous plates support the bronchi, whereas bronchioles and alveoli are completely devoid of cartilage. Consequently, the lack of support renders the smaller distal airways more susceptible to collapse. This occurs in emphysema in which increased extraluminal pressure generated during exhalation causes dynamic airway narrowing and subsequent "air trapping" in the small distal airways. This phenomenon contributes to the characteristic "hyperinflated" lungs associated with this disease.

Chest Wall and Respiratory Muscles

The active and passive aspects of breathing involve a close interaction among the mechanics of the lung, the chest wall, and the muscles of respiration. Air movement results from the establishment of a pressure gradient between the atmosphere and the thoracic cavity. In order to generate a pressure gradient, the chest wall must be intact. During inspiration, the *diaphragm* contracts and descends, whereas other inspiratory muscles move the ribs and sternum outward. This downward and outward expansion of the rib cage increases thoracic cavity volume, thereby adding to the negative intrathoracic pressure generated by diaphragmatic contracton. Air flows down the pressure gradient to inflate the lungs. During expiration the diaphragm relaxes and elevates and the rib cage moves inward; therefore, thoracic cavity volume decreases and the lungs deflate.

The diaphragm alone can provide adequate ventilation during normal, quiet breathing. It is when larger volumes of air movement are required, such as during exercise, that the *external intercostal* muscles assist the diaphragm during inspiration by pulling the rib cage upward and outward. Other *accessory muscles* of respiration (the scalenes and the

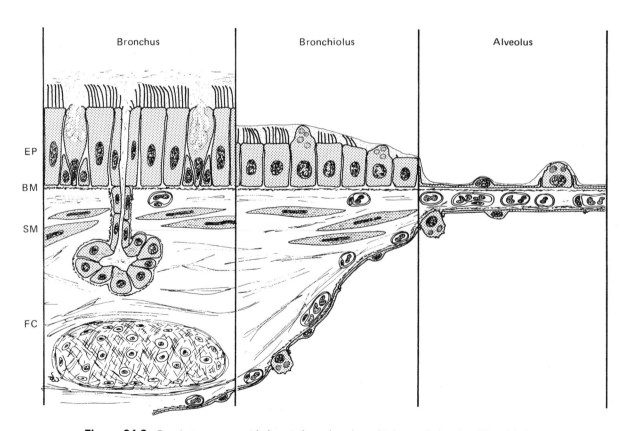

Figure 24-2 Respiratory tract epithelium in bronchus, bronchiolus, and alveolus. EP, epithelium; BM, basement membrane; SM, smooth muscle; FC, fibrocartilage. (From Weibel ER, Taylor CR. Design and structure of the human lung. In: Fishman AP, ed. *Pulmonary diseases and disorders*, Vol 1., 2nd ed. New York: McGraw-Hill, 1988:14, with permission.)

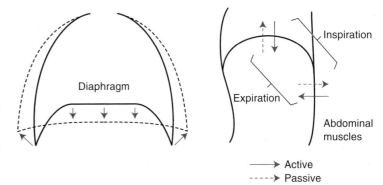

Figure 24-3 On inspiration, the dome-shaped diaphragm contracts, the abdominal contents are forced down and forward, and the rib cage is widened. Both increase the volume of the thorax. On forced expiration, the abdominal muscles contract and push the diaphragm up. (From West JB. *Respiratory physiology: the essentials*, 7th ed. Philadelphia: Lippincott Williams & Wilkins, 2005, with permission.)

sternocleiodomastoids) in the neck are also active during forced inspiration, moving the rib cage and sternum upward and outward to further increase thoracic cavity volume. Forced expiration recruits the *internal intercostal* muscles to pull the rib cage downward and inward, and the *abdominal wall muscles* may also be activated to push the diaphragm upward into the chest (see Fig 24-3). In this manner the chest wall and muscles of respiration adapt and coordinate changes in thoracic cavity volume to meet the constantly fluctuating ventilatory requirements of the human body.

Mechanics of Ventilation

The mechanics of breathing are based upon a balance between the opposing outwardly directed forces of the chest wall and the inwardly directed recoil forces of the lung. The lung and chest wall both possess elastic properties, giving them the capability to stretch and recoil. The rigidity of the ribs and cartilage of the chest wall are responsible for its inherent outward elastic force. This is opposed by a resting inward elastic recoil force generated by the elastin and collagen fibers embedded in the alveolar septal interstitium. Elastin can stretch to 130% of its length while retaining its elasticity, whereas collagen fibers resist stretch and thus limit lung expansion at high volumes. Elasticity is essential to lung function and is the factor that makes exhalation a passive event. At end inspiration, recoil forces generated within distended alveoli increase alveolar pressure, thereby creating a pressure gradient that results in passive air movement out of the lung when the diaphragm and chest wall muscles relax. Loss of this fibroelastic tissue, as in emphysema, leads to a reduction of the inward recoil force and subsequent hyperexpansion of lung tissue. The relationship of the two opposing forces of the lung and chest wall is best illustrated when their equilibrium is disrupted, as in the case of pneumothorax. In this situation, the loss of negative intrathoracic pressure caused by air in the thorax abolishes the outward pull of the chest wall on the lung. The inward recoil forces of the alveoli, now unopposed, cause the lung to collapse; similarly, the chest wall, unopposed by the inward elastic force of the lung, expands outward (Fig. 24-4).

At all times during the respiratory cycle, air movement is goverened by pressure gradients. At end expiration, the alveolar and atmospheric pressures are equal; there is no pressure gradient and thus no air movement. This point on the flow–volume loop is defined as the functional residual capacity (FRC). At FRC the outward recoil force of the chest wall and the inward recoil force of the lung are in equilibrium, and the average pleural pressure is −5 cm H₂O. As the diaphragm contracts to initiate inspiration, the thoracic cavity volume increases, thereby resulting in a decrease in intrathoracic pressure. The alveoli, in conjunction with Boyle's law ($P_1V_1 = P_2V_2$), expand and alveolar pressure drops. This establishes a pressure gradient between the atmospheric and alveolar pressures and air inflates the lung. End inspiration is achieved when the summed force of the elastic recoil of the inflated lung and expanded chest wall equal the force generated by the inspiratory muscle contraction. At this point, alveolar and atmospheric pressures are again equal and there is no air flow. Expiration is a passive process during quiet breathing. Relaxation of the inspiratory muscles causes a decrease in thoracic cavity volume, and the elastic recoil of the lungs results in a decreased alveolar volume and positive intraalveolar pressures. Again, a pressure gradient is established and the lung deflates until alveolar and atmospheric pressures equalize and FRC is achieved.

The *compliance* of the lungs (defined as the change in volume for a given change in pressure) is a measurement of the resistance of the lungs to expansion. It is clinically significant because a lung with decreased compliance requires the development of a larger pressure gradient to achieve the same tidal volumes. Therefore, patients with decreased lung compliance have an increased work of breathing. Diseases that affect lung parenchyma (e.g., pulmonary fibrosis and sarcoidoisis) or any condition that causes lung consolidation (e.g., pneumonia and atelectasis) reduce compliance and result in "stiff" lungs. In contrast, patients with emphysema experience destruction of

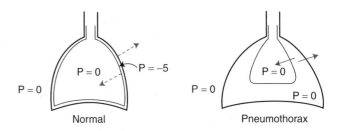

Figure 24-4 The tendency of the lung to recoil to its deflated volume is balanced by the tendency of the chest cage to bow out. As a result, the intrapleural pressure is subatmospheric. Pneumothorax allows the lung to collapse and the thorax to spring out. (From West JB. *Respiratory physiology: the essentials*, 7th ed. Philadelphia: Lippincott Williams & Wilkins, 2005, with permission.)

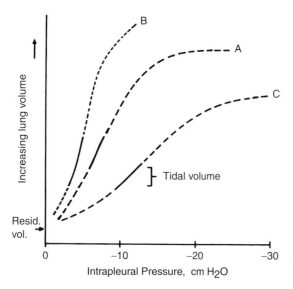

Figure 24-5 Compliance (change in volume divided by change in pressure) in **(A)** normal individuals, **(B)** patients with emphysema, and **(C)** patients with pulmonary fibrosis. (From Shields. *General thoracic surgery*, 3rd ed. Philadelphia: Lea & Febiger, 1989:111, with permission.)

elastic alveolar tissue, which would normally oppose lung expansion. This results in lungs that have increased compliance (Fig. 24-5). These patients have increased work of breathing for different reasons: alterations in lung volumes resulting in respiratory muscles that are forced to operate at a disadvantage and increased expiratory resistance.

An important component of lung compliance is the body's means of reducing surface tension in the alveoli. The alveolar membrane is moist and acts as a large air–water interface. Water molecules have a strong attraction to one other and, therefore, inward forces are generated that tend to reduce alveolar surface area. If these inward forces were unopposed, the resulting surface tension would cause alveolar collapse. However, type II alveolar cells produce *surfactant*, a dipalmitoyl phosphatidylcholine, which reduces alveolar surface tension and prevents alveolar collapse. This decrease in surface tension also helps equalize pressures within alveoli of differing sizes that would have otherwise resulted in the emptying of smaller alveoli into larger ones and subsequent collapse of smaller alveoli. In normal individuals, surfactant has the beneficial effect of reducing the lung's elastic recoil forces, which increases lung compliance and ultimately decreases the work of breathing. An example of a pathologic state in which surfactant is reduced is adult respiratory distress syndrome (ARDS). The loss of surfactant contributes to the "stiff" lungs that are characteristic of this disease.

Lung Volumes and Pulmonary Function Tests

The information provided by lung volumes and pulmonary function tests can aid in the diagnosis of pulmonary disease and give valuable preoperative information about surgical patients, particularly those undergoing pulmonary resection. The three different methods that are used to measure static lung volumes are spirometery, helium dilution, and body plethysmography. *Spirometry* can measure tidal

volume (VT), vital capacity (VC), inspiratory reserve volume (IRV) and expiratory reserve volume (ERV). VT is the volume of air inspired or expired during normal breathing, and is approximately 500 mL in the average adult. VC is the amount of air that can be expelled from the lungs during a maximal forced expiration following a maximal forced inspiration. IRV is the additional volume of gas that is inhaled during a maximal forced inspiration measured from the end of an inhaled VT. Correspondingly, ERV is the additional volume expelled from the lung during a maximal forced expiration measured from the end of an exhaled tidal volume. From these measurements, inspiratory capacity (IC) can be calculated (IC = VC − ERV).

As mentioned previously, FRC is the volume of air remaining in the lungs after exhalation during normal breathing. FRC is the sum of ERV and residual volume (RV). RV is the volume of gas in the lungs after a maximal forced expiration, but cannot be measured by spirometry and requires for measurement the use of either helium dilution or body plethysmography methods. Once RV is measured, FRC and total lung capacity (TLC), which is the volume of air in the lungs following maximal inspiration (5 to 6 L in the average adult) can be calculated (Fig. 24-6).

In addition to the measurement of static lung volumes, *pulmonary function tests* (PFTs) can measure dynamic characteristics of the lungs, which can be quantified and compared to predicted normal values as a measure of pathologic states. The measurements taken from these tests are based on flow–volume curves. One of the most important of these tests is the forced expiratory volume (FEV), often expressed as "FEV_1," which is the maximum volume of gas exhaled in one second. The relationship between FEV_1 and forced vital capacity (FVC) can define normal, restrictive, or obstructive patterns. In both restrictive and obstructive lung disease, the FEV_1 and FVC are reduced; however, in obstructive disease, the FEV_1/FVC ratio is markedly reduced (less than 70%) in contrast to restrictive disease states, where the ratio may be normal or increased. FEF of 25% to 75% (forced midexpiratory flow) is another test that gives evidence of obstructive airway disease. This measurement is defined by the slope (volume versus time) of the line between the points at 25% and 75% on the

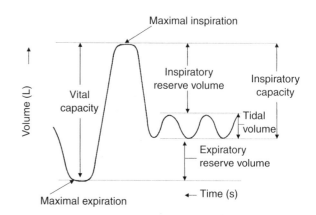

Figure 24-6 Determination of the tidal volume, vital capacity, inspiratory capacity, inspiratory reserve volume, and expiratory reserve volume from a spirometer. (From Levitzky MG. *Pulmonary physiology*, 3rd ed. New York: McGraw-Hill, 1991:57, with permission.)

expiratory curve. To perform these flow measurements, the patient is asked to inspire maximally to TLC, and then with maximal forced expiratory effort, air is blown out of the lungs to RV. With use of a spirometer, one can measure air volumes as a function of time, and FEV_1, FVC, FEF of 25% to 75% and other volumes can be determined.

PFTs are used selectively in the preoperative evaluation of the general surgical patient and routinely in the preoperative evaluation of patients undergoing lung resection. Any elective surgical patient with a history of chronic obstructive pulmonary disease (COPD) or symptoms of respiratory insufficiency should undergo pulmonary function testing several weeks prior to major surgery. This allows time for intervention (bronchodilators, antibiotics, and pulmonary rehabilitation, among others) and the chance to improve pulmonary function preoperatively. Furthermore, general surgery patients with COPD have an increased risk of pulmonary complications postoperatively and so their pulmonary toilet must be managed aggressively. In patients undergoing lung resection, several criteria have been identified as indicators of increased risk: FVC less than 2 L or 50% predicted , FEV_1/FVC less than 50%, and a diffusion capacity for carbon monoxide less than 50% of predicted. In addition, PFTs can help define the amount of lung that may be resected with a low likelihood of postoperative respiratory insufficiency. In general, pulmonary resection can be tolerated if the postoperative FEV_1 is anticipated to be greater than 800 mL per second. Patients who have an FEV_1 measurement greater than 2 L per second can usually tolerate most pulmonary resections, including pneumonectomy. Quantitative perfusion studies can complement the preoperative PFTs in those patients with FEV_1 measurements less than 2 L per second and can be used to predict postresection lung function. The test can determine how much of the area of planned resection contributes to overall lung function, and, therefore, postoperative lung function can be predicted by subtracting that quantity from initial baseline values.

Despite these guidelines, it must be noted that many of our previous concepts of adequacy of pulmonary reserve for emphysema patients undergoing pulmonary resection have been revised according to experience derived from lung volume reduction surgery (LVRS). The rationale behind LVRS is that removal of a portion of the most diseased lung in emphysema improves pulmonary function by decreasing FRC and RV, and, therefore, (i) restores the diaphragm to its natural position, which improves its function, and (ii) improves the elastic recoil of the lung. On the basis of this new concept, if one removes a lung cancer in an emphysematous lobe, that patient's pulmonary function may actually improve. If valid, this concept renders any predictions of postoperative morbidity and mortality according to preoperative pulmonary function unreliable in this population.

PULMONARY VASCULATURE

The lung has a *dual vascular supply*: the bronchial circulation and the pulmonary circulation. The *bronchial circulation* arises from branches off the descending aorta to supply the first 17 generations of the airway tree (conducting zone) and drains into the pulmonary veins. The *pulmonary circulation* brings mixed venous blood from the right ventricle into close contact with the respiratory zone of the lung so that gas exchange may occur. This is a unique circulatory system that is physiologically different than the systemic circulation and will be the focus of the following discussion.

The main pulmonary trunk divides into the right and left main pulmonary arteries, which subsequently branch into the lobar, segmental, and subsegmental branches. The arteries continue to divide in a manner similar to but more extensive than that of the airways, and they progressively narrow in caliber, moving from artery to arteriole until finally the capillary level is reached. The capillary network is an extensive plexus of vessels that completely envelops the alveoli and functions as a continuous sheet of blood. This design produces a large surface area so that the red blood cell may pass by many alveoli during its transit through the pulmonary microcirculation, thereby ensuring adequate gas exchange. Blood returns from the capillary network to the left atrium through the pulmonary venous system, which lacks valves and converges into distinct superior and inferior pulmonary veins bilaterally.

It is important to realize that the pulmonary circulation is a low pressure, low resistance system. Pulmonary arterial vessels contain less elastin and less smooth muscle, and they have thinner walls than systemic arteries; consequently, pulmonary vascular resistance is much less than systemic vascular resistance, and normal pulmonary arterial pressures (15 to 30/6 to 12 mm Hg) are approximately one fifth of their systemic counterparts. During exercise, when cardiac output increases, the pulmonary circulation maintains lower pressures by two mechanisms: *capillary recruitment* and *distension*. As blood flow increases, pressure rises and opens capillaries that are normally closed during low-flow states. *Capillary distension* occurs because the thin-walled capllaries are highly compliant and are able to distend in response to increased flow, which also helps to maintain lower pressures. The importance of maintaining low pulmonary capillary pressures is realized in the case of pulmonary edema, when high capillary pressures lead to leaky capillaries and impaired gas exchange.

In the upright human, blood flow is not uniformly distributed because gravity and alveolar pressures affect perfusion differently in different regions of the lung. Classically, the lung has been divided into three zones on the basis of the relationships among alveolar pressure (P_A), pulmonary arterial pressure (Pa), and pulmonary venous pressure (Pv), as affected by gravity (Fig. 24-7). Zone 1 conditions ($P_A > Pa > Pv$) occur at the theoretical apex of the lung. There is no blood flow in this region because alveolar pressures exceed pulmonary arterial pressures. Because this area therefore contains alveoli, which are ventilated but not perfused, it is considered *alveolar dead space*. Normally, zone 1 conditions do not exist; however, in situations where pulmonary arterial pressures are low (e.g., hypovolemia) or when alveolar pressures are elevated [e.g., mechanical ventialtion with positive end-expiratory pressure (PEEP)], this physiology may be present. Zone 3 conditions ($Pa > Pv > P_A$) are present at the theoretical base of the lung. The driving pressure for flow in this zone is the difference between the pulmonary arterial and venous pressures. Zone 2 conditions ($Pa > P_A > Pv$) prevail in the middle of the lung. The driving pressure for flow in this zone is the difference between the pulmonary arterial and

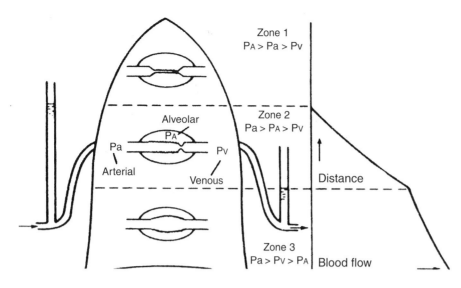

Figure 24-7 Lung zones. (From West JB. *Respiratory physiology: the essentials*, 4th ed. Baltimore: Williams & Wilkins, 1990, with permission.)

alveolar pressures. These zones do not have specific anatomic boundaries but are dependent upon the physiologic conditions of the individual at a given point in time. For example, regional differences in perfusion diminish during exercise. Exercise causes an increase in cardiac output and pulmonary artery pressures. Elevated pulmonary ateriolar pressures result in the opening of previously collapsed capillaries in zones 1 and 2, and thereby provide a more uniform distribution of blood flow when compared to the perfusion pattern of the lungs at rest (Fig. 24-7).

The relationship between ventilation (V) and perfusion (Q) determines PaO_2 and $PaCO_2$. Ideally alveolar ventilation and perfusion should allow for complete hemoglobin saturation and removal of sufficient carbon dioxide to result in a normal arterial pH level. However, this does not occur uniformly within the lung because, as described previously, V/Q mismatches occur in different regions of the lung. Apical regions have decreased perfusion in relation to ventilation (high V/Q ratio), whereas basilar regions have increased perfusion in relation to ventilation (low V/Q ratio) (Fig. 24-8). The extremes of V/Q mismatching are *alveolar dead space* (lung that is ventilated but not perfused) and *pure shunt* (lung that is perfused but not ventilated). Both of these

extremes lead to hypoxemia (low PaO_2). The pulmonary circulation has the capacity to recognize hypoxia (low PaO_2) and autoregulate to optimize the V/Q relationship. Pulmonary arterioles, which are dilated under normal conditions, have the unique ability to vasoconstrict in conditions of hypoxia, hypoxemia, and/or hypercarbia. This process, known as *hypoxic pulmonary vasoconstriction*, results in the redistribution of blood flow from regions that undergo minimal gas exchange (low V/Q ratio) to regions that are better ventilated (improved V/Q matching). In patients with COPD, who have chronic hypoxia, this autoregulatory process can become pathologic over time; prolonged pulmonary arteriolar vasoconstriction causes vascular smooth muscle cell hypertrophy and subsequent narrowing of the arteriolar lumen, thereby resulting in pulmonary hypertension. The ventilatory status of patients with pulmonary hypertension undergoing an operation must be monitored closely because acute episodes of hypoxia or hypercarbia may exacerbate already elevated pulmonary artery pressures and cause a pulmonary hypertensive crisis.

Although the pulmonary circulation's primary function is to deliver blood to the alveolar–capillary membrane for gas exchange, it also serves the body by acting both as a filter and a metabolic organ. Surgical patients are at an increased risk for developing pulmonary emboli. Pulmonary emboli occur when blood clots, or air or fat globules, gain access to the systemic venous circulation. These emboli have the potential to cause obstruction of vital systemic arteries (e.g., coronary, cerebral, and renal arteries) if they gain access to the systemic arterial circulation. The large network of pulmonary arteries and capillaries protect the sytemic circulation from obstruction by trapping these emboli. Small- to moderate-sized air emboli are gradually absorbed, whereas small blood clots can be dissolved by fibrinolytic substances released from pulmonary endothelial cells. Many of the pulmonary emboli are, therefore, relatively benign; however, a massive pulmonary embolus, or a large number of smaller emboli, can significantly affect gas exchange and hemodynamics, and result in death. The pulmonary vasculature is also involved in the metabolism of vasoactive hormones. Angiotension-converting enzyme (ACE) is located on the surface of pulmonary endothelial cells and converts angiotension I to angiotensin II.

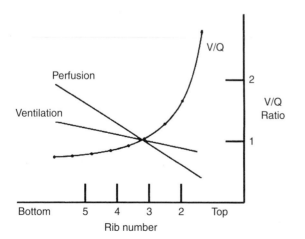

Figure 24-8 Distribution of ventilation and perfusion. (From West JB. *Ventilation blood flow and gas exchange*, 3rd ed. Oxford: Blackwell Science, 1977, with permission.)

Angiotensin II is a potent vasoconstrictor and affects salt regulation in the body by stimulating aldosterone release in the kidneys. The pulmonary endothelium affects different hormones in different ways. Some (vasopressin and epinephrine) flow through unaltered, whereas others (bradykinin and serotonin) are inactivated. By regulating vasoactive hormones, the pulmonary circulation provides an important contribution to the preservation of homeostasis.

GAS EXCHANGE

Gas exchange occurs at the alveolar level at the *interface of the alveolar epithelium and the capillary endothelium*. The alveoli are outpouchings of the respiratory bronchioles, alveolar ducts, and alveolar sacs. The alveolar septa are made up of a continuous flattened epithelium comprising type I and type II alveolar epithelial cells covering a thin layer of interstitial tissue (Fig. 24-9). Type I alveolar cells cover approximately 95% of the alveolar surface and are functionally involved in resorbing pathologic alveolar fluid or ingesting intraalveolar particulate material. The type II epithelial cells are the source of alveolar surfactant and are also involved in the renewal of the alveolar surface by differentiation into type I cells. A continuous basal lamina underlies both type I and type II cells and is in apposition to the underlying endothelial cell. The alveolar septal interstitium is also composed of a proteoglycan matrix that is embedded with elastin and collagen, which is responsible for the elastic properties of the lung as previously

discussed. Alveolar macrophages are important in clearance of intra-alveolar material, production of inflammatory mediators, and antigen presentation.

After oxygen is delivered to the alveoli, it diffuses through the alveolar–capillary interface. This enormous biologic membrane represents a convergence of the airway and vascular trees, and consists of approximately 500 million alveoli with a combined internal surface area of 100 m^2, each enveloped by a plexus of capillaries. This provides a surface area equivalent to the size of a tennis court over which gas exchange can occur. For oxygen to be delivered to the blood, it must first dissolve into the layer of pulmonary surfactant, thereby moving from the gas phase to the liquid phase. Once in the liquid phase, oxygen diffuses through the alveolar epithelium, intersitium, and capillary endothelium and into the plasma. Approximately 5% of oxygen remains dissolved in the plasma; the remainder enters the erythrocytes and binds to hemoglobin. The blood carries the oxygen out of the lung and delivers it to the tissues where it is used for energy production to drive metabolic processes.

Fick law of diffusion governs the flow of oxygen and carbon dioxide across the blood–gas interface. Fick law of diffusion states that that the volume of gas per minute diffusing across a membrane (V_{gas}) is directly proportional to the surface area (A), the diffusion coefficient of the gas (D), and the pressure gradient across the diffusion barrier ($P_1 - P_2$), and is inversely proportional to the thickness of the diffusion barrier (Table 24-1). Under normal conditions, P_{AO_2} is 100 mm Hg and P_{ACO_2} is 40 mm Hg. The mixed venous blood in the pulmonary arterial system has a P_{aO_2} of approximately 40 mm Hg and a P_{aCO_2} of approximately 45 mm Hg. Therefore, the gradients at the alveolar–capillary interface that drive diffusion are 60 mm Hg for oxygen to diffuse from the alveoli to the plasma and 5 mm Hg for carbon dioxide to diffuse from plasma to the alveoli. Because the alveolar–capillary membrane has such a large surface area and is extremely thin (0.2 to 0.5 μm), gas exchange occurs within about 0.25 seconds, which is

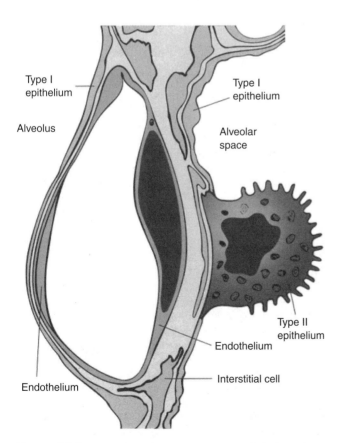

Figure 24-9 Alveolar septum. (Robbins RB. *Pathologic basis of disease*, 6th ed. Philadelphia: WB Saunders, 1999:698, with permission.)

TABLE 24-1	
IMPORTANT PULMONARY PHYSIOLOGY EQUATIONS	
Alveolar gas equation[a]	$P_{AO_2} = P_{IO_2} - P_{ACO_2}/0.8 + F$
A-a gradient (Nrl 15–20 mm Hg)[b]	$P(A-a)_{O_2} = P_{AO_2} - P_{aO_2}$
Shunt equation[c]	$Q_s/Q_T = C_{CO_2} - C_{aO_2}/C_{CO_2} - C_{vO_2}$
Pulmonary vascular resistance[d]	$PVR = PA_m - LA_m/CO$
Fick law of diffusion[e]	$V_{gas} = A \times D \times (P_1 - P_2)/T$

[a] P_{AO_2}, alveolar partial pressure of oxygen; P_{IO_2}, partial pressure of oxygen in inspired air; P_{ACO_2}, alveolar CO_2 = arterial CO_2; F, correction factor (ignored).
[b] P_{AO_2}, alveolar partial pressure of oxygen; P_{aO_2}, arterial partial pressure of oxygen.
[c] Q_s/Q_T, shunt; C_{CO_2}, content of capillary oxygen; C_{aO_2}, content of arterial oxygen; C_{vO_2}, content of venous oxygen.
[d] PA_m, mean pulmonary artery pressure; LA_m, mean left atrial pressure; CO, cardiac output.
[e] A, area available for diffusion; D, diffusion coefficient; $P_1 - P_2$, pressure gradient of the gas across the diffusion barrier; T, thickness of the barrier.

approximately one third of the time required for the blood to transit the pulmonary capillary. Pathologic states such as interstitial edema [e.g., congestive heart failure (CHF)] and fibrosis (e.g., idiopathic pulmonary fibrosis) cause thickening of the diffusion barrier and impair gas exchange. The *diffusing capacity* of the lung is a valuable measurement that can assist in the diagnosis and treatment of pulmonary diseases. It is technically difficult to measure the lung's diffusing capacity using oxygen, so carbon monoxide is used (DL_{CO}). The DL_{CO} can be determined by dividing the uptake of carbon monoxide by its arterial partial pressure by using the single breath technique in the pulmonary function laboratory. Some authors have found that a low DL_{CO} is as important a prognostic indicator of risk following pulmonary resection as a low FEV_1. Certainly patients with a DL_{CO} less than 50% of predicted are at a significantly increased risk following pulmonary resection and those with a DL_{CO} less than 20% of predicted are a prohibitive risk.

Hypoxemia

Gas exchange is best understood by examining the factors that cause *hypoxemia*, which is defined by an arterial Po_2 less than 85 mm Hg. Normally, the Pao_2 is approximately 100 mm Hg. When oxygen diffuses across the capillary–alveolar interface, it completely saturates hemoglobin in the erythrocyte and the Pao_2 becomes equal to the partial pressure of oxygen in the in the capillary. However, by the time the blood enters the left atrium, the Po_2 has dropped to an 85 to 95 mm Hg, resulting in an A–a gradient of 10 to 15 mm Hg. The *A–a gradient* exists in normal individuals primarily because of normal regional V/Q mismatching (physiologic dead space and shunting), and anatomic shunting when the bronchial venous circulation joins the venous admixture in the pulmonary veins. The five main causes of hypoxemia are listed in Table 24-2. When confronted with a patient with a low arterial Po_2, determining the the A–a gradient is very useful in diagnosing and treating the underlying cause of hypoxemia.

Surgical patients are prone to develop hypoxemia from a reduction in alveolar ventilation. This usually occurs during the postoperative period after patients have been extubated but the effects of general anesthesia persist, or their ability to breathe is limited by pain. *Hypoventilation* has numerous causes; the most common ones seen in the surgical population are (i) respiratory depression secondary to general anesthesia or pain medications (especially opiates, narcotics, and benzodiazepines); (ii) respiratory muscle dysfunction secondary to paralytic medications or phrenic nerve injuries; (iii) splinting, especially in patients postthoracotomy; (iv) traumatic injuries to the thorax impairing chest wall mechanics, such as a flail chest; and (v) upper airway obstruction from tumor invasion. Unfortunately hypoxemia is usually not the major concern in the case of hypoventilation. Arterial partial pressure of carbon dioxide is inversely related to the volume of alveolar ventilation; halving alveolar ventilation results in a doubling of arterial partial pressure of carbon dioxide. Consequently, hypercarbia is a key diagnostic feature of hypoventilation. Often these patients are treated only with oxygen, which resolves their hypoxemia but fails to correct the hypercarbia. This may lead to respiratory acidosis and further depression of the respiratory centers in the brainstem, which ultimately requires intubation and mechanical ventilation.

Hypoxemia may also be caused by an increased diffusion gradient. Normally the red blood cell has fully equilibrated with alveolar oxygen after about one third of its transit time through the capillary. However, any condition that compromises the alveolar–capillary interface may affect the diffusing capacity of the lung and cause hypoxemia. This type of pathology occurs in parenchymal lung diseases such as sarcoidosis and idiopathic pulmonary fibrosis, but can also be caused by the presence of interstitial edema secondary to CHF. In these states, the red blood cell is unable to equilibrate with alveolar oxygen because of an underlying *diffusion impairment*. According to Fick law, the diffusion rate of oxygen is signicantly reduced because of an increased thickness or decreased permeability of the blood-gas membrane (Table 24-1). At rest, these patients may not have hypoxemia because they have time in reserve and are able to equilibrate over the course of 0.75 seconds. However, Pao_2 will drop in these patients with exertion, as the increased cardiac output causes the erythrocyte to transit through the capillary bed in a shorter time. The elimination of carbon dioxide is less severely affected in patients with impaired diffusion, and increasing Pao_2 with 100% fraction of inspired oxygen, Fio_2, will usually correct the hypoxemia.

Ventilation/perfusion (V/Q) mismatch is the most common cause of hypoxemia. As discussed previously, at the extreme ends of V/Q mismatching are *physiologic dead space* (lung that is ventilated but not perfused) and *shunt* (lung that is perfused but not ventilated). Physiologic dead space does not usually result in hypoxemia, but a large shunt can cause severe hypoxemia and overt cyanosis. Intrapulmonary shunts can be arteriovenous fistulas, but usually consist of regions of consolidated lung secondary to pneumonia or atelectasis, which are bypassed when the pulmonary circulation autoregulates. The majority of extrapulmonary shunts are intracardiac congenital defects in which blood flows from the right heart to to the left heart without passing through the lungs via atrial or ventricular septal defects. Shunts are relatively easy to diagnose as the cause of hypoxemia; this is the only cause of hypoxemia that does not improve with the administration of 100% oxygen. In patients with pulmonary disease, the lung will have alveoli with varying V/Q ratios, which lie somewhere between the two ends of the spectrum of V/Q inequality, and can be considered "partial shunting." The hyperventilatory response to hypoxia, which results from chemoreceptors at the carotid bifurcation and below the aortic arch, is more effective in correcting hypercarbia than hypoxia. Therefore, the net result of V/Q mismatch is often hypoxemia and hyperventilation. V/Q mismatching is the mechanism of hypoxemia for most forms of COPD and is generally diagnosed by excluding all of the other etiologies.

TABLE 24-2
CAUSES OF HYPOXIA

Ventilation-perfusion mismatch
Shunt
Decreased alveolar Pao_2
Hypoventilation
Increased diffusion gradient

ASSISTED VENTILATION

The normal mechanics of breathing in an individual with an intact respiratory pump occurs by *negative pressure ventilation*. Augmenting ventilation requires the initiation of *positive pressure ventilation* by either a face mask (noninvasive) or intubation of the trachea (invasive). Most patients undergoing major surgery receive positive pressure ventilation during the operation, and they may require ventilatory assistance postoperatively. Therefore, it is important for the surgeon to understand when a patient requires ventilatory assistance, the different modes of ventilation available, and the principles of weaning a patient from mechanical ventilation.

Noninvasive Assisted Ventilation

For patients who are breathing spontaneously but who are hypoventilating, noninvasive positive pressure ventilation can often correct the hypercarbia and prevent the need for intubation. CPAP (continuous positive airway pressure) and BiPAP (bilevel positive airway pressure) are two modes of ventilation that can be delivered via a tightly fitting face mask that covers the nose and mouth. CPAP delivers positive pressure to the airways continuously throughout the respiratory cycle. This ventilatory mode (also used with invasive ventilatory support) decreases the overall work of breathing by recruiting previously unventilated, atelectatic alveoli, increasing FRC, and enhancing overall lung compliance. The use of CPAP is beneficial to patients who have restrictive and neuromuscular lung diseases, and it has been shown to reduce the need for intubation when compared to conventional therapy in patients with acute exacerbations of COPD. CPAP is also commonly used in the treatment of obstructive sleep apnea, where positive pressure provides the necessary support to maintain airway patency against the compressive forces of the collapsing pharynx. BiPAP delivers a set volume of positive pressure air with inhalation while maintaning a separate amount of PEEP during exhalation. This mode is most beneficial to hypoventilating patients with hyperinflated lungs as in emphysema. It is also used in obstructive sleep apnea when patients cannot tolerate CPAP. By preserving the natural airway and competence of the glottis, noninvasive ventilatory assistance preserves important physiologic functions such as cough, speech, and oral alimentation, all of which are lost once the trachea is intubated.

Invasive Assisted Ventilation

Although a number of criteria have been proposed as guidelines, it should be emphasized that indications for the institution of mechanical ventilatory are subjective and require clinical judgement. Support may be indicated secondary to derangements in any component of the respiratory system: central nervous system (CNS), chest wall, airway, respiratory muscles, or alveoli. Patients with CNS depression secondary to narcotic overdose or closed head injury often require intubation for airway protection and respiratory support. Abnormalities of the chest wall such as a flail chest, open pneumothorax, or marked scoliosis may require mechanical support. Respiratory muscle fatigue is thought to play a role in respiratory failure requiring support in COPD. Intubation is often required in patients with facial trauma, anaphylaxis,

or atelectasis from endobronchial masses or foreign bodies. Respiratory failure due to alveolar dysfunction may be caused by a variety of causes including chronic lung disease, cardiogenic or noncardiogenic pulmonary edema, and extensive pneumonia. Mechanical support may be indicated in the setting of hypercarbia ($PaCO_2$ >45 mm Hg) or life threatening hypoxemia (PaO_2 <55 mm Hg) despite maximal noninvasive oxygen therapy. Others have suggested a respiratory rate greater than 35 as a criterion. However, the most common indication for intubation and mechanical ventilation is the decision by an experienced clinician that the patient's respiratory system is in jeopardy and requires support.

There are two main categories of ventilatory support: volume control and pressure control. Volume control ventilation delivers a preset volume of gas to the patient with each breath. The two most commonly used modes of volume control ventilation are *assist-control (AC)* and *intermittent mandatory volume (IMV)*. In the AC mode, the ventilator is triggered to deliver a preset volume of gas with each patient breath. As a safety against hypoventilation or apnea, a respiratory rate is also preset, thereby ensuring a sufficient minute volume is delivered to the patient. AC is considered maximal ventilatory support because ventilation is assisted with every breath. In IMV ventilation, the patient is allowed to breathe without assistance from the ventilator. In this mode, respiratory rate and tidal volume are set and delivered to the patient intermittently between spontaneous breaths. The main difference between the two modes is that in IMV, a patient-initiated breath does not trigger the ventilator. *Synchronized intermittent mandatory ventilation (SIMV)* is a variation of IMV, which synchronizes the ventilator with the patient so that delivered breaths are initiated only after the patient exhales completely. IMV ventilation allows a wide range of levels of ventilatory support, as the preset number of breaths can be titrated to provide maximal or minimal ventilation to the patient. Many feel that this is the mode of choice when weaning a patient from the ventilator.

The selection of ventilatory mode is often dependent upon the lung compliance. AC and IMV modes are very effective in supporting patients with compliant lungs. However in disease states that cause reduced compliance (e.g., ARDS), volume control venitilatory modes may cause parenchymal damage secondary to barotruama. When ventilating patients with "stiff" lungs, the ventilator must generate high airway pressures to deliver the preset volume of gas. One acute danger of elevated airway pressures is alveolar rupture and pneumothorax. There is also increasing evidence that more subtle barotrauma may occur that results in less dramatic, chronic parenchymal injury and failure to wean.

A more suitable ventilatory approach in these patients is the use of *pressure control ventilation* (PCV). In this mode, the peak inspiratory pressure rather than volume is preset, and tidal volumes vary depending on lung compliance. Respiratory rate is also preset, and gas flow in this mode is either time-cycled (preset inspiratory time) or flow-cycled (gas flow stops when the flow rate drops below a preset percentage of the initial flow rate). *Pressure support ventilation* (PSV) is a variation of the PC mode that requires a spontaneously breathing patient. In this mode, every patient breath triggers the ventilator to deliver a preset amount of positive pressure. Tidal volumes again depend on lung compliance. PSV is often combined with IMV or CPAP when attempting to wean patients from ventilatory support. This type of *mixed-mode* ventilation strategy allows patients to spontaneously breathe with just enough positive pressure support to overcome the airway resistance caused by the breathing circuit.

The main function of PEEP is to prevent alveolar collapse at end expiration. The addition of PEEP to any mode of ventilation can help decrease V/Q mismatch by increasing FRC and subsequently allow for a reduction in inspired oxygen. It is important to remember that a prolonged FiO_2 greater than 70% can result in oxygen toxicity and damage to the alveolar–capillary membrane.

The previously described general ventilatory principles and practices can be applied to the majority of lung diseases. The notable exception is *acute respiratory distress syndrome* (ARDS). The pathophysiology behind this disease is thought to be diffuse alveolar damage and increased capillary permeability, which results in consolidated, noncompliant lungs and hypoxemia. Three characterisitcs are usually present in the setting of ARDS: (i) diffuse bilateral infiltrates on chest x-ray; (2) P_aO_2/FiO_2 ratio greater than 300 mm Hg; (iii) no clinicial evidence of elevated left atrial pressure, or PCWP less than 18 mm Hg. Mechanical ventilation is virtually the only treatment of ARDS, and the recommended ventilatory strategy is unique to this disease. The goals of support are to correct the profound hypoxemia while minimizing barotrauma, alveolar distension, and oxygen toxicity. These goals are achieved by the use of low tidal volumes, high PEEP, and *permissive hypercapnea*. Permissive hypercapnea, also know as controlled hypoventilation, is a consequence of low tidal volumes that is accepted as long as oxygenation is sufficient. Hypercarbia is a stimulant for respiration, and high spontaneous or set respiratory rates are therefore common in these patients. The current general ventilatory recommendations are (i) tidal volumes of 6 cc per kg (normal 10 cc per kg); (ii) optimal use of PEEP, up to 22 cm H_2O, depending on the FiO_2; (iii) pleateau airway pressures less than 30 cm H_2O;

(iv) respiratory rate less than or equal to 35 breaths per minute. For patients with refractory hypoxemia, there are adjunct measures such as prone ventilation and extracorporeal membrane oxygenation (ECMO), which may prove beneficial, but these have failed to show a reduction in mortality.

The weaning of mechanical ventilation is as much trial and error as science. Weaning involves incremental decreases in ventilatory support, allowing the patient to gradually regain the ability to support his or her own minute ventilation. Usually patients on AC mode are switched to IMV mode as the initial step of the process. Progressive decreases in the respiratory rate in the IMV and PC modes require the patient to maintain adequate minute venitlation with more unsupported breaths. In PSV, the level of pressure support is slowly decreased until the patient is providing adequate minute ventilation with minimal support. Most weaning protocols converge into a final CPAP trial, with only enough pressure support (5 to 7 cm H_2O) to overcome the resistance of the breathing circuit. There are mulitple factors, especially in the chronically ill, which can affect a patient's ability to wean from the ventilator including: mental status, respiratory muscle atrophy, secretions, acute processes (e.g., CHF) which impair diffusion, overfeeding with carbohydrate-rich elemental diets that elevate the respiratory quotient greater than 1.0, and any process that would prevent optimal lung expansion (e.g., abdominal distension or pleural effusion). General objective criteria that support extubation include (i) PaO_2 greater than 65 mm Hg, P_aCO_2 less than 50 mm Hg with FiO_2 less than or equal to 40%; (ii) spontaneous tidal volume greater than 5 mL per kg or FVC greater than 10 mL per kg; (iii) negative inspiratory force (NIF) greater than or equal to -25 cm H_2O; and (iv) respiratory rate less than 25 per minute. Neurologic status is extremely important as patients must be able to protect their airways from both collapse and aspiration. The ultimate decision to extubate should be based on both the objective respiratory data and the overall clinical condition of the patient and requires mature judgement.

KEY POINTS

▲ Etiologies of Hypoxemia
Hypoventilation
V/Q Mismatch
Shunt
Diffusion gradient

▲ Widely Cited Criteria for Operative Risk for Pulmonary Resection
Postoperative predicted FEV_1:

>1 L = Little increased operative risk
<0.8 L = Increased risk of severe pulmonary complications
DL: >70% predicted = Little increased risk
<50% predicted = Increased risk
<20% predicted = Prohibitive risk
Mortality of Pneumonectomy: 5% to 10%
Mortality of Lobectomy: <2%

▲ Tension pneumothorax causes hypotension and possible sudden death by mediastinal shifting resulting in compression of the vena cava. This causes decreased venous return and thus decreased cardiac output.

▲ Definitions of Pulmonary Function Tests
V_T = The amount of air inspired or expired during normal breathing
FRC = The amount of air contained in the lungs after normal expiration
VC = The amount of air exhaled following maximal inspiration and forced expiration.
RV = The amount of air remaining in the lungs after maximal expiration
FEV_1 = The volume of air exhaled in one second with a maximum expiratory effort.

▲ Positive End-Expiratory Pressure (PEEP)
Physiologic effects
Increases FRC, PaO_2 and compliance
Increases V/Q ratio
Decreases shunting

Adverse effects
Decreases cardiac output
Pneumothorax secondary to barotrauma, uncommon if less than or equal to 20 cm H_2O

SUGGESTED READINGS

Artigas A, Bernard GR, Carlet J, et al. The American-European consensus conference on ARDS, part 2. Ventilatory, pharmacologic, supportive therapy, study design strategies, and issues related to recovery and remodeling. *Am J Respir Crit Care Med* 1998;157:1332.

Brochard L, Mancebo J, Wysocki MW, et al. Noninvasive ventilation for acute exacerbations of chronic obstructive pulmonary disease. *N Engl J Med* 1995;333:817.

Ginsberg RJ. Preoperative assessment of the thoracic surgical patient: a surgeon's viewpoint. In: Pearson FG, Deslauriers J, Ginsberg RJ et al., eds. *Thoracic surgery*. New York: Churchill Livingstone, 1995:29–36.

Shrager JB, Kaiser LR. Lung volume reduction surgery. In: *Current problems in surgery*, Vol. 37, No. 4. St. Louis: Mosby, 2000:253–320.

West JB. *Respiratory physiology—the essentials*, 4th ed. Baltimore: Williams & Wilkins, 1990.

West JB. *Pulmonary pathophysiology—the essentials*, 5th ed. Baltimore: Williams & Wilkins, 1998.

Thoracic Pathophysiology and Malignancy

25

Michael J. Wilderman   *Larry R. Kaiser*

Alterations in the mechanics of breathing or pulmonary physiology can cause significant and sometimes catastrophic effects. Surgeons must understand and be able to address and treat conditions that affect breathing and respiration or those that may have an influence on lung function.

BENIGN LUNG DISEASE

Pulmonary tuberculosis (TB) is the most common infectious cause of death in the world. For many years, the incidence of TB had been decreasing in developed and industrialized nations. However, that progressive decline has been slowed by the emergence of human immunodeficiency virus (HIV) infection. Moreover, atypical mycobacterial disease is on the rise secondary to HIV, transplantation patients taking immunosuppressants, patients with various other autoimmune diseases, and cancer patients using chemotherapy. Among all the mycobacteria, *Mycobacterium tuberculosis* is the most commonly seen pathologic organism in the lung.

Mycobacterial infection is communicated via aerosolization. Patients infected initially present with a necrotizing pneumonia (primary tuberculosis). The mycobacteria eventually propagate to the hilar lymph nodes, where the response results in the classic picture of caseating granulomas. In a patient with a competent immune system, a robust cell-mediated immune response usually retards disease progression. However, the mycobacteria can enter the bloodstream, leading to disseminated or miliary tuberculosis in certain rare circumstances, especially in patients who are immunocompromised. The therapy for pulmonary tubercular infections has long been and continues to be antimycobacterial agents. There are various regimens but most include either 2 months treatment with isoniazid, rifampin, and pyrazinamide followed by 4 months of treatment with isoniazid and rifampin or 9 months of isoniazid and rifampin (for individuals who can not take pyrazinamide).

Ethambutol is usually included in most regimens until drug sensitivities can be determined. In children, streptomycin rather than ethambutol is used because of the ototoxicity associated with this drug and the difficulty in effectively monitoring the pediatric population. Operative intervention rarely is needed and only indicated in the following situations: (i) positive sputum samples plus cavitary lung lesions after more than 5 months of treatment with two or more drugs, (ii) severe or recurrent hemoptysis, (iii) bronchopleural fistula not responsive to treatment with chest tube drainage, (iv) a persistently infected space (empyema), (v) a mass found in the area of the lung infected with *M. tuberculosis*, and (vi) disease caused by drug-resistant atypical mycobacteria such as *M. avium-intracellulare*.

Bronchiectasis usually results from a chronic smoldering infection and is characterized by abnormal dilation of the bronchi. This condition is usually found in the more distal bronchial tree, usually presenting in subsegmental bronchi. In the current era of effective antibiotic therapy, the condition is less frequently seen than in the past but rarely may be seen after a severe pneumonia or other pulmonary infections, especially if recurrent, which may lead to decreased clearance of airway secretions and thus bronchial injury. Bronchiectasis has also been associated with certain congenital disorders, such as primary ciliary dysmotility (Kartagener syndrome), α_1-antitrypsin deficiency, and cystic fibrosis, which also lead to decreased clearance of secretions. The most common presenting findings of bronchiectasis, no matter the etiology, include a persistent productive cough of purulent sputum and not infrequently hemoptysis, and a history of recurrent pulmonary infections. Physical examination may reveal crackles or rales over the involved areas, osteoarthropathy, and clubbing. Chest radiographs usually show nonspecific findings such as atelectasis, increased lung markings, pneumonia or cystic areas. Computerized tomographic (CT) scans of the chest demonstrate more specific findings of bronchial dilation within the lung parenchyma, which are especially well visualized on high resolution scans with 2-mm slices. Patients who present with this spectrum of signs and symptoms should also have a bronchoscopy to rule out a mass or obstructing lesion. In addition, a complete evaluation should include pulmonary function tests to assess the adequacy of pulmonary reserve. The majority of patients with bronchiectasis can be treated successfully with antibiotics, cessation of cigarette smoking, and pulmonary toilet during periodic exacerbations. Pulmonary resection of the involved lung parenchyma is reserved for patients with localized disease who fail medical therapy and lifestyle alterations. Patients who have bilateral disease may improve with a surgical resection on the more severe side. This alone may improve the contralateral lung and overall function.

THORACIC TRAUMA

Twenty-five percent of all trauma-related deaths occurs secondary to thoracic injuries, via either penetrating or blunt mechanisms. A penetrating injury to the chest, via a bullet or impaled object such as a knife, usually leads to a pneumothorax or hemothorax. A thorough evaluation of all of the intrathoracic and mediastinal structures must be carried out in these cases. Some injuries, such as those involving the heart or great vessels, may present as life-threatening hemorrhage, whereas injuries involving the trachea, bronchi, esophagus, or smaller blood vessels such as intercostal or internal mammary arteries may be more subtle, although they may still result in considerable blood loss. Blunt injury to intrathoracic structures results from either a direct blow to the chest or from rapid deceleration. The initial evaluation of any patient presenting with chest trauma should include examination of the airway to determine patency, an evaluation of the mechanics of respiration, and demonstration of adequacy of hemodynamics by assessing peripheral perfusion. Patients who appear anxious, combative, or who demonstrate poor oxygenation may require supplemental oxygenation or more likely endotracheal intubation. Careful examination and auscultation of the chest should be performed, assessing any change in breath sounds. In addition, the chest should be palpated to assess soft tissue and bone injury and to determine if there is evidence of subcutaneous emphysema, signaling a possible airway injury or parenchymal injury. Evidence of decreased breath sounds over either hemithorax should alert the physician to the possibility of a pneumothorax, and if there is alteration of the hemodynamics, particularly if the patient is hypotensive, the possibility of a tension pneumothorax must be entertained. Immediate tube thoracostomy should be performed if there is significant concern. Any patient with rapid hemodynamic compromise and a difficulty ventilating because of high peak airway pressures should trigger concern about the likelihood of a tension pneumothorax. All patients with thoracic trauma should have a chest x-ray (upright if possible) performed promptly, if sufficiently stable, because at times the presentation of a pneumothorax or hemothorax is not obvious. Throughout the examination and resuscitation, airway patency and oxygenation should be continuously monitored. In a patient who presents to the emergency department following penetrating chest trauma with vital signs still present who then goes on to lose vital signs, an emergency thoracotomy has been shown to be beneficial in some circumstances. For patients who present after sustaining blunt thoracic trauma, situations requiring an emergency department thoracotomy have been associated with a near 100% mortality. An emergency department thoracotomy is performed through the anterior left chest, usually in the fourth intercostal space. This desperate procedure is performed to accomplish four main objectives: (i) evacuation of pericardial blood that could be causing acute cardiac tamponade, (ii) control of any exsanguinating thoracic hemorrhage, (iii) cross-clamping of the descending aorta to increase coronary and cerebral perfusion, and (iv) open cardiac massage. If a patient does not respond to any of these maneuvers, he or she should be transported immediately to the operating room for definitive surgical repair of their injuries and closure of the chest.

Rib fractures are the most common chest wall injury incurred following blunt chest trauma, and their significance is often overlooked. The diagnosis can be made with a combination of physical examination and a chest radiograph. On examination breath sounds may be decreased because of splinting secondary to the pain, point tenderness may be present, and crepitus with palpation may be appreciated. Rib fractures should not be looked upon as trivial, since their presence implies significant force of injury. More importantly, they should alert the physician to the possibility of injury to underlying or nearby structures, with the most common such structure being the lung parenchyma with a resultant pulmonary contusion. Another sometimes overlooked injury following blunt chest trauma to the left side is the spleen. Twenty percent of patients with fractures of the left ribs 9 through 11 will have a splenic injury. Fractures of the first rib, a situation indicative of very significant force, often are associated with major vessel injuries. The major morbidity associated with rib fractures is the diminished respiratory mechanics resulting from splinting and the subsequent development of atelectasis or pneumonia. This is usually the result of inadequate pain relief and the inability to adequately clear secretions. Significant pain leads to a decreased inspiratory effort and cough, resulting in atelectasis, retained secretions, and sometimes pneumonia. This is especially true in elderly patients or in patients with underlying pulmonary disease. The mainstay of treatment for rib fractures is pain control, pulmonary toilet, and prompt recognition of any infectious pulmonary process. Epidural analgesia and patient-controlled analgesia have been shown to greatly decrease morbidity caused by rib fractures, especially when multiple ribs are injured. Unlike other fractures that are typically treated with immobilization, the practice of "taping" the fractured ribs is of historical interest only and should no longer be used. Moreover, it can actually be harmful by further limiting chest expansion and pulmonary mechanics. Patients without significant comorbid medical conditions who have adequate analgesia on oral pain regimens usually do not require hospital admission.

Flail chest is defined as an unstable portion of the thoracic cavity created by unilateral anterior and posterior fractures of four or more ribs or bilateral anterior or costochondral fractures of four or more ribs. These fractures result in paradoxical movement of the flail segment during inspiration. These can be diagnosed by x-rays or inspection of the chest during respiration. In the past, this type of injury was treated with operative stabilization of the rib fractures in an attempt to improve respiratory mechanics. However, it is now known that the major cause of respiratory embarrassment or failure in a patient with a flail chest is the coexisting pulmonary contusion, not the rib fractures themselves. Pulmonary contusions are seen in most patients with severe chest trauma and are particularly associated with flail chest. The pathophysiology of this involves the rupture of capillaries and subsequent hemorrhage into the pulmonary parenchyma and alveoli. Most pulmonary contusions appear as haziness over the involved lung, usually seen even on the first diagnostic chest radiograph. However, some injuries may not be visible for 4 to 5 hours, so a high index of suspicion is required. The treatment of a flail chest follows the same guidelines as for all significant chest wall injuries: pain control and pulmonary toilet. Epidural analgesia may be useful for pain control. If the injury results in less than adequate oxygenation and ventilation, then the patient may need to have an endotracheal tube placed and be mechanically ventilated. The use of positive end-expiratory pressure (PEEP) to maintain lung inflation and the judicious use of intravenous fluids are both helpful in supporting this type of trauma patient. With early diagnosis and aggressive pulmonary support, the mortality rate due to flail chest has been reduced to 5%. Mortality in a patient with a flail segment usually is caused by associated injuries, rather than the flail segment itself.

Sternal fractures can occur when a significant force, such as a steering column is applied to the anterior chest. Only 5% of trauma patients with chest wall injuries present with a sternal fracture. The major morbidity and mortality associated with this type an injury is concomitant injury to a neighboring structure such as the heart, aorta, or the tracheobronchial tree. A sternal fracture can be diagnosed by palpation (the classic finding of crepitus or an unstable chest) and radiographs of the lateral chest or sternum, with a specific request for sternal views. As is the case with rib fractures, the primary treatments for a fractured sternum are pain control and pulmonary toilet. Occasionally, sternal fractures with severe posterior displacement may require an operative repair with an open reduction and fixation, but this is distinctly unusual.

An *open pneumothorax*, also known as a "sucking chest wound," occurs when an injury creates a large defect in the chest wall with the associated loss of the physiologic negative intrathoracic pressure. When the cross-sectional area of the wound is greater than the cross-sectional area of the larynx, air will begin to preferentially enter the chest wound. An open pneumothorax is an immediate life-threatening injury because it will quickly lead to inadequate ventilation and a rising blood $Paco_2$. Once this injury is diagnosed, the first step in the treatment plan is coverage of the wound with an impermeable, sealed dressing. Following coverage of the wound a chest tube is placed on the affected side. Definitive operative treatment with repair of the chest wall defect may be carried out a soon as the patient is stable from both a respiratory and hemodynamic standpoint.

Pulmonary parenchymal injuries can appear as lacerations, hematomas, and pneumatoceles. Lacerations are usually caused by penetrating trauma. Occasionally they may result from the sharp edge of a fractured rib. Most lacerations can be treated by placement of a chest tube followed by a period of careful observation. The bleeding associated with a pulmonary laceration will usually stop spontaneously, since the pulmonary circulation is a low-pressure circuit. Persistent or massive hemorrhage (greater than 1,500 instantly or greater than 200 mL per hour for 4 to 6 hours) signals a more severe injury and operative exploration is required. In addition, patients with hemoptysis or large air leaks require a diagnostic bronchoscopy to rule out a ruptured bronchus. Surgical repair of a parenchymal injury, if required, can usually be performed by a simple wedge resection of the injured area of lung by using a surgical stapler. A formal anatomic lobectomy is required in less than 1% of all penetrating lung injuries. Bleeding from a bullet hole in the lung parenchyma may be managed by creating a tractotomy with a mechanical stapler. This opens the tract and allows for direct ligation or cauterization of bleeding vessels. Pulmonary hematomas usually occur from mechanisms similar to those involved with pulmonary contusion. Most of these injuries can be managed conservatively with pain control and pulmonary toilet. When patients with pulmonary hematomas develop a fever, an infected clot or abscess needs to be ruled out. CT scan of the chest should be performed to look for any pulmonary collections. Antibiotic therapy combined with drainage via the bronchial tree often facilitated by bronchoscopy usually results in resolution. Occasionally percutaneous catheter drainage or a surgical washout with a lung resection is required. A pneumatocele forms when significant trauma leads to the rupture of a small airway, forming an air-filled cavity. This diagnosis can be made with a chest x-ray demonstrating a round air-filled lesion. A CT scan is more helpful in further defining the cavity. Once other disease processes, such as tuberculosis, abscess, and cancer, have been ruled out, a pneumatocele can be diagnosed and managed by pulmonary toilet and observation. Most pneumatoceles will resolve spontaneously within 4 months.

Tracheobronchial injuries occur in less than 1% of patients with blunt trauma and are more commonly seen in penetrating injuries to the neck and chest. Deceleration injuries, caused by a rapid stop as occurs during a motor vehicle collision, can cause disruption of one or both of the main bronchi or the carina. Compression of the thorax against a closed glottis can lead to a "blow out" type injury. Patients with tracheobronchial injuries may present with hemoptysis, dyspnea, stridor, and crepitus over the neck and chest. Chest x-ray often reveals subcutaneous emphysema accompanied at times, but not always, by a pneumothorax. The treatment depends on the severity of the injury and the condition of the patient. Patients with a pneumothorax should undergo immediate chest tube placement on the affected side. All patients suspected of having a tracheobronchial injury should undergo urgent bronchoscopy. In a stable patient, an injury that involves less than one third of the tracheal circumference can be managed conservatively, depending on the location of the injury. Larger injuries, manifest by massive continuous air leak or large pneumothorax unresponsive to chest tube drainage, require surgical repair. Occasionally the larynx or trachea may be too distorted from the injury for an endotracheal tube to be placed. In these situations, either endotracheal intubation over a bronchoscope or emergent cricothyroidotomy may be necessary. Cricothyroidotomy is the emergency procedure of choice to establish an airway in the patient with significant head or neck trauma. All surgeons should be familiar with the technique of performing a life-saving cricothyroidotomy.

A *tension pneumothorax* can occur anytime the normal negative intrathoracic pressure is lost but is usually caused by a lung injury with an ongoing air leak with air escaping from the lung into the hemithorax. It may also occur with chest wall injuries that act as one-way valves, allowing air to enter the chest without being able to exit the chest through the same opening. As more air enters the thoracic cavity, the affected lung and the mediastinum shift to the opposite side, leading to a decrease in lung ventilation and, most significantly, a decrease in venous return to the heart, thereby decreasing cardiac output with resultant hypoperfusion and shock. A patient with a tension pneumothorax presents with hypotension, cyanosis, tracheal deviation away from the affected side, and absent breath sounds over the involved hemithorax. The initial as well as life-saving treatment involves converting the tension pneumothorax to an open pneumothorax by placing a large-bore catheter into the affected chest, usually at the second or third intercostal space at the midclavicular line. Once the hemithorax has been decompressed and the hemodynamics are stabilized, a conventional chest tube can be placed and the catheter removed.

Traumatic diaphragmatic injuries present as lacerations much more commonly than ruptures. The herniation of abdominal viscera into the chest may occur either at the time of injury or months to years later. If herniation occurs at the time of injury, the diagnosis can be made with the initial chest radiograph. Classically, the radiograph demonstrates opacification of the involved hemithorax along with an intestinal gas pattern. If the stomach has herniated, a nasogastric tube may be seen within the chest. However, when the herniation presents late, these injuries are found inadvertently during an abdominal exploration or on a chest radiograph while looking for something else. Before the use of CT scanning, most of these injuries were thought to occur on the left side with only a rare injury seen on the right. Several more recent studies using abdominal and chest CT scans have shown that diaphragmatic injuries may be more evenly distributed between the right and the left sides than previously thought. Injuries on the right side, however, tend to lead to less herniation because of the presence of the liver on the right side, which often prevents herniation of abdominal hollow viscera. The treatment of a diaphragmatic hernia involves placing abdominal viscera back into the peritoneal cavity and closure of the diaphragmatic defect. This usually can be best accomplished via an abdominal approach. This procedure also allows other intraabdominal injuries to be ruled out. Even in a chronic diaphragmatic hernia, the abdominal approach often is preferred, although these may be approached via the chest as well, especially if there is concern about significant adhesion formation that would make it difficult to "pull" the abdominal viscera back into the peritoneal cavity.

BENIGN LUNG TUMORS

Benign lung masses may arise from epithelial, mesenchymal, or endothelial tissue. The most common of the benign lesions is a hamartoma. Hamartomas usually present as asymptomatic solitary pulmonary nodules discovered incidentally on a chest x-ray or CT scan which was performed for another reason. These masses exhibit a slow rate of growth. On chest radiographs, hamartomas are usually noted to be discrete rounded nodules, often with "popcorn calcifications." Rarely, hamartomas cause symptoms secondary to obstruction or erosion into a bronchus. More often, however, these lesions present as diagnostic dilemmas and sometimes need be resected to rule out malignancy. The presence of a fat density within the nodule seen on CT scan provides a significant diagnostic clue that the lesion may be a hamartoma. Needle biopsy may rarely demonstrate the presence of a benign lesion unless a "positive" finding is obtained, that is, cartilage and fat indicative of a hamartoma, or distinct organisms from a granulomatous lesion. A "negative" needle biopsy is not helpful; it does not rule out the possibility that malignancy may be present and it does it make the diagnosis that the lesion is benign. There are a number of other benign neoplasms that occur rarely but deserve mention. These include hemangiopericytoma, sclerosing hemangioma, granular cell tumor, pseudolymphoma, fibroma, lipoma, leiomyoma, and clear cell (sugar) tumor of the lung. Other than hamartoma these lesions are distinctly uncommon.

LUNG CANCER

Lung cancer is the most common cause of cancer-related deaths in both men and women, and is second in prevalence only to breast cancer in women and prostate cancer in men. Although men comprise more than 60% of all patients with lung cancer, the percentage of women being seen with lung cancer is quickly climbing owing mainly to the increased incidence of smoking among women. Although smoking is a clearly defined risk factor, the majority of people who smoke do not develop lung cancer, and occasionally individuals with no history of tobacco use develop the disease. The mechanism behind the development of lung cancer appears to be multifactorial. Epidemiologic studies show an increase in familial cases, whereas environmental toxins, such as asbestos, chromium, and radon gas have also been linked to the development of lung cancers. Several genetic mutations have been linked to the development of the disease. K-ras mutations are the most common oncogene abnormalities seen in non–small cell lung cancer (NSCLC) and have been associated with a decreased survival rate. Mutations in the tumor suppressor genes, p53 and Rb, have also been associated with the development of lung cancer. Other genetic links with lung cancer include the growth factors, epidermal growth factor receptor (EGFR), vascular endothelial growth factor (VEGF), transforming growth factor-β (TGF-β), along with the lack of A- and H-related blood group antigens and nonexpression of the bcl-2 protein.

Seventy five percent to 80% of primary lung cancers are NSCLC, with small cell lung cancer (SCLC) making up the remaining 25% to 30%. The most common histologic type of NSCLC is adenocarcinoma, followed by squamous cell, and then large cell carcinomas. Two thirds of patients who develop lung cancer present initially to the physician with disseminated, and, thus, inoperable, disease. Of the remaining one third of patients, approximately two thirds have potentially resectable disease.

NSCLC is staged according to the tumor node metastasis (TNM) staging criteria, which is summarized in Table 25-1. The most common presentation is a patient with an asymptomatic pulmonary nodule found on a chest radiograph. Although benign lesions may occur and present as an asymptomatic nodule on chest radiograph, a solitary pulmonary nodule should be assumed to be lung cancer until proved otherwise. This is especially true if the patient is a smoker and has had a previous film within the last 2 years where the lesion in question was not present. The management of a patient with an asymptomatic solitary pulmonary nodule depends on many risk factors including age, history of cigarette use, the size of the nodule, and change in size of the nodule. In younger patients or in patients with nodules that have been stable in size over many years a biopsy is not necessarily warranted. These patients can be followed with serial chest radiographs with intervention only warranted if the lesion is noted to be increasing in size. However, older patients, those with a history of cigarette use, and those in whom the nodule has increased in size warrant a definitive tissue diagnosis. Symptomatic patients who present with a chronic nonproductive cough, pneumonia, hemoptysis, or chest pain also warrant a thorough evaluation.

The presence of a new solitary nodule in a patient with a smoking history must be assumed to be a lung cancer until proved otherwise, and resection of the lesion is indicated. Neither preoperative bronchoscopy nor a transthoracic needle biopsy is required, since the patient fulfills criteria for operation. Obtaining a tissue diagnosis prior to operation is not mandatory and if the needle biopsy is negative the patient needs an operation anyway. Needless to say a positive needle biopsy also mandates operation; therefore, if the needle biopsy results do not alter the plan that is in place what is the purpose for doing it? It is important to restate what may not be obvious. A negative needle biopsy does not rule out the presence of carcinoma. Needle biopsy is indicated for the patient with multiple nodules, especially with a previous history of malignant disease; for the patient who is inoperable because of presumed disseminated disease where it is necessary to establish a tissue diagnosis; and for the rare patient who is physiologically not a candidate for operation. Patients who come to the operating room without a tissue diagnosis often have a videothoracoscopy and wedge excision to confirm a malignant diagnosis followed by an anatomic resection of the involved lobe.

Bronchoscopy, along with bronchial brushing, washing, and biopsy, is another technique that may be used to obtain a tissue diagnosis from pulmonary nodules, but there should be a good indication to perform this procedure before doing it. If the results of the procedure will not influence what needs to be done to the patient then there is no indication to proceed with the procedure prior to operation. Bronchoscopy should be performed routinely by the surgeon at the time of the operative procedure. Bronchial washings and brushings can supply a diagnosis 75% of the time when a tumor is visible via a bronchoscope versus 50% of the time when the tumor is not visible. When tissue biopsy is added to this procedure, the diagnostic yield is increased to 94% for visible tumors and 60% for tumors that are not visible. Magnetic resonance imaging (MRI) and positron emission tomographic (PET)

TABLE 25-1

CLASSIFICATION OF LUNG CANCER

Stage	TNM classification
Ia	T1 N0 M0
Ib	T2 N0 M0
IIa	T1 N1 M0
IIb	T2 N1 M0, T3 N0 M0
IIIa	T1 N2 M0, T2 N2 M0, T3 N1 M0, T3 N2 M0
IIIb	Any T N3 M0, T4, Any N M0
IV	Any T Any N M1

Primary tumor

T1	Tumor ≤3 cm
	No bronchoscopic evidence of invasion into main bronchus
T2	Tumor >3 cm
	Involvement of main bronchus
	≥2 cm from the carina
	Invasion of visceral pleura
	Associated atelectasis or obstructive pneumonitis extending into the hilar region but not entire lung
T3	Any size tumor invading chest wall (includes superior sulcus tumors), diaphragm, mediastinal pleura, parietal pericardium
	Tumor ≥2 cm from the carina, without carinal involvement
	Atelectasis or pneumonitis of the entire lung
T4	Any size tumor invading mediastinum, heart, great vessels, trachea, esophagus, vertebral body, or carina
	Separate tumor nodules in the same lobe
	Malignant pleural effusion

Regional lymph Nodes

N0	No lymph node metastases
N1	Ipsilateral peribronchial or hilar metastases
	Ipsilateral intrapulmonary nodes involved by direct extension
N2	Ipsilateral mediastinal and/or subcarinal lymph node metastases
N3	Contralateral mediastinal or hilar lymph node metastases
	Ipsilateral or contralateral scalene or supraclavicular lymph node metastases

Nodal levels

N	Level/nodes
N2	1/highest mediastinal
	2/upper paratracheal
	3/pretracheal and retrotracheal
	4/lower paratracheal, including azygous nodes
Aortic	5/subaortic (aortopulmonary window)
	6/paraaortic (ascending aortic or phrenic)
	Inferior 7/subcarinal
	8/paraesophageal (below carina)
	9/inferior pulmonary ligament
N1	10/hilar
	11/interlobar
	12/segmental
	13/subsegmental

Distant metastases

M0	No distant metastases
M1	Distant metastases, including synchronous nodules in a different lobe

scanning have also been used in the preoperative workup of a patient with a solitary pulmonary nodule. MRI is used primarily to evaluate a chest mass and nodal involvement in a patient who can not tolerate intravenous contrast. PET scanning uses fluorinated glucose uptake to differentiate benign from malignant masses. This technique is highly sensitive, with rates ranging from 90% to 95%, but it is limited in specificity. False-positive results occur mainly with inflammation from mycobacterial or other pulmonary infections.

Once a diagnosis of NSCLC has been made, a preoperative evaluation of the needs to be carried out. This includes a complete history and physical examination, an antero-posterior (AP) and lateral chest x-ray, a complete blood count, chemistry panel, liver function tests, and CT scan of the chest and upper abdomen. On the abdominal CT scan the adrenal glands need to be assessed for the presence of metastatic disease. Other studies that may help rule out metastatic disease include an MRI scan of the brain along with a bone scan, although a PET scan obviates the need for a separate bone scan.

Mediastinoscopy is an invasive procedure that is extremely useful in staging the cancer. Mediastinoscopy can be used in conjunction with CT scanning to definitely identify tumor or the absence of tumor in mediastinal lymph nodes. A patient with a peripheral lesion and a CT scan with lymph nodes smaller than 1.5 cm has only a 10% chance of having tumor spread to lymph nodes. Typically, this type of patient does not require a mediastinoscopy, especially if the PET scan is negative in the mediastinum as well. However, a patient with a more centrally located tumor or mediastinal lymph nodes larger than 1.5 cm, should have mediastinoscopy to rule out nodal involvement. Approximately 90% of mediastinal lymph nodes can be sampled via mediastinoscopy. Another essential study for patients who may undergo a lung resection is pulmonary function testing, which is used to determine whether the patient is a candidate for resection. The parameters that may have predictive value relative to postoperative morbidity include the forced expiratory volume at 1 second (FEV_1), the maximal ventilatory ventilation, and the ratio between FEV_1 and the forced vital capacity, and the diffusing capacity. Patients with marginal lung function require a quantitative ventilation-perfusion (V/Q) scan to determine how much the lung parenchyma that is planned to be removed contributes to overall lung function. In addition, a preoperative Pco_2 level greater than 50 mm Hg also identifies patients at higher risk for postoperative morbidity.

The therapy for lung cancer, including the use of adjuvant and neoadjuvant therapy, is complex and dependent on many factors, such as the physical condition of the patient, tumor size, and lymph node status. *Surgical resection* is the *mainstay* of therapy for stage I and II NSCLCs (Fig. 25-1A–D). Most patients will undergo a lobectomy or pneumonectomy to achieve negative margins, depending on the location of their tumor. Segmentectomy and wedge resection may be appropriate for patients with marginal lung reserve who cannot tolerate larger resections, but these procedures are associated with higher recurrence rates than either lobectomy or pneumonectomy. *Resection for stage IIIa* is performed with the objective of resecting all

pulmonary disease and lymph node disease (Fig. 25-1E). Survival rates of 25% to 40% can be achieved in patients with resected T3 or N1 (hilar or peripheral nodal) disease. The current practice regarding N2 (mediastinal lymph node) disease centers on the use of neoadjuvant chemotherapy or chemoradiotherapy followed by surgical resection for those patients for whom the disease does not progress during treatment. This aggressive method of treatment has been associated with an increase in the median survival of patients with N2 disease, although large prospective randomized trials are lacking. Patients with *stage IIIb disease* are generally *not considered operative candidates* (Fig. 25-1F). This is particularly true in patients with involved contralateral or supraclavicular lymph nodes. One study, however, reported by the Southwest Oncology Group, did show a benefit to surgical resection in these patients that was essentially equivalent to results obtained in patients with N2 disease. They were able to achieve a 63% resectability rate and a 39% 2-year survival rate in patients with stage IIIb disease who received neoadjuvant chemotherapy/radiation therapy.

Preoperative treatment with either chemotherapy or chemotherapy combined with radiation therapy is not indicated for any patient with stage Ia disease. Although there have been several recent trials looking at a potential role for preoperative chemotherapy in patients with early stage NSCLC (Ib, IIa, IIb), these trials have failed to show a difference in overall survival between treated and non-treated patients. Therefore, preoperative therapy for these patients is not warranted outside of a clinical trial at the present time.

There has been renewed interest recently in postoperative adjuvant therapy for patients with resected lung cancer with any stage other than Ia based on the results of several large scale randomized trials that showed a significant, albeit small, difference in survival between those receiving postoperative chemotherapy and those not receiving therapy. At this time all resected patients other than those with stage Ia disease should be referred to a medical oncologist, at least for an opinion regarding postoperative treatment.

Postoperative radiation therapy has been evaluated in multiple studies and despite the possibility of reducing the risk of locally recurrent disease none of these studies has ever shown a survival advantage. The role of postoperative radiation therapy remains controversial despite the lack of survival advantage. There is something intuitively attractive about optimizing control of local disease that continues to cause postoperative radiation therapy to be recommended to select patients following resection.

Patients with lung cancer die because of disseminated disease that may be, but is not always, associated with local recurrence. In fact most patients with resected disease do not recur locally. Most patients with stages II and III lung cancer who develop recurrences do so within 2 years. Nearly 100% will develop recurrences within 5 years of their initial diagnosis. Although the brain is the most common site of distant disease for tumors of all stages, recurrences may be found in almost any organ including most commonly bones, adrenal glands, lung, and liver.

The pathologic stage of a patient's tumor is the best predictor of survival, with lymph node status having the greatest effect on long-term survival. Five-year survival rates

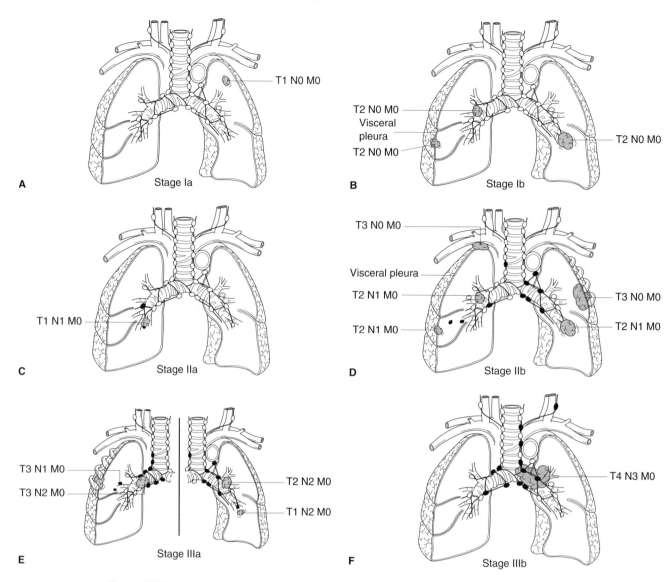

Figure 25-1   Staging of lung cancer. **A:** Stage Ia disease (T1 N0 M0) identifies a small (less than 3-cm) tumor surrounded by lung parenchyma. **B:** Stage Ib disease (T2 N0 M0) includes larger tumors that invade the visceral pleura or the main bronchi, or that have evidence of atelectasis/pneumonitis extending to the hilar regions. No metastatic disease is present with stage I tumors. **C:** Stage IIa (T1 N1 M0) identifies small tumors with TI characteristics (less than 3 cm) involving the peribronchial or hilar nodes by extension or metastasis. **D:** Stage IIb disease includes larger tumors (more than 3 cm) involving the peribronchial or hilar lymph nodes (T2 N1 M0) or tumors with limited extrapulmonary extension such as involvement of the chest wall or the pericardium (T3 N0 M0) but no evidence of metastasis. **E:** Stage IIIa describes tumors with localized extrapulmonary extension and involvement of peribronchial or hilar lymph nodes (T3 N1 M0) as well as any T1, T2, or T3 tumor with metastasis to the ipsilateral mediastinal and subcarinal lymph nodes (T1, T2, or T3 N2 M0). **F:** Stage IIIb describes either extensive extrapulmonary tumor invasion (T4 any N M0) or metastasis to the contralateral mediastinal and hilar lymph nodes as well as ipsilateral and contralateral supraclavicular/scalene lymph nodes. (From Mountain CF. The international system for staging lung cancer. *Semin Surg Oncol* 2000;18:106–115, with permission.)

range from 60% to 85% for stage I tumors, 40% to 50% for stage IIa tumors, 22% to 30 percent for stage IIIa tumors, and 5% for stage IIIb tumors and stage IV tumors. The effect of lymph node status can be seen in stage IIb tumors. Stage IIb (T3 N0) tumors have a greater than 40% 5-year survival rate while IIb patients with N1 disease have a 30% to 40% 5-year survival rate.

SCLCs can be classified as APUD (amine precursor uptake, decarboxylase) tumors because of their ability to produce and secrete neuroendocrine peptides. These aggressive tumors usually present on chest x-ray or CT scan

with bulky mediastinal lymph node disease and are assumed to be systemic at the time of presentation. Rarely do they present as pulmonary nodules that may be resectable, with fewer than 10% of all patients presenting with T1 to T2 or N0 to N1 lesions. The mainstay of treatment of SCLC is systemic chemotherapy. Up to 80% of patients respond to chemotherapy, regardless of the stage disease, but the response is not durable for the most part. Patients with SCLC are stratified according to limited disease within the chest, or extensive disease. Despite the positive response of SCLC to chemotherapy, the overall 5-year survival rate is a dismal 10%. Most patients presenting with limited disease SCLC receive a combination of chemotherapy and radiation therapy, even though the addition of radiation only improves disease-free and not overall survival. The role of operation in patients with limited disease SCLC remains controversial and operation in this group rarely is offered.

The lungs are a site for metastases from various tumors. Pulmonary metastatectomy, initially performed in the late 1920s, has now become an accepted adjunct to the overall treatment of many cancers. Most patients with pulmonary metastases present with asymptomatic lesions on follow-up chest radiographs. Further investigation of the lesions with CT scans is necessary to determine the location, number, and extent of involvement. CT scans often are unreliable in assessing the number of metastases; up to 25% of pulmonary metastases may be missed by standard chest CT scanning. Although particular contraindications to resection are under debate, several guidelines for resection include control of the primary cancer, absence of extrathoracic metastases, adequate health and pulmonary function, and lack of an efficacious systemic therapy. One of the largest series of patients to undergo pulmonary metastatectomy was collected by the International Registry of Lung Metastases. The study reported on more than 4,000 resected cases of metastatic disease from a variety of primary tumors 5-, 10-, and 15-year actuarial survival rates for completely resected metastases were 36%, 26%, and 22%, respectively. This contrasted to 5- and 10-year actuarial survival rates of 13% and 7%, respectively, for incompletely resected tumors. A better prognosis was seen in patients with germ-cell tumors, with a disease-free interval of more than 36 months, and single metastases. Among all patients with metastatic lung tumors, those with resections for metastatic Wilms tumors had the best prognosis, whereas those patients with melanoma had the worst survival.

Carcinoid tumors are neuroendocrine tumors that arise from bronchial epithelial cells and are classified as carcinomas, although they rarely metastasize to distant sites. They make up only 2% of all lung carcinomas and more than 80% of all pulmonary adenomas. Although usually associated with serotonin production, these tumors can produce and secrete various neuroendocrine peptides, such as bradykinin, glucagon, insulin, vasopressin, melanocyte-stimulating hormone, and calcitonin, but the majority of pulmonary carcinoids do not secrete active peptides. Unlike typical carcinoids, which rarely metastasize, atypical carcinoids are associated with lymph node metastases in up to 50% of patients. Patients with bronchial carcinoid tumors usually present with symptoms such as hemoptysis, dyspnea, or recurrent pulmonary infections. Only 2% of patients will present with true carcinoid syndrome and mostly these are patients with metastatic disease. The treatment centers on a complete surgical resection of the tumor. Five-year survival is 90% for typical carcinoids and 60% for atypical carcinoids. Carcinoid tumors may also present as asymptomatic peripheral nodules with no endobronchial component, and anatomic resection is the treatment of choice.

Bronchial adenomas encompass a group of tumors that include adenoid cystic carcinoma, mucoepidermoid carcinoma, and mucous gland adenoma (some sources will include carcinoid tumor in this group). The last of these, mucous gland adenoma, represents the only benign tumor in the group. These tumors are very slow growing, requiring years of growth to produce pulmonary symptoms.

Adenoid cystic carcinomas, formerly known as "cylindromas," arise from the submucosal glands in the bronchi and trachea and resemble salivary gland tumors. These tumors, although slow growing, invade the submucosal plane along perineural lymphatics. Because of this, these tumors typically extend well past their gross margin. The mainstay of therapy for adenoid cystic carcinomas is resection of the tumor and involved airway followed by postoperative radiation therapy. When lesions are truly unresectable, palliation can be obtained with endobronchial laser therapy and radiation. The slow growth of these tumors allows for long-term survival, even in patients with unresectable tumors.

Mucoepidermoid carcinomas are rarely seen and account for less than 5% of all bronchial adenomas. These tumors can vary in degree of malignancy from low to high grades, and have features of salivary glands on histologic evaluation. Treatment for these lesions involves surgical resection. High-grade lesions can be treated as bronchogenic carcinomas with regard to resection and survival.

CHEST WALL TUMORS

Chest wall tumors are relatively uncommon tumors that may arise from bone, cartilage, or soft tissue. More than one half of these are primary tumors, with the remainder being metastatic lesions from a variety of primary sites. Approximately 60% of chest wall tumors are malignant. In decreasing frequency, these tumors typically are chondrosarcomas, fibrosarcomas, plasmacytoma, Ewing sarcomas, or osteosarcomas. Fibrous dysplasia of bone, chondromas, and osteochondromas comprise the majority of the benign chest wall tumors. Most patients present to their physician with an enlarging chest wall mass. Typical preoperative workup includes anteroposterior and lateral chest radiographs to look for rib involvement, metastases, or pleural effusion, a chest CT scan to evaluate the relationship of the chest wall mass to other thoracic structures, as well as evaluate adenopathy or pulmonary lesions. An abdominal CT scan should also be obtained to rule out hepatic metastases and to search for a possible primary source such as the kidney or colon. A bone scan is also an essential study to rule out the involvement of other bony sites in the event of that the chest wall mass is a metastatic lesion.

The definitive treatment for tumors smaller than 4 cm is a wide local excision. Larger lesions should be approached via an incisional biopsy as the initial procedure, with the incision made with definitive resection in mind. An incisional biopsy can provide adequate tissue for a diagnosis and does not increase the risk of local recurrence or distant spread, and obviates a large resection in the case of a "medical" chest wall tumor such as plasmacytoma, lymphoma, or Ewing tumor. The biopsy incision should be placed to allow for its excision upon definitive resection of the mass.

Most rib tumors are malignant, with the most common of these being chondrosarcomas. Chondrosarcomas usually are seen in adult patients and present as a painful slowly growing solitary mass involving one or more of the first four ribs. Chest radiographs may show a lobulated mass with poorly defined margins, along with bony destruction. The treatment for these lesions is a local excision with a 4- to 5-cm margin. A complete resection can achieve 10-year survival rates of greater than 90%. Negative predictors of survival include distant metastases at the time of presentation, age greater than 50 years old, and an incomplete surgical resection.

Ewing sarcoma is a vascular tumor that is usually seen in male children or adolescents. Patients commonly present with a painful chest wall mass. A chest x-ray often shows a pleural effusion. Patients may also experience fever, leukocytosis, and an elevated erythrocyte sedimentation rate. Radiographically these lesions take on an "onion skin" appearance owing to periosteal elevation and new bone formation. Radiographs may also demonstrate areas of bone destruction. A patient presenting with these radiographic findings in conjunction with a fever can be mistaken to have osteomyelitis. Therefore, a tissue sample is required for a definitive diagnosis. Treatment for Ewing sarcoma involves a combination of radiation, surgical resection, and chemotherapy, with the combined therapy usually given prior to resection. This multimodality therapy yields a 10-year survival of 40% to 50%. Approximately one half of patients with Ewing sarcoma present with metastases to the lungs or brain, findings obviously associated with a poorer prognosis.

Osteogenic sarcoma, like Ewing sarcoma, usually affects male children or adolescents. Typically, patients present in a similar fashion to that with Ewing sarcoma, with a painful rapidly growing chest wall mass. Chest radiographs may show a characteristic "sunburst" pattern along with bony destruction and soft tissue involvement. Patients commonly present with pulmonary metastases secondary to vascular invasion. The treatment typically consists of an excision with wide margins and may or may not involve chemotherapy. The optimal treatment for metastatic disease to the lungs, when possible, is resection once the primary tumor is controlled. Even with this combined approach, the 5-year survival rate is a disappointing 15% to 20%.

Plasmacytoma, most commonly seen in men in their 40s to 60s usually is associated with the development of multiple myeloma, but this diagnosis may not be made prior to the presentation of the chest wall mass. Patients commonly present with chest pain. An associated mass may or may not be present. Patients typically have fever, malaise, anemia, elevated erythrocyte sedimentation rates, an abnormal serum protein electrophoreses, hypercalcemia, and Bence Jones proteinuria. The classic chest radiograph findings of multiple myeloma are lytic "punched out" rib lesions and soft tissue involvement, but a plasmacytoma presents as a discrete chest wall mass. A biopsy specimen demonstrating plasma cells clinches the diagnosis. Because these tumors usually occur in patients with multiple myeloma, treatment involves chemotherapy, prednisone, and radiation therapy. Surgical resection is reserved for the rare isolated chest plasmacytoma. The 5-year survival rate in these patients has been reported at 20% to 40%.

Soft tissue sarcomas comprise 20% of chest wall tumors and include fibrosarcomas, leiomyosarcomas, liposarcomas, synovial sarcomas, neurofibrosarcomas, and malignant fibrous histiocytomas. Ten percent of these tumors will recur locally after excision, and early metastases, almost always to the lungs, is the rule.

Osteochondromas are the most common benign bony chest wall tumors. These tumors typically present in childhood, most commonly in boys, and tend to grow slowly. Because of their slow growth, osteochondromas may be observed for a period. Painful tumors in children may

signify malignant degeneration and should be evaluated and resected. Osteochondromas arising in adults should also be resected because of the possibility of malignancy. *Chondromas* are slow-growing tumors that usually arise from the costochondral junction. These tumors may be difficult to differentiate from chondrosarcomas and therefore require excision for definitive diagnosis.

Fibrous dysplasia is a cystic disease of the rib caused by replacement of the rib marrow with fibrous tissue. These tumors occur with equal prevalence in men and women but may also present as part of Albright syndrome along with other bone cysts, dark pigmentation, and precocious puberty in girls. These tumors occur most commonly on the posterolateral aspect of a given rib. Resection is reserved for symptomatic tumors or tumors found in adults. Asymptomatic tumors in children can be observed and usually stop growing by puberty. *Histiocytosis X* is one of several reticuloendothelial disorders that include eosinophilic granuloma, Letterer-Siwe disease, and Hand-Schueller-Christian disease. All of these diseases may present with rib tumors. The most common bone tumors in histiocytosis X occur in the skull, but rib tumors can also be seen. The histology of these tumors demonstrates eosinophilic and histiocytic infiltration into the bone marrow. Solitary lesions can be treated with excision, whereas radiation therapy is reserved for multiple lesions.

Regardless of which tumor is present, the dominant principle in any chest wall resection is complete resection of all tumor with at least 4-cm margins and one normal rib above and below the tumor (Fig. 25-2). All biopsy incisions should be included in the resection. Reconstruction may involve the use of polypropylene mesh, PTFE (polytetrafluoroethylene), or methyl methacrylate sandwiched between polypropylene mesh. Muscle flaps can also be used to provide coverage of chest wall defect. Posterior defects that underlie the scapula may not require any coverage. The goals of chest wall reconstruction are to provide protection

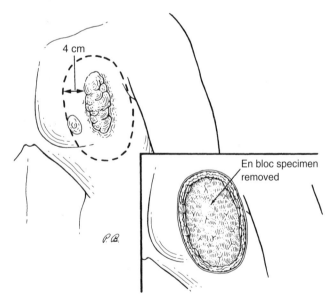

Figure 25-2 Planned *en bloc* resection of a chest wall tumor should include a 4-cm margin of tissue and one normal rib above and below the tumor. (From Miller JI. Surgical resection of the chest wall including sternum. In: Kaiser LK, Kron IL, Spray TL, eds. *Mastery of cardiothoracic surgery*, Philadelphia: Lippincott Williams & Wilkins, 1998:190, with permission.)

of the intrathoracic organs, a good cosmetic result, and, perhaps, most importantly, for anterior chest wall defects, the prevention of paradoxical chest wall motion.

DISEASE OF THE PLEURA AND THE PLEURAL SPACE

The pleural surface is a mesothelial layer that is composed of two layers. One is the parietal pleura, which covers the chest wall, diaphragm, and mediastinum. The other is the visceral pleura, which covers the lungs. The arterial and venous blood supply of the parietal pleura is derived from the intercostal, internal mammary, superior phrenic, and anterior mediastinal arteries. The visceral pleural receives its blood supply from the bronchial and pulmonary arteries while its venous flow is via the pulmonary veins alone. There is also an extensive lymphatic network within the pleura. The pleura and its components are subject to the same benign and malignant processes that affect epithelial tissues throughout the body.

A *pleural effusion* can be a sign of a localized or systemic process stemming from a wide variety of etiologies. Classically, effusions are divided into exudates and transudates. Exudates are indicative of pleural disease or pleural lymphatic disease, whereas a transudative effusion is caused by either increased production or decreased absorption of pleural fluid. It is not necessarily indicative of a primary pulmonary process. The need to differentiate an exudative from a transudative effusion is crucial because almost one half of exudates result from malignant processes, whereas most transudates are secondary to congestive heart failure. Generally, pleural fluid from a transudate will have a specific gravity less than 1.016 and a protein content of less than 3 g per dL. This may not be true for long-standing transudate effusions. Most transudate effusions are either clear or straw-colored and odorless. Ninety percent of bloody effusions, not secondary to trauma or pulmonary emboli, are caused by malignancy. Findings that may also be seen include elevated fluid amylase levels in patients with concomitant pancreatitis, malignancy or esophageal rupture, and a glucose level in the pleural fluid of greater than 60 mg per dL is typically seen in patients with tuberculosis, malignancy, rheumatoid disease, or parapneumonic effusions. Additional tests that may be performed on the fluid include microbiology cultures, cell counts, lactate dehydrogenase (LDH) level, cytology, and chylomicron/fat content. Effusions can usually be diagnosed by chest radiograph, but, occasionally, ultrasonography or CT scan may be necessary to differentiate an effusion from a mass. Moreover, a CT scan can help to further characterize the extent of the fluid collection and determine if it is loculated. Any treatment modality focuses on diagnostic thoracentesis followed by attempts to reverse the underlying process. In the case of malignant pleural effusions, the only reasonable therapy to prevent the fluid from returning may be tube thoracentesis and instillation of talc, doxycycline, or with talc or bleomycin to effect a chemical pleurodesis.

Another condition affecting the pleural space is a *spontaneous pneumothorax*. It has an incidence of approximately 10 cases per 100,000 people with a male-to-female ratio of 3:1. Classically patients have a tall, thin body habitus and are often in their early 20s or 30s. The source of the pneumothorax is usually rupture of a bleb located in the apex of the upper lobe or the superior segment of the lower lobe and occurs more commonly in the right lung. Although the exact etiology of a spontaneous pneumothorax is unknown, people who smoke cigarettes are at an increased risk. Occasionally, pneumothoraces are diagnosed in relation to women's menstrual cycles, so-called catamenial pneumothorax. These pneumothoraces are thought to be caused by endometrial implants on the lung or diaphragm. Patients who experience a spontaneous pneumothorax complain of a sudden onset of pleuritic chest pain accompanied by shortness of breath. These patients may subsequently develop subcutaneous emphysema, pneumomediastinum, a continuous air leak, hemopneumothorax, and, rarely, a tension pneumothorax. Approximately 30% of these patients will have a recurrence after their initial presentation and more than 60% of those who experience a second pneumothorax will experience a subsequent one. Spontaneous pneumothoraces are treated successfully in most patients with chest tube placement. Most air leaks will stop within 24 hours. Surgical intervention is mandated by a persistent air leak (3 to 5 days), a massive air leak for 24 hours, failure of the lung to reexpand, history of previous pneumothorax, bilateral pneumothoraces, patients with occupations that could lead to life-threatening pneumothoraces (pilot, diver), location far from any medical facility, and large pulmonary bullae. In these situations, the treatment is modified to include either open or preferably thoracoscopic mechanical pleurodesis alone or in combination with blebectomy. Occasionally, young patients who have a spontaneous pneumothorax are asymptomatic. They can be watched and followed with serial chest x-rays until the lung completely reexpands.

A *hemothorax* refers to a collection of blood in the pleural space. This usually occurs secondary to a traumatic injury of the chest, but it may also occur with pulmonary emboli/infarction, tumors, systemic heparinization, and following thoracic surgery. Diagnosis can usually be made with an upright chest radiograph considered along with the patient's history, physical examination, and vital signs. Small hemothoraces, which may not even be recognized, usually resolve without intervention. Larger collections can be treated successfully with tube thoracostomy in up to 85% of patients if the tube is placed early. Depending on the mechanism of injury surgical intervention is required for hemothoraces that drain more than 1,500 mL upon tube thoracostomy placement or for ongoing chest tube output greater than 250 mL per hour for 3 or more hours.

Problems that can arise from undrained or incompletely drained hemothorax include empyema and fibrothorax with entrapped lung. Empyema requires definitive drainage, often surgical, which is discussed later in this chapter. Fibrothorax and trapped lung result from undrained blood in the chest that organizes as a fibrous peel, encasing the lung and leading to a functional reduction in the volume of the hemithorax. Therapy involves removing the fibrous peel from both the chest wall and lung, that is, the visceral and parietal pleural peel, to allow the lung to fully reexpand. Although this procedure classically is performed through a thoracotomy, video-assisted thoracoscopy may at times be used, especially if early in the course. A well-developed fibrous peel requires an open pleurectomy and decortication to assure that the lung fully expands to fill the space.

Chylothorax is caused by a leakage of chyle from an injured thoracic duct or one of its branches. The thoracic duct, the structure through which the lymphatic drainage from the gut and lower body drains, originates in the abdomen as the cisterna chyli, just to the right of the aorta. From here, the duct traverses the diaphragmatic hiatus and enters the chest. Once in the chest, the thoracic duct crosses over to the left of the aorta, at the level of T4 to T5, ultimately emptying into the left subclavian vein near the confluence of the left subclavian and internal jugular veins. Although often depicted as a single conduit, the thoracic duct has a variable course that involves many branches and connections with the azygous vein. Chyle is a milky white, alkaline, odorless liquid with a specific gravity of 1.012 to 1.025 and a lymphocyte count of 400 to 6,800 cells per mL. Approximately 50% of chylothoraces in adults are secondary to tumors, of which lymphoma far and away predominates. Other etiologies may include trauma, violent coughing, iatrogenic injury (thoracic surgery, central line placement), or an infection; they are occasionally idiopathic. Once the thoracic duct has been injured, chyle leaks either into the mediastinum until it ruptures into one or both of the pleural spaces or directly into the pleural space. A chylothorax can be identified by a cholesterol-to-triglyceride ratio of less than 1 and a triglyceride level of greater than 110 mL per dL in the pleural fluid. In addition, fat in the chyle can be stained with Sudan red to secure the diagnosis. In a postoperative patient with persistent high-volume serous chest tube output, a chyle leak can be diagnosed quickly by feeding the patient a high-fat substance and observing if the color of the chest tube output changes to a milky white color and confirmed by a fluid triglyceride level. The treatment of a chylothorax can involve either conservative or invasive management depending on the amount of drainage. Conservative therapy uses chest tube drainage along with a low-fat hyperalimentation regimen. The chest tube output will gradually decrease with time. This is more often successful for isolated branch injuries of the thoracic duct than for leaks secondary to tumor infiltration where congestion and multiple leakage sites can be seen. Conservative therapy can be attempted initially, but if the output remains elevated for more than 5 to 7 days, this condition can lead to severe nutritional depletion and lymphopenia. For adults with chyle leaks greater than 1 L per day for greater than 1 week, conservative management should be aborted. The goal of surgical therapy is ligation of the duct at the level of the diaphragm and not an attempt to locate the precise area of the leak. Proceeding via a low right thoracotomy all of the tissue along the spine between the aorta and the azygous is ligated to ensure that the thoracic duct is included. Olive oil or cream may be given via a nasogastric tube to aid in identifying the duct if that is desirable. The ligation should be done as close to the diaphragmatic hiatus as possible to avoid missing any early branches.

An *empyema* is defined as the accumulation of pus in the pleural space. A sample of the fluid from one of these collections usually will have a pH level of less than 7.0, a glucose of less than 40 mg per dL, an LDH of more than 1,000 IU per L, and a positive gram stain. Additional findings include a white blood cell (WBC) count of greater than 15,000 cells per mL, a protein level of greater than 3 g per dL and a specific gravity greater than 1.016. Most empyemas occur secondary to a pneumonic infiltrate, whereas others are attributed to surgical procedures involving the chest, mediastinum, the thoracic extension of subphrenic abscesses, or chest trauma. The most common organism cultured from an empyema is *Staphylococcus aureus*, but Streptococcus species and gram-negative and anaerobic organisms can also be found in these infections. An empyema can present in any of three phases, as defined by the American Thoracic Society: acute/exudative, transitional/fibrinopurulent, and chronic/organizing. The fluid of the acute/exudative phase is thin and has a low WBC count, low LDH level, and low glucose level with a normal pH. The next phase is the transitional/fibrinopurulent phase, which is characterized by turbid fluid with a chemistry profile that resembles classic empyema fluid. During this phase, a fibrinous layer forms on both the parietal and visceral pleura that can begin to limit lung expansion. The third and final phase, the chronic/organizing phase, is seen after 4 to 6 weeks of the infection. The fibrinous layer eventually becomes infiltrated with new blood vessels and the fluid contains a large amount of sediment. Patients with an empyema may present with any array of symptoms including overt sepsis, pleuritic chest pain accompanied by cough, fever, pneumonia, or a lung abscess. In the later stages, patients can develop empyema necessitans, in which the empyema erodes through the chest wall and presents as a soft tissue abscess, a draining sinus, or a disseminated infection. The diagnosis is made with an anteroposterior and lateral chest x-ray and a thoracentesis to confirm the presence of infected fluid. A chest CT scan may be helpful in defining the size and location of the empyema and ruling out invasion of the chest wall, mediastinum, and other adjacent structures. Treatment of empyema involves eradicating the primary infection, evacuating the infected fluid, and reexpanding the lung. When the pleural fluid has a pH level of greater than 7.20, glucose of greater than 40 mg per dL, and an LDH level of less than 1,000 IU per L, thoracentesis alone may prove therapeutic and chest tube placement may not be required but these patients have to be closely followed. Purulent collections, reaccumulation of the aspirated fluid, and inability to completely drain the fluid with a needle or systemic toxicity, on the other hand, will require the placement of a large-bore chest tube for ideal drainage. Some patients are not able to be adequately drained by tube thoracostomy alone and require more extensive procedures such as video-assisted thoracoscopic drainage, decortication, or rib resection along with vigorous irrigation and a chest tube (empyema tube) placed for drainage of the abscess. In this latter procedure, the chest tube is then gradually removed over a period of 3 to 4 weeks to allow the infected cavity to close around the tube. If the lung fails to expand once the chest tube has been removed, decortication or marsupialization (Eloesser flap) of the cavity may be required. Lytic agents, first introduced in the 1950s, have regained some popularity for the treatment of an empyema owing to a rising emphasis on less-invasive approaches toward treatments. Streptokinase, the most widely used agent can be mixed with saline with a concentration of 250,000 U per 100 mL of normal saline and inserted into the thoracic cavity via a chest tube. The chest tube is then clamped for several hours at a time. This procedure is performed daily for 2 weeks. Success rates of up to 90% have been reported with minimal systemic absorption and toxicity.

Pleural malignancies most commonly present as metastases from lung, breast, stomach, and pancreas cancers.

Primary malignant tumors of the pleura also occur but are far less common than metastatic lesions. The most common primary pleural tumor is *malignant mesothelioma*. It is most commonly found in the chest, although it may also occur in the pericardium, peritoneum, testes, and ovaries. In the United States, there are approximately 3,000 cases of malignant pleural mesothelioma diagnosed each year. The biggest risk factor for developing mesothelioma is prior asbestos exposure. Approximately 20% of patients with malignant mesothelioma are either unaware of or deny exposure to asbestos. Malignant mesothelioma can be separated into three subtypes based on histology: epithelial, sarcomatous, and a mixed/biphasic tumor, a mix of the two other subtypes. The epithelial variant is most commonly seen followed by the mixed, and then the least common is the sarcomatous subtype. The disease usually affects older men who are more likely to have occupational exposure. Most likely, this is because the latency period from time of asbestos exposure to onset of the disease is approximately 30 to 40 years. Patients typically present with nonpleuritic chest pain, dyspnea, cough, fever, and weight loss. Chest radiographs may show classic pleural plaques or pleural thickening, and most patients either present with or will develop a pleural effusion at some time during the course of their disease. Mesothelioma may be difficult to distinguish from adenocarcinoma that has metastasized to the pleural cavity. A definitive diagnosis is achieved only by obtaining a sample of the tumor. Certain characteristics that distinguish malignant mesotheliomas from other tumors include: large length to diameter ratio of the microvilli on electron microscopy, negative test results for carcinoembryonic antigen (CEA), positive staining results for keratin, negative staining results for LEU M1 antigen, and the presence of hyaluronic acid in the absence of any other acid mucins. Patients diagnosed with malignant mesothelioma have a dismal prognosis with the median survival being 8 to 14 months. Positive prognostic indicators include early stage disease, epithelial subtype, age less than 55 years, female sex, and the absence of malignant cells in the pleural fluid. Surgical treatment options include biopsy with pleurodesis, pleurectomy/decortication, and extrapleural pneumonectomy and some combination of radiation therapy and chemotherapy. The lack of response to single modality therapy has created interest in multimodal therapy. Trimodal therapy combining extrapleural pneumonectomy and postoperative chemotherapy and radiation therapy has been used with some success in selected patients. A 5-year survival rate of 45% has been achieved in patients with the epithelial subtype and no nodal disease. However, the perioperative morbidity and mortality from this approach are 30% and 4.6%, respectively. The poor response to treatment in malignant mesothelioma has led to research efforts evaluating adenoviral-based suicide gene therapy, photodynamic therapy, and immunotherapy. None of these approaches have yet proved efficacious. However, trials are ongoing.

MEDIASTINAL DISEASE

The mediastinum can be thought of as three anatomic entities: anterosuperior, middle, and posterior divisions, according to their relation to the pericardium (Table 25-2). The anterior mediastinum has been further divided into a

TABLE 25-2
MEDIASTINAL STRUCTURES

Anterior	Middle	Posterior
Thymus	Heart	Esophagus
Aorta/great vessels	Pericardium	Vagus nerves
Lymphatics plexus	Phrenic nerves	Sympathetic nerve
Fatty areolar tissue	Carina	Thoracic duct
Upper trachea	Main bronchi	Descending aorta
Upper esophagus	Pulmonary hilum lymph nodes	Azygous vein
		Hemiazygous vein
		Paravertebral lymphatics
		Fatty areolar tissue

separate superior section. The anterior mediastinum includes all structures anterior to the pericardium and the great vessels. The middle mediastinum is bounded by the anterior and posterior pericardial reflections, whereas the posterior mediastinum includes everything posterior to the posterior pericardial reflections.

One pathologic condition that can affect any division of the mediastinum is *mediastinitis*. Bacterial contamination of the mediastinum can lead to a rapidly progressive infection that has a high morbidity and mortality rate, especially if it is not recognized and treated immediately. Mediastinitis may be secondary to esophageal perforation, contamination after a surgical procedure, or it may descend from an infectious process in the posterior pharynx. Patients often present with fever, tachycardia, chest pain, or overt sepsis. Subcutaneous emphysema may also be present if the source is a perforation in the esophagus, the trachea, or a bronchus. Pharyngeal abscesses can also spread to the mediastinum and present in patients as erythema and pain over the anterior neck and chest (Ludwig angina). A standard chest x-ray series of AP and lateral chest radiographs often shows air or an air–fluid level in the mediastinum or chest. A chest CT scan is helpful in identifying fluid and gas in the mediastinum and in localizing infectious sources in the neck or chest. Bronchoscopy, esophageal endoscopy, and water-soluble contrast studies are the definitive diagnostic studies used in identifying tracheal and esophageal perforations. The successful treatment of mediastinitis requires rapid identification of the process followed by reversal of the inciting cause usually with a drainage procedure, in conjunction with broad-spectrum antibiotic therapy. Gross contamination due to an esophageal perforation requires wide débridement and drainage usually accompanied by definitive repair of the esophageal perforation. On occasion, the esophagus has to be divided and excluded with a distal staple line and a cervical esophagostomy in the event of marked delay in recognition of the perforation that, at operation, proves to be unable to be repaired primarily. A postoperative sternal infection with mediastinitis usually requires sternal débridement along with flap closure (usually with the pectoralis major muscle). A rare cause of mediastinitis results from granulomatous disease in the mediastinal lymph nodes. Histoplasmosis, the most common pathogen identified in this disease, is treated with antimycobacterial drugs and occasionally it may require surgical debridement of the involved lymph nodes.

Although controversial, some surgeons have recommended the routine resection of all acutely inflamed lymph nodes to avoid granulomatous mediastinitis.

The most common mediastinal masses include neurogenic tumors, thymomas, primary cysts, lymphomas, and germ-cell tumors. The most common site for these masses is the anterior mediastinum (54%), followed by the posterior mediastinum and then the middle mediastinum. Between 25% and 40% of mediastinal masses in adults are malignant and these most commonly are found in the anterior mediastinum (Table 25-3). Patients may present with symptoms due to localized compression of neighboring structures or with syndromes associated with specific tumors. The diagnosis of a mediastinal mass can often be made with AP and lateral chest radiographs. Chest CT scan or MRI definitely establish the presence of a mediastinal mass and define the origin of the mass. Either of these studies will also demonstrate whether the mass is cystic or solid. Other tests that may also be useful include arteriography (rarely used unless a vascular lesion is suspected), endoscopy, radioisotope scanning, and needle biopsy.

Thymomas are the most common tumors found in the anterior mediastinum and rank only behind neurogenic tumors, found in the posterior mediastinum, as the second most common of all mediastinal tumors. Thymomas are more common in adults and rarely seen in children. Patients usually present with local symptoms such as dyspnea, cough, hemoptysis, or chest pain that may be accompanied by one of many paraneoplastic syndromes including myasthenia gravis, Cushing syndrome, lupus, rheumatoid arthritis, or hypercoagulopathy. These tumors may appear as irregular central masses on chest radiograph, but either a CT scan or an MRI is more useful at delineating the tumor. Thymomas have been classified histologically as either epithelial or lymphocytic. Importantly, though, is the presence of either gross or microscopic invasion of either the capsule or adjacent structures. When seen at operation this defines whether a thymoma is "invasive," the thymic equivalent of malignant. (Table 25-4). Although 65% of thymomas are encapsulated (or benign), it may be possible to overlook occult invasion in an otherwise benign-appearing thymoma. This is obviously true for the assessment of microscopic invasion of the capsule. During the resection of any thymoma, the surgeon must take care not to violate the capsule as "drop metastases" primarily to the pleural space have been reported. Whether pleural metastatic disease results from tumor spillage remains a matter of

TABLE 25-4

STAGING AND 5-YEAR SURVIVAL RATES FOR MALIGNANT THYMOMAS

Stage	5-year survival
I (encapsulated, no evidence of gross or microscopic capsular invasion)	85%–100%
II (pericapsular invasion into mediastinal fat, pleura, or pericardium)	60%–80%
III (invasion into adjacent organs or intrathoracic metastases)	40%–70%
IV (extrathoracic metastases)	50%

conjecture, although effort should be made to remove the tumor without disrupting the capsule. The treatment of patient with a thymoma is total thymectomy via either a median sternotomy or thoracotomy. Adjuvant radiation therapy is recommended for stages II (microinvasive) and III (gross invasion of adjacent structures) tumors, whereas chemotherapy is reserved for patients with stage IV disease or those with recurrent disease.

Myasthenia gravis occurs in approximately 35% of patients who have thymomas, but only 10% to 20% of patients with myasthenia gravis will have a thymoma. The disease is thought to result from the stimulation of thymic lymphocytes leading to the production of acetylcholine antibodies to acetylcholine receptor–like antigens in the thymus. Clinically, patients present with progressive skeletal muscle weakness that tends to involve the ocular muscles first. It may progress to involve a patient's respiratory muscles, leading to respiratory failure. The diagnosis is suggested by clinical muscle weakness and usually confirmed with a Tensilon test in which transient muscle strength is regained after the administration of a short-acting acetylcholinesterase inhibitor. Single fiber electromyography may be required in some cases to confirm the diagnosis. The mainstays of treatment for myasthenia gravis are acetylcholinesterase inhibitors and immunosuppressants. A thymectomy is also beneficial in many patients with myasthenia gravis, with more than 80% of patients having some clinical improvement in their disease after resection. When followed over time, more than 40% of patients will go into complete remission with no continuing requirement for medication. Positive predictors of response to thymectomy include a short duration of the disease process prior to a thymectomy, female sex, milder forms of myasthenia, and absence of a thymoma.

Neurogenic tumors, most commonly originating from neural crest cells, are the most common mediastinal tumor and usually are located in the posterior mediastinum. These tumors have the ability to secrete various hormones but rarely do. The tumors can arise from any of the mediastinal neural tissue including sympathetic ganglia, paraganglia cells, and intercostal nerves. Most neurogenic tumors that occur in adults are benign. Those that are found in children are more likely to be malignant. Neurogenic tumors that arise in the posterior mediastinum include *neuroblastomas, ganglioneuroblastomas, ganglioneuromas, neurilemomas (schwannomas), neurofibromas, neurosarcomas,* and *paragangliomas,* with *neurilemomas* being the most common. Patients usually present asymptomatically

TABLE 25-3

MEDIASTINAL MASSES

Anterior	Middle	Posterior
Thymoma (31%)	Cysts (61%)	Neurogenic (52%)
Lymphoma (23%)	Lymphoma (20%)	Cysts (32%)
Germ cell tumors (17%)	Mesenchymal (8%)	Mesenchymal (10%)
Carcinoma (13%)	Carcinoma (6%)	Endocrine (2%)
Germ cell tumors (17%)	Other (5%)	Other (4%)
Cysts (6%)		
Other (10%)[a]		

[a] Includes teratoma, lipoma, lymphangioma, hemangioma, parathyroid adenoma/carcinoma, thyroid adenoma/carcinoma/goiter.

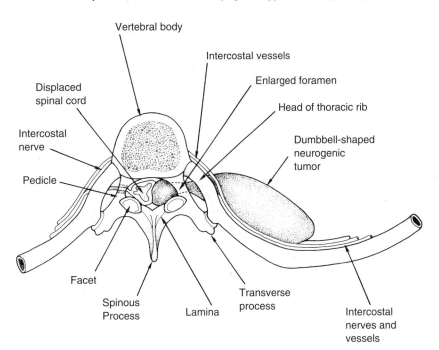

Figure 25-3 A neurogenic dumbbell tumor resulting in spinal cord compression, enlargement of the neural foramen, and a large posterior mediastinal mass. (From Kern JA, Daniel TM. Resection of posterior mediastinal tumors. In: Kaiser LK, Kron IL, Spray TL, eds. *Mastery of cardiothoracic surgery*, Philadelphia: Lippincott William & Wilkins 1998:114, with permission.)

with a mass having been noted on a chest radiograph obtained for some other reason. Respiratory and neurologic symptoms may arise from local compression or invasion of the spinal canal via the neural foramen ("dumbbell tumors" because of the characteristic appearance of their intraspinal and extraspinal portions) (Fig. 25-3). Any patient with a posterior mediastinal mass and either radicular pain or symptoms of vertebral destruction should be evaluated for a dumbbell tumor with either a myelogram or preferably an MRI. The failure to recognize a tumor invading into the spinal canal by way of a neural foramen can result in disastrous complications at the time of resection. If the tumor is transected and bleeding occurs in the intraspinal portion, spinal cord compression and paraplegia may result. Neurilemomas arise from Schwann cells and represent the most common neurogenic tumors. These tumors are most commonly seen in adults. Along with neurofibromas, neurilemomas can occur as part of the spectrum of the disease neurofibromatosis. The treatment for both of these tumors is surgical resection.

Neurosarcomas can arise in children with neurofibromatosis as well as in adults with no other associated illnesses. These tumors tend to be very aggressive, and if not completely resected they carry a very poor prognosis. Neuroblastomas are most commonly seen in children younger than 4 years of age. Although most of these tumors arise in the retroperitoneum, 10% to 20% are found in the posterior mediastinum. Neuroblastomas have been known to be aggressive and tend to metastasize early. Many patients present with neurologic symptoms due to spinal cord compression. Occasionally, one of the several paraneoplastic syndromes is also seen with these tumors. Surgical resection is the mainstay of therapy for noninvasive (stage I) disease. Invasive tumors (stage II) require resection plus radiation therapy, whereas tumors with spread to the opposite hemithorax or distant metastases (stages III and IV) are treated with a combination of surgical debulking, radiation therapy, and chemotherapy. Positive prognostic indicators for neuroblastoma include patients younger than 1 year old and lack of the N-*myc* amplification.

Ganglioneuroblastomas can be broken down into two types according to their cellular composition. *Composite ganglioneuroblastomas* are made up mostly of well-differentiated neuroblasts, whereas *diffuse ganglioneuroblastomas* contain a mixture of well-differentiated and poorly differentiated neuroblasts. Patients with the composite type of tumor have a much worse prognosis, with more than 60% developing metastatic disease. Surgical resection is reserved for patients with stage I or II diffuse type disease. Patients who are older than 3 years, who have stage III/IV disease, or who have composite type tumors are treated with chemotherapy. Ganglioneuromas are benign tumors that arise from the sympathetic chain. These tumors are less common than neurilemomas and are treated with complete surgical resection. Pheochromocytomas are tumors derived from chromaffin cells that actively secrete catecholamines. Ninety percent of these tumors are found in the adrenal medulla, whereas only 2% are found in the chest. Extra-adrenal pheochromocytomas, also called "paragangliomas," most commonly are found in the organ of Zuckerkandl. Mediastinal paragangliomas usually develop in the paravertebral area in the posterior mediastinum, but they may also be found in the pericardium in the middle mediastinum. Unlike adrenal pheochromocytomas, which usually produce epinephrine and norepinephrine, extraadrenal tumors rarely produce epinephrine and often do not produce any hormones. Patients who do present with symptoms typically have uncontrollable hypertension along with palpitations and weight loss. Urinary catecholamines, metanephrines, and vanillylmandelic acid levels usually are elevated and clinch the diagnosis. Tumor localization can be accomplished with chest CT. If hormonally active, iodine-131 MIBG scan can further localize the lesion. The treatment for these tumors is a complete surgical resection. In the 3% of patients who present with metastatic disease, α-methyltyrosine can be used to prevent catecholamine synthesis and reduce some of the symptoms.

The mediastinum is frequently the site for *lymphoma*, either focal or diffuse disease. Patients with Hodgkin and non-Hodgkin lymphomas can present with dyspnea, hoarseness, chest pain, and superior vena cava (SVC) obstruction, as well as fever, chills, and weight loss. A chest x-ray often identifies an anterior or anterosuperior mass in the patient, but MRI and CT scan are necessary to further delineate the lesion. The definitive diagnosis must be made with tissue obtained usually from an open biopsy because fine needle aspirates typically do not supply sufficient material. Hodgkin disease is further subdivided by histologic features into nodular sclerosing, lymphocytic predominant, lymphocyte depleted, and mixed cellularity disease. Stages I and IIa may be treated with radiation therapy with a 10-year survival rate of 90%. Stages IIb, III, and IV are treated primarily with chemotherapy. The treatment for non-Hodgkin lymphoma is systemic chemotherapy. Surgery occasionally is of value for a subset of patients who present with primary mediastinal lymphoma of the B-cell type confined to the mediastinum. Surgical resection is used in combination with chemotherapy for these patients.

Primary *mediastinal germ-cell tumors* are extremely rare tumors usually found in the anterior mediastinum but occasionally seen in the posterior mediastinum. These tumors are histologically identical to tumors that arise in the gonads. They are further separated into teratomas/teratocarcinomas, seminomas, embryonal cell carcinomas, choriocarcinomas, and endodermal cell tumors. Teratomas are tumors comprising cells derived from multiple embryonic germ-cell layers. More than 80% of teratomas are benign, dermoid cysts being the most common. Those that are malignant are often associated with elevated CEA and α-fetoprotein (AFP) levels. Teratomas felt to be benign require resection to rule out malignancy and to prevent local compressive symptoms. Malignant teratomas can be diagnosed with needle biopsies and then treated with a combination of neoadjuvant chemotherapy followed by resection. Preoperative CEA and AFP levels should be obtained on all patients with malignant teratomas. Malignant germ-cell tumors can be further classified as seminomatous and nonseminomatous. These tumors usually arise in men in their 20s and 30s. On presentation, these individuals may complain of chest pain, cough, dyspnea, or hemoptysis. Lesions visualized on chest x-ray are further characterized on MRI and CT scan. A male patient diagnosed with a mediastinal germ-cell tumor should have a thorough physical examination of the testes as well as testicular ultrasonographic evaluation. Any mass identified should be sampled to rule out a primary gonadal cancer. Patients suspected of having a germ-cell tumor should also have β-hCG (human chorionic gonadotropin) and AFP levels ascertained. Elevation of one or both of these markers makes the diagnosis and provides the oncologist with a means to follow the response of the tumor to treatment. Seminomas comprise about one half of all malignant germ-cell tumors. These tumors rarely secrete β-hCG or AFP, and thereby can be distinguished from nonseminomatous lesions. Seminomas usually spread locally within the mediastinum, although late metastases may occur via the lymphatic and blood vessels. The most common sites of metastases are the lung and bone followed less frequently by the brain, spleen, tonsils, and subcutaneous tissue. Surgical resection alone is the treatment for these tumors whenever possible. When tumors are deemed unresectable, radiation therapy is used for tumors confined to the mediastinum, whereas chemotherapy is used in patients with distant metastases, large intrathoracic tumors unlikely to respond to radiation therapy alone, and recurrences.

Malignant nonseminomatous tumors, including choriocarcinoma, embryonal cell carcinoma, malignant teratoma, and endodermal sinus tumors (yolk sac), tend to be significantly more aggressive tumors than seminomas. They tend to produce β-hCG or AFP and are less radiosensitive. Patients usually present with cough, dyspnea, chest pain, fevers/chills, and occasionally SVC syndrome if the tumor is sufficiently large. Similar to patients with seminomas, most patients with nonseminomatous tumors are men in their 30s and 40s. These tumors occasionally are found in association with chromosomal abnormalities (Klinefelter and trisomy syndromes) as well as rare hematologic malignancies. Nonseminomatous tumors often invade the chest wall and tend to metastasize early to the brain, lung, liver, and bone. Surgical resection is rarely possible as initial therapy. The function of the surgeon is typically to make a tissue diagnosis. Often patients have residual disease resected following chemotherapy, to which most patients respond. A patient is a candidate for resection if the level of marker noted to be elevated prior to treatment has returned to a normal value. Chemotherapy followed by surgical resection has yielded up to a 40% long-term survival rate in some studies, but patients with recurrent or persistent disease have a mean survival time of less than 6 months regardless of therapy. Some nonseminomatous tumors may also contain a focus of adenocarcinoma or sarcoma that is not responsive to chemotherapy. This too is associated with a worse prognosis.

Primary mediastinal carcinoma makes up approximately 5% of all mediastinal masses. Although the origin of the tumors is unknown, most of these masses are composed of undifferentiated large cells. The most important aspect in diagnosing these tumors is to differentiate them from other mediastinal tumors such as lymphomas and metastatic cancer. Most patients have symptoms secondary to local mass effect. When found, these tumors tend to have thoracic spread as well as distant metastases. Most lesions are not resectable and even with chemotherapy and radiation therapy, patients' survival time is less than 1 year. In this category thymic carcinoma must be distinguished from thymoma, a different neoplasm altogether. Whereas the microscopic appearance of a thymoma is that of bland thymocytes, a thymic carcinoma comprises frankly malignant cells with nuclear and cytologic findings characteristic of a malignancy.

Cysts can also be seen in the mediastinum. The most common *mediastinal cysts* include *bronchogenic cysts and esophageal duplication cysts*, which are part of the spectrum of bronchopulmonary foregut abnormalities, a category that also includes pulmonary sequestration. These cysts contain cartilage and mucous glands and are lined with epithelium, the exact type being responsible for the cyst classification. They almost never communicate directly with the bronchus or esophagus. Most patients are asymptomatic upon presentation. When symptoms do occur, they usually do so secondary to local compression or infection. Surgical resection is required to rule out malignancy and to prevent complications later in life. Malignant degeneration is often mentioned but probably occurs rarely if ever in these cysts. Pericardial cysts are the next most frequently found lesions in the middle mediastinum.

They usually occur at the pericardiophrenic angles with a predilection for the right side. Some patients have been managed with simple needle aspiration, but surgical resection is generally recommended to rule out malignancy. Usually, this may be accomplished with a video-assisted thoracoscopic procedure. Care must be taken to avoid injury to the phrenic nerve during resection.

CONGENITAL CHEST WALL DEFORMITIES

The most common congenital abnormality of the chest wall is *pectus excavatum*, a concave depression of the lower sternum. The pathophysiology of this condition is thought to result from an overgrowth of costal cartilages during chest wall development. The cartilages have a greater than normal longitudinal growth phase. Because of this, the sternum becomes depressed more posterior than normal. If a deformity is significant, it is apparent by 3 years of age. Over the years, the significance of pectus excavatum has been a subject of debate. Most suggest that pulmonary function studies performed at both stress and rest are either normal or mildly abnormal. Even children with some of the most severe defects have only mildly decreased pulmonary function tests. Children typically present with an abnormal physical deformity of their chest but appear otherwise well. They are typically active and sometimes have a vague complaint of chest pain. Most are concerned about the cosmetic appearance. A physical examination will demonstrate the obvious defect. Serial chest x-rays have been useful in documenting the progression or compression/displacement of the heart or lungs. CT scan has been used to grade severity via a measurement of the depth of the depression compared to the overall thoracic cavity. The ratio of the distance between the sternum and vertebral bodies and the overall transverse diameter of the chest has been used to create an index of severity. A child without the deformity will have a ratio less than 2.5, whereas children with severe deformities can reach ratios as high as 6. Indications for an operative repair include exercise intolerance, cosmetic concerns, cardiac abnormalities, psychological distress or the future need for a median sternotomy (Marfan syndrome). The timing of the operation has been controversial. Surgeons have reported good results in both school age children and after puberty and a child's growth spurt. The operation has been performed via open and minimally invasive techniques. Because the abnormality resides at the level of the costal cartilage, the operation involves resection, or partial resection, of all involved costal cartilage, a sternal osteotomy to allow the sternum, now freed of attachments, to be brought back to a normal anatomic position, and fixation of the sternum in the normal position by one of various techniques. (6 to 8 weeks). A support bar may need to be removed at a subsequent operation. Results are generally excellent with patient satisfaction very high.

Pectus carinatum, conversely, is an anterior displacement of the chest wall also caused by an overgrowth of the costal cartilage. This is seen much less commonly than the excavatum deformity and individuals tend to present for evaluation for repair at an older age. There have been no clinically significant physiologic defects associated with pectus carinatum. The indication for operative repair has been one of cosmesis.

KEY CONCEPTS

▲ Prethoracotomy pulmonary function tests need forced expiratory volume at 1 second (FEV_1) >2 L, >1 L, >600 mL for pneumonectomy, lobectomy, wedge resection, respectively. Need postoperative $FEV_1 > 0.8$.

▲ Adenocarcinoma is the number one cause of malignancy.

▲ Signs of inoperability in lung cancer are bloody pleural effusion, Horner syndrome, vocal cord paralysis, superior vena cava (SVC) syndrome, distant metastases.

▲ Tension pneumothorax in the operating room presents as:
  ● Increasing inspiratory pressures
  ● Hypoxia
  ● Hyper capnia
  ● Hypotension
  ● Tracheal deviation

  ● Distended neck veins
  ● Decreased breath sounds
  ● Arrest and death if not recognized and treated

▲ Resection of the thymus in myasthenia improves symptoms in more than 80% of cases, regardless of the presence of a thymoma.

▲ Diaphragmatic rupture from blunt trauma: left > right; diagnosis via chest x-ray, treat with a laparotomy

▲ Indications for thoracotomy for hemothorax:
  ● Instability
  ● $>1,500$ mL output initially
  ● >200 mL per hour for 4 to 6 hours
  ● Incompletely drained hemothorax despite two functioning chest tubes

---

SUGGESTED READINGS

Cameron JL, ed. *Current surgical therapy*. St Louis: Mosby, 2001.

Kaiser LK, Kron IL, Spray TL, eds. *Mastery of cardiothoracic surgery*. Philadelphia: Lippincott Williams & Wilkins, 1998.

Oldham KT, Colombani PM, Foglia RP, eds. *Surgery of infants and children*. Philadelphia: Lippincott Williams & Wilkins, 1998.

Pass HI, Mitchell JB, Johnson DH, et al., eds. *Lung cancer: principles and practice*. Philadelphia: Lippincott Williams & Wilkins, 2000.

Sabiston DC, Lyerly HK eds. *Surgery: the biological basis of modern surgical practice*. Philadelphia: WB Saunders, 1997.

Genitourinary System 26

C. William Schwab II   Keith N. Van Arsdalen

ANATOMY

The *kidneys* are derived embryologically from the metanephric blastema. They are paired, bean-shaped organs obliquely positioned in the high retroperitoneum along the lateral border of the psoas muscle and are protected by the lower rib cage and overlying musculature. The hilum of the kidney is located medially and is the entry and exit point for the renal pelvis, artery, and vein. The right kidney is closely related to the liver, right adrenal gland, psoas muscle, duodenum, and the ascending colon. The left kidney is closely related to the spleen, left adrenal gland, the tail of the pancreas, and the descending colon (Fig. 26-1). The right kidney is usually more caudal than the left because of the large size of the liver. The kidneys and the perirenal fat are contained within the Gerota fascia, a layer that also invests the adrenal gland superiorly and the ureter and gonadal vessels inferiorly. This fascia serves as a possible barrier to the spread of infection and malignancy from the kidney to other retroperitoneal structures. It may also act to tamponade potentially life-threatening hemorrhage originating from the kidney or the adrenal gland.

The arterial supply to the kidneys is derived directly from the aorta, inferior to the superior mesenteric artery. The right renal artery takes off from the aorta superior to the left renal artery and travels in a caudal direction posterior to the vena cava to reach the hilum. The left artery is shorter than the right because of the kidney's proximity to the aorta. The renal artery is usually single but may be paired, leading to considerations during cadaveric or living renal donation. The renal artery branches into the segmental, lobar, arcuate, and interlobular arteries. The interlobular arteries in turn supply blood to the glomeruli via the afferent arterioles (Fig. 26-2). The renal arteries are all end arteries.

Glomerular blood drains from the efferent arterioles into interlobular, arcuate, interlobar, and segmental veins, which join to form the main renal vein. The renal vein is located anterior to the artery and is shorter on the right side because of the kidney's proximity to the vena cava. The left renal vein typically drains the left adrenal vein, the left gonadal vein, and lumbar branches. Failure to ligate these branches can lead to considerable intraoperative hemorrhage during nephrectomy. Lymphatic drainage of the kidneys follows the venous drainage. The *adrenal* gland usually is located within Gerota fascia superomedially to the kidney. However, it is derived independently

from neuroendocrine origins, and, in cases of renal ectopia, the adrenal gland will preserve its absolute location rather than its relation to the kidney. Similarly, congenital absence of the kidney is not associated with absence of the ipsilateral adrenal gland. The adrenal gland is composed of a cortex and medulla. The cortex is divided into three zones: the zona glomerulosa, the zona fasciculata, and the zona reticularis. These zones produce mineralocorticoids, glucocorticoids, and sex steroids, respectively. The adrenal medulla produces epinephrine under the control of the sympathetic nervous system. Each adrenal gland may receive an artery from the aorta, the renal artery, and/or the phrenic artery. The adrenal vein on the left drains into the renal vein, and, on the right, it drains directly into the vena cava. The branch on the right may be difficult to control and can be a source of significant intraoperative bleeding. Lymphatic drainage follows the venous channels.

Urine drains from the collecting ducts through the pyramids emptying at the renal papillae into minor calyces. These unite to form the major calyces, which drain via infundibula to form the renal pelvis. The renal pelvis is located posterior to the renal vein and artery, and it drains into the ureter at the ureteropelvic junction. The ureter is an approximately 30-cm long tubular structure the function of which is the low-pressure transfer of urine in an antegrade fashion to the bladder. The collecting system and ureter are lined with a transitional cell epithelium. Surrounding this layer is a muscular layer and an adventitial layer. The ureter courses along the posterior psoas muscle and enters the bony pelvis at the level of the bifurcation of the iliac vessels. It passes posterior to the cecum and ascending colon on the right and to the sigmoid and descending colon on the left, and then enters the bladder posterolaterally. There are three relative narrowings of the ureteral lumen: at the ureteropelvic junction, at the level of the iliac vessels, and at the ureterovesical junction. It is at these three sites that ureteral calculi will most commonly lodge.

The blood supply to the ureter is derived from many arteries, most commonly the renal artery, the gonadal artery, the aorta, the hypogastric artery, and the vesical arteries. The blood supply approaches the ureter from the medial side proximally and from the lateral side distally. When the ureter is mobilized, care must be taken not to disrupt the adventitia, where distal branches of the blood supply of the ureter anastomose.

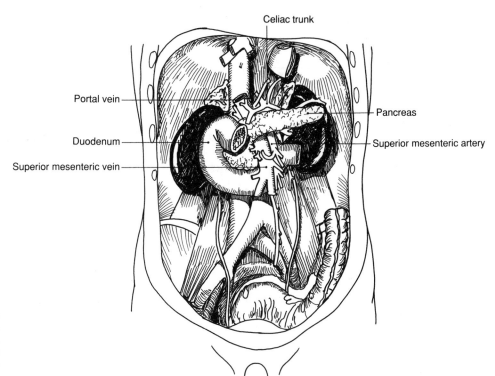

Figure 26-1 Relations of the kidney to adjacent organs. (From Scott-Connor C, Dawson DL, eds. *Operative anatomy.* Philadelphia: JB Lippincott, 1993:511, with permission.)

The *urinary bladder* is a hollow muscular pelvic organ the function of which is twofold: (i) low-pressure storage of urine and (ii) expulsion of urine at a socially opportune time. The adult bladder typically stores 350 to 550 mL. The bladder is derived from the urogenital sinus. During early development it is connected to the umbilicus by the urachus. This subsequently obliterates to form the median umbilical ligament. The umbilical arteries likewise obliterate to form the lateral umbilical ligaments. The bladder is lined with a transitional epithelium and has a thick muscular

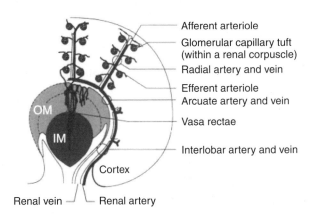

Figure 26-2 Schematic diagram of the major blood vessels supplying the kidney. All the glomeruli are located in the cortex and are supplied by the afferent arteriole arising as a branch of the renal artery. The peritubular capillary network arising from the glomeruli in the outer regions of the cortex remains confined to the cortex, whereas the capillary network of the glomeruli located next to the corticomedullary junction penetrates deep into the medulla in a series of hairpin loops known as "vasa recta." OM, outer medulla; IM, inner medulla. (From Johnson LR. *Essential medical physiology.* Philadelphia: Lippincott Williams & Wilkins, 1998:309, with permission.)

layer made up of inner and outer longitudinal and middle circular layers. The serosa of the bladder is surrounded by the perivesical fat and fascia, which is proximate to the peritoneum cephalad, the space of Retzius anteroinferiorly, and the rectum posteriorly in men. In women, the vagina is posterior, with the uterus lying posterior and superior. The bladder has a rich blood supply derived mainly from the superior, middle, and inferior vesical arteries, branches of the internal iliac (hypogastric) artery. Obturator, gluteal, uterine, or vaginal branches may also supply the bladder. Venous drainage is via the vesical plexus into the internal iliac (hypogastric) vein. Lymphatic drainage is primarily to the external iliac chain but may also include the obturator and internal iliac chains. The innervation of the smooth muscle of the bladder is autonomic, with sacral parasympathetic innervation initiating the contraction of the bladder. Extensive perivesical dissection during pelvic surgery (e.g., abdominoperineal resection) can lead to bladder atony and resultant urinary retention.

The *prostate* is a small organ located deep in the male pelvis. It abuts the bladder at its outlet and surrounds the prostatic urethra. Its anatomic relations are the bony pelvis anteriorly (puboprostatic ligaments), the rectum and seminal vesicles posteriorly, and the bladder cephalad. The verumontanum is the exit point of the ejaculatory duct, which empties sperm and seminal fluid from the vas deferens and the seminal vesicles, respectively.

The prostate can be divided into several zones. The most common sites of pathology are the transition zone [most frequent site of benign prostatic hyperplasia (BPH)] and the peripheral zone (most frequent site of adenocarcinoma of the prostate).

The blood supply of the prostate is mainly from the inferior vesical artery, and the venous drainage is via the pelvic plexus of Santorini. The venous drainage of the penis, the deep dorsal venous complex, travels anterior to the prostate, and its careful ligation is necessary during radical retropubic prostatectomy. The lymphatic drainage of the prostate is to the obturator and external iliac lymph nodes. This explains the common practice of pelvic lymph node dissection prior to radical prostatectomy. Lying posteriorly and cephalad to the prostate are the seminal vesicles. These paired organs join the ipsilateral vas deferens to form the ejaculatory duct, which traverses the prostate.

The *penis* is composed of the two erectile bodies, the *corpora cavernosa* and the *corpus spongiosum*, which contains the urethra and is contiguous with the glans penis. The corpora derive their blood supply from the internal pudendal artery.

The *male urethra* can be divided into two portions: posterior (prostatic and membranous) and anterior (bulbar, penile, and glanular). The prostatic urethra includes the portion from the bladder neck to the verumontanum. The membranous urethra continues to just past the external urinary sphincter and is the most common site of urethral disruption in pelvic trauma. These portions are derived from mesodermal origin and are lined with transitional cell epithelium. The bulbous urethra is the most common site of postgonococcal urethral stricture. It is somewhat dilated and continues until the corpus spongiosum becomes adherent to the underside of the fused corpora cavernosa. The penile urethra continues along the length of the penile shaft, where the glanular urethra dilates at the fossa navicularis. The bulbar and penile urethra are derived from endodermal origins and are lined with stratified columnar epithelium, and the fossa is derived from ectodermal origins and is lined with squamous cell epithelium. The blood supply to the posterior urethra is from the inferior vesical artery, and the anterior urethra from the bulbar branch of the internal pudendal artery. Lymphatic drainage of the posterior urethra is to obturator and iliac nodes, and the anterior urethra to superficial and deep inguinal nodes.

The *scrotum* (male equivalent of labia majora) is a pouch-like structure inferior to the penis that serves to maintain the homeostasis of the testes, which are contained in the two separate compartments of the scrotum. The muscular dartos layer of the scrotum is continuous with the Colles fascia in the perineum and with the Scarpa fascia in the abdominal wall. Fournier gangrene may track via these fascial planes but virtually never affects the testes. Blood supply to the scrotum is via the external pudendal artery. The scrotum is innervated by the ilioinguinal and genitofemoral nerves. Inadvertent injury of the genitofemoral nerve during inguinal hernia repair presents as numbness of the lateral scrotum and medial thigh.

The *testes* are paired ovoid-shaped organs normally located in the scrotum, the function of which is the production of sperm for transport through the epididymis and vas deferens into the urethra during ejaculation. The tubules of the testis are surrounded by a dense layer of tissue called the tunica albuginea. The blood vessels and nerves supplying the testis travel in the spermatic cord. The blood supply to the testis includes the gonadal (testicular) artery, deferential artery, and cremasteric artery.

The parenchyma of the testis consists of Leydig cells and seminiferous tubules. Leydig cells are responsible for the production of testosterone under the influence of gonadotropins. The seminiferous tubules contain Sertoli cells and germ cells. The Sertoli cells function as support cells in spermatogenesis. The seminiferous tubules are the site of spermatogenesis and connect to the rete testis, which connects to the epididymis. Sperm travel through the epididymis into the vas deferens, until they are expelled into the posterior urethra during emission.

RENAL PHYSIOLOGY

The kidney is an organ with myriad functions. Its main purpose is homeostatic, and the kidney is integral in the regulation of intravascular volume, salt and water balance, and control of blood pressure. It acts to rid the body of acids and other byproducts of normal metabolism, and it degrades exogenous substances, including many pharmacologic agents. It serves as an endocrine organ, secreting several hormones, including erythropoietin and renin.

The most obvious function of the kidney is urine production. The kidneys receive about 20% of the resting cardiac output, approximatley 1,440 L of blood per day. Approximately 20% of this plasma is filtered at the glomeruli to create a glomerular filtrate of about 170 L per day. Unfiltered plasma leaves the glomerulus via the efferent arteriole into the postglomerular capillaries. Approximately 99% of the filtrate is reabsorbed by passive and active forces along the length of the nephron ultimately creating 1 to 2 L of urine per day.

Renal blood flow (RBF) travels through the renal artery into the interlobar, arcuate, interlobular, and afferent arterioles before entering the glomerulus, where the plasma is filtered. The filtration fraction, or renal plasma flow (RPF) divided by glomerular filtration rate (GFR), is dependent on the oncotic and hydrostatic forces acting in the glomerulus (g) and Bowman space (bs), which determine the pressure for ultrafiltration (P_{uf}). Increased hydrostatic forces (P) within the glomerulus increase P_{uf}, and increased P within the Bowman space decreases P_{uf}. Because the glomerulus is located between the afferent and efferent arterioles, changes in the arteriolar resistances can have a significant impact on the filtration fraction. The glomerular basement membrane is impermeable to most proteins; therefore, oncotic forces play a role in filtration. Increased oncotic pressure (π) within the glomerulus decreases P_{uf}, whereas increased π within Bowman space increases P_{uf}. In general, $P_{uf} = [(P_g-P_{bs})-(\pi_g-\pi_{bs})]$. Because the act of filtration changes the P and π along the glomerulus, the fraction of the plasma filtered per unit length decreases.

The GFR is the volume of plasma that is filtered into Bowman space per unit time. Given a substance that is freely filtered at the glomerulus and neither secreted nor absorbed, the GFR is equal to the clearance of that solute, defined as the volume of plasma that is cleared of that substance per unit time. Creatinine is a plasma solute that is for practical purposes neither secreted nor absorbed, and thus creatinine clearance ($U_{cr}V/P_{cr}$) is an excellent proxy for GFR. Knowing the patient's age, weight (in kilograms), and plasma creatinine concentration, an alternative to estimate creatinine clearance can be done with a simple formula: GFR = $[(140-age) \times (body\ weight)]/(72 \times P_{cr})$.

The glomerular filtrate flows through the various segments of the nephron, where all but a fraction of 1% of the filtrate is reabsorbed. In the proximal convoluted tubule

(PCT), almost three fourths of the glomerular filtrate is reabsorbed by passive diffusion. In the loop of Henle, energy is consumed to reabsorb salt in greater proportion than water in order to make a relatively dilute, hypoosmotic urine and to create the hyperosmotic medullary gradient necessary for countercurrent exchange and urine concentration. In the distal convoluted tubule (DCT), the fine tuning of salt and water reabsorption occurs, and the final urine may be as dilute as one third or as concentrated as fourfold the osmolality of plasma.

Several hormones and neural stimuli act on the nephron to regulate electrolytes and blood pressure. The *renin-angiotensin-aldosterone* series of hormones is interdependent and sensitive to volume status. Renin is produced in the juxtaglomerular apparatus (a specialized group of cells located at the afferent arteriole of each nephron) in response to stimuli caused by decreased intravascular volume, namely decreased hydrostatic pressure in the afferent arteriole, decreased salt delivery to the macula densa of the distal tubule, and increased sympathetic tone. Renin cleaves angiotensinogen to form angiotensin I. This peptide is metabolized to form angiotensin II in the lung. Angiotensin II is a powerful peripheral vasoconstrictor. In the kidney its effect is mainly on the efferent arteriole. It reduces renal sodium excretion by increasing its reabsorption by proximal tubules. Angiotensin II also acts on the zona glomerulosa of the adrenal gland to stimulate secretion of aldosterone, a potent mineralocorticoid that increases sodium reabsorption and potassium secretion in the collecting duct. The net effect is an increase in intravascular volume.

Increased *sympathetic tone* causes afferent arteriolar vasoconstriction, leading to decreased RBF and GFR. Furthermore, increased sympathetic tone promotes renin secretion and proximal tubular reabsorption of sodium. These changes cause decreased delivery of salt and water to the distal nephron.

Atrial natriuretic factor (ANF) is a polypeptide secreted by the atrium in response to stretch, increased sodium concentration, and other stimuli related to hypervolemia. It causes a salt and water diuresis as well as a significant peripheral vasodilation, and it inhibits renin secretion and antidiuretic hormone (ADH) action.

ADH is released by the posterior pituitary gland (neurohypophysis), mainly in response to osmotic stimuli on the hypothalamus, although some regulation by volume stimuli has also been recognized. ADH makes the collecting duct permeable to water, which is reabsorbed into the medulla because of the high concentration of medullary solutes. Without the medullary concentration gradient, ADH cannot function and the concentrating ability of the kidney is hampered. The syndrome of inappropriate ADH secretion causes an inappropriately concentrated urine in the face of plasma hyposmolality. Diabetes insipidus, or a lack of ADH action, leads to polyuria from a defect in renal concentration ability.

HOMEOSTASIS

The aforementioned agents act in concert with several other factors to regulate the electrolyte homeostasis. The balance of *sodium* is regulated by factors affected primarily by intravascular volume. An increase in intravascular volume triggers baroreceptors and receptors in the juxtaglomerular apparatus, leading to the following changes, which increase the excretion of sodium:

1. Increased RBF, RPF, and glomerular hydrostatic pressure, all of which lead to increased GFR.
2. Decreased renin and aldosterone levels, which cause decreased reabsorption of sodium in the PCT and collecting duct, respectively.
3. Increased ANF level, which leads to increased sodium excretion by increasing delivery of salt to the distal tubule and by inhibiting ADH action.
4. Decreased sympathetic tone, which leads to increased GFR, decreased PCT sodium reabsorption, and increased delivery of sodium to the distal nephron.

Water balance is responsible primarily for the sodium concentration and osmolality of the plasma, and it is appropriately regulated by osmoreceptors in the hypothalamus. The osmolality of the plasma is a function of the concentration of solutes that do not freely cross the cell membrane. The main determinants of the osmolality of plasma are sodium and glucose. Plasma osmolality can be estimated using the simple formula $(2 \times [Na^+]) + ([glucose]/18) + ([urea]/2.8)$.

Increased osmolality triggers the osmoreceptors, leading to increased thirst for free water, as well as the release of ADH from the anterior pituitary. ADH acts to make the collecting duct permeable to water, thereby allowing the urine to equilibrate with the medullary concentration gradient. This causes reabsorption of free water and concentration of the urine.

Potassium is mainly an intracellular ion. Plasma potassium concentration in the short term is mainly dependent on shifts of the extracellular store of potassium into and out of the intracellular store. Factors that cause a shift of potassium into cells, thus decreasing the plasma potassium level are as follows:

1. Alkalosis, by driving protons out of the cell. This increases the positive charge gradient for potassium to move into the cell.
2. Insulin level, by increasing the active cotransport of glucose and potassium into cells.

Factors that may cause a shift of potassium out of the intracellular space, thereby increasing plasma potassium, include the following:

1. Acidosis, by driving protons into the cell. This decreases the positive charge gradient for potassium to move into the cell.
2. Cell lysis, by rapidly releasing intracellular potassium. This may occur during certain pathologic states such as transfusion reaction and rhabdomyolysis.

The total body store of potassium is dependent on intake and excretion. The excretion of potassium by the kidney occurs primarily in the distal tubule and collecting duct. It is almost solely dependent on two factors. They are as follows:

1. Aldosterone level. Aldosterone makes the collecting duct permeable to potassium, leading to passage of potassium from the cells of the collecting duct into the urine.

2. Urine flow rate in the collecting duct. The increased flow of urine leads to a washout of the potassium gradient in the collecting duct, causing an increase in the secretion of potassium at this site.

Byproducts of normal metabolism lead to a significant *acid load*, which must be excreted each day. This is accomplished by the secretion of hydrogen ions, the reabsorption of bicarbonate, and the buffering of the urine with ammonium in the distal tubule. In response to acid loads, the body maintains *acid–base homeostasis* in several ways. The pH level of the plasma is dependent on the concentration of bicarbonate and carbon dioxide. In response to an acid load, the body has a short-term and a long-term response. In the short term, the acid load is buffered by the bicarbonate buffer system. Furthermore, increased ventilation causes a decrease in plasma carbon dioxide concentration. In the long term, acid loads are neutralized by increased bicarbonate reabsorption in the kidney, a process that is dependent on a sodium-proton exchange and on carbonic anhydrase.

The kidney is responsible for significant regulation of calcium balance. It metabolizes 25-hydroxy vitamin D to its highly active form, 1,25-dihydroxy vitamin D. Furthermore, under the regulation of parathyroid hormone (PTH), it excretes most of the daily calcium load. PTH increases renal tubular reabsorption of calcium, thereby increasing the serum calcium level.

Erythropoietin is secreted by the kidney in response to decreased oxygen delivery to the renal cortex. This hormone acts on the bone marrow to increase the production of erythrocytes. Patients with chronic renal failure may have anemia responsive to exogenous erythropoietin because of their decreased viable renal parenchyma. Erythropoietin secretion by renal cell carcinoma may cause a paraneoplastic polycythemia.

DIURETICS

Diuretics cause the excretion of salt and water in addition to what the kidney would excrete under normal physiologic conditions. There are several classes of diuretics. *Loop diuretics* (such as furosemide) work by inhibiting the active transport of sodium in the thick ascending limb. This deactivates the medullary concentration gradient (rendering ADH ineffective) and increases the delivery of salt to the collecting duct. The result is a salt and water diuresis. Chronic use of loop diuretics can cause hypokalemia because of the increased secretion of potassium secondary to increased urine flow in the collecting duct.

Thiazide diuretics (such as hydrochlorothiazide) act in the distal nephron. Their mechanism of action is incompletely understood. *Osmotic diuretics* (such as mannitol) are osmotically active particles that are filtered but not reabsorbed by the kidney. The osmotic pressure within the nephron causes an obligate loss of free water.

Potassium-sparing diuretics (such as spironolactone and amiloride) inhibit aldosterone action. This causes an increase in sodium excretion and a decrease in potassium excretion. Often a loop diuretic is formulated with a potassium-sparing diuretic to mitigate the potassium wasting effects of the former.

ACUTE RENAL FAILURE

Acute renal failure is a precipitious deterioration in renal function that results in the retention of nitrogenous wastes and/or a failure to regulate the extracellular fluid volume/composition. Renal failure may be classified according to its various causes as prerenal, intrarenal, or postrenal. *Prerenal failure* (prerenal azotemia) is caused by a decreased blood flow to the kidneys. This may be secondary to decreased intravascular volume, decreased cardiac output, or relative vasodilation of the peripheral vasculature. Decreased renal blood flow leads to the conservation of salt via an increased sympathetic tone and increased renin/angiotensin II/aldosterone activity by decreasing the amount of glomerular filtrate but increasing the filtration fraction, and thus the reabsorption in the PCT. The increase in resorption by the PCT [which passively resorbs blood urea nitrogen (BUN) but not creatinine] is greater than the decrease in GFR; therefore, the BUN level rises faster than the creatinine level. A BUN-creatinine ratio of greater than 20:1 is typical in prerenal azotemia.

Intrarenal failure is caused by reversible or irreversible insults to the kidneys. Common medical etiologies include acute glomerulonephritides, acute vasculidities, or acute interstitial nephritidies. The vast majority of hospital-acquired intrarenal failure is caused by acute tubular necrosis. Etiologies include: hypoxia, drug toxicity, myoglobinuria, profound hypotension, and sepsis. Intrarenal failure may cause oliguria but rarely causes complete anuria.

Postrenal failure is caused by urinary tract obstruction. This obstruction may occur at any level of the collecting system, ureter, or bladder outlet. Causes of obstruction include stones, tumors, extrinsic compression by tumor or retroperitoneal fibrosis, and bladder outlet obstruction from prostatism, urethral stricture, or detrusor failure. The cause and completeness of the obstruction, the rapidity of onset, and the duration of obstruction are important determinants of reversibility. Complete acute obstruction of one ureter usually leads to a temporary increase of the serum creatinine level followed by a gradual return to the baseline caused by contralateral renal compensation. True anuria in a patient with two normal kidneys suggests bladder outlet obstruction or bilateral ureteral obstruction, which is rare. In cases of suspected postrenal failure, the passage of a Foley catheter should confirm or exclude the possibility of bladder outlet obstruction. Renal ultrasonography can suggest upper tract obstruction by showing hydronephrosis and hydroureter. Obstruction can be confirmed by diuretic renogram, intravenous urogram, or by antegrade/retrograde pyelography. Upper tract obstruction may be relieved percutaneously or by retrograde placement of ureteral stents. Bladder outlet obstruction may be relieved by placement of a Foley or suprapubic catheter. Prompt relief of acute obstruction usually leads to a return to normal renal function, although it may sometimes require several weeks for the serum creatinine concentration to reach its nadir.

Relief of bilateral upper tract obstruction may lead to a brisk postobstructive diuresis. A temporary concentrating defect in the kidney leads to derangements in serum electrolytes and volume status. Most patients who are alert and have relatively short-term obstruction may be followed as outpatients, as their thirst and hunger mechanisms will compensate for renal losses of sodium, potassium, and water. Obtunded, elderly, or demented patients, as well as those with long-term obstruction, require intravenous fluids and close monitoring of electrolytes.

IATROGENIC INJURIES

Ureteral iatrogenic injury occurs most commonly during abdominal hysterectomy or vascular procedures, but it may also occur during other operations for inflammatory bowel disease, diverticulitis, pelvic malignancy, or during ureteroscopy. Uncontrolled blood loss and inflammatory or neoplastic processes are obvious risk factors. Preoperative imaging and ureteral stenting can reduce risk of injury and improve intraoperative recognition of ureteral injuries. Principles of repair are similar to those for external trauma, and, as always, the condition of the patient as well as other complicating factors should be considered.

When a ureteral injury is detected early, surgical repair should be attempted. If a clip is placed on the ureter and immediately recognized, it may be removed and treated with only ureteral stenting. If there is any question about the severity of a crush injury to the ureter, urology consultation should be obtained. Excision of the affected segment and reanastomosis may be necessary. Upper and middle ureteral injuries can be managed with débridement and end-to-end anastomosis. Distal injuries should be managed with ureteral reimplantation with a psoas hitch or a Boari flap. In case of multiple injuries or loss of a large segment of ureter, nephrectomy should be considered. A ureteral injury during a vascular procedure with fresh prosthetic material should prompt serious consideration of ipsilateral nephrectomy, particularly if the contralateral kidney has normal function. In certain situations (i.e., a patient with a solitary kidney) one might consider an ileal-ureter interposition, autotransplantation, or ureteral ligation with subsequent placement of a nephrostomy tube to allow for delayed/staged repair. Transureteroureterostomy should be performed rarely because of the risk it may place on the unaffected renal unit, particularly in patients with a history of kidney stone disease or transitional cell carcinoma of the ipsilateral unit. All ureteral repairs should be coupled with urinary diversion with a ureteral stent or a percutaneous nephrostomy tube.

Treatment of recognized *iatrogentic injuries to the bladder* depends on severity of injury as well as the presence of other injuries that may require exploration. Small cystotomies at the dome of the bladder can be primarily repaired in two layers. Larger injuries require exploration. The bladder must be opened widely in order to inspect its entire mucosal surface and ureteral orifices. All devitalized tissue should be débrided and the bladder wall should be closed in two layers with absorbable suture. A suprapubic tube ensures maximal drainage of the healing bladder, and a surgical drain should be used until the healing of the injury can be confirmed with a cystogram 1 to 2 weeks postoperatively.

EMERGENCY ROOM UROLOGY

Urologic emergencies are rare but torsion of the testis (more properly, torsion of the spermatic cord), priapism, and Fournier gangrene can often present in an acute fashion and lead to significant morbidity if not treated properly. Torsion of the testis is a surgical emergency. It typically occurs in young adolescents, but it may occur in any age group. The underlying etiology is a congenital defect of the gubernaculum of the testis and of the insertion of the spermatic cord on the testis (the "bell clapper" deformity). The typical patient will present in the emergency room with a brief history of the sudden onset of unilateral testis pain relieved by nothing. The pain is often associated with nausea and vomiting. Physical examination is difficult because of the pain but will show a tense testis that is high riding in the scrotum, as well as a "knot" in the spermatic cord secondary to volvulus. The cremasteric reflex is invariably absent in torsion of the testis. Urinalysis is typically negative for blood or white blood cells.

The differential diagnosis of acute scrotal pain includes intermittent torsion, torsion of an appendix testis, epididymoorchitis, and trauma. History of fevers, sexually transmitted diseases (STDs), urethral discharge, or white blood cell on urinalysis strongly suggest an infectious process but do not rule out torsion. Patients with torsion of an appendix testis will have point pain and tenderness and may have a dark spot on the testis visible through the scrotal skin (the "blue dot sign"). Radiographic imaging may be useful in cases where the diagnosis is in question. Doppler ultrasonography will show a lack of blood flow to the torsioned testis. Nuclear scan will show a photopenic area in the hemiscrotum of the torsed testis.

Although manual detorsion may be attempted in the emergency room, the definitive treatment of testicular torsion is immediate exploration. The affected side is explored first and detorsion performed. If there is question of viability of the testis, it is placed to the side in a moist sponge while the other testis is exposed. The contralateral testis is fixed to the scrotum in three spots with nonabsorbable suture because of the risk of subsequent contralateral torsion. After the contralateral orchiopexy, the torsioned testis is either removed (if nonviable) or fixed to the scrotal wall in a similar fashion.

Priapism is defined as a prolonged erection, not necessarily related to arousal, that will not detumesce in response to climax. It generally involves only the corpora cavernosa. It can occur at any age. There are two types of priapism: low flow and high flow. Low-flow priapism is an ischemic state caused by venous congestion and may be idiopathic or due to sickle cell trait/disease, malignancy, drugs, neurologic disorders, or even total parenteral nutrition administration. The patient usually complains of a painful erection of several hours' duration. Timely detumescence is important because of a rising risk of corporal fibrosis in untreated priapism.

The immediate treatment involves aspiration of hypoxic blood from the corporal bodies and injection of an alpha agonist (often phenylephrine) to cause vasoconstriction of the corporal arteries. A 19-gauge butterfly needle is inserted laterally into the corpora cavernosa and aspiration of blood from the corpora is performed until bright red blood is aspirated. The perforated septum between the corpora will allow effective drainage of both bodies. Blood gas analysis of an aliquot of the initial aspiration should be obtained to diagnose and document low or high flow priapism. Blood obtained from low flow priapism will reveal hypoxia and acidosis. Irrigation of the corpora with sterile saline can be useful. A dilute solution of phenylephrine (1 mg in 40 mL of normal saline) is prepared and injected into the cavernosa in boluses of approximately 250 μg. This may be repeated at 3 to 5 minute intervals. Detumescence should quickly ensue. Failure to respond to treatment with aspiration/irrigation/alpha-agonist therapy is approached with the surgical creation of one of a variety of shunts from the corpus cavernosum to the corpus spongiosum.

High-flow priapism is usually caused by trauma and results from rupture of a cavernous artery. Treatment involves angiography and embolization of the involved artery. Because this is a nonischemic state, aspiration will reveal bright red blood and fibrosis is usually not a complication.

Fournier gangrene is a rapidly spreading, gangrenous infection arising in the external genitalia and/or the perineal tissues. Most patients are older than age 50 and have some type of systemic disease, most commonly diabetes. The infection is typically an extension from a urinary, abdominal, perianal or retroperitoneal source. Both aerobic and anerobic organizms may be involved. The patient usually presents with fever and progressive scrotal swelling. The scrotum is markedly swollen and ecchymotic, and areas of necrosis or crepitus may be present. Plain film, ultrasonography, or computerized tomographic (CT) scanning may show air in the affected areas. If allowed to progress, the infection tracks along the Colles fascia of the perineum and may extend to Scarpa fascia of the abdomen. Broad-spectrum antibiotics are helpful, but surgery is the definitive treatment and consists of aggressive débridement and drainage, with repeated trips to the operating room as needed for further débridement. The prognosis for these patients is poor, and mortality rates as high as 50% may be expected.

UROLOGIC NEOPLASMS

Many benign and malignant neoplasms arise from the genitourinary organs. Those that are encountered most frequently by the general surgeon include benign and malignant renal masses, transitional cell carcinoma, tumors of the testis, adenocarcinoma of the prostate, and benign prostatic hypertrophy.

Renal masses may be found during imaging for hematuria or flank pain or more commonly as incidental findings during imaging for nonurologic reasons. The incidence of renal mass increased several-fold after the advent of cross-sectional imaging. Most renal masses are cysts, which may be simple, with an imperceptible wall and without septations, or complex, a term describing cysts with wall thickening, septations, or calcifications. Increasing complexity of a cyst correlates with an increasing probability of malignancy. Simple cysts are derived from proximal tubular epithelium and are truly benign entities that need no followup. Complex cysts must be followed with cross-sectional imaging; either thin-section CT scanning with and without intravenous contrast or with magnetic resonance imaging (MRI) with gadolinium.

Although most solid renal masses are malignant, benign tumors, including *angiomyolipoma* and *oncocytoma* are seen as well. Angiomyolipoma is a hamartoma of the kidney, the hallmark of which is the presence of fat within the tumor. It may occur sporadically, usually in women, or as a part of

the syndrome of *tuberous sclerosis,* which in its most serious form consists of mental retardation; seizure disorder; hamartomas of the brain, lung, and kidney; and adenoma sebaceum. Angiomyolipoma may be an incidental finding or may present with flank pain with or without hypotension from an acute retroperitoneal hemorrhage. CT scan will show a well-circumscribed mass containing fat (less than 0 Hounsfield units). Treatment of angiomyolipoma is based on the size of the lesion and the symptomatology. Asymptomatic lesions may be treated conservatively, but lesions that are symptomatic, particularly those larger than 4 cm, should be treated with angioinfarction or partial nephrectomy when possible. Furthermore, asymptomatic lesions that grow significantly during follow-up should be considered for excision.

Oncocytoma is a benign tumor that may be difficult to distinguish from renal cell carcinoma by imaging alone. It is a tumor thought to be derived from distal tubular cells and it tends to be asymptomatic and discovered incidentally. Grossly, it may be large and have a central scar that extends to the periphery in a stellate pattern. Histologically, oncocytoma is well differentiated and highly eosinophilic, with significant mitochondrial hyperplasia and rare mitoses. On cross-sectional imaging, there is no reliable way to differentiate this tumor from renal cell carcinoma, but angiography may show a typical "spoke wheel" appearance caused by the stellate scar. Although these tumors are benign, excision remains the standard of care because of the difficulty in definitive diagnosis. For small lesions or in patients with large or bilateral lesions, partial nephrectomy may be attempted, whereas radical nephrectomy remains the standard of care for large (more than 4 cm) unilateral lesions.

Renal cell carcinoma is the most common primary renal malignancy but is relatively rare compared to other adult solid tumors. Approximately 30,000 new cases of renal cell carcinoma are reported each year, and there are more than 10,000 deaths a year from the disease. The tumors, thought to occur from cells of the proximal convoluted tubule, are usually sporadic but may be familial or associated with von Hippel–Lindau disease. Known risk factors for renal cell carcinoma include smoking (twofold increase in risk), male sex, and acquired cystic kidney disease associated with hemodialysis in end-stage renal disease patients (30-fold increased risk). Most patients are affected in the fifth through seventh decades of life, although patients who are considerably younger have been reported.

Patients with renal cell carcinoma may be asymptomatic at the time of presentation or may present with one or more of the symptoms of the "classic triad," namely flank pain, abdominal mass, and hematuria. Only 10% of patients will present with all three of these symptoms. Fever, weight loss, and hypertension may also be presenting features. Certain paraneoplastic syndromes have been associated with renal cell carcinoma. Hypercalcemia may be related to tumor production of parathyroid hormone–related peptide. *Stauffer syndrome,* hepatic dysfunction not related to metastatic disease, is a transient elevation of liver enzymes that resolves following tumor excision. Reappearance of the abnormality may herald recurrence of tumor. Polycythemia may be related to inappropriate production of erythropoietin by the tumor.

Physical examination is rarely useful in the diagnosis, as most patients will have a normal physical examination until the tumor is locally advanced. Radiography is the mainstay of diagnosis. Renal ultrasonography will show a solid renal mass. CT scanning should be performed before and after intravenous contrast administration. A solid mass that enhances more than 20 Hounsfield units after administration of intravenous contrast is pathognomonic for renal cell carcinoma. For patients who are unable to receive contrast or in those in whom CT is nondiagnostic, MRI with gadolinium may be used in a similar fashion. CT and MRI have the added advantage in detecting extension into the renal vasculature or surrounding structures as well as distant metastases to the liver or bone.

Staging of renal cell carcinoma is commonly based on the tumor, node, metastasis (TNM) staging system or the modified Robson classification and is based on local extent of the tumor as well as on spread to local lymph nodes, vascular involvement, and distant metastases (Table 26-1).

The most common sites of metastases are lung, liver, and bone. Staging workup includes CT scan of the abdomen to evaluate for local extent and evaluation of the abdominal organs. Any question of involvement of the renal vein or vena cava with thrombus should be imaged with MRI. Chest x-ray is used to screen for lung metastases. Bone scan is often used to evaluate for bony metastases, although its use in patients without bone pain is controversial. Chemistry panel and liver function studies are performed as well, and patients with abnormal renal function may benefit from split-function renal scan if partial nephrectomy is considered.

Renal cell carcinoma is truly a surgical disease. The only effective treatment is extirpation of all tumor mass. Surgery is usually reserved for those with tumor localized to the kidney. Radical nephrectomy is the most effective treatment and consists of removal of the entire kidney with the surrounding Gerota fascia and the adrenal gland. Partial nephrectomy may be considered in patients with small tumors, particularly if they are exophytic and do not invade the collecting system. Partial nephrectomy is especially attractive for patients with a solitary kidney, poor renal function, or bilateral disease. Large tumors are occasionally

treated with angiographic embolization prior to surgery. Patients with thrombus extending as far as the right atrium may be treated with radical nephrectomy and removal of the tumor thrombus. This may involve consultation with vascular or cardiothoracic surgeons and can require cardiopulmonary bypass. Select patients with a single metastasis may benefit from concomitant radical nephrectomy and excision of the metastasis.

Patients with widely metastatic disease at the time of diagnosis have a poor prognosis. Cytoreductive surgery has been shown to lengthen survival time in patients with good preoperative functional status. There is no effective medical therapy for renal cell carcinoma although limited success (about 15% complete response) has been seen with immunotherapy using IL-2 and interferon α (IFN-α) with 5-fluorouracil chemotherapy. There is no role for pre- or postoperative radiotherapy.

Transitional cell carcinoma may occur anywhere in the urinary tract, from the collecting system of the kidney to the proximal urethra. Transitional cell carcinoma is diagnosed in approximately 50,000 new patients a year and causes about 11,000 deaths. It is about three times more prevalent in men than in women. The disease is thought to be the result of multiple epithelial mutations caused by carcinogens in the urine. As the entire urothelium is bathed by the same urine, transitional cell carcinoma is often multifocal, an example of a "field change." Known bladder carcinogens are nitrosamines and aromatic amines from cigarette smoke, aniline dyes and several aromatic amines from occupational exposure, and phenacetin. Furthermore, cyclophosphamide chemotherapy is a risk factor for transitional cell carcinoma because of the mutagenic properties of a metabolite, acrolein. This risk can be minimized by the concomitant administration of mesna, a substance that complexes with acrolein. External beam radiation to the pelvis is also a risk factor for transitional cell carcinoma. Substances suspected but never proven to cause bladder cancer are caffeine, artificial sweeteners, and metabolites of tryptophan.

Greater than 70% of patients with transitional cell carcinoma present with hematuria. Intravenous urography (IVU), urine culture and cytology, and cystoscopy should be performed in all patients with hematuria. Intravenous pyelography (IVP) evaluates the upper urinary tracts for filling defects (3% of patients with transitional cell carcinoma of the bladder will have an upper tract lesion). Positive urine culture results do not eliminate the possibility of malignancy. The sensitivity of urine cytology increases as the grade of the lesion increases. Cystoscopy will identify most lesions in the bladder or urethra.

Patients with upper tract lesions should have brush biopsy or ureteroscopic biopsy of the tumor. Patients with bladder lesions should undergo complete transurethral resection including a portion of the underlying detrusor muscle. When the diagnosis is confirmed, staging workup consists of IVU, chest x-ray, CT scan of the abdomen and pelvis, and bone scan. The commonly used staging systems for bladder cancer are outlined in Table 26-2.

Treatment of transitional cell carcinoma depends on the grade, stage, and location of the lesion, as well as the overall health of the patient. In general, superficial disease (Ta and T1) is treated conservatively with resection, surveillance cystoscopy, and intravesical therapy when needed.

TABLE 26-1

ROBSON AND TNM CLASSIFICATIONS FOR RENAL CELL CA

Robson	TNM	
I	T1	Tumor ≤2.5 cm, limited to the kidney
I	T2	Tumor >2.5 cm, limited to the kidney
II	T3a	Tumor extends into perirenal fat or ipsilateral adrenal gland within Gerota fascia
IIIa	T3b	Renal vein involvment
IIIa	T3c	Renal vein and IVC involved
IIIa	T4b	IVC involved above diaphragm
IIIb	N1	Single ipsilateral node
IIIb	N2	Multiple regional/contralateral or bilateral nodes involved
IIIc	T3,4 N1,2	Combination of IIIa and IIIb
IVa	T4a	Spread to contiguous organs
IVb	M1	Distant metastases

IVC, inferior vena cava.

TABLE 26-2

STAGING FOR BLADDER CANCER

Extent of Involvement	Stage
Marshall Modification of Jewett-Strong Classification	
Mucosa	0
Lamina propria	A
Superficial muscle	B1
Deep muscle	B2
Perivesical tissue	C
Pelvic lymph nodes	D1
Distant metastases	D2
Union Internationale Contrel le Cancer Classification	
Carcinoma *in situ*	Tis
Mucosa	Ta
Submucosal invasion	T1
Superficial muscle invasion	T2
Deep muscle invasion	T3a
Perivesical fat invasion	T3b
Invasion of contiguous organs	T4
Regional lymph nodes involved	N1-3
Distant metastases	M1

When superficial disease recurs, it usually remains noninvasive. Muscle invasive bladder cancer, on the other hand, is generally treated more aggressively with partial or radical cystectomy, or with a bladder-sparing protocol of external beam radiation and chemotherapy.

In the bladder, unifocal superficial lesions (Ta) can be treated with surveillance cystoscopy every 3 to 6 months. Intravesical chemotherapy [bacille Calmette-Guérin (BCG), mitomycin, thiotepa] and surveillance cystoscopy every 3 to 6 months are used for multifocal tumors, as well as those associated with carcinoma *in situ*, a flat lesion that is at high risk for disease progression. Higher grade superficial lesions and those with invasion of the lamina propria (T1) are treated similarly with intravesical therapy but tend to be more aggressive than Ta lesions and thus need careful follow-up. Although it is not currently the standard of care, some advocate early cystectomy for T1 lesions (particularly if recurrent or multifocal) because of the high risk of progression and death from bladder cancer.

The mainstay of truly invasive disease without distant metastases (T2+, NX, M0) is radical cystectomy with pelvic lymph node dissection and urinary diversion. Patients with solitary invasive tumors away from the trigone may be treated with partial cystectomy with a 2-cm cuff of normal bladder around the tumor. Patients who refuse cystectomy or who are poor anesthetic risks may be treated with a bladder-sparing protocol of radiation therapy and MVAC chemotherapy (mitomycin, vinblastine, adriamycin, and cisplatin). Patients with metastatic disease (M1) at the time of diagnosis have a poor prognosis and should be treated with MVAC chemotherapy.

There are several methods of urinary diversion used following radical cystectomy. These include jejunal, ileal or colon conduit, continent catheterizable pouch, and orthotopic neobladder, which is connected to the native urethra and most closely approximates the normal anatomy. Stomal stenosis, ureteral stricture, pyelonephritis, and stone formation can complicate urinary diversion. In addition, several metabolic abnormalities have been observed in patients with intestinal urinary diversion. The type and severity of the metabolic abnormality depends on the segment of intestine used and the type of diversion. Jejunal segments typically cause a hyperkalemic, hypochloremic metabolic acidosis, whereas ileum and colon cause a hyperchloremic metabolic acidosis. Although not commonly used for primary urinary diversion, gastric segments are sometimes used for bladder augmentation and may be complicated by a hypokalemic, hypochloremic metabolic alkalosis. Continent reservoirs have an increased contact time with the urine and therefore lead to more severe metabolic abnormalities. These diversions should not be used in patients with significant preoperative renal insufficiency.

Transitional cell carcinoma of the upper urinary tract is usually treated with nephroureterectomy or partial ureterectomy, except in those patients with lesions in a solitary kidney, those with chronic renal insufficiency, those who are poor surgical risks, or those in whom endoscopic or percutaneous resection is feasible. Transitional cell carcinoma limited to the renal pelvis or proximal ureter is generally treated with nephroureterectomy, as there is a significant risk of downstream recurrence. Transitional cell carcinoma of the distal ureter can be managed with distal ureterectomy and ureteral reimplantation. Depending on the length of ureter excised, a psoas hitch, Boari flap, or ileal ureter may be necessary to bridge the gap from the kidney to the bladder.

Postoperative management of patients with transitional cell carcinoma includes interval IVU, chest x-ray, and urinary cytology. Positive surgical margins or lymph nodes and recurrent disease are typically treated with MVAC chemotherapy.

Other bladder neoplasms include squamous cell carcinoma, which is associated with indwelling urinary catheters and *Schistosoma haematobium* infection. Small cell carcinoma and carcinosarcoma are rare and have a poor prognosis. Rhabdomyosarcoma is typically a pediatric disease and is usually treated with radiation and chemotherapy with good results.

Testicular cancer is relatively rare, but because it affects a young patient population and because it is one of the most treatable cancers, its early diagnosis and effective treatment is of obvious social and economic benefit. The incidence of testis tumors is about 5,000 to 6,000 per year in the United States. Despite this number, fewer than 300 patients die per year of the disease, largely because of the effectiveness of available treatment. Testis tumors most often affect young men in their 20s and 30s, although young children and older men may also be affected.

The main risk factor for testis cancer is cryptorchidism, and the risk correlates with the severity of maldescent. The risk of developing cancer in a high scrotal testis is approximately 1 in 100, whereas the risk in an intraabdominal testis is about 1 in 20. There is an associated but smaller risk in the contralateral testis if it is normally descended, and although the risk of malignancy is not diminished by orchiopexy, the operation is recommended in part because it aids in future self-examination for tumor.

Testis tumors are almost always (more than 95%) derived from germinal elements, and *germ-cell tumors* are classified as *pure seminoma* or as *nonseminomatous germ-cell tumors* (NSGCTs). NSGCTs are further characterized as embryonal carcinoma, yolk sac tumor, teratoma, or choriocarcinoma. NSGCT also includes mixed seminoma with nonseminomatous elements. This distinction is important in treatment, as pure seminoma tumors are highly sensitive to radiation, whereas NSGCTs are highly sensitive to chemotherapy. A testis tumor usually presents as a hard, painless scrotal mass in a young man. The differential diagnosis of testis mass includes hydrocele, hernia, hematoma, orchitis, and spermatocele. Scrotal ultrasonography should easily differentiate among these diagnoses if the history and physical examination leave any doubt. In case of testis tumor, ultrasonography will show a hypoechoic, often hypervascular mass in the testis.

Patients with testis tumors should undergo inguinal orchiectomy as soon as possible. Scrotal orchiectomy is not performed because of the theoretical risk of contamination of scrotal lymphatics with tumor cells. Because testis tumors metastasize most commonly to the retroperitoneum and mediastinum via lymphatics and to the lungs hematogenously, the staging workup includes CT scan of the retroperitoneum and chest. Staging is based on the histology of the primary specimen and on the imaging results and is outlined in Table 26-3. Tumor markers α-fetoprotein (AFP) and human chorionic gonadotropin (hCG) are useful in the determination of tumor type, tumor volume, and response to treatment. AFP (half-life about 6 days) is produced by yolk sac tumors but not by choriocarcinoma or by seminoma. Presence of AFP rules out a pure seminoma. hCG (half-life about 24 hours) is produced by choriocarcinoma and

embryonal carcinoma. Although hCG is not produced by seminoma directly, it is produced by syncytiotrophoblasts within the tumor. Elevation of hCG thus can be seen in seminoma, but this elevation is rarely greater than two times the normal level.

Treatment consists of removal of the primary tumor with prophylactic sterilization of the retroperitoneum in stage 1 and early stage 2 disease. This is accomplished with radiation therapy for seminoma and with *retroperitoneal lymph node dissection* (RPLND) for NSGCT. Patients who are well motivated and willing to undergo surveillance may be followed for recurrence of NSGCT. However, the schedule for surveillance (chest x-ray every month, CT scan and tumor markers every 2 months) is so rigorous that few patients actually comply. Persistently elevated markers following RPLND suggest distant metastases that should be treated with adjuvant chemotherapy.

In both seminoma and NSGCT, bulky retroperitoneal disease should be treated first with chemotherapy. Residual NSGCT should be treated with RPLND if markers normalize and with salvage chemotherapy if they do not normalize. The treatment of residual seminoma is controversial.

Retroperitoneal lymph node dissection is performed through a midline incision. Pericaval and periaortic nodes are dissected from the level of the renal vessels to the bifurcation of the iliac vessels. The main long-term risks of the procedure are absence of emission and retrograde ejaculation from disruption of sympathetic nerve fibers. Through the use of modified templates of dissection based on the side of the tumor and by using a nerve-sparing approach, these effects have been minimized.

Prostate cancer is the most common tumor and the second most common cause of cancer death in men. Approximately 220,000 new cases of prostate cancer are diagnosed each year, and approximately 29,000 men die each year of the disease. Ninety-five percent of cancers are detected in men between ages 45 and 89 years, although the disease may occur in younger men. It certainly occurs commonly in older men who eventually die *with* prostate cancer rather than *of* prostate cancer. Major risk factors include advancing age, history of prostate cancer in a first-degree relative, and race (blacks have a 30% higher incidence than whites). Potential minor risk factors include high-fat diet and high serum testosterone level, although neither of these has been definitively proved. Certain vitamins such as vitamins A and D and selenium have been proposed as possible preventatives.

Because low-stage prostate cancer is asymptomatic, screening for prostate cancer using the prostate-specific antigen (PSA) and digital rectal examination is used widely. More prostate cancer is detected with the use of both of these tests than with either test alone. PSA has a sensitivity of 80% and a specificity of 35% to 50%. Other serologic markers are being investigated to improve the specificity. Although there is some controversy surrounding the utility of screening for prostate cancer, the American Cancer Society, the American Urological Association, and the American Radiological Association recommend annual screening in men between the ages of 50 and 70. African Americans and those with a family history of prostate cancer generally begin screening at age 40. Patients with an abnormal serum PSA level (usually greater than 4.0 ng per mL although this may be lower on an age-adjusted basis) or an abnormal digital

TABLE 26-3

TNM CLASSIFICATION FOR TESTIS CARCINOMA

Primary Tumor (T)

TX	Cannot be assessed
T0	No evidence of primary tumor
Tis	Intratubular germ cell neoplasia (CIS)
T1	Limited to the testis and epididymis, no vascular invasion
T2	Invades beyond the tunica albuginea or has vascular invasion
T3	Invades spermatic cord
T4	Invades scrotum

Regional Lymph Nodes (N)

Nx	Cannot be assessed
N0	No regional lymph node metastasis
N1	Lymph node metastasis = 2 cm, = 5 nodes
N2	Metastasis in >5 nodes, nodal mass 2–5 cm
N3	Nodal mass >5 cm

Distant Metastasis (M)

Mx	Cannot be assessed
M0	No distant metastasis
M1	Distant metastasis present

Serum Tumor Markers (S)

Sx	Markers not available
S0	Within normal limits
S1	LDH <1.5 × normal and hCG <5,000 mIU/mL and AFP <1,000 ng/mL
S2	LDH 1.5–10 × normal or hCG 5,000–50,000 mIU/mL or AFP 1,000–10,000 ng/mL
S3	LDH >10 × normal or hCG >50,000 mIU/mL or AFP >10,000 ng/mL

rectal examination (DRE) undergo transrectal ultrasound-guided biopsy of the peripheral zone of the prostate, the most common site of tumor formation. Biopsies are graded using the Gleason scoring system. The tumor growth pattern is graded from 1 to 5 (least dysplastic to most dysplastic) and a score of 2 to 10 is assigned by adding the two most common patterns. A Gleason score of 7 or higher suggests a poor prognosis.

The TNM staging system of prostate cancer is shown in Table 26-4. The most common sites of metastasis of prostate cancer are bone and pelvic lymph nodes. The staging workup for prostate cancer is somewhat controversial and may involve several radiographic examinations. Radionuclide bone scan may detect bony metastases. CT scan of the pelvis may detect obturator or iliac lymph node metastases in the pelvis. MRI with an endorectal coil can be useful in the detection of extension of the tumor beyond the capsule of the prostate, a finding that significantly alters the treatment of choice. Elevation in the PSA level alone is useful for predicting stage, as most men with low PSA levels (less than 10) have organ-confined disease, whereas those with significant elevations in PSA have extraprostatic disease.

The treatment of prostate cancer depends on the grade and stage of the lesion, as well as on the overall condition of the patient. The various treatments, from least to most invasive, are as follows:

1. Watchful waiting consists of following the PSA level and DRE for signs of progression with treatment only for advancing lesions. This is used predominantly in patients older than 70 years with minimal disease or in patients with a life expectancy of less than 10 years.
2. Antiandrogen therapy consists of either injection of a luteinizing hormone-releasing hormone (LHRH) agonist (Zoladex, Lupron) or surgical castration. This therapy is usually reserved for older patients, patients with widely metastatic disease, or for treatment failures. Side effects include impotence, decreased libido, and hot flashes.
3. External beam radiation. This modality of therapy can be curative for organ-confined disease but may also be used for T3, T4, and N+ disease. It has potential side effects on adjacent structures resulting in bladder and bowel symptoms, and erectile dysfunction.
4. Brachytherapy with radioactive seeds composed of palladium, iodine, or gold may be curative for patients with low-grade organ-confined disease. Its advantage over external beam therapy is that the entire potential radiation dose is placed at one time and does not require an open procedure. Its side effects include irritative bowel and urinary symptoms but with limited effects on continence. There may be symptoms of erectile dysfunction.
5. Transperineal cryoablation of the prostate is an experimental therapy that is fraught with complications and today is rarely used.
6. Radical prostatectomy is the definitive surgical treatment in men with a life expectancy of more than 10 years with organ-confined disease. It is statistically the most durable cure for localized disease. It may be performed via a retropubic or perineal approach. Major complications include bleeding, rectal injury, impotence, and incontinence.

There is no effective chemotherapy for prostate cancer, although strontium may be palliative for patients with bone metastases and bony pain. Follow-up for treated prostate cancer consists of serial PSA determinations and DRE with repeated radiographic imaging performed as clinically indicated. Most patients with PSA recurrences following definitive treatment can receive antiandrogen therapy. Although this therapy will reduce the serum PSA level, there is no definite evidence that it will extend life.

BPH is a common condition resulting from adenomatous hyperplasia of the transition zone of the prostate. Although it is by definition a benign process, it may cause significant lower urinary tract obstruction, which if left untreated may lead to life-threatening complications such as urosepsis or renal failure. BPH affects men with an increasing frequency as they age. The prevalence in autopsy studies ranges from less than 20% in men younger than 40 to more than 90% in men older than 80. A large portion of men with BPH are asymptomatic and therefore never come to the attention of a clinician.

There are several theories as to the etiology of BPH and the bladder outlet obstruction that results. Most would agree that hyperplasia is largely mediated by the action of dihydrotestosterone (DHT), and indeed inhibitors of the

TABLE 26-4

TNM CLASSIFICATION FOR PROSTATE CARCINOMA (1997)

Stage	Definition
Primary Tumor (T)	
TX	Primary tumor can not be assessed
T0	No evidence of primary tumor
T1	Clinically inapparent tumor not palpable or visible by imaging
T1a	Tumor incidental histologic finding in 5% or less of tissue resected
T1b	Tumor incidental histologic finding in more than 5% of tissue resected
T1c	Tumor identified by needle biopsy (e.g., because of elevated prostate-specific antigen)
T2	Tumor confined within the prostate
T2a	Tumor palpable by DRE or visible on TRUS on 1 side only
T2b	Tumor palpable by DRE or visible on TRUS on both sides
T3	Tumor extends through the prostatic capsule
T3a	Unilateral or bilateral extracapsular extension
T3b	Seminal vesicle involvement
T4	Tumor is fixed or invades adjacent structures other than the seminal vesicles (bladder neck, external sphincter, rectum, levator muscles, or pelvic sidewall)
Regional Lymph Nodes (N)	
NX	Regional lymph nodes cannot be assessed
NX	No regional lymph node metastasis
N1	Metastasis in a single regional lymph node or nodes
MX	Presence of distant metastasis cannot be assessed
M0	No distant metastasis
M1	Distant metastasis
M1a	Nonregional lymph node(s)
M1b	Bone(s)
M1c	Other site(s)

DRE, digital rectal exam; TRUS, transrectal ultrasound.

production of DHT have been shown to decrease and even reverse BPH. Finasteride, a 5α-reductase inhibitor, inhibits the formation of DHT from testosterone and has been shown to significantly decrease the volume of the prostate in men with BPH. Bladder outlet obstruction results from increased prostate size as well as from an increased amount and tone of smooth muscle in the prostate and bladder neck. This muscle is rich in α_1-adrenergic receptors, and α_1-adrenergic antagonists such as terazosin, doxazosin, and tamsulosin can cause significant improvement in lower urinary tract symptoms.

Symptoms of prostatism result from many factors, including detrusor hypertrophy, increased voiding pressures, and incomplete emptying. Lower urinary tract symptoms can be separated into obstructive symptoms (such as hesitancy, straining, decreased stream, postvoid dribbling) and irritative symptoms (such as urgency, frequency, and nocturia). The American Urologic Association symptom index scores total symptomatology based on the severity of several obstructive and irritative symptoms and ranges from 0 to 35, with higher scores indicating more severe symptoms. This score can be valuable in assessing the effects of treatment.

Treatments of symptomatic BPH include the following:

1. Watchful waiting for mildly symptomatic cases.
2. Medical therapy, including α_1 blockade and antitestosterone agents such as finasteride and LHRH agonists.
3. Clean intermittent catheterization for patients with elevated postvoid residuals complicated by infection or significant symptoms, who have failed or refused medical and surgical therapies. This may be the only viable option for some with detrusor failure from long-standing obstruction.
4. Transurethral resection of the prostate (TURP) is a highly effective treatment reserved for patients who have failed medical therapy or for those who present with significant complications including upper tract degeneration, gross hematuria, acute urinary retention, and/or bladder stones. This operation requires a 1- to 2-day hospital stay and has a side-effect profile including bleeding, infection, incontinence, and retrograde ejaculation. Extended TURP lasting more than 1 hour may lead to significant absorption of irrigant used during the procedure. The post-TURP syndrome that results consists of a combination of hyponatremia, fluid overload, and mental status changes. Alternative techniques to debulk the surgical outlet have been developed more recently and may be considered less invasive. These include microwave therapy, thermotherapy, laser ablation, and transurethral incision of the prostate. All must be compared to TURP, the gold standard.
5. Open prostatectomy. The indications for open prostatectomy are similar to those for TURP, but open surgery is performed in those with glands too large for TURP (usually more than 60 g). The operation is performed suprapubically by opening the bladder or retropubically by incising the capsule of the prostate. This operation causes the greatest relief in symptomatology of all treatments but also requires a 4- to 6-day hospital stay and may have significant complications, as can all major pelvic surgery.

Many patients, particularly men, will experience urinary retention following nonurologic procedures. This retention may be result from several factors, including underlying BPH, anticholinergic effects of certain medications, and bladder atony secondary to the effects of anesthesia. Furthermore, certain radical surgeries, most notably abdominal perineal resection (APR), may interrupt autonomic pathways mediating normal voiding function. The treatment of postoperative urinary retention consists of assisted bladder drainage (Foley catheter, or preferably clean intermittent catheterization) with or without adjuvant pharmacologic therapy until emptying function has returned. In rare instances, normal voiding will not resume, and surgical therapy or prolonged catheter drainage is required.

KEY CONCEPTS

▲ The pathologic separation of testicular cancer into seminoma and nonseminomatous germ cell tumors is important in determining treatment because pure seminoma tumors are highly sensitive to radiation, whereas nonseminomatous germ-cell tumors (NSGCTs) are highly sensitive to chemotherapy.

▲ Radical prostatectomy is the definitive surgical treatment in men with organ-confined prostate cancer and a life expectancy of more than 10 years

▲ The scrotum is innervated by the ilioinguinal and genitofemoral nerves. Inadvertent injury of the genitofemoral nerve during inguinal hernia repair presents as numbness of the lateral scrotum and medial thigh.

▲ Postoperative retention may be caused by several factors, including underlying benign prostatic hypertrophy (BPH), anticholinergic effects of certain medications, and bladder atony secondary to anesthesia. Pelvic surgeries, most notably APR, may interrupt autonomic pathways mediating normal voiding function.

▲ Repair of iatrogenic injuries to the bladder requires thorough inspection of bladder mucosa, excision of devitalized tissue, and two-layer closure. Suprapubic tube placement may be required to ensure complete postoperative bladder decompression and urinary diversion.

SUGGESTED READINGS

Gillenwater JY, Howards S, Grayhack JT et al., eds. *Adult and pediatric urology*, 4th ed. Philadelphia: Lippincott Williams & Wilkins, 2002.

Hanno PM, Malkowicz SB, Wein AJ, eds. *Clinical manual of urology*, 3rd ed. New York: McGraw-Hill, 2001.

Walsh PC, Retik AB, Darracott Vaughn E Jr et al., eds. *Campbell's urology*, 8th ed. Philadelphia: WB Saunders, 2002.

Female Reproductive System

27

Raffi Ara Chalian   *Thomas J. Bader*

Obstetricians and gynecologists specialize in diseases of the female reproductive tract. The female reproductive tract is in proximity to both the genitourinary and the gastrointestinal tracts. Therefore most complaints relating to the female genital tract can reflect either a gynecologic or surgical disease process. As a result, general surgeons must be aware of the anatomy and pathophysiology of the female reproductive tract.

EMBRYOLOGY

The female reproductive tract is derived from the Müllerian duct system (paramesonephric duct) and the male reproductive tract is derived from the Wolffian duct system (mesonephric duct). During the first 8 weeks of development the embryo is ambisexual, after which time differentiation to male and female reproductive organs begins. If the embryo possesses a Y chromosome, differentiation from the indifferent gonad to male reproductive organs begins during gestational weeks 6 through 9. The testes produce testosterone and Müllerian inhibiting factor (MIF), which leads to regression of the Müllerian system during the eighth week of gestation. In the absence of testicular differentiation and the production of testosterone and MIF, the Müllerian duct system persists and the Wolffian system regresses leading to female reproductive organs. By 10 weeks of gestation, the Müllerian ducts fuse and form the three distinct zones of the female reproductive tract: the fallopian tubes, the uterus, and the upper two thirds of the vagina (Fig. 27-1). The lower third of the vagina is derived from the urogenital sinus, which is an inclusion of the ectoderm. Failure of complete regression of the Wolffian system in the developed female reproductive tract can result in paratubal cysts anywhere along the length of the fallopian tubes.

The two major kinds of defects related to the embryologic development of the female genital tract are defects in fusion and defects in canalization. Fusion defects are responsible for duplications in the organs such as a bicornuate uterus, and uterus didelphys. Canalization defects are responsible for transverse vaginal septi and incomplete formation of the uterine cavity or cervical canal. This pres-

ents most commonly as primary amenorrhea, an abdominal mass, and/or cyclical pain. A buildup of sloughed endometrium and blood in the vagina (hematocolpos) and the uterus (hematometra) results as an occlusion of the vagina. Magnetic resonance imaging (MRI) of the abdomen and pelvis demonstrates an enlarged vagina and uterus filled with blood.

ANATOMY

The external genitalia consist of the vulva, which is the hair-bearing skin and adipose tissue underneath the skin. The vulva consists of two portions, the labia majora and the labia minora. Between the labia minora are the vestibule of the vagina, the urethra, and the clitoris. The erectile bodies and their associated muscles lie underneath the subcutaneous tissue and above the fascial layer.

The perineal membrane is the underlying fascial layer. It consists of a dense sheet of fibromuscular tissue that spans the anterior portion of the pelvic outlet. Posteriorly, the perineal body is a condensation of connective tissue that separates the lower vagina and the anus. The perineal membrane connects the vagina and the perineal body. The perineal membrane supports the pelvic floor against increases in intra-abdominal pressure.

The external genitalia have a rich blood supply. The vasculature and nerves travel through the pelvis together, and these are responsible for the innervation and blood supply of the anterior and posterior triangles of the external genitalia. The pudendal nerve (S2-4) contains both sensory and motor components. The internal iliac vessels branch within the pelvis to form the pudendal artery and vein. The nerve, artery, and vein leave the pelvis through the greater sciatic foramen, and wrap around the ischial spine and the sacrospinous ligament. They subsequently re-enter the pelvis through the Alcock canal and the lesser sciatic foramen. Both vessels and the nerve have three branches: clitoral, perineal, and inferior hemorrhoidal.

The inguinal system is the lymphatic drainage of the external genitalia. Tissues external to the vaginal vestibule are drained by a series of lymphatics that coalesce into a

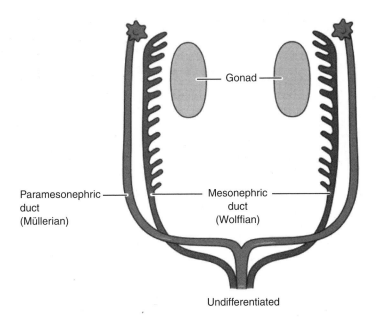

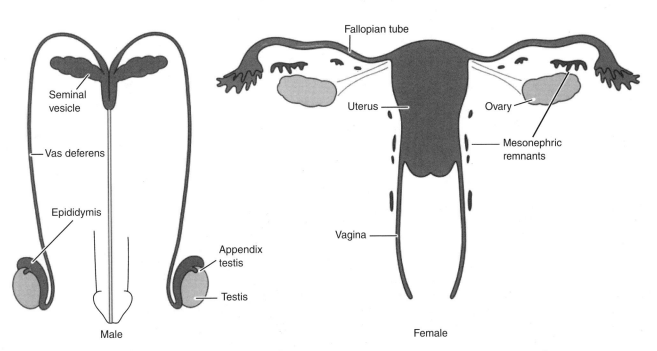

Figure 27-1 Development of the normal male and female reproductive tract. (From Speroff L, Glass RH, Kase N, eds. *Clinical gynecologic endocrinology and infertility*, 5th ed. Baltimore: J.B. Lippincott, 1994:323, with permission.)

few trunks lateral to the clitoris, which in turn drain into the superficial inguinal nodes. The urethral lymphatics also drain into the superficial inguinal nodes. These superficial lymph nodes drain and communicate into deep inguinal lymph nodes, which are found under the fascia cribrosa in the femoral triangle.

The bony *pelvis* is formed by the union of the sacrum and coccyx with the ilium, the ischium, and the pubis (Fig. 27-2). The sacrospinous and sacrotuberous ligaments delineate the margins of the greater and lesser sciatic foramina. The pelvic floor consists of muscles and fascia. The principal muscles are the levator ani, which consist of the pubococcygeal, iliococcygeal, puborectal,

and coccygeal muscles form the pelvic diaphragm. The urethra, vagina, and rectum run through the defect that is formed in the pelvic diaphragm. The region of the levator ani between the anus and the coccyx is the raphe anococcygea. The raphe forms a supportive shelf on which rest the rectum, upper vagina, and uterus (Fig. 27-3). Defects in pelvic support can result in pelvic organ prolapse. The most commonly attributed risk for pelvic organ prolapse is pregnancy. Symptoms of pelvic organ prolapse include the sensation of an intravaginal mass, urinary stress incontinence, and difficulty in the defecation.

The *female genital organs* consist of the vagina, uterus, fallopian tubes, and ovaries. The vagina is effectively horizontal

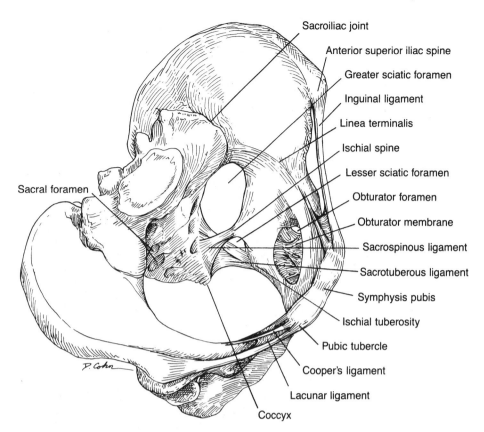

Sacroiliac joint
Anterior superior iliac spine
Greater sciatic foramen
Inguinal ligament
Linea terminalis
Ischial spine
Lesser sciatic foramen
Obturator foramen
Obturator membrane
Sacrospinous ligament
Sacrotuberous ligament
Symphysis pubis
Ischial tuberosity
Pubic tubercle
Cooper's ligament
Lacunar ligament
Coccyx
Sacral foramen

Figure 27-2 The female pelvis. (From Berek JS, Adashi EY, Hillard PA, eds. *Novak's gynecology,* 12th ed. Baltimore: Lippincott-Raven, 1996:72, with permission.)

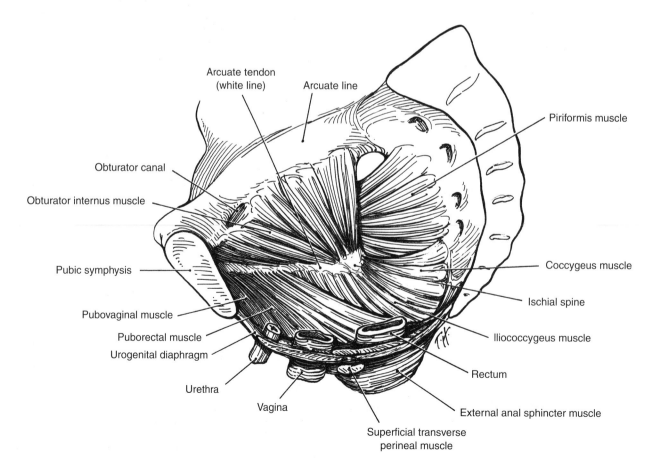

Arcuate tendon (white line)
Arcuate line
Piriformis muscle
Obturator canal
Obturator internus muscle
Pubic symphysis
Pubovaginal muscle
Puborectal muscle
Urogenital diaphragm
Urethra
Vagina
Coccygeus muscle
Ischial spine
Iliococcygeus muscle
Rectum
External anal sphincter muscle
Superficial transverse perineal muscle

Figure 27-3 Muscles of the pelvic floor. (From Berek JS, Adashi EY, Hillard PA, eds. *Novak's gynecology,* 12th ed. Baltimore: Lippincott-Raven, 1996:77, with permission.)

when a woman is standing; this orientation occurs by the obtuse angle formed by the pelvic diaphragm on the retroperitoneal margin on the vagina. This angle is used to delineate the margin of the lower third and upper two thirds of the vagina. The uterus consists of smooth muscle and connective tissue. The uterine corpus consists of mainly smooth muscle, whereas the cervix is composed of fibrous tissue. The uterus is anteverted in the majority of women and lies over the dome of the bladder. The fallopian tubes are paired structures projecting from either side of the uterine fundus and consist of four portions: from medial to lateral these are named the interstitial, isthmic, ampullary, and fimbria. The fimbria ovarica is a band of fibrous tissue that keeps the fimbria apposed to the ovary.

Other organs in the pelvis have important anatomic relationships to the female reproductive organs. The rectum lies behind the uterus and posterior to the cul-de-sac, the intraperitoneal cul-de-sac formed is called the pouch of Douglas. The bladder rests anterior to the lower uterine segment, cervix, and upper vagina. The ureters are intimately associated with many components of the female pelvis as they traverse the female reproductive organs to reach the bladder. The ureter passes over the bifurcation of the common iliac vessels at the pelvic brim and descends into the pelvis. A connective tissue sheath is attached to the lateral pelvic sidewall and to the medial leaf of the broad ligament. The ureter then runs in the cardinal ligament beneath the uterine artery and lies 1 cm from the anterolateral surface of the cervix. The ureter then passes on the anterior vaginal wall and proceeds for another 1.5 cm through the bladder wall (Fig. 27-4).

The *ligaments of the internal pelvic organs* provide structural support and are formed by the condensation of the peritoneum on either side of the pelvic organs. Through these ligaments most of the major blood vessels of the pelvis are situated. The broad ligament is the largest ligament and covers the fallopian tubes, uterus and the ovaries. The broad ligament is separated into the mesosalpinx and the mesovarium, which cover the fallopian tubes and the ovaries, respectively. The round ligament is encased within the anterior broad ligament. It is the remains of the lower half of the gunbernaculum and is the extension of the uterine musculature. Arising at the anterolateral aspect of the uterus, this ligament enters the inguinal canal at the internal inguinal ring and exits the canal to insert into the subcutaneous tissue of the labia majora. The infundibulopelvic ligaments attach the ovary and fallopian tubes to the pelvic sidewall. The ovarian artery and vein run through these ligaments. The uterosacral ligaments are a condensation of ligaments from the second, third, and fourth segments of the sacrum to the cervix. These ligaments hold the cervix posteriorly over the levator plate. Finally, the cardinal ligaments (transverse cervical) run from the lateral wall of the cervix and vagina to the pelvic sidewall and provide the primary support for the uterus in the pelvis. The uterine artery and vein reside within the cardinal ligaments.

The arterial supply to the ovaries *arises* from the aorta just below the level of the renal arteries, thereby forming the ovarian arteries. These vessels course the infundibulopelvic ligaments. The right ovarian vein follows the course of the artery and drains into the inferior vena cava, whereas the left ovarian vein drains into the left renal vein.

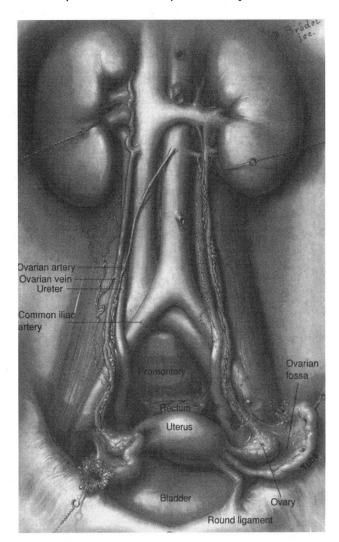

Ovarian artery
Ovarian vein
Ureter
Common iliac artery
Promontory
Rectum
Uterus
Bladder
Round ligament
Ovarian fossa
Tube
Ovary

Figure 27-4 The relationship of the ureters to the female reproductive organs. (From Rock J, Thompson JD, eds. *TeLinde's operative gynecology*, 8th ed. Philadelphia: Lippincott-Raven, 1997:82, with permission.)

The main arterial supply to the uterus is from the right and left uterine arteries, which are branches of the anterior division of the right and left internal iliacs. These vessels course through the cardinal ligaments at the junction of the uterine corpus and cervix at a 90-degree angle. They subsequently divide into superior and inferior branches. The marginal arteries run lateral to the uterus and anastomose with the ovarian arteries in the mesosalpinx (Fig. 27-5).

The lymphatic drainage of the upper two thirds of the vagina and the uterus drain into the obturator, internal, and external iliac lymph nodes, which then proceed to the common iliac lymph nodes and the paraaortic lymph nodes. Accessory channels also include uterine drainage along the round ligaments to the superficial inguinal lymph nodes and from the posterior surface of the uterus along the uterosacral ligaments to the lateral sacral lymph nodes. Lymphatic channels from the ovaries follow the course of the ovarian vessels and drain into the paraaortic lymph nodes.

The *autonomic nerves of the pelvis* lie in the presacral space. The uterus receives its innervation from the uterovaginal plexus (Frankenhäuser ganglion), which is

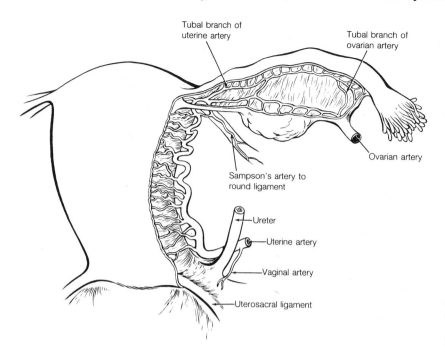

Figure 27-5 The vascular supply of the female pelvis. (From Rock J, Thompson JD, eds. *TeLinde's operative gynecology*, 8th ed. Philadelphia: Lippincott-Raven, 1997:73, with permission.)

one of the three divisions from the superior hypogastric plexus. This plexus runs within the connective tissue of the cardinal ligament. The fallopian tubes and ovaries receive their innervation from the plexus of nerves that accompany the ovarian vessels having originated from the renal plexus.

ENDOCRINOLOGY OF THE HYPOTHALAMUS/PITUITARY/OVARIAN AXIS

The menstrual cycle is mediated centrally via gonadotropin-releasing hormone (GnRH). GnRH is produced in the hypothalamus and transported to the pituitary gland via the local portal blood system. The amplitude and frequency of the pulsatile secretion of GnRH vary throughout the menstrual cycle and are the essential components in the control of the cycle. Follicle-stimulating hormone (FSH) and luteinizing hormone (LH) are secreted from the anterior pituitary. They are responsible for estrogen and progesterone production from the ovary and the corpus luteum (after ovulation). Depending on the time of the cycle, FSH and LH may have negative and/or positive feedback relationships with the hypothalamus and the pituitary, which result in regulation of hormone levels.

The *normal menstrual cycle* lasts 21 to 35 days with 2 to 6 days of flow and an average blood loss of 20 to 60 mL. The cycle consists of two phases: the follicular phase and the luteal phase. During the follicular phase, hormonal feedback promotes the recruitment of follicles and ultimately the development of a single dominant follicle. This phase lasts on average 10 to 14 days. During the luteal phase, the endometrium is prepared for the possibility of pregnancy. This occurs by production of progesterone from the corpus luteum, which leads to coiling and folding of secretory glands and blood vessels. This phase lasts approximately 14 days and encompasses the events from ovulation to the first day of menstrual flow.

The hormonal, ovarian, and endometrial changes of the menstrual cycle are illustrated in Fig. 27-6. The cycle begins with the demise of the corpus luteum at day 25 and a rising FSH level. The rise in FSH level recruits a cohort of ovarian follicles. These follicles secrete estrogen, which serves as the stimulus for endometrial proliferation. Increased estrogen levels during this phase have a negative feedback on pituitary FSH secretion and a positive feedback on pituitary LH secretion. The negative feedback results in the selection of the dominant follicle. After sufficient estrogen stimulation, there is an LH surge, which causes ovulation to occur 24 to 36 hours later. Simultaneous with the development of a dominant follicle, there is progressive mitotic growth of the superficial two thirds of the endometrium in response to increasing levels of estrogen. During this period, the endometrial glands become elongated and tortuous.

The estrogen level declines through the early luteal phase and rises again at the end of the luteal phase as a result of corpus luteum secretion. In addition to estrogen secretion, the corpus luteum also secretes significant amounts of progesterone. Both estrogen and progesterone levels remain elevated throughout the lifespan of the corpus luteum, and their levels wane with its demise. This fall in gonadal steroids permits the increase in FSH level and the beginning of the next cycle.

The corpus luteum develops immediately after ovulation and the endometrial secretory phase begins. The rise in progesterone leads to the progestational stage, which causes the release of the glycogen vacuoles into glandular lumina. On day 21 the spiral arteries lengthen and coil and there is an increase in stromal edema. If pregnancy does not ensue then the hormone levels decrease as the corpus luteum dies. Two days prior to menstruation, polymorphonuclear cells infiltrate the vascular system. These falling hormone levels cause the breakdown of the superficial endometrium and the beginning of menstrual flow.

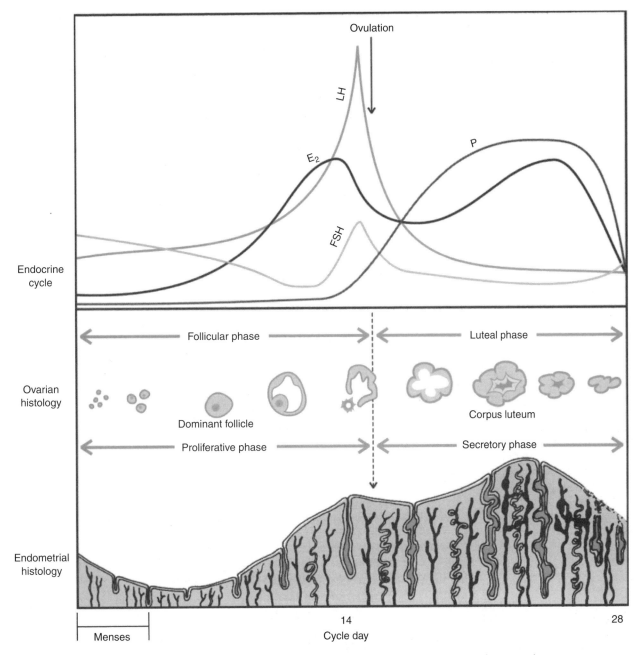

Figure 27-6 The menstrual cycle. (From Berek JS, Adashi EY, Hillard PA, eds. *Novak's gynecology*, 12th ed. Baltimore: Lippincott-Raven, 1996:160, with permission.)

INFECTIOUS DISEASES

The majority of vaginal infections are *lower genital tract infections* such as cervicitis and vaginitis and are readily treatable with minimal long-term sequelae. In contrast, *pelvic inflammatory disease* (PID) results from the infection of the endocervix with bacteria that ascend to the endometrium and the fallopian tubes. Approximately one half of all PID is caused by an infection due to *Neisseria gonorrhoeae* or *Chlamydia trachomatis*. The cervicitis allows anaerobic and aerobic vaginal organisms to ascend to the upper genital tract, which causes polymicrobial infection and inflammation. These organisms include normal vaginal flora such as *Escherichia coli* and group B streptococcus.

The symptoms of PID are pelvic pain, purulent vaginal discharge, fever, nausea, and vomiting. Gonococcal PID typically has an abrupt onset of the pain and fever, and worsens with movement. Associated arthralgia has been reported with gonococcal infection. Chlamydial PID can have a more insidious course. The diagnosis of PID is usually based on the triad of signs: abdominal tenderness with or without peritoneal signs, cervical motion tenderness, and adnexal tenderness. Other softer markers for PID include pyrexia, elevated leukocyte count, Gram stain of the cervical discharge and the presence of a pelvic or adnexal collection on ultrasound and/or bimanual examination. A physician should have a low threshold to treat PID, as the consequences of

TABLE 27-1
CURRENT RECOMMENDATIONS FOR TREATMENT OF PELVIC INFLAMMATORY DISEASE

Outpatient
  A. Cefoxitin 2 g i.m. plus probenecid 1 g p.o. or ceftriaxone 250 mg i.m. and doxycycline 100 mg p.o. b.i.d. for 14 days
  B. Ofloxacin 400 mg p.o. b.i.d. for 14 days and clindamycin 450 mg p.o. q.i.d. or metronidazole 500 mg p.o. b.i.d. for 14 days

Inpatient:
  A. Cefoxitin 2 g IV q6 hours or cefotetan 2 g IV q12 hours *and* doxycycline 100 mg IV q12 hours
  B. Clindamycin 900 mg IV q8 hours and gentamicin 2 mg/kg IV load then 1.5 mg/kg IV q8 hours

i.m., intramuscular; p.o., per os; b.i.d., twice a day; q.i.d., four times a day; IV, intravenous.
From Berek JS, Adashi EY, Hillard PA, eds. *Novak's gynecology*, 12th ed. Baltimore: Lippincott-Raven, 1996, with permission.

untreated PID can be devastating and include infertility and chronic pelvic pain.

Treatment of this disease requires broad-spectrum antibiotics. Both outpatient and inpatient treatment options exist (Table 27-1). Indications for inpatient therapy include nulliparity with the desire for future childbearing, pregnancy, presence of an intrauterine device, persistent nausea and vomiting precluding compliance with oral medication, and failure to respond to an outpatient regimen after 48 hours of treatment. Intravenous therapy is continued until there is complete resolution of abdominal pain and the patient has been afebrile for 48 hours.

PID may occur early in the first trimester of pregnancy. However by 12 weeks of gestation, the fetal membranes have sealed over the internal cervical os, protecting the upper genital tract from infection. Gonorrhea and chlamydia may cause cervicitis throughout pregnancy.

A *tuboovarian abscess* (TOA) is a variant of acute PID. The agglutination of inflamed fallopian tubes, ovaries, and sometimes bowel with inflammatory exudates forms a palpable complex. Diagnosis requires finding a palpable mass in a woman with PID. This finding is usually confirmed by ultrasound. A TOA is treated initially with a parenteral combination of ampicillin, gentamicin, and clindamycin Seventy-five percent of patients treated with triple antibiotics will respond to therapy with resolution of fever and abdominal pain. Treatment failure requires surgical exploration for possible abscess drainage or hysterectomy and bilateral salpingo-oophorectomy. With current antibiotic regimens and early initiation of treatment, and with the development of other modalities such as percutaneous drainage, the need for surgical exploration has decreased considerably.

PATHOLOGY

Endometriosis is the ectopic growth of endometrial tissue outside the uterine cavity. There are two main theories which explain this phenomenon: (i) metaplastic transformation of peritoneal tissue and (ii) retrograde menstruation, back flow of menses, and subsequent peritoneal implantation. The most prevalent site for endometriosis is the pelvis. Other sites include the ovary, bowel, bladder, omentum, umbilicus, and lungs. Endometriosis is found in 7% of reproductive-age women and may present as pelvic pain, infertility, dysmenorrhea, dyschezia, or dyspareunia. Endometriosis may also be asymptomatic. There does not appear to be a correlation between the degree of endometriosis and the severity of pelvic pain, dyspareunia, and infertility. The typical lesions present as black, brown, or blue nodules surrounded by various degrees of fibrosis. In addition, ovarian cysts, called "chocolate cysts," containing thick, viscous brown fluid may occur as a result of endometriosis.

Extrapelvic endometriosis is uncommon and is suspected when a palpable mass, associated with pain that occurs in a cyclic monthly pattern, is found outside the pelvis. The most common site for extrapelvic endometriosis is the intestinal tract, particularly the colon and rectum. These patients usually present with abdominal pain, back pain, abdominal distension, and cyclic rectal bleeding. Other less common sites of involvement include the ureters, bladder, umbilicus, and lungs.

Endometriosis can be treated medically and surgically. Medical treatment involves hormonal manipulation that suppresses estrogen synthesis and promotes atrophy of the endometrial implants. Drugs that have been used with variable success include continuous low-dose oral contraceptive pills, progesterone, and GnRH agonists. Surgical therapy includes both laparoscopy and laparotomy. Laparoscopy involves the ablation of the endometrial implants using bipolar coagulation, excision, or laser. The goal is to remove all implants and adhesions in an attempt to restore the pelvis to its normal anatomy. Laparotomy is reserved for severe cases in which fertility is not a concern. In extreme cases, a total abdominal hysterectomy and bilateral salpingo-oophorectomy with lysis of adhesions is performed.

Benign Pelvic Masses

Adnexal tumors frequently occur in women during their reproductive years (19 to 40 years of age). Eighty percent to 85% of adnexal masses are benign. Masses that are unilateral, cystic, mobile, and smooth are usually benign, whereas masses that are solid, fixed, irregular, and associated with ascites and cul-de-sac nodules may be malignant. These masses can cause abdominal distension, pain, pelvic pressure, urinary symptoms, or gastrointestinal tract symptoms. Acute abdominal pain and peritoneal signs in the presence of an adnexal mass can result from adnexal torsion, rupture of a cyst, or bleeding into a cyst.

The most common adnexal mass is a functional ovarian cyst. Functional ovarian cysts include follicular cysts and corpora lutea. Follicular cysts are more common and are usually less than 8 cm. They are often asymptomatic, found incidentally during a pelvic examination, and resolve within one or two menstrual cycles. Occasionally they can rupture and cause acute abdominal pain and peritoneal signs. A corpus luteum is called a cyst when its size exceeds 3 cm. If a luteal cyst does not resolve in subsequent menstrual cycles, it can also rupture, causing hemoperitoneum and sometimes requiring surgical intervention. These masses usually resolve spontaneously.

In addition to functional cysts, the differential diagnosis of an adnexal mass includes other benign ovarian neoplasms and ovarian carcinoma. Until age 19, the most common benign pelvic mass is a benign cystic teratoma. The differential diagnosis of benign pelvic masses in this age group includes a Wilms tumor and neuroblastoma. Benign cystic teratomas remain common in woman aged 20 to 44. The other common mass in this age group is serous cystadenomas; from age 45 to 74, the most common adnexal mass remains is a serous cystadenoma Intraoperatively, a frozen section must be performed to distinguish between benign, borderline, and malignant tumors, which determines further surgical management.

In women older than 45, the incidence of malignant lesions, both primary and metastatic to the adnexa, increases. Other less common adnexal tumors are mucinous cystadenomas, adenofibromas, endometriomas, and Brenner tumors. Mucinous cystadenomas may become quite large—tumors greater than 300 pounds have been reported. On gross inspection, they are smooth and loculated with a clear viscid fluid. Of major concern is on removal of these tumors, spillage of the cyst contents into the peritoneum can result in pseudomyxoma peritonei. Pseudomyxoma peritonei results in the transformation of peritoneal epithelium to mucin-secreting epithelium and results in the gradual accumulation of gelatinous material.

Benign cystic teratomas (dermoids) result from neoplastic growth of totipotent cells, which cause a mass composed of any or all of the following: skin, bone, teeth, hair, and dermal tissue. They are characterized by having calcium deposits and fat. Dermoids are bilateral in 10% of cases and have a relatively high incidence of torsion. Malignant transformation occurs in less than 2% of these masses. More than 75% of these transformations will occur in women older than 40. In all women for whom fertility is an important consideration, the surgical procedure of choice is an ovarian cystectomy with conservation of as much normal ovarian cortex as possible.

In addition to masses of ovarian origin, adnexal masses can also originate from tubal elements. Tuboovarian abscesses, ectopic pregnancies, and remnants of the Wolffian ducts can all present as adnexal masses.

Uterine neoplasms are predominately benign in origin and are extremely common in women of all age groups, the most common being leiomyomas (fibroids). They increase in incidence with age until menopause. Because leiomyomas are estrogen sensitive there is a gradual decrease in size after menopause. Their incidence is higher in the African American population, affecting approximately 50% of the population at age 50 and is lowest in the Asian population. Fibroids can present in many ways, which include lower abdominal pain, urinary symptoms, and abnormal vaginal bleeding.

Treatment of fibroids can vary depending on the presentation, age, position, number, and desire to preserve fertility in the individual patient. The treatment modalities include surgical and medical management. Surgical management can include hysteroscopy, laparoscopy and laparotomy. Surgical management results in either resection of the fibroids or hysterectomy. Medical management is predominately using a GnRH agonist, which inhibits the hypothalamic- pituitary axis and results in the inhibition of estrogen production by the ovaries. Nonsteroidal anti-inflammatory drugs (NSAIDs) have also been used for symptomatic pain in fibroids. Bleeding due to myomas can also be treated with NSAIDS, oral contraceptives (OCPs), GnRH analogs, or surgery.

Uterine Malignancies

Endometrial carcinoma is the most common pelvic malignancy in the United States. There are approximately 340,000 new cases and 6,000 deaths due to endometrial carcinoma annually. This malignancy is primarily a disease of postmenopausal women and becomes increasingly lethal with increasing age at presentation. In general, exposure to unopposed estrogen increases a woman's risk for endometrial carcinoma. More specifically, the most common risk factors for endometrial carcinoma include nulliparity, menopause after age 52, obesity, prolonged estrogen exposure, use of estrogen replacement without concurrent use of progesterone during menopause, tamoxifen use, and diabetes. Oncologists have broadly categorized the disease into two categories: those patients who are usually younger and have been exposed to hyperestrogenic states and those patients in whom endometrial carcinoma develops from an atrophic postmenopausal endometrium. The former group tends to have a more favorable histology and prognosis.

The classification of endometrial carcinoma includes eight different variants: endometrioid, adenocarcinoma, mucinous carcinoma, papillary serous carcinoma, clear cell carcinoma, squamous carcinoma, undifferentiated carcinoma, and mixed type. The endometrioid variant accounts for 80% of all endometrial carcinoma, and these tumor glands resemble normal endometrial glands. Less-differentiated tumors contain more solid elements and less glandular elements.

Ninety percent of women with endometrial carcinoma present with vaginal bleeding or discharge; however, only 10% of postmenopausal women with these symptoms actually have endometrial carcinoma. Other diagnoses to consider in these patients include endometrial atrophy, endometrial polyps, irregular bleeding from estrogen-replacement therapy, and endometrial hyperplasia. The first diagnostic study to perform is an office endometrial biopsy, where a small piece of endometrial tissue is removed from the uterus. This biopsy has a diagnostic accuracy of 98%. It is a manual curetting of the endometrial cavity by a disposable suction device approximately 5 mm in diameter. Approximately 5% of the uterus is sampled. Transvaginal ultrasonography is also highly accurate and may be helpful as an adjunctive study. Ultrasonography may be the best option for women who cannot tolerate an endometrial biopsy. A sonographic endometrial thickness of greater than or equal to 5 mm or a polypoid endometrial mass are considered suspicious findings for endometrial pathology in postmenopausal woman who are not taking exogenous hormones. One must also be cautious when interpreting results of patients who are taking tamoxifen as there can be alterations in the thickness of the endometrial lining. The Papanicolaou (Pap smear) test is an unreliable diagnostic test for endometrial pathology with a diagnostic accuracy of only 30% to 40%.

If an endometrial biopsy returns with a diagnosis of hyperplasia, the next diagnostic study is a hysteroscopic dilation and curettage to ensure the absence of carcinoma. If the endometrial biopsy results return with carcinoma, the patient begins evaluation for future surgical staging. The initial preoperative evaluation includes a chest roentgenogram and routine laboratory tests. MRI may provide preoperative information regarding the degree of myometrial invasion and may assist in the decision to proceed with lymph node sampling. In endometrial carcinoma, elevated CA125 levels may be used as a marker for extrauterine disease.

Endometrial carcinoma is surgically staged (Table 27-2). The procedure requires sampling of peritoneal fluid for cytology, excision of any extrauterine lesions, total abdominal hysterectomy, and bilateral salpingo-oophorectomy. The uterus is examined for tumor size and the extent of myometrial invasion, and a frozen section is performed to determine histologic type and grade. Clear cell carcinoma, papillary serous carcinoma, squamous carcinoma, any grade 3 lesion, myometrial invasion greater than one half of the myometrial thickness, isthmic/cervical extension, tumor size greater than 2 cm, or extrauterine disease are indicators of poor disease prognosis. Following surgical staging and treatment, some women may require adjuvant radiation therapy.

Treatment decreases the risk of local recurrence from 15% to 1% or 2%. External beam radiation therapy is indicated for cervical involvement, pelvic lymph node metastases, or pelvic disease outside the uterus. Women with paraaortic lymph node metastases receive extended field radiation therapy to include the common iliac and paraaortic lymph nodes. Abdominal radiation therapy is reserved for women with stage III or IV disease. Chemotherapy is not indicated as a primary treatment but reserved for palliation of recurrent disease.

Posttreatment surveillance is performed by serial examinations and imaging. Disease recurrence is found in 25% of patients with endometrial carcinoma. Greater than 50% of the recurrences are discovered within the first 2 years after diagnosis. The most common sites of recurrence include local pelvic recurrence, lung, abdomen, lymph nodes, liver, brain, and bone. Patients with isolated regional recurrence are best treated with external beam radiation therapy followed by vaginal radiation brachytherapy. Progesterone therapy is currently recommended for all patients with recurrent endometrial carcinoma, even though there is greater response in estrogen and/or progesterone receptor positive tumors, since 5% of tumors that are receptor-negative respond. Progesterone can be administered orally or intramuscularly and is continued indefinitely unless progression of disease is noted.

Sarcomas represent a small percentage of uterine malignancies, with an annual incidence of 1.7 per 100,000 women older than 20 years old. Sarcomas present with abdominal pain and a rapidly enlarging uterus. They are commonly diagnosed preoperatively as uterine leiomyomas. Women who have received pelvic irradiation are at increased risk for developing uterine sarcomas. There are three histologic variants: endometrial stromal sarcoma, leiomyosarcoma, and malignant mixed Müllerian tumor. Endometrial stromal sarcoma produces an enlarged uterus with a soft yellow-gray necrotic and hemorrhagic mass. Leiomyosarcoma originates from uterine smooth muscle and is differentiated from a leiomyoma by the number of mitotic figures per high-power field. Uterine sarcoma is treated with total abdominal hysterectomy, bilateral salpingo-oophorectomy, and either lymph node dissection or radiation therapy. Adjuvant chemotherapy with doxorubicin or dimethyl triazeno-imidazole carboxamide as the main component decreases the risk for distant metastases. Fifty percent of the recurrences are localized to the pelvis. The most common site of distant disease is the lung. The overall prognosis is poor regardless of stage.

Cervical Malignancies

The squamocolumnar junction is the boundary of the columnar epithelium of the cervical canal with the squamous epithelium of the ectocervix. During the reproductive

---

TABLE 27-2

STAGING AND GRADING OF ENDOMETRIAL CARCINOMA

1988 FIGO surgical staging for endometrial carcinoma

Stage Ia	G123	Tumor limited to endometrium
Ib	G123	Invasion to less than one half of the myometrium
Ic	G123	Invasion to more than one half of the myometrium
Stage IIa	G123	Endocervical glandular involvement only
IIb	G123	Cervical stromal invasion
Stage IIIa	G123	Tumor invades serosa and/or adnexa and/or positive peritoneal cytology
IIIb	G123	Vaginal metastases
IIIc	G123	Metastases to pelvic and/or paraaortic lymph nodes
Stage IVa	G123	Tumor invasion of bladder and/or bowel mucosa
IVb		Distant metastases including intraabdominal and/or inguinal lymph nodes

1971 FIGO clinical staging for endometrial carcinoma

Stage 0	Carcinoma *in situ*
Stage I	The carcinoma is confined to the corpus
Stage Ia	The length of the uterine cavity is 8 cm or less
Stage Ib	The length of the uterine cavity is more than 8 cm
Stage 1	Cases should be subgrouped with regard to the histologic grade of the adenocarcinoma as follows:
Grade 1	Highly differentiated adenomatous carcinoma
Grade 2	Moderately differentiated adenomatous carcinoma with partly solid areas
Grade 3	Predominantly solid or entirely undifferentiated carcinoma
Stage II	The carcinoma has involved the corpus and the cervix but has not extended outside the uterus
Stage III	The carcinoma has extended outside the uterus but not outside the true pelvis
Stage IV	The carcinoma has extended outside the true pelvis or has obviously involved the mucosa of the bladder or rectum. A bullous edema as such does not permit a case to be allocated to stage IV
Stage IVa	Spread of the growth to adjacent organs
Stage IVb	Spread to distant organs

FIGO, International Federation of Gynecology and Obstetrics.
From Berek JS, Adashi EY, Hilland PA, eds. *Novak's gynecology*, 12th ed. Baltimore: Lippincott-Raven, 1996:1069, with permission.

years, the columnar epithelium undergoes squamous metaplasia, and this region is known as the "transformation zone." Most neoplastic changes of the cervix occur in the transformation zone. The premalignant changes of the cervix are considered a continuum from mild-to-severe cytologic atypia. The predominant descriptive pathologic system used to describe these changes is the Bethesda system. The Bethesda system classifies premalignant changes into low-grade squamous intraepithelial lesion (LGSIL) and high-grade squamous intraepithelial lesion (HGSIL). LGSIL includes koilocytotic change and mild dysplasia. HGSIL includes moderate to severe dysplasia. Carcinoma *in situ* (CIS) indicates malignant disease.

The major risk factors for cervical neoplastic changes include early age at first sexual intercourse, multiple sexual partners, early marriage, early childbearing, prostitution, sexually transmitted diseases, and immunocompromised states. The common denominator for all these factors may be human papillomavirus (HPV), which plays a major role in premalignant conditions of the cervix. HPV subtypes 16, 18, 31, 33, 35, 39, 45, 51, 52, 56, and 58 are more virulent and have been associated with cervical carcinoma.

The Pap smear is the primary screening test for cervical dysplasia. Because of the relatively low sensitivity of a single pap (approximately 50%), the full benefit of cervical cancer screening is seen in individuals who have had regular screening. If a Pap smear demonstrates abnormal cytology or the presence of high risk HPV subtypes, a colposcopy is usually performed accompanied by cervical biopsies. The colposcope is a binocular microscope that can magnify the cervix 10 to 16 times. The cervix is prepared with acetic acid and the colposcope is used to identify the abnormal lesions that require biopsy. The Pap smear, findings on colposcopy, and histology from the cervical biopsies are used together to form a diagnosis. Lesions that are LGSIL have a spontaneous regression rate of 70% and can be watched by regular Pap smears with colposcopic examinations if warranted. If lesions are HGSIL or if there is a discrepancy between the cytologic impression and the biopsy results, then excision therapy or destructive therapy must be performed. The goal of therapy is complete eradication of all abnormal tissue. There are multiple techniques that can be used for excision therapy such as cold knife cone biopsy or loop electrocautery excision. Laser, electrocautery, and freezing can be used to destroy certain lesions. HIV-positive patients and other immunosuppressed patients usually get more aggressive disease and can experience unpredictable progression. Therefore, curative surgery is initiated sooner in these patients.

Cervical carcinoma is the third most frequently occurring gynecologic malignancy in the United States. There are 16,000 new cases and 5,000 deaths due to cervical carcinoma annually. Most women present with abnormal bleeding, classically postcoital bleeding or brown vaginal discharge after intercourse or between menstrual cycles. The diagnosis of cervical carcinoma is made by biopsy of the tumor, and the extent of cervical involvement is determined by a cone biopsy of the cervix.

Eighty-five percent to 90% of cervical carcinomas are squamous cell carcinoma. This malignancy infiltrates locally and disease spreads laterally and inferiorly from the cervix to the vagina and paracervical and parametrial tissues. Hematogenous metastases are a late complication of cervical carcinoma and most commonly involve lung, liver, and bone.

Cervical carcinoma is staged clinically (Table 27-3). The stage is primarily determined by physical examination and the status of the ureters. This system has been adapted, as most of cervical cancer occurs in areas where advanced imaging technology is not available. Initial evaluation of cervical carcinoma includes the history and physical examination, laboratory studies, an intravenous pyelogram, or computerized tomography (CT), and a chest x-ray. An examination under anesthesia, cystoscopy, and sigmoidoscopy are then performed. These examinations provide information about the spread of disease to the parametrial tissues, bladder, and rectum. Once the evaluation has been completed, the patient is assigned a clinical stage and therapy is determined by this stage.

Women with stage Ia$_1$ or Ia$_2$ cervical carcinoma have microinvasive disease and are treated with a simple hysterectomy. Women with stage Ib or IIa are treated with either radical hysterectomy and lymph node dissection or radiation therapy. If examination of the lymph nodes demonstrates metastatic disease, then postoperative external pelvic radiation is required. As a primary treatment, radiation therapy consists of both external beam radiation and brachytherapy. Women with stage IIb or greater are treated with radiation therapy as definitive treatment. Recently released results from the National Cancer Institute have demonstrated that adding cisplatin-based chemotherapy regimens to radiation therapy decreases the death rate from cervical cancer by 30% to 50%.

One third of patients have recurrence of disease 6 months or more after primary treatment. Fifty percent of recurrences occur in the pelvis. Other common sites for recurrent disease include periaortic lymph nodes, lung, liver, or bone. Surgical failures are treated with radiation alone or chemotherapy in combination with radiation therapy. If the cervical carcinoma was treated initially with radiation therapy, surgical resection should be considered, because further radiation is usually contraindicated. Palliative chemotherapy regimens that include cisplatin and 5-fluorouracil may also be used as treatment for recurrent disease. Pelvic exenteration may be considered for patients with a central pelvic recurrence and a preoperative evaluation that fails to demonstrate metastatic disease.

Ovarian Malignancies

In the United States, ovarian carcinoma is the second most common gynecologic malignancy after endometrial carcinoma. However, ovarian carcinoma is the most frequent cause of death from any pelvic malignancy. The higher death rate is due to the late stage at which ovarian carcinoma is typically detected.

There are many risk factors that increase the chance of developing ovarian cancer. In general, prolongation of a woman's number of ovulatory cycles increases the risk of developing ovarian carcinoma. For example, frequent ovulation, late menopause, nulliparity, and late childbearing increase a woman's risk of this malignancy. In contrast, breastfeeding, the use of OCPs, tubal ligation, and hysterectomy with ovarian conservation decrease a woman's risk for this disease.

TABLE 27-3
STAGING OF CARCINOMA CERVIX UTERI

Preinvasive carcinoma

Stage 0   Carcinoma *in situ*, intraepithelial carcinoma (cases of stage 0 should not be included in any therapeutic statistics).

Invasive carcinoma

Stage I[a]   Carcinoma strictly confined to the cervix (extension to the corpus should be disregarded).
Stage Ia   Preclinical carcinomas of the cervix, i.e., those diagnosed only by microscopy.
Stage Ia1   Lesions with ≤3-mm invasion.
Stage Ia2   Lesions detected microscopically that can be measured. The upper limit of the measurement should show a depth of invasion of >3–5 mm taken from the base of the epithelium, either surface or glandular, from which it originates, and a second dimension, the horizontal spread, must not exceed 7 mm. Larger lesions should be staged as Ib.
Stage Ib   Lesions invasive >5 mm.
Stage Ib1   Lesions ≤4 cm.
Stage Ib2   Lesions larger than 4 cm.
Stage II[b]   The carcinoma extends beyond the cervix but has not extended onto the wall the carcinoma involves the vagina, but not the lower one third.
Stage IIa   No obvious parametrial involvement.
Stage IIb   Obvious parametrial involvement.
Stage III[c] The carcinoma has extended onto the pelvic wall. On rectal examination, there is no cancer-free space between the tumor and the pelvic wall. The tumor involves the lower one third of the vagina. All cases with hydronephrosis or nonfunctioning kidney.
Stage IIIa   No extension to the pelvic wall.
Stage IIIb   Extension onto the pelvic wall and/or hydronephrosis or nonfunctioning kidney.
Stage IV[d]   The carcinoma has extended beyond the true pelvis or has clinically involved the mucosa of the bladder or rectum. A bullous edema, as such, does not permit a case to be allotted to stage IV.
Stage IVa   Spread of the growth to adjacent organs.
Stage IVb   Spread to distant organs.

[a] The diagnosis of both stages Ia1 and Ia2 should be based on microscopic examination of removed tissue, preferably a cone, which must include the entire lesion. The depth of invasion should not be more than 5 mm taken from the base of the epithelium, either surface or glandular, from which it originates. The second dimension, the horizontal spread, must not exceed 7 mm. Vascular space involvement, either venous or lymphatic, should not alter the staging but should be specifically recorded as it may affect treatment decisions in the future. Lesions of greater size should be staged as Ib. As a rule, it is impossible to estimate clinically whether a cancer of the cervix has extended to the corpus. Extension to the corpus should therefore be disregarded.
[b] A patient with a growth fixed to the pelvic wall by a short and indurated, but not nodular, parametrium should be allotted to stage IIb. At clinical examination, it is impossible to decide whether a smooth, indurated parametrium is truly cancerous or only inflammatory. Therefore, the case should be assigned to stage III only if the parametrium is nodular to the pelvic wall or the growth itself extends to the pelvic wall.
[c] The presence of hydronephrosis or nonfunctioning kidney due to stenosis of the ureter by cancer permits a case to be allotted to stage III even if, according to other findings, it should be allotted to stage I or II.
[d] The presence of the bullous edema, as such, should not permit a case to be allotted to stage IV. Ridges and furrows into the bladder wall should be interpreted as signs of submucous involvement of the bladder if they remain fixed to the growth at palpation (i.e., examination from the vagina or the rectum during cystoscopy). A cytologic finding of malignant cells in washings from the urinary bladder requires further examination and a biopsy specimen from the wall of the bladder.
From Berek JS, Adashi EY, Hilland PA, eds. *Novak's gynecology*, 12th ed. Baltimore: Lippincott-Raven, 1996:1120, with permission.

There are three major histologic types of ovarian carcinoma: epithelial, germ cell, and sex cord stromal. Epithelial tumors arise from ovarian surface epithelial cells and account for 65% of all ovarian malignancies. Germ-cell tumors originate from embryonic and extraembryonic tissues and are responsible for 20% to 25% of ovarian malignancies. They have the capacity to stimulate sex steroid hormone secretion or may themselves be hormonally inactive. Sex cord stromal tumors contain elements that recapitulate the ovary or the testes and account for 6% of ovarian malignancies. Gonadoblastomas are tumors composed of both sex cord elements and germ-cell elements. They are found in dysgenic gonads, particularly when a Y chromosome is present in the patient's karyotype. Women with these genotypic abnormalities require removal of their gonads to prevent this rare tumor.

Ovarian carcinoma spreads along peritoneal surfaces to both parietal and visceral surfaces of the abdomen. Because the ovaries are intrapelvic organs and ovarian tumors are usually asymptomatic, the disease has usually spread beyond the ovaries before any signs or symptoms of the malignancy are present. Patients may complain of a distended abdomen and physical examination may reveal ascites and a pelvic mass. The preoperative evaluation includes basic laboratory studies, a CA125 level, CT scan of the abdomen and pelvis, and a barium enema.

Staging of ovarian carcinoma requires a surgical procedure (Table 27-4). During this procedure, ascites or peritoneal washings are sent for cytologic examination, the undersurface of the diaphragm is sampled, all suspicious nodules are removed, and a total abdominal hysterectomy, bilateral salpingo-oophorectomy, and infracolic omentectomy are performed. If there is no gross disease outside of the pelvis, a pelvic and paraaortic lymph node dissection is completed. It is critical that staging is correctly performed at the time of the initial exploratory laparotomy to provide important prognostic information so that the appropriate postoperative treatment may be carried out.

Twenty percent of all ovarian epithelial carcinomas are borderline. These tumors consist of malignant cells that

TABLE 27-4

STAGING OF PRIMARY CARCINOMA OF THE OVARY[a]

Stage I	Growth limited to the ovaries
Stage Ia	Growth limited to one ovary; no ascites containing malignant cells
	No tumor on the external surface; capsule intact
Stage Ib	Growth limited to both ovaries; no ascites containing malignant cells
	No tumor on the external surfaces; capsules intact
Stage Ic[b]	Tumor either stage Ia or Ib but with tumor on the surface of one or both ovaries; or with capsule ruptured; or with ascites present containing malignant cells; or with positive peritoneal washings
Stage II	Growth involving one or both ovaries with pelvic extension
Stage IIa	Extension and/or metastases to the uterus and/or tubes
Stage IIb	Extension to other pelvic tissues
Stage IIc[b]	Tumor either stage IIa or stage IIb but with tumor on the surface of one or both ovaries; or with capsule(s) ruptured; or with ascites present containing malignant cells or with positive peritoneal washings
Stage III	Tumor involving one or both ovaries with peritoneal implants outside the pelvis and/or positive retroperitoneal or inguinal nodes; superficial liver metastasis equals stage III; tumor is limited to the true pelvis, but with histologically proven malignant extension to small bowel or omentum
Stage IIIa	Tumor grossly limited to the true pelvis with negative nodes but with histologically confirmed microscopic seeding of abdominal peritoneal surfaces
Stage IIIb	Tumor of one or both ovaries with histologically confirmed implants of abdominal peritoneal surfaces, none exceeding 2 cm in diameter; nodes negative
Stage IIIc	Abdominal implants >2 cm in diameter and/or positive retroperitoneal or inguinal nodes
Stage IV	Growth involving one or both ovaries with distant metastasis; if pleural effusion is present, there must be positive cytologic test results to allot a case to stage IV; parenchymal liver metastasis equals stage IV

[a] These categories are based on findings at clinical examination and/or surgical exploration. The histologic characteristics are to be considered in the staging, as are results of cytologic testing as far as effusions are concerned. It is desirable that a biopsy be performed on suspicious areas outside the pelvis.

[b] In order to evaluate the impact on prognosis of the different criteria for allotting cases to stage Ic or IIc it would be of value to know if rupture of the capsule was (a) spontaneous or (b) caused by the surgeon and if the source of malignant cells detected was (i) peritoneal washings or (ii) ascites.

From Berek JS, Adashi EY, Hilland PA, eds. *Novak's gynecology*, 12th ed. Baltimore: Lippincott-Raven, 1996:1170, with permission.

are not invasive. Women with this condition require an appropriate staging procedure. A unilateral salpingo-oophorectomy can be performed if the tumor is confined to one ovary, the contralateral ovary appears normal, and biopsy results of the omentum and peritoneal surfaces are negative. This is particularly important for young patients when preservation of fertility is desired. With resection

alone, the 5-year survival rate approaches 90%. Adjuvant chemotherapy and radiation therapy are reserved for patients whose malignancy is invasive or has cytologic atypia.

The primary management for all stages of epithelial ovarian carcinoma is removal of all resectable disease and reduction of nonresectable lesions to less than 1 cm during the staging laparotomy. Patients with stage IC disease or higher or for whom histologic evaluation demonstrates poorly differentiated carcinoma benefit from adjuvant postoperative chemotherapy. This chemotherapeutic regimen consists of Taxol and cisplatin administered every 3 weeks for six cycles. Patients are followed with serial physical examinations, CT examinations, and CA125 tests. Exponential regression of a patient's CA125 level suggests response to this regimen.

Germ-cell tumors comprise 20% to 25% of all ovarian tumors; however, only 2% to 3% are malignant. These tumors originate from the primitive germ cells and differentiate into embryonic (endoderm, mesoderm, and ectoderm) or extraembryonic (yolk sac or trophoblast) tissues. Dysgerminomas account for 45% of all malignant germ-cell tumors, and immature teratomas and endodermal sinus tumors are the next most frequently occurring malignant germ-cell tumors.

Dysgerminomas are composed of primitive germ cells infiltrated by lymphocytes. They represent approximately 1% of all ovarian malignancies. Dysgerminomas are found primarily in women younger than 30 years old. In 10% of the patients, they are found on both ovaries. These tumors are very sensitive to both radiation therapy and multiagent chemotherapy with cisplatin and bleomycin plus etoposide or vinblastine. Chemotherapy generally is used as the first line of treatment.

Endodermal sinus tumors (yolk sac tumors) account for approximately 10% of malignant germ-cell tumors. This tumor resembles the extraembryonic tissue of the yolk sac and secretes α-fetoprotein (AFP), which is used as a marker to follow disease progression and response to treatment. Before the development of multiagent chemotherapy, endodermal sinus tumors were universally fatal. At present, they may be successfully treated with vincristine, actinomycin D, 5-fluorouracil, and cyclophosphamide.

Choriocarcinoma of the ovary is a highly malignant rare form of germ-cell tumor. This tumor resembles the extraembryonic tissue of the cytotrophoblast and the syncytiotrophoblast. Human chorionic gonadotropin (hCG) is the tumor marker used to follow disease progression and response to treatment. In the past, choriocarcinoma was also a universally fatal disease; however, multiagent chemotherapy now provides improved response rates for this disease.

The histology of *sex cord stromal tumors* resembles the sex cord and specialized stroma of the developing gonad. In the ovary, the granulosa cells represent the sex cord tissue and the theca cells represent the specialized stroma. Granulosa theca cell tumors are a low-grade malignancy, and these tumors often secrete estrogen. This additional supply of estrogen can be responsible for a range of symptoms from precocious puberty to postmenopausal bleeding. These tumors are identified histologically by the presence of Call-Exner bodies, which are eosinophilic bodies surrounded by granulosa cells. Sertoli-Leydig tumors are also low-grade malignancies that replicate testicular elements. In 75% to 80% of patients these tumors produce androgens. As a result, women present with amenorrhea, breast atrophy, acne, hirsutism, clitoromegaly, deepening of the voice, and male pattern baldness. Treatment for both of these tumors requires surgical excision followed by multiagent chemotherapy. Once a patient has completed child-bearing, the contralateral ovary should be removed.

Malignancies Metastatic to the Ovary

Most tumors metastatic to the ovary originate from malignancies of other pelvic organs such as the uterus or the fallopian tube. The most common distant sites of origin include the breasts and the gastrointestinal tract. A Krukenberg tumor is a specialized type of gastrointestinal tumor metastatic to the ovary. This tumor contains signet ring cells filled with mucin in an acellular stroma. The stomach and the large intestine are the most common sites of origin.

Vaginal Carcinoma

Vaginal carcinomas are rare and make up less than 2% of all gynecologic malignancies. Eighty percent of these carcinomas are squamous cell and the remaining are adenocarcinomas, melanomas, and sarcomas. For women with a history of cervical or vulvar carcinoma, a vaginal lesion appearing at least 5 years after the initial malignancy is considered a primary vaginal cancer and not a recurrence of their original disease. Most women present with abnormal vaginal bleeding or abnormal vaginal discharge. This malignancy spreads by direct extension to the pelvic soft tissues. Hematogenous dissemination to the lungs, liver, and bone occurs late in the disease. The diagnosis is confirmed by a biopsy of the vaginal lesion. The mainstay of treatment is radiation therapy to the vagina with surgical therapy, an option only for young women whose disease is limited to the upper vagina.

Vulvar Carcinoma

Squamous cell carcinoma accounts for 90% of vulvar malignancies. Five percent of vulvar malignancies are melanomas. Another 5% are adenocarcinomas, verrucous carcinomas, basal cell carcinomas, and sarcomas. Most women complain of perineal bleeding, a lesion that fails to heal and pruritus. On physical examination, a polypoid mass may be found on the vulva; clinically suspicious lesions should be biopsied as early treatment can be curative and considerably less morbid. This tumor spreads via the lymphatic system to the superficial inguinal femoral lymph nodes and to the deep pelvic, obturator, and iliac lymph nodes. The diagnosis is confirmed by a directed biopsy of the lesion. Treatment consists of a radical vulvectomy and bilateral inguinal lymph node dissection. If the superficial lymph nodes are found to contain metastatic disease, then a course of radiation therapy is given to the deep pelvic and iliac lymph nodes.

Carcinoma of the Fallopian Tube

Primary fallopian tube malignancy is the rarest gynecologic cancer and represents only 0.3% to 1.1% of all gynecologic cancers. These lesions usually are adenocarcinomas when they originate from the tube; however, 80% to 90%

of fallopian tube malignancies are metastatic from other sites, which include the ovary, uterus, and gastrointestinal tract. The classic signs and symptoms in women with this malignancy include abnormal vaginal bleeding and discharge, lower abdominal pain, and an adnexal mass. The diagnosis is made during surgical exploration. The operative strategy and staging for this disease are identical to those for epithelial ovarian carcinoma. Adjuvant chemotherapy with platinum-containing regimens or radiation therapy are appropriate for advanced stage disease.

Gestational Trophoblastic Disease

Gestational trophoblastic disease (GTD) is composed of a rare spectrum of tumors that includes complete hydatidiform mole, partial hydatidiform mole, placental site trophoblastic tumor, and choriocarcinoma. In the United States, the incidence of GTD is 0.6 to 1.1 per 1,000 pregnancies. Risk factors for GTD include maternal age less than 15 and greater than 40 years, a low dietary intake of carotene, and vitamin A deficiency. A higher incidence is seen in the Japanese population.

Complete hydatidiform moles contain chorionic villi with hydatidiform swelling and trophoblastic hyperplasia, and lack fetal tissue. The karyotype is 46XX; however, all of the chromosomes are of paternal origin, either by fertilization of an egg by a single sperm cell or two sperm cells in an ovum devoid of maternal DNA. Partial hydatidiform moles have chorionic villi with focal hydatidiform swelling and trophoblastic hyperplasia. Identifiable fetal parts may be present with this form of GTD. Partial moles have a triploid karyotype and the extra set of chromosomes is of paternal origin. Complete and partial molar pregnancies usually present with abnormal bleeding. Molar pregnancies may also present with excess uterine size, hyperemesis gravidarum, hyperthyroidism, and prominent theca lutein ovarian cysts. An abnormally elevated β-hCG level and transvaginal ultrasound usually confirm the diagnosis. A complete mole has a characteristic vesicular sonographic pattern "snowstorm appearance," whereas a partial mole has cystic spaces in the placental tissue and an increase in the transverse diameter of the gestational sac. Treatment begins with evacuation of the uterine contents by suction curettage. Women are followed after uterine evacuation with serial β-hCG levels. Concurrent contraception is prescribed to prevent a subsequent pregnancy which will interfere with the monitoring of the disease. If the β-hCG level does not fall to zero or begins to increase, the patient is presumed to have persistent disease and may be at risk for distant metastases. In complete moles, local invasion occurs in 15% of the patients and metastases occur in 4% of the patients. In contrast, partial molar gestations will have a persistent nonmetastatic tumor in 4% of the patients. GTD is considered the most treatable gynecologic malignancy and is treated with methotrexate. Persistent and high risk disease is treated by using a combination of etoposide, actinomycin D, cyclophosphamide, and vincristine.

Ectopic Pregnancy

In the United States, there are 16 *ectopic pregnancies* per 1,000 pregnancies annually. Ectopic pregnancy is responsible for 15% of all maternal deaths in this country, with adolescents having the highest mortality rate. After a woman has one ectopic pregnancy, there is a 50% to 80% chance of subsequent intrauterine pregnancy and a 10% to 25% risk of another ectopic pregnancy at the next conception. The major risk factors for ectopic pregnancy are tubal damage from tubal inflammation, infection, use of tobacco, or prior abdominal surgery. Therefore, previous PID, prior ectopic pregnancy, previous tubal surgery (tubal ligation or tubal reanastomosis), and current intrauterine device use are risk factors for ectopic pregnancy. Some chlamydial infections of the cervix are indolent and can cause a silent, ascending salpingitis without the clinical features of PID. This type of chlamydial infection leads to tubal inflammation and damage, which predisposes the patient to future tubal pregnancy. The presentation of this disease is variable, ranging from no symptoms to hemorrhagic shock. However, common symptoms include amenorrhea, abdominal cramping, and abnormal vaginal bleeding. Serial β-hCG measurements and transvaginal ultrasound are helpful in establishing the diagnosis. In a normal intrauterine pregnancy, the β-hCG level increases by at least 66% every 48 hours. If the β-hCG level fails to rise appropriately, ectopic pregnancy must be suspected. If the β-hCG level does rise appropriately, ultrasound should be performed at a β-hCG of 1,500 to 2,000 IU per mL. This is the earliest that an intrauterine pregnancy can be visualized by transvaginal ultrasound. This β-hCG level is known as the discriminatory zone. If the diagnosis remains uncertain following these tests in a hemodynamically stable patient, serial β-hCG levels may be followed and ultrasound examinations repeated until the condition of the pregnancy is clear by the demonstration of fetal pole and or demonstration of an intrauterine yolk sac. However, emergent laparotomy or laparoscopy is indicated for evidence of hemodynamic instability. The differential diagnosis includes early normal intrauterine pregnancy, abnormal intrauterine pregnancy, and completed abortion. The natural progression for an ectopic pregnancy may lead to expulsion from the fimbriated end of the fallopian tube (tubal abortion), involution of the conceptus within the tube, or tubal rupture.

Treatment for an ectopic pregnancy can be either medical or surgical therapy. Medical management with methotrexate requires fulfillment of strict clinical criteria. Surgical intervention includes linear salpingostomy or salpingectomy via laparoscopy or laparotomy. After diagnosis and treatment of an ectopic pregnancy it is imperative that β-hCG levels are followed until they are undetectable in the blood, as there are failure rates with both medical and surgical management. If the entire ectopic pregnancy is removed by salpingectomy, β-hCG levels do not need to be followed.

KEY CONCEPTS

▲ Post menopausal bleeding is endometrial cancer until proved otherwise.

▲ The best diagnostic test for evaluating the female reproductive organs is transvaginal ultrasonography.

▲ Pregnancy must be excluded in all reproductive age women who complain of abdominal pain.

▲ The majority of premenopausal adnexal masses are benign and resolve spontaneously.

▲ Pelvic inflammatory disease can mimic a myriad of surgical diseases.

SUGGESTED READINGS

Bankowski B, Hearne A, Lambrou N, eds. *The Johns Hopkins manual of gynecology and obstetrics,* 2nd ed. Baltimore: Williams & Wilkins, 2002.

Berek JS, Adashi EY, Hillard PA, eds. *Novak's gynecology,* 12th ed. Baltimore: Williams & Wilkins, 1996.

Gabbe SG, Niebyl JR, Simpson JL, eds. *Obstetrics normal and problem pregnancies,* 3rd ed. New York: Churchill Livingstone, 1996.

Mishell DR Jr, Stenchever MA, Droegemueller W et al., eds. *Comprehensive gynecology,* 3rd ed. St. Louis: Mosby, 1997.

Rock J, Thompson JD, eds. *TeLinde's operative gynecology,* 8th ed. Philadelphia: Lippincott-Raven, 1997.

Speroff L, Glass RH, Kase N, eds. *Clinical gynecologic endocrinology and infertility,* 5th ed. Baltimore: Williams & Wilkins, 1994.

Otorhinolaryngology

28

Jeffrey M. Shaari   Ara A. Chalian

SALIVARY GLAND ANATOMY, PHYSIOLOGY, AND PATHOLOGY

There are three paired groups of major salivary glands: parotid, submandibular, and sublingual. The largest of these is the *parotid gland* located over the masseter muscle of the cheek. The parotid gland is enclosed by deep cervical fascia and extends from its superior most point at the zygoma to an inferior point that curves around the angle of the mandible (Fig. 28-1). Saliva produced by this gland is mostly serous and is directed through Stensen duct into the oral cavity through an orifice located opposite the second upper molar. The parotid gland is divided into superficial and deep lobes by the facial nerve, which exits the stylomastoid foramen as a single trunk before dividing

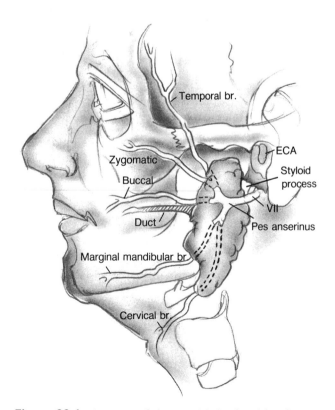

Figure 28-1 Anatomy of the parotid gland and facial nerve. (From Bailey BJ, ed. *Head and neck surgery: Otolaryngology.* Philadelphia: Lippincott Williams & Wilkins, 2001, with permission.)

into two principal divisions at a point called the "pes anserinus" (goose's foot), from where it further divides into five named branches. All surgery performed on the parotid gland places the facial nerve at risk. The temporal and mandibular divisions are injured most frequently in surgery.

The *submandibular gland* courses around the mylohyoid muscle and mandible and is enclosed by the deep cervical fascia. The mandibular division of the facial nerve lies superficial to the submandibular gland and must be identified during any procedure involving the gland. Saliva produced in this gland is mostly seromucous and is directed via Wharton duct to an orifice on the ipsilateral side of the floor of the mouth adjacent to the frenulum (the midline attachment between the ventral tongue and the floor of the mouth).

The *sublingual gland* is the smallest of the major salivary glands and secretes mostly mucous saliva through approximately 10 small ducts that drain directly into the floor of mouth along the sublingual fold. The remainder of saliva is produced by approximately 500 minor salivary glands distributed in the cheek, lips, and hard and soft palates. The quantity of saliva produced daily is influenced by various cues but normally ranges between 500 and 1,500 mL.

Dysfunction within the salivary glands can be divided into nonneoplastic and neoplastic groups. The former includes multiple infectious processes. Acute suppurative infections typically affect the parotid and submandibular glands, causing induration, tenderness, and swelling. Purulent discharge can frequently be expressed intraorally with gentle massage of the gland. Bacterial organisms responsible for acute infections commomly include *Staphylococcus aureus, Streptococcus pneumoniae, Escherichia coli,* and *Haemophilus influenzae;* anaerobic organisms may also be invloved. These disorders may be observed in the debilitated, dehydrated, elderly nursing home population, as well as in the postoperative patient. Management includes appropriate antibiotics, hydration, and sialagogues (oral agents that promote the production and flow of saliva, for example lemon slices). Removal of obstructing calculi, when present, are also indicated to restore salivary flow. Incision and drainage of an associated abscess and/or removal of the affected gland (in the case of the submandibular gland) may also be indicated. Viral inflammation may involve the parotid gland (viral parotitis or mumps). Additional infectious disorders include granulomatous agents and actinomycosis; these disorders are more prevalent in the human immunodeficiency virus (HIV)–positive population.

Nonneoplastic salivary disease also includes sialolithiasis, or ductal stones, which are commonly found in the submandibular glands (80% to 92%). Of parotid calculi, 65% to 90% are radiolucent, whereas 65% to 90% of submandibular gland stones are radiopaque on conventional plain films. Painful swelling is temporally associated with meals; obstructing calculi may also lead to acute suppurative infections (see preceding text). Methods for removing stones include lithotripsy and surgical extraction; however, recurrent sialolithiasis may necessitate gland removal. Autoimmune processes frequently involve the salivary glands. *Sjögren syndrome* is a disorder seen in the middle-aged and the elderly, with women outnumbering men by a ratio of nine to one. Symptoms include *xerostomia* (dry mouth), *keratoconjunctivitis sicca* (dry eyes), glandular swelling, and papillary atrophy of the tongue. Sjögren syndrome frequently presents as a symptom within a larger group of connective tissue disorders. Diagnosis is made on the basis of salivary gland biopsy, usually from the lower lip, which demonstrates plasma cell and histiocytic infiltration with acinar atrophy. Other causes of xerostomia, and, therefore, increased susceptibility to suppurative infections, include previous irradiation to the head and neck as well as a variety of pharmacologic agents (anticholinergics, diuretics, antihistamines, psychotropics, antispasmodics, and parkinsonian agents).

Neoplastic disorders include benign and malignant lesions of the salivary glands and account for approximately 3% to 5% of tumors arising in the head and neck. Approximately 70% of tumors arise from the parotid gland, 15% to 20% from the submandibular gland, and the remaining 8% to 15% from minor salivary glands of the head and neck. As a general rule, the larger the gland, the more likely the neoplasm is to be benign. Benign entities progress slowly, are painless, and rarely cause facial nerve dysfunction. In contrast, malignant tumors are suspected in cases of rapid growth, facial nerve paresis, or pain (associated with perineural invasion). Mitotic nuclei have been identified at all levels within the ductal apparatus, suggesting that neoplasms may arise from any portion of the glandular unit. Many of these cells are pluripotential in nature, and, as a result, histologic classification is complicated with at least 30 described neoplasms identified in the pathology literature. With respect to parotid masses, preoperative imaging is not mandatory for simple, well-circumscribed lesions of the superficial lobe, although it is often performed. In cases where malignancy is suspected or deep lobe or parapharyngeal space extension is anticipated, preoperative imaging is well-advised to evaluate tumor extent and potential nodal metastases. Preoperative fine needle aspirate (FNA) is highly sensitive and specific for the diagnosis of salivary neoplasms. It is particularly useful to differentiate inflammation from tumor and to limit the extent of surgery, or to avoid surgery if the diagnosis is lymphoma. Some surgeons utilize FNA on every case to aid in preoperative counseling, treatment planning, and scheduling.

With respect to benign entities, the *pleomorphic adenoma* (benign mixed tumor) is the most common salivary tumor (approximately 50% of all salivary neoplasms). There is a slight female preponderance, with peak occurrence in the fifth and sixth decades. Surgical management includes removal of the mass with an adequate cuff of normal surrounding tissue (often superficial parotidectomy). Simple enucleation of the tumor can result in unacceptably high rates of recurrence secondary to the presence of microscopic extensions through the tumor capsule. A second group of benign tumors includes *monomorphic adenomas*, which are identified in 4% of parotid masses. Histologically, they resemble pleomorphic tumors, however, only a single morphologic class is present.

Warthin tumors (papillary cystadenoma lymphomatosum) represent the second most common type of benign salivary neoplasm. They represent 5% to 10% of all salivary tumors and are found predominantly in the parotid gland (10% to 15% of parotid tumors) with a marked male-to-female predilection (five to one). Again, they are most commonly identified in the fifth and sixth decades. Warthin tumors are multicentric in 12% of individuals and bilateral in 2% to 10%. Warthin tumors have been associated with cigarette smoking. Microscopically, they possess a biphasic composition with lymphoid sheets interspersed with oncocytic cells demonstrating high concentrations of mitochondria. The *oncocytoma* is the fourth most frequently identified benign salivary tumor (less than 2%) and is localized most commonly to the parotid gland. The oncocytoma exhibits a slow growth rate, and multicentricity is common. A fifth entity affecting the salivary glands is the *benign lymphoepithelial lesion of Godwin*. This disorder is characterized by lymphocytic infiltration of the glands causing bilateral cystic masses that require frequent aspiration or gland excision. Association with HIV infection has been noted, and a 10% incidence of lymphoma has been reported in these cystic lesions.

The malignant tumors of the salivary gland constitute approximately 35% to 46% of all salivary masses. The likelihood of malignancy is inversely proportional to the size of the salivary gland: parotid (approximately 20%), submandibular (approximately 50%), and minor (approximately 80%). Of the minor salivary gland neoplasms, approximately 40% arise in the palate. The most common malignant tumor of the salivary glands is the *mucoepidermoid carcinoma*. These unencapsulated neoplasms arise in the third through fifth decades. Patients note a slowly enlarging painless mass with rare cranial nerve (CN) VII involvement; 30% to 40% of patients have lymph node metastases. Mucoepidermoid carcinoma is the most common malignancy of the parotid gland (80% to 90% of mucoepidermoid carcinomas occur in the parotid gland) and the second most common malignancy of the submandibular and minor glands. Of the salivary malignancies, this group is most commonly associated with prior exposure to radiation. High-grade, low-grade, and intermediate histologic patterns are described, with poor prognosis carried by high-grade tumors (poorly differentiated).

Adenoid cystic carcinoma is the most common tumor of the submandibular and minor salivary glands. Classically, this tumor is associated with bone involvement and aggressive spread along nerves (perineural invasion). *Acinic cell carcinoma* arises almost exclusively in the parotid gland. Additional malignant tumors include *malignant mixed tumors* and *adenocarcinoma*. The latter group demonstrates frequent facial nerve involvement (20%) and pain (15%). The remaining 1% of parotid malignancies fall within various cell types including squamous cell carcinoma, salivary duct carcinoma (which resembles breast cancer), and lymphomas. Metastases to the parotid gland are rare and are often secondary to metastases from facial cutaneous melanoma and squamous cell carcinoma.

The diagnosis of parotid neoplasms incorporates elements of patient history (pain, paresis, and progress of growth), physical examination (tenderness, compressibility, fixation, erythema, and edema), pathology (histologic evidence from FNA), and radiologic evaluation on computerized tomographic (CT) scanning and magnetic resonance imaging (MRI) (enhancing, cystic, and perineural tracking). Additional diagnostic studies of salivary function have been described (sialography and radiosialography) but are less frequently employed. Despite these factors, uncertainty with respect to malignancy may exist and most salivary tumors are ultimately excised. Superficial parotidectomy is indicated for all parotid tumors, unless deep lobe extension is noted, in which case, total parotidectomy is performed with sparing of the facial nerve. Because of the presence of pseudopod extensions from neoplasms, enucleation alone carries a higher rate of recurrence. Malignant neoplasms may require excision of all or part of the mastoid bone if retrograde tracking along facial nerve branches is noted. Submandibular and minor salivary gland tumors require gland excision. Management of minor salivary gland tumors also requires wide surgical margins. Neck dissection is indicated for patients with obvious cervical node metastases. The role of elective neck dissection in the clinically negative neck is more controversial, with indications being larger tumors (greater than 4 cm), undifferentiated carcinoma, high-grade mucoepidermoid carcinoma, squamous cell carcinoma, and malignancies arising in the submandibular gland.

Postoperative radiation is recommended for intermediate and high-grade mucoepidermoid carcinoma, malignant mixed tumor, adenocarcinoma, adenoid cystic carcinoma, high-grade acinic cell carcinoma, squamous cell carcinomas, and malignant tumors greater than 2 cm in diameter. Protocols involving adjuvant chemotherapy are currently under investigation. Local failure is common among all salivary gland malignancies; distant failure is highest for adenoid cystic and adenocarcinomas, both of which frequently exhibit lung metastases. Overall, parotid malignancies have the best prognosis, followed by minor salivary gland tumors and then by submandibular malignancies.

Complications of salivary gland surgery typically occur as sequelae of surgery on the parotid gland. Temporary facial nerve paresis is not unusual and most often involves the temporal and mandibular branches; this usually relates to neuropraxia from dissection on the facial nerve branches. The integrity of the nerve may be assessed at the termination of the procedure with a nerve stimulator. If intact, return to normal function can be predicted with confidence. When tumor involvement requires sacrifice of CN VII, nerve grafting to distal branches is recommended. Grafts are obtained from the sural nerve, or, alternatively, CN XII to CN VII anastomoses can be performed. Time to maximal recovery is approximately 6 to 12 months, although complete return of function is rare. *Frey syndrome,* or gustatory sweating, arises after parotidectomy when severed parasympathetic fibers initially supplying the parotid gland aberrantly reinnervate sweat glands on the skin. Therefore, actions that would normally trigger firing of these parasympathetic fibers (for example, salivation) instead produce sweating. Its incidence is unknown although estimated to be 35% to 60%. Gustatory sweating that is clinically noticeable to patients is probably less than that present by objective testing for the disorder. Treatment includes topical anticholinergic creams (scopolamine), antiperspirants, and injection of botulinum toxin.

ORAL CAVITY AND PHARYNX

The oral cavity is involved in three principal functions: phonation, food ingestion, and breathing. Anatomically, it is defined as the area including the lips, upper and lower alveolar ridges, buccal mucosa, floor of the mouth, retromolar trigone, hard palate, and anterior two thirds of the tongue (bordered posteriorly by the circumvallate papillae). The oral cavity contains 20 deciduous teeth in the child and 32 permanent teeth in the adult. Motor functions of the oral cavity are provided by the tongue and the masticatory muscles. The muscles of mastication, which include the masseter, temporalis, medial pterygoid, and lateral pterygoid, are innervated by the mandibular division of cranial nerve five (CN V^3). The tongue receives motor innervation from the *hypoglossal nerve* (CN XII). Tactile sensation of the tongue is provided by the *lingual nerve* (a branch CN V^3), whereas taste is provided by the *chorda tympani nerve* (from CN VII) (anterior two thirds of the tongue) and the *glossopharyngeal nerve* (CN IX) (posterior two thirds of the tongue). Two pairs of named ducts (Stensen and Wharton) open into the oral cavity from the parotid and submandibular (submaxillary) glands, respectively, whereas numerous small ducts drain the sublingual glands directly into the floor of mouth or the Wharton duct. Up to 1,500 mL of saliva is produced each day.

The pharynx includes three distinct regions. The *nasopharynx* extends from the base of the skull to the level of the junction of hard and soft palates. Anteriorly, it begins at the most posterior extent of the nasal septum. Laterally, it includes the region defined by the fossae of Rosenmuller adjacent to the openings to the eustachian tubes. Proceeding inferiorly, the *oropharynx* begins at the undersurface of the soft palate. The lateral walls encompass the palatine tonsils and tonsillar fossae. The posterior or base of tongue is defined as tissue posterior to the circumvallate papillae and is included in the oropharynx. The *oropharynx* also includes the vallecula (the recess located between the base of tongue and epiglottis). The final division of the pharynx is the *hypopharynx,* which extends from the level of the floor of the vallecula and pharyngoepiglottic folds to the inferior border of the cricoid cartilage. Important structures of the hypopharynx include the pharyngoesophageal junction and pyriform sinuses (the funnel-shaped recessed areas located on either side of the larynx).

Multiple benign processes may produce inflammation of the oral cavity and pharynx. These include bacterial, viral, and fungal infections, autoimmune disorders, nutritional deficiencies, and toxin or chemical exposure. Certain entities are rarely seen in developed countries. Oral candidiasis, or thrush, is seen frequently in the HIV population and in postirradiation patients with diminished salivary production.

The most concerning infections are those that can lead to airway compromise. Odontogenic infections can spread

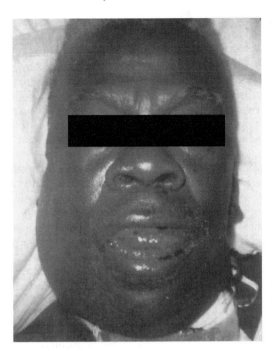

Figure 28-2 Ludwig angina. Note the cuff of bilateral submandibular and submental swelling enveloping the upper neck and elevation of the floor of the mouth causing protrusion of the tongue. (From Bailey BJ, ed. *Head and neck surgery: Otolaryngology*. Philadelphia: Lippincott Williams & Wilkins, 2001, with permission.)

rapidly to the floor of the mouth, tongue base, and submandibular space (*Ludwig angina*), sometimes necessitating tracheostomy to secure the airway until the infection has resolved (Fig. 28-2). Bacterial collections adjacent to the palatine tonsils within the tonsillar capsule (*peritonsillar abscess*) can cause airway compromise if submucosal extension proceeds inferiorly toward the larynx. Common signs and symptoms of peritonsillar abscess include *trismus* (decreased jaw range of motion), odynophagia, dysphagia, dehydration, "hot potato" voice, uvular deviation to the contralateral side and bulging of the anterior tonsillar pillar secondary to infection. Management includes bedside needle aspiration of the abscess after topical anesthesia is applied. This is often followed by making a mucosal incision in the anterior tonsillar pillar and spreading into the abscess cavity with a blunt instrument. Care must be taken laterally, where the great vessels are located in the parapharyngeal space. Broad-spectrum antibiotics effective against the Gram-positive, Gram-negative, and anaerobic flora of the oral cavity are instituted for 14 days. The preferred time for tonsillectomy is approximately 6 weeks postinfection, after acute inflammation has subsided. Although bloody and more technically challenging, a *quinsy tonsillectomy* can be performed in the acute setting. Other noninfectious lesions that can lead to dehydration include recurrent aphthous ulcer, erythema multiforme, pemphigus vulgaris (intraepidermoid bullae), and pemphigoid (subepidermoid bullae).

Malignant Lesions of the Oral Cavity and Pharynx

Approximately 31,000 new cancers of the oral cavity and pharynx are diagnosed each year in the United States

(representing 2.7% of newly diagnosed cancers in men and 1.6% in women). Overall, these tumors constitute 65% of all malignancies of the head and neck. More than 90% of these neoplasms are squamous cell carcinomas. Despite advances in radiotherapy and chemotherapy protocols, survival rates are little improved from those of the 1960s, with a generalized 5-year survival rate of 50% documented for the oral and pharyngeal cancer patient. Factors implicated in the etiology of these carcinomas include tobacco use (cigarettes, cigars, and chewing products), excessive alcohol consumption, and human papillomavirus exposure. Exposure to ultraviolet light has been associated with carcinomas of the lower lip. In parts of the world where other oral stimulants are used (e.g., betel nut in India), significantly higher incidences of the disease are noted.

Lesions of the oral cavity present at varying levels of differentiation. Commonly identified lesions include leukoplakia, which presents as a superficial, hyperkeratotic, mucosal plaque. These white lesions demonstrate epithelial hyperplasia in approximately 80% of cases and should be biopsied to rule out carcinoma *in situ* or frank invasion. The overwhelmingly predominant histology identified in tumors of these areas is squamous cell carcinoma (greater than 90%). These cancers can exhibit high, low, or moderate degrees of differentiation. Molecular biologic techniques have demonstrated a high percentage with mutations of the tumor suppressor gene p53. Clinically, the level of differentiation does not significantly influence management when compared to factors such as location of primary tumor and nodal status. Distant metastases (lung, liver, and bone) may be evident in advanced disease, and diagnostic workup should include chest x-ray and liver function tests (LFTs). In more advanced disease, a CT scan of the chest and abdomen, as well as a bone scan, are warranted. Operative evaluation is performed in two stages: panendoscopy for staging followed by definitive resection. Direct laryngoscopy, bronchoscopy, and esophagoscopy (or barium swallow) are advocated because of the 5% to 8% incidence of synchronous primary lesions of the aerodigestive tract. Postoperatively these patients carry an elevated risk of developing a second tumor (approximately 4% per year) most commonly in the head and neck (50%) and lung (20%). If extensive resection is anticipated, or if radiation therapy to the head and neck region is planned, many surgeons advocate tracheotomy, insertion of gastric feeding tube, and teeth extraction before performing a definitive resection or starting radiation therapy. These procedures are indicated because of concern over radiation-induced edema of the airway and esophagus and induction of dental caries and osteoradionecrosis of the mandible and maxilla. Moreover, reconstruction of the airway and pharynx may limit oral intake.

Early carcinomas of the oral cavity and pharynx exhibit comparable responses to either radiation or surgical treatment. However, carcinoma of the oral cavity and pharynx frequently present as advanced disease. Prolonged exposure of tobacco and alcohol in the gingivobuccal sulcus and the floor of the mouth regions are thought to contribute to the distribution of these cancers. Lesions are frequently painless, and abundant soft tissue of the tongue and floor of the mouth permit considerable tumor growth before detection. Presenting symptoms may include altered tongue mobility, dysphagia, and dysarthria. However, more commonly, the patient will present with a mass in the neck that represents advanced nodal disease. In tumors of the hypopharynx, more than one half of patients will complain of referred ear pain.

Management of cancers of the oral cavity and pharynx are among the most challenging of surgical oncologic procedures. Resection typically includes partial or complete glossectomy and resection of involved mandibular segments. Neck dissection, which is routinely performed with oral cavity and pharynx neoplasms, will be discussed in subsequent text.

Advances have been made in reconstructive surgery, allowing the creation of bulky or pliable surfaces and contours in the oral cavity with pedicled and free flaps to permit deglutition. In addition, mandibular reconstruction can be accomplished with titanium plates or osteocutaneous free flaps from the fibula and iliac crest. Nevertheless, the inability to recreate delicate motor movements performed by the tongue can carry considerable morbidity with respect to swallowing competency; speech is most often articulate.

Adjuvant radiation is used in cancers of the oral cavity and pharynx, with the general indications including positive or close margins, extracapsular lymph node spread, perineural invasion, and multiple lymph node involvement.

Nasopharyngeal Carcinoma

An interesting subset of pharyngeal tumors occurs in the nasopharynx. These cancers comprise only 0.2% of newly diagnosed malignancies in the United States. However, in certain regions of China, these cancers represent 25% of all diagnosed cancers. This disparity in incidence is thought to be related to environmental exposure to specific types of Epstein-Barr virus (EBV), food-preserving nitrosamines, and to the prevalence of specific human leukocyte antigen genotypes. Demographically, peak incidence occurs in the fifth and sixth decades, although 20% of patients are younger than the age of 30 at diagnosis.

Tumors located in the fossa of Rosenmuller, immediately adjacent to the eustachian tube orifice, may cause obstruction of the eustachiam tube (Fig. 28-3). For this reason, persistent unilateral serous otitis media in the adult represents nasopharyngeal carcinoma until proved otherwise. Delayed diagnosis can have considerable negative impact with respect to prognosis. The presence of a neck mass, which represents cervical metastasis, is a common presenting complaint owing to the silent nature of this malignancy early-on. Other presenting symptoms may include nasal congestion, eye pain, hyperesthesia in the CN V^1 or V^2 distribution, epistaxis, and headache secondary to intracranial extension. Diplopia secondary to abducens (CN VI) paresis is the most commonly observed of the cranial neuropathies. Endoscopic nasopharyngoscopic examination may not detect submucosal spread, therefore, MRI examination should be ordered if uncertainty persists. The mainstay of treatment is radiation with chemotherapy. The cisplatin-based chemotherapy regimen increases disease-free survival time and overall survival. Surgery may be employed for patients with radiation failure or tumor recurrence. Because nasopharyngeal tumors frequently present with palpable nodal disease (87%), postirradiation neck dissection is recommended for persistent neck disease.

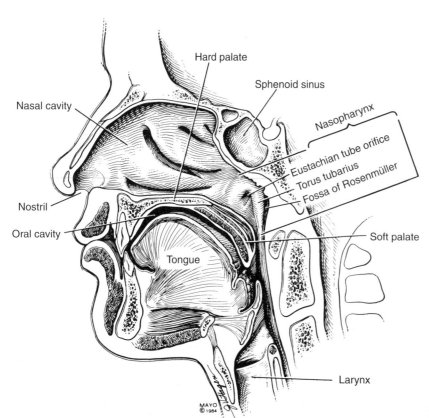

Figure 28-3 The nasopharynx and its anatomic relationships. (From Bailey BJ, ed. *Head and neck surgery: Otolaryngology*. Philadelphia: Lippincott Williams & Wilkins, 2001, with permission.)

OTHER HEAD AND NECK NEOPLASMS

Additional cancers of the head and neck include lymphomas. Extranodal sites commonly include the lypmhoid tissue of Waldeyer ring (adenoid, palatine tonsil, and lingual tonsil); however, other sites may include the paranasal sinuses, nasal cavity, oral cavity, salivary glands, and larynx. Non-Hodgkin lymphoma of the head and neck commonly presents as cervical adenopathy, although extranodal disease is present in 10% to 25% of patients. In contrast, it is unusual for Hodgkin disease of the head and neck to present in extranodal sites; rather, cervical adenopathy is the rule. When FNA is inconclusive, diagnosis is made on the basis of excisional lymph node biopsy or open biopsy of an extranodal site. Specimens should also be sent for flow cytometry to identify atypical lymphocytes, the presence of which increases diagnostic accuracy.

In the pediatric population, developmental anomalies can account for additional neck masses. *Branchial cleft cysts* (types I to IV) are typically found along the anatomic line that extends inferiorly from the external auditory canal along the anterior border of the sternocleidomastoid muscle. A patent ductal remnant frequently communicates with the aerodigestive tract, thereby resulting in intermittent swelling associated with upper respiratory tract infections. Treatment involves excision of the cyst along with its tract. Branchial cleft cysts may also initially present in the adult. The thyroglossal duct cyst represents a midline ductal remnant, which is found along the course of descent of the thyroid gland from the foramen cecum at the tongue base to the anterior neck. These congenital masses may present initially in the adult. As with other congenital masses, swelling and tenderness may occur with upper respiratory tract infections. Management includes removal of the cyst, its tract, and the midportion of the hyoid bone, which is intimately associated with the gland's descent. A preoperative ultrasounographic study of the neck should be ordered to ensure that normal thyroid tissue is present. In rare instances, the thyroglossal duct cyst represents the only functioning thyroid tissue in the individual; in these individuals preoperative counseling regarding the need for thyroid hormone replacement postoperatively must be discussed with the patient. Carcinomas have been rarely found within thyroglossal duct cysts. In fact, any cystic mass in the adult, either midline or lateral, may represent a cystic metastasis from a primary head and neck malignancy, most commonly tonsil and tongue base. This should be considered in the adult population with appropriate diagnostic workup, including FNA of the cyst, prior to definitive surgical excision.

LYMPHATICS OF THE HEAD AND NECK

Management of tumors involving the head and neck requires an understanding of staging algorithms that incorporates size of primary tumor, nodal status, and presence of metastases. Review of surgical pathology of head and neck malignancies indicates that neoplasms localized to each region of the head and neck have a predictable pattern of spread to specific lymph node chains (Fig. 28-4). This pattern is influenced by size and location of the tumor. By utilizing MRI or CT scanning, it is frequently

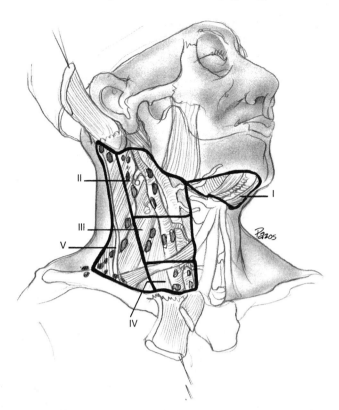

Figure 28-4 Lymph node regions of the neck. Level VI (central compartment) is not shown. (From Bailey BJ, ed. *Head and neck surgery: Otolaryngology.* Philadelphia: Lippincott Williams & Wilkins, 2003, with permission.)

possible to identify pathologic lymph nodes that may be undetectable clinically. (Normal nodes in the neck should not exceed 1 cm in greatest dimension, with the exception of the jugulodigastric lymph node, which may be as large as 1.5 cm). By identifying suspicious nodes, and by having a knowledge of metastatic patterns, the surgeon can plan tumor resection with the associated lymph nodes most likely to be involved.

The term *neck dissection* refers to procedures for surgical excision of lymph nodes and surrounding fibrofatty tissue from any or all of the six nodal groups in the neck. Multiple procedures have been described to accomplish resection. The most extensive procedure is the *radical neck dissection*, which requires sacrifice of lymph node levels I to V (see subsequent text) and (i) internal jugular vein, (ii) sternocleidomastoid muscle, and (iii) accessory nerve (CN XI). Predictably, this procedure carries the highest morbidity. In recent years, efforts have been made to spare one or more of these vital structures to lessen morbidity (*modified radical neck dissection*). Furthermore, attention has focused on limiting nodal dissection to only those groups most likely to be involved in tumor (*selective neck dissection*). Six lymph node groups or levels have been defined in the neck (Fig. 28-4). Level I nodes are located in the submental and submandibular triangles and drain the oral cavity and submandibular gland. The next three nodal groups are closely associated with the internal jugular vein. The most superior group, level II, extends from skull base to carotid bifurcation at the hyoid bone. Drainage from nasopharynx, oropharynx, the parotid gland, and supraglottic structures first involves these nodes. Intermediate, or level III, nodes are located between the carotid bifurcation and the intersection of the omohyoid muscle with the internal jugular vein at the level of the cricothyroid membrane. Level III nodes drain the oropharynx, hypopharynx, and supraglottic larynx. Level IV nodes are present inferior to level III and extend to the level of the clavicles. These nodes drain the subglottic larynx, hypopharynx, esophagus, and thyroid. The level V (posterior triangle) nodal group is bounded anteriorly by the posterior border of the sternocleidomastoid muscle and posteriorly by the anterior border of the trapezius muscle. This nodal group is a frequent site of metastases from tumors of the nasopharynx and oropharynx. The level VI (central compartment) nodes are located between the medial borders of the carotid sheath and drain thyroid and parathyroid malignancies.

Therapeutic neck dissection is performed when nodal disease is clinically apparent. *Elective neck dissection* is performed in patients with cancers where the risk of occult cervical metastases is high (e.g., tongue, floor of the mouth, and piriform sinus cancers have approximately a 30% risk of cervical metastases). In tumors associated with a lower risk (such as buccal mucosa, with a 9% incidence of occult nodes), some would recommend close observation in the postoperative period, rather than elective neck dissection.

Radiation therapy is directed at the site of the primary tumor and bed of involved lymph nodes when indicated. The role of chemotherapy as an adjuvant to surgery and radiation is currently under investigation. Although squamous cell carcinomas do not respond as well as certain other carcinomas, chemotherapy may enhance survival for patients with extracapsular tumor spread.

THE LARYNX

The larynx is composed of a cartilaginous tube that projects into the hypopharynx. Anatomically, the larynx is described as having three divisions: *supraglottis, glottis,* and *subglottis* (Figs. 28-5 and 28-6). The supraglottis is

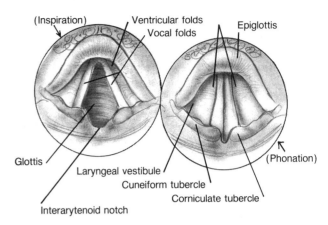

Figure 28-6 Endoscopic view of the larynx. (From Bailey BJ, ed. *Head and neck surgery: Otolaryngology.* Philadelphia: Lippincott Williams & Wilkins, 2001, with permission.)

bounded superiorly by the tip of the epiglottis and inferiorly by the floor of the laryngeal ventricle (the space between the true and false vocal folds). The glottis contains the true vocal folds. The subglottis arbitrarily begins 5 mm below the free edge of the true vocal folds and extends to the inferior border of the cricoid cartilage. The glottis serves as a sphincter to protect the airway from aspiration and to provide phonation. These structures are enclosed by the cricoid and thyroid cartilages, to which the intrinsic muscles of the glottis are attached. The actions of these intrinsic muscles serve to abduct and adduct the vocal folds, as well as to modulate vocal fold tension, thereby permitting ventilation and cord vibration. The superior laryngeal nerve (a branch of the vagus nerve) provides sensory innervation to the supraglottic area; stimulation in this region triggers a strong cough reflex. Inability to detect sensation in this area places an individual at great risk for aspiration. The superior laryngeal nerve also provides motor innervation to the cricothyroid muscle, which lengthens and tenses the vocal folds.

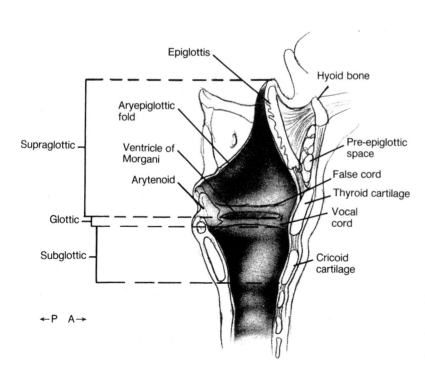

Figure 28-5 Midline sagittal section of the larynx, demonstrating the supraglottic, glottic, and subglottic regions, as well as the pre-epiglottic space. A, anterior; P, posterior. (From Bailey BJ, ed. *Head and neck surgery: Otolaryngology.* Philadelphia: Lippincott Williams & Wilkins, 2001, with permission.)

The remaining intrinsic muscles of the larynx are innervated by the recurrent laryngeal nerve (also a branch of the vagus nerve).

Unilateral vocal fold paralysis/paresis usually manifests as hoarseness and may be caused by a variety of pathologic conditions. Laryngeal cancer can present with hoarseness from vocal fold paralysis, as can a variety of neck and chest masses and tumors that may compress the recurrent laryngeal nerve. For this reason, unless an identifiable etiology is known (for example, sacrifice of the recurrent laryngeal nerve during chest surgery), imaging (chest x-ray plus contrast enhanced CT scanning or MRI) from the base of skull to the aortic arch is indicated to follow the course of the recurrent laryngeal nerve. Iatrogenic causes include surgical trauma that may have injured the recurrent laryngeal nerve anywhere along its course, for example from cardiothoracic surgery, anterior approaches to the cervical spine, and thyroid surgery. Other causes include stroke, intubation trauma, and viral infections. When a definitive etiology cannot be identified, the diagnosis of *idiopathic vocal fold paralysis* is given; these cases are most likely caused by a viral infection and may spontaneously resolve. Several surgical options exist to medialize a paralyzed vocal fold if a glottic gap exists. Injection thyroplasty involves injecting one of several available materials into the true vocal fold to bring it toward the midline. This is usually performed in the operating room by using direct laryngoscopy with the needle inserted directly into the vocal fold. Office injections under local anesthesia are also employed where the needle is inserted externally though the thyroid cartilage or cricothyroid membrane with visualization provided by flexible nasopharyngolaryngoscopy (see subsequent text).

Hoarseness does not always imply vocal fold paralysis or paresis. Lesions of the larynx, such as glottic tumors (both benign and malignant) and vocal cord nodules, may cause voice changes without impairing overall vocal cord mobility; rather *apposition* of the true vocal cord surfaces is impaired. Chronic changes of the larynx from gastroesophageal reflux (discussed in subsequent text) or postnasal drip may also cause voice changes secondary to laryngeal irritation and inflammation. In addition to history, office endoscopy is essential in the workup of hoarseness. Flexible nasopharyngolaryngoscopy (NPL) is relatively quick and well tolerated. No topical preparation is needed, although decongestant and anesthetic sprays are often administered to aid in patient comfort. This office procedure allows examination of the nasal cavities, nasopharynx, oropharynx, hypopharynx, and larynx down to and including the true vocal folds. If suspicious lesions are seen, more extensive evaluation may be performed in the operating room with direct laryngoscopy (using rigid laryngoscopes); biopsies may also be taken at this time to aid in diagnosis.

With respect to the sudden onset of stridor, principal causes include infectious etiologies, foreign bodies, and angioedema. The first step in management is securing the airway. Flexible NPL can be extremely helpful in assessing the patency of the upper airway and the possible need for intubation or awake tracheotomy. Viral or bacterial infections can be managed with humidification, appropriate antibiotics, and steroids. Angioedema is an unusual entity presenting as a rapid onset of swelling in some or all parts of the upper airway, (e.g., lips, tongue, or larynx). Swelling of other body parts may also be involved in cases of angioedema, including the extremities and gastrointestinal

tract. It occurs most commonly in response to food allergy or medications (particularly angiotensin-converting enzyme inhibitors). Management includes high-dose systemic steroids, histamine blockers [e.g., diphenhydramine (H1-receptor antagonist) and ranitidine (H2-receptor antagonist)], subcutaneous epinephrine and airway observation in a monitored bed. Securing the airway in these patients can be a challenge beccause of airway swelling, and is often achieved via fiberoptic nasotracheal intubation by someone skilled in the technique; if this fails, emergent tracheotomy may be necessary. An additional cause of acute-onset stridor is an aspirated foreign body. More common in the pediatric population, airway foreign bodies may be pieces of food, toy parts, or other animate or inanimate objects. Because organic matter is often radiolucent, plain films are of little use, although they may demonstrate air trapping with lung hyperinflation. Direct laryngoscopy and bronchoscopy are often employed to rule out foreign bodies as a source of wheezing or stridor when a suggestive history exists.

Gastroesophageal reflux disease may manifest itself in the larynx, sometimes as its sole presentation. The pathophysiology of this entity, termed reflux laryngitis, involves intermittent reflux of gastric acid into the cervical esophagus that spills over into the larynx. Only small amounts of episodic regurgitation are required to cause laryngeal inflammation, and laryngeal symptoms may be present in the absence of gastrointestinal complaints in up to one third of patients. Common symptoms of reflux laryngitis include hoarseness, chronic cough or throat clearing, and *globus sensation* (feeling of a lump in the throat). Findings on flexible NPL include arytenoid erythema and interarytenoid edema or fullness. Significant reflux may cause more diffuse supraglottic inflammation. Treatment consists of reducing stomach acid production with H2 blockers or proton pump inhibitors, dietary and lifestyle modification, head of bed elevation while sleeping, and avoiding eating within 3 hours of going to sleep. Patients who fail conservative medical management may need gastrointestinal referral for further workup, with the possibility of surgery if pathology is identified (e.g., hiatal hernia).

With respect to the pediatric population, noisy breathing and respiratory obstruction can be the result of supraglottic, glottic, or subglottic pathology. (It is important to note that in children, the cricoid cartilage represents the narrowest diameter of the upper airway.) A common cause of neonatal airway distress, usually manifested as "noisy breathing," is laryngotracheomalacia. In these patients, immature cartilage of the larynx and trachea is unable to maintain its shape and collpases with breathing, particularly when forceful. Laryngomalacia may exist separately from tracheomalacia, and each presents differently. With laryngomalacia, inspiratory stridor is noted as the eipglottis and arytenoids collapse into the glottic airway with inspiration. During expiration, these structures are propelled back to their normal supraglottic positions. Conversely, with tracheomalacia, expiratory stridor is heard as the tracheal cartilage collpases as air is expelled; with inspiration, inspired air fills the trachea and stents it open. In most cases, management of these conditions is observation; as the child matures and the cartilage becomes more sturdy, breathing becomes quieter and more comfortable. In severe cases of laryngomalacia with respiratory distress, supraglottoplasty may be performed to release the epiglottis from the aryepiglottic folds and to prevent collapse. For severe tracheomalacia with respiratory distress, tracheotomy may be required. Other causes of chronic respiratory distress and noisy breathing in pediatric patients include vascular malformations that compress the trachea, subglottic cysts, hemangiomas, and subglottic stenosis. Cardiothoracic surgery may be required to repair vascular rings or anomalous vessels, whereas cysts are usually resected by using direct laryngoscopy/bronchoscopy and lasers. Hemangiomas, which typically enlarge during the first few months of life, may produce symptoms of airway compromise. Continued growth occurs for approximately 3 to 4 years before involution. The preferred treatment involves observation; steroids may be required for episodes of respiratory distress exacerbated by viral croup, for example. In cases of severe airway compromise, tracheotomy or laser resection of the hemangioma can be used to improve the airway. Subglottic stenosis, which may be primary or acquired (e.g., from prolonged intubation), typically causes biphasic stridor. For patients with respiratory distress, tracheotomy may be necessary until laryngotracheoplasty (widening of the stenotic area using cartilage grafts) can be performed.

Cancers of the Larynx

Approximately 11,000 laryngeal cancers are diagnosed each year in the United States. Peak incidence occurs in the fifth through seventh decades, with men affected more commonly than women. As with other head and neck cancers, principal risk factors include tobacco and alcohol products. Presenting symptoms include hoarseness, dyspnea, hemoptysis, dysphagia, and odynophagia. Referred ear pain (otalgia) is also observed secondary to overlapping afferents from the vagus nerve supplying both the ear and larynx. The overwhelming majority of laryngeal lesions are squamous cell carcinomas (greater than 90%), with the remaining tumors including verrucous carcinoma, adenocarcinoma, sarcoma, and rare metastases (renal cell, breast, prostate, and melanoma).

Anatomically, the larynx is described as having three divisions (see descriptions in preceding text and Fig. 28-5). Extensive lymphatics from the supraglottic larynx drain anteriorly to the pre-epiglottic space and to bilateral cervical lymph nodes. Metastases to lymph nodes is relatively high at the time of diagnosis and tends to be bilateral. Glottic cancers represent the majority of laryngeal tumors. These tumors are frequently detected early in the course of the disease as persistent hoarseness often prompts further investigation. Lymph node involvement tends to be relatively low at presentation, and when present tends to be ipsilateral. Although the rarest of the laryngeal cancers (less than 5%), subglottic tumors carry a poor prognosis because patients develop symptoms late in the disease; nodal metastases at presentation is common.

Treatment for laryngeal cancer includes surgical approaches (both organ-preserving and more extensive procedures), radiation, and chemotherapy. Extensive surgical resections (partial and total laryngectomy) carry the significant morbidity associated with voice loss or hoarseness. Voice-conservative procedures, such as supracricoid laryngectomy and partial laryngectomy (either open or laser), are used to preserve functional levels of phonation while providing successful cancer treatment. Discrete

mapping of tumor location allows for preservation of portions of the glottis that might have been resected previously. In instances in which total laryngectomy is performed, a permanent stoma is created in the lower neck. Postoperative communication can be accomplished with the electrolarynx, through esophageal speech, or via creation of a tracheoesophageal fistula with placement of a voice prosthesis. This last method uses a one-way plastic valve that allows air to flow from t he trachea into the neopharynx while the tracheostoma is temporarily occluded by the patient. Pharyngeal and oral cavity vibration creates sound, which takes time and practice to convert into intelligible speech.

ANATOMY OF THE NOSE AND PARANASAL SINUSES

The external nose consists of a bony skeleton forming the upper one third of the nose and a cartilaginous skeleton forming the lower two thirds. The internal nose is divided by the septum, which is composed of four structures: the perpendicular plate of the ethmoid bone, the vomer bone, the quadrilateral cartilage, and the crest of the maxillary bone. All of these structures are covered by mucoperichondrium or mucoperiostium. The term *deviated septum* refers to folding or bending of the midline septum. An asymptomatic deviation is present in many individuals. In severe instances in which unilateral nasal obstruction is present, the cartilage and bone can be excised, trimmed, or reshaped to increase air flow (*septoplasty*).

Four paired sinuses communicate with the nasal cavity. All sinuses begin development *in utero*; however, adult dimensions are not attained until late adolescence. Each sinus produces mucus, which serves to warm and humidify inspired air, as well as to trap inspired allergens and fine particulate matter. The maxillary sinuses develop beneath the orbits, the frontal sinuses anterosuperior to the orbits, and the sphenoid sinuses midline and posterior to the orbits. The ethmoid sinuses consist of two groups of eight to twelve cells arranged in a honeycomb configuration between the orbits. The inferior, middle, and superior turbinates represent the terminal extensions of the lateral nasal wall. These turbinates project into each nasal cavity and direct air flow and mucus posteriorly into the nasopharynx. Ciliary beating directs mucus to the natural sinus openings (ostia), into the nasal cavity, and then posteriorly to the nasopharynx, where the mucus is swallowed.

Rhinitis

Most complaints related to the nasal cavity concern symptoms of rhinitis and sinusitis, collectively referred to as rhinosinusitis. Symptoms of rhinitis occur secondary to engorgement of nasal mucosa and hypersecretion of glands and include nasal congestion, rhinorrhea, nasal itching, and postnasal drip. Numerous etiologies exist and are first categorized as either nonallergic or allergic. Nonallergic causes include infections, environmental irritants, medications, pregnancy, and systemic disease states. Allergic rhinitis may be perennial or seasonal, depending on the particular allergen involved. Treatment of nonallergic rhinitis is directed at the cause of the disease. Infectious rhinitis, which may be viral, bacterial, or both, may require antibiotics; removal of environmental irritants, such as second-hand smoke, industrial chemicals, and cosmetic products, may alleviate symptoms; medications, most commonly sympathetic-blocking agents and birth control pills, may need to be changed. Additional pharmacotherapy for nonallergic rhinitis includes nasal and systemic decongestants. Caution must be used in patients with uncontrolled hypertension, as decongestants are alpha agonists. In addition, nasal decongestant sprays must not be used for more than 3 days, as prolonged use can cause *rhinitis medicamentosa*, a rebound nasal congestion that becomes a challenge to treat effectively. The pathophysiology of allergic rhinitis involves a Gel & Coombs Type I hypersensitivity reaction involving immunoglobulin E (IgE), basophils, and mast cells. Histamine, prostaglandins, and leukotrienes are several mediators implicated in the pathogenesis and cause nasal obstruction, rhinorrhea, and itching. Therefore, treatment is aimed at controlling these pathways. Nasal steroids are first-line therapy for allergic rhinitis and blunt the allergic response by stabilizing mast cells, inhibiting formation of inflammatory mediators, and blocking chemotaxis of inflammatory cells. Topical administration has little systemic absorption, and side effects are usually local, including nasal irritation, crusting, and epistaxis. Other treatment modalities include antihistamines, the newer of which have less central nervous system penetration and are, therefore, less sedating. Leukotriene antagonists, used in the management of reactive airways disease, are finding a more-defined role in the treatment of allergic rhinitis. Systemic decongestants also play a role in decreasing nasal congestion, as in nonallergic rhinitis. In addition to pharmacotherapy for allergic rhinitis, identification of allergens through allergy testing is essential. Once identified, immunotherapy, which is aimed at desensitization of the immune system against a particular allergen, may be employed as a treatment.

Paranasal Sinus Infections

The development of sinus infections stems from impaired sinonasal mucociliary transport and/or blockage of sinus ostia. The former may occur from a viral infection that damages ciliary action, whereas the latter may be secondary to blockage from a deviated septum, turbinate hypertrophy, or allergic nasal polyps. In either case, sinus infection may result, manifesting as facial pain or pressure, nasal obstruction, postnasal drip, rhinorrhea, and fever. Diagnosis is based on history and physical examination. Imaging is not indicated for acute sinusitis unless a complication extending beyond the sinuses is suspected (see subsequent text). First-line therapy for acute bacterial sinusitis involves decongestants and antibiotics.

Acute sinusitis is defined as sinusitis for which symptoms last less than 4 weeks. Chronic sinusitis is defined as sinus disease for which symptoms last more than 12 weeks and are persistent. In between is arbitrarily defined subacute sinusitis. Chronic sinusitis, for which symptoms are persistent, should be differentiated from recurrent sinusitis, in which patients get recurrent attacks of acute sinusitis, each lasting less than 4 weeks, with symptom-free intervals between acute attacks.

Management of chronic sinusitis includes nasal steroid sprays, antibiotics, and treatment of allergy when present. In patients who fail medical management, endoscopic sinus surgery may be indicated to enlarge natural sinus ostia and to resect areas of obstructing bony overgrowth and sinonasal polyps, when present. In this manner, egress of mucus and pus from the sinuses is improved.

Complications of Sinusitis

The most serious complications of sinus infections involve spread of infection to the orbits and central nervous system (CNS). Orbital complications of sinus disease most commonly originate from the ethmoid sinuses, and this is most commonly seen in the pediatric population (Fig. 28-7). The mode of spread from all sinuses is by means of the bloodstream or direct extension. The degree of orbital involvement ranges from periorbital cellulitis to orbital abscess, with cavernous sinus thrombosis being the most severe on the disease spectrum. Symptoms may include proptosis, *chemosis* (conjunctival edema), extraocular muscle entrapment, and

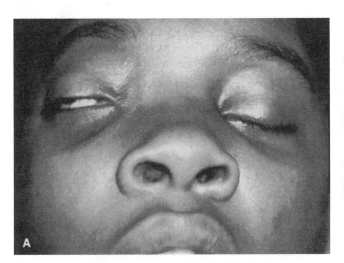
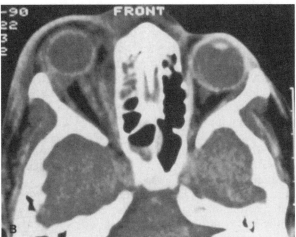

Figure 28-7   A: Patient with asymmetric proptosis secondary to a subperiosteal abscess. **B:** Axial computerized tomographic scan of the same patient. (From Bailey BJ, ed. *Head and neck surgery: Otolaryngology.* Philadelphia: Lippincott Williams & Wilkins, 2001, with permission.)

vision loss. Diagnosis is based upon physical examination and contrast-enhanced imaging. Patients with periorbital cellulitis typically can be managed successfully with broad-spectrum intravenous antibiotics. More advanced stages with abscess formation usually require surgical drainage and opening of the involved sinuses (either endoscopically or externally). An ophthalmology consultation is necessary to document vision and any progression of visual compromise or ocular muscle entrapment, which would prompt surgical intervention.

Intracranial spread of sinusitis most commonly stems from the frontal sinuses, especially in male adolescents; this is thought to be related to the rich vascularity of the diploic veins in this patient population. Intracranial involvement may present as meningitis, epidural abscess, subdural empyema, intracerebral abscess, venous sinus thrombosis, and osteomyelitis. Diagnosis is again determined by physical examination plus contrast-enhanced imaging, often employing MRI. Treatment is multidisciplinary consisting of an otolaryngologist and neurosurgeon and involves drainage of the involved sinuses (either endoscopically or externally) as well as any intracranial collection when appropriate.

Epistaxis

Epistaxis represents a potentially serious medical emergency. Global questions need to be addressed, such as airway patency and hemodynamic stability. Information regarding prescription and nonprescription medications [Coumadin, aspirin, nonsteroidal anti-inflammatory drugs (NSAIDs)], history of hypertension, myelodysplasias, coagulopathy, hemodialysis, hepatic disease, prior bleeding episodes, and recent trauma should be elicited. Duration and quantity of bleeding, as well as unilateral versus bilateral nature, should be determined. Pharmacologic control of blood pressure should be initiated in the hypertensive patient. Intravenous access should be established if there is evidence of significant epistaxis or hemodynamic instability. Laboratory studies should be ordered, including complete blood count and coagulation panels. In the presence of considerable bleeding with anemia, blood products should be available, particularly for the elderly patient.

Epistaxis can be categorized as either anterior or posterior in origin. Anterior nosebleeds tend to be unilateral in nature, whereas posterior nosebleeds are more likely to be bilateral as blood makes its way around the nasal septum posteriorly and drains out of the contrateral nare (although profuse anterior bleeds may also do this). Of all nosebleeds, approximately 90% originate from the anterior septum in a region called Kiesselbach plexus, which represents a rich anastomotic network of vessels. Local irritative factors predispose to bleeding from this area, including digital or mechanical trauma, dry indoor heat in the wintertime, and chemical irritants. Anterior rhinoscopy (using either nasal speculum and headlight or an otoscope) will often reveal excoriated septal mucosa with exposed vessels. If pressure applied across the nose, along with correction of coagulopathy and control of hypertension, does not stop the bleeding, point cauterization with silver nitrate sticks may suffice. However, care must be taken with cauterization on the contralateral side at the same level, as this may lead to septal perforation. If cauterization does not work, anterior

nasal packing will usually halt persistent bleeding. For posterior bleeding, endoscopic evaluation may reveal the bleeding source. If accessible, cauterization with silver nitrate may be sufficient. Alternatively, placement of a small nasal pack under endoscopic visualization may be necessary. If this is not possible secondary to copious bleeding or patient discomfort, placement of a posterior nasal pack may be required. Packs are left in place for 3 to 5 days, antistaphylococcal antibiotics are administered (to guard against toxic shock syndrome), and blood-thinning agents are discontinued if medically possible.

In the extreme case, ligation of the internal maxillary artery or anterior or posterior ethmoid arteries may be required, either transnasally or externally. Angiography and embolization are becoming more successful in identifying involved vessels and controlling bleeding.

ANATOMY AND PHYSIOLOGY OF THE AUDITORY SYSTEM

The anatomy of the ear serves to transduce disturbances in atmospheric pressure into electrical impulses that are carried to the CNS. The human auditory system is capable of hearing sounds from 20 to 20,000 Hz, with typical speech exhibiting frequencies in the 500 to 4,000 Hz range. Sound intensities are measured on a logarithmic scale from 0 to 120 decibels (dB). An individual with normal hearing has a threshold for perception of sounds at an intensity of 0 to 20 dB. Normal conversational speech is in the 20 to 50 dB range. Painful levels of noise occur in excess of 80 dB and exposure to elevated sound intensity for prolonged periods may result in permanent sensorineural hearing loss. The system responsible for perception of auditory stimuli consists of a *conductive* portion (external ear, external auditory canal, tympanic membrane, and ossicles) and a *sensorineural* portion [cochlea and cochlear nerve (CN VIII)]. Acoustic stimuli produce vibrations of the tympanic membrane, which are transferred via the ossicles (*malleus, incus,* and *stapes*) to the footplate of the stapes (Fig. 28-8). Amplification of sound is accomplished according to the ratio of vibrating tympanic membrane area to stapes footplate area (17:1). The acoustic impedance matching is also enhanced by the ratio of the lengths of the long processes of the malleus and incus (1.3:1). These two factors yield an approximate 25-fold amplification of signal intensity delivered at the footplate, which rests in the oval window of the cochlea.

Conductive hearing losses may occur secondary to cerumen ("ear wax") impaction, tympanic membrane perforation, middle-ear effusion, or ossicular discontinuity. *Otosclerosis,* another cause of conductive hearing loss, is caused by fixation of the stapes footplate at its articulation with the oval window. Otosclerosis is a disorder that affects predominantly middle-aged, white patients with a familial propensity. Women are affected roughly twice as often as men. For surgical candidates, the stapes is removed and replaced with a prosthetic implant. As in the case of otosclerosis, other defects in the conduction system are often amenable to improvement or correction (e.g., cerumen disimpaction, repair of tympanic membrane perforation, or drainage of middle ear fluid).

An audiogram (hearing test) is a valuable diagnostic test in the evaluation of the auditory system. Conductive hearing

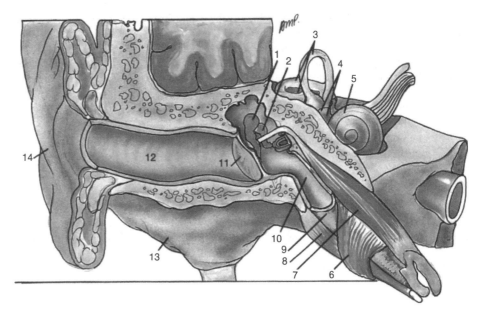

Figure 28-8 Structures of the ear: *(1)* malleus, *(2)* incus, *(3)* semicircular canals, *(4)* utricle and saccule, *(5)* cochlea, *(6)* dilator tubae muscle, *(7)* tensor tympani muscle, *(8)* levator veli palatini muscle, *(9)* cartilaginous auditory tube, *(10)* eustachian tube, *(11)* tympanic membrane, *(12)* external auditory canal, *(13)* mastoid, and *(14)* pinna. (From Bailey BJ, ed. *Head and neck surgery: Otolaryngology.* Philadelphia: Lippincott Williams & Wilkins, 2001, with permission.)

losses can be differentiated from sensorineural hearing losses on routine audiometry. Additional information about conductive losses can be gained by *tympanometry*. Tympanometry is a test that measures the compliance of the tympanic membrane, which in turn represents the status of the middle ear (for example, middle ear fluid will decrease the compliance of the tympanic membrane and result in a flattened tympanogram).

In contrast to conductive hearing loss, sensorineural hearing loss is more difficult to diagnose and correct. This type of hearing loss can be diagnosed on a standard audiogram. An additional form of sensitivity testing involves delivery of stimuli to the ear while recording regional brain activity via surface electrodes (auditory brainstem response). This form of testing is valuable for auditory screening in the neonate with suspected hearing loss, in whom interactive means of testing are not possible. Evidence of an asymmetric sensorineural hearing loss on audiogram merits workup to exclude pathology of the vestibulocochlear nerve and cerebellopontine angle. This pathology, when present, is typically an acoustic neuroma, which most commonly represents a schwannoma of the vestibular portion of CN VIII. Meningiomas are less common. Diagnosis is determined from MRI examination of the internal auditory canals; treatment options include observation, surgery, or radiotherapy.

The differential diagnosis for sensorineural hearing loss is extensive. A variety of infections, both bacterial and viral, can affect the cochlea and cochlear nerve, whereas meningitis can have drastic effects on sensorineural hearing. Head trauma can result in sensorineural hearing loss, either through fracture of the otic capsule or from concussive effects. Noise-induced hearing loss, which is the most common etiology after infancy and before old age, can result from a single, significant loud noise exposure or more commonly from repeated exposure to loud noises. Neurologic and autoimmune conditions can cause hearing loss, as can neoplasms and bone disorders (for example, narrowing of bony foramenae and canals that transmit cranial nerves, as in Paget disease). Among medications,

several are known to be ototoxic and/or vestibulotoxic, including aminoglycoside antimicrobials, vancomycin, loop diuretics (furosemide), salicylates, NSAIDs, and several chemotherapeutic agents, such as cisplatin. Of the various ototoxic medications, antibiotics and diuretics are the most common offenders. With respect to antimicrobial ototoxicity, the hearing loss is typically bilateral (although can be unilateral), begins after several days of treatment (although it may occur after one dose or even several months after the completion of therapy) and may be permanent. Patients who require long-term treatment with ototoxic antibiotics should, therefore, undergo baseline audiometry prior to treatment. In children, numerous congenital anomalies can manifest as hearing loss, either as the sole symptom or as part of a clinical syndrome. In the elderly, when an identifiable etiology is unapparent, the disorder is termed *presbycusis*, or age-related hearing loss.

Treatment of hearing loss depends upon the etiology. In the case of bacterial infection (such as syphilis or Lyme disease), appropriate antibiotic therapy is initiated, which may result in partial recovery of hearing. Autoimmune hearing loss may improve with treatment of the underlying disorder (for example, use of steroids and/or immunosuppressives). Ototoxic medications should be discontinued to prevent further damage, as should exposure to loud noise. Tumors may require surgical excision, and congenital deafness may be improved with cochlear implantation (see subsequent text) or hearing aids. A special case of hearing loss is sudden sensorineural hearing loss (SSNHL). Patients rapidly develop hearing loss over 12 hours or less, and this is often noticed upon awakening in the morning. The hearing loss is usually isolated to one ear, and tinnitus or vertigo may also be present. The etiology is usually unknown, however the workup for sensorineural hearing loss is completed before it is assumed to be idiopathic. Treatment usually consists of high-dose steroids to reduce presumed inflammation of the cochlear nerve, and many clinicians use antivirals to treat presumed viral agents, which may be responsible for idiopathic cases.

In cases of stable, idiopathic, sensorineural hearing loss (such as presbycusis in the elderly), hearing amplification devices can be worn in one or both ears. In specialized cases (such as congenital deafness or trauma in the adult), serious sensorineural hearing loss can be improved by the use of cochlear implants. In a simplified description, these devices employ a wire electrode that is threaded into the cochlea and attached to a receiver that is anchored to the skull under skin flaps. The receiver converts sound into electrical impulses that are transmitted along the wire electrode into the cochlea, where they stimulate spiral ganglion neurons. Specific channels activated along the length of the wire transmit electrical impulses to hair cells corresponding to the desired frequencies for amplification. Activation of selected channels can be tailored to accommodate the deficits identified in a particular individual. Success in cochlear nerve implants is influenced by the candidates; optimal candidates are the postlingual deaf adult and the prelingual deaf child.

BALANCE AND THE VESTIBULAR SYSTEM

The perception of position, spatial orientation, acceleration, and rotation is accomplished through synthesis of sensory input from peripheral muscles and ocular cues, as well as from the vestibular structures of the inner ear. The *otolithic organs* refer to the *saccule* and *utricle*, which are filled with *endolymph* produced by the *stria vascularis*. The sensory component of each organ (*macula*) is made up of hair cells attached to a membrane composed of crystals of calcium carbonate (*otoconia*). Changes in gravity and linear acceleration result in displacement of the membrane, producing discharge in hair cells and a neural impulse. This information is processed with impulses generated in the *ampulla*, or in the sensory component of the *right* and *left semicircular canals*. These three structures are oriented at 90 degrees to each other in x, y, and z planes. The semicircular canals respond to angular acceleration. Movement of endolymph within a semicircular canal produces traction on a gelatinous membrane (*cupula*), resulting in discharge in vestibular hair cells. Because the right and left canals exist in a mirror orientation, changes in inertia will produce deflection of endolymph toward the ampulla on one side and away from the ampulla on the contralateral side. Proportional discharge of right and left vestibular systems allows assignment of motion direction. Asymmetric firing of right and left vestibular systems produces the subjective sensation of rotation, or vertigo. This firing pattern can be the result of viral infection (*vestibular neuritis*), vascular compromise, or displacement of otoconia in the posterior semicircular canal. The latter event results in episodic vertigo over a period of weeks elicited when the head assumes specific positions (e.g., lying down with head to the right). This syndrome is called *benign paroxysmal positional vertigo*, or cupulolithiasis, which can be reversed by a series of head motions (Dix-Hallpike maneuvers) that direct the crystals back to the utricle. An additional entity associated with vertigo is Menière disease, which represents a "diagnosis of exclusion." The syndrome consists of sudden attacks of vertigo, tinnitus, aural fullness, and hearing loss lasting 30 to 120 minutes. Seventy percent of cases are unilateral,

whereas 30% develop contralateral symptoms within several years. Progressive sensorineural hearing loss occurs. Many medical and surgical treatments have been described to address the most distressing symptoms associated with intractable vertigo and include gentamicin injections into the middle ear, laryrinthectomy, and vestibular nerve section.

Otologic Infection

Infections of the external, middle, and inner ear are common. Otitis externa is an inflammatory condition that typically affects the external auditory canal. Etiologic factors include water exposure (hence the layman's term "swimmer's ear") and local trauma to the canal, which typically occurs when patients insert objects in the canal in an attempt to remove wax. The patient presents with symptoms of ear pain (*otalgia*) and ear drainage (*otorrhea*). On physical examination, the auricle and external canal may be erythematous and tender upon manipulation. Canal edema is typically present, sometimes impairing visualization of the tympanic membrane, and otorrhea with debris in the canal is usually seen, further obstructing one's view of the tympanic membrane. The causative organisms are usually *Pseudomonas aeruginosa* and *Staphylococcus aureus*. Management includes débridement of the ear canal (usually performed in the office using micro-otoscopy) and application of steroid-containing antibiotic drops; severe cases (for example, when an overlying cellulitis and chondritis of the auricle is present) may warrant the addition of oral antibiotics. In patients with significant canal edema, a cotton wick may be inserted into the canal; this serves to both stent-open the canal and provide a means for topical drops to penetrate the entire canal. The wick may be removed in follow-up after several days.

More severe infections may be seen in the immunocompromised patient. Seen in the patients with poorly controlled diabetes or in the immunocompromised patient, *malignant otitis externa* represents a serious infection of the external auditory canal. Infection spreads beyond the external auditory canal to involve the skull base, which may lead to osteomyelitis of the skull base, cranial neuropathies, meningitis, venous sinus thrombosis, and death. Diagnostic studies include CT scan to document bony destruction, bone scan to evaluate for osteomyelitis and gallium-67 scan to track active inflammation. Management includes diabetic control, long-term antibiotics, and surgical drainage of any associated abscesses.

Inflammation of the middle ear is broadly referred to as *otitis media*, with modifiers added to refer to specific conditions, for example *acute* otitis media and *serous* otitis media. Briefly, the middle ear space houses the ossicles and is connected to the mastoid air cells posteriorly and to the nasopharynx via the eustachian tube anteriorly. This connection to the nasopharynx is what allows ventilation of an otherwise sealed space. When the eustachian tube is blocked (for example, from adenoid hypertrophy) or its function impaired (for example, during an upper respiratory infection), ventilation of the middle ear is disrupted and fluid accumulates it this space. When noninfected, this condition is referred to as *serous otitis media*. This fluid may become secondarily infected and result in *acute otitis media*. In either case a conductive hearing loss may be apparent with the sensation of aural fullness. In the acute infectious state, pain, fever, and possibly otorrhea from tympanic membrane rupture may be reported. Treatment consists of oral antibiotics, and is directed at the usual pathogens (*Streptococcus pneumoniae*, *Haemophilus influenzae*, and *Moraxella catarrhalis*). Acute otitis media in children is a common problem and is caused by several factors. Adenoidal hypertrophy is not uncommon in children; this tissue not only blocks the eustachian tube orifice but also serves as a reservoir for bacteria, which may travel retrograde into the middle ear. This is further facilitated by anatomic differences in the pediatric eustachian tube that make this retrograde travel easier. In children who experience recurrent bouts of acute otitis media or who have persistent sterile middle ear fluid (which may cause a conductive hearing loss and cause speech and language delays), pressure equalization tubes may be indicated. This is a common surgical procedure in which an incision is made in the tympanic membrane (*myringotomy*) into which a small tube is placed. This improves ventilation of the middle ear and relieves the build up of fluid. Serious complications of acute otitis media can involve local structures and may lead to facial nerve paralysis, meningitis, venous sinus thrombosis, or brain abscess. These potentially serious complications require aggressive medical and surgical management, often requiring mastoidectomy to drain infection.

Chronic ear infections can lead to the development of a *cholesteatoma*, which is an epithelial-lined cyst containing desquamated keratin. Growth of this histologically benign lesion can lead to erosion of bone and local structures, including the ossicles. Destruction may proceed to involve the semicircular canals, the facial nerve, and the brain. Surgical resection of the cholesteatoma with reconstruction of ossicles and tympanic membrane is required to restore functional hearing.

Additional infections of the ear include viral infections harbored in cranial nerve ganglia. The most serious is caused by the reactivation of the herpes virus leading to herpes zoster oticus, which is associated with Ramsay Hunt syndrome. Herpetic lesions are seen in the external canal and in the distribution of CN VII. Facial nerve edema with associated paresis is often noted. The infections typically respond well to antiviral agents and oral steroids.

Otologic Neoplasms

Neoplastic processes affecting the inner ear and cerebellopontine angle are rare. Benign tumors (neuromas) arising in the internal auditory canal can compress any of four nerves that travel via this canal to the central nervous system: the facial nerve, the cochlear nerve (a division of CN VIII), or the inferior and superior vestibular nerves (divisions of CN VIII). Other tumors of the cerebellopontine angle include gliomas, meningiomas, epidermoid cysts, and arachnoid cysts. Compression of CN VII or the divisions of CN VIII can produce various symptoms, necessitating diagnostic evaluation. Surgery includes excision of tumors with an attempt at preserving nerve function. Paragangliomas (commonly referred to as glomus tumors) are benign neoplasms of chromaffin-producing cells located within the head and neck, most commonly at the carotid bifurcation, jugular bulb, and middle ear. Growth of these neoplasms can result in hearing loss and cranial neuropathies. Rare malignant transformation of paragangliomas has been reported, as has catecholamine-secreting ability. Multiple or bilateral lesions occur in about 10% of patients, and those with a positive family history of these neoplasms should undergo genetic counseling. The treatment options for these neoplasms are observation for growth or change, surgery and/or radiation. Counselling regarding possible cranial nerve injury from resection needs to be discussed with patients before surgery. Preoperative assessment for urine metanephrines and vanillylmandelic acid (VMA) is also indicated. Angiography with possible embolization of feeding vessels is usually performed in conjunction with surgery; ideally this is performed within 24 hours of the planned resection. Radiation, which provides growth arrest and some decrease in tumor size, is reserved for patients who are poor surgical candidates but who need treatment.

Although cutaneous malignancies of the auricle are not uncommon, neoplasms of the external auditory canal and temporal bone do occur. Of tumors of the auricle, the overwhelming majority are squamous cell and basal cell carcinomas that develop secondary to sun exposure. Management includes wide-margin resection of involved portions of the auricle. Tumors of the external auditory canal and temporal bone are mostly squamous cell carcinomas, although adnexal tumors are also possible. Surgical management is the mainstay of treatment. This may range from a sleeve resection of the ear canal for small, nonbony tumors to more extensive temporal bone resections for larger tumors. Most cases require postoperative radiation therapy.

TRAUMA

Otologic Trauma

The temporal bone is one of the hardest bones in the human body and fractures affecting this structure are rare. Those that do occur are typically the result of high-speed motor vehicle accidents, falls, or assault. Two principal classifications have been described with the diagnosis made on the basis of noncontrast temporal bone CT scans. Longitudinal fractures (70% to 90%) are caused by lateral trauma to the squamous portion of the temporal bone. The fracture line extends from the posterosuperior portion of the external auditory canal, through the eardrum, to the otic capsule and petrous apex. Delayed paresis of the facial nerve occurs in approximately 10% to 20% of cases and is caused by edema of the seventh nerve. If the nerve is intact, this weakness should resolve with time. Physical examination findings may include mastoid hematoma (Battle sign), blood in the external auditory canal, cerebrospinal fluid (CSF) otorrhea, and tympanic membrane perforation. Conductive hearing loss is common because of disruption of middle-ear ossicles and eardrum perforation. Vestibular symptoms and sensorineural hearing loss are uncommon and are usually caused by the concussive effect on the cochlea and inner ear.

Transverse fractures represent 10% to 20% of injuries and occur with trauma to either the posterior occiput or to the frontal area. Transverse fractures typically are associated with higher mortality secondary to severe associated head trauma. The fracture line extends across the petrous pyramid, through the foramen spinosum or foramen lacerum, and through the internal auditory canal. Facial nerve injury occurs in approximately 50% of cases and is caused by crush injury or laceration of the nerve. Evidence of immediate facial nerve injury warrants middle-ear exploration to identify compressed or transected areas. Sensorineural loss is severe and is usually caused by direct cochlear injury or cochlear nerve damage. The eardrum is usually not torn, but blood is often present behind the tympanic membrane (*hemotympanum*). Vestibular complaints including vertigo occur because of concussion of the semicircular canals. CSF leak may not manifest as otorrhea caused by an intact eardrum but rather as clear rhinorrhea as the leaking CSF gains access to the nose through the eustachian tube. When present, CSF leaks are usually managed conservatively with bed rest, head of bed elevation, and possible lumbar drain placement. Exploration and surgical repair are indicated when these conservative measures are unsuccessful. It is important to note that although longitudinal and transverse fractures are described separately, temporal bone fractures may represent a combination of these patterns.

Management strategies for temporal bone trauma depend on the nature of the defect. As stated in the preceding text, immediate facial nerve paralysis warrants exploration but is often delayed owing to concomitant severe injuries that take precedence. Sensorineural hearing loss is rarely reversible. Conductive hearing loss resulting from tympanic membrane perforation may heal spontaneously or require tympanoplasty later on, whereas ossicular chain disruption often requires surgical repair at a later date.

Trauma can also be localized to the external ear and canal. Blunt trauma is common in athletes (wrestling and boxing). Typically, a subperichondral hematoma can develop between the cartilage and the anterior perichondrium. The cartilage has no intrinsic blood supply but rather relies on the overlying perichondrium. Therefore, if the hematoma is not drained, the cartilage is deprived of its blood supply, which leads to necrosis, scar formation, and loss of the helical shape (cauliflower or wrestler's ear). Treatment involves hematoma evacuation and placement of a bolster to maintain approximation of cartilage and perichondrium. Additional injuries or lacerations may expose cartilage to infection. Treatment involves surgical débridement of devitalized cartilage and repositioning of perichondrium and skin. Antibiotics are required to prevent cartilage infection.

Mandibular Trauma

The mandible is the largest and strongest of the facial bones. However, because of its prominent location, it is frequently fractured in facial trauma. It is the second most fractured facial bone after the nasal bone. The classification of mandibular fractures is based on location and tendency for displacement or distraction. Affected regions of the mandible include the body (36%), angle (20%), condylar head (35%), ramus (3%), coronoid process (2%), symphysis (1%), parasymphysis (14%), and alveolus (3%). The sites of weakness that are predisposed to fracture include the third molar (particularly when impacted), the

parasymphysial region at the mental foramen between the first and second bicuspid teeth, and the condylar neck. Thirty-two teeth are present in adults, whereas twenty teeth are present in children. In the pediatric population, areas of unerupted teeth represent potential areas of fracture. Examination should determine the degree of maxillomandibular occlusion. Normal class I occlusion has the mesiobuccal cusp of the maxillary first molar meeting the buccal groove of the first mandibular molar. This condition exists in 73% of the population. Class II occlusion (24%) suggests an overbite or mandibular retrognathism, whereas class III occlusion (3%) suggests an underbite or mandibular prognathism. Presence of teeth on both sides of the fracture facilitates interdental wire fixation. An intact molar in the fracture line should be left untouched to maximize repositioning surface. A mobile tooth is usually removed. Trismus suggests injury to the condyles. Condylar fractures may be associated with external auditory canal laceration or bloody otorrhea.

A simple fracture does not communicate with the oral cavity, whereas a complex fracture is associated with violation of mucous membranes or skin and carries increased risk of infection. A complex fracture is suggested by the presence of blood in the oral cavity. The panorex x-ray provides a complete view of the mandible and is optimal for diagnosing fractures. Although isolated fractures occur in children, most fractures in adults are multiple; in fact, when one fracture is identified on radiography, a search should ensue for a second fracture. In general, surgical management for mandibular fractures, when indicated, includes intermaxillary fixation (wiring the mandible to the maxilla) with or without open reduction and internal fixation of involved bone fragments.

Additional factors influence healing and morbidity. The elderly, edentulous population or patients with poor dentition represent a greater challenge to fixation owing to the lack of repositioning surface areas provided by the teeth. In certain cases fixation can be performed with dentures in place to ensure adequate height of the mandibular ramus.

In general, any form of compression plating increases the risk of intraoperative damage to the inferior alveolar nerve, which runs in the mandibular canal and exits the mental foramen as the mental nerve. Damage to this nerve can result in hypesthesia of the ipsilateral anterior chin and lower lip. Other complications, such as infection and osteomyelitis, are unlikely to occur in the presence of a solid reduction.

Emergencies resulting from mandibular fractures are rare. One such emergency is airway collapse caused by bilateral body fractures or multisegment fractures as the tongue base falls posteriorly. A jaw thrust or pulling the tongue anteriorly can relieve the obstruction and open the airway. An airway should be established with intubation or tracheostomy. If one is unable to intubate a patient with major facial fractures or suspected cervical spine injury, emergent tracheotomy or cricothyroidotomy is indicated. As a general rule, cricothyroidotomy offers the advantage of rapid airway access with a decreased risk of thyroid hemorrhage. However, there is a greater likelihood of injury to the recurrent laryngeal nerve, which pierces the cricothyrohyoid membrane. In addition, there is an elevated risk of subglottic stenosis. Therefore, cricothyroidotomy should be considered only as a temporizing measure, and a revision tracheotomy should be performed as soon as possible in the operating room.

Zygomatic, Maxillary, and Orbital Trauma

High-velocity blunt trauma to the head can result in fractures of the zygomatic arch, the maxilla, and the orbits. An understanding of management issues requires review of the structural support systems of the face. The middle one third of the facial skeleton consists of an intersecting system of buttresses that distribute forces generated through mastication. The vertical dimensions are maintained by the (i) nasomaxillary, (ii) zygomaticomaxillary, and (iii) pterygomaxillary buttresses. These vertical supports are interconnected via the lesser horizontal buttresses, which include the orbital rims, maxillary alveolus and palate, zygomatic process, greater wing of the sphenoid, and medial and lateral pterygoid plates. If sufficient force is directed at the anterior face, predictable patterns of structural collapse are observed.

In 1901, René Le Fort described these patterns, which bear his name (Fig. 28-9). Each of the three classifications involves a fracture of the pterygoid plates. The Le Fort I fracture line passes horizontally along the palate inward to the pterygoid plates. The Le Fort II fracture line incorporates the nasofrontal suture line, traverses the lamina papyracea (medial orbital wall) of the ethmoid bone, proceeds across the orbital floor, and proceeds inferiorly beneath the zygomatic arch to the palate. The Le Fort III fracture is the most serious and involves each of the three vertical buttresses, resulting in craniofacial dysjunction. The fracture line extends from the nasofrontal suture line

posteriorly along the cribriform plate/anterior skull base, travels through the root of the zygoma, and disrupts the junction of pterygoid plates with skull base.

The classic finding indicative of a Le Fort fracture is a palate that is mobile to traction. Le Fort II and III fractures are commonly associated with CSF rhinorrhea, profound epistaxis, visual loss, and upper airway obstruction necessitating tracheostomy. Nasal intubation is contraindicated secondary to risk of intracranial injury. Typically, trauma with force sufficient to produce facial fractures will result in extensive cerebral injury (52%). Most of these Le Fort fractures are repaired in a delayed fashion (days) following stabilization of the patient. Poor candidates are those with Glasgow coma scale scores of less than 6, evidence of intracerebral hemorrhage, midline shift, intracerebral pressures of more than 15 mm Hg, and basal cistern effacement. Correction is directed at open reduction with miniplating to reestablish vertical and horizontal buttresses. Common postoperative complications include malocclusion, and, less frequently, facial asymmetry.

The *tripod fracture* is the most common fracture of the midface. The principal fracture sites include the frontozygomatic suture line, the zygomatic arch, and the maxilla extending from inferior orbital rim to palate. Posterior displacement of the complex produces a flattened appearance of the malar eminence. Compression of the infraorbital nerve may produce hypesthesia in the CN V^2 distribution, whereas impingement upon the coronoid process, which courses deep to the zygomatic arch, may cause trismus. The tripod fracture and isolated fractures of the zygomatic arch are easily identified on head CT scan. Surgical correction of the tripod fracture requires reapproximation and plating of the orbital rim, zygomatic arch, and maxilla. Stable fixation is achieved by methods that involve the use of miniplates and that incorporate the frontozygomatic suture line as one of the points of fixation. Ideally, these procedures are performed within 7 to 10 days of the traumatic insult.

An additional group of facial fractures involves the orbit. The blowout fracture is caused by blunt trauma to the malar or frontal regions. Inferiorly directed forces produce a fracture of the thin orbital floor along the infraorbital canal. Palpation along the inferior orbital rim may detect irregularity of contour, or "step off," if the orbital rim is involved. Inferior displacement of orbital contents into the maxillary sinus may result in enophthalmos and entrapment of the inferior rectus muscle resulting in restriction of upward gaze. Diplopia on upward gaze may also be noted. A coronal CT scan may reveal the inferior rectus muscle and orbital fat herniating into the maxillary sinus. Edema of extraocular muscles caused by trauma from bony spicules can also be seen. The CT scan assists in identifying intraorbital free air, which suggests violation of the bony orbit. Material to reconstruct the orbital floor can be in the form of autologous bone, titanium mesh, silastic, or gelfilm. If orbital injury is suspected, an ophthalmology consultation is mandated to assess ocular entrapment, globe projection, and to document visual acuity. Most fractures should be repaired within 7 to 10 days, prior to scar formation and bone fusion. However, optic nerve compression, nerve sheath hematoma, and suspected orbital hemorrhage are indications for emergent exploration. Unrecognized orbital

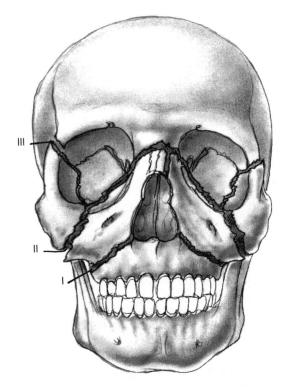

Figure 28-9 Le Fort fracture levels. (From Bailey BJ, ed. *Head and neck surgery: Otolaryngology*. Philadelphia: Lippincott Williams & Wilkins, 2001, with permission.)

floor fractures can result in late presentation (after 6 weeks) of enophthalmos and diplopia owing to slow, inferior herniation of orbital contents. Delayed surgical correction is technically more complicated.

An additional facial injury requiring surgical repair involves the region located between the eyes, the naso-orbital-ethmoid region. The ethmoid sinus, located between the orbits, represents a delicate lattice of bones, which incorporate the medial orbital walls and floor of the anterior cranial fossa (cribriform plate). Collapse of this area can occur with posteriorly directed force applied to the bridge of the nose. Again, fine-cut axial and coronal CT imaging is the preferred examination to assess the integrity of the orbits and ethmoid sinus. Clinically, the patient has a flattened appearance of the nasal bridge. The distance between the medial canthi is increased, as is the interpupillary distance. Telecanthus (increased distance between medial canthi) is associated with diplopia and cosmetic defects that are extremely difficult to correct. Functionally, disruption of the attachment of the medial canthal tendons causes epiphora (excessive tearing) secondary to dysfunction of the lacrimal system. Tears normally drain via the nasolacrimal duct into the nose, where they exit in the anterosuperior region of the inferior meatus. If necessary, recanalization of the nasolacrimal duct with a silastic stent can be performed at a later date.

Nasal Fracture

The most common trauma to the facial bones involves the nose. The nasal bones are located at the insertion of the nose between the eyes. These small bones (less than 1 cm in length) provide superior support for the nose. However, most structural support is provided by the bony septum, which extends from the maxilla to connect with the cartilaginous septum. Presenting symptoms of nasal fractures may include epistaxis, which is typically self-resolving. In certain instances, reduction of fractures is required for hemostasis. Simple fractures of the nasal bones are corrected by repositioning with an elevator and then placing an external nasal splint with internal nasal packs. In all cases of nasal trauma, an inspection of the nasal cavity is required to rule out a septal hematoma. This bluish swelling of the midline septum represents dissection of blood between the mucoperichondrium and septal cartilage. As there is no intrinsic blood supply to the cartilage, the presence of hematoma predisposes to infection and cartilage necrosis. This combination may result in delayed collapse of the nose and lead to significant cosmetic defects. If identified, the hematoma should be evacuated and the patient placed on antibiotics. In rare instances, nasal trauma is associated with CSF rhinorrhea resulting from fracture of the cribriform plate of the ethmoid bone, which is connected to the bony septum. In most of these patients, spontaneous resolution will occur with bed rest and head of bed elevation.

Penetrating Trauma of the Pharynx

Penetrating trauma of the oropharynx is relatively rare in the adult population but not uncommon in the pediatric age group. Children who fall while an object is in the mouth may sustain injury to the soft palate. Impalement is most dangerous when it occurs in the lateral soft palate near the course of the internal carotid artery, which can sustain either puncture or blunt injury. Radiographic imaging of the great vessels is indicated in cases where parapharyngeal space violation has occurred or is suspected. Regardless, most such injuries are associated with a minimal amount of self-limited bleeding, and the lacerations themselves usually heal by secondary intention.

Laryngeal Trauma

Laryngeal injury should be considered in all patients who sustain blunt or sharp trauma to the neck. Signs of acute laryngeal trauma include voice change, stridor, respiratory distress, dysphagia, odynophagia, and hemoptysis. Physical examination may reveal edema, subcutaneous emphysema, hematoma, ecchymosis, loss of thyroid cartilage prominence, or palpable laryngeal cartilage fracture. Initial management consists of securing an adequate airway. When laryngeal or tracheal injury is apparent and airway compromise is imminent, a controlled tracheostomy should be performed. Ideally, the trachea is entered below the cricoid cartilage with an incision between tracheal rings three and four. A cricothyroidotomy (access through the cricothyroid membrane) should not be used because of potential injury to the larynx and upper trachea. Oral endotracheal intubation is not recommended because additional laryngeal injury may result.

In cases in which trauma has occurred but the airway is stable, the mainstay of treatment includes flexible fiberoptic laryngoscopy to assess vocal cord motion, mucosal integrity, and any evidence of laryngeal swelling or ecchymosis. In the absence of obvious injury, management should include elevation of the head of bed, humidified oxygen, and steroids with airway observation in a monitored bed. If there is evidence of significant or airway-threatening mucosal edema, a tracheostomy is performed emergently, as the stable airway can be lost rapidly with progression of edema. Most mucosal lacerations can be expected to heal primarily. Following stabilization of the airway, a CT scan is obtained to identify fracture of the thyroid and cricoid cartilages. If a fracture is present, open exploration of the neck is performed with reduction and internal fixation, employing nonabsorbable suture, wires or miniplates.

Facial Nerve Injury

Injury to CN VII frequently accompanies trauma to the head. The portion of the facial nerve proximal to the stylomastoid foramen is composed of motor, sensory, and autonomic fibers. The nerve is divided into the meatal, labyrinthine, tympanic, and mastoid segments. In addition, the nerve exits at the stylomastoid foramen and is composed almost entirely of motor fibers. The nerve courses posteriorly around the angle of the mandible and enters the parotid gland. At this point the nerve divides into superior and inferior divisions and is referred to as the pes anserinus (goose's foot). From here the nerve splits into five main branches: (i) temporal, (ii) zygomatic, (iii) buccal, (iv) marginal mandibular, and (v) cervical (Fig. 28-1). All head trauma patients should undergo full cranial nerve evaluation. With respect to the facial nerve, each subdivision should be assessed.

Penetrating trauma to the face that results in loss of facial nerve function may be repaired surgically if the injury is proximal to the lateral canthus. Distal to this point, nerve fibers are too narrow to be surgically approximated; in addition, extensive arborization between buccal and zygomatic branches limits paresis affecting these divisions and regeneration should occur spontaneously within months. Direct end-to-end anastomosis of nerve branches is performed after exploration of the nerve. If sections of the facial nerve are missing, interposition grafting using the greater auricular nerve or sural nerve can be performed at the time of exploration or at a later date. If larger segments of nerve are missing, some innervation can be restored with the hypoglossal-facial nerve anastomosis (XII to VII) or the cross-facial nerve (VII to VII) technique. Both procedures may result in synkinesis (single axon innervating widely separated facial muscles, resulting in nonlocalized muscle contraction with nerve stimulation) and limited movement; however, tone is preserved and muscle atrophy avoided.

Aside from cosmetic asymmetry, facial nerve paresis is a concern because of potential corneal dessication caused by incomplete eye closure. This problem can be addressed with lubricants, surgical implantation of upper-lid gold weights to assist closure, or lid-shortening procedures to prevent lagophthalmos. In cases of permanent nerve injury, additional surgical suspension procedures are available to address function of the oral commissure (to prevent drooling) and closure of the eye.

Salivary Gland Trauma

Injury to the salivary gland may be blunt, penetrating, intraoral, or extraoral. Of the major salivary glands, the parotid is the most commonly injured. Lacerations of the face posterior to the anterior margin of the masseter muscle may injure the parotid (Stensen) duct. If a lacerated or transected duct is identified during wound exploration, end-to-end anastomosis over a stent is indicated. Identification of the injured duct can be facilitated by passing a probe intraorally through the duct orifice and identifying it within the wound. Postoperative stenosis of the duct may require dilation with ophthalmic lacrimal probes. Smaller lacerations to salivary gland parenchyma can be repaired with careful closure of the gland capsule. The principal complications of salivary gland trauma include sialocele (cystic collection of saliva) and salivary-cutaneous fistula. Facial nerve injury is also possible, and is discussed in the preceding text. Management includes aspiration of the cyst and application of a pressure dressing; repeat aspirations are often required in the case of sialocele, and recurrent cases may indicate ductal obstruction. Persistent collections are best addressed by gland excision. Similar management strategies apply to the submandibular and sublingual glands; however, ductal injuries are much less common owing to the protective effects of the mandible.

KEY POINTS

▲ Salivary gland infections have numerous etiologies; those of the submandibular gland and associated floor of mouth have the potential to spread rapidly and cause airway obstruction and respiratory compromise.

▲ Salivary gland neoplasms may be benign or malignant. As a general rule, the larger the gland, the more likely the pathology is to be benign.

▲ The majority of cancers of the upper aerodigestive tract are squamous cell carcinomas. Tobacco and alcohol are implicated in their pathogenesis. Malignancies from different subsites within the head and neck tend to metastasize to specific cervical lymph node chains, and understanding lymphatic drainage is important in management.

▲ Paranasal sinus infections are common. Surrounding structures, such as the eye, cavernous sinus, and brain, rarely may be involved in untreated or inadequately treated cases.

▲ Trauma to the face, mandible, and larynx can be associated with airway obstruction and often poses a challenge to intubation; in addition, concomitant cervical spine injury must be assumed. In these cases a surgical airway (e.g., tracheotomy) may be required.

▲ Sound is converted from pressure disturbances to electrical signals through the conductive (external and middle ears) and sensorineural (inner ear, cochlear nerve) components of the ear. Hearing loss is characterized as conductive, sensorineural, or mixed.

SUGGESTED READINGS

Bailey BJ, ed. *Head and neck surgery: Otolaryngology*, 3rd ed. Philadelphia: Lippincott Williams & Wilkins, 2001.

Cummings CW, ed. *Otolaryngology: Head and neck surgery*, 3rd ed. St. Louis: Mosby, 1998.

Lee KJ, ed. *Essential otolaryngology*, 8th ed. New York: McGraw-Hill, 2003.

Paparella MM, Shumrick DA, Gluckman JL et al., eds. *Otolaryngology.* Philadelphia: WB Saunders, 1991.

Ruckenstein MJ. *Comprehensive review of otolaryngology.* Philadelphia: WB Saunders, 2004.

Orthopaedic Surgery

29

Lisa D. Khoury   *John L. Esterhai, Jr*

Orthopaedics is the study of musculoskeletal injury and disease and its medical and surgical treatment. Like any medical specialty, orthopaedics relies on a knowledge of underlying principles of disease, a complete history and physical examination, careful evaluation of laboratory data, and the examination of radiologic studies. To fully understand the theories of musculoskeletal disease and injury management, it is essential to understand the biology and biomechanics of bone, cartilage, and muscle.

BASIC SCIENCE OF ORTHOPAEDICS

Bone Structure and Formation

The long bone is divided into the epiphysis, metaphysis, and diaphysis (Fig. 29-1). Bone formation consists of a combination of two microscopic forms, lamellar and woven bone. *Woven bone* (primary bone) is composed of a randomly distributed collagen matrix and has a higher cellular concentration. It is weaker and more flexible than lamellar bone because the matrix is not stress-oriented. Woven bone is either immature bone, which will be remodeled, or pathologic bone. *Lamellar bone* (mature bone) largely replaces woven bone as a person matures and consists of a highly organized collagen matrix in which the fibers are stress-oriented or distributed parallel to the direction of force application.

Lamellar bone is further divided into *cancellous* and *cortical* bone. *Cancellous bone* (also known as "trabecular" or "spongy" bone) is most abundant in the epiphysis and metaphysis and consists of a branching lattice pattern (Fig. 29-1). Cancellous bone is less dense and undergoes a higher turnover, and, therefore, more remodeling in response to lines of stress. Cortical bone makes up 80% of the skeleton. It is most commonly arranged in osteon units, which are composed of haversian canals (vascular channels) surrounded by lamellar bone (Fig. 29-2).

The major cell types of bone are the osteoblasts, osteocytes, and osteoclasts. *Osteoblasts* are involved in the synthesis and secretion of bone matrix. They are derived from undifferentiated mesenchymal cells and line trabecular bone and the Volkmann canals and canaliculi of cortical bone. Disruption of this lining cell layer activates these cells. In addition, they are the primary responders to extracellular signals such as bone morphogenic protein (BMP), parathyroid hormone (PTH), 1,25(OH)$_2$D, prostaglandins, estrogen, and glucocorticoids.

Once bone is mineralized with hydroxyapatite crystals and osteoblasts are surrounded by bony matrix, the intracellular makeup of the osteoblast changes, and the cells are now termed "osteocytes." *Osteocytes* are embedded within the bone in lacunae and are arranged concentrically

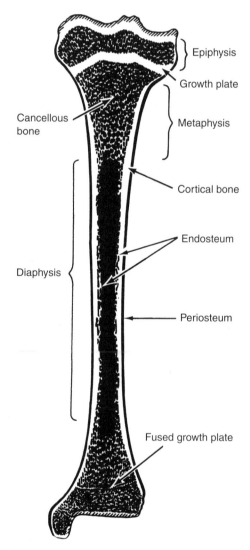

Figure 29-1 Schematic view of a long bone. The growth plate (physis) is present only in the growing child. (From Favus MJ, et al., eds. *Primer on the metabolic bone diseases and disorders of mineral metabolism*, 4th ed. Philadelphia: Lippincott Williams & Wilkins, 1999:3, with permission.)

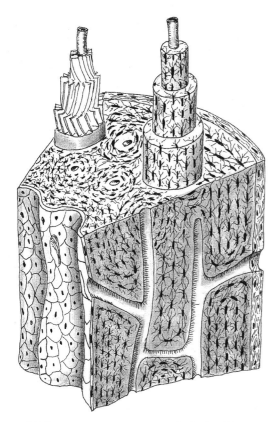

Figure 29-2 Cortical bone consists of cylindrical haversian systems oriented parallel along the shafts of long bones. (From Vigorita VJ. *Orthopaedic pathology.* Philadelphia: Lippincott Williams & Wilkins, 1999:37, with permission.)

around the center of the osteon. They are stimulated by calcitonin, inhibited by PTH, and help to regulate extracellular calcium and phosphorous concentration.

Osteoclasts, which lie in bony pits known as Howship lacunae, are multinucleated giant cells derived from *hemopoietic* macrophage precursors. They have a ruffled border, which increases the area, through which they can bind to bone surface to break down bone matrix. Bone remodeling consists of a highly organized interaction of osteoblasts and osteoclasts (Fig. 29-3). Osteoclasts have receptors for calcitonin by which they can regulate bone resorption directly. Estrogen prevents bone resorption and has been found to increase bone density, specifically in the femoral neck, thereby reducing the rate of hip fracture.

Bone is composed of 60% to 70% inorganic tissue, 5% to 8% water, and organic tissue. The inorganic tissue is largely *hydroxyapatite crystals,* which consist mainly of calcium phosphate salts. The organic bone matrix undergoes mineralization with these salts and provides extra strength and support to the bone structure. The organic phase of bone is composed chiefly of *type I collagen* and matrix proteins such as osteocalcin and osteonectin. The bone *blood supply* to long bones consists of three systems: diaphyseal, metaphyseal, and periosteal. The diaphysis is supplied by a variable number of nutrient arteries that enter the bone through foramina and branch into a vast network of intraosseous arterioles. The metaphyseal regions are supplied by a periarticular or geniculate complex that penetrates the bone. Finally, the outer 15% to 20% of cortical bone, the periosteal tissue, and muscular attachments to the bone are supplied by a periosteal capillary system.

These three systems are ultimately interconnected, and the intermediate watershed areas become very important in situations in which one vascular system is insufficient (such as when the bone is fractured).

Biomechanics and Patterns of Fracture

Bone is formed by either *intramembranous ossification* or *endochondral ossification.* During intramembranous ossification, seen during the development of the skull, maxilla, mandible, and clavicle, the bony trabecula is laid down directly by the mesenchymal cells. In endochondral ossification, which is responsible for interstitial (lengthwise) growth of the bone, an initial cartilaginous framework is followed by bony deposition and cartilage resorption. Active growth occurs at the epiphysis, which is separated from the metaphysis by the cartilaginous growth plate (physis) in the growing child. Once the skeleton reaches maturity, the growth plate closes and the epiphysis fuses with the metaphysis (Fig. 29-1).

Bone formation is dependent on *calcium metabolism,* which is finely balanced by the kidney, osteoclasts, osteoblasts, PTH, vitamin D, and calcitonin. Calcium is absorbed from the duodenum [regulated by $1,25(OH)_2D$, which is activated in both the kidney and liver] and by passive diffusion through the jejunum. In addition, the skeleton serves as a reservoir of the body's calcium. PTH, secreted by the chief cells of the parathyroid glands, stimulates an increase in serum calcium level by stimulating absorption and activation of vitamin D, promoting urinary excretion of phosphate and stimulating osteoclastic resorption of bone. Calcitonin, secreted by the parafollicular cells of the thyroid in response to elevated calcium levels, inhibits osteoclast resorption and thus lowers serum calcium levels.

A bone fractures when it is overloaded, as a result of either abnormal stresses on normal bone or normal stresses on abnormal bone (which results in a pathologic fracture). As bone absorbs more kinetic energy from a traumatic insult, it is forced to release the energy it cannot sustain by undergoing structural change. Bone is an anisotropic material, meaning that it reacts differently to different stresses. This is reflected in bone fracture patterns, which vary depending on the severity of the force, the direction of the force, and the age of the patient. Bending forces place tensile stresses on bone, which are poorly tolerated compared to compressive forces. Uneven bending forces can cause an oblique fracture, whereas pure bending forces result in transverse fracture formation commonly with a butterfly fragment. Torsional and rotatory forces cause *spiral fractures* (Fig. 29-4) in which the oblique fracture line circles longitudinally along part of the length of a bone. A fracture can be simple (one fracture line) or comminuted (more than two fragments). Severely comminuted fractures, which involve destruction of bone into multiple small pieces, can result from a severe crush injury by heavy machinery or a high-velocity motor vehicle accident. *Compression fractures* occur in trabecular bone and are common in osteopenic vertebrae. In the *open fracture,* which usually signifies a higher energy injury, there is communication between the fracture and the outside environment. The size of the skin laceration can range from a pinprick-size puncture to a grossly contaminated degloving injury.

Repetitive trauma over time results in *stress fractures* of cortical bone such as a long-distance runner developing a

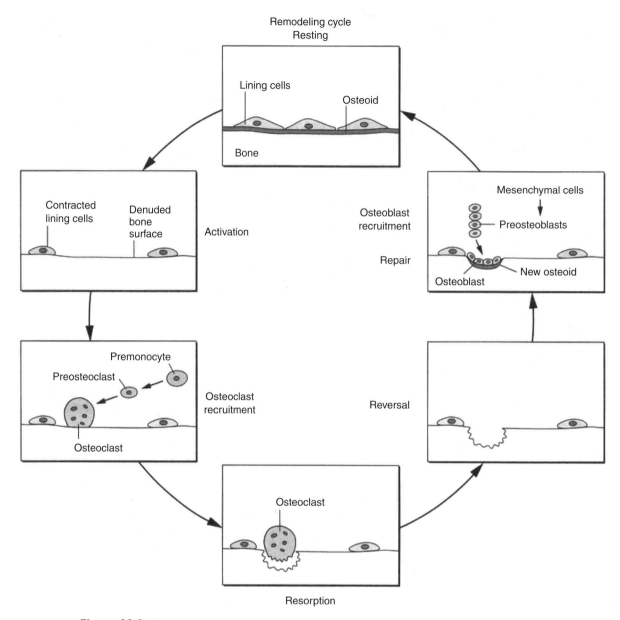

Figure 29-3 The bone remodeling cycle involves a highly organized interaction of osteoblasts and osteoclasts. (From Vigorita VJ. *Orthopaedic pathology.* Philadelphia: Lippincott Williams & Wilkins, 1999:32, with permission.)

stress fracture of the metatarsi. With increased load over time, the stiffness and strength of the bone decrease, and microfractures develop. Although microfractures do not progress easily to complete full-thickness fractures, with continued fatigue, they become so numerous that a complete fracture is inevitable.

Because of the thicker periosteum and the open growth plates, children are susceptible to two unique fracture patterns—greenstick fractures and physeal injuries. In the *greenstick fracture,* there is an incomplete fracture because a significant portion of the thick periosteum usually remains intact on the concave (compression) side of the injury (Fig. 29-5). *Physeal injuries* occur when the fracture involves the epiphysis or the physis (growth plate). Active growth occurs at the epiphysis, which is separated from the metaphysis by the cartilaginous growth plate (physis) in the growing child. Once the skeleton reaches maturity,

the growth plate closes and the epiphysis fuses with the metaphysis, as previously mentioned (Fig. 29-1). Physeal injuries can be devastating if growth plate arrest occurs prematurely as a consequence of fracture.

Bone and Fracture Healing

Fractures caused by increased energy generally heal with greater incidence of complications than fractures produced by less stress. Fracture healing is completed in five stages (Fig. 29-6). *Induction* involves fracture hematoma development and proceeds with local bone necrosis and the release of factors that attract inflammatory cells. *Inflammation* involves the migration of polymorphonuclear neutrophils, macrophages, and other inflammatory cells to the fracture site and the eventual initiation of bone and cartilage formation with fibroblast recruitment. In the

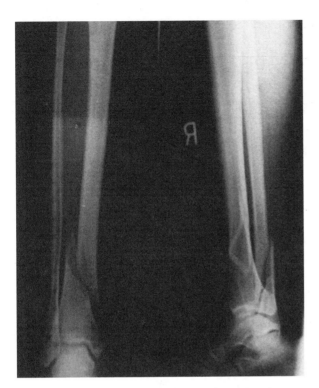

Figure 29-4 Spiral fracture of the distal tibia. Note the accompanying fibula fracture. (From Rockwood CA Jr, et al., eds. *Rockwood and Green's fractures in adults*, 4th ed. Philadelphia: Lippincott-Raven, 1996:2135, with permission.)

soft callous stage, which can be seen by 2 weeks, bone and cartilage formation continues until fracture motion is considerably limited and involves subperiosteal bone formation at the fracture ends. By 4 weeks, there is a significant increase in the stiffness of the healing bone. The *hard callous stage* involves conversion of the soft callus to hard woven bone by endochondral ossification. At this point, there is a gradual disappearance of the radiolucent line, signifying radiographic healing. *Bone remodeling*, the final stage, refers to the eventual replacement of woven bone with structurally stronger lamellar bone and is guided by the *law of Wolff* (which states that bone formation and resorption is influenced by mechanical stresses on the bone). Remodeling can be fast and extensive in the child owing to the higher osteogenic potential, but in the adult, it can take many years.

For the first several hours to days after the fracture, the vascular supply to the bone is decreased owing to the initial trauma and small vessel disruption. After this point, vascular supply increases to supranormal levels until approximately 12 weeks postfracture when it returns to prefracture levels. Disruption of the medullary blood supply by the insertion of an intramedullary rod or disruption of the periosteal blood supply by periosteal stripping during surgical fixation may delay bone healing.

Bone growth factors have recently been discovered to play an important role in normal fracture healing and therapy for poorly healing fractures. *BMP* has been shown to induce bone formation by causing transformation of mesenchymal cells into osteoblasts. BMP-3, which is also known as "osteogen," is particularly effective in promoting this transformation and is now being studied for potential therapeutic use. Other factors important in fracture as well as wound healing are insulin-like growth factor-I and -II, transforming growth factor-β, and platelet-derived growth factor.

A *nonunion* is defined as a fracture that has not healed in a 6-month period. Several factors that increase the risk of nonunion include systemic states such as poor nutritional status and tobacco use, as well as local determinants such as soft tissue trauma, bone loss, infection, vascular injury, and insufficient stabilization. Nonunion occurs in three varieties: (i) atrophic, characterized by little or no callous formation because of poor vascularity; (ii) hypertrophic, characterized by lack of union despite rich vascularity and the formation of a large amount of callus; and (iii) pseudoarthrosis, characterized by joint-like synovial tissue surrounding the unhealed ends.

Treatment of the nonunion fracture involves open resection of interposed fibrous or synovial tissue, reduction of the fracture, and rigid fixation. Autogenous iliac crest bone graft is often used, along with recombinant BMP in certain circumstances, to increase healing of nonunions. An alternative or adjunct to surgery is the use of electrical or ultrasound stimulation for healing of a nonunion fracture. The electrical current may function by stimulating cyclic adenosine monophosphate and angiogenesis while encouraging fibrocartilage calcification. It may also alter the ionic status of the bone.

Bone grafting promotes osteogenesis and structural support. Allograft mainly serves as a framework for chondrocytes and angiogenic cells (*osteoconduction*). It is often freeze-dried, stored at −70°C, and sterilized by gamma

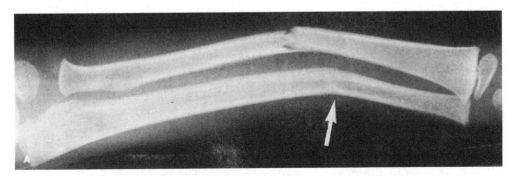

Figure 29-5 Greenstick fracture of the forearm in a child. Note that the radial cortex is completely fractured, whereas the ulnar cortex is still intact. (From Rockwood CA Jr, et al., eds. *Rockwood and Green's fractures in children*, 4th ed. Philadelphia: Lippincott-Raven, 1996:28, with permission.)

Stages of callus formation

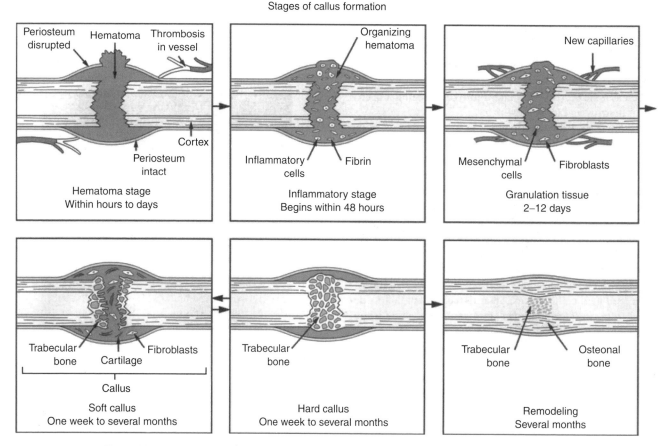

Figure 29-6 Stages of fracture healing. (From Vigorita VJ. *Orthopaedic pathology*. Philadelphia: Lippincott Williams & Wilkins, 1999:87, with permission.)

irradiation or ethanol. These processes decrease the availability of osteoinductive factors. Protection against human immunodeficiency virus 1 (HIV-1) and hepatitis is effectively ensured by careful screening of donors. With osteoinduction by local growth factors, the graft is eventually incorporated into native bone by the transformation of local mesenchymal cells to osteogenic cells and remodeling of the graft. Autograft, most commonly harvested from the iliac crest is both osteoinductive and osteoconductive.

Articular cartilage

Composed of *hyaline cartilage*, articular cartilage provides joints with the characteristics of remarkably decreased friction, excellent lubrication, and shock absorption. It consists of chondrocytes (10% dry weight), proteoglycans (40% dry weight), collagen (50% dry weight), and water (65% to 80% of the wet weight of the cartilage). The water content of articular cartilage increases with osteoarthritis, thereby leading to increased permeability and decreased strength. Chondrocytes are highly differentiated cells that maintain the extracellular matrix (ECM), and that respond to biochemical signaling and biomechanical forces to adapt cartilage structurally to the local and systemic environment. Chondrocytes are also responsible for producing collagen and proteoglycans.

The predominant type of collagen in articular cartilage is type II, which consists of three identical alpha chain proteins formed into a triple helix. These small type II helices interact and eventually form large fibrils that are the functional molecules of active cartilage. The collagen in cartilage is organized in a cross-linked network, which is thought to provide tensile strength to the articular cartilage.

Proteoglycans consist of a large protein core to which are attached 1 to 150 carbohydrate side chains known as "glycosaminoglycans" (GAGs). The structure of the ECM is strongly dictated by the interactions between the large proteoglycan molecules. By interacting with collagen in a porous-permeable collagen-proteoglycan solid matrix, proteoglycans help to provide the articular cartilage with structural rigidity.

Blood vessels do not pass the *tide mark*, which is the area separating the articular cartilage from the subchondral bone. As a result of this arrangement, *articular cartilage* receives minimal to no blood supply. Instead, it receives its nutrients from the circulating milieu of synovial fluid that surrounds the joint space. A laceration of the cartilage above the tide mark does not result in the formation of a fibrin clot because there is no blood supply to the tissue. Because there are no mobile undifferentiated cells, minimal tissue replacement occurs by chondrocytes, and the non-healing injury gap remains in the cartilage for the lifetime of the patient. In addition, softening of the cartilage around the injury creates more surface gaps, and intermittent sloughing of surrounding cartilage leads to the eventual complete wear down to subchondral bone.

Lacerations extending into the subchondral bone beyond the tide mark result in bleeding into the cartilage and formation of a fibrin clot. This allows access of undifferentiated cells and materials necessary for healing. However, much of the new cartilage formation is fibrocartilage, instead of hyaline cartilage. Therefore, the collagen is not deposited in its original ordered configuration, and the cartilage rapidly loses elasticity with abnormal increases in permeability.

Osteoarthritis (OA) is a disease that involves the destruction of articular cartilage and changes in bone structure. In OA, the cartilage undergoes a sequence of fibrillation, extreme fissuring of the tissue, and finally a total loss of cartilage with exposure of the subchondral bone. Underlying bony changes include the formation of bone cysts, sclerotic bone formation, extraosseous deposition of collagen, and osteophyte formation. Loss of cartilage from OA is associated with a substantially diminished amount of proteoglycans (particularly keratan sulfate), which is directly proportional to the severity of the disease. The poor healing capacity of the cartilage explains the high incidence of post-traumatic arthritis after intraarticular fractures.

Muscle

The most basic unit of muscle is the myofibril, which is composed of an organized matrix of actin and myosin. Several myofibrils associate to make up a multinucleated cell, the muscle fiber. The muscle fiber is enclosed by the connective tissue endomysium, and several fibers join to form the most basic unit of muscle visible to eye, the fascicle. Fascicles combine to form muscle, which is covered by a layer of epimysium (Fig. 29-7). Muscles originate in bone or cartilage and have tendinous insertions.

Each myofibril is made up of *actin thin filaments* and *myosin thick filaments* organized into the basic muscle unit, the sarcomere (Fig. 29-8). The binding of calcium and cleavage of adenosine triphosphate results in myosin cross bridges interacting with actin to shorten the sarcomere and, if propagated on a larger scale, to shorten the associated muscle fiber (contraction). The stimulus for muscle contraction is signaled by the nerve fibers that branch to supply several fibers.

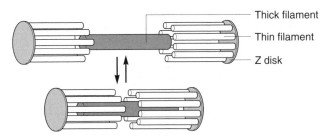

Figure 29-8   The sarcomere is made up of actin thin filaments and myosin thick filaments. When the muscle contracts, the actin and myosin filaments slide past one another.

Each nerve terminal releases acetylcholine upon stimulation by an action potential. The acetylcholine crosses the synaptic cleft and binds to acetylcholine receptors, which allows depolarizing currents to enter the cell. As an action potential is conducted down the muscle fiber cytoplasm (sarcoplasm), the sarcoplasmic reticulum is depolarized, resulting in intracellular calcium release from the sarcoplasmic reticulum. The calcium, which is integral in muscle contraction, binds to troponin, thereby allowing myosin–actin interaction. Several pharmacologic agents including tubocurarine (inhibitory agent) and succinylcholine (depolarizing agent) act on the acetylcholine receptor and induce paralysis.

Muscle fiber types include types I, IIA, and IIB. Type I fibers (red fibers), which are more common in muscles with smaller motor units, are highly aerobic, less fatigable, and contract slowly. In contrast, type IIA fibers (white fibers) are fast contracting, more anaerobic, fatigable, and common in muscles with large motor units. Type IIB muscle fibers are the fastest contracting and have the quickest rate of fatigue. Recruitment of contracting muscle fibers is based on the size of the motor unit, with the smaller motor units activated first. Sprinting and heavy weight lifting involve recruitment of larger motor units, most often type II fibers.

With muscle *disuse* and *immobilization,* structural changes that occur result in muscle weakness and dysfunction. Among the first changes is atrophy with a decrease in both fiber size and fiber number. Changes have also been demonstrated within the fibers as the organization of the sarcomere is disrupted and fiber metabolism is altered. The fatigability and weakness of the affected muscle is also increased.

Muscle laceration by a sharp object results in incomplete healing via scar tissue and fibrosis when the cut ends are reapproximated. Although fiber regeneration across the scar tissue is rare, much of the muscle function can return depending on the severity of injury. Contusion of a muscle by blunt force injury results in hematoma formation, inflammation, and muscle cell injury and death. Recovery is dependent on hematoma clearance and revascularization of the injured tissue. This process can be promoted by initial rest in flexion and early muscle movement and rehabilitation.

Indirect muscle injury occurs most often at the myotendinous junction. This refers to failure of muscle by excessive stress rather than by direct trauma and includes muscle strains and tears. The forces responsible for the tear are often eccentric contractions, as these contractions place more strain on involved muscle. Healing involves muscle cell necrosis followed by some muscle fiber regeneration and

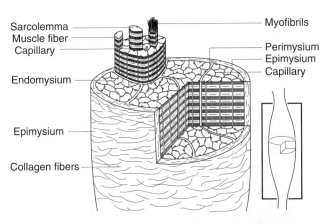

Figure 29-7   Schematic drawing of skeletal muscle.

the reconstitution of the vascular supply. Decreasing inflammation and ensuring minimal vascular injury improves healing time.

ORTHOPAEDIC ONCOLOGY

The diagnosis and treatment of musculoskeletal neoplasms require a team of doctors, which includes a radiologist, oncologist, pathologist, radiation oncologist, and general and orthopaedic surgeon. In addition to thorough history, physical examination, and laboratory workup, radiographic studies can be extremely useful in diagnosing a lesion. X-rays in two planes are helpful in evaluating bone tumors as well as some soft tissue masses and should be performed routinely. Radiographic features of malignant tumors include either an osteolytic or osteosclerotic lesion, poorly demarcated borders (signifying the aggressive nature of the tumor), and periosteal reaction, which can form a triangular shape (Codman triangle) (Fig. 29-9).

Computerized tomographic (CT) scans are helpful both in screening the lungs and head for metastases as well as evaluating the integrity of cortex or examining bone formation. Magnetic resonance imaging (MRI) is the best study for determining both the consistency of tumors and the boundaries of bone and soft tissue tumors in and outside bone. Nuclear bone scans highlight areas of increased metabolic activity within bone and can be useful in identifying metastases as well as determining the relative aggressiveness of a lesion. Indium-tagged white blood cell scans indicate areas of inflammation suggestive of infection.

Ultimately, in instances where musculoskeletal neoplasm is suspected, histologic examination is necessary. Lesions can be sampled by percutaneous needle biopsy by using fine needle aspiration, which provides samples for cytology or by using Tru-cut or large-bore needles, both of which can provide samples for histology as well as cytology. The gold standard for definitive diagnosis of a bony lesion is the *open incisional biopsy*. The open biopsy of a tumor must be carried out carefully to prevent seeding of the tumor by violating soft tissue or muscle planes. Immunohistochemical analysis is very useful in differentiating the various tumors.

Neoplasms can have a clinical presentation similar to that of an infection, so it is important to send all specimens for pathologic as well as microbiologic analysis to prevent mistaking a neoplasm for a simple infection.

Marginal excision involves excision through the pseudocapsule of the tumor and is used for some benign tumors such as lipomas. In the *wide excision*, the pseudocapsule, as well as several more centimeters of the surrounding normal tissue, is removed. *Radical excision* (such as an amputation) involves the removal of the entire compartment or compartments that the tumor occupies and is used to treat tumors that have multiple local satellites or that are recurrent. *Wide excision* (with or without salvage reconstruction) is used for most malignant tumors today. Adjuvant chemotherapy has had a significant impact on limb salvage and long-term survival for patients with osteosarcoma and Ewing sarcoma as well as metastases to the musculoskeletal system. Radiation therapy is utilized for local control of Ewing tumor, lymphoma, myeloma, and metastatic disease. Postradiation sarcoma and late stress fracture are known complications of radiation therapy.

The *most common malignant neoplasms* affecting bone are metastatic tumors. After the lung and liver, bone is the third most common site of metastatic disease. Breast, prostate, lung, kidney, and thyroid tumors account for 80% of the metastasis. The most common bones affected are the spine (lumbar vertebrae), ribs, pelvis, and the proximal ends of long bones. Metastasis to the facial bones and to the skeleton distal to the elbows and knees is rare.

All primary musculoskeletal tumors can be staged with the Enneking system, which categorizes tumors as benign (G0), low grade malignant (G1), and high grade malignant (G2). Anatomic setting is designated as intracapsular (T0), extracapsular/intracompartmental (T1), and extracapsular/extracompartmental (T2). Metastases are either present (M1) or absent (M2). (Table 29-1)

Primary bone neoplasms are generally classified according to the normal cell or tissue type from which they originate (Tables 29-2, 29-3). Those lesions that do not have normal tissue counterparts are grouped according to clinicopathologic features. We will begin with osteogenic, or bone-forming tumors, which (with the exception of

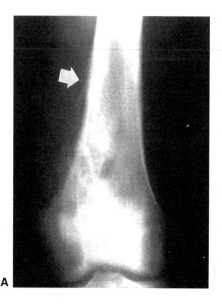

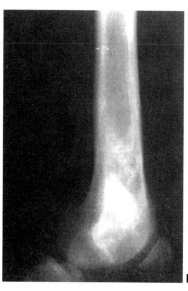

Figure 29-9 Anteroposterior radiograph demonstrating osteosarcoma of the distal femur. Aggressive periosteal reaction is noted along the medial cortex of the distal femoral metaphysis with a proximal Codman triangle (*arrow*). (From Levesque J, Marx R, Bell RS, et al. *A clinical guide to primary bone tumors*. Lippincott Williams & Wilkins 1998:190, with permission.)

A   B

TABLE 29-1

ENNEKING GRADING SYSTEM OF SARCOMAS

Stage[a]	Grade[b]	Tumor[c]	Metastasis[d]
Ia	G1	T1	M0
Ib	G1	T2	M0
IIa	G2	T1	M0
IIb	G2	T2	M0
IIIa	G1 or G2	T1	M1
IIIb	G1 or G2	T2	M1

[a] These factors are combined to give an overall stage, designated in Roman numerals from I to III. Each stage is also subdivided into a or b.
[b] The grade (how likely the cells are to grow and spread, based on their appearance under the microscope) is divided into low grade (G1) and high grade (G2).
[c] The extent of the primary tumor is classified as either intracompartmental (T1), meaning it has basically remained in place, or extracompartmental (T2), meaning it has extended into other nearby structures.
[d] Tumors that have not spread to the lymph nodes or other organs are considered M0, whereas those that have spread are M1.

osteomas) generally produce woven, variably mineralized bone. *Osteomas* are sessile tumors that project from the subperiosteal or endosteal surface of the cortex. Multiple osteomas can be seen in Gardner syndrome of intestinal familial polyposis.

Osteoid osteomas are another benign bone tumor which is typically seen in the second to third decades of life. They commonly arise in the appendicular skeleton and cause pain through the release of prostaglandins. They can be treated symptomatically with nonsteroidal anti-inflammatory medications and will typically "burn out" over time or they can be treated with conservative resection or ablation. *Osteoblastomas* occur in the same age group and have a similar histologic appearance. Like osteoid osteomas they have little to no chance of transformation and can, therefore, be treated with resection.

Osteosarcoma is a malignant mesenchymal tumor with a bimodal age distribution. Approximately three fourths of osteosarcomas occur in patients younger than 20 years. The majority of the other 25% occur in the elderly, who generally develop osteosarcoma in concert with Paget disease,

TABLE 29-2

BENIGN TUMORS OF BONE

Tumor	Age of Onset	Location	Diagnosis	Treatment	Miscellaneous
Osteochondroma (exostosis) 40% of benign bone tumors	Childhood	Out-of-bone lesion connected to metaphysis by trabecular stalk	Palpable mass; the stalk blends into metaphyseal trabecular bone; has cartilaginous cap	Marginal excision if symptomatic; for example, nerve irritation, bursitis; no treatment if asymptomatic	Low rate of malignant transformation to chondrosarcoma; multiple osteochondromas in hereditary multiple exostoses with 1% risk of malignant transformation
Giant cell tumor 20% of benign bone tumors	Third and fourth decades	Metaphysis and epiphysis of long bones, most commonly around knee	Expansile and radiolucent lesions of bone; osteoclast-like giant cells on histology	Intralesional curettage with cementation or bone grafting; adjuvant cryotherapy reduces recurrence	Benign but aggressive lesion; can metastasize to the lungs
Unicameral bone cyst (simple bone cyst)	Childhood	Metaphysis, 90% in proximal humerus or femur	Cystic lesion that abuts but does not involve the growth plate; usually diagnosed after pathologic fracture through the cyst	Immobilization until fracture healing followed by steroid (methylprednisolone acetate) injection into the cyst or curettage and bone grafting	The fracture itself may stimulate the cyst to heal on its own
Nonossifying fibroma	Childhood	Metaphysis	Eccentric lucent lesions, sometimes multiloculated, bubbly, usually incidental plain film findings	Smaller lesions will heal, no treatment; large lesions, curettage and bone grafting to prevent pathologic fracture	
Enchondroma	Childhood and adulthood	Central metaphysis, 53% in phalanges	Well-circumscribed lucent lesion with punctate calcifications	Inactive enchondroma, no treatment; active enchondroma or low-grade chondrosarcoma, curettage with adjuvant cryotherapy	Chondrosarcoma can be distinguished from enchondroma by increased pain, variable lucency on plain films, and endosteal erosion

TABLE 29-3

PRIMARY MALIGNANT TUMORS OF BONE

Tumor	Age of Onset	Location	Diagnosis	Treatment	5-year Survival
Multiple myeloma (plasma cell tumor), most common	Adulthood after age 40	Spine (most common), ribs, skull, long bones; often presents with vertebral compression fractures	Multiple discrete lytic lesions; bone scan may be cold; monoclonal gammopathy on serum and immunoelectrophoresis; Bence-Jones proteinuria; sheets of plasma cells on histology	Chemotherapy is the mainstay of therapy; supportive orthopaedic care (treat pathologic or impending pathologic fractures)	
Osteosarcoma, second most common bone tumor after myeloma	Adolescence 75% occurs at 10–30 y of age	56% involving the metaphysis of the distal femur or proximal tibial	Bone pain with palpable mass, increased alkaline phosphatase; radiodense lesion with bony destruction and soft tissue extension on radiographs	High grade tumor adjuvant preoperative and postoperative chemotherapy and wide resection with limb salvage reconstruction or amputation	>50%
Chondrosarcoma, 10%–20% of malignant bone tumors	Adulthood 50–70 y	Metaphysis of proximal femur or pelvis	May arise from preexisting enchondroma or osteochondroma; on x-ray, lucent lesion with punctate calcifications	Usually slow growing and low grade, so no chemotherapy or x-ray therapy; usually treated with wide surgical resection	Good
Ewing sarcoma (primitive neuroectodermal tumor), 5% of malignant bone tumors	Childhood 5–15 y	Pelvis and diaphysis-metaphysis of large long bones (lower extremity)	Radiologically destructive bone-forming lesion with raised periosteum (Codman triangle), soft tissue extension, and onion skinning; histologically, sheets of blue small round cells, which are derived from mesenchymal stem cell or neural crest origin; associated with 11:22 translocation	Often high grade with rapid growth; treat with neo-adjuvant chemotherapy, wide-resection with limb salvage (if possible), and possibly x-ray therapy; must not be confused with osteomyelitis	65%
Malignant fibrous histiocytoma	>50 y of age	Metaphysis or diaphysis of lower extremities	Predominantly lytic lesion; pleomorphic malignant cells on histology; commonly presents as a primary soft tissue tumor	Often high grade; treatment is wide surgical resection with adjuvant chemotherapy	60%

bone infarct, or prior radiation. They are more likely to occur at the metaphyseal region of, in order of decreasing frequency, the femur, tibia, or humerus. More than 12 subtypes exist, which are grouped according to anatomic location, multicentricity, preexisting disorders, and histologic variation. Osteosarcomas typically present as painful, rapidly growing masses. Radiographs demonstrate a mixed lytic and blastic picture with permeative margins that may have a sunburst pattern.

Cartilage-forming tumors are characterized by the production of hyaline, myxoid, elastic, or fibrocartilage. The principal benign cartilage lesions are *enchondromas, osteochondromas, chondromyxoid fibroma,* and *chondroblastoma.* Enchondromas are exceedingly common and are generally discovered incidentally. Radiographically they appear as an area of lucency with or without associated stippled calcification. They can be monitored radiographically without biopsy or surgery. Multiple enchondromas are associated with Ollier disease and Maffucci syndrome. These patients are at an increased risk for both chondrosarcoma as well as visceral malignancies.

Osteochondromas are benign surface lesions thought to be derived from aberrant cartilage. They are attached to the cortical bone by a stalk with a cartilage cap, which at its base is contiguous with the underlying cortex. There is an entity known as multiple hereditary exostosis which has an autosomal dominance pattern of heredity. The risk of malignant transformation in patients with single osteochondromas is less than 1%; however, the risk approaches 10% in patients with multiple hereditary exostosis. Chondromyxoid fibroma and chondroblastoma are both rare benign lesions that show a predilection for long bones.

Chondrosarcomas span a wide spectrum of relatively benign to aggressive tumors. Differentiating grade I chondrosarcomas from enchondromas requires histologic analysis. Both are composed of hyaline cartilage cells; however, low-grade malignant tumors are more cellular, contain more binucleate cells, and possess giant cartilage cells with clumps of chromatin. Low- and intermediate-grade chondrosarcomas are treated most reliably with wide excision. Patients with dedifferentiated chondrosarcoma are additionally treated with multiagent chemotherapy.

Three common fibrous neoplasms of bone include *nonossifying fibroma* (NOF), *desmoplastic fibroma* and *fibrous histiocytoma*, and *fibrosarcoma*. Nonossifying fibromas are painless metaphyseal, lytic, eccentric lesions that resolve spontaneously prior to skeletal maturity. Desmoplastic fibroma is a rare, low-grade malignancy best treated with wide resection. with periosteal reaction, which can form a triangular shape (Codman triangle). Malignant fibrous histiocytoma and fibrosarcoma arise in the pelvic and long bones of adults and often have extended into the soft tissues prior to diagnosis. They are both characterized by a herringbone pattern of malignant fibroblasts seen on histology.

Chordoma is a tumor for which the cell of origin is primitive notochordal tissue. These neoplasms are seen within the spine and more commonly the sacrum. Treatment of choice is wide resection, which is very difficult owing to the location of these tumors. *Lymphoma and myeloma* are two malignant hematopoietic tumors, which can both be single or multifocal. Both conditions can result in extensive bone destruction and resulting hypercalcemia. Myeloma and lymphoma are both treated with external beam radiation as well as surgical fixation to prevent impending fracture when necessary.

Giant cell tumors, *Ewing tumor*, and *adamantinoma* are three important tumors of unknown origin that affect bone. Giant cell tumors are distinctive neoplasms that are benign but aggressive and even rarely (less than 2%) metastasize to lung. These tumors commonly affect the epiphysis of long bones, 50% of the time about the knee. Radiographs demonstrate lucent lesions often bordering subchondral bone. These tumors are treated with evacuation, aggressive curettage, chemical cauterization (generally with phenol), and reconstruction with methyl methacrylate or bone graft. Ewing tumor is an aggressive round cell sarcoma, which may have an onion skin appearance on x-ray owing to layers of reactive new bone formation around the lesion. Tumors often have a large soft tissue component seen on MRI. There is a consistent chromosomal translocation (11:22) seen in tumor cells. Treatment involves a multimodal approach utilizing radiation therapy and chemotherapy to shrink lesions prior to wide excision. Finally, adamantinoma is a rare tumor characteristically seen on the anterior tibia, although other long bones may be involved. Histologically cells have an epithelial or glandular pattern.

Many lesions affect bone that simulate neoplasms and must be included in any differential diagnosis for unidentified bone lesion. These include osteomyelitis, fibrous dysplasia, bone cysts (aneurysmal and unicameral), histiocytosis X, eosinophilic granuloma, Paget disease, and many other conditions that are beyond the scope of this text.

GENERAL CLINICAL PRINCIPLES OF ORTHOPAEDIC SURGERY

Evaluation and Treatment

The evaluation and treatment of the trauma patient demands a large amount of overlap between the role of the trauma surgeon and that of the orthopaedic surgeon. Patients can present with multiple musculoskeletal injuries, and the rapid assessment, diagnosis, and provisional treatment by the trauma team can prevent permanent neuromuscular disability and even death. Initial evaluation of the polytrauma patient should focus on stabilizing the patient according to Advanced Trauma Life Support (ATLS) guidelines. A coordinated team approach between the trauma team and the orthopaedic surgeons is crucial. A complete history will offer invaluable clues about the mechanism of injury, which will help with clinical diagnosis and treatment. Although some fractures or dislocations can be obvious on physical examination, nondisplaced fractures, distracting injury, or head trauma can make the diagnosis more difficult. Localized pain and tenderness, swelling, shortening, deformity, loss of function of the affected extremity, and abnormal motion are indicative of a possible fracture or dislocation. It is important to examine carefully and radiograph the joint above and joint below the fracture site. Neurovascular examination is also vital, particularly before performing a reduction maneuver. CT scans may be useful in evaluating a comminuted intraarticular fracture; an MRI is helpful to look at soft tissue structures such as ligaments; and bone scan and an MRI both may identify occult fractures not visible on plain radiographs. Patients are reexamined from head to toe in a tertiary survey 12 to 24 hours after the primary survey to look for additional injuries that may have been overlooked initially.

The goal for the treatment of all orthopaedic fractures is fracture union, early mobilization, and rapid return to baseline activity level. In the polytrauma patient, there is a special emphasis on rigid fixation of fractures to facilitate earlier mobilization. In most cases, definitive treatment should be delayed until the patient has been medically stabilized. There are a few exceptions in which emergent operative intervention is required within 6 hours of the initial injury: open fractures, fractures with vascular injuries, amputations, and compartment syndromes. In cases in which soft tissue swelling can seriously compromise the wound healing (e.g., calcaneus fractures and tibial plateau fractures), waiting 1 to 2 weeks to allow the swelling and fracture blisters to resolve may be preferable.

The fracture or dislocation can be treated with either closed reduction, closed reduction with percutaneous internal fixation, or open reduction with internal fixation. For many fractures and dislocations, closed reduction will be successful if attempted acutely with adequate muscle relaxation. However, certain circumstances such as soft tissue interposition, comminuted fractures, and inadequate muscle relaxation will require open reduction.

There are four broad categories of *fixation methods* to hold the fracture: (i) splinting and casting, (ii) traction, (iii) external fixation, and (iv) internal fixation. The choice of treatment depends on many factors, including the inherent stability of the fracture. For the most part, the initial injury, particularly the amount of displacement and comminution, will determine the maximal degree of fracture instability. There are many fractures in which splinting or casting is the treatment of choice (e.g., clavicle, humerus, distal radius, and foot). In addition, most pediatric fractures can be treated successfully in a cast because of the rapid healing and remodeling potential in that patient population.

When splinting or casting a fracture, the physician must immobilize the joints above and below the fracture site. The main disadvantages of this form of stabilization are the inability to rigidly hold a reduction, joint stiffness from

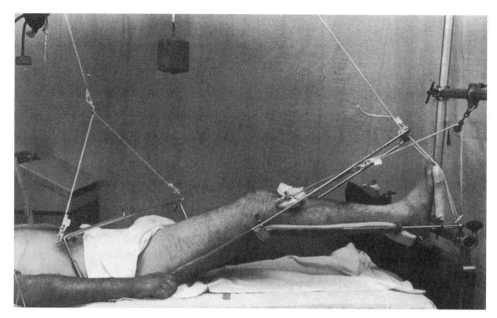

Figure 29-10 Skeletal traction for a femoral fracture using a tibial traction pin. (From Rockwood CA Jr, et al., eds. *Rockwood and Green's fractures in adults*, 4th ed. Philadelphia: Lippincott-Raven, 1996:45, with permission.)

prolonged immobilization, and danger of skin ulcerations at bony prominences. Traction is currently used mostly in the lower extremity, in which longitudinal traction is applied through a pin inserted either through the distal femur or through the proximal tibia (Fig. 29-10). It is generally used as a temporizing measure in patients with unstable fractures who cannot tolerate surgery, or in children whose fractures cannot be internally fixated without risk of physeal trauma. The main drawbacks are suboptimal fracture fixation (tendency for shortening and rotational malunion) and the need for prolonged immobilization (greater than 6 weeks), which can lead to development of sacral ulcers, joint stiffness, and pneumonia. External fixation is indicated in fractures with segmental bone loss, associated vascular injuries, and massive soft tissue injuries with a high risk of infection. In addition, because of the speed with which it can be applied, external fixation is also indicated in the unstable patient with extremity injuries and in the hemodynamically unstable patient. The main complications of external fixator are the risk of pin tract infection and less rigid fixation when compared with internal fixation.

The five main types of internal fixation devices are pins (such as K wires), screws (such as lag screws), plates, intramedullary (IM) rods, and prosthetic replacements. Pins, which can be inserted percutaneously, are often used to hold fractures in the hand and foot and to supplement fixation elsewhere. Lag screws, which provide compression across a fracture site, are used to fix simple transverse or oblique fractures such as the femoral neck fracture. Plates such as the dynamic compression plate and locking plates are useful in long-bone fractures and provide rigid fixation and compression across the fracture site. The IM rod, which is commonly used for femur and tibia fractures, provides rigid fixation and acts as a load-sharing device. The rod is inserted from one end of the bone down the intramedullary canal, thereby transfixing the fracture site and providing translational and angular stability.

Rotational motion is controlled by the interlocking screws at the proximal and distal ends. The smaller incision used to insert the IM rod avoids extensive soft tissue dissection and allows rapid healing and early return to function. Sometimes the intramedullary canal is reamed to allow for insertion of a larger (and hence, stiffer) rod. However, there have been reports of embolization of fat and marrow elements during IM reaming and rodding. Lastly, prosthetic replacement such as the hemiarthroplasty of the humeral head and femoral head is used in situations in which there is comminution of the bone and cartilage is so severe that anatomic reduction can not be restored.

ORTHOPAEDIC COMPLICATIONS AND ASSOCIATED INJURIES

Posttraumatic arthritis is a common complication that occurs after an intraarticular fracture. Articular displacement of greater than 2 mm is associated with an increased risk of subsequent arthritis. Anatomic reduction and fixation of the fracture can help to minimize the risk.

Malunion results from inadequate fracture alignment or later loss of fixation. Although children have the potential for a great deal of remodeling, very little spontaneous correction can be expected in the adult bone, and it is unlikely that the malunion will resolve without intervention. There are many possible causes of *delayed union* and *nonunion*: (i) poor fixation leading to motion at the fracture site, (ii) large gap at the fracture site, (iii) infection, (iv) poor vascular supply, (v) soft tissue interposition, (vi) significant bone loss, and (vii) host factors such as nutritional status and smoking habits. The tibia, ulna, scaphoid, and femoral neck are particularly susceptible to delayed unions or nonunions.

Loss of fixation after either closed or open treatment can lead to malunions and nonunions and is related to several factors. Patient risk factors include obesity, noncompliance with the weight-bearing limitations, increased age, and medical conditions such as osteopenia. In addition, infection and inherent fracture instability caused by fracture comminution can lead to a loss of fixation. Lastly, poor casting technique or inappropriate choice of internal fixation might also result in a loss of fixation.

Postoperative *wound infections* and *osteomyelitis* are usually related to high-energy injuries, which are associated with significant wound contamination and osseous devascularization. Other risk factors include prolonged open wound time, inadequate fixation, and extensive surgical dissection and periosteal stripping, which compromise blood flow to the wound. Leaving a skin bridge less than 7 cm wide will also compromise the vascular status of the soft tissue and increase the incidence of infection. *Staphylococcus aureus* is the most common offending organism (90% of cases). Treatment for osteomyelitis consists of incisional drainage followed by intravenous antibiotics. Temporary implantation of antibiotic-impregnated cement beads and hyperbaric oxygen can help with more resistant cases of infection.

Heterotopic ossification, the formation of ectopic (extra) bone adjacent to the fracture site and within the soft tissues, can be a debilitating posttraumatic complication because of pain and loss of motion that may occur if the ectopic bone crosses the joint. It is mainly associated with fractures of the elbow, acetabulum, and hip. Although the exact causes of heterotopic ossification are not known, risk factors include head trauma, burns, extensive surgery, immobilization, and passive range of motion. Use of indomethacin for 4 to 6 weeks posttrauma can help reduce the chances of developing heterotopic ossification. In the trauma patients in whom indomethacin would be contraindicated, low-dose single-fraction limited field radiation (800 cGy) in the postoperative period is another alternative. (Although long-term effects are not fully known, there is a theoretical risk of future radiation-induced sarcoma.) To be most effective, indomethacin or radiation treatment must be started within 5 days of the injury.

Avascular necrosis (AVN), which is also known as "osteonecrosis" or "aseptic" necrosis, describes the death of bone cells due to impairment in circulation. Posttraumatic AVN occurs when the amount of displacement from the fracture or dislocation is sufficiently severe to disrupt the blood supply to the bone. Sites that are more susceptible to AVN are the scaphoid, femoral head, talus, and odontoid. Other causes of AVN include (i) arterial and venous obstruction due to thrombosis, (ii) fat embolism, (iii) nitrogen gas (decompression sickness, Caisson disease), (iv) radiation therapy, (v) corticosteroid use, and (vi) ethanol abuse. Radiographic changes include sclerosis of the bone on x-ray and edema of the bone marrow on MRI.

Trabecular bone repair from necrosis involves formation and deposition of osteoid and mineral matrix on top of the existing structural framework, a process that increases the density of the cancellous bone. Cortical bone must be largely resorbed by osteoclasts before osteoblastic deposition of new cortical bone, a process that can take up to 2 years. During resorption of the cortical matrix, the necrotic bone becomes very susceptible to fracture because the bone framework is weakened. If osteonecrosis occurs under a region of articular cartilage, eventual fracture and permanent damage to the cartilage is likely. This phenomenon

may be caused by an increased stress within the area, an inability to repair microfractures, or an increased vascularity in the area leading to more extensive resorption of necrotic bone. The end result of AVN is collapse of the articular surface, which leads to osteoarthritis.

Deep venous thrombosis (DVT) can occur in up to 50% to 60% of trauma patients and is most frequently seen in patients with spinal cord injury and fractures of the pelvis, femur, or tibia. Venography is the diagnostic gold standard, but Doppler ultrasonography has been shown to be effective and reliable. Although iodine-labeled fibrinogen is good for diagnosing thrombosis below the popliteal fossa, it is unreliable in detecting clots in the upper thigh or pelvis or in the vicinity of a deep wound. Prophylaxis against DVT and the potential sequelae of pulmonary embolism is important in all trauma patients. If there are no contraindications, subcutaneous heparin, Lovenox, or low-dose warfarin can be used, along with compression or pneumatic stockings. In patients with contraindications to anticoagulation or with proximal venous thrombosis with major pelvic, acetabular, or multiple long bone fractures, vena cava filters should be placed.

In the polytrauma patient, *fat embolism* is an important cause of acute respiratory distress syndrome (ARDS) and a major source of morbidity and mortality. Fat embolism syndrome is clinically apparent in 10% of polytrauma patients, although the actual incidence (which includes subacute presentation) is probably much higher. The risk factors include trauma, long-bone (femur or tibia) fractures, myeloplastic disorders, collagen vascular disease, osteoporosis, and immobilization. Fat embolism has also been documented after intramedullary reaming and rodding and after prosthetic hemiarthroplasty of the hip. It may not appear until 2 to 3 days after the injury and may present as respiratory distress (shortness of breath and tachypnea), arterial hypoxemia, tachycardia, fevers, and a deterioration of neurologic status (restlessness, confusion, or coma). In addition, petechiae (which may be short lived) can appear across the chest and axilla. Treatment consists of pulmonary support and early orthopaedic care. Corticosteroids, heparin, and hypertonic glucose have also been used with variable amounts of success.

Compartment syndrome is a true orthopaedic emergency because of the potential for irreversible muscular and neurologic compromise within 6 hours of onset. Compartment syndrome after a closed injury can result from swelling of the extremity after a fracture, blow, severe crush injury, vascular injury, or tight cast. Stab wounds resulting in arterial puncture or hemophiliac bleeding can also lead to compartment syndrome. The mechanism of compartment syndrome involves fluid exudation at the capillary level within a tight fascial space, leading to venous obstruction. Because the compliant venous system is obstructed before the arterial system, compartment syndrome perpetuates itself.

The most commonly involved extremities are the lower leg and the forearm. The lower leg contains four compartments (anterior, lateral, posterior, and deep posterior). The most frequently affected compartments are the anterior compartment (which contains the deep peroneal nerve and the ankle/toe dorsiflexors such as the tibialis anterior, extensor digitorum longus, and extensor hallucis longus) and the deep posterior compartment (which contains the posterior tibial nerve, posterior tibial artery, peroneal artery, and ankle/toe plantar flexors such as the tibialis posterior, flexor hallucis longus, and flexor digitorum longus).

Diagnosis is based on a high index of suspicion and a careful physical examination. On examination the patient has pain out of proportion to the injury and will generally experience pain with passive motion of adjacent joints. The compartment will be hard and tense on palpation. The classic findings of paralysis, pulselessness, pallor, and paresthesias are typically very late findings. It is important to remember that pulses may continue to be palpable and strong despite the onset of compartment syndrome. Although the diagnosis of compartment syndrome should be made clinically, compartment pressure measurements may be helpful, particularly in the unconscious patient. Absolute compartment pressures of greater than 40 to 45 mm Hg have classically defined the criteria for compartment syndrome (normal pressures are about 0 mm Hg). However, comparing the compartment pressures with the systemic blood pressure is more accurate because hypotension can exacerbate ischemia. Therefore, another criteria for compartment syndrome is a pressure rise in the extremity to within 30 mm Hg of the patient's diastolic blood pressure.

The treatment of compartment syndrome is a fasciotomy of all affected compartments (four in the lower leg and three in the forearm) along with thorough débridement of the involved muscles. The skin is closed secondarily, and a skin graft may be needed for the wound closure. Untreated compartment syndrome leads to muscular and neurologic dysfunction, as well as contractures and clawing of the fingers (Volkmann ischemic contracture) or toes.

Open fractures and *open joint wounds* are surgical emergencies because of the increased risk of infection, which can result from the grossly contaminated wound, extensive soft tissue and skeletal injury, and a delay in treatment. Open fractures are also at a greater risk of nonunion. The Gustilo open fracture classification reflects the severity of the soft tissue injury (Table 29-4). Treatment is surgical débridement within 6 hours of the injury. Repeated débridement in 48 hours and delayed primary closure when the wound is clean are recommended. Antibiotic coverage for grade I and II open fractures consists of 48 hours of intravenous cephalosporin to treat *S. aureus*. For grade III open fractures, an aminoglycoside is added to cover Gram-negative organisms. In open fractures with significant contamination such as a barnyard injury, penicillin is added to cover anaerobes such as *Clostridium perfringens*. Although external fixation is commonly used for severely contaminated fractures, internal fixation as well as external fixation can be used in most grade I, grade II, and grade IIIA fractures. Low-velocity gunshot wounds do not require formal irrigation and débridement of the deeper soft tissues unless the bullets have passed through bowel prior to bone. They can be treated with local wound care and immediate internal fixation. High-energy gunshot wounds (close-range shotgun or military rifle wounds) are more serious and should be managed as a grade IIIB open injury.

Because many of the major nerves run in proximity to the bones, neurologic injuries are commonly associated with fractures and dislocations. For example, radial nerve injuries are associated with humerus fractures, sciatic nerve injuries are associated with hip dislocations, and peroneal nerve injuries are associated with knee injuries. The initial treatment for acute neuropathy is gentle reduction of the fracture or dislocation. Because most nerve injuries sustained in fractures, dislocations, and gunshot wounds are a result of neurapraxia (contusion to the nerve), recovery over a few weeks or months often occurs spontaneously, and immediate surgical exploration is not indicated. However, in cases where nerve examination findings worsen after reduction or when nerve injuries are caused by sharp trauma such as a knife wound, surgical exploration and repair of the lacerated nerve is indicated.

To prevent irreversible muscle and nerve injury, the surgeon must treat *fractures associated with vascular injury* (Gustilo grade IIIC fractures) within 6 hours. Immediate reduction and stabilization of the fracture in the emergency room may alleviate any arterial compromise associated with a kinked or entrapped vessel. If the presence and location of the vascular injury is obvious based on the mechanism of injury, the patient should be brought directly to the operating room instead of going to interventional radiology for an angiogram. To avoid injury to the

TABLE 29-4

CLASSIFICATION OF OPEN FRACTURES[a]

Type	Wound	Level of Contamination	Soft Tissue Injury	Bone Injury
I	<1 cm long	Clean	Minimal	Simple, minimal comminution
II	>1 cm long	Moderate	Moderate, some muscle damage	Moderate comminution
III[a]				
A	Usually >10 cm long	High	Severe with crushing	Usually comminuted; soft tissue coverage of bone possible
B	Usually >10 cm long	High	Very severe loss of coverage	Bone coverage poor; usually requires soft tissue reconstructive surgery
C	Usually >10 cm long	High	Very severe loss of coverage plus vascular injury requiring repair	Bone coverage poor; usually requires soft tissue reconstructive surgery

[a] Segmental fractures, farmyard injuries, fractures occurring in a highly contaminated environment shotgun wounds, or high-velocity gunshot wounds automatically result in classification as a type III open fracture.
From Chapman MW. The role of intramedullary fixation in open fractures. *Clin Orthop* 1986;212:27, with permission.

vascular repair, the surgeon must place a *temporary vascular shunt* to allow débridement and stabilization of the bone before definitive vascular repair. In addition, *fasciotomies should be routinely performed after reperfusion* of the ischemic limb to avoid a subsequent compartment syndrome.

With modern advances in microvascular surgery, the treatment of *traumatic amputations* has become more successful. Replantation is more commonly performed in the upper extremity. Because of the difficulties presented by an insensate foot and the good functional results of a lower extremity prosthesis, replantations are less frequently performed for lower extremity injuries. One of the most important determining factors for a successful replantation is the allowable ischemia time, which is inversely related to the volume of muscle in the amputated part. In general, acceptable ischemia times are 6 hours for warm ischemia and 10 to 12 hours for cool ischemia. Smaller parts such as a digit may be viable after a warm ischemia time of more than 12 hours. Replantation after prolonged ischemia time may lead to acute renal failure secondary to muscle necrosis.

Initial care of an amputated extremity consists of loosely dressing the stump. A tourniquet should not be used if there is any possibility of microvascular repair. The amputated part should be wrapped in a moist gauze and placed in a sterile container or plastic bag, which in turn should be placed in ice water (4° to 10°C). Placing the amputated part directly on ice may lead to frostbite injury. The general sequence for replantation is skeletal fixation, tendon repair, arterial and nerve repair, and lastly venous reanastomosis. Immediate postoperative care includes elevation, keeping the room warm, and avoidance of nicotine and caffeine, which can cause arterial constriction. Venous congestion can be relieved by the application of leaches. A compromise of arterial flow within 48 hours warrants reexploration. Aspirin, Persantine, low-molecular-weight dextran, heparin, and a sympathetic blockade may also prevent arterial thrombosis and spasm.

INJURIES OF THE UPPER EXTREMITY

Sternoclavicular Injuries

Injuries of the sternoclavicular (SC) joint are rare because of the strong ligamentous support of the SC joint. Because of the strong forces involved and the proximity of the SC joint to the great vessels and other mediastinal structures, SC dislocations can be very serious and potentially life-threatening. Signs of potentially dangerous and life-threatening associated injuries to the trachea, esophagus, brachial plexus, and vascular structures include breathing difficulties, dysphagia, paresthesias, and vascular congestion in the upper extremity. Anterior dislocations are more common (73% to 95% of dislocations) than posterior (retrosternal) dislocations. Retrosternal dislocations are associated with much higher complication rates than anterior dislocations (Fig. 29-11). *Intrathoracic injuries* involving the trachea, esophagus, brachial plexus, and great vessels occur in 30% of retrosternal dislocations.

Clinical suspicion is the most important factor in diagnosing an SC injury because this injury is often dismissed as a soft tissue injury or contusion owing to an equivocal deformity or a negative radiograph. *Nonoperative management,*

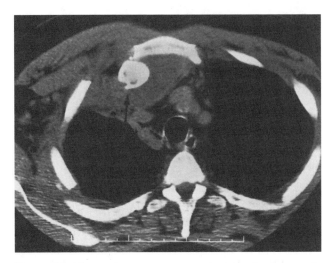

Figure 29-11 Computerized tomographic scan showing a right retrosternal sternoclavicular dislocation (*arrow*). (From Rockwood CA Jr, Wilkins DP, Beaty RW et al., eds. *Rockwood and Green's fractures in adults*, 4th ed. Philadelphia: Lippincott-Raven, 1996:1422, with permission.)

consisting of benign neglect and closed or percutaneous reduction and immobilization in a sling-and-swath dressing is the treatment of choice for most SC injuries. Because of the potential for iatrogenic surgical injury to the underlying neurovascular structures, open reduction is reserved for cases in which the posterior displacement of the medial clavicle is associated with complications caused by mediastinal compression.

Fractures of the Scapula

Fractures of the scapula (most commonly involving the scapular body) usually occur as a result of a direct high-energy impact to the scapular region. Scapular fractures are often seen incidentally on chest radiographs. Because of the large amount of energy required to fracture the scapula, associated injuries are found in up to 96% of patients. Associated injuries include pulmonary injuries (hemopneumothorax and pulmonary contusion), head injuries, ipsilateral clavicle fractures, cervical spine injuries, and brachial plexus injuries.

Fractures of the scapular body, even with severe displacement, usually do well with conservative care. Nonunion is rare. Displaced fracture of the scapular neck, spine, and glenoid have a high rate of associated disability because of shoulder abduction weakness, rotator cuff dysfunction, and subacromial pain. Surgical management may be warranted in these cases.

Fractures of the Clavicle

Clavicle fractures are common injuries in both adults and children and result from direct trauma or a fall on an outstretched arm. Because there is usually superior displacement of the fracture, the diagnosis is easily made both clinically and radiographically. Because of the proximity of the underlying neurovascular structures, a complete neurovascular examination of the upper extremity is essential. On the radiograph, it is important to look for an associated injury such as a pneumothorax.

Because most fractures will heal with minimal treatment, *initial management* usually consists of immobilization in either a sling or a figure-eight harness. Delayed union and nonunion rates of between 0.1% and 23% have been reported. Although conservative management is usually the rule, indications for acute surgical stabilization include injury to underlying vascular structures, open fractures, and impending open fractures indicated by tenting of the skin. The initial management for an associated brachial plexus injury should be observation, because as many as 66% of these cases will resolve spontaneously.

INJURIES OF THE SHOULDER

Acromioclavicular (AC) sprains (also known as "shoulder separations") are commonly caused by a direct impact to the AC joint. Depending on the severity of the sprain, the AC joint capsule is disrupted, the coracoclavicular ligament may be partially or completely disrupted, and the distal end of the clavicle is displaced relative to the acromion. Diagnosis can be confirmed by an anteroposterior (AP) stress radiograph of the AC joint (in which downward traction is applied to the affected arm to accentuate the AC joint separation). In the absence of severe displacement (more than 100% displacement), the treatment is most often conservative, consisting of a sling and mobilization when comfortable.

Dislocations of the shoulder (glenohumeral joint) are common injuries that affect all age groups. They are caused by a direct blow to the shoulder or indirect trauma such as a fall onto an outstretched arm. The *most common direction for shoulder dislocations* is *anterior*. Less than 5% of dislocations are posterior, which can be associated with epileptic seizures. On clinical examination, severe pain and deformity involving the affected shoulder and arm are present. In a thin person, the anteriorly dislocated humeral head is often noticeable and palpable, but in a heavier patient, the soft tissue and swelling may often obscure the humeral head and make the diagnosis less evident. A careful neurovascular examination to rule out associated brachial plexus injuries is also important.

Three views of the shoulder are essential for evaluation of the shoulder. Although the anterior dislocation may be easily seen on the AP view and the lateral view (Y view of the scapula), the axillary view more reliably demonstrates a dislocation, particularly a posterior dislocation. It is also important to look for associated fractures of the proximal humerus, which may change the treatment protocol.

Urgent reduction of the acute dislocated shoulder under sedation or general anesthesia, followed by immobilization in a sling for 3 weeks, is the initial treatment of choice. Open reduction may be necessary in an irreducible dislocation, such as in a shoulder that is chronically dislocated or that has an associated humerus fracture.

Because of the proximity of the brachial plexus, neurologic injuries are relatively common. *Axillary nerve palsy* following shoulder dislocations is 10%. Another complication is chronic (recurrent) instability, which is more often seen in the younger patient who has sustained a high-energy trauma. Inability to abduct the arm should raise suspicions for an associated rotator cuff injury, which is particularly common in elderly patients.

Fractures of the Proximal Humerus

Fractures of the surgical neck of the humerus are commonly seen in the elderly osteoporotic patient and can occur following a simple fall. In the younger patient, these fractures are usually seen following more serious trauma. Evaluation and diagnosis of the proximal humerus fracture is similar to that of the shoulder dislocation. Again, it is important to look for associated injuries to the brachial plexus. In addition, in the severely displaced fracture, an expanding axillary hematoma or diminished or absent distal pulses requires immediate evaluation for axillary artery laceration.

The three radiographic views (AP, lateral, and axillary) will demonstrate the displacement and angulation of the fracture. These are considered significant if they are greater than 1 cm and 45 degrees, respectively. CT scans may also be helpful to evaluate the exact nature of the fracture. In 80% of fractures, the fragments are relatively nondisplaced and nonangulated, and these fractures can be treated simply by *immobilization in a sling* and early motion exercises once the patient is comfortable. Early motion is essential to prevent stiffness because loss of significant shoulder range of motion can lead to a very poor outcome.

In fractures with significant displacement or angulation, surgical intervention is usually necessary to help restore function. Surgical options include closed reduction and percutaneous pinning or open reduction and internal fixation. Surgical treatment for displaced fractures of the humeral head and severely comminuted proximal humerus fractures is prosthetic replacement of the humeral head because of the high risk of osteonecrosis of the head (Fig. 29-12).

Fractures of the Humeral Shaft

Humeral shaft fractures are relatively simple fractures to diagnose and treat. Special attention must be taken to examine the function of the radial nerve because it is the neurovascular structure that is most at risk as it courses in the spiral groove at the junction of the middle and distal thirds of the humerus. The inability to extend the wrist or thumb may indicate a *radial nerve palsy.*

In the isolated closed injury, the treatment of choice is nonsurgical management in a splint or brace because rigid fixation and perfect alignment are not necessary to achieve healing and good functional results (Fig. 29-13). *Absolute indications for surgery* are open fractures and fractures with associated vascular injuries. Relative indications include failure of closed treatment to achieve acceptable alignment, poor patient compliance, ipsilateral humeral shaft and forearm fractures (floating elbow), fractures associated with brachial plexus injuries, and ipsilateral lower extremity fractures. In the polytrauma patient, rigid fixation of fractures is important to facilitate earlier mobilization. This helps to prevent the onset of secondary pulmonary and vascular complications. Surgical options for fixing the humerus include plating and IM rodding. External fixation is rarely used except in severe open fractures or when rapid stabilization is essential.

Fractures of the Distal Humerus

Fractures of the distal humerus are complex injuries that include fractures of the supracondylar region of the elbow and the articular surface of the elbow. In more severe

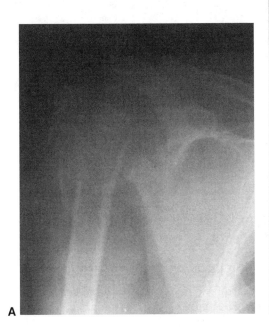
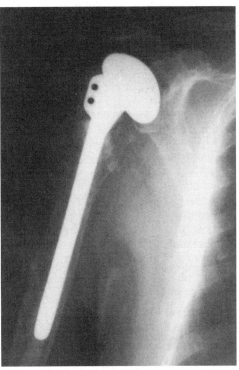

Figure 29-12 **A:** Comminuted fracture of the proximal humerus. **B:** Because of the high risk of avascular necrosis in comminuted proximal humerus fractures, the treatment is prosthetic replacement. (From Rockwood CA Jr, Wilkins DP, Beaty RW et al., eds. *Rockwood and Green's fractures in adults*, 4th ed. Philadelphia: Lippincott-Raven, 1996:1080, with permission.)

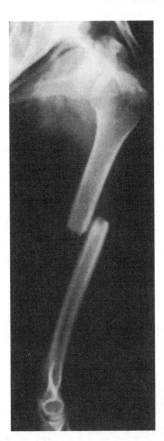

Figure 29-13 A simple transverse fracture of the humerus midshaft, which can be treated in a splint or brace. (From Rockwood CA Jr, Wilkins DP, Beaty RW et al., eds. *Rockwood and Green's fractures in adults*, 4th ed. Philadelphia: Lippincott-Raven, 1996:16, with permission.)

fractures, CT scans are helpful to evaluate articular comminution. Because this fracture is often a result of a high-energy injury, associated soft tissue injury is common.

Because closed reduction and casting or bracing are usually incapable of restoring the anatomy of the supracondylar humerus and the articular surface of the elbow, the only indication for nonoperative treatment is a nondisplaced distal humerus fracture. The treatment of choice for most distal humeral fractures is open reduction and plate fixation, followed by early mobilization. In grossly contaminated open fractures, an external fixator that spans the elbow joint may be used to temporarily stabilize the fracture.

Although fractures of the distal humerus account for only 2% of adult fractures, they account for a large number of poor outcomes and complications such as pain, deformity, instability, stiffness, nonunion, and malunion. *Ulnar nerve injury* is also a common complication, which can be caused by the injury itself or by impinging hardware. Ulnar neuropathy can be minimized by performing an ulnar nerve transposition during surgery. As with all elbow injuries, *heterotopic ossification* is another potential complication and is seen in 4% of distal humerus fractures.

Injuries of the Elbow

Injuries of the elbow are common and include elbow dislocations, olecranon fractures, and radial head fractures. Physical findings can be variable, ranging from a small effusion seen in a nondisplaced radial head fracture to gross deformity seen in an elbow dislocation. Radiographs may show an obvious fracture or dislocation. However, in the absence of an obvious finding, the presence of a posterior fat pad sign signifies an elbow effusion, suggesting an occult injury such as a nondisplaced radial head fracture.

The most common elbow dislocation is the posterior dislocation. Good anesthesia and traction usually allow easy closed reduction with minimal force. The elbow is then placed in a posterior splint at 90 degrees of elbow flexion for 7 to 10 days, followed by progressive mobilization. Nondisplaced fractures of the olecranon can be treated with casting or splinting. However, most olecranon fractures are displaced because of the pull of the triceps and require operative fixation with tension-band technique or plating.

Neurovascular complications include ulnar and radial nerve injuries in elbow dislocations, ulnar nerve injuries in olecranon fractures, and radial nerve injury in radial head fractures. For all elbow fractures, stiffness (exacerbated by prolonged immobilization for more than 3 weeks) and *heterotopic bone formation* are other potential complications.

Fractures of the Forearm

Fractures of the radial and ulnar shafts are commonly caused by high-energy trauma from a direct blow (e.g., nightstick fracture of the ulna) or from a fall from a height. In evaluating the forearm fracture, it is particularly important to examine both the wrist and the elbow for an associated fracture. A common injury that may be missed is the Monteggia fracture, in which an ulna fracture is accompanied by a radial head dislocation (Fig. 29-14).

Because of the difficulty of maintaining anatomic alignment of the forearm fracture in a cast, there is a limited role for conservative care in forearm fractures. Isolated nondisplaced ulna fractures are usually treated in a cast, but most fractures of the radius, as well as combined radius and ulna fractures, are treated by open reduction and internal plate fixation. For comminuted fractures, additional bone grafting may be necessary.

Associated injuries include radial head dislocation (Monteggia fracture) and injuries to the distal radial ulnar joint (DRUJ). Both are easily seen on routine radiographs. In the elbow x-ray, the radial head should align with the capitellum in both AP and lateral views. In the

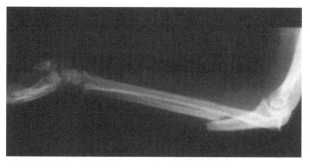

Figure 29-14   Monteggia fracture in which there is a radial head dislocation associated with an ulna fracture. Notice that the radial head lies posterior to the capitellum. (From Rockwood CA Jr, Wilkins DP, Beaty RW et al., eds. *Rockwood and Green's fractures in adults*, 4th ed. Philadelphia: Lippincott-Raven, 1996:916, with permission.)

wrist x-ray, injury to the DRUJ results in widening of the joint space.

Fractures of the Distal Radius

Fractures of the wrist are one of the most common orthopaedic injuries (1:500 people). Although wrist fractures are mainly seen in young adolescents and in the elderly, they are becoming more common in young adults as a result of activities such as in-line skating.

In the common extraarticular distal radius fracture with a dorsally angulated distal fragment (also known as the "Colles fracture") (Fig. 29-15), closed reduction and cast immobilization is the treatment of choice. Unstable injuries with extensive comminution and open injuries are best treated surgically with external fixation. Open reduction and pinning or internal plating is also useful in unstable fractures and in intraarticular fractures.

The most common complication following the distal radius fracture is nerve injury. *Median nerve injury* is the most common, followed by ulnar neuropathy. Radial nerve injury is usually a result of external fixator pin placement. Acute neuropathy is usually caused by a contusion from the initial injury, but subsequent swelling and immobilization

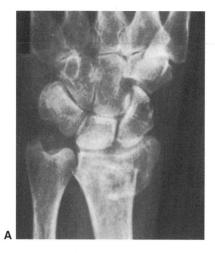
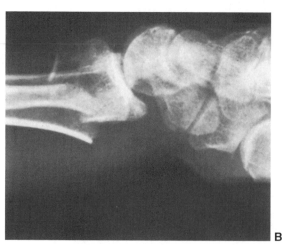

Figure 29-15   Anterior-posterior **(A)** and lateral **(B)** view of the wrist showing a Colles distal radius fracture with characteristic shortening and dorsal angulation of the distal fragment. (From Rockwood CA Jr, Wilkins DP, Beaty RW et al., eds. *Rockwood and Green's fractures in adults*, 4th ed. Philadelphia: Lippincott-Raven, 1996:776, with permission.)

in excessive wrist flexion can also lead to neurapraxia. Initial treatment is reduction of the fracture, but if there is no improvement, then nerve decompression (such as a carpal tunnel release for median neuropathy) may be necessary. Scaphoid fractures are also associated with distal radius fractures.

Fractures of the Hand

Common fractures of the hand include scaphoid fractures, fractures of the base of the thumb metacarpal, fractures of the fifth metacarpal neck (boxer's fracture), and phalangeal fractures. It is particularly important to diagnose and treat the scaphoid fracture because of the high risk of nonunion and AVN. Pain to palpation over the anatomic snuffbox of the wrist, even in the absence of an apparent scaphoid fracture on the radiograph, is suggestive of a scaphoid fracture, and the wrist should be immobilized in a thumb spica cast. If there are any questions, a bone scan or MRI will definitively reveal a scaphoid fracture. In boxer's fracture it is important to look for penetrating wounds to the metacarpal phalangeal joint resulting from a punch to a mouth, because this may represent an open fracture requiring operative incisional drainage.

In general, most fractures of the hand can be treated by closed reduction and buddy taping, splinting, or casting. Although residual angular deformity in the hand may be well tolerated (e.g., 45 degrees of angulation is acceptable in fifth metacarpal neck fractures), rotational deformity is never acceptable. Unsuccessful attempts at nonsurgical treatment necessitate operative intervention, usually in the form of closed reduction and percutaneous pinning. However, other techniques such as plating, screw fixation, or external fixation can be used in certain situations.

The risk of AVN in scaphoid fractures is related to the level of the fracture. Because the vascular supply enters the scaphoid distally, fractures involving the proximal pole have a higher incidence of AVN than fractures of the distal or middle third. AVN presents radiographically as sclerosis and fragmentation, typically at the proximal pole of the scaphoid.

Other complications of hand fractures include capsular or collateral ligament contractures (particularly in the metacarpophalangeal joint following immobilization in extension), decreased motion, and extensor and flexor tendon adhesions. Prolonged immobilization (more than 3 weeks) can aggravate the stiffness. Because of the abundant vascular supply of the hand, infections following open fractures in the hand are less common than those in other areas of the body.

Injuries of the Hand

Although it is now possible to reattach most amputated parts of the hand with microvascular techniques, reattachment may not always lead to a better cosmetic or functional outcome. Specific indications for replantation include (i) injury to multiple digits; (ii) amputations of the thumb; (iii) most amputations in children; and (iv) sharp amputations at the level of the hand, wrist, or distal forearm. Relative contraindications include (i) contaminated or severe crush or avulsion injury, (ii) single-digit amputations in adults, and (iii) a history of smoking. Absolute contraindications include (i) severe medical problems, (ii) multilevel injury of the amputated part, and (iii) a psychiatric patient with a self-inflicted injury.

Peripheral nerve injuries to the upper extremity are common and disabling injuries. The most important aspect of the diagnosis of the injury is the knowledge of the distribution and motor function of the major nerves (Table 29-5). The three major nerves in the upper extremity are the radial, median, and ulnar nerves. Both the median and the ulnar nerves innervate muscles in the forearm (extrinsic muscles) and in the hand (intrinsic muscles), although the radial nerve does not innervate any muscles in the hand (Fig. 29-16). The digital nerves, which supply sensation to

TABLE 29-5

NERVES OF THE WRIST AND HAND

	Radial Nerve	Median Nerve	Ulnar Nerve
Location	Posterior compartment of the forearm, entering the wrist dorsally	Volar surface of the forearm between the FDP and FDS, entering the wrist through the carpal tunnel	Behind the medial epicondyle of the elbow, along the ulnar aspect of forearm between the FDP and FCU, entering the wrist through the Guyon canal (ulnar to the carpal tunnel) ulnar to the ulnar artery
Motor function	Wrist extension (ECRB, ECRL), thumb extension (EPL), extension of fingers at MCP joint (ED)	Extrinsic: wrist flexion (FCR), finger and thumb flexion (FDS, FDP for index finger, FPL) Intrinsic: thumb abduction (APB) and opposition (OP), MCP flexion (radial lumbricals)	Extrinsic: wrist flexion (FCU), ring and little finger flexion (FDP for ring and little finger) Intrinsic: finger abduction/adduction (interosseous), intrinsic hand movements (hypothenar muscles, ulnar lumbricals)
Sensory innervation	See Fig. 29-16	See Fig. 29-16	See Fig. 29-16
Specific areas of sensory innervation	First dorsal web space (between thumb and index finger)	Palmar aspect of the tip of the index finger	Palmar aspect of the tip of the little finger

FDP, flexor digitorum profundus; FDS, flexor digitorum superficialis; ECRB, extensor carpi radialis brevis; ECRL, extensor carpi radialis longus; ED, extensor digitorum; EPL, extensor pollicis longus; FCR, flexor carpi radialis; FPL, flexor pollicis longus; MCP, metacarpophalangeal; APB, abductor pollicis brevis; OP, opponens pollicis; FCU, flexor carpi ulnaris.

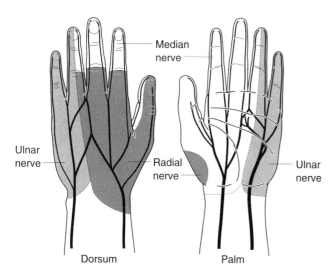

Figure 29-16 Sensory innervation of the hand.

the fingers, are terminal branches of these three nerves. Because most nerve injuries sustained in fractures, dislocations, crush injuries, and gunshot wounds result in neurapraxia, immediate surgical exploration is not indicated. However, in sharp trauma, surgical exploration and primary nerve repair or nerve grafting is the treatment of choice.

Flexor tendon lacerations will result in severe disability if not treated. Although extensor tendon lacerations may be repaired in the emergency room, flexor tendon injuries are best repaired in the operating room under more controlled circumstances. Repair within 1 to 2 weeks is acceptable and will not compromise the outcome.

FRACTURES OF THE PELVIS AND ACETABULUM

Pelvic Fractures

Fractures of the pelvic ring are life-threatening injuries that result from high-energy trauma such as a car accident or a fall from a height. The overall mortality rate is 9%, with hemorrhage accounting for 60% of the deaths. Open pelvic fractures have a mortality rate of up to 50%.

External clues to an underlying pelvic fracture are scrotal or labial swelling, ecchymosis, abnormal positioning of the lower extremity, unexplained hypotension, and instability and pain of the pelvis on examination. Rectal and perineal examination is essential to look for open communication with the vagina or rectum. Evaluation should include an abdominal CT scan and diagnostic peritoneal lavage (DPL) to assess the sources of bleeding. For the DPL, the needle must be inserted supraumbilically to avoid inadvertent puncture and decompression of a large intrapelvic hematoma. Urogenital injuries will present as bleeding from the urethral meatus, a high-riding prostate, or difficulty with passing a urinary catheter into the bladder. If this occurs in the trauma bay, a retrograde urethrogram is indicated.

As with all multitrauma patients, the first priority is aggressive resuscitation and stabilization of the patient according to ATLS protocol. The orthopaedic issues must

be addressed concurrently: retroperitoneal hemorrhage, pelvic ring instability, and associated injury to the urogenital and gastrointestinal system. The most common sources of retroperitoneal bleeding are from low-pressure sources such as cancellous bone bleeding from the fracture site and retroperitoneal venous bleeding. Because only 15% of the hemorrhage-related deaths are a result of the high-pressure arterial bleeds (most commonly injured artery is the superior gluteal artery), emergent angiography before pelvic stabilization may not be helpful. In the hypotensive patient suspected of retroperitoneal bleeding, the pelvis must be immediately stabilized by application of a T-pod corset, an external fixator, pelvic clamp, or even a sheet tied around the pelvis. A stabilized pelvis will help with tamponade of the retroperitoneal bleeding by reducing pelvic volume. For continued uncontrollable blood loss and a rapidly expanding or pulsatile retroperitoneal hematoma, emergent angiography with embolization is warranted. Pelvic fractures that communicate with the rectum or perineum are open fractures by definition and must be managed surgically with a *diverting colostomy*. Early treatment of a vaginal laceration can minimize formation of a pelvic abscess.

Definitive management of the unstable pelvic injury consists of surgical stabilization. Posterior instability (such as with disruption of the sacroiliac joint) is associated with increased patient mortality. Indications for external fixation include pelvic instability, hemodynamic instability, and associated pelvic soft tissue injuries. In certain situations, open reduction and internal fixation may be another option. Pubic symphysis disruptions (diastasis of more than 2.5 cm) can be plated through an anterior Pfannenstiel incision. Posterior sacroiliac joint injuries can be fixed with plates, sacral bars, or iliosacral lag screws. Pubic rami fractures generally do not need to be surgically repaired. Because of the complexity of the repair, the surgery should be delayed until the patient is stable and the entire surgical staff is fully prepared.

Associated injuries are common in patients with pelvic fractures: hemodynamic instability (20%), urogenital injury (12% to 20%), and injury to the lumbosacral plexus (8%). A very high risk of injury to the lumbosacral nerve roots is seen with associated sacral foraminal fractures. In addition, 60% to 85% of patients have other associated fractures. Lastly, the risk for DVT is also significant because of injury to the pelvic veins.

Acetabular Fractures

Most acetabular fractures result from high-energy blunt trauma, which may involve other significant life-threatening injuries. The diagnosis can be made on the plain radiograph (Fig. 29-17), but the fracture can be best evaluated by the CT scan. Nondisplaced fractures can be treated with protected weight bearing. For fractures with a greater than 2-mm articular step off, open reduction and plate fixation is preferred to help decrease the likelihood of posttraumatic arthritis. Skeletal traction can be used as a temporary measure or as definitive treatment in the patient who cannot undergo surgery. Complications include heterotopic ossification, sciatic nerve injury, and posttraumatic arthritis, as well as osteonecrosis of the femoral head if there is a concomitant posterior hip dislocation.

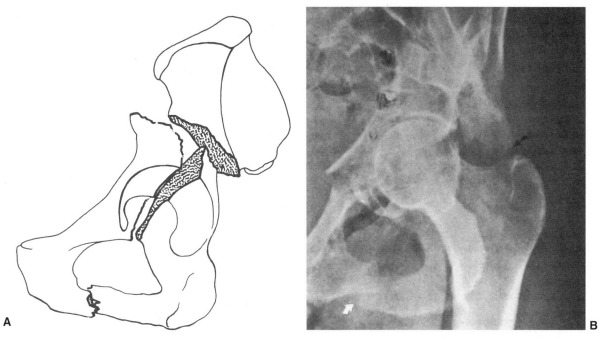

Figure 29-17 **A,B:** Fracture of the acetabulum (*arrows*). (From Rockwood CA Jr, Wilkins DP, Beaty RW et al., eds. *Rockwood and Green's fractures in adults*, 4th ed. Philadelphia: Lippincott-Raven, 1996:1632, with permission.)

INJURIES OF THE LOWER EXTREMITY

Hip Dislocations

Because of the intrinsic stability of the hip joint, an isolated hip dislocation is an uncommon injury and is usually caused by a high-energy trauma such as in a motor vehicle accident in which the hip is driven posteriorly by the dashboard. In the classic clinical presentation of the more common posterior hip dislocation, the leg is adducted, internally rotated, and shortened (Fig. 29-18). Special attention must be paid to the neurologic examination, particularly the sciatic nerve. The dislocation is usually evident in the standard AP pelvis and hip radiograph.

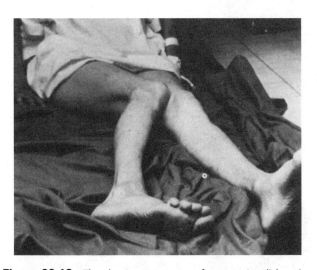

Figure 29-18 The classic appearance of a posterior dislocation of the right hip. (From Rockwood CA Jr, Wilkins DP, Beaty RW et al., eds. *Rockwood and Green's fractures in adults*, 4th ed. Philadelphia: Lippincott-Raven, 1996:1771, with permission.)

In the posterior dislocation, the femoral head lies superiorly out of the acetabulum.

Prompt reduction within 24 hours (and preferably within 6 hours) is important to minimize the risk of AVN of the femoral head and permanent sciatic nerve injury. Closed reduction may not be possible if there is entrapment of a tendon, a capsule, or a fracture fragment, and open reduction will be necessary. After reduction, the hip should be tested for stability. In addition, a CT scan may be useful to confirm a congruent reduction. When comfortable, the patient may begin ambulation with full weight bearing.

AVN of the femoral head, which usually presents 1 to 5 years after the injury, is a devastating complication and has been reported in up to 17% of patients. Prompt reduction has been shown to decrease the risk of AVN. The most frequent long-term complication is posttraumatic arthritis and is related to the severity of the injury. Because of the proximity of the sciatic nerve, sciatic nerve injuries (more commonly the peroneal branch) occur in 8% to 19% of posterior hip dislocations. However, 50% of the time, the patient eventually recovers full function.

HIP FRACTURES

Femoral neck fractures are common injuries that result from low-energy trauma (such as a fall) in the elderly and high-energy trauma in young adults. Hip fractures are more common in women, and risk factors include poor balance and vision, smoking, lack of physical activity, medications such as sedatives, and neurologic impairments. In the classic clinical presentation, the leg is abducted, externally rotated, and shortened (distinct from the hip dislocation). AP and cross-lateral radiographs of the hip are required for evaluation. In the patient who has negative findings on the radiograph but who has examination results suspicious for a hip fracture, a bone scan performed 48 hours after the injury or an MRI will be diagnostic.

Because early mobilization in patients with hip fractures can help prevent deep venous thrombosis (DVT) and pneumonia, the *treatment of choice* is surgical stabilization. The technique is dictated by the amount of displacement of the fracture. In patients with femoral neck fractures, disruption of the blood supply to the femoral head is proportional to the amount of displacement. In nondisplaced or minimally displaced fractures, the *risk of AVN* is less than 10%, compared to a rate of 25% in displaced fractures. Nondisplaced or minimally displaced fractures can be treated by closed or open reduction and fixation with multiple screws (Fig. 29-19). Other complications include nonunion and failure of fixation.

Prosthetic replacement of the femoral head (hemiarthroplasty) is preferred in displaced fractures. Patients with preexisting osteoarthritis and rheumatoid arthritis should be treated with a prosthetic total hip replacement. Although hip fractures do not need to be fixed emergently, fixation within 2 days has been shown to decrease the risk of mortality within the first year after the fracture.

The evaluation and diagnosis of the *intertrochanteric hip fracture* is similar to that of the femoral neck fracture. Although isolated avulsion fractures of the greater or lesser trochanter can be managed by protected weight bearing, surgical stabilization in the form of a compression hip screw and side plate or IM fixation are the treatment of choice for the intertrochanteric fractures. In contrast to femoral neck fractures, there is no increased risk of AVN with the intertrochanteric hip fracture. The major complication is the loss of fixation.

Fractures of the Femur

Fractures of the femoral shaft and distal supracondylar femur are generally high-energy injuries that are easily diagnosed on physical examination because of the obvious swelling, shortening, deformity, and pain in the thigh. Radiographs should include views of the knee, hip, and pelvis. It is particularly important to look for an associated femoral neck fracture, which is often missed.

Immediate stabilization of femoral shaft fractures, particularly in a patient with multiple injuries, has been shown to decrease the incidence of pulmonary complications (such as ARDS) and the length of stay in the hospital. *IM rodding* either antegrade (from a starting point at the hip) or retrograde (from a starting point at the knee) is the treatment of choice for most femoral shaft fractures. Results are excellent, with a 99% union rate and only a 0.9% infection rate. Traction and external fixation can be used as a temporary measure in patients with open fractures, in patients awaiting medical stabilization, or in patients too ill to undergo surgery. Unlocked plate fixation is not optimal in most cases because of the extensive exposure required. In patients with gunshot wounds, IM rods can be inserted in concert with local wound care.

Minimally displaced distal femur fractures can be treated nonoperatively in a knee immobilizer or a long leg cast. Displaced fractures and fractures with articular involvement are best treated surgically with devices such as an IM nail, condylar screws and plates, or lag screws and buttress plates.

Femoral neck fractures are found in 2.5% to 5% of femoral shaft fractures. However, because the femoral neck fracture is often nondisplaced and the femoral shaft fracture is obvious, the femoral neck fracture is missed 30% of the time. In these cases when both are fractured, fixation of the femoral neck fracture is prioritized owing to the risk of AVN over the femoral shaft fracture. Infections, nonunion, and malunion following IM nailing for femoral shaft fractures are rare. Compartment syndrome of the thigh is also rare. Heterotopic ossification can occur in 25% of patients following IM nailing, but the long-term

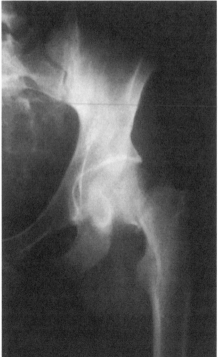
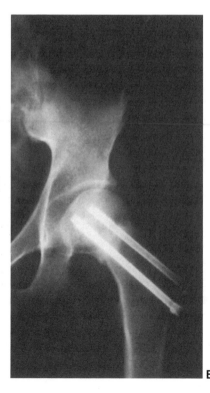

Figure 29-19 A: Fracture of the femoral neck with minimal displacement. **B:** The fracture has been fixed by lag screw fixation. The treatment for completely displaced fractures is prosthetic replacement of the femoral head. (From Rockwood CA Jr, Wilkins DP, Beaty RW et al., eds. *Rockwood and Green's fractures in adults*, 4th ed. Philadelphia: Lippincott-Raven, 1996: 1698, with permission.)

A   B negative impact is minimal. Complications following distal femur fractures include infection, nonunion, malunion, loss of fixation, knee stiffness, and posttraumatic arthritis.

Soft Tissue Injuries of the Knee

Isolated sprains and ruptures of the ligaments of the knee are common injuries and can be caused both by minor and major trauma. The anterior cruciate ligament (ACL) and the posterior cruciate ligament (PCL) provide anterior and posterior stability to the knee, respectively. The medial collateral ligament (MCL) and the lateral collateral ligament provide stability in the medial-lateral plane. ACL ruptures are often associated with MCL and medial meniscus injuries. The MRI is the radiographic study of choice to evaluate the status of the ligaments. Treatment of isolated injuries to any of the four ligaments is bracing. For the younger and more active patient, surgical reconstruction of the ACL or PCL may be recommended.

Meniscal tears are very common injuries and can be traumatic or degenerative in nature. Treatment is symptomatic unless there are mechanical symptoms such as knee catching or locking, in which case, arthroscopic partial meniscectomy may be indicated.

Knee Dislocations

Knee dislocations can be devastating because of associated injuries to the neurovascular bundle as it passes posteriorly through the popliteal fossa. Anterior dislocations are usually caused by hyperextension, and posterior dislocations can be caused when the proximal tibia is driven posteriorly, such as when the proximal tibia strikes the dashboard during a car accident. Although knee dislocations are usually clearly seen on routine radiographs, it is important to remember that spontaneous reductions can sometimes occur. Injuries that involve a suspicious mechanism or multiligamentous instability should be treated as knee dislocations until proved otherwise. Evaluation of the neurovascular status of the involved extremity is particularly important. Although distal pulses may be present, they do not rule out vascular injury such as an intimal tear. Therefore, arteriography is recommended in all patients with a history of abnormal ankle–brachial indices (ABIs) or diminished pulses. Status of the four major knee ligaments should be determined, and in most patients, the ACL and PCL are both ruptured.

Immediate closed reduction can restore the neurovascular status of the leg. The vascular surgery team should be consulted immediately, as increased rates of amputation are seen with delays in vascular repair after more than 6 hours. Reverse saphenous vein interposition graft is the treatment of choice for occlusive vascular injuries. Four-compartment fasciotomy is also recommended for ischemia times greater than 4 hours. Attention is then directed toward the associated ligamentous injuries. If there is a vascular injury, any associated ligamentous repair should be delayed a few weeks or should be performed without a tourniquet. Because the use of a tourniquet may aggravate an underlying vascular repair, arteriography should be performed before tourniquet use.

Associated injuries include vascular injury (30%), neurologic injury typically involving the peroneal nerve (23%), open injury (5%), and fractures (10%). Meniscal

injury is also common (40%), but compartment syndrome is rare. Knee stiffness is the most common complication, but surprisingly, instability is rarely a major complaint.

Fractures of the Tibial Plateau

Tibial plateau (proximal tibia) fractures are most commonly seen in high-energy trauma in middle-aged men and in osteopenic fractures in elderly women. The mechanisms of injury include falls, motor vehicle accidents, and pedestrian accidents (such as when the car bumper hits the lateral aspect of the pedestrian's knee). On physical examination, the status of soft tissue and skin and the neurovascular structures should be carefully documented. Although standard radiographs will show the fracture (most commonly involving the lateral tibial plateau), a CT scan will better delineate the comminution and depression of the articular surface.

For nondisplaced fractures with minimally depressed articular fragments, the fracture can be treated with casting or bracing and early range of motion. In fractures with a significant amount of articular depression (5 to 10 mm) or with significant ligamentous laxity, surgical reduction and fixation with lag screws and buttress plates is preferred (Fig. 29-20). Joint spanning external fixation can be used in markedly comminuted fractures or open fractures.

The most common complications are posttraumatic arthritis (meniscal preservation is important to prevent arthritis) and knee stiffness (prevented by early mobilization). Surgical complications include infection and skin sloughing secondary to poor skin condition in high-energy traumas and extensive surgical dissections in complex fractures.

Fractures of the Tibia

Fractures of the tibial shaft are the most common long-bone fractures. Because of the subcutaneous location of the tibia, the deformity is usually evident. Intraarticular fractures of the distal tibia (also known as a "tibial plafond

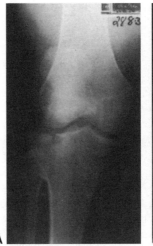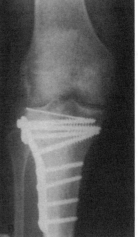

A   B

Figure 29-20 Intraarticular fracture of the **(A)** lateral tibial plateau, which has been stabilized by a **(B)** buttress plate. (From Rockwood CA Jr, Wilkins DP, Beaty RW et al., eds. *Rockwood and Green's fractures in adults*, 4th ed. Philadelphia: Lippincott-Raven, 1996:1933, with permission.)

fracture" or "pilon fracture") are usually high-energy injuries that result from axial loading and are accompanied by significant soft tissue swelling. Although radiographs are adequate in most cases, bone scan or MRI can be used to diagnose occult stress fractures in the tibial shaft.

For minimally displaced and angulated tibial shaft fractures (less than 10 degrees of angulation), cast immobilization is an acceptable treatment option. For unstable and comminuted fractures, surgical fixation in the form of IM rodding is the preferred treatment. External fixation is useful in grossly contaminated open injuries. In grade IIIC open tibial fractures, amputation may be preferable to leg salvage because of poor results following neurovascular repair.

Delayed unions and nonunions are relatively common complications of tibial shaft fractures. For nonsurgical treatment, the delayed union rate is 19% and the nonunion rate is 4%. Malunions are also more common with nonsurgical treatment. Complications specific to IM rodding include implant failures and anterior knee pain (because of the entrance point of the rod in the anterior knee). Pin tract infections can occur in up to 50% of patients treated with external fixation. Because compartment syndrome is also more common in the lower leg, close observation and frequent neurovascular checks essential.

The nondisplaced tibial plafond fracture is treated nonsurgically. Because the fracture usually involves comminution of the articular surface, surgical fixation is generally preferred. In addition, because of the high risk of wound infection and sloughing, it may be prudent to wait 7 to 10 days to allow swelling and blistering to subside before surgery is performed. Surgical options include plate fixation, although the potential for wound complications makes external fixation an attractive alternative. Because of the intraarticular injury in the pilon fracture, posttraumatic arthritis of the ankle joint is an expected complication. However, the most feared complication is wound infection and dehiscence.

Fractures of the Fibula

The fibula bears only a small percentage of the body weight as compared to the tibia; therefore, isolated fractures of the fibula are generally successfully managed conservatively except when associated with displaced or unstable ankle fractures. Symptomatic treatment and splinting for comfort are the mainstays of treatment. There usually are no long-term complications. Fractures of the proximal fibula near the level of the fibular head may result in peroneal nerve neurapraxia.

Achilles Tendon Ruptures

In the acute rupture of the Achilles tendon, pain is localized at the posterior calf and there is an absence of ankle plantar flexion even with passive squeezing of the calf muscles (Thompson test). Nonsurgical treatment consists of casting with the ankle in plantar flexion. For the more active patient, open repair will allow for quicker return to activities and a lower rerupture rate. However, because of the thin soft tissue envelope around the Achilles tendon, postsurgical wound infection is seen in up to 13% of open repairs.

Fractures of the Calcaneus

Fractures of the calcaneus are caused by a high-energy axial load, such as a fall from a height. A common presentation is a patient who has fallen from a building who presents with severe foot pain and deformity as well as lower back pain. Careful examination of the spine is essential because of the risk of associated compression fractures of the lumbar vertebrae. In addition to plain radiographs, CT scan of the calcaneus is useful in evaluating the integrity of the articular surface. Slices of 3 to 5 mm in the coronal plane perpendicular to the posterior facet and then perpendicular to that in the transverse plane allow the surgeon to evaluate the injury. Treatment is nonsurgical for extraarticular fractures (25% of fractures) and open reduction and internal fixation for intraarticular fractures. Because massive soft tissue swelling is usually present, surgical fixation is best performed in 7 to 10 days to allow the swelling to subside.

Complications are posttraumatic arthritis to the subtalar joint, which may cause significant pain. Compartment syndrome of the foot occurs in up to 10% of fractures. Wound infection and dehiscence and injury to the sural nerve are potential risks related to the surgical repair.

KEY CONCEPTS

▲ Orthopaedic injuries that require emergent operative intervention within 6 hours of the initial injury include: open fractures, fractures with vascular injuries, amputations, and compartment syndromes

▲ External fixation is indicated in fractures with segmental bone loss, associated vascular injuries, and massive soft tissue injuries with a high risk of infection. In addition, because of the speed with which it can be applied, external fixation is also indicated in the patient with unstable extremity injuries and in the hemodynamically unstable patient.

▲ Compartment syndrome is a clinical diagnosis, made when a patient experiences symptoms such as pain with passive stretch, pain out of proportion to injury, and tense compartments. However, compartment pressure measurements may be helpful, particularly in the unconscious patient. Absolute compartment pressures of over 40 to 45 mm Hg define compartment syndrome (normal pressures are approximately 0 to 15 mm Hg). Comparing compartment pressures with systemic blood pressure offers a more accurate picture of limb perfusion, since hypotension can exacerbate ischemia in the case of tense compartments. Therefore, another criteria for defining compartment syndrome is a pressure rise in the extremity to within 30 mm Hg of the patient's diastolic blood pressure.

▲ *Dislocations of the shoulder* (glenohumeral joint) are common injuries that affect all age groups. They are caused by a direct blow to the shoulder or indirect trauma such as a fall onto an outstretched arm. The *most common direction for shoulder dislocations* is *anterior.* Less than 5% of dislocations are posterior, and these are commonly associated with epileptic seizures.

▲ In the classic clinical presentation of the more common posterior hip dislocation, the leg is adducted, internally rotated, and shortened. In the posterior dislocation, the femoral head lies superiorly out of the acetabulum. Prompt reduction within 24 hours (and preferably within 6 hours) is important to minimize the risk of AVN of the femoral head and permanent sciatic nerve injury.

SUGGESTED READINGS

Rockwood CA Jr, Wilkins DP, Beaty RW et al., eds. *Rockwood and green's fractures in adults,* 4th ed. Philadelphia: Lippincott–Raven, 1996.

Rockwood CA Jr, Wilkins KE, Beaty JH, eds. *Fractures in children,* 4th ed. Philadelphia: Lippincott–Raven, 1996.

Simon SR. *Orthopaedic basic science.* Rosemont: American Academy of Orthopaedic Surgeons, 1994.

Thyroid, Parathyroid, and Adrenal Glands

30

Giorgos C. Karakousis   **Rachel Rapaport Kelz**   **Douglas L. Fraker**

THYROID

Embryology

The thyroid gland, derived from endodermal cells, develops between the third and fourth weeks of gestation. The first endocrine organ to originate in the body, the thyroid initially develops between the first two pairs of pharyngeal pouches on the median surface of the primitive pharyngeal floor. Initially an endodermal thickening, the native thyroid develops from a diverticulum at the base of the tongue, the *foramen cecum*. The gland then descends along the thyroglossal duct anterior to the pharyngeal gut, hyoid bone, and laryngeal cartilages, to arrive at its final position at about the seventh gestational week ventral to the trachea. As the gland matures in its descent, two lateral lobes form, which are connected through a midline bridge of tissue, the isthmus. Thyroid follicles can be observed to form around this time. The parafollicular cells or C cells of the thyroid, which secrete calcitonin, an important hormone in calcium regulation, originate from neural crest cells, which migrate into the ultimobranchial body. It is these cells that give rise to medullary cancer of the thyroid. The ultimobranchial body develops from the ventral portion of the fourth pharyngeal pouch, and fuses posteromedially with each thyroid lobe. By the tenth week of gestation, the thyroid gland is competent in the concentration and organification of iodine.

An appreciation of the normal embryologic formation of the thyroid gland is helpful to the clinician in understanding variations in thyroid anatomy and anomalies in thyroid development. By approximately the eighth week of gestation, the thyroglossal duct has solidified and becomes obliterated. A remnant of the distal duct can be seen in approximately 50% of the population as a midline structure, known as the *pyramidal lobe*, extending superiorly from the isthmus of the gland. Failure of the duct to disappear completely can also result in the formation of thyroglossal duct cysts. Clinically, these are the most common manifestations of anomalous thyroid development and frequently present as midline neck masses in children. Although these cysts may develop anywhere along the course of the thyroglossal duct (Fig. 30-1), the majority

(50% to 75%) are found inferior to the hyoid bone. Ruptured cysts may result in thyroglossal duct sinuses or fistulas. Thyroglossal duct cysts may be the source of infection or even malignancy, usually in the form of papillary thyroid cancer, and their excision is, therefore, generally recommended. To prevent cyst recurrence, full excision of the cyst along the ductal tract to the base of the tongue, with excision of the central portion of the hyoid bone (Sistrunk procedure) is typically required.

Complete failure of the thyroid gland to descend results in a *lingual thyroid* at the base of the tongue, a condition more common in women and representing the most common site of ectopic thyroid tissue. Management of this is frequently medical with use of thyroid stimulating hormone (TSH), although surgery is indicated in instances of bleeding, dysphagia, or dyspnea. Incomplete descent of the thyroid can result in thyroid tissue superior or just inferior

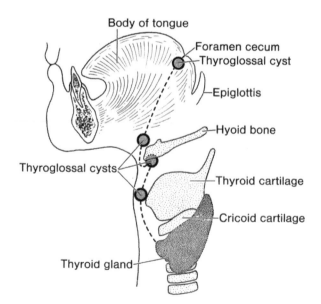

Figure 30-1 The location of thyroglossal cysts parallels embryologic thyroid descent. These cysts are most frequently found in the thyroid region and are always located close to the midline. (From Sadler TW. *Langman's medical embryology*, 5th ed. Baltimore: Williams & Wilkins, 1985:294, with permission.)

to the hyoid bone. Overdescent of the thyroid can result in ectopic thyroid tissue in the inferior neck or anterior mediastinum. Excision of ectopic thyroid tissue can result in hypothyroidism. Masses in the lateral neck very rarely correspond to aberrant thyroid tissue because the fusion of the lateral thyroid anlages with the median thyroid anlage during development and should, therefore, raise the suspicion for well-differentiated metastatic thyroid carcinoma.

Anatomy

The thyroid gland can vary considerably in size and weight, particularly as a function of the dietary iodine content, but in the United States, the gland weighs on average between 10 and 20 g. The largest of the endocrine organs, the thyroid gland is a bilobed structure (each lobe approximately 5 cm in greatest dimension) with an isthmus that connects the two lobes. The thyroid is encapsulated in a layer of connective tissue, the *fibrous capsule*, which is in turn invested in a false capsular layer arising from the sheaths of the deep cervical fascia, the pretracheal fascia. This fascial attachment between the gland and the upper two or three tracheal rings is also known as the *ligament of Berry*. As mentioned, a pyramidal lobe may exist in about one half of the population, extending superiorly from the isthmus. Anterior to the lobes of the gland reside the strap muscles, including the sternothyroid and more-ventral sternohyoid muscles. After division of the superficial platysma muscle and the formation of subplatysmal flaps superiorly and inferiorly, dissection is typically carried down through the midline to separate the strap muscles and expose the underlying gland. The thyroid itself wraps around the trachea and the esophagus, which define the posteromedial borders of the gland. Posterolateral to each lobe of the

thyroid lies the common carotid artery, the internal jugular vein and the vagus nerve. Lateral to these structures lies the omohyoid muscle. This muscle, along with the anterior strap muscles, is innervated by the ansa cervicalis, and can be divided or resected if necessary during thyroid surgery with little consequence. The parathyroid glands have a variable location but typically reside near the posterolateral surface of the thyroid lobes and can sometimes be embedded within the thyroid sheath. The recurrent laryngeal nerve typically lies posteromedial to each thyroid lobe, in the cleft between the trachea and esophagus, lying beneath or embedded in the ligament of Berry.

The thyroid is a highly vascularized gland, receiving its blood supply predominantly from the paired superior and inferior thyroid arteries. Figure 30-2 displays the thyroid from a posterior view and its relationship to some of the important neurovascular structures. The superior thyroid artery is the first branch of the external carotid artery and descends toward each superior pole of the gland, where it divides into anterior and posterior branches. These branches anastomose with branches of the inferior thyroid artery just deep to the pretracheal fascia. The inferior thyroid artery is a branch of the thyrocervical trunk and travels posterior to the carotid sheath before it reaches the posterior surface of the midportion of the gland. This artery is closely associated with the recurrent laryngeal nerve during part of its course, and great care must be taken in its dissection. The inferior thyroid artery also represents the principal blood supply to all four parathyroid glands in approximately 80% of people and, therefore, should be ligated close to the thyroid gland to prevent ischemia to the parathyroid glands. Present in only about 5% to 10% of the population, the *thyroid ima artery* can provide some of the blood supply to the thyroid. This artery can arise

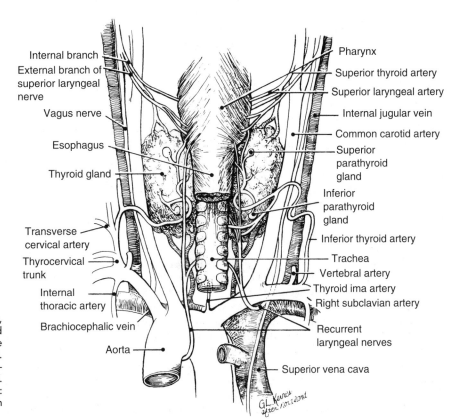

Figure 30-2 Posterior view of the larynx, trachea, thyroid, parathyroid glands, and the recurrent laryngeal nerve illustrates the anatomic relationship of these structures. (From Black S. Surgical anatomy of the thyroid gland. In: Nyhus LM, Baker RJ, eds. *Mastery of surgery*, 2nd ed. New York: Little, Brown and Company, 1992:193, with permission.)

Internal branch
External branch of superior laryngeal nerve
Vagus nerve
Esophagus
Thyroid gland
Transverse cervical artery
Thyrocervical trunk
Internal thoracic artery
Brachiocephalic vein
Aorta

Pharynx
Superior thyroid artery
Superior laryngeal artery
Internal jugular vein
Common carotid artery
Superior parathyroid gland
Inferior parathyroid gland
Inferior thyroid artery
Trachea
Vertebral artery
Thyroid ima artery
Right subclavian artery
Recurrent laryngeal nerves
Superior vena cava

from the brachiocephalic trunk or directly from the aortic arch and courses anterior to the trachea as it ascends toward the isthmus. A number of smaller unnamed arteries supplying the trachea and pharynx also contribute to the blood supply of the thyroid and can be the source of bleeding if not recognized.

The venous drainage of the thyroid gland is supplied primarily by three pairs of veins: the superior, middle, and inferior thyroid veins. The superior and middle veins drain the superior poles and lateral aspects of the thyroid, respectively, and drain into the internal jugular veins. The middle thyroid veins are frequently the first vessels ligated, as the thyroid lobes are retracted anteriorly and medially during thyroidectomy. The inferior thyroid veins arise from the inferior poles of the thyroid and course anterior to the trachea, draining into the brachiocephalic veins.

The thyroid gland has a rich and complex lymphatic drainage, an appreciation of which is important in the context of thyroid cancer. Interlobular subcapsular lymphatics connect the two lobes of the gland through the isthmus and provide some explanation to the relatively high frequency of multifocal tumors. Interlobular lymphatics communicate with intracapsular lymphatics, which in turn drain to various regional nodal beds including the pretracheal lymph nodes, paratracheal lymph nodes, and the tracheoesophageal lymph nodes along the recurrent laryngeal chain. These regional nodal basins are a frequent site of metastatic disease for thyroid cancer, particularly of the papillary and medullary type. The supra-isthmic pretracheal nodes that run alongside the pyramidal lobe are also known as the *Delphian nodes*. Cancers of the upper thyroid gland can also drain into the nodes anterior and lateral to the internal jugular vein, whereas those of the mid and lower thyroid can drain beyond the regional nodes to the middle and lower jugular veins and brachiocephalic veins in the anterior mediastinum.

The innervation to the thyroid gland is from postganglionic fibers that originate from the cervical sympathetic ganglia and travel alongside the arteries supplying the gland. A thorough appreciation of the anatomy of two other nerves, the recurrent laryngeal nerve (RLN) and the external branch of the superior laryngeal nerve, is essential for the safe performance of a thyroidectomy. The RLN innervates all the intrinsic laryngeal muscles except for the cricothyroid. Injury to one RLN results in hoarseness in voice and difficulty in phonation secondary to paralysis of the ipsilateral vocal cord. Bilateral RLN injury can result in abduction of both vocal cords with complete airway obstruction necessitating emergent intubation or tracheostomy. The recurrent laryngeal nerve can typically be found in the tracheoesophageal groove. Less commonly, it may lie lateral or even rarely (approximately 5% of cases) anterolateral to the trachea. On the right, the RLN branches from the vagus nerve and loops around the origin of the right subclavian artery to ascend in the tracheoesophageal groove. The left RLN branches from the vagus nerve and loops around the aortic arch near the ligamentum arteriosum. The RLN can pass anterior, posterior, or between branches of the inferior thyroid artery. Great care must, therefore, be taken in dissecting and ligating this artery to avoid nerve injury. The RLN in approximately one half of the cases is embedded within the ligament of Berry and should be carefully identified before division of this fascial attachment. A nonrecurrent laryngeal nerve on the right can be seen in approximately 1% of the population, often associated with an aberrant subclavian artery. A nonrecurrent left laryngeal nerve is much less common, often seen with a right-sided aortic arch.

The external branch of the superior laryngeal nerve travels in proximity to the superior thyroid artery for part of its course, and great care must, therefore, be taken when ligating this artery. Typically, the artery is ligated in proximity to the superior pole of the gland to avoid injuring the nerve. The external branch of the superior laryngeal nerve innervates the cricothyroid muscle, and damage to this nerve can result in a monotonous voice with inability to increase pitch.

Physiology

The thyroid gland synthesizes and secretes two groups of metabolically active hormones: *thyroid hormones* [triiodothyronine (T_3) or thyroxine (T_4)] and *calcitonin*, which is discussed in more depth in subsequent text along with calcium metabolism.

Thyroid hormone is synthesized at the apical border of the follicular cell and is important for normal growth and development. Essential for the formation of thyroid hormone is *iodine*, the daily requirement of which is approximately 100 to 200 μg. Ingested iodine is converted to iodide and absorbed in the upper gastrointestinal tract. It reaches the thyroid gland via the bloodstream, where it is trapped by the thyroid follicular cells through an adenosine active [adenosine triphosphate (ATP)-dependent] transmembrane transport mechanism. Approximately 90% of the total body iodine is stored in the thyroid gland in organic form.

In the follicular cell, iodide is rapidly oxidized to a free radical form by thyroid peroxidases. This activated form of iodine binds to tyrosine in the *thyroglobulin* molecule (a glycoprotein, which is the predominant component of colloid), forming either monoiodotyrosine (MIT) or diiodotyrosine (DIT). MIT and DIT molecules then combine with each other to form T_3 or T_4.

T_4 is the iodothyronine found in highest concentration in the plasma but is the less biologically active form of hormone. Because there is no conversion of T_3 to T_4 in the periphery, T_4 arises exclusively from secretion from the thyroid gland. Conversely, peripheral T_3 is largely derived by cleavage of the 5'-iodine from the outer ring of T_4 by 5'-monodeiodinase in the liver, muscle, and kidney (direct T_3 secretion from the thyroid gland normally accounts for approximately 20% of T_3 present in the periphery, although this may be increased in certain hyperthyroid conditions). If the 5'-iodine is removed from the inner ring of T_4, this results in *reverse* T_3, which is metabolically inactive. Only a small amount of thyroid hormone (less than 1%) circulates unbound in the plasma in a metabolically active form. Most thyroid hormones are bound to thyroxine-binding globulin (TBG), with the remainder bound to prealbumin and albumin. Pregnancy and oral contraceptives increase the levels of TBG and, therefore, the levels of total T_3 and T_4 but not the levels of free T_3 or free T_4. On the other hand, androgens and anabolic steroids decrease serum levels of TBG and total T_4. Free thyroid hormone levels remain within normal limits and these patients are euthyroid.

The cellular effects of thyroid hormone are dependent on binding of thyroid hormone to an intracellular receptor, which migrates to the nucleus to regulate transcription and translation. Excess thyroid hormone upregulates the activity and number of ATP-dependent sodium pumps, which increases the basal metabolic rate and oxygen consumption of most cells. Mitochondrial oxidative phosphorylation is upregulated as well, the combined effects leading to increased heat production. T_3 may increase or decrease fat formation depending on the caloric status of the individual. Overall, the lipolytic effect of thyroid hormones predominates, as evidenced by decreased triglyceride and cholesterol levels and elevated levels of free fatty acids and glycerol in hyperthyroid patients.

Thyroid hormone production is regulated by the hypothalamic-pituitary-thyroid axis. Thyroid stimulating hormone (TSH) is secreted by the anterior pituitary gland and leads to increased production of thyroid hormone (Fig. 30-3). TSH regulates iodine trapping by the thyroid gland and stimulates the synthesis of iodothyronines, acting via a second messenger cyclic adenosine monophosphate (cAMP) system. TSH also causes proteolytic separation of T_3 and T_4 from thyroglobulin. Under normal circumstances, thyroglobulin is too large to be transported across the follicular cell membrane. It therefore stimulates the release of thyroid hormones into the circulation. Secretion of TSH is stimulated by thyrotropin-releasing hormone (TRH), a tripeptide that is synthesized by the hypothalamus and carried to the anterior hypophyseal lobe via the hypophyseal portal system. Increased plasma levels of free T_3 or T_4 decrease secretion of TSH directly and also inhibit the action of TRH. Large amounts of ingested iodine can also decrease thyroid hormone production.

Thyroid hormone production can be inhibited in hyperthyroid states by the thionamide class of drugs, which include propylthiouracil (PTU), methimazole (Tapazole),

and carbimazole, which is converted *in vivo* to the active metabolite methimazole. These drugs act by inhibiting the oxidation of iodide to iodine, through inhibition of thyroid peroxidases, and thereby preventing the incorporation of iodine into the tyrosine residues of thyroglobulin. PTU also blocks the peripheral conversion of T_4 to T_3 by decreasing the activity of 5'-monodeiodinase. Methimazole can cross the placenta and its use is generally restricted in pregnant women. A serious but rare side effect of the thionamides is agranulocyotsis. Patients using these agents who have a rash, fever, or sore throat should be evaluated with a white blood cell count.

Thyroid Function Tests

Measurement of *serum TSH* levels has been recommended as the single most efficient test for assessing thyroid function. A normal TSH level in a healthy ambulatory patient essentially excludes the possibility of thyroid dysfunction. Unlike total T_4 or T_3 levels, which can vary depending upon the plasma levels of TBG, albumin, and prealbumin, serum TSH levels are independent of the concentration of carrier proteins in the circulation. Free (unbound) T_4 levels can be measured, but this test is generally more expensive, and TSH levels are thought to be the most sensitive indicator of thyroid dysfunction in mild or early stages of disease. TSH levels can also be used to titrate thyroid hormone–replacement therapy. Because the half-life of T_4 is approximately 1 week, at least 4 to 8 weeks must be allowed between alteration of oral T_4 dosage and serum TSH measurement. In addition, TSH measurement can be used to optimize hormone levels for suppressive therapy in benign and malignant disease. TSH levels are not reliable indicators of thyroid dysfunction in patients who have neuropsychiatric disorders or diseases of the pituitary gland (such as with pituitary adenomas).

Other tests of a patient's thyroid state include the T_3 resin uptake, the free T_4 index, and total T_3 and T_4 levels. The T_3 *resin uptake* indirectly measures the level of thyroid hormone and of carrier proteins by assessing the amount of radiolabeled T_3 absorbed on a resin after being mixed with the patient's serum. High T_3 resin uptake may result from decreased carrier protein levels or increased T_3 levels in the serum, or both. The *free T_4 index* can be estimated by calculating the ratio of the patient's T_3 resin uptake and a mean T_3 resin uptake of a control population and then multiplying this ratio by the total serum T_4 concentration. *Total* T_3 measures both free T_3 and protein-bound T_3. This test reflects peripheral metabolism of thyroid hormone, rather than thyroid function, and should be obtained in patients in whom hyperthyroidism is suspected but whose T_4 levels are normal.

The *TRH stimulation test* determines the functional status of the anterior pituitary TSH secretion, although its role has diminished owing to increased sensitivity of TSH assays. It is performed by checking a baseline TSH level, administering synthetic TRH intravenously, and measuring TSH after 30 and 60 minutes. Normally, a rise in TSH from the baseline is observed after TRH administration. Patients with hypothyroidism have a blunted response or no rise in TSH. This test can also determine whether TSH secretion is decreased in patients with pituitary tumors.

The *serum thyroglobulin* assay can be applied for the surveillance of patients treated for differentiated thyroid

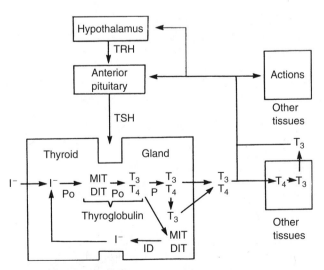

Figure 30-3 The regulation and feedback pathway of the hypothalamic-pituitary-thyroid system and intrathyroidal thyroid hormone synthesis and release. DIT, diiodotyrosine; I, inorganic iodide; ID, iodotyrosine deiodinase; MIT, monoiodotyrosine; P, proteolytic enzymes; Po, thyroid peroxidase; T_3, triiodothyronine; T_4, thyroxine; TRH, thyrotropin-releasing hormone; TSH, thyroid-stimulating hormone. (From Utiger RD. Disorders of the thyroid gland. In: Kelley WN, ed. *Textbook of internal medicine*, 3rd ed. Philadelphia: Lippincott-Raven, 1997:2205, with permission.)

carcinoma to detect recurrent or metastatic disease. This test is complementary with iodine-131 (^{131}I) scintiscanning for this purpose. In most cases, a high thyroglobulin level, even with negative thyroid scan results, indicates metastatic disease.

Thyroid Imaging

A functional assessment of the thyroid gland can be achieved through *radionuclide imaging*. This modality allows for localization of thyroid tissue, for detection of functional metastatic lesions from thyroid cancer, and for an estimation of the size of the thyroid gland. Several radioisotopes are in clinical use for scanning of the thyroid gland. Technetium-99m (^{99m}Tc) pertechnetate is the most commonly available radionuclide scan for the thyroid. In a normal thyroid gland, the tracer should be seen uniformly in both lobes on anteroposterior and oblique views. Any defect in tracer uptake represents a nonfunctional or hypofunctional ("cold") nodule, whereas areas of increased tracer uptake represent functional ("hot") nodules. Cold nodules are associated with an approximately 12% to 15% of thyroid cancer, although this incidence may be even higher in younger patients and patients with calcified nodules evident on ultrasonography. Nuclear medicine scans are less reliable at diagnosing hypofunctional than autonomously hyperfunctional nodules. An iodine-123 (^{123}I) scan permits assessment of the trapping and organification capacity of the thyroid gland. The study is more expensive and less convenient to obtain compared to ^{99m}Tc. ^{131}I results in much higher radiation exposure to the patient and the images obtained are inferior to those for ^{99m}Tc or ^{123}I. This is the study of choice, however, to assess the distribution of functioning metastatic thyroid tumors which concentrate radioiodine, and to determine the potential effectiveness of cancer therapy with ^{131}I.

Ultrasonography of the thyroid is a noninvasive and inexpensive technique for differentiating solid and cystic lesions. This technique is particularly useful for detection and fine needle aspiration (FNA) of nodules that can not be palpated and for recurrent tumor in the thyroid bed or regional lymph nodes. *High resolution ultrasound* can detect areas of calcification and *ultrasonography with power Doppler* can evaluate regions of increased vascularity. Both of these features may lead to a higher incidence of malignancy. *Computerized tomographic* (CT) scanning and *magnetic resonance imaging* (MRI) can detect subclinical cervical lymphadenopathy and substernal goiters. These studies can not differentiate benign from malignant thyroid lesions and, therefore, play only a limited role in the evaluation of thyroid nodules. These studies may be used preoperatively in patients with anaplastic tumors to assess involvement of adjacent structures, and also occasionally posttreatment in patients with thyroid carcinoma to follow for recurrent disease. They should be obtained after radionuclide imaging studies because the iodine in the contrast blocks the uptake of radionuclides by the thyroid for at least 6 weeks.

Indications for thyroid surgery include treatment of benign conditions of the thyroid (thyrotoxicosis and goiter), excision of thyroid nodules (benign and cancerous), and palliation of symptoms (e.g., airway obstruction from large metastatic thyroid tumor).

Benign Conditions of the Thyroid

Hyperthyroid Conditions

Hyperthyroidism results from excess plasma thyroid hormone. Three causes that more commonly require surgical intervention are Graves disease (or toxic diffuse goiter), which accounts for more than 80% of cases, toxic nodular goiter, and solitary toxic nodule. Other rarer causes of hyperthyroidism that may require surgery are postpartum thyroiditis, iodine-induced hyperthyroidism, iatrogenic hyperthyroidism, struma ovarii, TSH-secreting pituitary tumors, and functioning metastatic carcinoma.

Graves disease is an autoimmune disorder characterized by the presence of a family of antibodies directed against the receptor of TSH on the follicular cell, leading to increased thyroid hormone production and secretion. It is six to seven times more common in women than in men. Genetic factors seem to play an important role, and various human leukocyte antigen (HLA) alleles have been associated with the disease. Clinical manifestations of Graves disease are generally those associated with hyperthyroidism. These can include fatigue, heat intolerance, weight loss, diarrhea, hair loss, irritability, tremor, arrhythmias, hypertension, osteoporosis, amenorrhea, and sweating. In some instances, dermopathy (up to 15% of cases) such as with pretibial myxedema, and ophthalmopathy with periorbital edema, proptosis, and upper lid twitching can be seen. Clinically significant eye involvement is seen only in a minority of patients with the disease, and since it is thought to be autoimmune mediated, whether thyroid ablation decreases the risk of progressive eye disease in these patients is controversial. In older patients, the initial presentation may include atrial fibrillation or congestive heart failure. If left untreated, one third of patients with Graves disease will improve to euthyroid states or even develop hypothyroidism, one third will remain chronically hyperthyroid, and one third will progress to thyroid storm, a serious condition characterized by tachycardia, fever, and even death. On examination, the thyroid gland is typically diffusely enlarged, symmetric, and smooth. The presence of nodularity warrants investigation, as there is about a 5% incidence of carcinomas in patients with Graves disease. Abnormal laboratory test results include elevated levels of T_4 or T_3, or both, and a suppressed serum TSH level. Diffuse, increased uptake of ^{131}I within a symmetrically enlarged gland is diagnostic of Graves disease.

There are three principal treatment options for patients with Graves disease: medical therapy, radioactive iodine thyroid ablation, and surgical thyroid ablation. The optimum treatment for a given patient will be based on age, health, severity of disease, size of the gland, and patient preference. Medical therapy is aimed at reducing thyroid hormone levels, and antithyroid drugs are the first line of therapy in most patients with Graves disease. Thionamide therapy must be continued for a prolonged period to control thyroid levels, with a hope of spontaneous remission. However, recurrent disease has been reported in up to 90% of patients after medication was discontinued. The success rate of therapy correlates inversely with gland size: 75% for small-to-normal-sized glands and less than 30% for large goiters. Patients with a high T_3 level or high T_3–T_4 ratio have a lower success rate. The benefit of thionamide therapy is that there is no risk of hypothyroidism when the drug is dosed appropriately. β-Blocking agents such as propranolol may be used in an adjuvant setting, particularly when symptoms of tachycardia are present in the hyperthyroid state.

Radioactive iodine (^{131}I) therapy provides lasting results to most patients, with relatively few side effects, and is the definitive treatment used for most adult patients with Graves disease in the United States. The primary advantage of this method is that surgery, with any associated morbidities, is not required. The disadvantage is the high incidence of hypothyroidism, which is an expected complication following effective therapy that can be easily diagnosed and treated with lifelong hormone replacement therapy. In some instances, radioiodine can also induce transient hyperthyroidism. Most patients can be treated with a single dose of radioactive iodine; however, a small percentage of patients will require a second or third dose. Once an initial response occurs, there is a less than 5% risk of recurrence. In general, there is still reluctance to treat children with radioactive iodine. Women of childbearing age, patients with concomitant thyroid nodules, those with very large glands, and patients opposed to the radioactive drug are also typically not treated with ^{131}I therapy.

Because of the success of nonsurgical therapy, *operative intervention* is generally reserved for patients who are noncompliant with or intolerant to antithyroid drug therapy, those who are refractory to medical therapy, patients with contraindications to ^{131}I therapy (such as pregnancy), and those with concurrent nodular disease with FNA biopsy results warranting surgery. Patients who are younger than 20 years of age with large goiters are unlikely to become euthyroid with drug therapy and often require thyroidectomy. Preoperatively, an euthyroid state should be achieved medically to minimize the risk of intraoperative or postoperative thyroid storm. Administration of PTU in combination with propranolol is typically initiated 4 to 8 weeks before surgery and continued during and after the surgery. Lugol solution (a combination of potassium iodide and iodine) can be given to patients to decrease the vascularity of the gland and make it firmer and easier to resect. Some surgeons believe that propranolol results in the same decrease in gland vascularity, making the use of Lugol solution unnecessary. The extent of thyroidectomy for Graves disease remains controversial. Operative approaches include subtotal thyroidectomy, near-total thyroidectomy, and total thyroidectomy. The former two approaches do not completely eliminate the risk of postoperative thyrotoxicosis. With total thyroidectomy, there is virtually no incidence of persistent hyperthyroidism; however, patients must receive lifelong thyroid replacement. With increased extent of thyroid surgery, there is concern for increased risk of injury to the recurrent laryngeal nerve or of transient or permanent hypoparathyroidism.

Autonomously functioning thyroid nodules are presumably independent of TSH for function and growth. They appear hot on radionuclide studies and the function of surrounding thyroid tissue is frequently suppressed with nodules that are large in size. Most patients with autonomously functioning nodules are euthyroid, although untreated hot nodules may progress to toxicity. The risk of developing hyperthyroidism is increased with large nodules. Approximately 20% of autonomous hot nodules enlarge sufficiently to result in hyperthyroidism. The majority of these nodules enlarge, develop central necrosis, and become nonfunctioning. Patients can have either solitary or multiple autonomously functioning nodules. The peak incidence of *solitary toxic nodules* is during the fifth decade and is much more common in women. *Toxic multinodular goiter* (Plummer disease) accounts for approximately 20% of patients with hyperthyroidism and is usually seen in women older than 50 years of age. Patients usually have a nodular goiter for some time before they develop symptoms of hyperthyroidism. Patients with a nodular goiter and subclinical hyperthyroidism may develop thyrotoxicosis following iodine-containing medication or after receiving an iodine-containing contrast media.

Treatment of solitary functional nodules is influenced by size and functional degree of the nodule, as well as by the patient's age and overall health. Toxic nodules that usually exceed 3 cm in diameter should be treated surgically with a thyroid lobectomy. Alternatively, radioiodine can be used. However, a prolonged treatment regimen may be required, as the nodule persists in approximately 20% of patients. Many surgeons recommend prophylactic excision of nontoxic large solitary nodules with secretory function in the upper range of normal in elderly patients. The standard treatment for toxic multinodular goiter is antithyroid drug therapy, followed by thyroidectomy. ^{131}I may be used as an alternative in high-risk surgical patients who have no evidence of airway compression. Surgery typically entails subtotal thyroidectomy, with removal of all autonomous nodules. Conservation of adequate remnant thyroid tissue is usually not a great concern, as patients are typically placed on thyroid hormone for thyroid suppression.

Hypothyroidism: Hashimoto Thyroiditis

Hypothyroidism results from deficient levels of thyroid hormone and can be seen in a variety of conditions, including iatrogenic (as in postsurgical ablation of the thyroid or following irradiation therapy) autoimmune disorders, as in Hashimoto thyroididitis, and endemic goiters. Clinically, hypothyroid patients may present with fatigue, weight gain, brittle nails, coarse hair, constipation, and psychiatric disturbances, such as depression, irritability, or decreased memory function. Typically, laboratory evaluation reveals decreased thyroid hormone levels with an elevation in TSH levels.

Hashimoto thyroiditis (also known as "chronic lymphocytic thyroiditis" or "struma lymphomatosa") is the most common inflammatory condition of the thyroid and the most frequent cause of spontaneous hypothyroidism. It is an *autoimmune disease* with apparent genetic predisposition, which is characterized by high levels of circulating antibodies against the microsomal fraction of the thyroid cell, thyroglobulin, T_3, T_4, and the TSH receptor. It can occur in any age group but is most common in middle-aged women. Hashimoto disease occurs more commonly in geographic areas with a high dietary iodine intake and is more common in patients who received radiation during infancy or childhood. Hashimoto disease results in impaired thyroid hormone synthesis, owing to a lack of organification of trapped iodine. Low T_4 and T_3 levels cause increased TSH secretion, which can result in a goiter. During the acute phase of the disease, transient hyperthyroidism may be seen. Clinically, patients may present with the signs and symptoms of hypothyroidism. Pain is typically not a common manifestation of Hashimoto thyroiditis but may occur at the initial onset of disease. On palpation, the gland is usually firm and rubbery with a lobulated surface. An elevated antimicrosomal antibody titer, along with the clinical examination, is usually sufficient to make the diagnosis. Treatment with thyroid hormone usually causes regression of the goiter. In some patients, the gland continues to grow despite thyroid suppression therapy, and, in these patients, partial thyroidectomy is indicated, particularly if symptoms of compression occur. If a solitary nodule is found in a patient with Hashimoto disease, it should be fully evaluated. Any rapid enlargement of the thyroid gland in a patient with a history of Hashimoto thyroiditis needs to be evaluated because of the increased incidence of *lymphoma*, including the mucosa-associated lymphoid tissue (MALT) type. FNA and cytologic evaluation should be undertaken if lymphoma is suspected. There is also a slightly increased risk of papillary thyroid cancer with Hashimoto thyroiditis.

Other Thyroiditis Conditions

Thyroiditis is generally classified based on the rapidity of onset into acute, subacute, and chronic types. *Acute thyroiditis* is an infectious disorder, which is more common in women. Bacteria such as *Streptococcus pyogenes*, *Staphylococcus aureus*, and *Pneumococcus pneumoniae* account for most cases, which usually spread via the lymphatics from local infectious foci. The risk of developing acute thyroiditis is increased in patients with nodular goiters or anatomic defects such as thyroglossal ducts. This condition presents with acute onset of neck pain and fever. Patients are typically euthyroid. The treatment of acute thyroiditis usually entails appropriate intravenous antibiotics and surgical drainage if abscess is present.

Subacute thyroiditis (granulomatous thyroiditis or *de Quervain thyroiditis*) is a disease that occurs in middle-aged women within weeks of an upper respiratory or other viral infection. Symptoms may include weakness, depression, easy fatigability, anterior neck pain, or referred pain to the ear or angle of the jaw. On examination, the patient is usually febrile and the thyroid is firm and extremely tender to palpation. The thyroid is swollen unilaterally and the overlying skin is occasionally erythematous. Laboratory evaluation and biopsy are usually not necessary. Transient mild hyperthyroidism can be observed during the initial phase of the disease in about half of these patients. This is thought to be caused by a release of preformed thyroid hormone from the inflamed gland into the circulation. The later course of disease can be complicated by hypothyroidism and some patients may require hormone replacement therapy. The disease is typically self limited and usually resolves within a few months. The discomfort can be managed with salicylates, nonsteroidal anti-inflammatory drugs (NSAIDS), or corticosteroids. Surgical therapy may be indicated only rarely if the disease is persistent despite several months of steroid therapy.

Riedel struma or "invasive fibrous thyroiditis," refers to a very rare chronic inflammatory thyroid condition in which the thyroid tissue and frequently the adjacent strap muscles and carotid sheaths are replaced by dense fibrous tissue. Its pathogenesis is largely unknown, although the disease is often associated with other fibrotic processes such as retroperitoneal fibrosis, mediastinal fibrosis, periorbital fibrosis, and sclerosing cholangitis. Similar to other forms of thyroiditis, Riedel struma is most commonly seen in middle-aged women. Patients with Riedel struma are generally euthyroid, although hypothyroidism may be seen in up to 30% of patients. An open biopsy should be obtained to rule out the presence of thyroid carcinoma or lymphoma. The goiter may result in considerable localized pain and compression of adjacent tissues. Treatment with steroids may sometimes be beneficial. If airway compromise is present, surgical therapy with isthmectomy is indicated.

Thyroid Nodules

Clinically apparent thyroid nodules are present in approximately 5% of adults and are more prevalent in women than in men. Both benign and malignant thyroid nodules have been associated with radiation exposure, occurring in some reports in up to one third of exposed individuals. The incidence of malignancy is approximately 10% in patients with palpable solitary thyroid nodules who have no history of neck irradiation. This incidence is increased several-fold in patients with prior radiation exposure (some studies report up to 50% incidence of cancer in thyroid nodules from this patient population). Men and patients at the extremes of age are also at a higher risk for malignancy. A solitary nodule is more worrisome than a thyroid with multiple nodules. However, any nodule that increases in size in the setting of a multinodular goiter needs to be evaluated to exclude carcinoma. The appearance of a new nodule, a rapid increase in the size of an existing nodule, and a painful nodule are worrisome for malignancy. New onset of hoarseness or the development of a Horner syndrome may indicate local invasion. On physical examination, the size, mobility, firmness, adherence to adjacent structures, and presence of adenopathy are all clues to the presence of carcinoma.

Very high serum levels of thyroglobulin in a patient with a small thyroid nodule may be suggestive of metastatic thyroid carcinoma. However, thyroid function tests generally don't play a role in differentiating benign from malignant nodules. Inhibition of TSH production with administration of thyroid hormone is based on the principle that benign lesions are less autonomous than malignant tumors and will therefore decrease in size over a period of several months of TSH suppression. However, because of issues such as patient compliance and lack of rigorously defined size criteria, this modality plays only a limited role in the diagnostic workup of thyroid nodules. Most benign and malignant thyroid nodules are hypofunctional when compared to normal functioning thyroid tissue, and therefore, the finding of a cold nodule on radionuclide scanning with ^{123}I or ^{99m}Tc is fairly nonspecific. Ultrasonography is useful for determining the size of nodules, number of nodules, and character of nodules (solid versus cystic), as well as to assist in FNA of nodules. Thyroid nodules that are greater than 3 cm in diameter, cystic/solid lesions, and cystic lesions that recur after three aspirations are more likely to be malignant and, therefore, should be biopsied.

FNA biopsy is safe, minimally invasive, inexpensive, and accurate in the diagnosis of thyroid nodules. It can be performed by direct palpation or with ultrasonographic guidance for nonpalpable nodules. It should be used to evaluate any new palpable thyroid nodule or any lesion greater than 1.5 cm identified by imaging. The four diagnostic categories of FNA are the following: (i) benign or negative, (ii) suspicious or indeterminate, (iii) malignant, and (iv) insufficient sample.

One of the main limitations of FNA is its ability to distinguish between benign follicular cell adenomas and follicular cell carcinomas. FNA biopsies of follicular neoplasms or those with extensive Hürthle cell changes are characterized as suspicious or indeterminate. Because 20% to 25% of these nodules are found to be malignant, they must be surgically resected. The false-negative rate of nodules with benign FNA biopsy results is less than 5%, and these patients can generally be followed medically. Nodules can be followed by physical examination or by ultrasonography, which is more precise at delineating changes in size. Any nodule with clinically worrisome features (fixed, firm, and painful) should be resected despite "negative" FNA biopsy results.

Thyroid Carcinoma

The reported incidence of thyroid carcinoma varies significantly worldwide by geography (particularly elevated in Iceland and Hawaii) and in the United States is approximately 10 per 100,000 (less than 1% of all malignancies). The actual incidence though may be significantly higher (approximately 2.5% or higher) according to results from autopsy series. The mortality rate is approximately 0.6 per 100,000, indicating that most thyroid cancers carry a favorable prognosis. Thyroid cancers are more common in females than in males (approximately 3:1 ratio), although the mortality ratio is significantly less than the incidence ratio (1.2-2:1, female to male). The incidence of thyroid cancer increases with age, and various environmental and genetic influences seem to be involved in its pathogenesis depending upon type, as discussed in subsequent text. Thyroid malignancies are derived from either thyroid follicular cells (as in *papillary, follicular, and anaplastic carcinomas*) or parafollicular cells (*medullary carcinoma*). Thyroid cancers can be further classified into those that are well-differentiated, those with intermediate differentiation, and those that are undifferentiated, depending upon their clinical aggressiveness.

Well-Differentiated Thyroid Carcinoma (Papillary and Follicular Carcinoma)

Well-differentiated thyroid cancers include *papillary* and *follicular thyroid carcinomas.* Thyroid tumors with papillary elements, even if follicular elements are present, are generally classified as follicular variant of papillary carcinomas, because pure papillary and mixed papillary-follicular have similar biology. Papillary carcinoma comprises approximately 80% to 90% of thyroid cancer in countries with sufficient dietary iodine intake. The majority of papillary carcinomas are intrathyroidal and are partially encapsulated. Cystic changes in these tumors are not uncommon. Histologically, they have distinctive nuclear features including large size, pale-staining appearance, intranuclear inclusion bodies, and deep "grooving." Diagnostic for papillary carcinoma are "psammoma bodies," which are laminated calcified bodies, found in approximately one half of the histologic specimens of this tumor type. Variants of papillary cancer include the follicular, the tall cell variant, the columnar variant, and the diffuse sclerosis variant.

Papillary carcinomas frequently spread through lymphatics to regional lymph nodes (approximately 30% to 40% of cases at presentation). The sclerosis variant has a 100% incidence of lymph node metastasis at the time of diagnosis.

Follicular carcinomas are defined as tumors with only follicular elements. Pure follicular thyroid carcinomas are rare, making up only 5% to 10% of thyroid malignancies in nonendemic goiter areas of the world. Follicular thyroid carcinomas are usually unifocal and thickly encapsulated, showing invasion into or through the capsule, frequently with vascular invasion. Lymph node involvement by follicular carcinoma is rare (1% to 10%).

Risk factors for well-differentiated carcinoma include both environmental and genetic influences. *Radiation exposure* to the thyroid has been shown to increase the incidence of benign thyroid nodules and of well-differentiated thyroid carcinoma, particularly of the papillary type. The latency period following exposure is at least 3 to 5 years. Previous radiation exposure accounts, however, for only less than 10% of cases in the United States. Intrachromosomal translocations of the *RET protooncogene* (a receptor tyrosine kinase the mutations of which are associated with familial medullary thyroid carcinoma syndromes) have been identified in some studies in more than 50% of papillary thyroid cancers. Other genetic mutations, including in the *Trk* and *BRAF* signaling molecules, in *APC* of familial colonic polyposis syndromes, and in *N-ras*, have been implicated in the development of papillary thyroid cancer. Recently, the fusion *PAX8/PPAR gamma1* oncogene has been implicated with follicular carcinoma, although it has been found to be present in some follicular adenomas as well. Well-differentiated cancers do not show a strong familial association and many questions still remain about the pathogenesis of most of these thyroid cancers.

Well-differentiated thyroid carcinoma typically presents as an asymptomatic thyroid nodule. Less commonly, patients present with palpable cervical lymphadenopathy without an identifiable thyroid primary. Other symptoms may include hoarseness, dyspnea, and dysphagia, reflecting local invasion of the recurrent laryngeal nerve, the trachea, and the esophagus, respectively. Most of these neoplasms are nonfunctional and patients with well-differentiated thyroid carcinoma are typically euthyroid.

Papillary and follicular cancers tend to be relatively indolent neoplasms with a favorable long-term survival rate. In contrast to other solid neoplasms, the presence of lymph node metastases has at best a very marginal influence on overall survival in most series. The overall 10-year survival rate for papillary cancer ranges from 74% to 93%, compared to 43% to 94% for follicular cancer. One of the most important prognostic factors for well-differentiated thyroid cancer is age at diagnosis based on many series, with the presence of distant metastases and size also being important predictors of outcome. Low-risk age categories have been defined as men younger than 40 years of age and women younger than 50 years of age. Recurrent malignant disease demonstrates a bimodal distribution with age, with younger patients exhibiting a more favorable outcome. The Lahey Clinic developed the AMES (age, metastases, extent of primary cancer, and tumor size) criteria to place patients into different risk groups with different prognoses. With this system, low-risk patients have a long-term overall survival of 98%, compared with 54% for high-risk patients. The Mayo Clinic group devised a similar scoring system called the AGES (age, grade of tumor, extent of tumor, size of tumor) system. A recent modification of this system is MACIS (metastasis, age, completeness of resection, invasion, and size). The survival rates for patients based on these prognostic factors are shown in Table 30-1. The TNM staging classification has also been used increasingly for thyroid cancers; for the well-differentiated carcinomas, two separate classifications exist based on age (for patients younger than 45 years, and for those older than 45 years).

The major decisions to be made in the surgical management of thyroid nodules and thyroid cancers are which patients should undergo surgery and how extensive a resection should be performed. Procedures for a thyroid neoplasm include a thyroid lobectomy, subtotal thyroidectomy, near-total thyroidectomy, and total thyroidectomy. A *subtotal thyroidectomy* leaves a rim of 2 to 4 g of tissue in the region of the ligament of Berry of the contralateral lobe. This decreases the risk of injury to the recurrent laryngeal nerve in that area and helps preserve the blood supply to the upper parathyroid gland on that side. A *near-total thyroidectomy* typically leaves less than 1 g of tissue adjacent to the ligament of Berry. More recently, video-assisted surgery has been employed in some centers for the thyroid surgical procedures discussed. Advocates of this approach point to smaller incisions or less conspicuous and more cosmetically favorable incisions in the lateral neck, the axilla, or below the clavicle. Opponents argue a potentially higher morbidity with this method. Video-assisted thyroidectomy requires surgeons highly skilled in endoscopy, and the true benefit of and the optimal patient population for this approach await large controlled studies.

The extent of resection for well-differentiated thyroid malignancies has been a significant point of controversy among endocrine surgeons. Some surgeons feel that for

patients with unilateral well-differentiated thyroid carcinoma defined as low-risk by AGES or AMES criteria, an ipsilateral thyroidectomy and isthmectomy with careful medical surveillance of the contralateral lobe is adequate therapy. Many surgeons generally agree with this approach for patients with papillary tumors that are smaller than 1 cm and follicular cancers with minimal capsular invasion. More controversial is the management of younger patients (those 40 years or younger) with thyroid lesions smaller than 1 to 2 cm because of the favorable prognosis of this group. Proponents of the less extensive unilateral resections for low risk well-differentiated thyroid carcinoma argue that this approach offers a lower risk of postoperative complications, such as permanent hypoparathyroidism or injury to the recurrent laryngeal nerve. However, patients undergoing more radical procedures have lower recurrence rates. Indications for total thyroidectomy for well-differentiated thyroid carcinoma include a history of prior head or neck irradiation or invasion of the neoplasm through the thyroid capsule. Many experienced endocrine surgeons generally recommend thyroidectomy for all patients with a papillary carcinoma of larger than 1.5 cm in diameter, and certainly among older patients (older than 40 years). Proponents of total thyroidectomy for all well-differentiated thyroid tumors feel that this more radical approach is indicated because of the high incidence of occult tumors in the contralateral lobe (multifocality of tumors can be seen in up to 30% to 80% of cases), decreased survival rates with recurrent disease, and more accurate surveillance for tumor persistence and recurrence with serum thyroglobulin levels. Unfortunately, most of the data comparing the extent of surgery for well-differentiated thyroid carcinomas is based on retrospective studies, and large controlled prospective studies are lacking. Patients with FNA cytology that is read as suspicious are recommended to undergo surgical resection owing to an incidence of follicular carcinoma of 20% to 25%. These patients typically undergo thyroid lobectomy on the side of the nodule with further management based on the final pathology report. If the lesion is a follicular carcinoma with characteristics that place the patient at high risk, then a completion total or subtotal thyroidectomy should be performed on reoperation.

Controversy exists over the surgical management of *cervical lymph node metastases from well-differentiated thyroid carcinoma*. Some surgeons perform selective resection for only grossly involved nodes, pointing to retrospective studies, which do not demonstrate any survival difference between this approach and more radical neck dissections. Others advocate prophylactic modified radical neck dissections in an attempt to remove asymptomatic metastatic disease. Because lymph node involvement is a marker for more aggressive papillary carcinoma, a formal neck dissection is generally recommended in patients with clinically evident adenopathy. If carcinoma is identified by frozen section of suspected lymph nodes at the time of thyroidectomy, then a complete dissection of lymph nodes in the central neck and the paratracheal region is indicated.

Radioiodine therapy with ^{131}I ablation is typically used as adjuvant therapy after surgical resection for well-differentiated carcinomas and is dependent on residual thyroid tissue concentrating iodine under the stimulation of elevated TSH levels. By uptake in and ablation of residual functional thyroid tissue, ^{131}I therapy plays a role in detecting metastatic

TABLE 30-1

SURVIVAL RATES IN PATIENTS WITH WELL-DIFFERENTIATED THYROID CANCER BASED ON VARIOUS PROGNOSTIC CLASSIFICATION SCHEMES

AMES Risk Group	Low	High
Overall survival rate	98%	54%
Disease-free survival rate	95%	45%

DAMES Risk Group	Low	Intermediate	High	
Disease-free survival rate	92%	45%	0%	
AGES PS	<4	4–5	5–6	>6
20-Year survival rate	99%	80%	33%	13%
MACIS PS	<6	6–7	7–8	>8
20-Year survival rate	99%	89%	56%	24%

AMES, age, metastases, extent of primary cancer, tumor size; DAMES, AMES system modified by DNA content; AGES, age, tumor grade, tumor extent, tumor size; PS, prognostic score; MACIS, metastasis, age, completeness of resection, invasion, size.

disease, in treating residual thyroid cancer, and in screening patients postoperatively for persistent or recurrent disease (^{131}I ablates thyroglobulin production by any remnants of normal thyroid, allowing this marker to be used to follow patients postoperatively). Patients with lymph node metastases should also be given ^{131}I ablation to decrease the risk of recurrence. The true efficacy of postoperative radioiodine therapy is less clear. Many studies have shown that ^{131}I ablation decreases cancer death, tumor recurrence, and the incidence of distant metastases, whereas other studies have failed to demonstrate an effect. ^{131}I ablation is generally performed at 6 weeks after near-total or total thyroidectomy. Thyroid hormone replacement is discontinued for 4 to 6 weeks and a low iodine diet is initiated 1 to 2 weeks before scanning, to optimize uptake and retention of ^{131}I by any residual normal and cancerous thyroid tissue. A post-therapy whole-body scan is obtained at 5 to 7 days to determine the extent of disease, with follow-up scanning at 6- to 12-month intervals. Radioiodine treatment is typically continued until there is no further ^{131}I uptake or serum thyroglobulin is in the athyrotic range, unless significant complications of ^{131}I arise. Serious side effects of ^{131}I are relatively uncommon, but sialadenitis, nausea, taste dysfunction, odynophagia, reversible impairment in spermatogenesis, temporary bone marrow suppression, and, rarely, vocal cord paralysis have been reported among some patients. Significantly elevated cumulative doses of ^{131}I therapy have been associated with a small increase in the incidence of leukemias, salivary carcinoma, and bladder carcinoma.

Distant metastases from well-differentiated thyroid carcinoma can be seen in approximately 10% to 15% of patients and portend a worse prognosis. For papillary carcinomas, they can be seen frequently in the form of pulmonary metastases. Follicular carcinomas more frequently metastasize to distant sites, including lung and bone. Less commonly, cerebral metastases are seen with differentiated thyroid cancer.

Intermediate Differentiation Thyroid Carcinomas (Hürthle Cell, Insular, and Medullary)

The *intermediate differentiation tumors* of the thyroid include Hürthle cell carcinoma, insular carcinoma, and medullary thyroid carcinoma. *Hürthle cell tumors* account for less than 5% of all thyroid carcinomas. They are considered to be variants of follicular tumors and cannot be classified as benign or malignant based on FNA. Compared to follicular tumors, Hürthle cell tumors are more often bilateral and multifocal and can spread to regional lymph nodes to a greater extent than can follicular lesions but much less than papillary carcinomas. Hürthle cell tumors do not take up radioiodine. Similar to the management of follicular tumors, patients who are found to have Hürthle cell neoplasm by FNA should undergo an ipsilateral lobectomy and isthmectomy. In addition, these patients should undergo an ipsilateral central neck dissection. Total completion thyroidectomy is indicated if the final pathology reveals a carcinoma. *Insular carcinomas* are tumors that histologically resemble pancreatic islets and contain small follicles that stain positively for thyroglobulin. Insular carcinomas invade lymphatics and veins and are commonly associated with nodal and distant metastases. In some series, the incidence of distant metastases with insular carcinomas is reported to be as high as 67%. Necrosis is common in the tumor and the only viable tumor may be near blood vessels. Treatment of insular carcinoma consists of surgical resection and radioiodine ablation.

Medullary thyroid cancer (MTC) accounts for 5% to 10% of thyroid cancers and arises from the calcitonin-producing parafollicular or C cells. C cells are derived from neural crest cells and have the typical characteristics of APUD cells (amine precursor uptake and decarboxylation) with high chromogranins and neuron-specific enolase content, as well as the ability to secrete various peptides. Unlike with papillary carcinoma, radiation exposure is not associated with the development of MTC. MTC is sporadic or nonfamilial in 60% to 70% of cases and is associated with a familial syndrome in the remainder of the cases [either multiple endocrine neoplasia (MEN) 2A or 2B or non-MEN familial MTC]. Sporadic tumors are usually unilateral and involve regional lymph nodes, whereas familial tumors are generally multifocal. Patients with non-MEN familial MTC have the least aggressive form of this tumor and MEN 2B is associated with the most aggressive variant. The characteristics of sporadic and familial forms of MTC are shown in Table 30-2. Immunostaining for calcitonin is typically required to make the diagnosis because of the various possible histologic patterns. Immunostaining also aids in prognosis, as tumors with less than 25% of cells staining for calcitonin typically metastasize early. MTC can secrete various peptide hormones including adrenocorticotropic hormone (ACTH) and serotonin and can also produce mucin or melanin.

It is important that family members of patients with medullary carcinoma (particularly for multifocal tumors) are screened early for disease. Defects in the *RET* protooncogene on chromosome 10 have been found to be responsible for MEN and non-MEN familial forms of MTC. Gene carriers can be identified by a blood test before development of overt disease and are candidates for prophylactic surgery at a young age. Patients with medullary carcinoma should also be evaluated for pheochromocytomas because of the relatively high concurrent incidence of these tumors.

Patients with sporadic MTC typically present with a mass in the thyroid. Some patients present with advanced cases with local invasion and symptoms of hoarseness, dysphagia, or cough. Those with extremely high levels of calcitonin may have severe secretory diarrhea. The basal and stimulated *serum calcitonin test* is an important tool for confirming the diagnosis of MTC. The test involves administering calcium gluconate and measuring serum calcitonin before and at multiple times after stimulation. An increase to more than 1,000 pg per mL (normal serum level 250 to 300 pg per mL) is distinctly abnormal and pathognomonic for MTC. Elevation to between 300 and 1,000 pg per mL is borderline and warrants close observation with sequential retesting. Measurement of serum calcitonin levels can been useful in the screening of MTC (though this is more commonly done now through genetic testing) and for following patients for recurrent disease post-treatment. Because MTC does not concentrate iodine, ^{131}I scans are of no use in MTC. Thallium and technetium scans have not proved to be beneficial. ^{131}I metaiodobenzylguanidine scans, which are useful in identifying pheochromocytomas and neuroblastomas, also fail to identify a large proportion of MTCs. A strategy to regionally localize occult lesions is selected venous sampling for serum calcitonin after stimulation with calcium.

TABLE 30-2

CHARACTERISTICS OF SPORADIC AND VARIOUS FAMILIAL FORMS OF MEDULLARY THYROID

| | Sporadic | Non-MEN | Familial | |
			MEN 2A	MEN 2B
Age at diagnosis (y)	42–45	43–45	24–27[a]	15–20
Gender	M = F	M = F	M = F	M = F
Associated diseases	None	None	(1) Pheochromocytoma (2) Hyperparathyroidism	(1) Pheochromocytoma (2) Marfanoid body habitus (3) Oral & eye mucosal neuromas (4) Gastrointestinal ganglioneuromas
Disease extent	Unilateral	Bilateral	Bilateral	Bilateral
Lymph nodes involved at diagnosis	40%–50%	10%–20%	14%	38%
Distant metastases at diagnosis	12%	0%	0%–3%	20%
Cured of MTC	14%–30%	70%–80%	56%–100%	0%
Dead due to MTC	30%	0%	0%–17%	50%
Mutations in RET on chromosome 10	MET 918 → Thr (33%) Glu 768 → Asp	Mutations in cysteines in extracellular domain near membrane	Mutations in cysteines in extracellular domain near membrane	MET 918 → Thr

MTC, medullary thyroid cancer; MEN, multiple endocrine neoplasia; Thr, thyroid.
[a]The age at diagnosis at centers doing genetic screening can be at or even before birth. Numbers reported reflect series based on biochemical screening of families at risk.

Surgical therapy is the only effective therapy for MTC. Chemotherapy and external beam radiation are of no benefit. Patients who present with sporadic MTC should undergo total thyroidectomy and central node dissection. If there is evidence of metastatic spread in the central neck nodes, a formal modified radical neck dissection is performed. Total thyroidectomy and central neck dissection should be performed for all cases of familial MTC. There is a direct correlation between lesion size and incidence of nodal metastases, with lesions greater than 2 cm having a 60% incidence of lymph node metastases. Therefore, some surgeons advocate a modified radical neck dissection for all lesions greater than 2 cm. The incidence of distant metastases at the time of diagnosis is the lowest for familial non-MEN MTC and MEN 2A (less than 5%) and the highest for MEN 2B (20%). Recent series show a 5-year survival rate between 80% and 90% and a 10-year survival rate between 70% and 80% for all MTCs. Persistently elevated calcitonin levels following resection are managed by close follow-up and reoperation only when clinically apparent disease is present.

Undifferentiated Thyroid Carcinoma (Anaplastic)

Anaplastic thyroid cancer (ATC) accounts for 1% to 2% of thyroid cancers and is one of the most aggressive and lethal human malignancies. A recent decline in incidence likely reflects reclassification of some of these tumors as lymphomas. The median survival time is 4 to 5 months, with a 5-year survival rate of approximately 5%. Patients who are diagnosed with ATC are typically in their seventh decade of life, and ATC has been associated with iodine deficiency in regions with endemic goiter. There is an equal gender distribution in patients with ATC. Patients with ATC commonly have a prior or concurrent diagnosis of well-differentiated thyroid cancer or benign thyroid disease, and there is evidence that ATC can arise from the dedifferentiation of well-differentiated thyroid cancer. Most patients with ATC have not had prior radiation. Patients with ATC typically present with a palpable mass that is growing, or with symptoms of dyspnea or hoarseness in voice. Synchronous pulmonary metastases are observed in up to 50% of patients at the time of diagnosis. Most patients with ATC die from aggressive local-regional disease, mostly from upper airway obstruction. Therefore, aggressive local therapy is indicated whenever possible. Aggressive resection should include removal of the strap muscles and any other structures with local invasion and tracheostomy if needed. Anaplastic carcinoma cells do not concentrate iodine and there is, therefore, no role for ^{131}I imaging or therapy in patients with ATC. External beam radiation has been used with limited success for recurrent ATC. Doxorubicin-based chemotherapy has also been shown to prolong survival.

Thyroid Lymphoma and Metastatic Disease to the Thyroid

Lymphoma of the thyroid constitutes approximately 4% of thyroid cancers and represents only 1% of all lymphomas and 2% of extranodal non-Hodgkin lymphoma cases. The most common histologic types include the small-cell non-cleaved type and the large cell non-cleaved follicular type. Thyroid lymphoma is usually seen in older women with Hashimoto thyroiditis. Patients virtually never have hyperthyroidism but frequently have hypothyroidism. Treatment of lymphoma of the thyroid is radiation therapy and chemotherapy, with typically no role for surgical resection. Clinically apparent metastases to the thyroid from other sites account for less than 1% of all thyroid malignancies, although autopsy studies identify metastases to the thyroid in 2% to 26% of people. In these series, the most predominant primary sites are breast, lung, melanoma, renal cell carcinoma, and gastrointestinal tract malignancies. In patients with premortem detection of metastasis to the thyroid, renal cell carcinoma accounts for most of the cases. Surgery tends to play a minimal role in the management of these patients, typically limited to palliation of symptoms.

PARATHYROID GLANDS

Embryology and Anatomy

The parathyroids are small yellowish brown usually flat and ovoid glands, typically 5 to 7 mm in greatest dimension and weighing on average 30 to 50 mg. Usually, there are four glands, two *superior* and two *inferior*, although supernumerary glands can be seen in about 5% to 15% of the population (often within the thymus). The location of the glands, particularly of the inferior parathyroids, can vary considerably and is better understood through an appreciation of their embryologic development. The parathyroid glands develop around the fifth to sixth weeks of gestation (Fig. 30-4). The superior glands are derived from the fourth pharyngeal pouch along with the lateral thyroid lobes. They migrate a shorter distance and, therefore, their final resting location is usually less variable, typically on the extracapsular posteromedial surface of the thyroid lobes just below the level of the cricoid cartilage. The inferior glands originate from the third pharyngeal pouch along with the thymus. Although they often can be found near the inferior poles of the thyroid, their location can vary depending on the extent of their migration from the pharynx to the mediastinum. The parathyroid glands are typically located deep to the pretracheal fascia just outside the thyroid capsule, although they can sometimes be intracapsular, embedded within the thyroid gland itself.

The blood supply to all the parathyroid glands is principally from the inferior thyroid artery, although they can sometimes be supplied in part from the superior thyroid artery or the *thyroid ima*. The venous and lymphatic drainage of the glands is typically shared with that of the thyroid gland and thymus. The innervation to the parathyroid glands is from cervical sympathetic ganglia.

Physiology

The parathyroid gland's primary physiologic role is the regulation of calcium and phosphate metabolism. Calcium is a critical ion for cellular homeostasis, participating in enzymatic reactions and mediating hormone metabolism. It is the major cation in bone and teeth, representing approximately 2% of the average body weight. The normal range of serum calcium is 9 to 10.5 mg per dL. About half of the total serum calcium is in an ionized, biologically active form. Forty percent is bound to serum protein (albumin), and the remaining 10% is complexed with citrate. Calcium is absorbed in its inorganic form from the duodenum and proximal jejunum, with absorption regulated according to body calcium status. Calcium reabsorption from the kidney under normal conditions is approximately 99% of the filtered load.

Phosphate is also an important component of many biologic systems, including the pathways of glycolysis. It is the functional group of ATP, and it is the major anion in crystalline bone. The normal range of serum phosphate ranges from 2.5 to 4.3 mg per dL, and the level varies inversely with that of the serum calcium. Unlike that of calcium, phosphate absorption from the diet is relatively constant, and excretion provides the major mechanism for the regulation of phosphate balance.

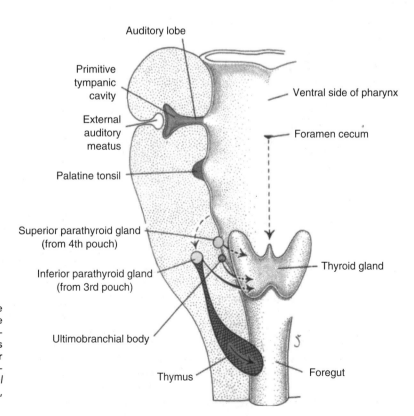

Figure 30-4 Schematic representation of the migration of the parathyroid glands. Although the inferior parathyroid gland arises from the third pharyngeal pouch, it migrates along with the thymus and ends its descent inferior to the superior parathyroid gland, which arises from the fourth pharyngeal pouch. (From Sadler TW. *Langman's medical embryology,* 5th ed. Baltimore: Williams & Wilkins, 1985:289, with permission.)

The primary hormonal regulators of calcium and phosphate homeostasis are parathyroid hormone (PTH), vitamin D, and calcitonin. Regulation depends on three organ systems: the gastrointestinal tract, the skeletal system, and the renal system.

PTH appears to be the most important regulator of calcium and phosphate metabolism. PTH is synthesized by the *chief cells* of the parathyroids as a precursor pre-proparathyroid hormone, which is then cleaved to form pre-PTH and ultimately PTH. Secretion of PTH is regulated by plasma calcium levels through a negative feedback mechanism. Secreted PTH is then cleaved by the Kupffer cells of the liver into *N-* and *C-*terminal fragments. The *N-*terminus contains most of the biologic activity. In target tissues, PTH binds to membrane receptors, activating the cyclic AMP pathway to regulate intracellular enzymes. In bone, PTH stimulates osteoclasts and inhibits osteoblasts, thereby stimulating bone resorption with the release of calcium and phosphate. In the kidney, PTH increases the reabsorption of extracellular calcium throughout the nephron, but particularly in the distal nephron. PTH also increases renal phosphate excretion. PTH acts indirectly on the gastrointestinal tract, by stimulating the hydroxylation of 25-hydroxy vitamin D to 1,25-dihydroxy vitamin D in the kidney.

Vitamin D has two major sites of action. It increases intestinal absorption of calcium and phosphate, and it promotes mineralization and enhances PTH-mediated mobilization of calcium and phosphate from bone. Vitamin D_3 is produced normally by the action of sunlight on 7-dehydrocholesterol in the skin. It then binds to plasma proteins and is transported to the liver where 25-hydroxylation occurs. In turn, 25-hydroxy vitamin D_3 undergoes a second hydroxylation in the renal tubular epithelial cell to form the active calcitriol or 1,25-dihydroxy vitamin D_3.

Calcitonin is a 32-amino-acid peptide, which is secreted in its pro-protein form by the parafollicular or C cells of the thyroid gland. Increased serum calcium levels stimulate secretion of calcitonin, which inhibits bone resorption and increases urinary calcium and phosphate excretion, both of which are mediated through cyclic AMP pathways. Although G-protein-coupled calcitonin receptors are located throughout the body, the absence of calcitonin (as can be seen in total thyroidectomy), or its overexpression (as in medullary thyroid carcinoma), do not result in significant changes in serum calcium levels and have little significant clinical impact.

Pathophysiology: Hyperparathyroidism

Clinical Presentation

Increased secretion of parathyroid hormone can be seen with *primary, secondary,* or *tertiary hyperparathyroidism. Primary hyperparathyroidism* is the most common cause of hypercalcemia in nonhospitalized patients, occurring in more than one half of the patients in this group (causes of hypercalcemia are listed in Table 30-3). The incidence has risen since the 1970s with the advent of the blood chemistry multichannel autoanalyzer. In familial disease, such as MEN-1 or MEN 2A, primary hyperparathyroidism is largely caused by multiglandular disease with multiple adenomas in all four parathyroids. In nonfamilial patients,

TABLE 30-3

CAUSES OF HYPERCALCEMIA

- **Hyperparathyroidism.** (Discussed in detail in the text.) Typically patients have elevated serum calcium and parathyroid hormone (PTH) levels, normal or elevated urine calcium excretion, and low or normal plasma concentration of phosphate.
- **Hypercalcemia of malignancy.** Patients with solid tumors often have elevated serum calcium levels, including those with lung carcinoma, breast carcinoma, and squamous cell carcinoma of the head and neck. The hypercalcemia is thought to be caused by PTH related protein secreted by the tumor. Patients with hematologic malignancies may also have increased serum calcium levels, but this is thought to result from cytokines causing increased osteoclastic activity in bone.
- **Excess vitamin D and vitamin A.** Patients will have normal or elevated serum phosphate levels associated with a low PTH level.
- **Thiazide diuretics.** Thiazides may increase serum calcium level, whereas serum phosphate may also be depressed.
- **Hyperthyroidism.** Hyperthyroidism may cause increased calcium by stimulating bone resorption. Serum calcium levels normalize when the patient becomes euthyroid.
- **Milk-alkali syndrome.** This syndrome typically occurs in patients with peptic ulcer disease who consume large amounts of milk and absorbable antacids. PTH levels are low.
- **Sarcoidosis.** Granulomas are hypertensive to vitamin D, converting the inactive vitamin into its active form. PTH levels are low.
- **Paget disease (osteitis deformans).**
- **Adrenal insufficiency.**

primary hyperparathyroidism is caused by a single adenoma in 90% to 92% of cases, a "double" adenoma in 4% to 5% of patients, hyperplasia in 3% to 4% of patients and parathyroid cancer in fewer than 0.1% of cases. The actual incidence of double adenomas may be as high as 10% according to recent series using intraoperative PTH monitoring. Approximately 50,000 to 100,000 cases of primary hyperparathyroidism are seen annually, and the disease is more commonly seen in postmenopausal women. Although the etiology of primary hyperparathyroidism is not completely understood, genetic influences seem to contribute at least to some degree to the development of this condition. Mutations in the *PRAD1/cyclinD1* oncogene are commonly seen (up to 40%) in patients with parathyroid adenoma. Parathyroid hyperplasia may also be frequently seen in conjunction with familial syndromes, including MEN type 1 or 2A, familial isolated hyperparathyroidism, and familial hypocalciuric hypercalcemia (FHH). In patients with FHH, an autosomal dominant disease, urinary calcium levels are relatively low, and parathyroidectomy is seldom helpful in reducing serum calcium levels and is not indicated.

Secondary hyperparathyroidism can be seen in disease states such as chronic renal failure or severe vitamin D deficiency, in which decreased levels of serum ionized calcium result in parathyroid hyperplasia and a physiologic elevation in parathyroid hormone levels. These patients may benefit from restrictions of phosphate and aluminum in their diet and dialysate, and from dietary supplementation of calcium, vitamin D, and phosphate-binding resins. Failure of medical measures may necessitate surgery. *Tertiary hyperparathyroidism* results when the overstimulated hyperplastic parathyroid glands of secondary hyperparathyroidism begin to autonomously produce PTH in a manner dysregulated from serum calcium levels. This condition is usually seen in patients following renal transplantation as serum calcium levels normalize.

Patients with primary hyperparathyroidism most commonly are asymptomatic on presentation. The diagnosis is usually established by elevated serum calcium levels in the setting of elevated levels of PTH. Twenty-four-hour urinary calcium levels are typically increased and are routinely measured to exclude the diagnosis of FHH. Other laboratory abnormalities may include an elevation in alkaline phosphatase, a decrease in serum phosphate levels, and a hyperchloremic metabolic acidosis. Patients may present with symptoms of hypercalcemia, which may be remembered from the mnemonic "painful bones, stones, abdominal groans, and psychic moans." Radiographic skeletal manifestations of hypercalcemia include subperiosteal resorption on the radial aspect of the middle phalanges of the second or third digits (most common), bone cysts of the skull and long bones, and in more advanced cases, *osteoclastomas* or brown tumors. Bone densitometric studies are frequently obtained in hyperparathyroid patients. Nephrolithiasis occurs more frequently in the setting of primary hyperparathyroidism secondary to increased calcium and phosphate excretion and from increased urinary pH. Gastrointestinal sequelae of hypercalcemia range from nonspecific gastrointestinal (GI) complaints (nausea, vomiting, and constipation) to increased incidences of pancreatitis, gallstones, and peptic ulcer disease. Hypercalcemia can also result in a wide variety of psychiatric symptoms ranging from anxiety, depression, and psychosis to fatigue, lethargy, and coma. Less commonly, patients can present with *hypercalcemic crisis*, a serious and rapidly deteriorating condition characterized by elevated serum calcium levels, nausea and vomiting, polyuria, polydipsia, weight loss, lethargy, and coma. Interestingly, symptoms do not always correlate with serum calcium levels. Initial treatment is aimed at reducing serum calcium levels with hydration (typically with normal saline) and loop diuretics. If these measures are unsuccessful, other strategies include the use of diphosphonates, calcitonin, or mithramycin. Ultimately, when calcium levels have been lowered to a safe range, therapy is aimed at eliminating the etiology of primary hyperparathyroidism, usually through surgery. Patients with primary hyperparathyroidism frequently have an unrevealing physical examination. Primary adenomas are seldom palpable and hypercalcemia frequently produces no evident clinical findings.

Preoperative Assessment of Patients with Hyperparathyroidism

The routine use of preoperative imaging and localization studies is not generally accepted for initial surgical management of primary hyperparathyroidism, since the success rate for surgical treatment of the disease approaches 95% in experienced hands. With the advent of intraoperative PTH testing, however, preoperative imaging for minimally invasive approaches is becoming more common. Localization studies typically play an integral role in reoperative surgery, either for persistent or recurrent disease. Ultrasonography is a relatively inexpensive and rapid method for identifying lesions in approximately 50% to 60% of reoperative candidates, and allows for the acquisition of pathologic information through FNA. CT scan has similar sensitivity, although it is more expensive and can be limited in distinguishing thyroid and parathyroid tissue. This modality is particularly beneficial in identifying ectopic parathyroids in the mediastinum. MRI imaging is even more expensive, but provides a greater sensitivity than does CT scan and avoids the contrast load. Sestamibi-technetium-99m imaging, which has largely replaced the older thallium-technetium scan has been shown to achieve sensitivity rates as high as 90% for parathyroid adenomas and has emerged as probably the single most useful localizing study. It has also demonstrated increasing utility preoperatively among patients who are initially presenting with primary hyperparathyroidism and electing to undergo *minimally invasive parathyroidectomy*, as discussed in greater detail in subsequent text. Angiography and selective venous sampling are other localization modalities for abnormal parathyroids, but are more invasive and are typically limited in their use in the rare instances when other methods have failed.

In general, patients with primary hyperparathyroidism and clinical symptoms are recommended for surgical intervention. Symptomatic response following surgery, particularly in those patients with bone disease, neuromuscular symptoms, or nephrolithiasis, is frequently seen as serum calcium levels normalize, although patients with psychiatric complaints or renal insufficiency may show less benefit. The surgical management of patients with documented primary hyperparathyroidism in the absence of symptoms is somewhat controversial. The 1990 NIH Consensus Development Conference Statement on Diagnosis and Management of Asymptomatic Primary Hyperparathyroidism outlines guidelines for potential surgical intervention among these patients. These guidelines include asymptomatic patients with (i) markedly elevated serum calcium levels (greater than 11.4 to 12 mg per dL); (ii) reduced creatinine clearance (greater than 30% compared to age-matched controls); (iii) elevated 24-hour urinary calcium level (greater than 400 mg); (iv) reduced bone mass (greater than 2 standard deviations below matched controls) or presence of nephrolithiasis by x-ray; (v) history of an episode of life-threatening hypercalcemia; and (vi) unsuitability for routine surveillance, including patients with poor medical compliance, patients requesting surgery, and young patients (younger than 50 years of age) where the unknown long-term effects of hypercalcemia and costs of long-term surveillance would favor surgical intervention.

Surgery for Hyperparathyroidism

Surgery provides definitive treatment for patients with primary hyperparathyroidism and is accomplished with relatively high initial success rates (90% to 95%) and low morbidity. Traditionally, experienced endocrine surgeons have advocated bilateral neck exploration at the time of initial surgery with identification of all four parathyroid glands because of the possibility of multiglandular disease. With the advent of the highly sensitive sestamibi scans (often in conjunction with ultrasonography), some endocrine centers have moved toward *minimally invasive radioguided parathyroidectomy* (MIRP) through small (less than 2.5 cm incisions) with unilateral neck dissections. Advocates of this method argue similar cure rates with reduced operative times, potentially shorter hospital stays and theoretically less chance for morbidity with the more limited dissection. The key component for this approach is the ability to measure PTH intraoperatively. Standard dogma is to do a bilateral exploration to identify all four glands to rule out double adenomas or hyperplasia. Normalizing levels of PTH upon excision of the lesion can prove the patient has only a single adenoma without an extensive dissection. Preoperative imaging allows a directed approach for parathyroid excision, but the use of an intraoperative radioprobe (as in MIRP) is typically not helpful to an experienced endocrine surgeon who can clearly identify the parathyroid adenoma.

A systematic identification of all four parathyroid glands usually reveals the superior parathyroids in a fairly constant location as discussed. If the evaluation of biopsy of these glands proves to be normal, the search for the abnormal inferior gland(s) may sometimes be more difficult. Frequently, ectopic inferior parathyroid glands are found in the thyrothymic ligament or in the thymus itself. If the inferior glands cannot be localized, the thymic pedicle should be carefully inspected and mobilized, and a transcervical thymectomy should be performed. If the gland is not located by this method, then mobilization of the thyroid lobe ipsilateral to the missing parathyroid gland is indicated, as a small percentage (2% to 5%) of glands are intrathyroidal. Intraoperative ultrasonography may be helpful in identifying these parathyroid glands, but thyroid lobectomy is sometimes indicated if the abnormal gland cannot be localized. If all these methods prove to be unsuccessful, it is generally recommended that the procedure be aborted and further localization studies be obtained prior to reexploration.

The surgical procedure indicated for primary hyperparathyroidism depends upon the etiology of the disease. For parathyroid adenomas, simple excision is sufficient. Success of the procedure depends upon careful visual inspection of the size of the glands by an experienced surgeon, and by histologic confirmation by frozen sections. Other methods, such as intraoperative PTH measurements and MIRP, can also help to ensure curative outcome. For parathyroid hyperplasia or four gland disease, the recommended surgical treatment is either subtotal parathyroidectomy (removal of 3.5 of the 4 glands), or total parathyroidectomy with immediate autotransplantation of parathyroid tissue, typically in the forearm muscle bed. The incidence of hypoparathyroidism is similar (approximately 5%) between these two surgical approaches. Recurrent disease in patients undergoing subtotal parathyroidectomy for sporadic parathyroid hyperplasia is up to 20%, and these patients typically require total parathyroidectomy with autografting. The incidence of recurrent disease is significantly higher in patients with MEN 1 or other familial parathyroid hyperplasia syndromes, and, therefore, total parathyroidectomy with cryopreservation and autotransplantation of parathyroid tissue is generally recommended in these patients to simplify reoperation. In some instances, subtotal parathyroidectomy or total thyroidectomy is indicated in patients with tertiary hyperparathyroidism, such as in prospective or postrenal transplantation patients or in those patients with severe clinical symptoms resulting from hypercalcemia refractory to medical management.

Complications of surgery for primary hyperparathyroidism are relatively rare. Persistent disease occurs in less than 5% of cases and usually results from a missed adenoma. Recurrent disease, characterized by a period of normocalcemia followed by a return of hypercalcemia is also uncommon, and is frequently the result of unrecognized hyperplasia, although may be the consequence of an incompletely excised adenoma, or spillage of tumor at the time of surgery. Reoperation should be performed only after exhaustive localization studies have been performed. The incidence of injury to the recurrent laryngeal nerve is approximately 1% for initial procedures, and 5% to 10% upon reexploration. Permanent hypoparathyroidism is relatively uncommon following initial procedures, but may occur in up to 20% of patients following reoperation.

Careful examination of patients postoperatively for the signs and symptoms of hypocalcemia that may result from hypoparathyroidism is important. Decreased plasma-ionized calcium levels result in increased neuromuscular excitability, which may also be seen in other conditions (Table 30-4). Patients may complain of circumoral numbness or tingling, or tingling in the fingers and toes. They may also present with more vague psychiatric symptoms of confusion or anxiety. On physical examination, hypocalcemia may be revealed by eliciting contraction of the fascial muscles by tapping anterior to the fascial nerve (*Chvostek sign*) or by eliciting carpal spasm by applying a blood pressure cuff for 3 minutes to occlude blood flow to the forearm (*Trousseau sign*). An electrocardiogram may reveal a prolonged QT interval. Generally, therapy is aimed at maintaining serum calcium levels greater than 8.0 mg per dL, which can usually be achieved by oral calcium supplementation. In some cases, administration of calcitriol

TABLE 30-4
CAUSES OF HYPOCALCEMIA

- **Postoperative hypoparathyroidism.** This most commonly occurs after total thyroidectomy for malignancy. The low calcium level probably represents contusion or temporary alteration of the blood supply to the parathyroids; the hypocalcemia is usually transient and is not treated unless significant symptoms develop. In patients with preoperative hyperparathyroidism and significant bone disease, removing the offending gland or glands may cause marked skeletal bone deposition ("hungry bone"), requiring calcium and vitamin D therapy.
- **Idiopathic hypoparathyroidism.** This occurs in both sporadic and familial forms and may have an autoimmune basis. DiGeorge syndrome is a congenital disorder involving the branchial pouches and produces agenesis of the thymus and parathyroids.
- **Vitamin D deficiency.** This may be caused by a dietary deficiency or lack of exposure to sunlight. There is a decrease in calcium absorption and an increased secretion of parathyroid hormone (PTH).
- **Pseudohypoparathyroidism.** A familial disease characterized by an unresponsiveness of the kidney to PTH. Elevated PTH levels cause bone resorption, but patients remain hypocalcemic and hyperphosphatemic.
- **Hypomagnesemia.** The defect appears to block the physical response to PTH as well as its release from the parathyroids.
- **Malabsorption.**
- **Pancreatitis.**

may be indicated if oral calcium supplementation alone is unsuccessful. Following parathyroidectomy, particularly in patients with preexisting metabolic bone disease, one may also see the development of the "hungry bone syndrome" characterized by hypocalcemia, hypophosphatemia, hypomagnesemia, and increased bone mineralization. Severe cases of hypocalcemia may result in convulsions and tetany, and rapid infusion of intravenous calcium solutions is warranted.

Parathyroid Carcinoma

Parathyroid carcinoma is an extremely rare functioning neoplasm, occurring in less than 1% of patients with primary hyperparathyroidism. There does not appear to be a gender predilection for this malignancy, which is more common in older patients (older than 30 years of age). Although the etiology is unknown, mutations in the retinoblastoma tumor suppressor gene (RB) gene, and more recently in the *HRPT-2* gene (seen in a particular type of familial hyperplasia), have been observed with higher frequency in patients with this cancer. Patients with parathyroid carcinoma often present with extremely high serum calcium levels and with significantly elevated PTH levels. In some patients, an elevated serum human chorionic gonadotropin (hCG) level may also be seen. Approximately one half of the patients will present with a palpable firm neck mass (in contrast to adenomas), and many patients may have an affected voice from RLN involvement. On the basis of preoperative and intraoperative findings, if parathyroid carcinoma is suspected, initial treatment should include radical resection of the involved gland, the ipsilateral thyroid lobe, and regional lymph nodes. Injury to the RLN in these operations may occur in more than one half of the cases. Management of parathyroid carcinoma that is metastatic is frequently oriented toward control of the resulting hypercalcemia, as chemotherapy or radiation have not been shown to provide any significant benefit in this situation.

ADRENAL GLANDS

Embryology

The *adrenal cortex* is derived from *coelomic mesoderm*, adjacent to the urogenital ridge. Aberrant adrenocortical tissue may be found near the kidney or in the pelvis, possibly along the bladder. The *adrenal medulla* is derived from the *neural crest*; consequently, the medulla and sympathetic nervous system develop together. During the fifth week of gestation, the neural crest cells migrate toward the adrenocortical cells and situate themselves within a capsule of mesodermal cortex. The chromaffin and neuronal cells are derived from the neural crest.

Anatomy

The adrenal glands are paired retroperitoneal organs, located on the superior medial aspect of the upper portion of each kidney. They are firm in texture and their dark yellow color distinguishes them from retroperitoneal fat. Each gland weighs approximately 4 to 5 g. The right adrenal

gland is situated among the inferior vena cava, the liver, and the right diaphragmatic crus. The left adrenal gland is situated near the aorta, the tail of the pancreas, and the spleen (Fig. 30-5). The glands receive blood from the inferior phrenic artery, the aorta, and the renal artery. The arterial branches form a subcapsular plexus, which explains why injuring the capsule can result in bleeding. A number of small vessels run from the cortex (outer layers) to the medulla. Some refer to this as an adrenal "portal venous" circulation. This relationship allows for fundamental catecholamine-glucocorticoid interactions. The venous blood drains via the central vein into the inferior vena cava on the right side or into the renal vein on the left side.

Functionally, the adrenal gland is divided into the adrenal cortex and the adrenal medulla. The cortex is organized into three distinct layers: the *zona glomerulosa*, the outer layer, situated beneath the outer capsule and making up 15% of the cortex; the *zona fasciculata*, the middle and largest layer (75%); and the *zona reticularis*, the most inner layer of the cortex surrounding the medulla. The three zones are the site of production of mineralocorticoids, glucocorticoids, and sex steroids, respectively. Glucocorticoids are required to sustain life. The adrenal medulla is similar to a peripheral sympathetic ganglia. It is the site of catecholamine production, primarily epinephrine.

Biologically Active Adrenal Products

All adrenal steroids have 19 or 21 total carbon molecules. They have a 17-carbon structure, made of three hexane rings and single pentane rings. Cortisol and aldosterone have an additional two-carbon side chain.

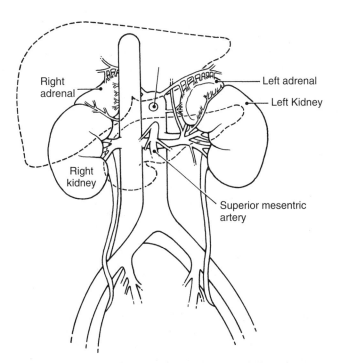

Figure 30-5 The right adrenal gland is situated among the inferior vena cava, the liver, and the right diaphragmatic crus. The left adrenal gland is situated near the aorta, the tail of the pancreas, and the spleen. (From Scott-Conner C, Dawson DL, eds. *Operative anatomy.* Philadelphia: JB Lippincott, 1993:499, with permission.)

Cortisol regulates the intermediary metabolism of carbohydrates, proteins, and lipids. It stimulates the release of glucagon and lactate from muscle and downregulates the sensitivity of insulin. Muscle cells undergo proteolysis and adipocytes undergo lipolysis, and the resulting amino acids and glycerol molecules are channeled to the liver for gluconeogenesis. In addition, cortisol acts directly on hepatic enzymes involved in gluconeogenesis. The combined effect of these processes is the production of a hyperglycemic state. It promotes an anabolic state in vital organs such as the brain and the liver at the expense of the lymphoid tissue, skin, muscle, and adipocytes, where a catabolic state predominates.

In addition to the effect on intermediate carbohydrate metabolism, cortisol regulates the intravascular volume and modulates the immune system. It has a positive chronotropic and inotropic effect on the heart. By stimulating angiotensin release and inhibiting prostaglandin I$_2$ (a potent vasodilator) synthesis, cortisol maintains blood pressure. To the detriment of surgical patients, the glucocorticoids retard wound healing by decreasing interleukin-2 production and release and lymphocyte activation, as well as by making mononuclear cells less responsive and less efficient for chemotaxis and phagocytosis. Osteoblast cell development necessary for bone growth and strength and fibroblast activity for collagen formation are also adversely affected. Chronic corticosteroid excess can cause emotional and psychologic disturbances.

Aldosterone is a mineralocorticoid that controls intravascular volume by stimulating the distal convoluted tubules (DCTs) of the kidney to reabsorb sodium, and, indirectly, free water, as well as to excrete potassium and hydrogen ion. An average individual secretes approximately 100 to 150 mg of aldosterone per day. The half-life of the mineralocorticoid is relatively short (15 minutes), and it is bound to transcortin and albumin much like cortisol. The majority (90%) of this steroid is cleared from the plasma after a single pass via the liver.

The major adrenal *androgens* are dehydroepiandrosterone, androstenedione, and testosterone. Estrogen is produced from androstenedione in the peripheral tissue. In adults, androgens promote the development of secondary sex characteristics such as deepening of the voice, producing a male hair distribution, coarsening of the skin, and promoting protein deposition in muscles. Estrogen has the opposite effects. In the fetus, the androgens stimulate Wolffian duct development, which results in male external genitalia. The lack of androgens in the female fetus allows the genital tubercle, labial folds, and urethral opening to remain in the normal female position. Adrenal androgen production and release is stimulated by adrenocorticotropic hormone (ACTH) and not by the gonadotropins.

Cells of the adrenal medulla secrete *biologically active amines*, including dopamine, norepinephrine, and epinephrine, in response to sympathetic nerve innervation. There are two general types of receptors, α and β, as well as subtypes α_1, α_2, β_1, and β_2, found in different concentrations in many groups of cells. The catecholamines that are released from secretory granules bind to receptors with different affinities that are based on the local concentration of each molecule and elicit different physiologic responses. For example, β_1-receptor stimulation causes an increased chronotropic and inotropic effect on the heart and stimulation of lipolysis, whereas β_2-receptor stimulation causes relaxation of smooth muscle. In contrast to steroids, catecholamines elicit physiologic responses in minutes, using cyclic AMP as a secondary messenger molecule.

Biosynthetic Pathways

The early steroid synthesis pathways are common to all adrenal hormones and steroids. The pathways begin with cholesterol, which is converted to pregnenolone by a desmolase enzyme in the cell mitochondria (Fig. 30-6). Pregnenolone is shuttled via a pathway for the direct synthesis of testosterone and is also shuttled via a pathway for the conversion to progesterone, which is an intermediate substrate for cortisol, aldosterone, and additional testosterone synthesis.

The adrenal medulla is the area of catecholamine synthesis, storage, and release, as well as reuptake of released steroids. Sympathetic stimulation of the chromaffin cells

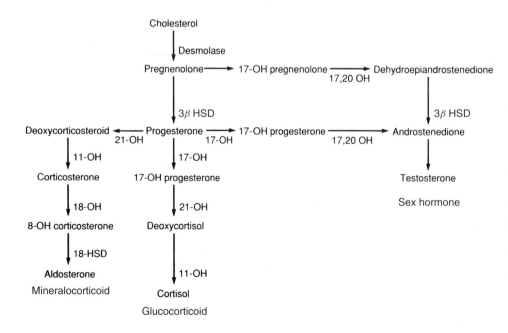

Figure 30-6 Steroidogenic pathways of the adrenal cortex include sex hormones, as well as glucocorticoid and mineralocorticoid hormones. A deficiency of 21-hydroxylase is the most common cause of congenital adrenal hyperplasia. This condition results in decreased cortisol and aldosterone production as well as an excess of progesterone, which is shuttled to increase androgen production. (From Newsome HH. Adrenal glands. In: Greenfield LJ, Mullholland MW, Oldham KT et al., eds. *Surgery: scientific principles and practice,* 2nd ed. Philadelphia: Lippincott-Raven, 1997:1334, with permission.)

increases the activity of the tyrosine hydroxylase, which converts the amino acid tyrosine into dihydroxyphenylalanine (DOPA) and ultimately leads to the sequential production of dopamine, norepinephrine, and epinephrine.

Regulatory Mechanisms for Hormone Secretion

Various regulatory mechanisms control the release of glucocorticoids, mineralocorticoids, and catecholamines. The production of cortisol is regulated by the hypothalamus-pituitary axis (Fig. 30-7). The central and peripheral nervous systems signal the hypothalamus during periods of emotional and physical stress to release corticotrophin-releasing hormone (CRH). CRH is delivered to the anterior pituitary via a rich blood plexus, and, in response, the pituitary releases ACTH and the adrenal glands synthesize and release cortisol. The resulting high level of cortisol signals the hypothalamus and pituitary to stop secreting CRH and ACTH, respectively. This regulatory negative-feedback system, which includes a short and long loop, ensures tight regulation.

Aldosterone secretion is regulated by multiple factors including the *renin–angiotensin system* and plasma sodium concentration. The juxtaglomerular apparatus of the kidney and the macula densa—a grouping of cells located near the afferent arteriole—detect decreased renal blood flow and low plasma sodium concentration (Fig. 30-8). In response, the juxtaglomerular apparatus releases renin that converts angiotensinogen to angiotensin I, a decapeptide

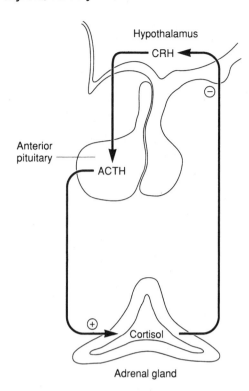

Figure 30-7 Feedback loop between the hypothalamus, the anterior pituitary, and the adrenal. (From Newsome HH. Adrenal glands. In: Greenfield LJ, Mullholland MW, Oldham KT et al., eds. *Surgery: Scientific principles and practice,* 2nd ed. Philadelphia: Lippincott-Raven, 1997:1334, with permission.)

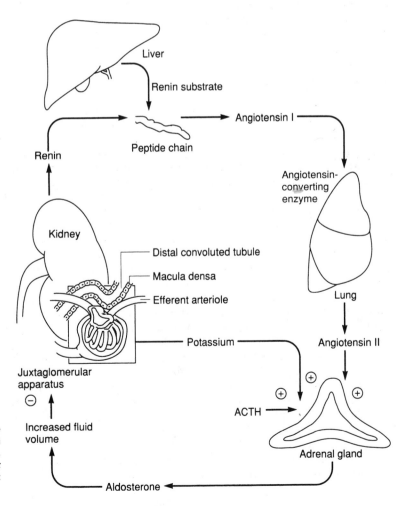

Figure 30-8 The renin–angiotensin–aldosterone system including their sites of production. (From Newsome HH. Adrenal glands. In: Greenfield LJ, Mullholland MW, Oldham KT et al., eds. *Surgery: Scientific principles and practice,* 2nd ed. Philadelphia: Lippincott-Raven, 1997:1335, with permission.)

derived from a large hepatic protein. Angiotensin I is converted to angiotensin II in the lung by an efficient carboxypeptidase. The newly formed protein signals aldosterone release. Conversely, a high sodium load, over-hydration, and the supine position result in decreased renin and aldosterone production. Two other minor factors that affect aldosterone release are plasma potassium concentration and ACTH. This hormone signals the adrenal glands to convert cholesterol into steroid products that are common to the mineralocorticoid and glucocorticoid synthesis pathway, but it favors the latter.

Catecholamine release is controlled by the *sympathetic nervous system*. The adrenal medulla is derived from the neural crest and is supplied by preganglionic sympathetic nerves from the greater splanchnic nerve and the celiac ganglion. Stimulation of the chromaffin cells moves the secretory granules to the cell membrane for release via exocytosis. The released catecholamines can be taken up by the chromaffin cells, enter the systemic circulation or neuronal cells, and undergo degradation or be excreted in the urine. The neuronal cells metabolize epinephrine and norepinephrine into vanillylmandelic acid (VMA) with monamine oxidase. Another enzyme, carboxy-O-methyltransferase converts extraneuronal epinephrine and norepinephrine into metabolic products, metanephrine and normetanephrine, respectively. A small portion will bind to receptor and elicit a physiological response.

Adrenal Imaging

CT scanning is the diagnostic study of choice to evaluate the adrenal gland with a sensitivity of approximately 95%. Simple cysts and myelolipomas can usually be identified by their CT characteristics. Intravenous contrast is not required. Benign lesions usually scan with less than 20 Hounsfield units (HU), whereas malignant lesions usually have a density greater than 30 HU. MRI also plays a role in evaluating adrenal pathology, especially for suspected pheochromocytoma. Enhancement on T2-weighted images generally depicts a functional adenoma or malignant focus. Radioisotope scans using iodocholesterol-labeled agents can help localize functional lesions such as aldosterone-producing adenomas and idiopathic aldosteronism; however, they are not widely available. Metaiodobenzylguanidine (MIBG) can be helpful for adrenal pheochromocytoma and neuroblastoma as ^{131}I-MIBG and ^{123}I-MIBG are concentrated in catecholamine storage vesicles. The positron emission tomography (PET) scan can be useful in identifying extraadrenal pheochromocytoma. Venous sampling may be required when anatomic studies do not definitively localize a pathologic lesion. When CT and MRI are unsuccessful in demonstrating a source in Cushing disease, petrosal sinus sampling may be performed to differentiate between a pituitary and an ectopic source of ACTH. This test involves bilateral sampling of the inferior petrosal sinus and peripheral veins for plasma ACTH levels before and after CRH administration. Similarly, when CT and MRI fail to confirm a unilateral adrenal adenoma, adrenal venous sampling can often be used to differentiate between an aldosterone producing adenoma and idiopathic aldosteronism. Samples from each adrenal vein are taken for aldosterone and cortisol levels before and after ACTH administration. The lateralization of high serum levels of aldosterone suggests a functional adenoma on the positive side.

Pathophysiology

The production, release, and metabolism of the glucocorticoids and mineralocorticoids are tightly regulated to maintain body homeostasis. However, both benign and malignant adrenal and extraadrenal tumors, adrenal hyperplastic states, and congenital enzymatic deficiencies can cause the overproduction and insufficiency of glucocorticoids and mineralocorticoids and result in pathologic conditions.

Cushing Syndrome

As described by Harvey Cushing, patients with an excess of cortisol have a characteristic syndrome characterized by moon facies, truncal obesity, glucose intolerance, hypertension, polycythemia, and pulmonary infections. In addition, these patients often present with hirsutism, osteoporosis, menstrual irregularity in women, and muscle weakness. There is also an increased incidence of peptic ulcer disease and pancreatitis among these patients. The most common cause is iatrogenic resulting from the excessive administration of exogenous glucocorticoid steroids. The most common cause of endogenous hypercortisolism is excessive pituitary ACTH secretion (Cushing disease) associated with a pituitary adenoma. Other causes include ectopic ACTH production, which is also ACTH-dependent, and then ACTH-independent etiologies such as an adrenal adenoma or carcinoma and micronodular pigmented hyperplasia.

The *evaluation* and *diagnosis of hypercortisolism* is to first determine whether hypercortisolism is indeed present by checking a 24-hour urinary-free cortisol and 17-hydroxycorticoid levels. Secondly, it must be determined whether the pathologic state is ACTH-dependent or ACTH-independent by using a dexamethasone suppression test. Finally, one should attempt to localize a lesion radiographically with CT scan or MRI. The dexamethasone test involves a single dose of steroid the night (11 o'clock) before the morning (8 o'clock) measurement of cortisol levels in plasma and urine. In a healthy person, the single dose of steroid suppresses additional release and patients have levels less than 5 μg per dL in the morning. A patient may be given CRH to help determine whether the hypercortisolism is dependent on the pituitary. Although patients with Cushing disease will have a rise in ACTH and cortisol levels in response to CRH, patients with adrenal or ectopic sources of cortisol production do not respond to the administration of CRH. Measurement of urinary 17-hydroxysteroid levels after administration of a high-dose of dexamethasone (8 mg per day) can also aid in determining the source of cortisol production. The urinary levels of 17-hydroxysteroid decrease significantly in patients with Cushing disease. On the other hand, there is no change in 17-hydroxysteroid levels in patients with adrenal or ectopic production of ACTH.

The treatment of the many causes of Cushing syndrome is surgical. In Cushing disease, transsphenoidal resection of the pituitary adenoma is the treatment of choice. Radiation or medical therapy may be used if the symptoms persist or recur after surgery. Likewise, patients with adrenal adenoma or carcinoma require adrenalectomy. Patients with adrenal adenomas may undergo laparoscopic adrenalectomy. The laparoscopic approach to adrenalectomy has resulted in decreased length of stay, morbidity, time to return of normal diet, and activity and costs. The approach to adrenal carcinomas and metastatic lesions remains controversial, with some authors advocating a laparoscopic approach for small to moderately sized tumors and others preferring a traditional open procedure for all malignant tumors. Both approaches can be performed transperitoneally or via the retroperitoneum. Lastly, for those patients with ectopic ACTH syndrome, the primary lesion must be surgically removed. Unresectable lesions or tumor recurrences may be debulked with or without bilateral adrenalectomy to provide palliation of symptoms. Drugs including metyrapone, aminoglutethimide, and mitotane can be used to suppress the production of cortisol. In the past, patients who underwent bilateral adrenalectomy for Cushing syndrome with an unknown cause developed a condition known as "Nelson syndrome," characterized by pituitary tumors with dark skin pigmentation, visual disturbances, and amenorrhea.

Hyperaldosteronism

Hypersecretion of mineralocorticoids can cause a syndrome of hypertension and hypokalemia. *Primary hyperaldosteronism* is generally caused by autonomously functioning adrenal cortex tumors (Conn syndrome). *Secondary hyperaldosteronism* can be caused by an elevated level of renin in patients with renal artery stenosis, cirrhosis, congestive heart failure, and normal pregnancy. Treatment of the latter conditions usually corrects the hyperaldosteronism. In addition to moderate diastolic hypertension and hypokalemia, hyperaldosteronism can cause impaired insulin sensitivity and hyperglycemia. Potassium depletion can produce muscle weakness, fatigue, polyuria, and polydipsia. For a diagnosis of primary hyperaldosteronism, the patient must have diastolic hypertension without edema, hyposecretion of renin despite low intravascular volume, and hypersecretion of aldosterone.

Confirmation of the diagnosis includes serum potassium levels less than 3.5 mEq per L, a 24-hour urinary excretion of potassium that exceeds 30 mEq, and a plasma aldosterone–renin ratio of greater than 30. Captopril, an angiotensin-converting enzyme (ACE) inhibitor may be given to the patient before measuring his or her aldosterone and renin levels. In healthy patients, the ACE inhibitor decreases aldosterone production and increases renin production, thereby lowering the aldosterone–renin ratio. However, a patient with primary hyperaldosteronism will have a continuous high level of aldosterone and a aldosterone–renin ratio of more than 50. Twenty-four-hour urinary aldosterone secretion of more than 14 μg following 5 days of high-sodium diet is highly suggestive of primary hyperaldosteronism. Measuring urinary sodium and aldosterone levels after intravenous saline infusion may also be helpful in the diagnosis of primary hyperaldosteronism. The measurement of plasma aldosterone and renin levels in the supine position and 2 hours later in the standing position and the measurement of serum 18-hydroxycorticosterone are two additional tests that may be obtained. Patients with functional adenomas demonstrate suppression of renin and aldosterone levels when they move from a recumbent to a standing position and have elevated levels of 18-hydroxycorticosterone. Once the diagnosis has been confirmed, localization studies such as CT, MRI, iodocholesterol scan, and venous sampling must be done in order to plan definitive therapy.

Patients with primary hyperaldosteronism localized to a unilateral gland are typically treated with laparoscopic adrenalectomy. Those with idiopathic adrenal hyperplasia are managed medically with spironolactone and other potassium-sparing diuretics.

Pheochromocytoma

Pheochromocytoma, a tumor arising from neuroectodermal—chromaffin—cells can be the cause of life-threatening hypertension. It occurs in 0.05% to 0.1% of the population, affecting men and women equally. Ten percent of the tumors are bilateral, extraadrenal, familial, or malignant, in children, or multicentric. In children, 35% of pheochromocytomas can be extraadrenal. Unfortunately, malignancy is not always obvious upon presentation; therefore, the initial surgery should result in complete excision, and long-term follow-up is mandatory. The tumor is associated with individuals with MEN types 2A and 2B, von Recklinghausen neurofibromatosis, and von Hippel-Lindau disease. Most tumors secrete norepinephrine, either continuously or episodically. Patients often present with episodes of headaches, sweating, and palpitations, often described as anxiety attacks. The diagnosis of a pheochromocytoma can be made by performing 24-hour urine collections of catecholamines and metabolites including dopamine, VMA, and metanephrine, and serum measurements of epinephrine and norepinephrine. Because of episodic secretion, repeated 24-hour urinary tests may be necessary. If the urinary and plasma measurements are equivocal for the diagnosis of pheochromocytoma, the patient may be given clonidine, a centrally acting antihypertensive. In normal patients, clonidine suppresses plasma concentrations of catecholamines; however, this would not be the case for patients with pheochromocytomas. As with other functional tumors, upon confirmation of diagnosis, pheochromocytomas must be localized using either CT scan, MRI, MIBG, and/or venous sampling.

Patients with pheochromocytomas require surgical excision of the tumor. Today, most pheochromocytomas are treated by a laparoscopic adrenalectomy. In preparation for surgery, patients are given phenoxybenzamine, an α-blocker, to reduce blood pressure and to restore intravascular volume for at least 1 to 4 weeks. After adequate α-blockade has been achieved, a β-blocker may be added if the patient has evidence of tachycardia. β-Blockers can precipitate malignant hypertension and cardiac failure in patients with pheochromocytomas who are not adequately α-receptor blocked. An alternative or additional preoperative medication is metyrapone, which blocks production of catecholamines in the tumor. This decreases blood pressure changes that occur with the manipulation of the tumor during operative resection.

Adrenocortical Carcinoma

Adrenocortical carcinoma is a highly lethal and rare malignant disease. Patients commonly present with metastatic or locally advanced disease. The majority of patients present with an endocrinopathy, either Cushing syndrome or virilization. There is a bimodal occurrence by age in the first 4 years and then later in the fourth to fifth decades of life. Women develop functional adrenocortical carcinomas more commonly than men. The tumors usually are larger than 6 cm and weigh between 100 and 5,000 g. Several studies have demonstrated that metastasizing or recurring tumors are associated with high mitotic activity, nuclear DNA ploidy, and production of abnormal amounts of androgens and 11-deoxysteroids. The only hope for cure is complete excision. Often this is not possible, but aggressive local resection is appropriate. Mitotane, a chemotherapeutic agent, has been used in conjunction with surgery with moderate success. The overall prognosis is poor.

Congenital Adrenal Hyperplasia

In addition to functional tumors, enzyme deficiencies of the steroid synthesis pathway in the adrenal gland can result in overproduction of sex steroids. These enzymatic deficiencies result in a syndrome known as "congenital adrenal hyperplasia." It is the most common adrenal disorder of infancy and childhood. The syndrome results in decreased cortisol production and an accumulation of intermediate steroid metabolites that are shunted to androgen production. Peripheral tissues convert the androgen to testosterone, which can cause virilization. Prenatal congenital adrenal hyperplasia in girls produces ambiguous external genitalia (female pseudohermaphroditism), but the reproductive organs develop normally. Postnatal congenital adrenal hyperplasia can cause virilization of girls. Moreover, both sexes develop short stature, premature closure of bone epiphyses, and advanced bone age.

The most common cause of congenital adrenal hyperplasia is 21-hydroxylase deficiency (Fig. 30-6). This enzyme is responsible for the conversion of progesterone to 11-deoxycorticosterone, and subsequently to corticosterone and aldosterone. Without the enzyme, there is an accumulation of progesterone and delta-5-pregnenolone, which are converted to androgen by 17α-hydroxylase, as well as a decreased production of aldosterone that results in dehydration, hyponatremia, and hyperkalemia. The other less common causes of the hyperplasia are 11β-hydroxylase and 3β-hydroxydehydrogenase deficiencies. 3β-hydroxydehydrogenase deficiency results in early infant death secondary to significant salt-wasting. The most severe form is congenital lipoid adrenal hyperplasia, which results from the deficiency of cholesterol desmolase. All the steroid synthesis pathways are inhibited, and, as a result, all affected infants are phenotypic girls with several salt-wasting symptoms. The treatment of the deficiency is surgical correction of the external genitalia in girls, and medical treatment of the excess androgens.

Adrenal Insufficiency

Primary adrenal failure is caused by an inherent disease of the adrenal gland, whereas secondary failure is caused by disorders of the pituitary or hypothalamus. Primary adrenal insufficiency (AI) is typically caused by an autoimmune disease (Addison disease), an infectious disease like tuberculosis or histoplasmosis, adrenal hemorrhage, metastases, or by surgical resection. The most common cause of secondary AI is exogenous steroids. The symptoms of low cortisol are nonspecific but can present as nausea, vomiting, weight loss, weakness, and lethargy. Rarely, hypocortisolism can produce a sudden episode of hypotension or shock (crisis) that is life-threatening. Biochemically, the condition can produce hyponatremia and hyperkalemia.

A short cosyntropin stimulation test can be performed to make the diagnosis of primary and secondary adrenal failure. Cosyntropin (ACTH) (250 μg intravenous or intramuscular) is administered and plasma cortisol is measured 30 minutes later. Patients with adrenal failure will not demonstrate an increase in cortisol levels. An ACTH level can help distinguish between primary and secondary adrenal failure. In primary failure, patients will have elevated levels of ACTH but insufficient levels of glucocorticoids. Moreover, serum potassium and sodium levels may also be helpful in making the diagnosis.

The treatment of adrenal failure is exogenous glucocorticoids given twice daily with a higher morning dose. In primary failure, the treatment also includes the administration of a mineralocorticoid (Florinef) because all adrenal hormone synthesis is affected. The treatment of an Addisonian crisis is volume resuscitation with appropriate crystalloids and intravenous glucocorticoids. If the diagnosis of primary adrenal failure is known, the patients may be given hydrocortisone (100 mg intravenous every 8 hours), otherwise dexamethasone should be administered. Hydrocortisone is detected by the plasma cortisol assay and may cause confusion in making the diagnosis. Patients who use glucocorticoids or recently discontinued them require increased doses of the medication during illness, injury, or surgery, as well as in the postoperative period (*stress dose steroids*).

Incidentaloma

The prevalent use of imaging studies for diagnostic purposes has increased the detection of asymptomatic adrenal masses, or *incidentalomas*. Incidentalomas are seen in 0.6% to 5.0% of abdominal CT scans. Incidentaloma can be approached by consideration of three questions: (i) Is the lesion functional, (ii) is it malignant, and (iii) is it metastatic?

Patients should undergo a thorough history and physical examination focusing on signs and symptoms of Cushing syndrome, aldosteronism, and pheochromocytoma. Traditionally, 24-hour collections of urine for cortisol, VMA, metanephrines, and catecholamines have been performed along with serum potassium levels. If the potassium levels are low and the patient is hypertensive, serum aldosterone and renin levels should be collected. Alternatively, recent NIH guidelines suggest a 1-mg dexamethasone suppression test and a measurement of plasma-free metanephrines in addition to the measurement of serum potassium and plasma aldosterone–plasma renin activity ratio in hypertensive patients.

All functional tumors and all tumors larger than 5 cm are treated with unilateral laparoscopic adrenalectomy. Some authors advocate unilateral adrenalectomy for any tumor larger than 4 cm. In addition, in a patient with a history of cancer, particularly lung cancer, and a negative biochemical workup, an FNA may be performed to help detect suspected metastatic disease to the adrenal or lymphoma. An alternative test to FNA in evaluating an incidentaloma in a patient with prior malignancy is a PET scan. In general, FNA should not be routinely performed, because it typically cannot distinguish between benign and malignant tumors. Masses that are smaller than 4 cm or that are nonfunctional can be followed with repeated CT scans every 6 months. Size increase between observation periods warrants surgical resection.

KEY CONCEPTS

▲ The thyroid is derived from endoderm except for the calcitonin-secreting parafollicular (C cells), which are of ectodermal neural crest origin. The thyroid is principally supplied by the superior thyroid artery (branch of external carotid) and inferior thyroid artery (branch of thyrocervical trunk).

▲ Complications of thyroid or parathyroid surgery include recurrent laryngeal nerve, marked by hoarseness of voice (unilateral) or possible airway obstruction (bilateral), hypoparathyroidism, and neck hematoma, which may require emergent evacuation at the bedside if there is evidence of airway compromise.

▲ A new or enlarging palpable thyroid nodule or thyroid nodule larger than 1.5 cm usually warrants fine needle aspiration (FNA); FNA is limited in its ability to distinguish between follicular adenomas and follicular carcinomas.

▲ Medullary thyroid carcinoma (MTC) is derived from parafollicular or C-cells. It is associated with familial syndromes in about one third of the cases (e.g., MEN 2A/B), which frequently have mutations in the *RET* proto-oncogene. Serum calcitonin levels can be helpful in the diagnosis, screening, and follow-up for recurrence of patients with MTC.

▲ The superior and inferior parathyroid glands are derived from the third and fourth pharyngeal pouches, respectively; the blood supply to the parathyroids is principally from the inferior thyroid artery.

▲ The most common cause of primary hyperparathyroidism is parathyroid adenoma. Most patients are asymptomatic and the diagnosis is confirmed by elevated serum calcium levels with elevated parathyroid hormone (PTH) levels.

▲ *Hypercalcemic crisis* is a serious condition that can result from hyperparathyroidism and is often characterized by elevated serum calcium levels, nausea and vomiting, weight loss, lethargy, and coma. Therapy is initially aimed at reducing calcium levels by hydration and loop diuretics. Hypocalcemia may result from hypoparathyroidism after thyroid or parathyroid surgery and may be evident clinically through the *Chvostek* and *Trousseau* signs.

▲ Incidentalomas are incidentally detected asymptomatic adrenal masses. They should prompt a workup to exclude Cushing syndrome, aldosteronism, and pheochromocytoma; lesions larger than 5 cm should be resected.

▲ Pheochromocytomas are tumors of the adrenal medulla and are characterized by the "rule of 10s." Ten percent of the tumors are bilateral, extraadrenal (commonly organ of Zuckerkandl-Ao bifurcation), familial, malignant, present in children, or multicentric.

▲ Patients with pheochromocytomas are treated preoperatively with phenoxybenzamine (α-blocker), and typically a β-blocker if tachycardia is present. Metyrapone is also frequently used preoperatively and blocks catecholamine production by the tumor.

SUGGESTED READINGS

Adrenal. *Selected readings in general surgery*, Vol. 26, No. 7. Dallas, Texas: University of Texas, Southwestern Medical Center of Dallas, 1999.

Baker RJ, Fischer JE, eds. *Mastery of surgery*, 4th ed. Philadelphia: Lippincott Williams & Wilkins, 2001:477–488.

DeVita VT Jr, Hellman S, Roseberg SA, eds. *Cancer: Principles and practice of oncology*, 7th ed. Philadelphia: Lippincott Williams & Wilkins, 2005:1629–1652.

Norton J, Bollinger R et al., eds. *Essential practice of surgery: Basic science and clinical evidence*. New York: Springer-Verlag, 2003:369–399.

Parathyroid Disease. *Selected readings in general surgery*, Vol. 23, No. 4. Texas: University of Texas, Southwestern Medical Center of Dallas, 1996.

The Pancreas

31

Kristoffel Dumon   Ernest F. Rosato

The pancreas is an enigmatic organ that continues to fascinate and challenge even the most experienced surgeons. Recent advances in outlining the molecular biology and physiology of this organ are allowing us to embark on new therapeutic approaches such as islet cell transplantation and novel cancer strategies.

EMBRYOLOGY

The pancreas begins development during the fourth week of gestation. Pancreatic tissue originates from the endodermal lining of the duodenum, from which two pouches develop into a large dorsal and a smaller ventral pancreatic primordium. The dorsal primordium normally forms the bulk of adult pancreatic tissue. The ventral pancreas maintains a close association with the common bile duct throughout development and contains the main pancreatic duct (duct of Wirsung). As the duodenum rotates to form a C-shaped configuration, the ventral primordium migrates dorsally in a clockwise direction to assume a position adjacent to the posterior inferior surface of the dorsal pouch. At the eighth week of gestation, the dorsal and ventral primordia fuse, as do their respective ductal systems. The ventral primordium forms the uncinate process and the inferior aspect of the head of the adult gland. The dorsal primordium becomes the superior aspect of the head as well as the entire neck, body, and tail of the pancreas (Fig. 31-1). The fusion of the pancreatic ductal systems during fetal development produces the most typical anatomic arrangement of the pancreatic duct structures. More than 85% of the time, the ventral pancreatic duct fuses with the more-distal dorsal pancreatic duct to create the duct of Wirsung, also known as the main pancreatic duct. This duct joins with the common bile duct in an intrapancreatic location and empties pancreatic exocrine secretions through the ampulla of Vater at the major duodenal papilla. The proximal aspect of the dorsal pancreatic duct (duct of Santorini) often remains in communication with the duct of Wirsung and may empty small amounts of exocrine pancreatic secretions through a separate minor duodenal papilla located on the second portion of the duodenum proximal to the major papilla. Possible malformations of pancreatic embryology include heterotopic pancreas, pancreas divisum, and annular pancreas.

Heterotopic pancreas is found most commonly in the stomach, duodenum, small bowel, or Meckel diverticulum.

Heterotopic pancreas clinically presents as intussusception, less commonly as intestinal obstruction. Other presentations include ulceration and hemorrhage. Surgical excision is indicated.

Pancreas divisum is an anatomic variant that occurs if the two primordial ductal systems fail to fuse. In pancreas divisum, the larger portion of the pancreas (superior head, neck, body, and tail) is drained by the duct of Santorini through the minor duodenal papilla, and only the ventral pancreas (inferior head and uncinate process) communicates with the duct of Wirsung into the major duodenal papilla. Five percent to 10% of patients undergoing endoscopic retrograde cholangiopancreatography (ERCP) are found to have pancreas divisum and its significance remains controversial. If pancreas divisum is associated with relative stenosis of the minor duodenal papilla, it can cause pancreatitis. This has been treated with endoscopic stenting or transduodenal sphincteroplasty of the minor papilla, with mixed results. Pancreas divisum in association with extensive pancreatic tissue injury or multiple ductular stenoses may need pancreatic resection or longitudinal pancreaticojejunostomy.

Annular pancreas is rare. It is caused by failure of normal clockwise rotation of the ventral pancreatic primordium. As a result, normal pancreatic tissue encircles the second portion of the duodenum. The tissue originating from the ventral primordium lies anterior to the duodenum, where it can fuse with the dorsal pancreas to form a complete ring, or it may remain as an incomplete ring. It presents with varying degrees of duodenal obstructive symptoms. In children, a common association exists with other serious congenital anomalies such as intracardiac defects, Down syndrome, and intestinal malrotation. Some patients have no symptoms until adulthood. Obstructive symptoms are an indication for operation. Resection or division of the annulus is not indicated because of the high incidence of fistula. Instead, a bypass procedure in the form of duodenojejunostomy is the preferred treatment.

ENDOCRINE PANCREAS EMBRYOLOGY

In humans, the first islets of endocrine tissue appear in the 54-mm fetus; islets appear initially and in greater number in the tail of the pancreas. The concept that pancreatic endocrine cells originate from migrating neural crest cells [amine precursor uptake and decarboxylation (APUD)

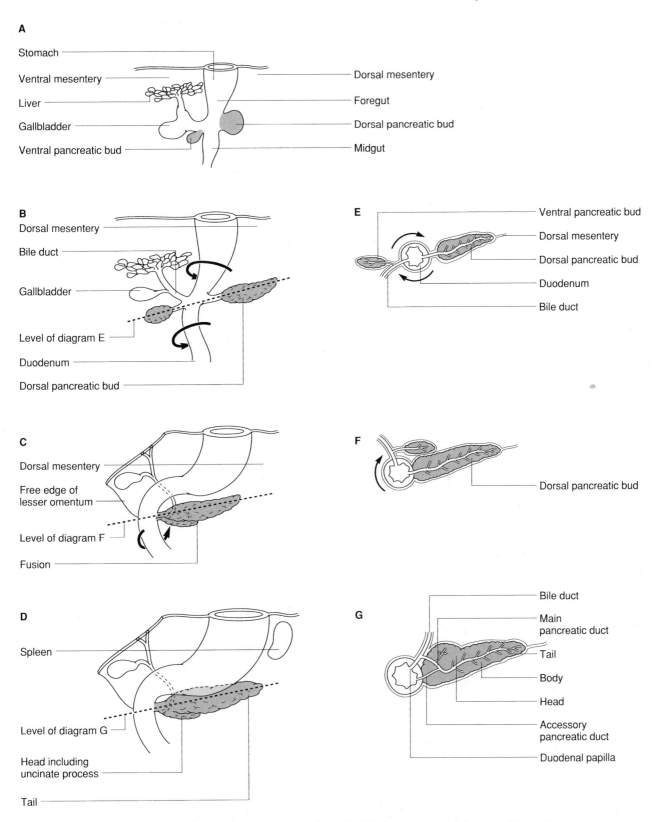

Figure 31-1 Development of the pancreas from the fifth through the eighth weeks. The smaller ventral pancreas rotates clockwise in a dorsal direction. The ventral pancreas is connected to the common bile duct and enters the duodenum at the major papilla. The dorsal pancreas enters the duodenum at the minor papilla. (From Moore KL. *The developing human,* 3rd ed. Philadelphia: WB Saunders, 1982, with permission.)

cells] is no longer widely accepted. The current view is that both endocrine and exocrine cells of the pancreas arise from embryonic foregut endoderm (not from the neural crest), with genetic mechanisms such as promotor regulation controlling the appearance of specific peptide hormones in designated islet cells. Initially the islet cells bud-off ductules followed by the appearance of β cells in the center of the islets with non-β cells on the periphery. In the final phase, β and non-β cells are distributed throughout the islet. Of note, 10% of islet cells consist of β cells outside discrete pancreatic islets.

ANATOMY

The pancreas occupies a retroperitoneal position in the abdomen, lying posterior to the stomach and lesser omentum. It extends obliquely from the duodenal C-shaped loop to a more cephalad position in the hilum of the spleen. The normal adult pancreas varies in weight from 75 to 125 g, in length from 10 to 20 cm, and in cephalad-to-caudad width from 3 to 5 cm. In the anteroposterior axis, the pancreas is thickest at the head, varying from 1.5 to 3.5 cm, and it is thinnest at the tail, from 0.8 to 2.5 cm. The gland is multilobulated. The pancreas is covered by peritoneum anteriorly, and posteriorly it lies in proximity to the inferior vena cava, the right renal vein, the aorta at the level of the first lumbar vertebra, the superior mesenteric vessels, and the splenic vein (Fig. 31-2).

The gland is divided into four portions: the head (which includes the uncinate process), the neck, the body, and the tail. That portion of the pancreas anterior to the superior mesenteric and portal veins is designated the neck. The head extends to the right of the neck and lies within the confines of the duodenal C-shaped loop; it includes the posteroinferior extension arising from the ventral primordium, designated the uncinate process. The uncinate process extends

posteriorly to the superior mesenteric vein and ends near the right margin of the superior mesenteric artery. The body of the pancreas lies immediately to the left of the neck; the tail of the pancreas extends to the left of the body into the splenic hilum. An extensive arterial system originating from multiple sources supplies the pancreas. The head of the pancreas is associated intimately with the second portion of the duodenum, and the anterior and posterior pancreaticoduodenal arteries jointly supply these two structures. These arteries originate from the superior and inferior pancreaticoduodenal vessels. The superior pancreaticoduodenal artery is a branch of the celiac axis, and the inferior pancreaticoduodenal is a branch of the superior mesenteric artery. The blood supply to the body and tail of the pancreas is through a more variable complex of arteries. Branches of the splenic and left gastroepiploic arteries, with the largest being the dorsal pancreatic and transverse pancreatic arteries, supply the distal body and tail of the pancreas. Within the posterosuperior and posteroinferior aspects of the body of the pancreas lay smaller arteries, the superior and inferior pancreatic arteries, respectively (Fig. 31-3).

The venous drainage of the pancreas corresponds with the arterial anatomy. Veins draining the pancreatic parenchyma eventually terminate in the portal vein, which arises posterior to the neck of the pancreas by the union of the splenic and superior mesenteric veins.

Multiple lymph node groups drain the pancreas. From the head of the gland, nodes in the pancreaticoduodenal groove communicate with subpyloric, portal, mesocolic, mesenteric, and aortocaval nodes. Lymphatic vessels in the body and tail of the pancreas drain to retroperitoneal nodes in the splenic hilum or to celiac, aortocaval, mesocolic, or mesenteric nodes.

Both sympathetic and parasympathetic fibers innervate the pancreas. Preganglionic sympathetic axons arise from cell bodies within the thoracic sympathetic ganglia and travel as splanchnic nerves to terminate within the celiac

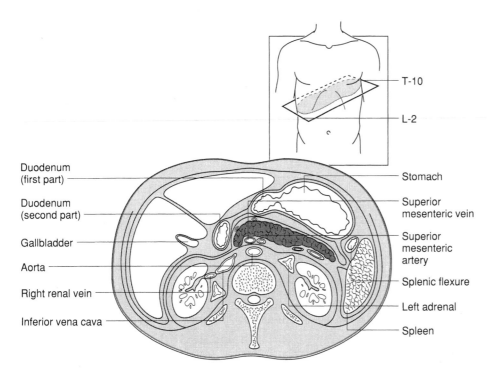

Duodenum (first part)
Duodenum (second part)
Gallbladder
Aorta
Right renal vein
Inferior vena cava

T-10
L-2

Stomach
Superior mesenteric vein
Superior mesenteric artery
Splenic flexure
Left adrenal
Spleen

Figure 31-2 Relationship of the pancreas to other abdominal organs and viscera. (From Mackie CR, Moosa AR. Surgical anatomy of the pancreas. In: Moosa AR, ed. Tumors of the pancreas. Baltimore: Williams & Wilkins, 1980, with permission.)

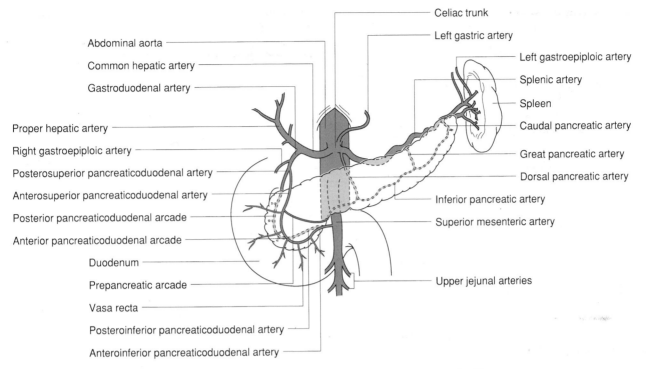

Figure 31-3   Arterial supply to the pancreas. (From Woodburne R.T. *Essentials of human anatomy.* New York: Oxford University Press, 1973, with permission.)

ganglia. From these structures, postganglionic sympathetic fibers traverse retroperitoneal tissue to innervate the pancreas and serve as the principal pathways for pain of pancreatic origin. This sympathetic pathway is the target during splanchnicectomy for the relief of pain of pancreatic origin. The parasympathetic innervation of the pancreas commences with preganglionic fiber cell bodies that reside within the vagal nuclei and travel through the posterior vagal trunk. These axons travel through the celiac plexus to terminate in parasympathetic ganglia within the pancreatic parenchyma. Postganglionic parasympathetic fibers then traverse a short course to innervate the pancreatic islets, acini, and ducts, and they serve an exclusively efferent function.

HISTOLOGY

The pancreas consists of both an endocrine and exocrine component. The acini and ductal systems constitute the exocrine portion of the pancreas. The exocrine pancreas is analogous to clusters of grapes (representing individual acini) on a vine (representing minor ducts). Each acinus has an approximately spheroid configuration and is composed of a single layer of acinar cells. Acinar cells contain zymogen granules in their apical portion and rest on a distinct basal lamina supported by reticular fibers. Acinar cells constitute about 80% of pancreatic mass. The pancreatic ductal system originates in the centroacinar cells of each individual acinus, includes intercalated duct cells and terminates in the main excretory duct of the pancreas. Duct cells constitute only 5% of pancreatic mass.

The endocrine cells of the pancreas reside in the islets of Langerhans. These are endocrine cells, diffusely scattered

in small clumps throughout the pancreas. Adult islets are composed of four major cell types (α, β, Δ, and PP) and two or more minor types. The α (alpha) cell secretes glucagon, the β (beta) cell secretes insulin, the Δ (delta) cell secretes somatostatin, $\Delta 2$ (delta-2) cell secretes vasoactive intestinal peptide (VIP), and the PP (or F) cell secretes pancreatic polypeptide (PP). Enterochromaffin cells are quite rare. Gastrin cells are normally only present in the fetal pancreas. Ectopic gastrin cells may give rise to gastrinomas in the pancreas, duodenum, or adjacent structures. Because of an accelerated growth of exocrine cells after birth, islets account for only 2% of the adult pancreatic mass and weigh approximately 1 g. The adult human pancreas contains about 10^6 islets scattered throughout the parenchyma. Islets vary greatly in size. Most islets are small, but the largest 15% of islets make up 60% of total islet volume. Location of cells within the islet itself is tightly regulated: beta cells occupy the center, and the peripheral mantle is composed of α, Δ, and PP cells. Any single cell may secrete more than one peptide; for example, the α cell may secrete cholecystokinin (CCK). Arterioles pierce the islet through short discontinuities of the mantle, entering directly into the β-cell core. Efferent capillaries pass through the mantle of non-beta cells. This portovenous islet flow has given rise to the concept that there is a simple β to α to Δ cell order of cellular perfusion, with resultant control of glucagon secretion, for example, depending on insulin output.

It is unclear whether all endocrine-to-endocrine cell signaling is carried out via the interislet circulation or whether some may be simply cell-to-cell paracrine effects.

There is a regional distribution of islet cells in the pancreas. The head of the pancreas is rich in PP cells. Glucagon-producing α cells predominate in the body and tail. β and Δ

cells are evenly distributed. The physiologic significance of this distribution is unknown.

Studies show a possible portovenous connection between endocrine islets and exocrine acini. Insulin and glucagon act antagonistically on the exocrine pancreas, with insulin stimulating and glucagon inhibiting exocrine pancreatic cell function. It is unclear if somatostatin acts via its inhibitory effect on islet β cells or acts directly on acinar cells via somatostatin receptors.

EXOCRINE PANCREAS PHYSIOLOGY

The final secretory product of the human exocrine pancreas is a clear isotonic solution with a pH in the range of 8. The two distinct components of pancreatic exocrine secretion are enzyme secretion originating from acinar cells and water and electrolyte secretion originating from the duct cells. Basal secretory rates of pancreatic exocrine products average 0.25 mL per minute, with rates approaching 5.0 mL per minute with maximal secretin stimulation. On a daily basis, the pancreas delivers between 6 and 20 g of digestive enzymes to the duodenum, in up to 2.5 L of bicarbonate-rich fluid.

Electrolyte Secretion

The secretion of water and electrolytes is under both vagal and humoral control. The electrolyte composition of exocrine pancreatic juice varies with the rate of pancreatic secretion. The sodium and potassium concentrations remain constant and are approximately equivalent to plasma concentrations. In contrast, the anion concentration of pancreatic exocrine secretion depends on the secretory rate. At low secretory rates, the concentrations of chloride and bicarbonate ions are equivalent to plasma, but with neurohumoral stimulation the bicarbonate component increases in concentration and the chloride anion concentration decreases (Fig. 31-4). The transport of bicarbonate from blood to duct lumen is an active process, with bicarbonate ions leaving the cell by a chloride-bicarbonate exchanger, the activity of which depends on the presence of chloride in the duct lumen. Secretin is the most potent endogenous stimulant of pancreatic bicarbonate secretion. Secretin is synthesized in the mucosal S cells of the crypts of Lieberkühn of the proximal small bowel and is released in the presence of luminal acid and bile. Secretin circulates in the blood and binds to secretin receptors on pancreatic ductal cells, effecting signal transduction through the intracellular adenylate cyclase system, with an increase in cyclic adenosine monophosphate (cAMP).

Enzyme Secretion

Total enzyme synthesis has been estimated at 10^7 enzyme molecules per acinar cell per minute. A stepwise sequence of intracellular events produces the final exocrine digestive enzyme products. Amino acids accumulate in the acinar cell through specific membrane transporters against a marked concentration gradient. Protein synthesis occurs in the ribosomes. The initial pre-proenzymes are released in the rough endoplasmic reticulum and pass through the Golgi apparatus, where they undergo posttranslational processing and are packaged within a glycoprotein vesicular membrane. The Golgi apparatus sorts the proteins destined for either lysosomes or zymogen granules. The zymogen granules contain a full complement of digestive enzymes. Zymogen granules then migrate to the acinar cell apex for extrusion of the granule into the luminal space (exocytosis) (Fig. 31-5). Specific enzymes synthesized and released include endopeptidases (trypsin, chymotrypsin, elastase, and kallikrein) and exopeptidases (carboxypeptidase A and B). Other synthesized enzymes include phospholipase, lipase, amylase, ribonuclease, and deoxyribonuclease. The peptidases synthesized by acinar cells are released into the pancreatic ductal system in inactive forms. In the duodenum, mucosal enterokinase cleaves trypsinogen to trypsin. Trypsin then activates the other peptidases. In contrast to the peptidases, ribonuclease, deoxyribonuclease, amylase, and lipase are released into the pancreatic ductal system in their active forms. Specific enzymes acting on acinar cell receptors mediate the control of pancreatic acinar cell secretion. CCK and acetylcholine stimulate acinar cell enzyme secretion by a membrane transduction process involving the activation of phospholipase C and the inositol pathway (I3P). CCK is the most potent endogenous hormonal stimulant of pancreatic enzyme secretion.

Phases of Digestion

The response of the pancreas to digestion is classically divided into three phases. During the *cephalic phase*, stimuli (smell and taste) activate vagal efferent signals, which

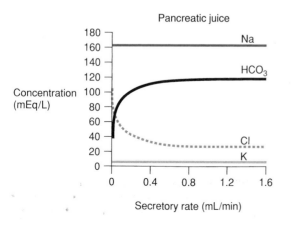

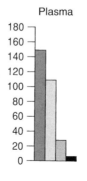

Figure 31-4   Relation of pancreatic electrolyte secretion and electrolyte concentration. (From Bro-Rasmussen F, Kilman SA, Thaysen JH. *Acta Physiol Scand* 1956;37:97, with permission.)

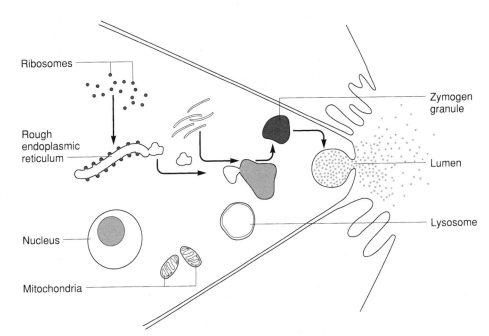

Figure 31-5 Normal acinar cell ultrastructure. Cytoplasmic processing of the proenzymes with apical discharge into the acinar ductule by means of zymogen granule exocytosis. (From Andersen DK, Brunicardi FC. Pancreas. In: Greenfield LJ, Mullholand MW, Oldham KT et al., eds. *Surgery: Scientific principles and practice*, 3rd ed. Philadelphia: Lippincott Williams & Wilkins, 2001, with permission.)

stimulate pancreatic enzyme release. In addition, cephalic-phase stimulation of gastric acid secretion causes duodenal acidification, which stimulates secretin release and subsequent pancreatic bicarbonate secretion. The net effect of cephalic-phase stimulation is the secretion of an enzyme-rich, bicarbonate-poor fluid. During the *gastric phase,* antral distention and antral protein stimulate the release of gastrin. Gastrin promotes gastric acid secretion and, because of the sequence homology between gastrin and CCK, also serves as a weak direct stimulator of pancreatic enzyme secretion. Gastrin-stimulated gastric acid secretion leads to pancreatic bicarbonate secretion by duodenal acidification and subsequent secretin release. Stimulation of vagal reflexes by antral distention also has a role in the gastric phase. During the *intestinal phase* of digestion (the most important phase), the hormones secretin and CCK serve a major function in mediating pancreatic exocrine secretion. Duodenal acid and bile stimulate secretin release, with pancreatic bicarbonate secretion from duct cells. Duodenal fat and protein release CCK, with release of pancreatic enzymes from acinar cells.

ENDOCRINE PANCREAS PHYSIOLOGY

The chief physiologic function of the endocrine pancreas can be starkly summarized as the regulation of body energy, which is largely achieved by hormonal control of carbohydrate metabolism. Simply stated, insulin is the hormone of energy storage and glucagon the hormone of energy release. Insulin stores energy by decreasing blood glucose level, increasing protein synthesis, decreasing glycogenolysis, decreasing lipolysis, and increasing glucose transport into cells (except beta cells, hepatocytes, and central nervous system cells). Glucagon releases energy by increasing blood glucose level via stimulation of glycogenolysis and stimulating gluconeogenesis and lipolysis.

Insulin

The insulin molecule is arranged into A and B chains connected by two disulfide bridges. In newly synthesized insulin, these chains are joined by means of a connecting (C) peptide. Patients with type I (insulin-dependent) diabetes have undergone loss of beta cells and have an absolute insulin deficiency. There is an abundant supply of beta cells: development of diabetes requires destruction of more than 80% of the beta cells. Insulin secretion is regulated by circulating levels of glucose and by humoral and neural factors. Beta cells have a very sensitive glucose-sensing mechanism with an immediate output of stored insulin that lasts about 5 minutes, followed by a longer sustained secretion of newly synthesized insulin. The insulin response to an oral ingestion of glucose is greater than the insulin response to an identical dose of glucose given intravenously, even though blood levels of glucose may be the same. Several gastrointestinal peptides have the capacity to augment nutrient-induced release of insulin. These insulinotropic factors act directly on beta cells and are called incretins. Gastric inhibitory peptide (GIP) is the best candidate for a physiologic incretin action, with CCK a distant second. Inhibitors of insulin release include somatostatin, pancreastatin, amylin, and the fatty tissue hormone leptin. Stating that the vagus stimulates release of insulin and the sympathetic nervous system inhibits it can summarize neural control of insulin release. However, alpha-sympathetic fibers inhibit insulin secretion, but beta fibers stimulate the secretion. In addition, the peptides released by nerve fibers modulate the secretion by both alpha and beta cells. Secreted insulin is transported rapidly to the portovenous system, and 50% is cleared by hepatocytes on first transit of the liver; insulin has a $t^{1}/_{2}$ of 7 to 10 minutes. All cells except cerebrocytes and red blood cells take up insulin. A major role of insulin is in promoting glucose transport into cells, and this transport may be enhanced by regulation of membrane-bound glucose transporter peptides. Insulin binds to a specific membrane receptor. Peripheral resistance to insulin may result from either a diminished number of receptors or a decreased receptor affinity for insulin. Type II diabetes is caused at least in part by receptor defects leading to insulin resistance. The complexity of control of insulin metabolism has been demonstrated repeatedly in normal individuals and in diabetic patients.

Glucagon

Glucagon, secreted by the α cells of the islet, is a straight chain, polypeptide, the main function of which is to promote conversion of hepatic glycogen to glucose. As with insulin, glucagon secretion is controlled by a complex interaction of neural, hormonal, and nutrient factors. As with insulin, the primary regulator of glucagon release is circulating glucose, high levels of which inhibit glucagon secretion. Glucagon and insulin exercise a reciprocal control of carbohydrate metabolism. Failure of glucagon secretion can cause hypoglycemia, and excess glucagon may bring about hyperglycemia. Insulin and somatostatin suppress glucagon release, probably via the islet portovenous system. Neural control of glucagon output is similar to that of insulin, but sympathetic neural transmitters and epinephrine stimulate the α cell, whereas they inhibit the β cell.

Somatostatin

Somatostatin, proposed to be a universal hormonal "off-switch," is a small, straight chain polypeptide that is secreted by Δ cells. Although it is assumed that somatostatin has a modulating influence on secretion of other islet hormones, its actual function within the pancreas is unknown. In addition, the question remains whether somatostatin acts through transport via the islet portovenous system or by simple paracrine effect. The full molecule has a short half-life, but the octapeptide analog octreotide has a longer life and has been used to treat secretory diarrhea, bowel fistulas, and endocrine hypersecretory syndromes.

Pancreatic Polypeptide

PP is a straight-chain molecule secreted by PP cells that are located primarily in the uncinate process and the head of the pancreas. The physiologic actions of PP are unknown, and its clinical usefulness is limited to its role as a marker for other endocrine tumors of the pancreas. Absence of PP may play a role in insulin resistant diabetes seen after pancreatic head resection or after chronic atrophic pancreatitis.

Other Peptides

VIP is secreted by the $\Delta 2$ cell of the pancreas and is found throughout the gastrointestinal tract. It stimulates insulin, inhibits gastric secretion, and causes vasodilation and bronchodilation. Amylin is secreted by the β cells and inhibits insulin secretion and uptake. Pancreastatin, part of the larger molecule chromogranin α, is found in the envelope of secretory granules and inhibits insulin secretion. Gastrin cells are present in fetal but not in normal adult islets. Other peptides (CCK, endorphin, etc.) have been reported in normal islets and in islet cell tumors.

ACUTE PANCREATITIS

Acute pancreatitis is an acute inflammatory process of the pancreas, with variable involvement of other organ systems. The disease encompasses a broad spectrum of disease, which varies from mild parenchymal edema to severe hemorrhagic pancreatitis with subsequent gangrene and necrosis. The clinical presentation varies, from episodes of mild abdominal discomfort to a severe illness associated with hypotension, metabolic derangements, fluid sequestration, multiorgan failure, sepsis, and death. Most patients experience mild-to-moderate symptoms and a self-limited course, and they improve with supportive care. In contrast, 10% of patients develop a life-threatening form of acute pancreatitis. In the initial phase, dehydration and hypotension, pulmonary edema, renal failure, and cardiac dysfunction contribute to most of the mortality, whereas patients who die after day 7 succumb to pancreatic abscess, infection, and multisystem organ failure.

In 90% of cases, the cause is related to excessive alcohol intake or biliary tract disease. The exact mechanism of *alcohol-related pancreatitis* is unknown but the association is undeniable. First, alcohol-related pancreatitis may be the result of pancreatic exocrine hypersecretion in the presence of partial ampullary obstruction. A second mechanism suggests that alcohol may initiate enzyme extravasation and cause pancreatic injury as a result of protein plugging of the pancreatic duct. A third mechanism involves the transient state of hypertriglyceridemia, which is known to occur after alcohol ingestion in some individuals. A fourth mechanism involves injury generated by oxygen-derived free radicals, such as the super oxide radical and the hydroxyl radical.

Gallstone pancreatitis is related to the anatomic existence of a common channel between the pancreatic and bile ducts, and it occurs in the setting of gallstone migration through the ampullary region. The migration of a gallstone, and not necessarily its impaction, initiates the pancreatic injury because it allows bile and duodenal contents into the pancreatic duct, which causes pancreatic cell injury. Acute pancreatitis affects between 3% and 8% of all patients with symptomatic gallstones and up to 30% of those with microlithiasis (stones smaller than 3 mm in diameter).

Many other causes of acute pancreatitis exist (Table 31-1). *Hyperlipidemia* may cause injury through free fatty acids liberated from triglycerides by lipase in the pancreatic microcirculation with subsequent microvascular ischemic injury. *Hypercalcemia* is occasionally associated with acute pancreatitis and generally is seen in the setting of hyperparathyroidism. The incidence of pancreatitis in hyperparathyroidism is less than 2%. The mechanism may involve calcium-induced trypsinogen activation, calcium-associated stone precipitation in the pancreatic duct, or calcium-stimulated pancreatic exocrine hypersecretion.

Patients with *hereditary pancreatitis* present with aspects of pancreatitis, often with a family history. This entity is caused by a mutation in the trypsin gene. The mutation prevents intracellular trypsin from being inactivated, with the subsequent likelihood of uncontrolled proteolytic activity in the pancreas. Acute pancreatitis may also occur after *pancreatic trauma* or may be caused by *ERCP* with pancreatic ductal over distention during retrograde

TABLE 31-1
CAUSES OF ACUTE PANCREATITIS

Alcohol	Ethanol
Biliary tract	Gall stones
	Biliary tract obstruction
Trauma	Direct impact
	ERCP
	Surgery
Metabolic disorders	Hyperparathyroidism
	Hyperlipidemia
	Hypercalcemia
Infection and ischemia	Viral and bacterial
	Hypotension, cardiopulmonary bypass
Mechanical obstruction	Pancreas, duodenal, bile duct tumor
	Duodenal obstruction
	Pancreas divisum, ampullary stenosis
Rare causes	Drugs
	Pregnancy
	Idiopathic

ERCP, endoscopic retrograde cholangiopancreatography.

pancreatography. *Pancreatic ischemia* as a result of systemic hypotension, visceral atheroembolism, or vasculitis can also cause acute pancreatitis. Many patients with presumed *"idiopathic pancreatitis"* harbor small biliary stones or sludge, termed microlithiasis, which can cause pancreatitis. Cholecystectomy or endoscopic sphincterotomy may prevent relapse. *Drug-induced* acute pancreatitis accounts for less than 5% of all cases of acute pancreatitis and is usually mild, with the exceptions of pancreatitis secondary to dideoxyinosine, pentamidine, and valproic acid.

The actual events on a cellular and molecular level responsible for the initiation of pancreatic parenchymal injury causing acute pancreatitis have not been fully elucidated. Studies suggest that prevention of zymogen-granule exocytosis causes fusion of the zymogen granules with intracellular lysosomes to create autophagosomes. Intracellular activation of trypsinogen to trypsin leads to activation of other proenzymes and cellular autodigestion.

Diagnosis

The clinical presentation, supported by appropriate laboratory determinations and radiographic findings normally leads to the diagnosis of acute pancreatitis. The predominant clinical feature of acute pancreatitis is abdominal pain. It is classically located in the midepigastrium, has a penetrating quality, and radiates to the back. Nausea and vomiting frequently accompany the abdominal pain. A diverse spectrum of illness is seen, varying from a mild, short-lived, self-limited disease to a severe toxic condition associated with shock, hypovolemia, multiple metabolic derangements, and death.

Typical findings on physical examination in patients with acute pancreatitis include fever, tachycardia, epigastric tenderness, and abdominal distention. Hemorrhage into the retroperitoneum may produce distinctive physical signs: the Turner sign (bluish discoloration in the left flank), the Cullen sign (bluish discoloration of the periumbilical region), and the Fox sign (bluish discoloration below the inguinal ligament or at the base of the penis). Fewer than

3% of patients present with these signs and they signal a severe episode of acute hemorrhagic pancreatitis with a mortality of up to 30%. Jaundice is not a frequent finding at the initial presentation of acute pancreatitis and suggests common duct stones with cholangitis. Acute pancreatitis can lead to a major systemic inflammatory response syndrome (SIRS) with hemodynamic alterations of a "sepsis-like syndrome." This is a hyperdynamic state with hypotension, elevated cardiac output, lowered systemic vascular resistance, and a lowered arteriovenous oxygen difference. Extraabdominal manifestations include left pleural effusion, left hemidiaphragm elevation or acute pulmonary failure. Acute renal failure may require dialysis. Other symptoms include subcutaneous fat necrosis and mental status changes. In severe cases disseminated intravascular coagulopathy can present.

Laboratory Determinations

Serum amylase is the most widely used laboratory test in the diagnosis of acute pancreatitis. Elevated amylase presents within 24 hours of the onset of symptoms and gradually normalizes in the following 7 days. Persistent high amylase levels may indicate ongoing acute pancreatic inflammation or the development of complications such as pancreatic ascites, pancreatic pseudocyst, or abscess. The actual amylase value is not a reliable predictor of the severity of pancreatitis. Higher amylase levels are more common in gallstone-associated pancreatitis. Serum amylase alone is limited as a marker for acute pancreatitis. Many other causes of hyperamylasemia exist (Table 31-2). In an acute hospital setting, 30% of elevated amylase is unrelated to acute pancreatitis (false-positive rate). The absence of hyperamylasemia does not exclude the diagnosis of acute pancreatitis (false-negative rate of 10%). Patients with hyperlipidemia-induced acute pancreatitis often present with normoamylasemia, possibly related to a circulating inhibitor of amylase activity. Measuring pancreatic isoenzymes may be beneficial in further elucidating falsely positive amylase levels. P-Type amylase arises from the pancreas and represents 40% of circulating amylase. The remaining 60%, S-type amylase, derives from salivary glands, fallopian tubes, ovaries, endometrium, prostate, breast, lung, and possibly liver. The urinary amylase excretion and the renal clearance of amylase are of limited clinical value. Elevated serum lipase is an indicator of acute pancreatitis and the duration of hyperlipasemia often

TABLE 31-2
HYPERAMYLASEMIA

Intraabdominal	Extraabdominal
• Pancreatic disorders	• Salivary gland disorders
• Nonpancreatic disorders	• Renal failure
• Biliary tract disorders	• Miscellaneous
• Intestinal disorders	• Pneumonia
• Intraabdominal vascular	• Trauma
• Peritonitis	• Burns
• Gynecologic disorders	• Diabetic ketoacidosis
	• Pregnancy
	• Drugs

exceeds that of hyperamylasemia. However, hyperlipasemia is also observed in other disease states such as perforated peptic ulcer, acute cholecystitis, and intestinal ischemia, and is not entirely specific for acute pancreatitis. Serum lactescence may be seen in patients with hyperlipidemia-associated pancreatitis or in alcohol-associated pancreatitis. Patients with lactescent serum usually have falsely normal serum amylase levels, and the finding of serum lactescence is one of the most specific indicators of acute pancreatitis. Standard laboratory tests such as hemoconcentration, elevated white blood cell (WBC) count, hyperglycemia, mild azotemia, and hypocalcemia may support the diagnosis. Abnormal liver function tests are more commonly found in gallstone-associated pancreatitis. Severe pancreatitis may also cause dramatic coagulation abnormalities marked by hypercoagulability, disseminated intravascular coagulation, and hypofibrinogenemia.

Abdominal radiographs may reveal nonspecific abnormalities. Most frequently seen is the presence of air in the duodenal loop, representing a local duodenal ileus. Also common is the *sentinel loop sign*, which represents a dilated proximal jejunal loop. The *colon cutoff sign* indicates distention of the colon to the level of the transverse colon, with absence of air present in the more distal colon. Abdominal ultrasonography (US) is used to detect gallstones. Although US has an overall accuracy of more than 95% for detecting gallbladder stones, its accuracy for gallbladder stones falls to only 70% to 80% in acute pancreatitis because of intestinal air and smaller stones. Currently, the most widely used method to confirm the diagnosis of acute pancreatitis is contrast-enhanced CT. Nearly all patients with acute pancreatitis have some abnormalities on computerized tomographic (CT) scan. A correlation exists between the degree of CT abnormality and the severity of acute pancreatitis. It is additionally useful for evaluating complications such as pancreatic abscess, pseudocyst, or necrosis. Generally, ERCP plays no role in the evaluation of acute pancreatitis. Elective ERCP may identify potentially correctable abnormalities in 50% of patients with recurrent episodes of acute pancreatitis without an obvious cause. These include findings such as pancreas divisum, stenosis of the ampulla of Vater, or focal pancreatic duct abnormalities.

Clinical Course

The clinical course in up to 90% of patients with acute pancreatitis follows a mild, self-limited pattern. However, in 10% to 15% of patients with acute pancreatitis, a severe form of illness develops, with significant associated morbidity and mortality. Predicting the severity of an attack of pancreatitis and determining the overall prognosis is possible using routinely available clinical and laboratory tests. The most widely used predictive criteria involve 11 prognostic signs identified by Ranson (Table 31-3). A modification of the Ranson score for patients with gallstone pancreatitis has been developed because the Ranson score is less accurate in that setting. The application of the Ranson prognostic scoring system allows early stratification of patients based on predicted outcome, and allows the triage of patients to the appropriate treatment plan. Patients who present with two or fewer prognostic signs have essentially no mortality, and simple supportive care suffices in their management. Patients with three or four

TABLE 31-3
RANSON CRITERIA FOR PANCREATITIS

	Pancreatitis	Gallstone Pancreatitis
Admission		
Age (y)	>55	>70
WBC count (per mm^3)	>16,000	>18,000
Glucose (mg/dL)	>200	>220
LDH (IU/L)	>350	>400
AST (IU/L)	>250	>250
Within 48 hours		
Hematocrit decrease (points)	>10	>10
BUN increase (mg/dL)	>5	>2
Calcium (mg/dL)	<8	<8
PaO$_2$ (mmHg)	<60	<60
Base deficit (mEq/L)	>4	>5
Fluid requirement (L)	>6	>4

AST, aspartate aminotransferase; BUN, blood urea nitrogen; LDH, lactate dehydrogenase; WBC, white blood cell.
From Ranson JHC, Rifkind KM, Roses DF, et al. Prognostic signs and the role of operative management in acute pancreatitis. *Surg Gynecol Obstet* 1974;139:69; and Ranson JHC. Etiological and prognostic factors in human acute pancreatitis. *Am J Gastroenterol* 1982;77:633.

prognostic signs have a mortality that approximates 15%, with nearly one half the patients requiring support in an intensive care setting. If five or six prognostic signs are present, intensive care is usually required, and mortality approaches 50%. Patients with seven or more prognostic signs have an even higher predicted mortality. Other scoring systems based on multiple laboratory and radiographic evidence have been evaluated. These include the APACHE II, the Medical Research Council Sepsis (MRCS) score, and the Simplified Acute Physiology (SAP) score, among others. In addition, some laboratory test may have some correlation with severity of disease such as C-reactive protein, phospholipase A 2, pancreatitis-associated protein, interleukin-6, elastase, methemalbumin, and serum ribonuclease.

Nonoperative Management

The initial management of patients with acute pancreatitis is nonoperative. Acute pancreatitis is commonly associated with massive fluid sequestration secondary to paralytic ileus, edema in the peripancreatic region, and emesis. Generous fluid resuscitation with crystalloid solutions is essential in restoring circulating plasma volume. The serum calcium concentration is often depressed secondary to hypoalbuminemia with normal ionized calcium levels. Calcium supplementation is indicated only in patients with low ionized calcium levels. Low magnesium should be corrected, because this will enhance the normalization of serum ionized calcium. Mild hyperglycemia is a frequent finding that improves with volume resuscitation but may require insulin therapy. Meperidine is the preferred drug for abdominal pain. Because morphine has the potential for causing spasm of the sphincter of Oddi, it is generally avoided. Percutaneous splanchnic nerve blocks and epidural analgesia can also be used. Oral intake is withheld completely. Nasogastric decompression is reserved for patients with significant ileus. Oral intake can generally be resumed during the first week when symptoms have improved. Premature return to oral intake has been associated with reactivation of pancreatic inflammation. In patients with severe pancreatitis and complications, nutritional support is indicated. Studies indicate that enteral alimentation may offer some advantages over total parenteral nutrition (TPN). Antibiotics are not indicated in the routine treatment of mild-to-moderate pancreatitis but accumulating data support the use of prophylactic antibiotic treatment in patients with severe pancreatitis, defined as more than three Ranson signs in association with CT evidence of pancreatic or peripancreatic necrosis. Respiratory and renal failure may require ventilation support and dialysis.

In addition to these standard supportive measures, specific therapies have undergone trial under experimental or clinical conditions. Therapeutic attempts to suppress pancreatic enzyme secretion have included nasogastric suction antacids, anticholinergics, glucagon, calcitonin, somatostatin, peptide YY, and CCK-receptor antagonists such as proglumide. None of these therapies are effective in shortening the duration of the disease, in reducing complications, or in reducing mortality. H 2-receptor antagonists or antacids are indicated as prophylaxis against upper gastrointestinal tract hemorrhage in patients with severe pancreatitis. Octreotide, a long-acting somatostatin analog, has no proven benefit in patients with acute pancreatitis.

Operative Management

Unexpected Finding During Exploratory Laparotomy

Because of the accuracy of current imaging studies, acute pancreatitis is only rarely encountered as an unexpected finding during exploratory laparotomy. In this setting, any ascitic fluid should be analyzed and cultured. In patients with evidence of cholelithiasis, cholecystectomy and intraoperative cholangiography is recommended. In patients with severe necrotizing pancreatitis without frank infection, cautious débridement of necrotic tissue with wide retroperitoneal drainage, tube gastrostomy to facilitate gastric decompression, and tube jejunostomy for early external feeding is recommended. If systemic toxicity and gross evidence of severe pancreatitis associated with large amounts of ascites is present, the placement of a peritoneal dialysis catheter should be considered.

Infectious Complications

Pancreatic abscess, infected pancreatic pseudocyst, and infected pancreatic necrosis are three life-threatening complications of acute pancreatitis that occur in up to 5% of patients. They occur in direct proportion to the severity of acute pancreatitis and correlate with the degree of pancreatic necrosis. In patients with six or more of Ranson prognostic signs, more than 50% develop a pancreatic septic complication. These are polymicrobial infections of enteric origin, which may arise from transmural migration of bacteria from adjacent inflamed bowel or from hematogenous seeding. Fungal infection is now recognized with increased frequency. The development of pancreatic septic complications should be suspected in patients with severe pancreatitis, in patients with documented bacteremia, and in patients with clinical deterioration or failure of resolution of the pancreatitis

within the first week to 10 days. Clinical manifestations include fever, tachycardia, abdominal pain, and abdominal distention. Associated laboratory abnormalities include persistent hyperamylasemia, nonspecific elevations of liver function tests, and leukocytosis. Plain abdominal films may show extraluminal retroperitoneal air, described as the *soap bubble sign*. Contrast-enhanced CT scanning is the most widely used and accurate procedure for evaluating potential pancreatic septic complications. In addition, CT is the "gold standard" for the noninvasive diagnosis of pancreatic abscess, with an accuracy of more than 90% when parenchymal necrosis is greater than 30%. The combination of abdominal CT scan and guided percutaneous needle aspiration is highly reliable in differentiating a pancreatic infectious process from a sterile peripancreatic phlegmon.

Treatment of secondary pancreatic infections combines antibiotic therapy with prompt surgical drainage. Only a few patients with solitary, well-defined pancreatic abscesses or infected pancreatic pseudocysts may be managed by percutaneous drainage techniques. In patients with infected pancreatic necrosis, operative débridement is indicated. The two currently accepted operative management strategies for infected pancreatic necrosis and some pancreatic abscesses are (i) laparotomy with débridement and wide sump drainage (often accompanied by postoperative retroperitoneal lavage), and (ii) laparotomy with débridement, open packing, and scheduled repacking.

Correction of Associated Biliary Tract Disease

Early surgical intervention is recommended in patients with gallstone pancreatitis because gallstone pancreatitis without early surgical intervention can lead to early recurrence in approximately 35% of patients. Most episodes of gallstone-associated pancreatitis are mild, and laparoscopic cholecystectomy at the time of the index admission has proved to be safe and cost-effective. This is normally performed after clinical resolution of the pancreatitis with normalization of the liver function tests.

For patients who present early with gallstone pancreatitis accompanied by either jaundice or cholangitis, the initial management includes urgent ERCP with endoscopic sphincterotomy (ES). For patients with severe gallstone pancreatitis, several weeks are allowed to elapse between the hospitalization for acute pancreatitis and readmission for laparoscopic cholecystectomy.

Deterioration of Clinical Status

The role of surgical intervention in patients with acute pancreatitis and a deteriorating clinical course remains controversial. Recommended operative procedures have ranged from local débridement of obviously necrotic tissue (necrosectomy) to formal total pancreatectomy. However, to date, no controlled randomized clinical trials allow realistic evaluation of the efficacy of such early resection therapies.

CHRONIC PANCREATITIS

Chronic pancreatitis presents as recurrent or persistent abdominal pain caused by pancreatic inflammation, and is characterized by exocrine and endocrine pancreatic insufficiency caused by irreversible destruction of pancreatic tissue. Pathologic findings in chronic pancreatitis include evidence of acinar loss, glandular shrinkage, proliferative fibrosis, calcification, and ductal structuring, with evidence of dense collagen and fibroblastic proliferation in the parenchyma. This fibroproliferative response separates large clusters of islet cells with normal features.

Etiology

Chronic pancreatitis is associated with alcohol abuse, hyperlipoproteinemia, hypercalcemia, cystic fibrosis, and congenital anomalies of the pancreatic duct such as pancreas divisum, pancreatic trauma, and hereditary pancreatitis. The most common cause of chronic pancreatitis in industrialized countries is alcohol abuse (60% to 80%). The exact etiology of alcohol-related pancreatitis is unknown, but alcohol is a weak toxin to the pancreas. Dietary factors such as protein and high-fat intake have a permissive role. In developing countries, tropical chronic pancreatitis appears to be related to nutritional deficiencies or toxin ingestion. Hyperparathyroidism and the associated hypercalcemia may overstimulate the exocrine secretions of the gland and induce precipitation of protein aggregates within the main pancreatic ductal system. Idiopathic chronic pancreatitis has been associated with social drinking, analgesic abuse, autoimmune diseases (primary sclerosing cholangitis, Sjögren syndrome, primary biliary cirrhosis), or genetic abnormalities.

Various mechanisms may play a role in the pathogenesis of chronic pancreatitis. These include hypersecretion of protein from acinar cells, plugging of the pancreatic ducts with protein precipitates, and pancreatic ductal hypertension. The genetic abnormalities found in cystic fibrosis (CFTR gene mutations) and hereditary pancreatitis (mutations in the cationic trypsinogen gene) were also found in up to 10% of patients with idiopathic pancreatitis.

Clinical Presentation

The incidence of chronic pancreatitis is 4 cases per 100,000 individuals per year. The tetrad of abdominal pain, weight loss, diabetes, and steatorrhea serves as a classic clinical presentation in patients with chronic pancreatitis. Many patients present with a history of narcotic abuse, used in an effort to control their abdominal pain. Anorexia and weight loss may be present. Insulin-dependent diabetes occurs in up to one third of patients. Up to one fourth have steatorrhea, indicative of a major reduction in pancreatic exocrine function.

Diagnosis

Before surgical intervention is warranted, mandatory evaluation of pancreatic disease involves parenchymal imaging by CT scan or MRI examination, as well as assessment of pancreatic ductal anatomy by ERCP or magnetic resonance cholangiopancreatography (MRCP). Routine laboratory tests are rarely helpful. Pancreatic calcifications on plain abdominal films are at least 95% specific for chronic pancreatitis but not sensitive. Abdominal US has a sensitivity that varies between 50% and 90%.

Important information can also be gained by endoscopic US and by the use of ERCP. Pancreatography can document ductal abnormalities not convincingly demonstrated by CT scan and has an essential role in guiding surgical therapy. Early changes observed by pancreatography include ductal dilation and filling of secondary and tertiary branches, which ordinarily are not visualized. The characteristic chain-of-lakes pancreatogram, representing ductal dilation in concert with ductal stricturing, is a classic finding in chronic pancreatitis, but it is not observed as frequently as uniform ductal dilatation. An entirely normal pancreatogram in a patient with abdominal pain eliminates the diagnosis of chronic pancreatitis. MRCP images in patients with chronic pancreatitis have results nearly comparable to the images obtained by ERCP. Pancreatic exocrine function tests such as the Lundh test meal are not essential for preoperative evaluation. A simple test to evaluate exocrine pancreatic function is measurement of fecal fat excretion with Sudan stain. Pancreatic endocrine function can be assessed by the glucose tolerance test. More than two thirds of all patients with chronic pancreatitis have abnormal results, but less than one third of patients are insulin dependent. Peripheral neuropathy is a common finding and appears to be related to both diabetes and the effects of alcohol. Endocrine function is generally unaffected by ductal drainage procedures but is reduced by resectional therapies.

Nonoperative Management

The nonoperative management of chronic pancreatitis is directed toward control of abdominal pain, treatment of endocrine insufficiency, and treatment of exocrine insufficiency. In addition, in some patients, endoscopic approaches may be applicable.

Therapeutic options for the control of abdominal pain include total abstinence from alcohol, dietary manipulation, and substitution of medium-chain triglycerides for long-chain fat and high-dosage regimens of exogenous pancreatic enzyme supplements. All of these measures have variable outcomes. Octreotide, the octapeptide analog of native somatostatin, may improve pain. Pain control often requires the early use of nonnarcotic analgesics, followed later by narcotic analgesics. Insulin therapy in patients with chronic pancreatitis–associated diabetes must be used cautiously because of poor nutrient absorption secondary to malabsorption or the irregular caloric intake typical of alcoholics. A 90% reduction in endogenous enzyme secretion is needed to produce malabsorption. Treatment includes low-fat diet and exogenous pancreatic enzyme supplementation. Proton pump agents are given to prevent the acid-induced degradation of exogenous enzyme preparations. Enteric-coated enzyme supplement preparations, particularly enteric-coated microspheres, are an alternative therapy. Various endoscopic techniques have evolved for the management of diverse clinical problems associated with chronic pancreatitis. These techniques include pancreatic sphincterotomy, pancreatic duct stenting, and pancreatic stone extraction. Although many novel endoscopic treatments are technically possible in patients with chronic pancreatitis, the long-term results of endoscopic therapy are largely unknown.

Operative Management

The goal of surgery for chronic pancreatitis is relief of pain with maximum preservation of endocrine and exocrine function. The different approaches to attain this goal include ampullary procedures, ductal drainage procedures, denervation procedures, and ablative procedures. Ablative procedures are usually considered the last step in surgical treatment for patients with chronic pancreatitis because of the fear of producing insulin-dependent diabetes mellitus.

Ampullary Procedures

The indication for ampullary procedures is limited. Transduodenal sphincteroplasty and pancreatic duct septoplasty is indicated for patients with a focal obstruction at the ampullary orifice. Transduodenal minor papilloplasty is successful in patients with pancreas divisum associated with recurrent acute pancreatitis but less effective in pancreas divisum and established chronic pancreatitis.

Ductal Drainage Procedures

The side-to-side pancreaticojejunostomy (Puestow procedure) is the most commonly applied pancreatic ductal drainage procedure, and it is recommended in patients with a dilated pancreatic duct in need of operative therapy for chronic pancreatitis (Fig. 31-6). It has widely replaced the former end-to-end caudal pancreaticojejunostomy of Duval. In patients with early disease, this procedure may delay the rate of progressive functional impairment of the pancreas.

Denervation Procedures

The results of denervation procedures are limited. Some approaches such as chemical splanchnicectomy can be used as an adjunct to other surgical interventions. Neuroablation in the treatment of pancreatic pain can be implemented in several ways including celiac ganglionectomy, thoracic splanchnicectomy, and chemical splanchnicectomy through infiltration of the celiac ganglion with ethanol.

Ablative Procedures

The operative treatment of chronic pancreatitis by surgical resection of the pancreas is associated with variable success rates (60% to 80% obtain adequate pain relief). Left-sided procedures, such as limited distal pancreatectomy (with or without splenectomy) may be indicated in patients with disease in the body and tail of the pancreas. Right-sided procedures such as Pylorus-preserving pancreaticoduodenectomy (modified Whipple operation) are indicated if the head of the pancreas is primarily affected. The modified Whipple procedure has the advantage of also providing relief of associated biliary or duodenal obstruction and preserving a substantial mass of islet cell tissue in the body and tail of the gland.

Total pancreatectomy, in essence, represents a procedure used for earlier surgical failures. However, the significant problems associated with labile insulin sensitivity, steatorrhea, and weight loss dictate that total pancreatectomy be applied as a last resort in carefully selected patients. Pancreatic autotransplantation should be considered in this setting.

Several alternative resection treatments exist with roughly equivalent results for pain relief and postoperative complications. The major advantage of using duodenum-sparing alternatives such as the Beger and the Frey procedure derives from the conservation of the endocrine capacity of the pancreas and the duodenum. The Beger procedure involves a duodenum-preserving resection of the

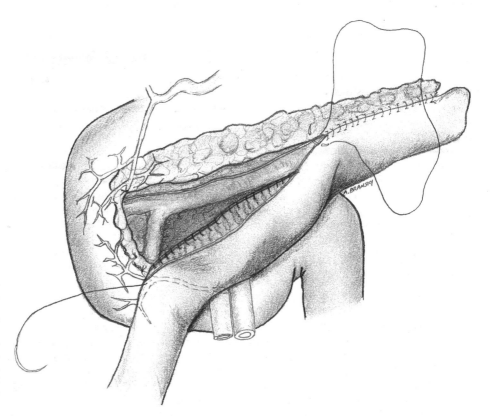

Figure 31-6 Longitudinal pancreaticojejunostomy (Puestow procedure). The main pancreatic duct is widely opened anteriorly and drained to a Roux-en-Y limb of the jejunum. (From Prinz RA, Deziel DJ, Bransky AS. Roux-enY lateral pancreaticojejunostomy for chronic pancreatitis. In: Baker RJ, Fischer JE. *Mastery of surgery*. Philadelphia: Lippincott Williams & Wilkins, 2001, with permission.)

pancreatic head combined with Roux-en-Y drainage of the retained main pancreatic duct in the neck of the gland. Frey popularized a modified side-to-side pancreaticojejunostomy with an anterior central resection or coring out of the pancreatic head.

DISRUPTIONS OF THE PANCREATIC DUCT

In adults, pancreatic duct disruptions are most commonly found in the setting of alcoholic pancreatitis. In children, trauma is the leading cause of pancreatic duct disruption. Disruptions of the main pancreatic duct can cause external or internal pancreatic fistulas. Pancreatic secretions may drain externally and create an external pancreaticocutaneous fistula. If adjacent tissues wall off the exocrine secretions, a pancreatic pseudocyst can develop. Pancreatic ascites occurs when the secretions drain freely from the pancreatic duct into the peritoneal cavity. A pancreatic pleural effusion can develop if secretions drain into the retroperitoneum and track through the diaphragm to enter the pleural space. Rarely, pancreatic secretions may erode into the intestine to form a pancreatic-enteric fistula.

External Pancreatic Fistula

Drainage of pancreatic exocrine secretions through an abdominal wound that persists for more than 7 days is, by definition, an external pancreatic fistula. Pancreaticocutaneous fistulas complicate pancreatic operations in as many as 25% of patients. Fistulas that drain less than 200 mL per day are termed low-output fistulas, whereas those draining in excess of 200 mL per day are high-output fistulas. Complications of pancreaticocutaneous fistulas include sepsis, fluid and electrolyte abnormalities, and skin excoriation. Sinography and CT are used to delineate the anatomy of the fistulous tract and to exclude the presence of undrained cavities. TPN is often used to avoid pancreatic stimulation. Octreotide has no clear benefit in external pancreatic fistulas. Most external pancreatic fistulas close with nonoperative management. Closure of external pancreatic fistulas may be assisted by endoscopic therapy including either sphincterotomy of the ampulla or pancreatic duct stenting. Refractory fistulas may require surgical management. Operative options include distal pancreatectomy with or without pancreaticojejunostomy for fistulas in the tail. Fistulas localized in the head, neck, or body of the gland can be managed by Roux-en-Y pancreaticojejunostomy to the fistula tract.

Internal Pancreatic Fistula

Pancreatic Pseudocyst

A pancreatic pseudocyst is a localized collection of pancreatic secretions in a cystic structure that lacks an epithelial lining. It is the result of walling-off a pancreatic duct disruption. Pancreatic pseudocysts may be located within the pancreatic parenchyma, but more often occur in one of the potential spaces that separate the pancreas from adjacent abdominal viscera. Pseudocysts contain a high concentration of pancreatic enzymes, including amylase, lipase, and trypsin. Pancreatic pseudocysts represent 75% to 80% of cystic lesions in the pancreas. Pancreatic pseudocysts develop in up to 10% of patients after an attack of acute alcoholic pancreatitis. Pseudocysts can also develop in the setting of other causes of acute or chronic pancreatitis, pancreatic trauma, and pancreatic neoplasms. By convention, collections of fluid containing pancreatic enzymes that occur within the first 3 weeks after an episode of acute pancreatitis are termed acute fluid collections and are not considered pseudocysts. Acute fluid collections should be termed pseudocysts if they persist beyond 4 weeks of the onset of acute pancreatitis. A 6-week period is generally allowed between the start of an episode of pancreatitis and elective operative intervention, to allow satisfactory internal drainage.

The mass effect of the pseudocyst can cause symptoms such as abdominal pain, early satiety, nausea, and vomiting secondary to gastroduodenal obstruction. Symptoms associated to complications include jaundice secondary to common bile duct obstruction, variceal bleeding secondary to either splenic vein or portal vein obstruction, sepsis secondary to pseudocyst infection, and intraabdominal hemorrhage secondary to bleeding from a pseudoaneurysm in adjacent visceral vessels. The initial study to evaluate a pancreatic pseudocyst is an abdominal CT. Laboratory findings in patients with pancreatic pseudocysts are nonspecific. Fluid analysis of a peripancreatic cystic structure may be helpful in further management. Asymptomatic pseudocysts are preferentially managed nonoperatively, with surgical intervention reserved for persistent abdominal pain, pseudocyst enlargement, or pseudocyst complications. Serial follow-up with CT or ultrasonography is performed to assess the size progression of the pseudocyst. Spontaneous resolution is observed in up to 60% of patients. Pseudocyst size still correlates with eventual need for operation: 67% of patients with pseudocysts larger than 6 cm will eventually required surgical therapy.

The preferred operative approach for an uncomplicated pseudocyst is internal drainage. This can be achieved by means of a cystojejunostomy or cystogastrostomy (Fig. 31-7). Surgical intervention should always include a biopsy of the pseudocyst wall to exclude a cystic pancreatic neoplasm. A cystogastrostomy is a faster and less technically demanding procedure than a Roux-en-Y cystojejunostomy but depends on the anatomic location of the pseudocyst. The indication for surgical excision is limited to distal pancreatic resections for pseudocysts in the tail of the gland. External drainage of pancreatic pseudocysts is indicated for infected pseudocysts, unstable patients, and for immature pseudocysts. A pancreaticocutaneous fistula occurs after external drainage, and it often closes spontaneously. Both percutaneous and endoscopic techniques have been used for the nonoperative management of pancreatic pseudocysts but the long-term efficacy of percutaneous catheter drainage has been poorly documented.

Pancreatic Ascites and Pancreatic Pleural Effusion

Pancreatic ascites and pancreatic pleural effusions are similar in presentation and management. Both entities result from a pancreatic duct disruption, in most cases related to alcohol. They can occasionally present in the absence of clinical pancreatitis. Pancreatic ascites occurs if the pancreatic secretions from a pancreatic duct disruption drain

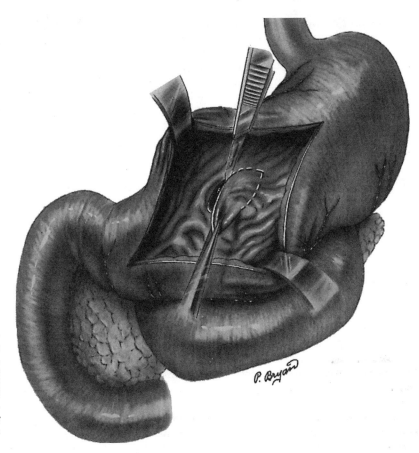

Figure 31-7 Drainage of pancreatic pseudocyst into the stomach. Once an incision has been made through the posterior wall of the stomach, through the cyst wall, and into the pseudocyst, a continuous locking suture is placed through and through the posterior wall of the stomach and the cyst wall. (From Bradley EL. Pancreatic cystenterostomy. In: Baker RJ, Fischer JE. *Mastery of surgery*. Philadelphia: Lippincott Williams & Wilkins, 2001, with permission.)

anteriorly into the peritoneal cavity. In pancreatic pleural effusion, the secretions drain posteriorly into the retroperitoneum and then into the mediastinum and pleural space. Patients with pancreatic ascites present with painless massive ascites and patients with pancreatic pleural effusion present with primary pulmonary symptoms. In both conditions, the serum amylase level may be elevated and paracentesis or thoracentesis will reveal a high fluid amylase and a high fluid albumin level. Up to 25% of patients can present with both conditions. The initial management is nonoperative including nil per os (NPO), TPN and paracentesis or thoracentesis, as appropriate, to evacuate the ascites or pleural fluid. Octreotide may be of benefit in some cases. Nonoperative management may resolve the clinical entity in 50% to 60% of patients. In patients not cured by nonoperative management, surgical therapy is indicated. ERCP usually shows a leak from an incompletely formed or ruptured pseudocyst or a direct duct leak. Sphincterotomy or pancreatic duct stenting have been used with some success. Surgical therapy includes distal pancreatectomy or Roux-en-Y pancreaticojejunostomy to the leak site.

Pancreatic-Enteric Fistula

Spontaneous decompression of a pancreatic pseudocyst (or abscess or acute fluid collection) into an adjacent hollow viscus is uncommon. Most enteric fistulas occur between the pancreas and the splenic flexure or transverse colon. In most cases, spontaneous rupture of a pseudocyst or abscess into a hollow viscus causes bleeding or sepsis, and appropriate operative intervention becomes necessary for correction of the disorder.

PANCREATIC TRAUMA

Pancreatic injury occurs in fewer than 2% of patients with abdominal trauma. Two thirds of pancreatic injuries are associated with penetrating abdominal trauma, and one third of these injuries are associated with blunt abdominal trauma. Given the retroperitoneal location of the pancreas, many patients will have injuries to adjacent organs and major vascular structures. Patients with pancreatic injury have an average of 3.5 other organs injured. In penetrating pancreatic injuries, the lowest mortality is associated with stab wounds (approximately 5% to 10%), with intermediate mortality associated with gunshot wounds, and the highest mortality (50%) observed with close-range shotgun wounds. Blunt pancreatic trauma is associated with mortality rates of 15% to 50%. The cause of early death is bleeding from nearby vascular structures. Delayed mortality from intraabdominal sepsis is the second most common cause of demise. In blunt abdominal trauma, the extent and location of pancreatic injury is determined by the mechanism of injury and the location of impact. The midline forces induced by the classic steering wheel injury are associated with pancreatic neck transections. No laboratory test is available for the diagnosis of pancreatic injury. Amylase levels are insensitive and nonspecific. Elevated amylase is present in 90% of patients with blunt pancreatic injury, but in only a few patients with penetrating pancreatic injury. In addition, elevated amylase is seen in 50% of patients with blunt abdominal trauma without pancreatic injury. Because of the retroperitoneal location of the pancreas and the existence of other sources for intraperitoneal amylase such as the bile duct, intestine, and fallopian tubes, peritoneal lavage is inaccurate and unreliable in the diagnosis of pancreatic trauma. Abdominal films and ultrasonography are not helpful in diagnosing pancreatic injury. In blunt abdominal trauma, CT scan is used for the serial evaluation of pancreatic injury. ERCP is rarely useful in the acute setting but can identify pancreatic ductal abnormalities in the delayed setting.

Stable patients with no other indication for laparotomy can be managed conservatively. These patients are followed for the development of complications such as acute fluid collections and pseudocyst formation. If a trauma laparotomy is performed, complete assessment of the pancreas is always indicated. All peripancreatic hematomas should be explored to exclude and repair major vascular injury. The goals of operative therapy for pancreatic injury include control of hemorrhage, débridement of nonviable tissue with maximal preservation of viable pancreatic tissue, and adequate drainage of exocrine secretions. According to severity, pancreatic injuries are categorized into five classes and operative therapy depends on the degree of pancreatic injury. More than two thirds of pancreatic injuries are class I or II.

Class I injuries consist of pancreatic contusion without capsular rupture and without injury to the main pancreatic duct. These injuries are treated by external drainage alone by using closed-suction drains.

Class II injuries represents pancreatic capsular and parenchymal rupture without injury to the main pancreatic duct. These injuries are treated by cautious débridement of devitalized tissue, hemostasis, suture closure of any major capsular disruption often assisted by omental patching, and external drainage of the injury site with closed-suction drains.

Class III injuries are severe pancreatic parenchymal injury with rupture of the main pancreatic duct. The treatment depends on the location and the associated injuries. Class III injuries to the body and tail of the pancreas are best treated by distal pancreatectomy, with or without splenectomy. Class III injuries to the head of the pancreas not associated with duodenal injury are uncommon and usually seen in penetrating trauma. Isolated injuries of the inferior head or uncinate process can be débrided and drained externally or via Roux-en-Y pancreaticojejunostomy. Injuries adjacent to the duodenal C-shaped loop in the central aspect of the pancreatic head are treated as class IV injuries.

Class IV-V injuries represent combined severe pancreatic and duodenal injuries. These lesions are rare, have a mortality of 45%, and are frequently associated with injuries to adjacent visceral or major vascular structures. Several surgical options exist, which all include débridement and external drainage of the pancreatic and duodenal injury. If the injury to the pancreatic head does not necessitate resection, discrete duodenal defects can be closed with the serosal patch technique. More extensive injuries to the duodenum and head of the pancreas can be treated by duodenal decompression with triple-tube intubation. This technique uses tube gastrostomy, retrograde tube jejunostomy for duodenal drainage, and antegrade tube jejunostomy for enteral feeding. Even more severe injuries to the duodenum and head of the pancreas may be managed by the pyloric exclusion procedure: the pylorus is closed from within the gastric lumen, a gastrojejunostomy is performed, and the injury to the duodenum is repaired primarily. The most severe devitalizing injuries require a Whipple resection and are associated with a mortality of up to 60%.

CANCER OF THE EXOCRINE PANCREAS

Epidemiological Features and Risk Factors

Pancreatic cancer continues to have a very grim prognosis, with surgery the only option for potential cure. Over the last 30 years the incidence rate has remained constant and almost equals the mortality rate. More than 28,000 Americans are expected to die of pancreatic cancer yearly, which makes this malignancy the fifth leading cause of cancer death in the United States. Demographic studies reveal an increased risk of pancreatic cancer with advancing age, black race, male gender, and Jewish ethnicity.

Six genetic syndromes are associated with an increased risk for pancreatic cancer: hereditary nonpolyposis colorectal cancer (HNPCC), familial breast cancer associated with the BRCA2 mutation, Peutz–Jeghers syndrome, ataxia-telangiectasia syndrome, familial atypical multiple mole melanoma syndrome (FAMMM), and hereditary pancreatitis. Low-level risk factors include chronic pancreatitis, cystic fibrosis, the use of estrogen hormones, and pernicious anemia. The apparent association between diabetes and pancreatic cancer is inconsistent. Environmental risk factors include cigarette smoking and increasing total energy intake. Chemists and coal gas workers are some of the occupational risk groups.

Pathologic Features

The most common type, *ductal adenocarcinoma*, is an epithelial, nonendocrine solid neoplasm that accounts for more than 80% of all primary pancreatic cancers. Approximately 65% of ductal adenocarcinomas arise in the head, neck, or uncinate process of the pancreas, 15% originate in the body and tail, and 20% diffusely involve the entire gland. Often the tumor arises close to the genu (or knee) of the main pancreatic duct and causes obstruction and dilation of the adjacent distal common bile duct or main pancreatic duct. At the time of discovery, most ductal adenocarcinomas have metastasized to peripancreatic lymph nodes. In addition to lymph node metastases, by the time of the patient's death, pancreatic ductal adenocarcinomas have frequently metastasized to the liver (up to 80% of cases), peritoneum (60%), lungs and pleura (50 to 70%), and adrenal glands (25%). Histologically identifiable precursor lesions such as intraductal papillary-mucinous neoplasms (IPMNs) can progress to infiltrating ductal adenocarcinoma. These abnormal ductal structures contain a mucin-producing proliferative epithelium with cytologic atypia. IPMN lesions are found adjacent to pancreatic cancer tissue and display some of the same genetic changes that infiltrating adenocarcinomas display, such as activating point mutations in codon 12 of k-ras, as well as mutations in the p16 and p53 tumor suppressor genes. *Adenosquamous carcinoma* is a rare variant of ductal adenocarcinomas that has a particularly poorer prognosis. *Acinar cell carcinoma* is a rare malignant tumor of the pancreas that may present as a bulkier tumor but with a better prognosis.

These tumors can present occasionally (20%) with subcutaneous fat necrosis, an erythema nodosum-like rash, peripheral eosinophilia, and polyarthralgia. Other rare exocrine malignancies of the pancreas include *giant cell carcinoma*, *giant cell carcinoma with osteoclast-like giant cells*, and the rare childhood neoplasm, *pancreatoblastoma*.

Genetics

Data from the National Familial Pancreas Tumor Registry (NFPTR) indicate that individuals with a positive family history have a 16- to 33-fold increased risk of the development of pancreatic cancer. More than 70% of pancreatic cancers have abnormal karyotypes, which include partial deletions (1p, 9p, 17p, 18q) and loss of whole chromosomes (18, 13, 12, 17, 6). The three tumor suppressor genes that are frequently inactivated in sporadic pancreatic cancer are Rb/p16, p53, and DPC4. The Rb/p16 gene residing on chromosome 9p is inactivated in up to 95% of all pancreatic cancers through methylation. The tumor suppressor gene p53 gene, which lies on chromosome 17p, is inactivated in 75% of pancreatic cancers. DPC4 on chromosome 18q is homozygously deleted in 30% and point mutated in 20% of pancreatic cancers. Oncogenes are also involved in pancreatic cancer. Activating point mutations in codon 12 of the k-ras oncogene occur in 90% of pancreatic cancers. Such activating mutations are more frequent in pancreatic cancers of smokers. The relative ease of detecting k-ras mutations makes this a potential candidate for the development of molecular-based screening tests for pancreatic cancer.

Specific genetic alterations have been identified for some of the clinical syndromes associated with pancreatic cancer. Germline mutations in the tumor suppressor gene BRCA2, the second breast cancer susceptibility gene, located on 18q, is found in only 7% of *sporadic* pancreatic cancers, but BRCA2 appears to be the most common *inherited* gene mutation in pancreatic cancer. Mutations in the mismatch repair genes are seen in HNPCC.

In addition, various growth factors and their receptors seem to be involved in the regulation of pancreatic cancer. Of note are the epidermal growth factor (EGF), the transforming growth factor-beta (TGF-β), the fibroblast growth factor (FGF), and insulin-like growth factor (ILGF).

Diagnosis and Clinical Staging

In practice, the diagnosis and staging of pancreatic cancer overlap. Physical examination and routine imaging studies such as CT or MRI/MRCP provide information regarding both diagnosis and staging.

Patients typically present with jaundice, weight loss, abdominal pain, and pruritus. Weakness, alteration of bowel habits, and anorexia may also be present. Unusual initial presentations include new-onset diabetes (10%) and acute pancreatitis. Physical examination may reveal a palpable gallbladder associated with jaundice (Courvoisier sign). Physical findings in patients with disseminated pancreatic cancer may include left supraclavicular adenopathy (Virchow node), periumbilical lymphadenopathy (Sister Mary Joseph nodes), and drop metastases in the pelvis encircling the perirectal region (Blumer shelf).

Laboratory studies are not specific: elevation of the total bilirubin and an elevation of liver function tests are often seen. Patients with localized cancer of the body and tail of the pancreas have normal laboratory values early in the course. Coagulation status should be assessed in patients presenting with bile obstruction because prolonged exclusion of the bile from the gastrointestinal tract leads to malabsorption of fat-soluble vitamins, with decreased hepatic production of vitamin K–dependent clotting factors.

At present, no accurate and reliable serum tumor marker is available for the diagnosis of pancreatic cancer. The best marker is the carbohydrate antigen 19-9 (CA 19-9). CA 19-9 is a Lewis blood group-related mucin. CA 19-9 approaches only 80% accuracy in identifying patients with pancreatic cancer. In addition to its use for diagnosis, CA 19-9 has been correlated both with prognosis and with tumor recurrence.

Among the many diagnostic imaging modalities available, high-quality spiral or helical CT scanning is the preferred noninvasive modality used for diagnosis and staging of pancreatic cancer. In addition to the assessment of the primary tumor, the CT scan is used to evaluate major vessels adjacent to the pancreas for neoplastic invasion or thrombosis and to evaluate for tumor spread to the liver, peripancreatic lymph nodes, or adjacent retroperitoneal structures. The quality of MRI/MRCP is evolving rapidly and has gained importance in diagnosing pancreatic cancer. With the current sophistication of spiral CT scanning or MRCP, the routine practice of diagnostic ERCP in pancreatic cancer is unsupported. Diagnostic ERCP is reserved for diagnostic dilemmas, such as patients with presumed pancreatic cancer and obstructive jaundice with no evident mass on CT, symptomatic patients without jaundice and no obvious pancreatic mass, or occasional patients with chronic pancreatitis with a clinical suspicion of pancreatic cancer. The role of PET scanning in pancreatic cancer will depend on further study results. In addition, three other techniques have been used for preoperative staging: angiography, endoscopic ultrasonography, and laparoscopy. CT, endoscopic ultrasonography, and MRI have largely replaced angiography in diagnosis and staging. Although endoscopic ultrasonography (EUS) can be particularly useful in providing staging information regarding the extent of the primary tumor (T stage), it cannot reliably assess metastatic involvement of the liver or distant lymph node involvement and is highly operator dependent.

Routine preoperative staging laparoscopy for patients with cancers of the head of the pancreas may be used. A small percentage of patients with obstructive jaundice caused by tumors in the head of the pancreas is found to have unexpected intraperitoneal metastases after routine staging studies. In contrast, staging laparoscopy is more beneficial for patients with cancer of the body or tail of the pancreas. These patients have unexpected metastases in up to 50% of cases and do not typically cause biliary or gastric outlet obstruction requiring palliative surgery.

Preoperative tissue diagnosis is not recommended in patients with a clinically resectable pancreatic mass. However, tissue diagnosis by means of percutaneous or ERCP-guided biopsy is indicated for an unresectable mass or for high-risk patients. These patients may be candidates for palliative chemoradiation therapy, for various neoadjuvant protocols, and may reveal less common entities such as pancreatic lymphoma.

Treatment

Pancreaticoduodenectomy for Tumors of the Head of the Pancreas (Whipple Procedure)

The initial portion of the operative procedure is dedicated to the assessment of resectability. This involves an extensive Kocher maneuver to elevate the duodenum and the head of the pancreas from the retroperitoneum. Distant metastasis and local extension to the mesenteric vessels preclude resection. After resection of the head of the pancreas, the reconstruction involves the anastomosis of the pancreas to the jejunum. The biliary-enteric anastomosis is typically performed in end-to-side fashion, approximately 10 cm down the jejunal limb from the pancreatic-enteric anastomosis. The third anastomosis is the duodenojejunostomy (or gastrojejunostomy), typically performed 10 to 15 cm downstream from the biliary-enteric anastomosis (Fig. 31-8). Several controversies remain pertaining to the surgical treatment. First, pylorus-preserving pancreaticoduodenectomy is more commonly performed than the classic pancreaticoduodenectomy (which includes distal gastrectomy). The pylorus-preserving procedure preserves the entire gastric reservoir and the pyloric sphincter, maintains more normal gastric acid secretion and hormone release, and does not appear to be associated with any consistent additional complications. Second, the issue of the safest technique of pancreatic-enteric reconstruction remains unsettled. Third, extended or radical pancreaticoduodenectomy has been reported by some groups but prospective, randomized studies did not demonstrate a consistent survival advantage for patients undergoing the extended resection.

The operative mortality rate for pancreaticoduodenectomy is currently less than 3% in major surgical centers with significant experience with the procedure. The leading causes of postoperative in-hospital death include

TABLE 31-4	
COMPLICATIONS OF PANCREATICODUODENECTOMY	

Common	Uncommon
Delayed gastric emptying	Fistula
Pancreatic fistula	Biliary
Intraabdominal abscess	Duodenal
Wound infection	Gastric
Metabolic	Organ failure
Diabetes	Cardiac
Pancreatic exocrine insufficiency	Hepatic
	Pulmonary
	Renal
	Pancreatitis
	Marginal ulceration

From Yeo CJ. Management of complications following pancreaticoduodenectomy. *Surg Clin North Am* 1995;75:913–924, with permission.

postoperative sepsis, hemorrhage, and cardiovascular events. Data indicate that hospital mortality rates after pancreaticoduodenectomy are six times higher in low-volume facilities as compared with those patients treated in high-volume surgical centers.

Although the mortality rate may be low, the incidence of postoperative complications remains 40% to 50%. The leading causes of morbidity include delayed gastric emptying, failure of the pancreatic anastomosis with subsequent pancreatic fistula formation, as well as intraabdominal abscess, hemorrhage, and wound infection (Table 31-4).

The prognosis for patients with resected carcinoma of the head of the pancreas yields an overall 5-year survival of between 15% and 21%. The median postresection survival

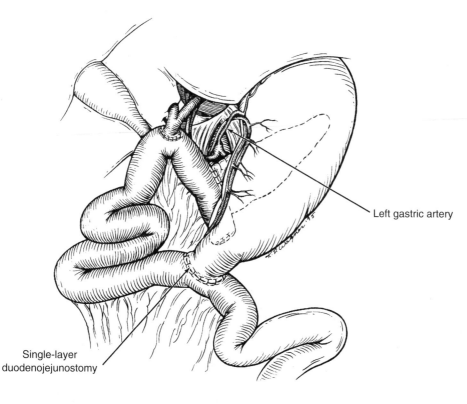

Left gastric artery

Single-layer duodenojejunostomy

Figure 31-8 Whipple procedure. After the end-to-end pancreaticojejunostomy and the end-to-side hepaticojejunostomy, the duodenum is anastomosed to the jejunum in an end-to-side fashion. (From Evans DB, Lee JE, Pisters PW. Pancreaticoduodenectomy (Whipple operation) and total pancreatectomy for cancer. In: Baker RJ, Fischer JE. *Mastery of surgery*. Philadelphia: Lippincott Williams & Wilkins, 2001, with permission.)

varies between 16 and 22 months. Factors that determine overall prognosis include clinicopathologic staging, tumor biologic features, molecular genetics, and the use of post-operative adjuvant therapy. Tumor characteristics found to be important predictors of survival include tumor diameter, lymph node status, and resection margin status.

Distal Pancreatectomy for Tumors of the Body and Tail

Adenocarcinomas of the body and tail of the pancreas represent up to one third of all cases of pancreatic cancer. Tumors in this location often have silent progression and present as large sized tumors with a much higher incidence of metastatic disease at initial diagnosis. The use of staging laparoscopy to identify metastases not visualized by CT appears to have improved the resectability rate in patients with body and tail tumors.

Splenic preservation is not indicated when the resection is performed for pancreatic adenocarcinoma. Patients undergoing resection for adenocarcinoma of the body and tail of the pancreas have median survival rates ranging from 7 to 13 months, with 5-year survival rates in the range of 10%.

Palliative Surgery

Palliative surgery for pancreatic cancer is designed to relieve biliary obstruction, to avoid or treat duodenal obstruction, to palliate tumor-associated pain, and to improve the patient's quality of life. The biliary obstruction is usually relieved through a hepatico- (choledocho-)jejunostomy with cholecystectomy. This method of biliary-enteric bypass has the lowest incidence of recurrent jaundice and the lowest rate of postoperative cholangitis. It is generally recommended to perform prophylactic gastrojejunostomy in patients who are undergoing operative palliation of pancreatic cancer. Postoperative acid suppression with histamine H 2-receptor antagonists or proton pump inhibitors may be used to prevent marginal ulceration. Chemical splanchnicectomy with 50% alcohol is designed to disrupt the transmission of afferent impulses to the celiac plexus and reduces postoperative abdominal and back pain, often associated with unresectable pancreatic cancer.

Nonoperative Management

Nonoperative management is indicated for patients with metastatic or unresectable disease or in patients with a prohibitive risk for surgery. In these patients, biliary decompression can be achieved either by endoscopic or percutaneous transhepatic techniques. Procedure-related morbidity of endoscopic approaches are less than 10% and the major late complication is stent occlusion. Patients with high-grade duodenal obstruction secondary to pancreatic cancer generally require an operative intervention to establish a gastrojejunostomy.

Radiation and Chemotherapy

The poor long-term results in patients who undergo resection for pancreatic cancer is believed to be related to the regional and systemic subclinical disease present at the time of surgery and supports the use of radiation therapy and chemotherapy in the *adjuvant* setting. Results of the Gastrointestinal Tumor Study Group (GITSG) and the Johns Hopkins Hospital showed that adjuvant chemoradiation therapy significantly improves survival. The role of *neoadjuvant* strategies is currently being investigated. In the *palliative* setting, the use of chemotherapy and radiation both alone and in combination may provide a marginal improvement in survival. Available data suggest that gemcitabine is an improvement over 5-fluorouracil (FU)-based chemotherapy. Gemcitabine is also a potent radiation sensitizer.

RARE NEOPLASMS OF THE EXOCRINE PANCREAS

Cystadenoma

Fewer than 10% of cystic pancreatic lesions are cystadenomas. Cystadenomas are difficult to differentiate from pancreatic pseudocysts, the most common cystic lesions of the pancreas. The two most common forms of these cystic tumors are serous neoplasms and mucinous neoplasms. Serous tumors are almost always benign and complete resection is curative. Mucinous tumors sometimes express carcinoembryonic antigen (CEA), are a more heterogeneous group, with a variable potential for malignant degeneration. Complete resection is curative for patients with benign mucinous cystadenomas and with an approximate 50% 5-year survival, resected mucinous cystadenocarcinomas have a much better prognosis than those with resected pancreatic ductal adenocarcinoma.

Solid and Papillary Neoplasms

Most of these tumors occur in the body or tail of the gland. These tumors tend to grow to a large size, and evidence of local invasion is observed frequently. These neoplasms can contain hemorrhagic areas, cysts, and necrosis. These tumors are usually curable by resection. Rare instances of lymph node and distant metastases have been reported.

Intraductal Papillary-Mucinous Neoplasms

IPMNs were first reported in Japan in the 1980s. ERCP may reveal mucin oozing from the ampulla of Vater. These villous tumors reside within mucus-filled, dilated pancreatic ducts and consist of columnar mucin-secreting cells lining papillary projections. IPMNs show varying degrees of cellular atypia, and they may contain areas of invasive carcinoma and are, therefore, an indication for surgical resection. Overall, most patients with these tumors have favorable outcomes after resection. Patients with areas that contain invasive carcinoma are at risk for recurrent disease.

Pancreatic Lymphoma

Primary involvement of the pancreas with non-Hodgkin lymphoma occurs rarely. Patients are treated with chemotherapy, and resection has no role in the management of patients with extensive pancreatic lymphoma. Patients with localized stage I or II pancreatic lymphoma may benefit from surgical resection.

ISLET CELL TUMORS

Pancreatic endocrine tumors are uncommon. The incidence of clinically significant tumors is estimated at about 5 to 10 cases per 1 million per year but autopsy studies show that nonfunctional and benign endocrine tumors are 1,000 times more common. Endocrine tumors of the pancreas vary greatly in mode of onset and severity of symptoms, location, and malignant potential. Only 10% of insulinomas are malignant but nearly all glucagonomas and somatostatinomas are malignant. By using light microscopy, there are no characteristics that separate benign from malignant tumors. Large aggressive tumors may invade adjacent structures and by such action proclaim their malignancy, but most tumors larger than 2 cm are potentially malignant. Individual tumors may vary greatly with time in secretion and biologic aggressiveness. A single tumor can produce multiple hormones, but the predominant endocrine agent identifies the syndrome. As many as 40% of patients with islet cell tumors have elevated levels of multiple hormones, not all of which produce symptoms. This feature may represent multiple clones of tumor cells or a common stem cell with multiple potentials for hormone production. Some tumors are frequently found in extrapancreatic locations, especially in the duodenum. Nearly all insulinomas, glucagonomas, and VIPomas occur within the pancreas itself, whereas most gastrinomas occur in the duodenum. Somatostatinomas are equally divided between the pancreas and the proximal small bowel. Patients with von Recklinghausen disease may have somatostatinomas or gastrinomas in the duodenum. The distribution of glucagonomas, insulinomas, and PPomas corresponded to the normal distribution of these endocrine cell types within the pancreas. Gastrinomas, PPomas, and somatostatinomas are preferentially (75%) located to the right of the superior mesenteric artery in the pancreatic head region. By contrast, about 75% of insulinomas and glucagonomas are located to the left of the superior mesenteric artery in the body and tail of the pancreas.

Pancreatic endocrine tumors may occur sporadically or in conjunction with the multiple endocrine neoplasia type 1 (MEN-1) syndrome (Table 31-5).

MEN-1

MEN-1 is characterized by tumors of the parathyroid, pituitary, and pancreas and occasionally the adrenal. A genetic defect on chromosome 11 is inherited in an autosomal dominant fashion. Because islet cell tumors in MEN-1 patients are always multiple, preoperative recognition of the MEN-1 status is necessary. Approximately 25% of patients with gastrinomas, 10% of those with insulinomas, and lesser percentages of those with glucagonomas and VIPomas have the MEN syndrome. Any patient with a pancreatic endocrine tumor syndrome should have a measurement of calcium level, and if that is elevated, the parathyroid and the pituitary should be studied.

Nearly all MEN-1 patients manifest hyperparathyroidism (95%), usually caused by hyperplasia of all four glands. Of all MEN-1 patients, more than 50% have gastrinomas, and 20% have an insulinoma. Nonfunctioning PPoma occurs in more than 80%. Pituitary adenomas are common, most of which are nonfunctioning, with prolactinomas being the next most common. A general principle is that in MEN-1 patients with islet tumors, the hyperparathyroidism should be surgically managed first, preferably by removing all four glands with immediate autograft.

Insulinoma

Insulinomas are the most common functioning tumors of the pancreas. Affected patients present with symptoms related to hypoglycemia such as autonomic nervous overactivity, fatigue and weakness, central nervous system depression, apathy, irritability, or convulsions. The Whipple triad of hypoglycemia, low blood glucose level, and relief of symptoms after intravenous administration of glucose, is the diagnostic hallmark but can be mimicked by factitious administration of insulin or hypoglycemic agents such as sulfonylurea, by rare soft tissue tumors, or occasionally by reactive hypoglycemia. The pathognomonic finding is an inappropriately high level of serum insulin during symptomatic hypoglycemia. The ratio of blood insulin to glucose has proved to be valuable in the diagnosis. The best way to induce hypoglycemia is with fasting. Provocative tests with tolbutamide or glucagon are usually not necessary and dangerous. Self-administration of insulin can be detected through low concentrations of C-peptide or proinsulin. Sulfonurea administration can be detected through blood tests and is not associated with inappropriately high insulin levels. Once diagnosed, severe hypoglycemia must be prevented to avoid permanent brain damage. Diet should be modified to include frequent meals. The drug diazoxide is helpful in about two thirds of patients but should be discontinued at least a week before operation because it may cause intraoperative hypotension. Preoperative fasting orders must be accompanied by intravenous administration of glucose. The long-acting somatostatin analog octreotide,

---

TABLE 31-5

PANCREATIC ENDOCRINE TUMORS

Tumor Syndrome	Cell of Origin	Malignant Potential	Anatomic Location	MEN-1 Association	Extrapancreatic
Insulinoma	β	Rare (10%)	Evenly distributed	10%	Rare
Gastrinoma	G	Most (>70%)	Gastrinoma triangle	25%	>50%
Glucagonoma	α	Most	Body and tail	Rare	Rare
VIPoma	$\Delta 2$	Most (>50%)	Body and tail	Rare	10%
Somatostatinoma	Δ	Most	Pancreatic head	Rare	Rare

VIP, vasoactive intestinal peptide.

although helpful in children with nesidioblastosis, is rarely effective in adults.

Most insulinomas are small (usually less than 1.5 cm), usually single (only 10% are multiple and those are usually associated with MEN-1 syndrome), usually benign (10% malignant) and may be difficult to locate. Success in localization often parallels the degree of invasiveness of the study. Contrast-augmented CT and MRI locate 50% to 60% of tumors. Selective arteriography is 50% to 90% accurate. Endoscopic ultrasonography has a higher rate of success in preoperative localization of insulinomas. Somatostatin receptor scintigraphy (SRS) is not successful because of lack of expression of somatostatin receptors by the beta cells. Selective portovenous sampling provides accurate information on the region of the pancreas from which high levels of insulin are released in approximately 75% of cases. Calcium is known to release insulin, and selective intraarterial calcium challenge is 94% accurate in localizing an insulinoma. Combinations of these studies identify most tumors before surgery. In addition, a surgeon unaware of the location by preoperative studies is successful in identifying the tumor by intraoperative ultrasound in approximately 85%.

Most insulinomas are benign and can be enucleated. If the pancreatic duct is injured, it should be sutured and drained. If malignant, the tumor should be resected in a cancer-type operation, and if metastatic, all primary and metastatic tumor tissue should be removed.

The 10% of patients with hyperinsulinism and MEN-1 syndrome have multiple islet tumors, one of which is usually dominant. These patients are probably best managed by resecting the area of the pancreas that shows the highest insulin output. Persistent hyperinsulinemia after operation for metastatic islet cell tumor may be managed by diazoxide (side effects are rare and are chiefly fluid retention and hirsutism) or by streptozotocin plus fluorouracil. Hyperinsulinism in infants is caused by nesidioblastosis, a nest-like increase in islet cells. Prolonged hypoglycemia leads to mental retardation in most of these children. A near-total (95% to 98%) pancreatectomy appears to offer the best results, with octreotide therapy reserved for preoperative preparation and those children not rendered euglycemic after operation.

Zollinger–Ellison Syndrome (Gastrinoma)

Gastrinomas are the second most common islet cell tumor and are the most common symptomatic malignant endocrine tumor of the pancreas. More than 50% of gastrinomas arise in the duodenum. Only the pancreas, the duodenum, and the ovaries can process progastrin to gastrin to cause signs of Zollinger–Ellison syndrome (ZES). Rare pulmonary, acoustic neuroma, and colon tumors may produce gastrin without causing hypergastrinemia.

The main symptoms are those caused by peptic acid hypersecretion. ZES must be excluded in all patients with intractable peptic ulcer, severe esophagitis, or persistent secretory diarrhea. A unique characteristic of this diarrhea is that it is halted by nasogastric aspiration of gastric secretion, a feature that separates it from all other secretory diarrheas. The diagnosis depends on the presence of hypergastrinemia concurrent with increased secretion of gastric acid. Other causes of hypergastrinemia must be ruled out. A secretin provocative test is useful in diagnostic dilemmas. Once the

diagnosis is established, acid secretion should be controlled with proton-pump inhibitors in order to prevent complications and to afford symptomatic relief.

Gastrinomas arise more frequently in the duodenum (greater than 50%) than in the pancreas. There is a pronounced proximal-to-distal gradient within the duodenum. Sixty percent to 90% are found in the so-called gastrinoma triangle, an area in the upper abdomen with its superior point at the junction of the cystic and common bile ducts, its inferior point at the junction or the inferior margin of the second and third parts of the duodenum, and its left lateral point at the junction of the head and neck of the pancreas (Fig. 31-9). Most gastrinomas are malignant (30% to 90%). Because the normal pancreas and duodenum contain no gastrin cells, the origin of gastrinomas remains elusive. Duodenal gastrinomas may arise from the ventral pancreatic bud, and tumors of the body and tail may arise from the dorsal bud. Liver metastasis is the dominant factor in survival. Lymph node involvement does not affect survival. Gastrinomas are usually slow growing, and some patients may live for years with metastatic disease. In 75% of patients with ZES, the gastrinoma is sporadic, whereas 25% have an associated MEN-1 syndrome. ZES patients with the MEN-1 syndrome have multiple tumors, often microadenomas, scattered throughout the pancreas. Attempts to localize gastrinomas by means of ultrasonography, arteriography, and enhanced CT and MRI have been only partly successful. Most gastrinomas have receptors for somatostatin and SRS is particularly sensitive in imaging both primary and metastatic gastrinoma tissue. Duodenal gastrinomas are usually small and are the most resistant to preoperative localization. Direct endoscopy and endoscopic ultrasonography are probably the most effective preoperative studies for detection of duodenal gastrinomas. Most patients with gastrinomas will need three or more localization techniques.

Pharmacologic control of acid secretion with proton pump inhibitors has rendered total gastrectomy unnecessary. Every ZES patient is a candidate for surgery. Most tumors are located in the gastrinoma triangle. Intraoperative

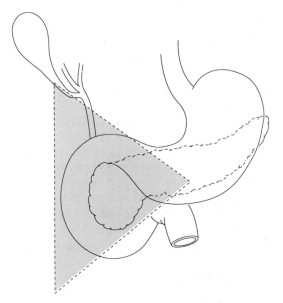

Figure 31-9 The gastrinoma triangle. (From Stabile BE, Morrow DJ, Passaro E. The gastrinoma triangle: operative implications. *Am J Surg* 1984;147:26, with permission.)

ultrasonography plus palpation is effective in localizing 95% of pancreatic gastrinomas but finding duodenal tumors is more difficult. Intraoperative endoscopy with transillumination of the duodenal wall facilitates visualization of many duodenal tumors. Duodenal tumors should be excised with a full-thickness elliptical incision. Tumors within the pancreas should be enucleated. If all apparent tumors are removed, the immediate cure rate approaches 90%, but with long follow-up nearly one half of the patients initially free of disease show symptomatic or biochemical (i.e., a positive secretin test result) recurrence by 5 years. Surgical treatment of distant metastases by cytoreduction procedures (debulking) appears useful. Radiation and chemotherapy are largely ineffective for the treatment of metastatic disease.

Verner–Morrison Syndrome (VIPoma)

VIPomas cause a syndrome of profound watery diarrhea, hypokalemia, and achlorhydria. The diarrhea persists despite fasting (which qualifies it as a secretory diarrhea) and despite nasogastric aspiration (which differentiates it from the diarrhea of ZES). It is unclear whether VIP is a normal islet hormone of $\Delta 2$ cells or whether it occurs only in islet tumors. Approximately 50% of patients have metastatic spread by the time of diagnosis. Surgical removal should be attempted. In patients with nonresectable tumors octreotide is helpful in the control of diarrhea. Most tumors are malignant.

Glucagonoma

A tumor of islet alpha cells, a glucagonoma, causes a syndrome of a characteristic skin rash (necrolytic migrating erythema), diabetes mellitus, anemia, weight loss, and elevated circulating levels of glucagon. Diabetes is usually mild. Glucagonoma is associated with a low level of amino acids, and parenteral administration of amino acid will resolve the skin lesions. One third of these patients have been reported to have thrombotic complications after surgery and perioperative heparin is indicated. Treatment is surgical excision of the tumor. Symptomatic relief can be achieved with octreotide. Most tumors are malignant.

Somatostatinoma

Somatostatinomas are rare. The clinical features are variable and consist of steatorrhea, diabetes mellitus or hypoglycemia, hypochlorhydria, and gallstones. Most tumors are malignant and surgical treatment is indicated.

Very Rare Tumors

Various functional tumors of the endocrine pancreas have been reported, some secreting GRF, some secreting neurotensin, some parathyroid hormone-related peptide, some PP, and some ACTHs. GRFomas are always associated with the MEN-1 syndrome. In addition, elevated levels of these hormones are often seen with other islet cell tumor syndromes.

Nonfunctioning Endocrine Tumors

Patients with nonfunctioning islet tumors present with symptoms of local tumor progression. Most such tumors are malignant and have metastasized by the time of diagnosis. Surgical resection should be attempted for cure when possible, since these tumors are often slow growing and compatible with prolonged survival.

KEY POINTS

▲ *Pancreas divisum* is an anatomic variant that occurs if the two primordial ductal systems fail to fuse. In pancreas divisum, the larger portion of the pancreas (superior head, neck, body, and tail) is drained by the duct of Santorini through the minor duodenal papilla, and only the ventral pancreas (inferior head and uncinate process) communicates with the duct of Wirsung into the major duodenal papilla.

▲ Secretin is the most potent endogenous stimulant of pancreatic bicarbonate secretion. Secretin is synthesized in the mucosal S cells of the crypts of Lieberkühn of the proximal small bowel and is released in the presence of luminal acid and bile. Secretin circulates in the blood and binds to secretin receptors on pancreatic ductal cells resulting in an increase in cyclic adenosine monophosphate (cAMP) through the signal transduction and intracellular adenylate cyclase system.

▲ The most widely used predictive criteria for acute pancreatitis involve 11 prognostic signs identified by Ranson. Antibiotics are not indicated in the routine treatment of mild-to-moderate pancreatitis but data support the use of prophylactic antibiotic treatment in patients with severe pancreatitis defined as more than three Ranson signs in association with computerized tomographic (CT) evidence of pancreatic or peripancreatic necrosis.

▲ Early surgical intervention is recommended in patients with gallstone pancreatitis because gallstone pancreatitis without early surgical intervention can lead to early recurrence in approximately 35% of patients. Most episodes of gallstone-associated pancreatitis are mild, and laparoscopic cholecystectomy at the time of the index admission has proved safe and cost-effective. This is normally performed after clinical resolution of the pancreatitis with normalization of the liver function tests.

▲ The operative mortality rate for pancreaticoduodenectomy is currently less than 3% in major surgical centers with significant experience with the procedure. Data indicate that hospital mortality rates after pancreaticoduodenectomy are six times higher in low-volume facilities as compared with those patients treated in high-volume surgical centers.

▲ The pathognomonic finding of insulinoma is an inappropriately high level of serum insulin during symptomatic hypoglycemia. Self-administration of insulin can be detected through low concentrations of C-peptide or proinsulin. Sulfonylurea administration can be detected through blood tests and is not associated with inappropriately high insulin levels.

▲ Sixty percent to 90% of gastrinomas are found in the so-called gastrinoma triangle, an area in the upper abdomen with its superior point at the junction of the cystic and common bile ducts, its inferior point at the junction or the inferior margin of the second and third parts of the duodenum, and its left lateral point at the junction of the head and neck of the pancreas.

▲ VIPomas cause a syndrome of profound watery diarrhea, hypokalemia, and achlorhydria. The diarrhea persists despite fasting (which qualifies it as a secretory diarrhea) and despite nasogastric aspiration [which differentiates it from the diarrhea of Zollinger–Ellison syndrome (ZES)].

▲ MEN-1 is characterized by tumors of the parathyroid, pituitary, and pancreas and occasionally the adrenal. It is associated with a genetic defect on chromosome 11, which is inherited in an autosomal dominant fashion. Any patient with a pancreatic endocrine tumor syndrome should have a measurement of calcium level, and if that is elevated, the parathyroid and the pituitary should be studied.

SUGGESTED READINGS

Brugge WR, Lauwers GY, Sahani D, et al. Cystic neoplasms of the pancreas. *N Engl J Med* 2004;351(12):1218–1226.

Moore EE, Cogbill TH, Malangoni MA, et al. Organ injury scaling, II: Pancreas, duodenum, small bowel, colon, and rectum. *J Trauma* 1990;30(11):1427–1429.

Norton JA, Fraker DL, Alexander HR, et al. Surgery to cure the Zollinger-Ellison syndrome. *N Engl J Med* 1999;341(9):635–644.

Takaori K, Hruban RH, Maitra A, et al. Pancreatic intraepithelial neoplasia. *Pancreas* 2004;28(3):257–262.

Yeo CJ. The Whipple procedure in the 1990s. *Adv Surg* 1999;32:271–303.

The Breast

32

Laura Kruper   Julia Tchou

EMBRYOLOGY

Early in fetal development, the ectodermal primitive milk streak develops from the axilla to inguinal region. This milk streak, or "galactic band," forms a mammary ridge in the area of the thorax, whereas the remainder of the band regresses. As the fetus develops during the second trimester, mesenchymal cells differentiate into the smooth muscle of the areola and nipple, and epithelial buds develop and then branch into epithelial strips. During the third trimester, these branched epithelial tissues undergo canalization as placental hormones enter the fetal circulation, eventually becoming secretory alveoli. Near term, there are approximately 15 to 25 mammary ducts with a fourfold increase in mammary gland mass. After birth, neonates of either sex can produce colostral milk owing to *in utero* exposure to maternal hormones.

The most common congenital breast abnormality seen is an accessory nipple (*polythelia*), which may occur anywhere along the milk line. Failure of complete regression of the milk streak leads to accessory mammary tissues in 2% to 6% of women. Rarely do true accessory mammary glands develop (*polymastia*). When found, they are located most frequently in the axilla and may swell during pregnancy and lactation. *Amastia* is the congenital absence of breast, whereas *amazia* refers to absence of breast tissue with a nipple present. In 90% of cases, amastia is associated with hypoplasia of the ipsilateral pectoralis muscle and rib cage, a syndrome first described by Poland in 1841.

ANATOMY

The breast lies on the anterior chest wall between the second and sixth ribs in the midclavicular line, and extends from the sternal edge to the midaxillary line laterally. Breast tissue also extends into the axilla as the axillary tail of Spence. It is important to note that the anatomic boundaries in relation to breast surgery follow less abstract landmarks. In a modified radical mastectomy, all breast tissue is removed, which extends from the inferior border of the clavicle, inferiorly to the superior rectus sheath, medially to the sternal lateral border, and laterally to the latissimus dorsi muscle. Three major structures comprise the breast: skin, subcutaneous tissue, and breast tissue. The skin of the breast contains hair follicles, eccrine sweat glands, and sebaceous glands, with the nipple containing abundant

sensory nerve endings and no hair follicles. Near the periphery of the areola sit the openings of Montgomery tubercles. These represent the openings of the Montgomery glands, which are large sebaceous glands, intermediate between sweat and mammary glands.

The breast tissue itself comprises stroma and parenchyma. The parenchyma is divided into 15 to 20 segments, each drained by a collecting duct. Each duct drains a lobe made up of 20 to 40 lobules, with each lobule comprising 10 to 100 alveoli (Fig. 32-1). Fat, connective tissue, lymphatics, nerves, and blood vessels comprise the stroma and subcutaneous fat of the breast. Enveloping the breast is the superficial pectoral fascia, which is continuous with the superficial abdominal fascia of Camper. The undersurface

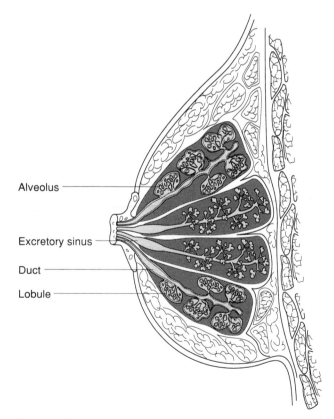

Figure 32-1 The basic lobular and ductal structure of the breast. (From August DA, Sondak VK. Breast. In: Greenfield LJ, Mulholland M, Oldham KT et al., eds. *Surgery: Scientific principles and practice*, 3rd ed. Philadelphia: Lippincott Williams & Wilkins, 2001:1334, with permission.)

of the breast lies on the deep pectoral fascia, which covers the serratus anterior and pectoralis major muscles. Representing the "natural" means of support for the breast, Cooper suspensory ligaments are fibrous bands that connect these two fascial layers. Dimpling of the skin occurs when an underlying breast cancer causes contraction of these ligaments.

The blood supply to the breast is mostly through the internal mammary and lateral thoracic arteries, with minor contributions from branches of the thoracodorsal and subscapular arteries, and perforating branches of the intercostal arteries. Sixty percent of the breast, mostly the medial and central part, is supplied by perforating branches of the internal mammary. The lateral thoracic artery supplies 30% of the breast, mostly the upper, outer quadrant.

Understanding the lymphatic anatomy of the breast is important because of the tendency of breast cancer to involve the regional lymph nodes. Injection studies of radioactive colloid have demonstrated that approximately 97% of the breast lymphatics drain to the axilla, whereas 3% flows to the internal mammary chain. Lymph flows in valveless vessels unidirectionally from the superficial to the deep plexus. Lymphatic vessels from the nipple and areola flow to the subareolar plexus, which then flow to the deep subcutaneous plexus. From the deep subcutaneous and intramammary lymphatic vessels, lymph flows to the axillary and internal mammary lymph nodes.

Axillary nodes are divided into three levels based on their anatomic relationship to the pectoralis minor muscle. Level I nodes are lateral to the pectoralis minor, level II are deep, and level III are medial to the pectoralis minor (Fig. 32-2). In axillary node dissection, level I and II nodal tissues are removed within the triangular boundaries as marked by the latissimus dorsi laterally, axillary vein superiorly, serratus anterior medially, and subscapularis posteriorly.

The medial pectoral nerve arises from the medial cord of the brachial plexus. It enters the deep surface of the pectoralis minor, supplying a branch to this muscle as well as providing motor supply to the lateral part of the pectoralis major. The terms medial and lateral pectoral nerves are confusing, for the standard terminology refers to their origin in the brachial plexus rather than their anatomic positions. The lateral pectoral nerve innervates the pectoralis major and enters the muscle medial to the medial pectoral nerve.

The long thoracic nerve of Bell is a motor nerve arising from the posterior roots of the brachial plexus. This important nerve innervates the serratus anterior and subscapularis, running posterior to the axillary vessels, and lying superficial to the deep fascia overlying the serratus. Because the serratus stabilizes the scapula on the chest wall, transection of this nerve results in a winged scapula, shoulder pain, and loss of shoulder power.

The thoracodorsal nerve is a motor nerve that arises from the posterior cord of the brachial plexus, supplying the latissimus dorsi muscle. It passes through the axilla, runs behind the subscapular artery, and is intimately involved with the subscapular lymph nodes. Resection of this nerve does not result in any cosmetic or functional defect, yet should be preserved when possible. Occasionally, when the latissimus dorsi muscle is used as an autologous tissue flap for breast reconstruction, the thoracodorsal nerve is deliberately severed.

The intercostobrachial nerve is a sensory nerve, which arises from the second intercostal and supplies the skin of the axilla and the inner aspect of the upper arm. Transection of this nerve results in upper arm numbness and paresthesia, but can also be seen in traumatic or intraoperative stretch injuries. Occasionally, sacrifice of this nerve results in the intercostobrachial nerve syndrome: hyperesthesias and severe pain in the shoulder, upper arm, axilla, and chest wall.

PHYSIOLOGY

Cyclic changes associated with the menstrual cycle have a major influence on breast morphology and physiology. The changes in response to hormones are mediated through steroid receptors or membrane-bound peptide receptors. Steroid receptors for estrogen and progesterone are present in the cytosol of breast epithelium and when these receptors are bound by hormone, they translocate into the nucleus. Increasing levels of estrogen stimulate breast epithelium proliferation during the follicular phase. During the luteal phase, progesterone induces changes in the mammary epithelium with differentiation of alveolar epithelial cells into secretory cells and dilation of mammary ducts. Under the influence of these sex steroid hormones and other hormones, lipid droplets are formed in the alveolar cells with some intraluminal secretion with resulting interlobular breast edema that results in premenstrual breast fullness. With the start of menstruation, the rapid decline in circulating levels of hormones leads to regression of the secretory activity of the epithelium and tissue edema slowly resolves.

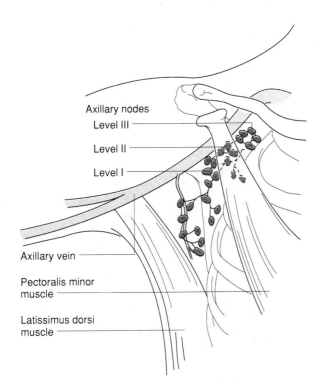

Figure 32-2 Axillary anatomy and distribution of axillary lymph nodes. (From August DA, Sondak VK. Breast. In: Greenfield LJ, Mulholland M, Oldham KT et al., eds. *Surgery: Scientific principles and practice*, 3rd ed. Philadelphia: Lippincott Williams & Wilkins, 2001:1335, with permission.)

Axillary nodes
Level III
Level II
Level I
Axillary vein
Pectoralis minor muscle
Latissimus dorsi muscle

During pregnancy, there are distinct changes in ductal, lobular, and alveolar growth under the influence of progesterone, estrogen, placental lactogen, prolactin, and chorionic gonadotropin. These hormones induce changes within the breast to enable milk production at parturition. Placental lactogen and sex hormones maintain the mammary epithelium in a presecretory phase by antagonizing the effect of prolactin during pregnancy. However, their abrupt withdrawal upon delivery leaves the breasts predominantly under the influence of the pituitary-derived prolactin. In the presence of growth hormone, insulin, and cortisol, prolactin converts the mammary epithelial cells to a secretory phase, resulting in the production of milk by alveolar cells. Initially, colostrum, which has significant nutritional value, is secreted; then by day 4 or 5, milk is produced. The release of prolactin is maintained and stimulated by suckling. Prolactin is secreted by the anterior pituitary and maintains milk production and secretion during lactation. Oxytocin, released from the posterior pituitary neurovesicles in response to nipple/areolar stimulation, causes the ductal myoepithelial breast cells to contract and eject milk.

Postlactational involution occurs typically 3 months after weaning. It is the glandular and ductal elements that atrophy, with regression of the extralobular stroma. In contrast, as ovarian function declines through premenopause into menopause, the breast epithelial structures regress, the lobules shrink and collapse, as the duct system remains. The postmenopausal breast consists predominantly of fat, connective tissue, and mammary ducts.

BREAST EXAMINATION

One of the first steps in a breast examination is eliciting a detailed history from the patient. Baseline information about menstrual status and breast cancer risk should be obtained, no matter the presenting reason for the examination. Each woman should be asked about the risk factors found to be major predictors of risk as defined by the Gail Model including age at menarche, age at first live birth, history of breast biopsies, and family history of breast cancer. For premenopausal women, questions specific to the date of the last menstrual cycle should be posed to aid in evaluating breast pain, nodularity, and cysts. Cycle regularity and use of oral contraceptives should also be ascertained. For postmenopausal women, it is important to inquire about use of hormone replacement therapy and date of menopause.

The patient should be examined in both the sitting and supine positions for the breast and nodal examinations. The examination should start with inspection of the breasts, first with the patient's arms in the raised position and then at her sides, to notice any skin changes or asymmetry between the two breasts. The clinician should then palpate the cervical, clavicular, and axillary nodes bilaterally. The breast examination in the sitting position is then performed by using the dominant hand to palpate and the nondominant hand to support the breast. The nipples are also assessed for nipple discharge. With the patient in the supine position and arms raised above the head, the breasts are palpated with the flat portions of the fingers systematically, either following the direction of spokes on a wheel fashion or concentrically moving in a peripheral to central direction. Abnormalities are noted by identifying the position of the area of concern as the position on the face of a clock and its distance from the areolar margin, that is, a 2 o'clock lesion 5 cm from the areolar margin of the left breast is located at the upper outer quadrant of the breast.

Current modalities for screening breast cancer include breast self examination (BSE), annual clinical breast examination (CBE) by a health care professional, and imaging modalities such as mammography. The current recommendations regarding the use of these modalities vary with different organizations, mostly because of lack of clear evidence regarding efficacy. Although there are no definite data supporting the use of BSE in lowering breast cancer mortality, BSE is viewed as a surveillance tool to detect breast changes as well as to increase awareness of the normal composition of the breasts.

The most common breast imaging modality is mammography, and several randomized controlled trials have supported its use for breast cancer screening. Other adjunct imaging modalities include ultrasonography and the increasingly utilized magnetic resonance imaging (MRI). There is evidence that breast ultrasonography complements mammography by enhancing mammography's sensitivity and specificity in the detection of mass lesion and has proved to be a useful adjunct breast imaging tool. Ultrasonography is especially useful in evaluating specific areas of concern raised either by mammography or by clinical examination, and breast ultrasound is the best tool to distinguish between cystic and solid lesions. For solid lesions, factors such as shape, borders, echogenicity, and acoustic shadowing might suggest a benign versus malignant lesion. Breast MRI is especially helpful in defining the extent of disease for infiltrating lobular breast cancer and clinically occult breast cancer. It is also useful in assessing breast implants integrity and rupture. Breast MRI, although highly sensitive, lacks the specificity to replace mammography as the future breast screening modality. However, there is increasing evidence to support its role in screening breast cancer in high-risk women such as those carrying deleterious breast cancer predisposition gene mutations. There is also interest in technetium-99m sestamibi imaging and positron emission tomographic (PET) scanning in some centers. However, their use is still in the investigative stages.

As mentioned previously, the only imaging modality that has proven efficacy for breast cancer screening is mammography. In randomized control trials (RCTs), screening of asymptomatic women to detect breast cancer earlier has been shown to reduce the death rate by 20% to 30%, presumably because of early detection. Previous screening controversy as to whether women ages 40 to 49 years benefit from earlier detection was mostly a result of the lack of properly conducted RCTs specifically designed to evaluate the efficacy of breast cancer screening in that particular age group. However, with systematic subgroup analysis of existing data, a statistically significant mortality reduction as high as 45% can be shown for screening women in their 40s. Subsequently, most organizations recommend that screening begin at age 40 with annual mammograms thereafter. Women at higher risk should consult with their physician about earlier screening. Although mammography can reduce the death rate by at

TABLE 32-1

MAMMOGRAPHY INTERPRETATIONS AND THE BREAST IMAGING REPORTING AND DATA SYSTEM CLASSIFICATION WITH RECOMMENDATIONS

Category 0   Needs additional studies
Category 1   Negative; routine screening mammogram
Category 2   Benign finding; routine screening mammogram
Category 3   Probably a benign finding; repeated mammogram in 6 months
Category 4   Suspicious abnormality; biopsy
Category 5   Highly suggestive of malignancy; biopsy if palpable or needle localization biopsy if nonpalpable

least 30%, it must be remembered that mammography neither finds all cancers nor finds all cancers early enough.

Screening mammography can detect a breast density, microcalcifications, or architectural distortion. The American College of Radiology developed the Breast-Imaging Reporting and Data System (BI-RADS) classification system to create a universal language for reporting mammographic findings. Findings are classified according to five categories 1 to 5 (Table 32-1), with category 0 representing an incomplete analysis with need for additional studies. Although mammography is sensitive, with a sensitivity of approximately 85%, only about 25% to 35% of mammographic abnormalities suspicious enough to biopsy are carcinomas.

EVALUATION OF SPECIFIC COMPLAINTS

Breast Mass Presenting as a Palpable Lesion

A *palpable breast mass* is one of the most anxiety-producing discoveries for a woman. Some of the important questions to answer in obtaining the patient's history concern the discovery and duration of the mass, any interval changes since first noticed, any associated pain, and its relation to menses. After the history and examination are obtained, the clinician should utilize the *"triple diagnosis"* approach to work up the mass. Triple diagnosis refers to the combination of physical examination, breast imaging such as mammogram and/or ultrasonography, and establishing a pathologic diagnosis using fine needle aspiration (FNA) cytology or core needle biopsy. If the results of all three studies are negative, the probability of a diagnostic error or false negative is less than 1%. Indications for excisional biopsy include any discordance between any of the three modalities, cytologic atypia on needle biopsy, or the patient's wish to eliminate a source for concern. The differences between FNA and core biopsy are noted in Table 32-2. If a patient chooses triple diagnosis, close follow-up is mandatory.

The management of benign or malignant breast masses (solid or cystic) will be discussed in separate sections in subsequent text. The differential diagnosis of a solid mass includes benign lesions such as fibroadenoma, a broad range of lesions grouped under "fibrocystic changes," hamartoma, fat necrosis, or malignant lesions such as infiltrating ductal or lobular carcinoma or rarely sarcoma.

Certain characteristics are more frequently associated with malignant lesions, such as hardness, indistinct borders, and attachment to skin or deep fascia. Benign lesions generally are mobile with well-demarcated borders. However, these characteristics can be seen with both types of lesions so definitive tissue diagnosis is necessary.

The appropriate imaging modality should also be somewhat tailored to the age of the patient and index of suspicion for the patient. For example, a solid mass in a woman in her 20s is more likely to be benign. Ultrasonography may be employed first to image the area of concern, and, if necessary, mammography may be obtained, even though the diagnostic value may be diminished, since younger women usually, but, not always, have dense breast tissue, which lowers the sensitivity of mammograms.

Breast Lesions Presenting as Abnormalities on Mammogram

Microcalcifications are the most frequent mammographic abnormalities prompting biopsy, with soft-tissue densities a close second. Evaluating calcifications involves systematic review of location, size, number, morphology, and distribution, with morphology as the most important element. Microcalcifications that tend to be benign are smooth and round, and they form in the acinar structures of the lobules. Other benign morphology includes solid or lucent-centered spheres or crescent-shaped calcifications that concave up. Often associated with ectatic ducts are rod-shaped or tubular calcifications. Calcifications that are classified as benign need no further evaluation, but if further analysis is required, magnification mammography in orthogonal views (cranial caudal, CC, or medial lateral, ML) is the primary technique used. Calcifications that vary in size and shape are a cause for concern. Almost all calcifications that form in breast cancers form in the intraductal portion of the cancer and are small and irregular. In many cases of ductal carcinoma *in situ* (DCIS), calcifications are pleomorphic and clustered. Although many cancer calcifications form in nonspecific clusters, clusters may also be caused by duct papillomas, hyperplasia, adenosis, and other benign processes; however, a biopsy, either by stereotactic core biopsy if feasible, or excisional biopsy, is required for an accurate diagnosis.

TABLE 32-2

COMPARISON OF FINE NEEDLE ASPIRATION AND CORE BIOPSY FOR NONPALPABLE LESIONS

	FNA	Core Biopsy
Needle size/gauge	20–22	11–14
Imaging modality for guidance	Ultrasound or stereotatic for both	
Pathologic evaluation	Cytology	Histology
Rate of inadequate samples	0%–37%	<1%
Able to differentiate between *in situ* and invasive	No	Yes
Cost	$	$$

From Harris JR, Lippman ME, Morrow M et al., eds. *Diseases of the breast*. Philadelphia: Lippincott Williams & Wilkins, 2000:150, with permission.

Mastalgia

Breast pain or *mastalgia* is a common problem seen in primary care settings and breast clinics. A survey indicated that up to 70% of women experience breast pain, but only 3% seek treatment. Most commonly, breast pain is cyclic, occurring premenstrually. A detailed history is essential to determine the relationship of the pain to the timing of the patient's menstrual cycle. Other important aspects of the history include type of pain, location, duration, other medical problems, and association with any masses or skin changes. Frequent causes of breast pain include fibrocystic changes, cysts, and infection. Breast pain is rarely a presenting symptom for cancer. Women older than the age of 35 should have a mammogram as part of their workup. Ultrasonography is often used to evaluate focal pain, but without a discrete lump or nodularity it is unlikely to yield any information of clinical value. For women with breast pain and benign disease, treatment includes eliminating caffeine, minimizing salt, and using anti-inflammatory drugs, evening primrose oil, and vitamins E and B6. In more severe cases, treatments that have been tried include danazol, tamoxifen (an antiestrogen agent), oral contraceptives, and Elavil.

Nipple Discharge

Nipple discharge accounts for approximately 5% of referrals to breast clinics. It is a symptom that heightens a patient's concern for breast cancer, even though 95% of women presenting to the hospital with nipple discharge have a benign cause. Overall, less than 10% of patients who have bloody nipple discharge have an underlying malignancy; however, the likelihood of nipple discharge being secondary to carcinoma increases with age. In patients younger than age 40, 3% were found to have cancers when presenting with nipple discharge as their only symptom, whereas it was 10% for women between ages 40 and 60, and 32% for patients older than 60. In addition to mammography, one of the first steps in evaluating nipple discharge is to determine whether it is pathologic or physiologic.

Physiologic discharge is usually nonspontaneous and bilateral and is induced from multiple ducts. Its color can be white, yellow, green, brown, or bluish-black. Copious bilateral milky discharge, when not associated with pregnancy or breastfeeding, can be indicative of galactorrhea. This condition may be secondary to medications (oral contraceptives, phenothiazines, and some antihypertensives) or a pituitary tumor (prolactinoma). The most common benign causes of bloody discharge are intraductal papilloma, periductal mastitis, and duct ectasia.

The most common cause of a bloody nipple discharge, as well as most common lesion causing a serous or serosanguineous discharge, is a *solitary intraductal papilloma*, which is a true polyp of epithelial-lined breast ducts. These lesions are most frequently observed in women 30 to 50 years of age. Because they are usually 3 to 4 mm in greatest dimension, they are frequently not palpable, although in one third of cases a small mass may be appreciated. Treatment consists of complete excision of the draining duct via a circumareolar incision.

Pathologic nipple discharge is usually spontaneous and unilateral and arises from a single duct. If clinical examination demonstrates a mass or a suspicious lesion is found on mammography, then cytology or core biopsy of the lesion should be performed. Spontaneous or inducible discharge that arises from a single duct warrants surgery if it has any of the following characteristics: bloody, persistent (at least two occasions per week), associated with a mass, or a new finding in a woman older than age 40. Prior to surgery, the draining duct and trigger point should be ascertained. During surgery, the terminal duct is excised with a biopsy of the surrounding breast tissue in the trigger point area.

Paget Disease

Paget disease indicates the presence of an underlying malignancy, *in situ* or invasive, and presents as a specific finding of the nipple. It initially presents with erythema and mild eczematous scaling of the nipple, often accompanied by itching and nipple discharge. Histologically, the Paget cell is a large, pale-staining cell with prominent nuclei. Diagnosis can be obtained by punch, shave, or wedge biopsy, scrape cytology, or nipple excision. In patients with clinical Paget disease and a mass, the majority of patients have invasive breast cancer, whereas in patients presenting without a mass, the number presenting with DCIS is higher. Before definitive treatment, it is important to rule out multicentric disease, for which MRI is gaining increasing utility. Treatment includes either simple mastectomy or breast conservation, which involves excision of nipple areolar complex and radiation.

Breast Abscess/Mastitis

Mastitis is a generalized cellulitis of the breast that occurs with relative frequency during lactation. The most common etiologic organism is *Staphylococcus aureus*, with streptococcal groups second. The treatment consists of heat/ice packs to the breast and oral antibiotics (first-generation cephalosporin or penicillin). If the patient is lactating, use of a breast pump is advised, since the infant commonly harbors the organism and can cause reinfection. If complicated by an abscess, repeated aspirations may be necessary. If these fail, or the patient is diabetic or systemically ill, incision and drainage with intravenous antibiotics is required.

BENIGN BREAST DISEASES AND THEIR MANAGEMENT

The College of American Pathologists has categorized benign breast diseases into those that are associated with no increased risk, slightly increased risk [relative risk (RR) 1.5 to 2.0), or moderately increased risk (RR ≥5) in breast cancer development as shown in Table 32-3.

Simple Breast Cysts

Simple breast cysts are epithelial-lined cavities that contain fluid. Clinically apparent cysts develop in approximately 7% of women. Cysts often fluctuate with the menstrual cycle, and occur at any age, but are most commonly seen in

TABLE 32-3

BENIGN BREAST DISEASE CATEGORIZED BY RELATIVE RISKS

No Increased Risk	Slightly Increased (1.5 to 2x)	Moderately Increased (5x)
Apocrine metaplasia	Hyperplasia, solid or papillary	Atypical ductal hyperplasia
Cysts	Papilloma with fibrovascular core	Atypical lobular hyperplasia
Duct ectasia	Sclerosing adenosis	
Fibroadenoma		
Fibrosis		
Hyperplasia, mild		
Mastitis		

From Morrow M, Jordan VC, eds. *Managing breast cancer risk.* Ontario: BC Decker, 2000:7, with permission.

the last decade of reproductive years. They tend to be firm, mobile, and well demarcated from the surrounding breast tissue, characteristics that mimic those of a solid lesion. The indications for aspiration are to confirm the diagnosis of a mass and, for some patients, to relieve symptoms. Complex masses that clearly have a solid component within a cyst require biopsy and should not be aspirated so as not to collapse the cyst, making the lesion more difficult to locate. Routine submission of cystic fluid for cytologic evaluation is not recommended, since the yield of a malignant result is less than 1%. If the fluid is bloody, or the mass does not resolve completely with aspiration (indicating a possible solid component), or if the same cyst recurs repeatedly in a short interval on follow-up clinical breast examination, then a biopsy is indicated to rule out intracystic carcinoma.

If ultrasonography was obtained and the results indicate a simple cyst, then no further intervention is necessary, unless the patient is symptomatic, then cyst aspiration is appropriate. In the absence of atypical pathologic findings, there is no increased risk of cancer. However, certain factors increase the suspicion for a cystic carcinoma, including an associated solid mass, a bloody aspirate, an irregular cyst wall on ultrasonography, or multiple recurrences after aspiration. If any of these factors are present, then a biopsy is warranted. Otherwise, for simple breast cysts, the treatment is reassurance.

Fibroadenoma

Fibroadenomas are the most common cause of breast masses in women younger than age 25. They are found in approximately 7% to 13% of patients examined in breast clinics and comprise approximately 50% of breast biopsies, up to 75% for biopsies in women younger than 20. Grossly, fibroadenomas are pseudoencapsulated and mobile, with smooth or slightly lobulated borders. Cytologically, the tumors comprise epithelial and stromal elements. They generally present as solitary painless masses and must be differentiated from cancer. Although the risk of cancer in a fibroadenoma is very rare, it is important that any solid breast mass in a woman older than 30 be biopsied for a

definitive diagnosis with an FNA, core needle biopsy, or excision biopsy. For suspected fibroadenomas, the general algorithm for women younger than the age of 40 is clinical examination, FNA, and ultrasonography. The combined accuracy is only 70% to 80%; however, they provide an accurate differentiation between a benign and a malignant lesion. If all three modalities confirm the diagnosis, the patient can be observed with close clinical follow-up.

The natural history of fibroadenomas is that 16% to 59% will resolve spontaneously, and of those that do not resolve, approximately 35% will remain stable or become smaller and about 30% will grow, at which time, they can be excised for pathologic confirmation. In 10% to 15% of cases, multiple adenomas are encountered. Juvenile fibroadenomas account for approximately 4% of all fibroadenomas and commonly present in adolescents and young adults. The most common time of presentation is within 1 to 3 years after the onset of menarche. These masses may grow rapidly and can cause marked breast asymmetry and vascular engorgement. The treatment is enucleation with special care taken to preserve the central breast bud.

Hamartomas

Hamartomas present as well-defined masses on clinical breast examination and on mammography. These lesions, microscopically, are composed of a combination of fibrous stroma, ducts, lobules and adipose tissue with occasional smooth muscle.

Fat Necrosis

Fat necrosis is important because, although benign, it can closely mimic carcinoma both clinically and on mammographic examination. The gross examination of fat necrosis depends on the age of the lesion. Early on, there is hemorrhage and indurated fat within the lesion. Later, a rounded, firm tumor is formed that may have areas of cavitation owing to liquefactive necrosis. On microscopic examination, early lesions have cystic space with lipid-laden macrophages, whereas later lesions have fibroplastic proliferation with deposition of collagen. This type of pathologic appearance may also appear after surgical trauma to the breast as well as after radiation therapy for cancer.

Mondor Disease

Mondor disease is a variant of thrombophlebitis involving the superficial veins of the anterior chest wall and breast. Patients present with local pain and a tender, palpable subcutaneous cord or skin dimpling. The etiology is unknown but there may be a history of trauma or inflammation in some women. Although generally considered a benign disorder, it is recommended that women older than the age of 35 have a mammogram when presenting with these complaints. This condition often resolves spontaneously, but anti-inflammatory agents and warm compresses may alleviate symptoms. If the condition is refractory to this treatment, then a complete excision of the involved vein can be performed.

Phyllodes Tumor

Phyllodes tumor represents a spectrum of lesions ranging from benign to malignant and accounts for less than 1% of all breast cancers. It usually presents as a painless mass that is rounded and multinodular. The mean age of women with this lesion is in the fourth decade, although it may appear in any age group. *Cystosarcoma phyllodes*, a malignant variant, presents with a similar clinical picture. One notable feature of phyllodes tumor is the absence of suspicious axillary lymph nodes despite the large sized-mass, unlike in breast cancer. Axillary nodes may be enlarged but are almost never the result of metastases. Like fibroadenomas, phyllodes tumors consist of epithelial elements and connective tissue stroma. Twenty-five percent to 50% are histologically malignant (increased mitotic activity, stromal cellularity with nuclear atypia, and overgrowth) with metastases in 6% to 22% of all cases. Regardless of their malignant potential, phyllodes tumors tend to have high recurrence rates, reported between 20% and 35%, especially if the tumor is simply enucleated during surgery. Recommended treatment includes wide excision with a 2- to 3-cm margin of normal tissue or total mastectomy without axillary dissection for large malignant lesions or lesions not amenable to breast conservation.

Inflammatory/Infectious Breast Disease

Breast abscess and mastitis are relatively common conditions for which women seek physician care, as mentioned in the preceding text. *Mammary duct ectasia* occurs primarily in perimenopausal and postmenopausal women and is characterized by dilation of the subareolar ducts. Nipple retraction can occur, with nipple discharge that is paste-like and sometimes green in color. A similar condition, seen more frequently in younger women, especially women who are heavy smokers, is periductal mastitis. This condition is characterized by episodes of periareolar inflammation, sometimes with accompanying nipple retraction and purulent discharge. There has been confusion between these two entities; however, they appear to be two separate clinical conditions based on differences among women with regards to age, clinical history, and smoking history.

MALIGNANT BREAST DISEASES AND THEIR MANAGEMENT

The annual incidence of breast cancer in the United States is estimated for the year 2003 to be 212,600 new cases, making it the most common cancer in women younger than age 60, with lung cancer being the most common cancer for those age 60 and older. The lifetime risk of being diagnosed with breast cancer is 12.5%, or 1 in 8 women. Moreover, in 2003, approximately 1,300 men were afflicted with 400 expected deaths. About 39,800 women died of breast cancer in 2003, making it the leading cause of death in women ages 40 to 49 and the overall second leading cause of cancer death in women after lung cancer. Although there was a slight increase in the absolute incidence of breast cancer during the 20th century, there was a decrease in the overall case-fatality rate.

PREINVASIVE (*IN SITU*) BREAST CARCINOMAS

Lobular Carcinoma *In Situ* and Treatment

Lobular carcinoma *in situ* (LCIS) arises from the lobular and terminal ducts of the breast and traditionally was considered to be, by most investigators, not a true cancer but instead a marker of increased risk. However, newer evidence supports that LCIS may be a direct precursor of invasive breast cancer. The true incidence of LCIS is not known because of the lack of clinical and mammographic signs. LCIS is almost always an incidental finding in breast tissue removed for another reason. Although the exact incidence of LCIS in biopsies varies, agreement exists that LCIS is an uncommon finding. However, the diagnosis of LCIS is increasing in frequency, thought mostly owing to the increasing use of screening mammography and partly because of greater recognition of LCIS as a pathologic entity.

Patients with LCIS carry an eightfold to tenfold increased risk of invasive carcinoma during their lifetime and a 1% per-year annual risk, a risk which persists indefinitely. Eighty percent to 90% of LCIS cases occur in premenopausal women. It is a risk factor for bilateral breast cancer, not limited to the side involved with LCIS. Most cancers that develop are invasive ductal carcinomas, but there is a higher incidence of invasive lobular carcinoma than in the general population. The current management of LCIS is surveillance, with annual mammograms and biannual CBEs along with the use of tamoxifen, a selective estrogen-receptor modulator (SERM). Bilateral prophylactic mastectomy is rarely indicated. The efficacy of tamoxifen in reducing the development of future breast cancer in patients with LCIS was shown in a landmark trial of 1993, the National Surgery Adjuvant Breast and Bowel Project (NSABP) P-1 Prevention Trial (also discussed in subsequent text). For women who had LCIS, the risk reduction in this study was 56% with 5 years of tamoxifen use.

Ductal Carcinoma *In Situ* and Treatment

Ductal carcinoma *in situ* (DCIS), is characterized by a clonal proliferation of presumably malignant epithelial cells within the lumens of the mammary ductal-lobular system, with no evidence of basement membrane invasion. DCIS lies along the spectrum of preinvasive lesions between atypical ductal hyperplasia and invasive ductal carcinoma. During breast tumorigenesis, there are dramatic changes in gene expression during the transition from normal breast tissue to DCIS. The estrogen receptor is expressed by more than 70% of ductal carcinoma *in situ* lesions. The HER2/neu protooncogene is overexpressed in approximately one half of DCIS lesions, but not in atypical hyperplasia. Loss of heterozygosity is found in more than 70% of high-grade DCIS lesions, compared to 0% in normal breast tissue and 35% to 40% of atypical hyperplasia lesions. In roughly 25% of DCIS lesions, the p53 tumor-suppressor gene is mutated, whereas in normal or benign tissue it is rarely mutated. Although the initiating steps and subsequent pathways are not completely understood, it seems that invasive breast cancers arise from *in situ* carcinomas, with both exhibiting shared chromosomal changes. Data suggests that in DCIS, most of the molecular changes that characterize invasive breast cancer are already present.

DCIS encompasses a pathologically heterogeneous group of lesions, with no universal agreement on a classification scheme. The traditional system classified lesions based on architecture with five subtypes: comedo, cribriform, micropapillary, papillary, and solid. Newer, alternative classification schemes are based on nuclear grade: high, intermediate, and low grade, and presence of necrosis. Some believe it useful to divide DCIS lesions into comedo and noncomedo, based on observations that the comedo type appears cytologically more malignant, with high-grade nuclei, architectural distortion, and necrosis. Although one system of classification is not universally endorsed, there is agreement that certain features must be reported in pathology reports of DCIS lesions: nuclear grade (low, intermediate, and high), presence of necrosis (comedo or punctate), cell polarization, and architectural pattern (Fig. 32-3).

The incidence, or detection rate, of DCIS has increased notably since the implementation of mammography as a screening tool, increasing by a factor of 10 in 2 decades. In the early 1980s, the incidence of DCIS was approximately 5,000 cases; now more than 50,000 cases are diagnosed annually. Of all breast cancers, DCIS accounts for 20% of those detected mammographically. Nearly 90% of DCIS lesions are diagnosed mammographically, with most lesions having microcalcifications (76%), soft-tissue densities (11%), or both (13%). DCIS may be associated with an occult microinvasive tumor (less than 0.1 cm), classifying the lesion as microinvasive disease, and is treated according to the guidelines for invasive disease. Microinvasion is most commonly found in DCIS lesions greater than 2.5 cm in diameter, those with high-grade DCIS or comedonecrosis, and in patients presenting with nipple discharge or palpable masses. Multicentricity, separate foci of DCIS in another quadrant, has been reported to range from 0% to 47%. More recent studies indicate that true multicentric disease is uncommon and that DCIS involves the breast in a segmental distribution; however, the segments involved might be quite large (greater than 3 cm). Nodal involvement in patients with radiographically detected DCIS is rare.

The goal in treating DCIS is prevention of progression to invasive cancer and local recurrence. The options for surgical treatment include mastectomy or breast-conserving therapy (BCT, i.e., lumpectomy with radiation), which will be described in greater detail. There have been no prospective, randomized trials comparing mastectomy versus BCT as treatment for DCIS; however, data from some surgical trials and large treatment registries suggest that there is no significant difference in overall survival, although local recurrence rate is lower after mastectomy. Traditionally, DCIS was treated with simple mastectomy, providing a highly effective cure rate of 98% of lesions. Still, breast cancer recurs in 1% to 2% of patients with DCIS who have undergone mastectomy. Currently, most women in the United States are treated with BCT for DCIS, owing in part to the shift toward breast-conserving surgery for invasive breast cancer. Also, most DCIS lesions are small and clinically occult, detected through mammography, which also explains the widespread use of breast conservation for DCIS.

Women with DCIS are at risk for a second tumor on the contralateral breast, at a rate of 0.5% to 1% per year. Neither axillary lymph node dissection nor sentinel node biopsy (described in subsequent text) is warranted in patients with DCIS, owing to the very low incidence of axillary metastases. However, SLN biopsy may be used in patients with a higher likelihood of occult invasive cancer, such as extensive, high-grade DCIS or DCIS associated with palpable masses, or those undergoing mastectomy, since SLN biopsy is no longer possible if invasive cancer is identified after surgery.

Women are at risk for recurrence after breast-conserving surgery for DCIS. Most recurrences in the ipsilateral breast are at or near the original site of the tumor, with one half of the recurrences being DCIS and one half being invasive tumors. The current management of DCIS in women who

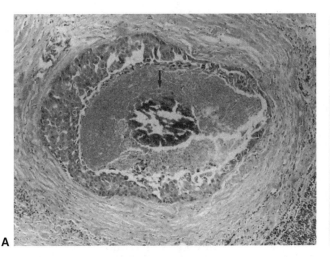 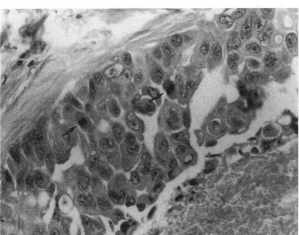

A **B**

Figure 32-3   A: Comedo-type ductal carcinoma *in situ* with prominent central necrosis and dense calcification. **B:** Considerable nuclear atypia and pleomorphism is consistent with poorly differentiated ductal carcinoma in situ. [From Harris JR, Lippman ME, Morrow M et al., eds. *Diseases of the breast.* Philadelphia: Lippincott Williams & Wilkins, 2000:384 (1A) and 387 (4C), with permission.]

have undergone breast-conserving surgery is based on several large, prospective, RCTs. Three of the trials directly compared excision alone versus excision with radiotherapy in patients with fully excised lesions and negative margins. The results show that radiotherapy consistently reduces the risk of recurrence in the ipsilateral breast by 40% to 60%. After 8 to 10 years of follow-up, there is an approximate 12% to 16% risk of recurrence in the ipsilateral breast with excision alone, whereas, radiotherapy reduces this risk to about 8%. At present, investigations are being conducted to identify patients with DCIS who may not require radiotherapy. According to a retrospective analysis, patients with low-grade, small tumors or lesions with clear margins greater than 10 mm have a very favorable prognosis, and may not necessarily gain additional benefit with radiotherapy. However, this finding has not been reproduced in prospective studies of wide excision alone for DCIS. Currently, it is not possible to identify women prospectively who are at low enough risk that radiotherapy may not offer at least some benefit in preventing recurrence.

In the NASBP B24 trial, tamoxifen was studied as adjuvant therapy in women with DCIS who had undergone excision and radiation treatment. In this study, it was shown that taking tamoxifen for 5 years will further reduce the likelihood of recurrence in the ipsilateral breast from 9% to 6% at 5 years. A detailed discussion about tamoxifen and its role in breast cancer follows later.

INVASIVE BREAST CANCER

Comprising a heterogeneous group of lesions, invasive breast cancers share one common feature: invasion into the breast stroma with potential for lymph node and distant metastases. Regardless of histologic type, most invasive breast malignancies arise in the terminal duct lobular unit. *Invasive* or *infiltrating ductal carcinoma* is by far the most common type of breast malignancy, and usually presents as either a palpable mass or radiographic abnormality (Fig. 32-4). Macroscopically, it is a gray-white mass with irregular spiculated edges. Microscopically, its appearance is highly heterogeneous with regard to mitotic activity, growth pattern, cytologic features, and extent of *in situ* component (Fig. 32-5A).

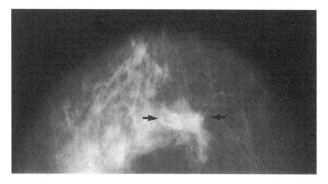

Figure 32-4 Typical mammographic appearance of a spiculated cancer (*arrows*). [From Harris JR, Lippman ME, Morrow M et al., eds. *Diseases of the breast*. Philadelphia: Lippincott Williams & Wilkins, 2000:124 (1B), with permission.]

The second most frequent type of invasive breast malignancy is *invasive lobular (infiltrating) carcinoma*, comprising about 5% to 10% of breast cancers. It may present as a palpable mass or mammographic abnormality, as with invasive ductal carcinoma. However, physical or radiographic findings may be subtle and underestimate the extent of disease. There is a significant incidence of multifocality in the ipsilateral breast, and often there are foci of LCIS within the tumor. Macroscopically, lobular cancer appears as firm, gray-white masses, indistinguishable from invasive ductal carcinomas, or the breast tissue can have a rubbery appearance. In other cases, there is no visible abnormality and only on microscopic examination is carcinoma apparent. On histologic examination, invasive lobular cancer usually appears as small, uniform neoplastic cells infiltrating the stroma in a single-file pattern, often growing around the duct concentrically (Fig. 32-5B).

A less common invasive breast carcinoma is *tubular carcinoma*, accounting for 7% to 27% of breast cancers detected in mammographically screened populations. They are typically small (less than 1.0 cm) tumors that are well differentiated and generally carry a good prognosis. The incidence of axillary lymph node metastasis ranges from 0% to 30%, depending on the size of the lesion, but on average, the incidence is 15%. There is controversy regarding the need for lymph node assessment for tubular carcinoma less than 1 cm. However, the standard of care continues to include either sentinel lymph node biopsy or axillary dissection.

Natural History and Staging of Breast Cancer

As early as the late 18th century, breast cancer had been described as a heterogeneous disease, characterized by a long natural history, when there was documentation of 250 patients with various stages of breast cancer and their subsequent clinical courses. The majority of these patients had advanced (stage IV) disease. The median survival in these patients was 2.7 years from onset of symptoms. Eighteen percent of the patients survived 5 years, and 4% survived 10 years, indicating that even patients with untreated, advanced disease can survive for long periods.

The majority of breast cancer tumors occur in the upper outer quadrant (approximately 50%). The spread of cancer through the breast occurs by direct extension into the breast parenchyma, along the mammary ducts and via the lymphatics. Tumor size and number of lymph node involvement delineate the prognosis for breast cancer patients. As the size of the primary tumor increases, so too does the frequency of distant metastases and axillary node involvement. Even after treatment, these patients are at risk for metastases for extended periods, so defining "cure" in this patient population remains a challenge.

The axillary nodes are the most common sites of regional involvement of breast cancer. For the purpose of staging and treatment planning, it is important to understand the likelihood of involvement of the axilla given the size of the tumor and tumor characteristics. Approximately 50% of patients with breast cancer detectable on physical examination will have axillary node involvement. In tumors smaller than 1.0 cm, the frequency of nodal involvement is 20%, indicating that even with small tumors, there is considerable chance of regional spread. In

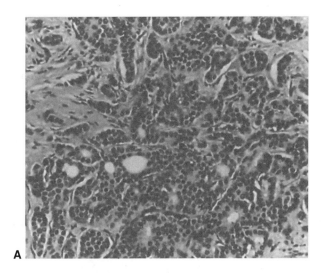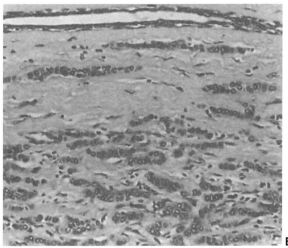

Figure 32-5 **A:** Infiltrating ductal carcinoma and **B:** infiltrating lobular carcinoma. [From Harris JR, Lippman ME, Morrow M et al., eds. *Diseases of the breast*. Philadelphia: Lippincott Williams & Wilkins, 2000:427 (2A) and 429 (4A), with permission.]

Table 32-4, 5-year breast cancer survival rates are shown according to the size of the tumor and axillary node involvement.

It is important to note that 20% to 30% of patients with negative axillary nodes develop distant metastases within 10 years. This suggests that metastases can occur hematogenously without first involving the lymph nodes. It is now known that one factor associated with an increased risk of distant relapse is the presence of bone marrow micrometastases, shown in one study to be associated with a sixfold increase in relative risk of relapse. The technique of immunohistochemical detection of epithelially derived cells in bone marrow is highly sensitive, but currently, bone marrow status does not have any role in patient management. The American College of Surgeons Oncology Group (ACOSOG) Z0010 Trial is investigating the prognostic significance of bone marrow micrometastases in women with stage I or IIa breast cancer.

Breast cancer treatment is aimed at controlling locoregional (breast and lymph nodes) and systemic disease. As outlined in the preceding text, treatment has evolved from radical mastectomies to lumpectomies with radiation and sentinel node biopsy. With the advancement of screening, breast cancer is detected at earlier stages with favorable 5-year survival rates. Tumor size, the presence of axillary node involvement, and tumor histology, not only influence the overall survival rates but also the time-course to distant metastases. Breast carcinoma can metastasize to a variety of organs, with bone, lung, and liver being the most common sites.

The American Joint Committee on Cancer (AJCC) has recently revised its recommendations for breast cancer staging (Table 32-5). The AJCC system is based on the TNM system: Tumor Node Metastasis. This new staging incorporates new areas regarding evaluation of the axilla and prognostic factors: the number of positive nodes, the relevance of micrometastatic disease, and the method used for detection, such as sentinel node biopsy or clinical examination.

Certain histopathologic results are not used for staging purposes, but instead for determining prognosis, such as tumor grade. Some investigators propose that tumor grade (well, moderately, or poorly differentiated) is a powerful predictor of the course of breast cancer; however, difficulties with grading include reproducibility and lack of agreement among different observers. Other factors that may help determine prognosis and guide therapy decisions include degree of tumor cell proliferation, presence of growth factors, hormonal receptor status, and measures of invasiveness. Proliferative activity of a tumor cell is quantified by mitotic index (MI), thymidine-labeling index (TLI), and flow cytometry. Flow cytometry can be performed on fresh or frozen tissue specimens or needle aspirates. Tumors with a high percentage of cells in the S-phase, or synthesis phase, correlate strongly with other prognostic factors such as poor histologic grade. In addition, cancers with a high DNA index have a considerable aneuploid cell population and are more poorly differentiated.

Inflammatory breast carcinoma is characterized by diffuse brawny induration of the skin, representing tumor embolization of the dermal lymphatics. Treatment includes local and

TABLE 32-4

5-YEAR BREAST CANCER SURVIVAL RATES ACCORDING TO TUMOR SIZE AND AXILLARY NODE INVOLVEMENT

Tumor Size in cm	Negative Nodes	1–3 Positive Nodes	>3 Positive Nodes
<0.5	99%	95%	59%
0.5–0.9	98%	94%	54%
1.0–1.9	96%	87%	67%
2.0–2.9	92%	83%	63%
3.0–3.9	86%	79%	57%
4.0–4.9	85%	70%	53%
>5.0	82%	73%	46%

From Harris JR, Lippman ME, Morrow M et al., eds. *Diseases of the breast*. Philadelphia: Lippincott, Williams & Wilkins, 2000:415, with permission.

TABLE 32-5

TNM CLASSIFICATION OF BREAST CANCER (AMERICAN JOINT COMMITTEE ON CANCER)

TNM	Tumor Size	Nodal Status	Metastasis
	In situ	N0	M0
Stage I	<2 cm	N0	M0
IIa	<2 cm	1-3 AN or IMN detected by SLN	M0
	2–5 cm	N0	M0
IIb	2–5 cm	1-3 AN or IMN detected by SLN	M0
	Or >5 cm	N0	M0
IIIa	Any size	Metastasis in 4–9 AN or clinical IMN	M0
IIIb	Any size plus skin involvement (edema, *peau d'orange*, satellite skin nodules, ulcers) or chest wall; inflammatory cancer	Any N	M0
IIIc	Any size (any T)	Metastasis in 10+ AN or infraclavicular node	M0
IV	Any size	Any N	Distant mets

AN, axillary node; IMN, internal mammary node; SLN, sentinel node biopsy.

systemic treatment. Metastatic workup is mandatory. Local control includes induction chemotherapy followed by modified radical mastectomy.

Male Breast Cancer

A special therapeutic problem that should be included under the heading of invasive breast cancer is male breast cancer (MBC). It accounts for approximately 1% of all breast cancers, with an estimated 1,300 cases and 400 deaths in 2003. The overall ratio of female breast cancer to MBC in the United States is 100:1 in whites and 100:1.4 in African Americans. The strongest risk for developing MBC is Klinefelter syndrome, which results in the inheritance of an additional X chromosome. Other risk factors include associated family history of breast or ovarian cancer, prior history of undescended testes, and chronic liver disorders such as cirrhosis. Men who are found to carry a BRCA-2 mutation are at an increased risk (up to 6%) for developing breast cancer. MBC usually presents as a painless, firm subareolar mass, or as a mass in the upper outer quadrant. As in the workup of a breast mass in women, mammography is used along with tissue sampling of suspicious lesions either by FNA, core biopsy, or open biopsy to rule out a benign process. Accounting for 85% of MBC cases is invasive ductal carcinoma. Breast conservation is not an option in men because of lack of breast tissue; consequently, a modified radical mastectomy (MRM) is the definitive treatment. Frequently tamoxifen, and occasionally adjuvant chemotherapy, is recommended based on the benefits of these therapies in clinical trials in women with early stage breast cancer, although the benefit in men is unproven at this time.

Treatment of Breast Cancer

Surgery

The multidisciplinary approach to the treatment of breast cancer has evolved over the years, requiring the collaborative effort of surgeons, radiologists, pathologists, and oncologists. The modern era of breast surgery began with Halsted in 1894 with the development of the radical mastectomy. This surgical approach was based on the theory of local spread of disease, especially through the lymphatics, and entailed an *en bloc* resection of the breast, overlying skin, pectoral muscles, and an axillary node dissection. It was effective in obtaining local control of the tumor, however, failed to cure many patients of breast cancer.

There was a switch to MRM as the operative therapy for invasive breast cancer when it became recognized that failure after treatment was usually caused by systemic dissemination of neoplastic cells before surgery rather than inadequate surgical resection. Although seemingly an almost identical procedure, MRM represented a major divergence from the Halstedian principle of *en bloc* surgery. MRM is used to define a variety of operative procedures, but all entail complete removal of the breast and some of the axillary nodes (Fig. 32-6). Further proof refuting the Halstedian concept of breast cancer came from the National Surgical Adjuvant Breast and Bowel Project's (NSABP) B-04 Trial. In this trial, clinically node-negative patients were randomized to radical mastectomy, simple mastectomy and nodal irradiation, or simple mastectomy with delayed dissection if positive nodes developed. There was no difference shown in survival between the groups, and, so today, there are rarely any indications for a radical mastectomy.

BCT developed from the same principles as did modified radical mastectomies. The strategy behind BCT is to surgically remove the tumor and eradicate any residual cancer by use of radiation. It consists of lumpectomy, axillary node dissection, and adjuvant radiation therapy. One of the major goals of BCT is to preserve the cosmetic appearance of the breast. There have been six modern prospective randomized trials, including the NSABP B-06 trial, comparing mastectomy with lumpectomy and radiation for stages I and II breast cancer. All trials demonstrated no significant differences in overall or disease-free survival rates between the two groups of treatment. The incidence of local recurrence was higher in the BCT arm in some of the trials (ranging from 3% to 20%); however, this may result from inappropriate patient selection (many patients with T2 tumors in the BCT arm), inadequate surgery or radiation therapy (trials including BCT patients with positive margins), or biologically aggressive disease. Overall the incidence of local recurrence in the BCT groups ranges from 3% to 20%, whereas in the mastectomy groups, the range is 4% to 14%, demonstrating that even mastectomy does not provide assurance against local recurrence.

A patient who is otherwise a good candidate for BCT should not be encouraged to have a mastectomy if the hope is to avoid a local recurrence. In a large meta-analysis of nine prospectively randomized trials comparing BCT and mastectomy, the 5-year rates for local recurrence were 5.9% and 6.2%, respectively. The majority of failures in a treated breast can be salvaged with mastectomy. Only a minority of patients has a contraindication to BCT (Table 32-6), which can be determined with a thorough history, physical examination, and detailed mammography

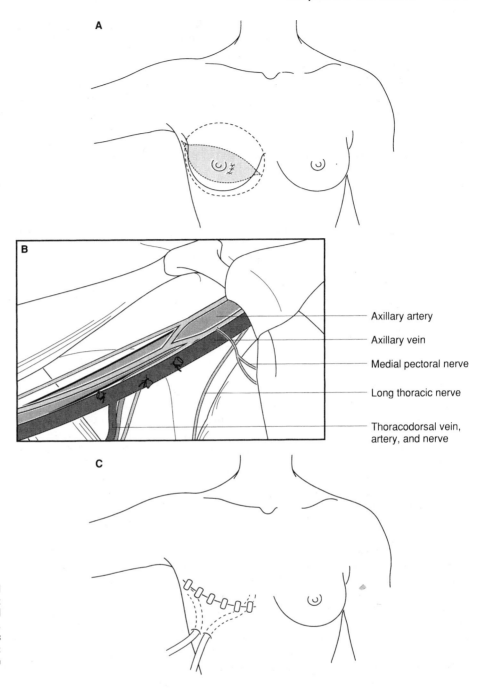

Figure 32-6 Technique of modified radical mastectomy. (From August DA, Sondak VK. Breast. In: Greenfield LJ, Mulholland M, Oldham KT et al., eds. *Surgery: scientific principles and practice*, 2nd ed. Philadelphia: Lippincott-Raven, 1997:1393, with permission.)

with magnification views. In one study, when these steps were taken and the cancer was determined to be localized, 97% of these patients could be treated with BCT. However, studies have shown that less than 50% of women with stages I and II breast cancer are treated with BCT, with considerable geographic variation. Some of the discrepancy between the percentage eligible versus actual percentage undergoing BCT is because of true contraindications to BCT, but other reasons include patient preference, inaccessibility to radiation facilities, and sometimes, inappropriate selection criteria by physicians.

Breast Reconstruction

Breast reconstruction has changed extensively over the last 15 years. Reconstruction may be immediate, occurring simultaneously with the mastectomy procedure, or delayed,

TABLE 32-6

CONTRAINDICATIONS TO BREAST-CONSERVATION THERAPY

Absolute	Relative
First/second trimester pregnancy as an absolute contraindication	Large tumor relative to size of breast
Multicentric disease	Anticipated poor cosmetic result
Diffuse microcalcifications	Tumor size >5 cm
History of prior x-ray therapy	Large breast size
	Central tumor under nipple requiring nipple excision
	History of collagen vascular disease

From Harris JR, Lippman ME, Morrow M et al., eds. *Diseases of the breast.* Philadelphia: Lippincott Williams & Wilkins, 2000:526, with permission.

carried out as a separate procedure sometime after the mastectomy. The most widely used form of reconstruction is the expander–implant reconstruction, with saline implants the dominant choice over silicone. The autogenous reconstructive method of choice is the transverse rectus myocutaneous flap (TRAM), first described in 1982. Use of flap reconstruction has been increasing steadily over the years as flap techniques have improved. Better methods for nipple reconstruction have also evolved.

Practically all patients undergoing mastectomy are potential candidates for immediate reconstruction, with the need for postoperative radiation only as a relative contraindication. Immediate reconstruction has now become the dominant choice over delayed reconstruction. One of its main benefits is that it provides the greatest psychological benefit for most women. For women who undergo postoperative radiation, autogenous flaps do better, but even for implants, one option is to place an expander and address final reconstruction after radiation therapy is completed. With some partial mastectomies and lumpectomies, partial reconstruction or reshaping is required leading to a new subset of breast reconstruction.

Sentinel Node Biopsy

The technique of SLN mapping and biopsy was developed on the observation that specific areas drain via afferent lymphatics to a sentinel node before draining to other lymph nodes in the basin. Radioactive colloids and/or isosulfan blue dye is injected into the region of the tumor, which then tracks through lymph channels to the first one or couple sentinel nodes. Either by visual inspection or by use of a hand-held gamma counter, the sentinel nodes are identified and removed for pathologic evaluation.

In experienced hands, the positive predictive value of a successful SLN biopsy approaches 100%. In general, patients with metastases in sentinel nodes should undergo complete levels I and II axillary dissection. If the SLN results are negative, then a patient is spared a full axillary dissection, thereby avoiding its associated complications such as lymphedema, neuropathies, and seromas. SLN biopsy is considered to be the standard practice when it is not contraindicated. Contraindications to SLN biopsy include clinically positive nodes, tumor size greater than 5 cm, locally advanced cancer, prior axillary surgery, or pregnant women. However, it must be noted that although there is a less than 5% false-negative rate in experienced hands, data on long-term follow-up is not complete.

Axillary Lymph Node Dissection

Axillary dissection remains the standard of care for invasive breast cancer for management of the axillary nodes if SLN biopsy is unavailable or contraindicated. Levels I and II axillary dissections (removal of nodes lateral and posterior to the pectoralis minor muscle) provide local control in the axilla. In addition, accurate staging information is obtained. The axillary dissection should be performed through the mastectomy ellipse in a patient undergoing a mastectomy. In a patient undergoing BCT, the axillary incision and breast incision should be separate. During the dissection, the long thoracic, thoracodorsal, and medial pectoral nerves should be preserved. With preservation of the intercostal brachiocutaneous nerve, numbness of the upper arm is less likely to

occur; however, if there are grossly involved lymph nodes, this nerve should be sacrificed.

Adjuvant therapy recommendations were traditionally made on the basis of the size of the tumor and lymph node status. Increasingly, recommendations take into account molecular markers, primary tumor features, and patient characteristics. This evolution in treatment practices can be explained by a better understanding of tumor-specific risk factors, especially when more and more women are presenting with stage I disease. Currently, ACOSOG is conducting a trial (Z0011) investigating whether observation of axillary nodes given a positive SLN has the same disease-free and overall survival as an axillary node dissection.

Adjuvant Therapy

Radiation

As discussed in the preceding text, radiation used in BST for DCIS decreased local recurrence in the ipsilateral breast from 16% to 8% in patients treated with excision alone. Similarly, radiation used in BCT for invasive disease shows decreased risk of recurrence with the use of radiation in a number of trials. One large trial with 20 years of follow-up, the NSABP B-06, demonstrated that breast irradiation decreased the risk of recurrence in the ipsilateral breast from 39.2% to 14.3% after 20 years. It is important to note that in this trial, 45% of the women had tumors larger than 2 cm and nearly 40% had positive nodes. Other trials comparing BCT with radiation to conservative surgery (CS) alone demonstrate recurrence rates for CS ranging from 18% to 35% and 2% to 15% for BCT. The trials differ in the patient populations (tumor size and nodal involvement), surgical techniques (extensive lumpectomies and tumor-free margins) as well as length of follow-up. The important fact to note is that all studies show a decrease in local recurrence with the use of radiation. However, that being said, there were no significant differences in overall survival rates.

Chemotherapy/Hormonal Therapy

Currently, all women with breast cancers larger than 1 cm or those with node-positive cancer are candidates for adjuvant chemotherapy. One commonly used regimen is cyclophosphamide, methotrexate, and 5-fluorouracil (CMF) with a duration in the range of 3 to 6 months. Other regimens commonly used are anthracycline, namely doxorubicin, and Cytoxan (AC). Newer agents shown to be as effective or more effective than older drugs in the treatment of advanced breast carcinoma are taxanes (paclitaxel and docetaxel), and vinca alkaloids, such as vinorelbine. One newer option includes Herceptin, a humanized antibody against the HER-2/neu oncoprotein (the c-erb-b2 oncogene product), which, when amplified, is associated with a worse prognosis for patients with node-positive breast cancer. Herceptin has activity in metastatic cancer, especially when used with doxorubicin and paclitaxel. However, its safety profile has yet to be established, especially with regard to cardiotoxicity.

Tamoxifen is widely used in the treatment of breast cancer today. As mentioned, it is a SERM and exhibits dual activities by binding to the estrogen receptor (ER), acting both as an estrogen antagonist and agonist. As an estrogen antagonist, tamoxifen binds competitively to ERs, which results in reduced transcription of estrogen-regulated genes. As an estrogen agonist, it has a favorable effect on blood lipid profiles and acts to preserve bone mineral density. Multiple trials have been conducted to determine the effectiveness of adjuvant tamoxifen in different subgroups. One large trial, the NSABP trial B-14, evaluated the role of tamoxifen in histologically node-negative patients. Patients, regardless of menopausal status, who had ER positive cancer and received tamoxifen, had significantly fewer recurrences and death than those given placebo. Not only did the tamoxifen-treated patients have fewer ipsilateral breast and distant recurrences, they also had a considerable reduction (nearly 50%) in contralateral breast cancer. In a large metaanalysis, tamoxifen given to patients with ER positive tumors resulted in an approximately 50% reduction in the annual odds of recurrence and 26% reduction in the annual odds of death. Metaanalysis data also suggest that adding tamoxifen to chemotherapy in premenopausal patients provides significant additional benefit, but only if the tumor is ER-positive. Recommendations for the use of adjuvant therapy are shown in Table 32-7.

Chemotherapy may also be used preoperatively, otherwise known as neoadjuvant therapy, in operable breast cancer. When used in patients with inoperable, locally advanced breast cancer for tumor reduction to facilitate irradiation or mastectomy, preoperative chemotherapy is referred to as induction chemotherapy. A phase II trial in Milan investigated neoadjuvant chemotherapy in tumors larger than 3 cm, with overall response rates of 80%, allowing breast-preserving surgery in 91% of patients. Three other trials had similar results, showing that preoperative chemotherapy may allow some patients with large tumors to be candidates for breast preservation when they would otherwise not qualify. However, with neoadjuvant therapy, control of distant micrometastases is not improved and pretreatment assessment of molecular markers is more complicated.

Treatment for metastatic disease includes endocrine therapy, chemotherapy, and radiation therapy, if indicated. Patients with metastatic breast cancer are not likely to be cured, with approximately 5% to 10% of patients surviving 5 or more years, so often the focus of treatment is palliative. Newly introduced therapies may further improve the disease-free interval over time. One such therapy is Herceptin, mentioned in the preceding text. Other promising agents include selective aromatase inhibitors (SAIs), which act to suppress postmenopausal estrogen levels by selectively inhibiting the enzyme, aromatase, which is involved in the production of estrogen. Some ER-positive patients develop resistance to endocrine therapy. There are newer SERMs under evaluation for the tamoxifen-resistant breast cancer.

For distant metastases, the most common sites are bones (40% to 50%); lung/pleura (20%); followed by liver, brain, and spine. Approximately 70% of patients who have recurrences are symptomatic, bringing their relapse to the attention of their physician. Fifteen percent to 40% of first recurrences are local-regional, involving the axillary/supraclavicular lymph nodes or chest wall. Thirty percent to 60% of first recurrences are in bone, with 10% to 15% involving bone in combination with some other site. There are therapeutic regimens that are specific to each site of metastases. The workup is also tailored to specific complaints. To evaluate bone pain, bone films and a bone scan should be obtained. However, results can vary depending on technical details, and, if further evaluation is needed, a CT or MRI scan would be the next imaging study. To evaluate liver complaints, first a hepatic panel should be ordered, then an abdominal CT scan if there are any enzyme abnormalities. To evaluate pulmonary complaints, first a chest x-ray should be ordered with follow-up thoracic CT scan only for further evaluation of suspicious findings. Central nervous system (CNS) complaints should be investigated with a CT scan or MRI of the head.

BREAST CANCER RISK ASSESSMENT AND PREVENTION

It is essential for early detection to identify patients at increased risk of developing breast cancer. Obtaining a detailed history from patients is one of the fundamental steps in determining risk. It provides an opportunity to plan preventive and diagnostic strategies as well as to enhance a patient's understanding of the disease. Increased risk of breast cancer is associated with intrinsic and extrinsic characteristics. Intrinsic risk factors include familial and genetic elements, benign breast lesions that are identified pathologically to confer high risk, and endogenous hormonal factors. Diet, environmental exposure, exogenous hormones, and geographic location comprise extrinsic factors. The factors that confer relative risks less than 2 are arbitrarily categorized as risk factors associated with a slightly increased risk of developing breast cancer. Those with relative risks between 2 and 4 and greater than 4 are typically categorized as those conferring a moderately increased risk and high risk of developing breast carcinoma, respectively. These risk factors are listed in Table 32-8; however, it is important to note that there is no agreement as to what level of risk classifies a patient as high risk.

One important risk factor is age. As a woman's age increases, so does the risk of breast cancer, although the rate of increase slows after menopause. The annual risk of developing breast cancer for a woman age 30 to 34 years is 1 in 4,000 women, compared to 1 in 200 women for a woman aged 70 to 74 years.

Patterns of endogenous and exogenous hormonal exposure are associated with relative risks less than 2. There is a

---

TABLE 32-7

RECOMMENDATIONS FOR USE OF ADJUVANT THERAPY IN BREAST CANCER

Patient Subset	Recommended Treatment
−Nodes, low risk	Physician judgement; no treatment; tamoxifen if ER+
−Nodes, higher risk	
ER+	Tamoxifen ± chemotherapy
ER−	Chemotherapy
+Nodes	
ER+	Chemotherapy + tamoxifen; or tamoxifen alone
ER−	Chemotherapy

ER, estrogen receptor.
[a] Low risk defined as negative axillary nodes and tumor ≤1 cm, nuclear grade 1; or 1–2 cm ER+ tumor with low proliferation index.
From Harris JR, Lippman ME, Morrow M et al., eds. *Diseases of the breast.* Philadelphia: Lippincott Williams & Wilkins, 2000:627, with permission.

TABLE 32-8

MAGNITUDE OF KNOWN BREAST CANCER RISK FACTORS

Relative Risk <2	Relative Risk 2–4	Relative Risk >4
Early menarche	One first-degree relative with breast cancer	Two first-degree relatives with breast cancer
Late menopause	Radiation exposure	Gene mutations
Nulliparity	Prior breast cancer	Ductal carcinoma *in situ*
Age >35 years at first birth	Dense breast	Lobular carcinoma *in situ*
Hormone replacement		
Obesity		
Proliferative benign breast disease		

From Morrow M, Jordan VC, eds. *Managing breast cancer risk.* Ontario: BC Decker, 2000:5, with permission.

modest increase in the lifetime risk of breast cancer from greater exposure to uninterrupted hormonal (menstrual) cycles. This includes women with early menarche (before age 12), women with late menopause (after 55), nulliparous women, and women whose first live-birth is after the age of 20. There is also an increase in risk from the use of postmenopausal hormone-replacement therapy (HRT).

As shown in Table 32-3, there are certain histologic factors that increase the risk of breast cancer. An important feature to note is that of atypical ductal or lobular hyperplasia, which has a highly increased risk (RR >5) of future breast carcinoma. As mentioned earlier, LCIS as well as DCIS increases risk to greater than 4. Women who develop a primary breast cancer before the age of 45 are five to six times more likely to develop a second breast cancer, with their annual risk of a second breast cancer being as high as 1% per year.

Inherited Causes of Breast Cancer

A positive family history of breast cancer is also a risk factor for developing breast cancer. In patients with one first-degree relative with breast cancer, the relative risk is between 2 to 4, whereas that risk increases to greater than 4 in patients with two first-degree relatives. For patients with a strong family history (i.e., at least two first-degree relatives with breast cancer before the age of 40), the lifetime risk is approximately 43%.

Positive family history of breast cancer increases a woman's own risk; however, that risk is substantially increased if there is a genetic component. In general, a personal or family history of breast cancer before age 40 years or any personal or family history of ovarian cancer or male breast cancer should suggest an increased risk of having a deleterious mutation of the breast susceptibilities genes, BRCA1 or BRCA2. When transmission of genetic risk is suggested by family history, counseling and testing programs should be offered to high-risk women and their families. Although high-risk women can potentially reduce their risk of cancer morbidity and mortality through increased surveillance and management, there still remain

many questions regarding cancer risks and the efficacy of certain strategies. In general, only 5% to 10% of all breast cancers are directly attributable to breast cancer susceptibility genes. It must be kept in mind that there are other breast cancer susceptibility genes that can increase a person's risk of developing breast cancer, which because of their low penetrance, have yet to be discovered.

Approximately 15% of all familial breast cancers are attributable to mutations in the high penetrance genes BRCA1 and BRCA2, with other rare syndromes accounting for less than 1% of all breast cancer cases. One such syndrome is *Li–Fraumeni syndrome,* an autosomal-dominant disease with an underlying mutation of the p53 tumor suppressor gene. It is associated with an increased incidence of breast cancer, often multiple breast cancers, and various sarcomas.

The BRCA1 gene is located on the long arm of chromosome 17. BRCA1 is a nuclear protein that most likely plays a role in response to DNA damage and in altering the expression of other genes. BRCA1 mutations are inherited in an autosomal-dominant fashion with high penetrance. Patients with this mutation have a 55% to 85% lifetime risk of developing breast cancer, a 65% risk of developing a second breast cancer, and a 15% to 60% risk of developing ovarian cancer. Approximately 20% of BRCA1 carriers develop cancer by age 40, and 50% of patients will develop breast cancer by age 50. In male patients with BRCA1 mutations, there is an increased risk of prostate cancer and colon cancer.

BRCA-2 is located on the long arm of chromosome 13. BRCA2 mutations contribute to fewer cases of early onset breast cancer than BRCA1. The lifetime risk of developing breast cancer from this autosomal-dominant mutation ranges 37% to 85%. There is still an increased risk of ovarian cancer with BRCA-2, but it is lower than that with BRCA-1. In contrast to BRCA1, with which all breast cancer occurs in women, BRCA2 mutations are associated with a 6% lifetime risk of male breast cancer. This represents a 100-fold increase over the general population.

Surveillance

As discussed, one of the first steps in evaluating a patient for breast cancer is to obtain a detailed history, with an emphasis on risk factors for breast cancer. The standard recommendation for breast cancer screening for most women, not considered to be high-risk, is annual mammogram and clinical breast examination, beginning at age 40, along with monthly SBE. Woman at moderate to high-risk should have more aggressive surveillance, with mammograms beginning before age 40 and annual CBE. Women with hereditary breast cancer have been shown to develop breast cancer in intervals between bi-annual mammograms, and MRI is used increasingly as a screening imaging modality in these women. When discussing surveillance with women, it should be emphasized that it is a means to detect disease at an early stage, even though there are few data to show that close adherence to a surveillance program will improve survival.

Chemoprevention with Tamoxifen

The aim of the 1993 National Surgery Adjuvant Breast and Bowel Project (NSABP) P-1 Prevention Trial was to evaluate the role of tamoxifen, a SERM, in the prevention of breast cancer. Participants in the trial were women considered to be at an increased risk for developing breast cancer, defined as those being at least 60 years old, those with a history of LCIS, or those with a 5-year Gail risk of developing breast cancer greater than 1.66%. By taking tamoxifen for 5 years, an overall 49% reduction in the risk of invasive breast carcinoma was demonstrated. For women who had LCIS, the risk reduction was 56% and for those with atypical ductal hyperplasia, the reduction was 86%. However, the study also demonstrated an increased risk of endometrial cancer with tamoxifen use of two- to threefold, especially in post-menopausal women, as well as an increased risk of thromboembolic events, such as deep vein thrombosis and pulmonary embolus. Other side effects included hot flashes and vaginal discharge. Nevertheless, women with a high risk of breast cancer should be counseled with regard to risk-reduction strategies and the possible role of tamoxifen, weighing its potential risks and benefits. Ongoing clinical trials are comparing tamoxifen with raloxifene, another SERM, as well as studying the efficacy of other potential chemoprevention agents in breast cancer, such as other SERMs, retinoids, and aromatase inhibitors.

Prophylactic Mastectomy

Prophylactic mastectomy with immediate reconstruction is a choice available to women at high risk for developing breast cancer. This option is most pertinent to women whose risk of breast cancer clearly exceeds that of the general population, including those testing positive for BRCA-1 and BRCA-2. Historically, patients with LCIS were also considered candidates for preventive mastectomy, since both breasts are at risk of developing invasive cancer. However,

given the clear reduction of risk when women with LCIS take tamoxifen for chemoprevention, prophylactic mastectomy is generally not the recommended treatment for LCIS. When considering prophylactic mastectomy as a treatment option, clinicians and women need to consider factors such as negative effects on quality of life, loss of normal breast functions, and complications of surgery.

Oophorectomy

One study has shown that when healthy BRCA-1 carriers underwent prophylactic bilateral oophorectomy, the overall risk of breast cancer was reduced by more than 70%. In BRCA-1 and BRCA-2 carriers, oophorectomy reduces the risk of ovarian cancer as well as the risk of breast cancer. Currently, there are no data regarding this procedure in women with a moderate-to-high risk of developing breast carcinoma.

SUMMARY

With our better understanding of the natural history of breast cancer, our treatments have evolved from the radical mastectomy developed by Halsted to the less-deforming surgical treatment of breast conservation, that is, lumpectomy with radiation. With the pending results of the ACOSOC Z11 trial, our management of positive SLNs and the role of axillary node dissections in breast cancer management may possibly change. As we gain further knowledge of the disease process of breast carcinoma, prevention and treatment of breast cancer will likely be customized for each individual patient.

KEY POINTS

▲ Tamoxifen is a selective estrogen receptor modulator and acts as estrogen agonist and antagonist.

▲ It is used for both chemoprevention (to decrease the risk of developing breast cancer in select patients) and for adjuvant hormonal therapy.

▲ Lobular carcinoma *in situ* (LCIS) is a risk factor for future bilateral breast cancer.

▲ With tumors larger than 5 cm (T3), axillary dissections are performed, not sentinel node (SLN) biopsy.

▲ Bone is the most common site of metastasis.

▲ BRCA1, one of the breast susceptibility genes, is associated with a high risk of developing breast and

ovarian cancer for women, and prostate and colon cancer for men. BRCA2 is associated with a high risk of developing breast cancer, increased risk for male breast cancer.

▲ Atypical ductal hyperplasia is a histologic feature associated with increased risk of breast cancer.

▲ The treatment for ductal carcinoma *in situ* (DCIS) is breast-conserving therapy (lumpectomy and radiation).

▲ Chemotherapy is recommended for all women with breast cancers larger than 1.0 cm and those with positive nodes.

SUGGESTED READINGS

Burstein HJ, Polyak K, Wong JS, et al. Ductal carcinoma in situ of the breast. *N Engl J Med* 2004;350(14):1430–1441.

Fisher B, Constantino JP, Wickerham L, et al. Tamoxifen for prevention of breast cancer: Report of the National Surgical Adjuvant Breast and Bowel Project P-1 Study. *J Natl Cancer Inst* 1998;90(18):1371–1388.

Grube BJ, Giuliano AE. Observation of the breast cancer patient with a tumor-positive sentinel node: Implications of the ACOSOC Z0011 trial. *Semin Surg Oncol* 2001;20:230–237.

Harris JR, Lippman ME, Morrow M et al., eds. *Diseases of the breast,* 2nd ed. Philadelphia: Lippincott Williams & Wilkins, 2000.

Jemal A, Murray T, Samuels A, et al. Cancer Statistics. *CA Cancer J Clin* 2003;53:5–26.

Morrow M, Jordon VC. Managing breast cancer risk. London: BC Decker Inc, 2003.

Index

Page numbers followed by *f* indicate figures; page numbers followed by *t* indicate tables